handbook of SURGERY

FIFTH EDITION

handbook of SURGERY

Edited By

JOHN L. WILSON, M.D.
Professor of Surgery
Stanford University School of Medicine
Palo Alto, California

Lange Medical Publications
Los Altos, California

1973

Italian Edition: *Piccin Editore, Padua, Italy*
Spanish Edition: *El Manual Moderno, S.A., Mexico, D.F.*
Serbo-Croatian Edition: *Medicinska Knjiga, Belgrade, Yugoslavia*
Turkish Edition: *Dr. Suha Demirtas, Ankara, Turkey*
Polish Edition: *Panstwowy Zaklad Wydawnictw Lekarskich, Warsaw, Poland*

International Standard Book Number: *0–87041–112–8*
Library of Congress Catalogue Card Number: *78–180540*

A Concise Medical Library for Practitioner and Student

Handbook of Surgery, 5th ed. $7.00

Current Diagnosis & Treatment 1973 (11th annual revision). Edited by M.A. Krupp and M.J. Chatton. 996 pp.	1973
Current Pediatric Diagnosis & Treatment, 2nd ed. Edited by C.H. Kempe, H.K. Silver, and D. O'Brien. 1008 pp, *illus.*	1972
Current Surgical Diagnosis & Treatment. Edited by J.E. Dunphy and L.W. Way. 1108 pp, *illus.*	1973
Review of Physiological Chemistry, 14th ed. H.A. Harper. 545 pp, *illus.*	1973
Review of Medical Physiology, 6th ed. W.F. Ganong. 580 pp, *illus.*	1973
Review of Medical Microbiology, 10th ed. E. Jawetz, J.L. Melnick, and E.A. Adelberg. 518 pp, *illus.*	1972
Review of Medical Pharmacology, 3rd ed. F.H. Meyers, E. Jawetz, and A. Goldfien. 688 pp, *illus.*	1972
General Urology, 7th ed. D.R. Smith. 436 pp, *illus.*	1972
General Ophthalmology, 6th ed. D. Vaughan, T. Asbury, and R. Cook. 316 pp, *illus.*	1971
Correlative Neuroanatomy & Functional Neurology, 15th ed. J.G. Chusid. 429 pp, *illus.*	1973
Principles of Clinical Electrocardiography, 8th ed. M.J. Goldman. 400 pp, *illus.*	1973
Handbook of Psychiatry, 2nd ed. Edited by P. Solomon and V.D. Patch. 648 pp.	1971
Handbook of Obstetrics & Gynecology, 4th ed. R.C. Benson. 774 pp, *illus.*	1971
Physician's Handbook, 17th ed. M.A. Krupp, N.J. Sweet, E. Jawetz, E.G. Biglieri, and R.L. Roe. 728 pp, *illus.*	1973
Handbook of Medical Treatment, 13th ed. Edited by M.J. Chatton. 648 pp.	1972
Handbook of Pediatrics, 10th ed. H.K. Silver, C.H. Kempe, and H.B. Bruyn. 693 pp, *illus.*	1973
Handbook of Poisoning: Diagnosis & Treatment, 7th ed. R.H. Dreisbach. 515 pp.	1971

Lithographed in USA

Table of Contents

Preface

The objective of this Handbook is to provide a concise summary of the essential features of the more common surgical disorders. An effort has been made to include basic information on diagnosis and management, including preoperative and postoperative care. Details of surgical technic have been omitted except in the discussion of those conditions where the nonspecialist may need guidance in an emergency.

Space limitations have posed difficult decisions about what to include and the relative emphasis each topic should receive. Fortunately, new editions of the Handbook are prepared at frequent intervals, so that it is possible to review each section and correct any disproportions or deficiencies that are found. At the same time, obsolete material can be eliminated and recent advances included. The suggestions and criticisms of readers are of much assistance in these revisions and are most welcome.

The authoritative contributions of the men whose names appear in the Table of Contents are much appreciated.

John L. Wilson

December, 1973

Authors

John E. Adams, MD, Guggenheim Professor of Neurological Surgery, University of California School of Medicine (San Francisco).

Stuart C. Cullen, MD, Professor of Anesthesia (Emeritus), University of California School of Medicine (San Francisco).

Francis L. DeBon, MD, Lecturer in Anesthesia, University of California School of Medicine (San Francisco).

Alfred A. deLorimier, MD, Associate Professor of Surgery, University of California School of Medicine (San Francisco).

John M. Erskine, MD, Associate Clinical Professor of Surgery, University of California School of Medicine (San Francisco).

Neri P. Guadagni, MD, Associate Professor of Anesthesia, University of California School of Medicine (San Francisco).

Harold A. Harper, PhD, Professor of Biochemistry, Departments of Biochemistry and Surgery, University of California School of Medicine (San Francisco).

Ernest Jawetz, PhD, MD, Professor of Microbiology and Chairman, Department of Microbiology; Professor of Medicine, Lecturer in Pediatrics, University of California School of Medicine (San Francisco).

Floyd H. Jergesen, MD, Clinical Professor of Orthopedic Surgery, University of California School of Medicine (San Francisco).

John H. Karam, MD, Assistant Professor of Medicine and Associate Director, Metabolic Research Unit, University of California Medical Center (San Francisco).

Eugene S. Kilgore, MD, Associate Clinical Professor of Surgery, University of California School of Medicine (San Francisco).

Albert E. Long, MD, Associate Clinical Professor of Obstetrics and Gynecology, University of California School of Medicine (San Francisco), and Associate in Gynecology and Obstetrics, Stanford University School of Medicine (Palo Alto).

John S. Najarian, MD, Professor and Chairman, Department of Surgery, University of Minnesota Medical School (Minneapolis).

William L. Newmeyer, MD, Assistant Clinical Professor of Surgery, University of California School of Medicine (San Francisco); Co-director, Hand Surgery Service, Department of Surgery, University of California at San Francisco General Hospital; Consultant, Hand Surgery Service, Veterans Administration Hospitals in San Francisco, Livermore, and Martinez.

Norman E. Shumway, MD, PhD, Professor of Surgery; Chief, Division of Cardiovascular Surgery, Stanford University School of Medicine (Palo Alto).

Richard L. Simmons, MD, Professor of Surgery, University of Minnesota Medical School (Minneapolis).

Donald R. Smith, MD, Professor of Urology and Chairman, Department of Urology, University of California School of Medicine (San Francisco).

Charles F. Steiss, MD. Assistant Clinical Professor of Surgery, University of California School of Medicine (San Francisco).

Edward B. Stinson, MD, Assistant Professor of Surgery, Stanford University School of Medicine (Palo Alto).

John L. Wilson, MD, Professor of Surgery, Stanford University School of Medicine (Palo Alto).

Walter P. Work, MD, Professor and Chairman, Department of Otorhinolaryngology, University of Michigan School of Medicine, Ann Arbor, Michigan.

HANDBOOK OF SURGERY

1...

Trauma & Emergencies

FIRST AID*

General Principles.

A. Determine the extent of injury quickly but thoroughly.

B. Treat immediately such life-endangering conditions as cardiac arrest, respiratory distress, serious external bleeding, and shock.

C. Improvise dressings, splints, and transportation and arrange for prompt, definitive treatment.

Evaluation of the Patient.

A. Take a sufficient history to ascertain the degree and type of damage and any serious underlying medical problems, e.g., cardiac disease or diabetes mellitus.

B. Examine the patient thoroughly after major trauma, with special attention to the following:

1. Cardiac arrest - In the unconscious apneic patient, check for carotid pulse immediately; if absent, begin mouth-to-mouth insufflation (see p. 8) and closed heart massage (see pp. 12-13) at once.
2. Respiratory distress or arrest - Stridor and suprasternal or intercostal retraction indicate airway obstruction. Cyanosis is due to poor oxygenation from any cause. Shortness of breath may be due to chest injury or shock. Respiratory depression may occur in head injury or in severe shock. In respiratory arrest, begin mouth-to-mouth insufflation immediately (see p. 8).
3. External wounds and bleeding - Control bleeding promptly (see below) and apply sterile dressing.
4. Shock - Typical signs are faintness, pallor, cool and moist skin, thirst, air hunger, and a weak, usually rapid pulse. Distinguish neurogenic shock from oligemic shock (see p. 19).
5. Fractures and dislocations - Palpate carefully from head to foot; move all joints cautiously; exert gentle pressure on the spine, chest, and pelvis. Pain, swelling, ecchymosis, deformity, and limitation of motion are classical signs of fracture and dislocation. Few or none of these may be apparent immediately after injury.
6. Brain and spinal cord damage - Assess CNS injury by noting the state of consciousness, gross skin sensation, and the ability to move extremities actively.
7. Internal injury - Overt localizing signs are often minimal.

*First aid for fractures and spine injuries is discussed in Chapter 19.

METHODS OF RELIEVING AIRWAY OBSTRUCTION*

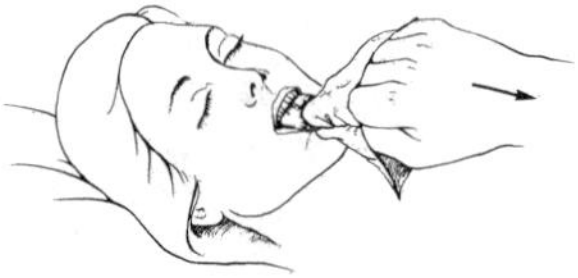

Pull Out Tongue

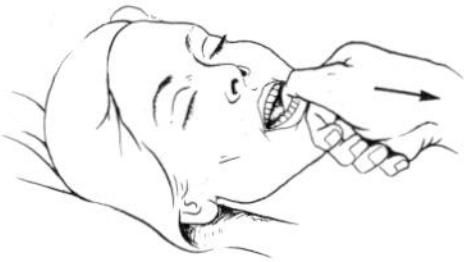

Pull Jaw Forward

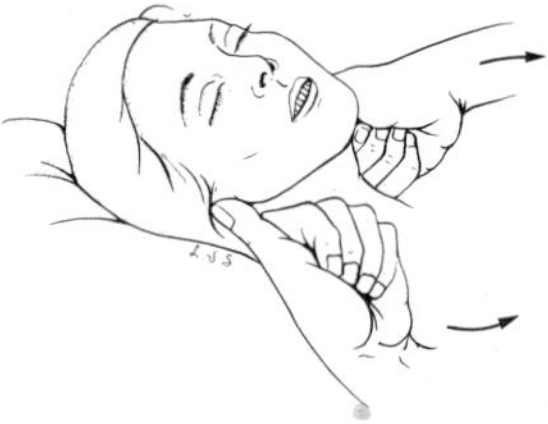

Lift Jaw Forward

TRACHEAL INTUBATION*

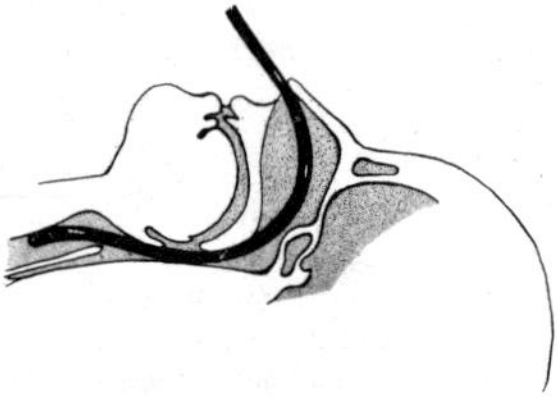

Nasotracheal Tube in Place
After Blind Insertion
Through the Nose

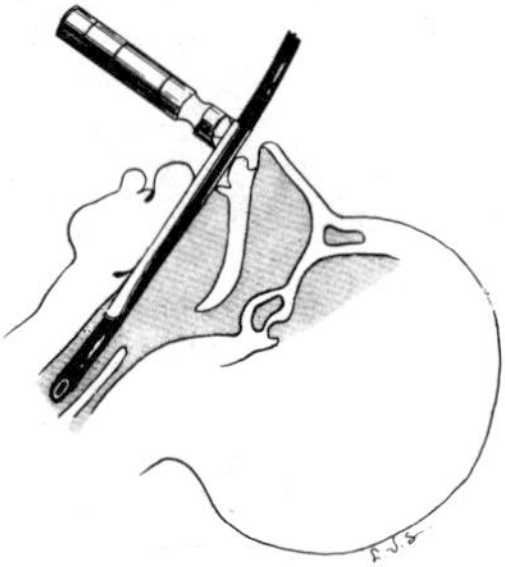

Endotracheal Tube Placement
With Laryngoscope

---

*Reproduced, with permission, from Dunphy and Way: Current Surgical Diagnosis and Treatment. Lange, 1973.

Hypovolemic shock in the absence of external bleeding or extensive soft tissue trauma suggests internal hemorrhage. Chest pain with respiratory distress and abdominal pain with signs of peritoneal irritation point to visceral injury.

Management of Cardiac Arrest.

See pp. 10-18.

Management of Respiratory Distress.

A. When Due to Airway Obstruction:
1. Remove secretions and foreign material from mouth and throat. Use suction if available.
2. Hold up the patient's chin, pull out his tongue, or force the mandible forward by pressure behind the angles when relaxation of the tongue and jaw obstruct the hypopharynx, as in comatose patients. Use an oropharyngeal airway if available. (See p. 2, top.)
3. Tracheal intubation with an endotracheal or nasotracheal tube may be required to establish an adequate airway. (See p. 2, bottom.)
4. Tracheostomy (see Chapter 8) may be necessary if a foreign body or edema obstructs the larynx.

B. When Due to Other Causes: Maintain a clear airway, treat the underlying cause, and administer oxygen if available.

C. In Respiratory Arrest: Clear the airway and institute artificial respiration by mouth-to-mouth insufflation (see p. 8).

Management of External Bleeding.

A. Venous and Minor Arterial Bleeding: These can be controlled by direct pressure on the wound with sterile gauze or a clean cloth and elevation of the part.

B. Major Arterial Bleeding: Serious bleeding is usually due to the laceration of a major artery. Speed is essential.
1. Direct pressure on the wound will reduce or stop the flow.
2. Compression of the major artery proximal to the wound may make local pressure effective, permit grasping of a bleeder with a hemostat, or allow time for fashioning a tourniquet.
3. A tourniquet is necessary when other methods fail. Do not use a tourniquet when direct pressure on the wound will control bleeding. **Caution:** Faulty use of a tourniquet may cause irreparable vascular or neurologic damage. Tourniquets can be made from rubber tubing, rope, neckties, belts, handkerchiefs, stockings, or strips of cloth. Keep the tourniquet exposed and release it briefly at least every 30 minutes.

Management of Shock.

Anticipate and prevent shock by the measures outlined below.

A. Control hemorrhage and such contributing causes as exposure and pain.

B. Keep the patient comfortably warm in the recumbent, slightly head-down position. Avoid rapid position changes.

C. Splint fractures and apply traction if necessary to relieve pain.

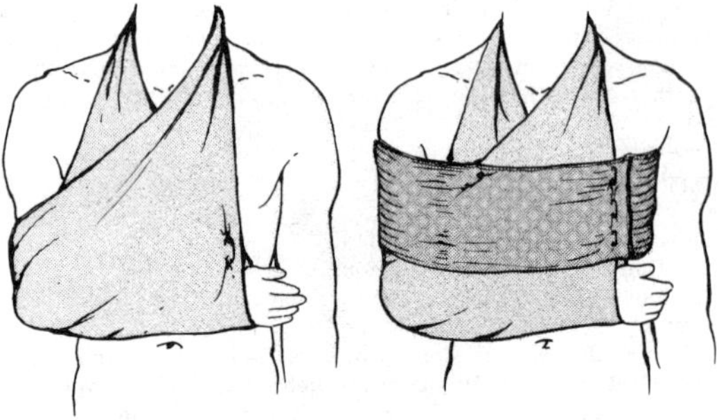

Method of Application of Sling and Swathe

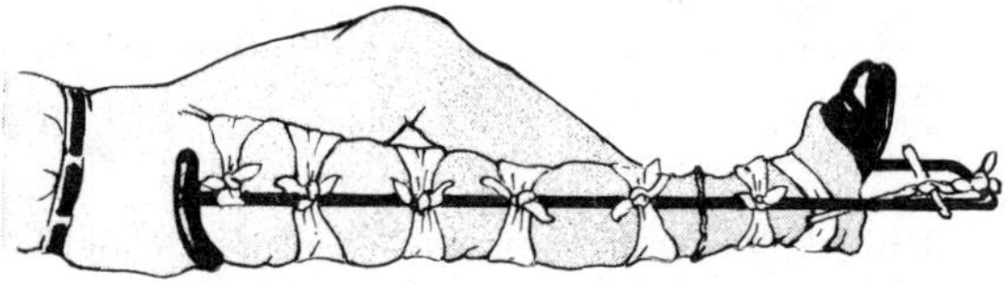

Keller-Blake Half-ring Splint for Transportation of Patient With Fracture of Thigh or Leg. Spanish windlass on a Collins hitch.

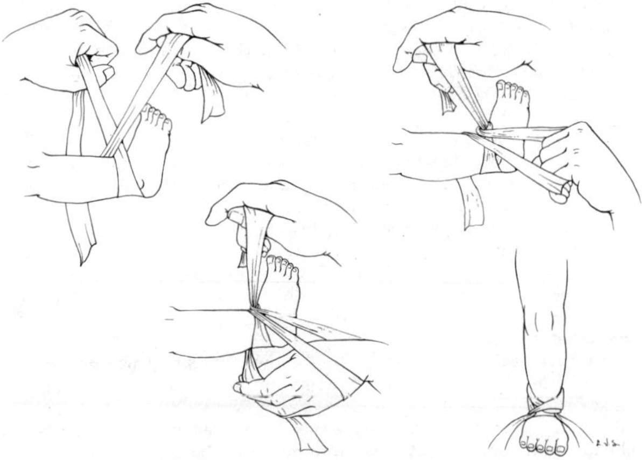

Method of Tying Collins Hitch

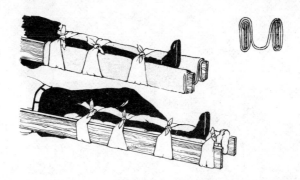

Padded Board Splints for Transportation of Patient With Fracture of Thigh and Leg. Outer board extends to axilla.

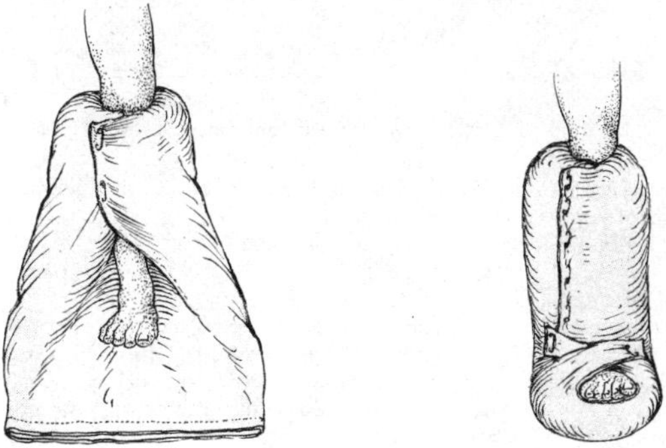

Method of Application of Pillow Splints

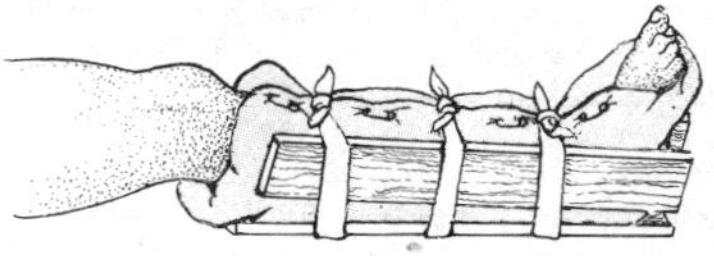

Reinforcement of Pillow Splint for Transportation of Patient With Injury of Ankle and Foot

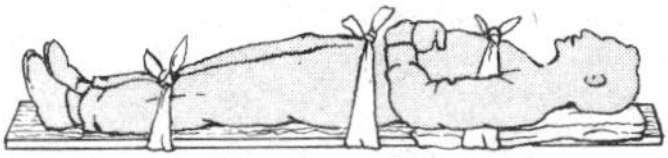

Board or Door Used for Transportation of Patient With Injured Spine

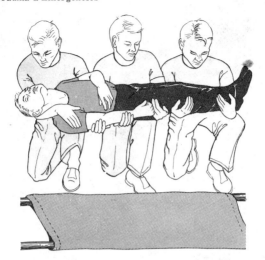

Method of Lifting Injured Patient Onto Stretcher

D. Transport as gently and as quickly as possible to a hospital.
E. If profound or progressive shock develops, give blood, plasma, or a plasma substitute as soon as possible.

Control of Pain.

Distinguish fear and excitement from real pain. Severe injuries frequently cause surprisingly little discomfort. Immobilization of injured parts often relieves distress. **Note**: Narcotics are contraindicated in coma, head injuries, and respiratory depression. Otherwise, when pain is severe, give morphine sulfate, 10-15 mg. ($1/6$-$1/4$ gr.) I.M. or slowly I.V. The I.V. route is quick and sure; peripheral vasoconstriction may delay absorption of a subcut. or I.M. injection, and will lead to overdosage if multiple injections are later absorbed at the same time. Inform the patient that he has received morphine, and record the time and dosage on a note or tag affixed to his wrist or ankle.

Care of Open Wounds.

A. Remove gross foreign debris; apply a dry, sterile dressing or a clean cloth and secure it firmly in place.
B. Do not place antiseptic solutions or antibacterial powders in the wound. It is not necessary to cleanse the skin around the wound with soap or antiseptic.
C. Arrange for the earliest possible cleansing, debridement, and closure under aseptic conditions.

Transportation of Injured Patients.

Improper methods of moving patients can increase injuries. Lift severely injured patients with care (see above), and improvise stretchers from blankets, boards, and doors (see p. 5) when necessary. Transport the following types of cases in the recumbent position, on a stretcher, preferably in an ambulance: head and internal injuries; fractures of the spine, pelvis, and the long bones of the lower extremities; shock; and major wounds in general. The physician administering first aid is morally and in some areas legally responsible for ensuring the transfer of the patient to a medical facility or to another physician.

EMERGENCY ROOM WORK-UP

Examine accident victims promptly and thoroughly. Record history and findings in accurate detail. Obtain the following information in cases of acute injury.

Identification.

A. Patient's name, address, phone number, age, sex, race, and marital status.
B. Date and exact time brought to emergency room.
C. Brought to emergency room by (give name, address, and phone number).
D. Referring physician (name, address, and phone number).
E. Next of kin (name, address, and phone number).
F. If injured at work, record the patient's occupation, the name, address, and phone number of his employer, and the name of the employer's insurance carrier.

History of Injury.

A. Date and exact time of accident.
B. Where and how it occurred.
C. Accurate description of the mechanism of injury, including symptoms, subsequent course, and treatment given.
D. In major injuries, take a complete general history.

Physical Examination.

A. In minor injuries, describe accurately the local findings. Line drawings are frequently helpful in showing the location and configuration of wounds. Measure and record dimensions.
B. In major injuries, perform a complete physical examination. Severe trauma commonly causes multiple injuries, and symptoms may not become manifest for many hours. Palpate such patients carefully and completely in order not to overlook occult fractures and visceral damage. Repeat the examination later in order to identify injuries in which delayed findings occur.

Laboratory Examination.

A. In major injuries determine the Hct., Hgb., WBC, and differential count, and perform a urinalysis.
B. Group and cross-match for blood transfusion as required.
C. Obtain appropriate x-rays. All sites of suspected fracture should be x-rayed as soon as the patient's condition permits.
D. Special laboratory tests as indicated.

TECHNIC OF MOUTH-TO-MOUTH INSUFFLATION

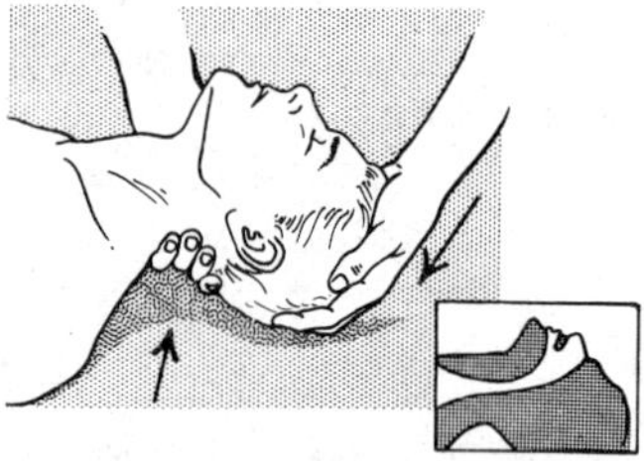

(1)

The operator takes his position at the patient's head.

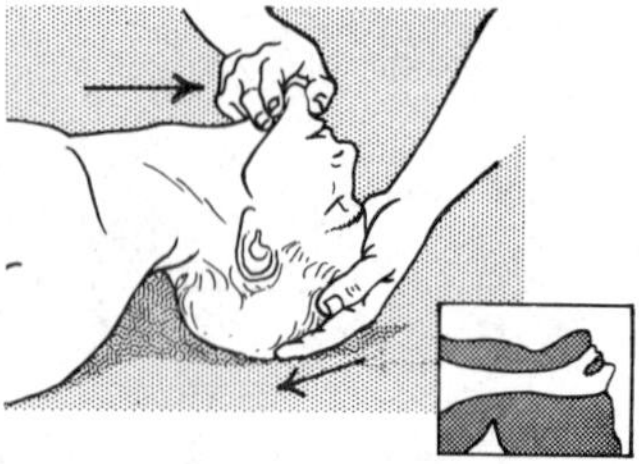

(2)

With the right thumb and index finger he displaces the mandible forward by pressing at its central portion (or by forward pressure at the angle of the jaw on both sides), at the same time lifting the neck and tilting the head as far back as possible.

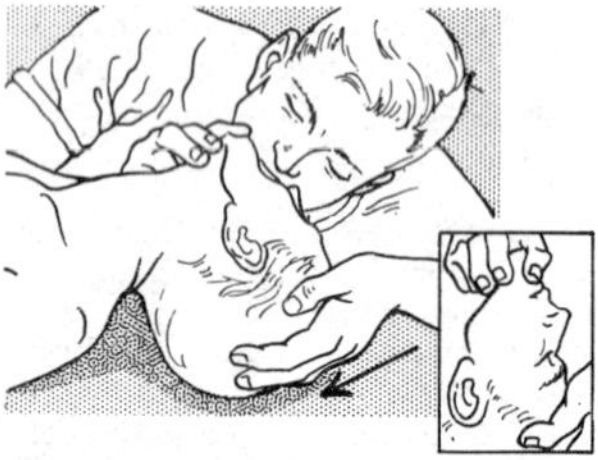

(3)

After taking a deep breath, the operator immediately seals his mouth around the mouth (or nose) of the victim and exhales until the chest of the victim rises.

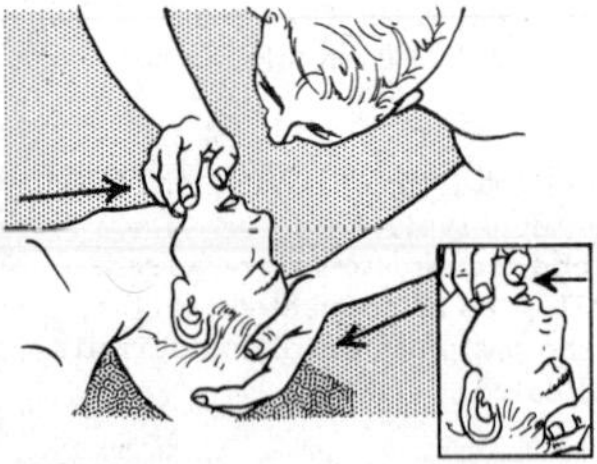

(4)

The victim's mouth is opened by pulling down slightly on the jaw or by pulling down the lower lip.

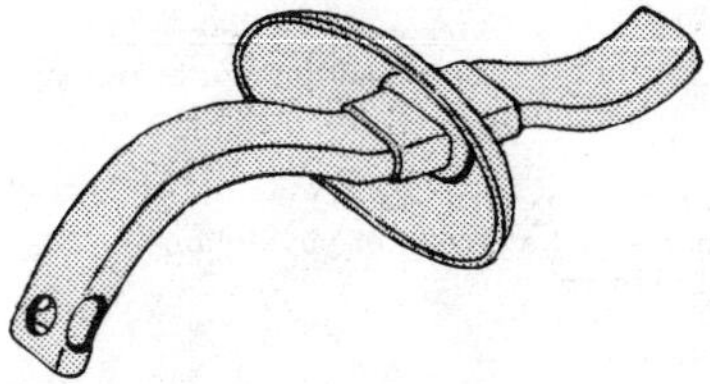

Airway for Use in Mouth-to-Mouth Insufflation. The larger airway is for adults. The guard is flexible and may be inverted from the position shown for use with infants and children.

PORTABLE MANUAL RESUSCITATOR

The manual resuscitator consists of a pliable bag, nonrebreathing valve, and face mask. Effective positive pressure ventilation can be achieved by applying the mask firmly over the nose and mouth and squeezing the bag, which recoils promptly to the full position when released. Oxygen can be administered if desired by attaching the oxygen tubing to the air intake valve at the end of the bag. The manual resuscitator should be available in ambulances, coronary care and intensive care units, and wherever there might be victims of heart attack, cardiac arrest, suffocation, drowning, etc.

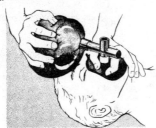

Instructions for Use of Manual Resuscitator.

1. Lift the victim's neck with one hand.
2. Tilt head backward into maximum neck extension. Remove secretions and debris from mouth and throat, and pull the tongue and mandible forward as required to clear the airway.
3. Hold the mask snugly over the nose and mouth, holding the chin forward and the neck in extension as shown in diagram.
4. Squeeze the bag, noting inflation of the lungs by the rise of the chest wall.
5. Release the bag, which will expand spontaneously. The patient will exhale and the chest will fall.
6. Repeat steps 4 and 5 approximately 12 times per minute.

Diagnostic Impression and Differential Diagnosis.

Signature of examiner
Date and hour of examination

Disposition.
A. Discharge; date of return visit.
B. Referral (name and address of physician).
C. Hospital admission.

ARTIFICIAL RESPIRATION

(See drawings on pp. 8-9.)

Begin artificial respiration immediately in any situation in which breathing has stopped, and continue efforts at artificial respiration as long as the heart is beating. Mouth-to-mouth insufflation should be employed for artificial respiration unless mask or endotracheal tube and bag for insufflation are available. A laryngoscope, endotracheal tubes, a bag for insufflation of air or oxygen under positive pressure, and suction equipment should be kept at hand wherever respiratory emergencies are apt to be encountered. If upper airway obstruction is present and cannot be promptly relieved manually or by instruments or suction, immediate tracheostomy should be performed.

CARDIAC ARREST

Cardiac arrest consists of the unexpected cessation of the heartbeat secondary to acute myocardial hypoxia, toxicity, or conduction disturbance. Cardiac arrest occurs most frequently in the operating room during induction of anesthesia or in the course of surgery. Normal hearts may be so affected, but the presence of heart disease increases the susceptibility to arrest under adverse conditions. The general health, state of nutrition, blood volume, and pulmonary reserve of the patient, when subnormal, are contributing factors insofar as they predispose to hypoxia or hypotension during a surgical procedure.

The commonest precipitating causes of cardiac arrest are as follows: (1) Shock, (2) hypoventilation, (3) airway obstruction, (4) overdosage of anesthetic, (5) drug effect or idiosyncrasy, (6) vagovagal reflex, (7) manipulation of the heart, (8) hypothermia, and (9) myocardial infarction. Other conditions producing cardiac arrest include drowning, electrocution, asphyxia, poisoning with carbon monoxide and other gases, air embolism, and heart block.

Cardiac arrest occurs about once in every 750-1000 operations, one-third of which are minor procedures. The highest incidence is in operations on the lung or heart. Cardiac arrest occurs either as a result of ventricular standstill (asystole) or ventricular fibrillation. After cardiac arrest has occurred, it is impossible to distinguish ventricular standstill from ventricular fibrillation unless the heart is in view or an Ecg. is taken. However, the distinction is of no immediate importance.

Prophylaxis.

A. Maintain adequate oxygenation at all times.
B. Maintain adequate coronary blood flow.
C. Prevent vagal effects. Preoperative administration of a vagal blocking agent (atropine or scopolamine) reduces the hazard of arrest. When bradycardia, A-V dissociation, or A-V nodal rhythm is produced during surgery by vagal stimulation, give atropine sulfate, 0.4-0.6 mg. (1/150-1/100 gr.) I.V. Avoid powerful traction on viscera, displacement of the heart, carotid sinus compression, etc.
D. Prevent hypotension and treat immediately when it occurs.

Diagnosis.

A. Premonitory Signs: The most constant signs of impending cardiac arrest are irregularity of rhythm, slowing of rate, and rapid fall of BP. Be alert for any or all of these premonitory changes during induction of anesthesia, intubation, or extubation; when re-positioning or moving the patient under anesthesia; after prolonged deep anesthesia; during periods of hypoxia or hypotension; when manipulating the heart; and when exciting vago-vagal reflexes (see above).
B. Pathognomonic Signs: **Verify cardiac arrest at once!** The following signs are pathognomonic:
   1. Absent pulse - Check for the pulse in a major vessel (e.g., carotid or femoral artery), or, when the abdomen is open, the aorta.
   2. Absent heart sounds - Listen to the precordium for the heart beat. An ear to the chest is often the quickest method. **Do not wait** for Ecg., BP apparatus, or special diagnostic equipment.

Principles of Treatment.

ACT IMMEDIATELY! Absence of pulse and heart sounds means cardiac arrest. Blood flow to the brain must be re-established within 4 minutes if permanent cerebral damage or death is to be avoided. Begin the following 2 procedures **simultaneously and immediately**:

A. Establish ventilation by mouth-to-mouth breathing until oxygen under pressure can be administered by mask or, preferably, endotracheal tube (see p. 2). Call for an anesthetist.
B. Start cardiac massage.
   1. **Closed chest cardiac massage is the procedure of choice; open chest massage is rarely required.**
   2. Open chest cardiac massage is undertaken only in an operating room or emergency room where team and equipment are available. Open massage may be required when the thorax is open or when chest wall damage, pneumothorax, hemorrhage in the chest, or other circumstances make closed chest massage unsatisfactory or unfeasible.

Closed Chest Cardiac Massage.

See pp. 12-13.

[Text cont'd. on p. 16.]

TECHNIC OF HEART-LUNG RESUSCITATION
(Modified after Safar.)

Phase I: First Aid (Emergency Oxygenation of the Brain).
Must be instituted within 3-4 minutes for optimal effectiveness and to minimize the possibility of permanent brain damage.

Step 1: Place patient in a supine position on a firm surface (not a bed). A 4 × 6 foot sheet of plywood should be available at emergency care stations.)

Step 2: Tilt head backward and maintain in this hyperextended position. Keep mandible displaced forward by pulling strongly at the angle of the jaw.

If Victim Is Not Breathing:

Step 3: Clear mouth and pharynx of mucus, blood, vomitus, or foreign material.

Step 4: Separate lips and teeth to open oral airway.

Step 5: If steps 2-4 fail to open airway, forcibly blow air through mouth (keeping nose closed) or nose (keeping mouth closed) and inflate the lungs 3-5 times. Watch for chest movement. If this fails to clear the airway immediately and if pharyngeal or tracheal tubes are available, use them without delay. Tracheostomy may be necessary.

Step 6: Feel the carotid artery for pulsations.

a. **If Carotid Pulsations Are Present:**

Give lung inflation by mouth-to-mouth breathing (keeping patient's nostrils closed) or mouth-to-nose breathing (keeping patient's mouth closed) 12-15 times per minute - allowing about 2 seconds for inspiration and 3 seconds for expiration - until spontaneous respirations return. Continue as long as the pulses remain palpable and previously dilated pupils remain constricted. Bag-mask technics for lung inflation should be reserved for experts. If pulsations cease, follow directions as in 6b, below.

b. **If Carotid Pulsations Are Absent:**

Alternate cardiac compression (closed heart massage) and pulmonary ventilation as in 6a, above. Place the heel of one hand on the sternum just above the xiphoid. With the heel of the other hand on top of it, apply firm vertical pressure sufficient to force the sternum about 2 inches downward (less in children) about once every second. After 15 sternal compressions, alternate with 3-5 deep lung inflations. Repeat and continue this alternating procedure until it is possible to obtain additional assistance and more definitive care. Resuscitation must be continuous during transportation to the hospital. Open heart massage should be attempted only in a hospital. When possible, obtain an Ecg., but do not interrupt resuscitation to do so. Have an assistant monitor the femoral or carotid pulse, which should be palpable with each cardiac compression as an indication of cardiac output.

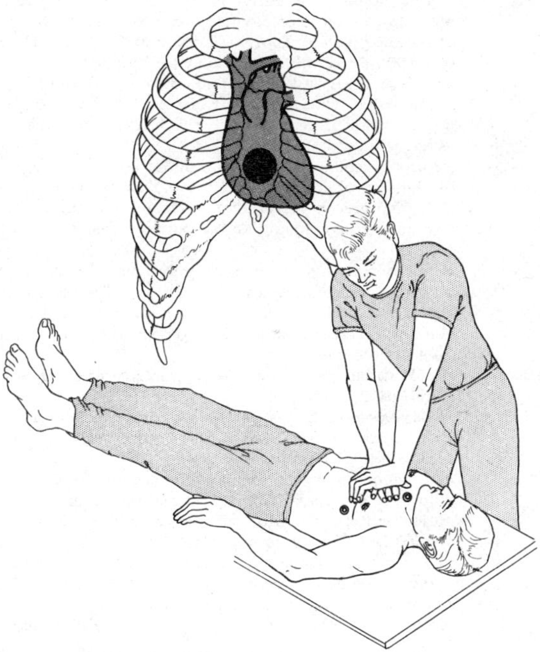

Technic of Closed Chest Cardiac Massage. Heavy circle in heart drawing shows area of application of force. Circles on supine figure show points of application of electrodes for defibrillation.

TECHNIC OF HEART-LUNG RESUSCITATION (Cont'd.)

Phase II: Restoration of Spontaneous Circulation. Until spontaneous respiration and circulation are restored, there must be no interruption of artificial ventilation and cardiac massage while steps 7-13 (below) are being carried out. Three basic questions must be considered at this point:

(1) What is the underlying cause, and is it correctable?
(2) What is the nature of the cardiac arrest?
(3) What further measures will be necessary? The physician must plan upon the assistance of trained hospital personnel,* an Ecg., a defibrillator, and emergency drugs.

Step 7: If a spontaneous effective heartbeat is not restored after 1-2 minutes of cardiac compression, have an assistant give epinephrine (adrenaline), 1 mg. (1 ml. of 1:1000 or 10 ml. of 1:10,000 aqueous solution) I.V. or 0.5 mg. (0.5 ml. of 1:1000 aqueous solution) by the intracardiac route. Repeat larger dose at 5-10 minute intervals if necessary. The intracardiac method is not without hazard.

Step 8: Promote venous return and combat shock by elevating the legs or placing patient in the Trendelenburg position, and give I.V. fluids as available and indicated. The use of tourniquets on the extremities may be of value.

Step 9: If the victim is pulseless for more than 5 minutes, give sodium bicarbonate solution, 3-4 Gm./50 ml. (1.5-2 Gm./50 ml. in children) I.V. to combat impending metabolic acidosis. Repeat every 5-10 minutes as indicated.

Step 10: If pulsations still do not return, suspect ventricular fibrillation. Obtain Ecg.

Step 11: If Ecg. demonstrates ventricular fibrillation, maintain cardiac massage until just before giving an external defibrillating shock of 440-1000 volts A.C. for 0.25 second with one electrode firmly applied to the skin over the apex of the heart and the other over the sternal notch. Monitor with Ecg. (A 50-400 watt-second D.C. shock is superior if a D.C. defibrillator is available.) If cardiac function is not restored, resume massage and repeat 3 shocks at intervals of 1-3 minutes. If cardiac action is reestablished but remains weak, give calcium chloride or calcium gluco-

*In the hospital, a physician able to intubate the trachea will quickly visualize the larynx, suck out all foreign material, pass a large, cuffed endotracheal tube, and attach the airway to an IPPB or anesthesia machine for adequate ventilation. Serial arterial blood gas, pH, and bicarbonate determinations are important.

nate, 5-10 ml. (0.5-1 Gm.) of 10% solution I. V. ; it probably should not be used in patients who have been taking digitalis.

Step 12: Thoracotomy and open heart massage may be considered (but only in a hospital) if cardiac function fails to return after all of the above measures have been used.

Step 13: If cardiac, pulmonary, and CNS functions are restored, the patient should be carefully observed for shock and complications of the precipitating cause.

Phase III: **Follow-Up Measures.** When cardiac and pulmonary function have been reestablished and satisfactorily maintained, evaluation of CNS function deserves careful consideration. Decision as to the nature and duration of subsequent treatment must be individualized. The physician must decide if he is "prolonging life" or simply "prolonging dying." Complete CNS recovery has been reported in a few patients unconscious up to a week after appropriate treatment.

Step 14: If circulation and respiration are restored but there are no signs of CNS recovery within 30 minutes, hypothermia at 30° C. for 2-3 days may lessen the degree of brain damage.

Step 15: Support ventilation and circulation. Treat any other complications which might arise. Do not overlook the possibility of complications of external cardiac massage (e.g., broken ribs, ruptured viscera).

Step 16: Meticulous postresuscitation care is required, particularly for the first 48 hours after recovery. Observe carefully for possible multiple cardiac arrhythmias, especially recurrent fibrillation or cardiac standstill.

Step 17: Consider the use of assisted circulation in selected cases. A few patients who cannot be salvaged by conventional cardiopulmonary resuscitation may be saved by the addition of partial cardiopulmonary bypass measures.

Open Chest Cardiac Massage.

A. Open the chest as soon as positive pressure ventilation with a mask or endotracheal tube has been started. Speed is essential; enter the chest in 30 seconds. Then send for surgical instruments, including a rib-spreader.
   1. A knife is the only necessary instrument.
   2. No skin preparation or gloves are required.
   3. Make a left submammary incision through the fourth or fifth interspace; spread the ribs wide enough so that the hand and wrist can be inserted.

B. Begin manual compression of the heart (cardiac massage) at once.
   1. Compress the heart rhythmically 70-80 times/minute, either against the sternum or between the thumb and fingers. Open the pericardium longitudinally if response is not immediate. Continue massage between the 2 hands.
   2. Establish coronary and brain circulation quickly. If manual compression is effective, a distinct peripheral pulse is felt. The pulse should be monitored constantly by an assistant palpating the femoral or carotid artery. Continue manual

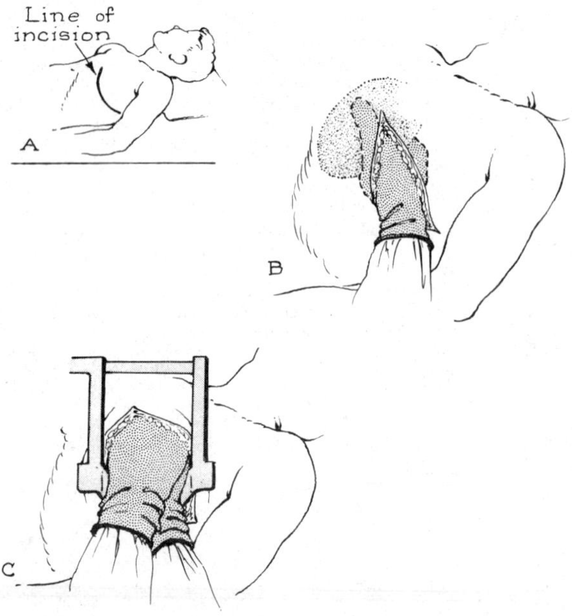

Open Chest Cardiac Massage. (A) Position of patient for cardiac massage. (B) and (C) Insertion of 1 hand or 2 hands for rhythmic compression of heart.

systole until the myocardium is oxygenated and pink; otherwise, strong contraction will not occur and defibrillation is impossible. The pupils should remain constricted if blood flow to the brain is adequate.

3. Be sure that the lungs are ventilating.
4. Intracardiac drugs - For the soft flabby heart (with or without fibrillation), inject epinephrine into the right ventricle; dilute 3 ml. of 1:1000 solution in 10 ml. saline; inject 2-5 ml.; and repeat p.r.n. If epinephrine is not available or is ineffective in the dilated, weakly beating heart, inject calcium gluconate or chloride, 3-10 ml. of 10% solution.
5. I.V. drugs - As soon as possible an I.V. infusion should be started, by cut-down or femoral, subclavian, or internal jugular puncture if necessary. Cardiac arrest and inadequate tissue perfusion during massage are accompanied by rapid development of metabolic acidosis. Correction of acidosis may have a very beneficial effect on cardiac function. As soon as the I.V. route is open, treat metabolic acidosis empirically by injection of 1-2 ampuls of sodium bicarbonate (44.6 mEq./ampul) in 50 ml. of saline over a period of several minutes. Reduce the dose appropriately in children. Injection may be repeated in 5-10 minutes if circulatory stasis persists. Determination of arterial pH will permit more accurate correction of acidosis.

C. Defibrillation: Ventricular fibrillation may be present at the outset or may develop during manual compression. It is rarely reversible except by electric shock. Proceed as follows:
   1. First have an oxygenated (pink) myocardium with good tone. It is futile and hazardous to attempt to defibrillate a cyanotic, flabby heart.
   2. Pericardium must be open.
   3. Apply defibrillator poles on opposite sides of ventricles.
   4. Set DC defibrillator for 20-60 watt-seconds over a period of 4-6 msec. and deliver a shock. The direct current defibrillator is more effective than the alternating current (AC) defibrillator which may also be used for defibrillation by delivery of 110-200 volts over 0.1-0.2 seconds.
   5. If fibrillation continues after the first shock, repeat quickly up to several times.
   6. If defibrillation is not successful, continue massage, administer intracardiac epinephrine if indicated, and repeat shock when the condition of the myocardium is optimal.

D. Continuation or repetition of resuscitative effort is indicated as long as the heart maintains tone, color, and responsiveness, and there is no evidence of irreversible brain damage such as widely dilated pupils, flaccid paralysis, and absence of spontaneous respiration for 15-30 minutes. Resuscitation may, rarely, be successful after as long as 6 hours of manual compression, and repeated resuscitations may be necessary, usually for recurrent ventricular fibrillation. Failures are usually due to delay in treatment, poor resuscitation technic, or inherent cardiac disease.

E. Chest closure is routine. Establish intercostal tube drainage and close with catgut. Begin intensive antibiotic therapy I.V. during operation.

Care After Resuscitation by Closed or Open Method.

Post-resuscitative care should, if possible, be carried out in an intensive care unit where continuous monitoring of Ecg. and frequent determination of central venous and arterial blood pressures are feasible. Equipment for external defibrillation should be immediately available. Recurrent cardiac arrest is common. Hypoxia and hypercapnia should be avoided by administration of oxygen and, if necessary, by ventilatory assistance with mask or endotracheal or tracheostomy tube. Determinations of arterial pH, pO_2, and pCO_2 are valuable when there is question of acidosis or inadequate ventilation. If acidosis is present, sodium bicarbonate may be indicated (see above). Hypovolemia is corrected by administration of blood and fluids as needed and urinary output is watched and maintained. Neurologic status must be closely followed, since cerebral damage is frequent. Complete CNS recovery has been reported in a few patients unconscious up to a week after cardiac arrest. Treatment of prolonged coma must be individualized. Sternal and rib fractures, ruptured liver, pneumothorax, or other complication of overly vigorous external massage should not be overlooked.

Prognosis.

Good results are proportional to the speed and skill of resuscitative efforts. When arrest occurs in the operating room, it is possible to save about 75% of patients. The percentage of successful resuscitations outside the operating room in cardiac arrest due to myocardial infarction and other causes is increasing with the wider application of closed chest massage. It is the responsibility of every physician to acquire the judgment, skill, and decisiveness needed to accomplish cardiac resuscitation. It is the responsibility of the hospital to provide resuscitation equipment, which should include a laryngoscope, endotracheal tubes, a mask and bag for artificial ventilation, and a D.C. defibrillator. Along with the necessary cardiac drugs, this equipment can be conveniently stored in a special cart. The cart can be kept available in the operating suite, or in those hospital units concerned with emergency, intensive, and coronary care.

SHOCK

Shock is a syndrome characterized by prostration and hypotension due to diminished circulating blood volume of such a degree that there is reduced capillary blood flow with tissue hypoxia.

NEUROGENIC SHOCK
(Primary Shock, Syncope, or Fainting)

This form of shock is due to a sudden outflow of autonomic impulses to the arterioles, producing vasodilatation or inhibition of constriction and rapid pooling of blood in the splanchnic bed and voluntary muscles. Cerebral blood flow is reduced and fainting occurs. Primary shock is usually caused by nervous or psychic stimuli, e.g., sudden pain, fright, fear, or vasodilator drugs (e.g., nitrites).

Prodromal signs and symptoms are pallor, cold sweat, weakness, lightheadedness, and occasionally nausea. Fainting occurs abruptly thereafter, with transient hypotension and bradycardia.

Neurogenic shock is self-limiting. Rest in the recumbent or head-down (Trendelenburg) position for a few minutes is usually sufficient. Elevation of the legs alone in the recumbent patient is useful. If the patient is sitting down and reclining is not possible, have him bend forward with his head between his knees. When faintness or prostration persists, other types of shock must be considered.

High spinal anesthesia may also induce a form of neurogenic shock, chiefly by paralyzing the vasoconstrictor nerves. Treatment consists of placing the patient in the Trendelenburg position and administering a vasopressor agent.

HYPOVOLEMIC SHOCK
(Oligemic, Hemorrhagic, Traumatic, Wound, or Surgical Shock)

In hypovolemic shock there is a true reduction in blood volume as a result of the rapid escape of whole blood or plasma from the vascular space. Blood pressure is maintained initially by vasoconstriction, which reduces the size of the vascular bed. When this mechanism proves inadequate, hypotension results and tissue hypoxia increases. Prolongation of this state leads to irreparable damage to vital centers and shock becomes "irreversible." For this reason, early recognition of hypovolemic shock is imperative and treatment must be intensive.

Rapid loss of 20% of blood volume produces mild shock; 35% loss produces moderately severe shock; 45% reduction causes severe shock; loss of over 50% of blood volume over a short interval is often fatal. (Blood volume is approximately 7% of body weight.)

Common Causes of Hypovolemic Shock.

A. Massive hemorrhage from wounds and internal injuries.
B. Severe crushing injuries, with extensive loss of blood and plasma into the tissues.
C. Major fractures, especially of the proximal half of the femur. The mechanism of blood and plasma loss is the same as in crushing injuries.
D. Extensive burns, with plasma loss and red cell hemolysis.
E. Nontraumatic hemorrhage, as from duodenal ulcer and esophageal varices; or reduction of plasma volume, as in severe peritonitis or dehydration with electrolyte imbalance.

Contributing Factors.

A. Age: The very young and the elderly tolerate loss of blood or plasma poorly.
B. Chronic Illness: The chronically ill often have a reduced blood volume. Relatively small diminution of circulating blood volume may cause failure of vascular compensation and precipitate shock. Blood volume determination is helpful in evaluating this group of patients (see p. 163).

C. Anesthesia: Paralysis of vasomotor tone by spinal or deep general anesthesia may precipitate shock in a patient who has previously compensated for a reduced blood volume.

D. Adrenal Insufficiency: Patients with Addison's disease suffer profound hypotension on minimal stress such as blood loss, trauma, or anesthesia. Patients who have been on regular therapeutic doses of corticosteroids (e.g., for arthritis or allergy) may have diminished adrenal cortical reserve and, unless supported by corticosteroids during and after surgery or other trauma, may develop resistant shock.

Clinical Findings.

The classical signs of shock are hypotension, tachycardia, pallor, and prostration accompanied by evidence of hyperactivity of the sympathetic nervous system (such as cold, sweaty skin). A precipitating cause of blood or plasma loss can usually be readily identified. From the standpoint of management, it is useful to recognize 3 stages of shock: compensated, established, and resistant.

A. Compensated Shock: When less than 20% of blood volume is lost, hypotension is usually prevented by compensatory vasoconstriction. During this stage, other manifestations of intense sympathetic activity may appear such as pallor; cool, moist skin; thirst; and mild tachycardia. Occasionally bradycardia or even mild hypertension may occur. There is generalized weakness. The patient may be comfortable and normotensive in the recumbent position, but become faint and hypotensive when sat up. Induction of general or spinal anesthesia at this stage may produce vasorelaxation and precipitate severe shock. It is important to suspect hypovolemia during the compensated phase of shock and to institute appropriate treatment.

B. Established Shock: Hypotension (systolic BP below 100 mm. Hg) is superimposed on the above early signs when blood volume deficit exceeds about 20%. Tachycardia (over 90) with small or "thready" pulse develops. Prostration is marked, and sympathetic activity is intensified. The patient may complain of thirst. Oliguria is present. Metabolic acidosis develops. The sensorium is usually clear until shock is moderately severe, although pain responses may be lessened. Air hunger, progressive dulling of the sensorium, coma, and unobtainable BP or pulse are all signs of severe shock, indicating loss of 40-50% of blood volume. Under these circumstances, immediate and massive blood replacement is required to prevent cardiac arrest and death.

C. Resistant Shock: Improvement in BP, pulse, mental state, and other signs usually occurs promptly or, at most, within 1-2 hours when blood volume has been restored. If shock is resistant to treatment or recurs after a transient remission, one of the following causes should be suspected and sought: (1) Inadequate blood replacement, (2) continued blood loss, (3) brain trauma, (4) thoracic injury interfering with ventilation or circulation, e.g., cardiac tamponade, tension pneumothorax, flail chest, (5) ruptured viscus with continued intraperitoneal or retroperitoneal leakage, (6) coincident disease, e.g., cardiac or pulmonary disease, sepsis, electrolyte imbalance (especially metabolic acidosis), adrenal insufficiency, and (7) prolonged hypoxia due to inadequate blood flow, which may produce "irreversible shock" due to brain, cardiac, and generalized tissue damage.

Preventive Measures.

Identify patients in whom shock is impending, and institute the following prophylactic steps without delay.

(1) Control and replace blood loss.
(2) Splint fractures.
(3) Relieve pain and apprehension.
(4) Keep patient recumbent.
(5) Avoid unnecessary movement. Rough handling and undue manipulation may precipitate shock.
(6) Treat all physiologic abnormalities which might intensify shock, e.g., dehydration, electrolyte imbalance, hypoxia, and infection.

Treatment.

Act rapidly. Shock is an acute emergency which takes precedence over all other conditions except gross hemorrhage and respiratory failure. **Correction of hypovolemia by restoration of effective blood volume is the primary goal of antishock therapy.** Begin at once to replace the volume of blood estimated to have been lost. In addition, identify and begin appropriate treatment of the underlying cause of the shock.

A. Recumbent or slightly head-down (Trendelenburg) position. Do not move the patient unnecessarily.

B. Monitor vital signs closely. Arterial and central venous pressure, pulse, respiration, temperature, urine output, specific gravity, osmolality, and hematocrit are recorded at appropriate intervals. Continuous Ecg. monitor is connected. Serum electrolytes and arterial blood gases are determined as required.

C. Maintain oxygenation. Clear the airway. Administer oxygen by nasal catheter, cannula, or mask at 5-10 L./minute. Rule out chest injury. Persistent dyspnea, cyanosis, or inadequate ventilation requires immediate control. Tracheal intubation or tracheostomy to permit suctioning of secretions or assisted respiration may be lifesaving. In severe shock and in patients with major chest injuries and chronic lung disease, it is necessary to obtain arterial pH and arterial blood gases (PO_2, PCO_2, HCO_3^-) in order to evaluate pulmonary status. Repeated determinations are indicated in suspected respiratory failure or in incipient posttraumatic pulmonary insufficiency.

D. Keep the patient comfortably warm. Excessive external heat produces undesirable vasodilatation.

E. Control pain promptly. Use all appropriate first aid measures, including splints, dressings, and careful transportation. Shocked patients often have little or no pain. When necessary, give morphine sulfate, 5-10 mg. ($^1/_{12}$-$^1/_6$ gr.) I.V., to ensure rapid action and to prevent delay in absorption from ischemic tissues. **Caution:** Do not give narcotics to patients in coma or to those who have head injuries or respiratory depression.

F. Allay apprehension. Reassure the patient. A sedative is often more suitable than a narcotic. Use pentobarbital sodium, 0.1

Gm. ($1\frac{1}{2}$ gr.) I.M., or diazepam (Valium®), 5-10 mg. I.M. or I.V.

G. Parenteral Fluids: Restore adequate blood volume at once with the fluids immediately available. Normal cardiac output and tissue perfusion is the goal. Whole blood is the most effective fluid available for this purpose. Plasma, plasma products, plasma expanders, lactated Ringer's injection, normal saline, and 5% dextrose solution are also effective, in that order.

When starting the initial infusion, obtain blood for Hct., CBC, typing, and cross-matching. When surface veins are unavailable because of peripheral collapse, it may be necessary to puncture the femoral vein so that a blood sample can be collected and a temporary infusion given until a cut-down can be made in the antecubital space or ankle for insertion of a polyethylene catheter.

In patients in whom intensive, difficult shock therapy is anticipated, do a cut-down on the brachial, cephalic, or external jugular vein and thread a plastic catheter into the subclavian or innominate vein or the superior vena cava for fluid administration and intermittent determination of central venous pressure. Alternatively, the central venous pressure line may be inserted by direct puncture of the internal jugular or subclavian vein (Daily, P.O., and others, Arch. Surg. 101:534-536, 1970). Observation of urine output and specific gravity is essential in such cases, and constant bladder drainage with a Foley catheter should be instituted if voiding is unsatisfactory.

1. Whole blood - When whole blood has been lost, use properly typed and cross-matched whole blood for replacement if possible. In severe shock after extensive trauma, it may be necessary to transfuse massively. Bank blood should be warmed to body temperature before administration in order to avoid hypothermia if large-volume replacement is anticipated. Transfusion of over 4000 ml. in one-half hour has been required for resuscitation. If overloading is feared, determine central venous pressure before and after each unit of blood is given. Venous pressure may be monitored with a simple side-arm connected to the needle and the infusion set. A calibrated glass manometer is attached to the side-arm whenever venous pressure is to be measured. Transfuse until the systolic pressure is above 100 mm. Hg or venous pressure is above 12 cm. water. Rh-negative universal donor (group O) blood with low anti-A titer may be used without cross-matching if necessary to save life. Pressure transfusion through multiple venipunctures may be advisable.
2. Plasma and serum albumin - Plasma and its products can be stored and made immediately available for emergencies. They are specifically indicated when plasma loss has led to hemoconcentration, as in burns and peritonitis. Pooled plasma is most likely to transmit homologous serum jaundice and should therefore be used only when other agents are inadequate or unavailable. Normal Human Serum Albumin, U.S.P., or salt-poor serum albumin contains 25 Gm. albumin/100 ml. and is equivalent in osmotic pressure to 500 ml. of plasma. It is expensive, but it will not transmit

homologous serum jaundice. Plasmanate® is a 5% human plasma protein fraction also free of the risk of hepatitis.

3. Electrolyte solutions - The rapid intravenous administration to a patient in shock of 1-2 L. of lactated Ringer's injection expands the blood volume and will often restore BP to normal. If the blood loss has been minimal, shock can be relieved without the use of blood or colloid solutions. Preliminary administration of lactated Ringer's injection allows time for proper typing and cross-matching of blood, and the balanced electrolyte solution serves to prevent depletion of the interstitial fluid, which may be markedly reduced in hypovolemic shock treated by blood or plasma alone. If lactated Ringer's injection is not available, 5% glucose, normal saline or, preferably, normal saline buffered with 45 mEq. of sodium bicarbonate per liter may be used. Oral administration of lactated Ringer's or salt solution may be helpful if shock must be treated where there is no access to intravenous fluids.

   Inadequate tissue perfusion in severe shock leads to anaerobic cellular metabolism with increased production of organic acids and metabolic acidosis. This may further reduce cardiac output and tissue perfusion, so that progressive metabolic acidosis leads to death, usually by ventricular fibrillation. Metabolic acidosis can be confirmed by blood electrolyte and pH studies and arterial blood lactic acid. Solution of sodium bicarbonate, available in ampules of 45 mEq., may be added to crystalloid, colloid, or whole blood infusions. If acidosis is present - as indicated by arterial pH of less than 7.35 - give sodium bicarbonate, 40-100 mEq. I.V. initially, and gauge further therapy by serial arterial pH and electrolyte determinations.

4. Dextran - Dextrans are effective plasma substitutes in the emergency treatment of shock. They are water-soluble biosynthetic polysaccharides of high molecular weight and oncotic pressure. Dextran 70 has an average molecular weight of 70,000 and is available as a 6% solution in either normal saline or 5% glucose. Dextran 40 (Rheomacrodex®) has an average molecular weight of 40,000 and is available as a 10% solution in either normal saline or 5% glucose. Dextrans have the advantage of ready availability, of compatibility with other intravenous solutions, and of not causing infectious hepatitis. They also reduce blood viscosity and red cell agglutination. Prolongation of bleeding time and a functional defect in platelets have been seen after administration of dextran.

   Dextrans should be used with caution in thrombocytopenic patients. Obtain blood for typing and cross-matching prior to giving dextran, which may interfere with these tests. A small percentage of individuals may experience a mild urticarial reaction, and rarely there may be tightness of chest, wheezing, vomiting, or other systemic symptoms of anaphylactoid type. Symptoms and signs of adverse systemic reaction may be relieved by parenteral administration of antihistamines, ephedrine, or epinephrine (see p. 31) and discontinuance of the dextran infusion. The usual dose is 500-

1000 ml. I.V., but this quantity can be increased to 1500 ml. if required to combat shock. The rate of injection should be from 20-40 ml./minute so that the time required for administration of 500 ml. averages 15-30 minutes. Since interstitial fluid deficits must be corrected, crystalloid in the form of Ringer's or saline solution should be given in addition to dextran. Whole blood is essential if blood loss has been great.

5. Drug therapy -
   a. Vasopressor drugs - These agents are of value in the management of hypotension not associated with decrease in blood volume. There is little place for vasopressors in hypovolemic shock, and they often cause harm by increasing the tissue ischemia through excessive vasoconstriction. Blood volume expansion by parenteral blood and other fluids is the primary treatment of hypovolemia. A vasopressor drug may occasionally be useful to sustain BP temporarily and to preserve blood flow to vital centers until parenteral fluid can be started, whereupon the vasopressor should be discontinued as soon as possible. Dosage levels for the various agents are empirical and must be adjusted to obtain the desired BP response, which should not exceed normotensive levels. It is preferable to try metaraminol (Aramine®) before using levarterenol (Levophed®), the most powerful vasoconstrictor. Both drugs are alpha-adrenergic and beta-adrenergic stimulators, with alpha stimulation predominating. They have vasopressor and cardiotonic (inotropic) effects that result in an increase in cardiac output, peripheral resistance, and blood pressure.
      (1) Metaraminol bitartrate (Aramine®) - Administer 4-16 mg. I.M., or 15-200 mg. in 250-1000 ml. of 5% dextrose, or 0.5-5 mg. I.V.
      (2) Levarterenol bitartrate (Levophed®) - Administer 4-16 mg. in 1 L. of 5% dextrose solution I.V. Avoid extravasation. Give in upper extremity or into a major central vein. Levarterenol may cause tissue necrosis if it leaks into the tissues or if the infusion is in the ankle vein. Constant supervision with regular determination of BP is essential. With concentrations greater than 4 mg./L., an inlying venous catheter is required.
   b. Vasodilator drugs - Vasodilator drugs may be useful in carefully selected patients who continue to have low arterial blood pressure, possibly associated with high central venous pressure, in spite of adequate blood volume replacement. Also, if vasoconstriction is still pronounced and the capillary circulation is sluggish, regional blood flow may be improved by the judicious use of a vasodilator. The most frequently used drug is isoproterenol. It is a beta-adrenergic stimulator with direct (inotropic) action on the heart. It does not produce a marked increase in blood pressure but causes an increase in myocardial contractility, cardiac output, and visceral blood flow and a decrease in peripheral resistance and central venous pressure. Because of its inotropic effect, an

increased incidence of cardiac arrhythmias makes the administration of isoproterenol hazardous when the heart rate exceeds 120/minute. Phenoxybenzamine hydrochloride (Dibenzyline®) is an alpha-adrenergic blocking agent which blocks the vasoconstrictor effects of endogenous epinephrine and norepinephrine, thus acting as a vasodilator. It is an experimental drug and is not available for general use. Blood volume should always be restored and central venous pressure raised to normal levels before giving a vasodilator drug.

(1) Isoproterenol - Administer **(cautiously)** 1 mg. diluted in 500 ml. of 5% dextrose in saline or dextrose in water I.V. Begin infusion at a rate of 4 μg. or 2 ml./minute (20-30 drops/minute). Increase as required for effect, usually not exceeding 10 μg. or 5 ml./minute. Monitor Ecg., CVP, BP, and urine output.

(2) Phenoxybenzamine hydrochloride (Dibenzyline®) - Administer 1 mg./kg. in 500 ml. dextrose in saline or dextrose in water I.V. over at least one hour. Monitor vital signs.

c. Hydrocortisone - There is no convincing evidence that corticosteroids are of significant value in hypovolemic shock.

H. Treatment of Oliguria: Normal urinary output (at least 40-50 ml./hour in the average adult) is a major objective and an important prognostic sign in the management of hypovolemic shock. Prompt and sufficient fluid therapy is the most important measure in prevention and treatment of oliguria. Effective circulating plasma volume is required to preserve renocortical blood flow, which is reduced in shock by compensatory sympathetic mechanisms. In the presence of severe hypovolemia, kidney damage leading to renal failure may result from diminished kidney perfusion secondary to the marked vasoconstriction which prevents a profound fall in blood pressure. Low urine output may also result in deleterious effects due to accumulation in the tubules of hemoglobin and myoglobin released into the circulation by tissue damage. When the patient does not respond to fluid replacement by satisfactory urine output, osmotic diuresis with mannitol or chemical diuresis with ethacrynic acid or furosemide should be considered. Although the effectiveness of these agents continues to be under study, it is probable that prevention of oliguria by osmotic or chemical diuresis serves to prevent acute tubular necrosis in some cases. If fluid replacement and osmotic and chemical diuresis fail, do not persist with fluid loading. Accept the probability that the patient has intrinsic renal insufficiency and begin conservative management by limiting fluids and, if necessary, using dialysis (see p. 172).

1. Osmotic diuresis - Mannitol is an inert 6-carbon polyalcohol which can be administered intravenously in 10-25% solution. Perhaps the best indication for its use is when measured urine output is low despite adequate fluid and blood replacement. It produces a marked increase in total osmolality of the plasma and is rapidly distributed throughout the extracellular fluid. The result is a sharp increase in plasma and

extracellular fluid by withdrawal of water from body cells. There follows a brisk osmotic diuresis due to the fact that mannitol is readily excreted by the kidney but is not absorbed from the glomerular filtrate. By inducing rapid urine flow, mannitol is said to prevent the acute renal failure which may follow major crushing injuries, severe shock, extensive burns, and transfusion reactions. In selected patients with these conditions in whom oliguria is present or anticipated, it may be of value to give mannitol. Mannitol must be accompanied by adequate fluid replacement and must be given within the first few hours after injury to be most effective. The drastic redistribution of body water caused by mannitol may produce undesirable side-effects such as hyponatremia, later hypernatremia, plasma volume over-expansion, and renal tubular changes. Mannitol is a plasma expander; it is therefore advisable to monitor central venous pressure and urine output during therapy. Mannitol may be kept conveniently available in sterile solution for I.V. injection as 50 ml. of 25% solution and 500 ml. of 20% solution. After preliminary resuscitative measures and fluid replacement have been instituted in severe crushing injuries and other conditions predisposing to acute renal failure, give 12.5-25 Gm. of mannitol immediately by syringe and follow with an infusion of an additional 50 Gm. in 500-1000 ml. balanced electrolyte or normal saline solution. Urine output, monitored by means of a Foley catheter in the bladder, should be in the range of 50-60 ml./hour if the response is good. In the presence of continued anuria or severe oliguria, a dose of 50-75 Gm. of mannitol should be considered maximum. The beneficial effects of mannitol are still under study and may be no greater than those of the diuresis produced by hydration with balanced electrolyte, normal saline, or 5% dextrose solution.

2. Chemical diuresis - If there is no response to mannitol administration and circulating blood volume has been restored, give furosemide (Lasix®), 10-20 mg. I.V. Alternatively, ethacrynic acid (Edecrin®), 50 mg. I.V., may be given. Dosage of either drug may be repeated in 1-2 hours. These drugs depend on adequate blood volume for effectiveness. Urine output and central venous pressure should be monitored. Chemical or osmotic diuresis may be repeated every 6-8 hours if necessary to assure adequate urine flow.

Evaluation of Antishock Therapy.

Constant observation is essential. Accurate determination of blood volume deficit is rarely feasible in an emergency. Fluid requirements must be estimated clinically, and the response of vital signs is the most dependable guide to therapy. When systolic BP rises above 100 mm. Hg, tachycardia lessens, and the skin becomes warm and dry, shock is abating and infusions may be slowed or stopped while progress is observed.

A. Record BP, pulse, and respirations every 15-30 minutes.
B. Measure fluid intake and output. Severe or prolonged shock frequently produces tubular damage and may cause acute renal failure (see p. 74).
C. Hct. should be repeated at appropriate intervals (e.g., every few hours if continued bleeding is suspected). Keep in mind

Variables Frequently Monitored in Shock

Measurement	Typical Normal Values	Typical Values In Severe Shock
Arterial blood pressure	120/180	< 90 mm. Hg systolic
Pulse rate	80/min.	> 100/min.
Central venous pressure	4-8 cm. saline	< 3 cm.
Hematocrit	35-45%	< 35%
Arterial blood:		
pH	7.4	7.3
pO_2	95 mm. Hg	85 mm. Hg
pCO_2	40 mm. Hg	< 30 mm. Hg
$-HCO_3$	23-25 mEq./liter	< 23 mEq./liter
Lactic acid	12 mg./100 ml.	> 20 mg./100 ml.
Urine:		
Volume	50 ml./hour	< 20 ml./hour
Specific gravity	1.015-1.025	> 1.025
Osmolality	300-400 mOsm./ Kg. water	> 700 mOsm./ Kg. water

that Hct. usually falls gradually over a period of 24-48 hours as hemodilution occurs. Determine blood volume by the radio-isotope or dye-dilution technic if possible and repeat as needed.

D. Listen to the patient's chest for signs of pulmonary edema and observe central venous pressure if excessive fluid administration is feared. Free fluctuation of the saline column on respirations when the manometer is held at the level of the right atrium indicates proper placement and patency of the CVP catheter. Normal range of CVP is 4-8 cm. of saline. CVP persistently below this range is consistent with inadequate volume replacement or, after presumed adequate replacement, of continuing occult blood loss. An elevated CVP (12-18 cm. of saline or above) in the presence of low arterial pressure suggests right heart failure or pericardial tamponade.

SEPTIC SHOCK
(Vasogenic, Toxic, or Endotoxic Shock)

Diagnostic Features.

Septic shock is characterized by onset of hypotension, tachycardia, and prostration in a febrile patient in whom hemorrhage or other cause for shock is not present. It is commonly caused by infection due to gram-negative organisms (Escherichia coli, klebsiella, proteus, pseudomonas, meningococci) and less frequently by gram-positive organisms such as pneumococci, staphylococci, and clostridia. Frequent predisposing factors include diabetes, hematologic malignancies, diseases of the genitourinary, hepatobiliary, and intestinal tracts, and corticosteroid, immunosuppressive, or radiation therapy. Immediate precipitating causes may be urinary, biliary, or gynecologic surgery or manipulations. Septic shock occurs predominantly in the very young and the very old and should always be suspected when a febrile patient has chills associated with hypotension. There may or may not be a known infection.

The hypotension associated with the toxemia of overwhelming infection is usually characterized by initial vasoconstriction followed by (or alternating with) vasodilatation, with venous pooling of blood. There may be increased, normal, or decreased cardiac output, central venous pressure, blood volume, and peripheral resistance. In the early stage, the skin may be warm and the pulse full, with peripheral vasoconstriction developing later. Hyperventilation may occur and may result in respiratory alkalosis. Sensorium and urine output may at first be normal and then deteriorate rapidly. There is a direct toxic effect on the heart and adrenals. The symptoms and signs of the inciting infection are not invariably present, particularly in the geriatric patient. Evidence of sepsis may be obscured by corticosteroid therapy or inadequate antibiotic therapy.

Hemoconcentration (increased hematocrit) and oliguria are common findings, and they usually respond poorly to parenteral fluids alone. Early leukopenia followed by leukocytosis may occur. Usually, a high white blood cell count (15,000 or more), with shift to the left, is found. Identification of the infecting organism is urgent. Blood and other appropriate cultures are taken immediately and repeated several times daily if necessary. Antibiotic sensitivity studies are crucial. Blood and other specimens for culture are also examined by Gram's stain in pursuit of early diagnosis.

Treatment.

As in other forms of shock, the objective is to improve tissue perfusion and metabolism by relieving hypotension and sluggish capillary blood flow. There may be slight or no hypovolemia. Measures to combat infection are instituted, including necessary surgical procedures for drainage of abscess or removal of infected tissue. Intensive antibiotic therapy should be started immediately.

A. General Supportive Measures: These include the administration of oxygen and the treatment of accompanying disorders. As in treatment of hypovolemic shock, tissue metabolism and urine output must be maintained by adequate fluid intake and control of BP and capillary perfusion. An indwelling bladder catheter may be essential for accurate observation of renal function, and monitoring of central venous pressure may be required as a guide to fluid administration. Continuous Ecg. monitoring is advisable.

B. Parenteral Fluids: These should include plasma if hemoconcentration is present, or whole blood if anemia is present. Dehydration and electrolyte imbalance must be corrected. Relieve acidosis by administration of sodium bicarbonate. If the central venous pressure is low, expand the blood volume to bring it to 10-15 cm. of saline.

C. Antibiotic Therapy: This should be intensive and specific if the infecting organism has been identified. The causative agent is frequently unknown at the time of onset of septic shock, however; therefore, prompt empirical treatment with antibiotics is indicated as soon as blood and other cultures have been obtained. In order to combat either gram-negative or gram-positive bacteria, kanamycin, 4 Gm. daily, and cephalothin, 12 Gm. daily (or other appropriate broad-spectrum combination), are administered I.V. initially. Specific antibiotics are substituted as soon as sensitivity data are available from cultures.

D. Corticosteroids: Corticosteroid therapy is generally considered to be indicated in septic shock. Its effectiveness is possibly due to its vasodilating effect, which results in improved tissue perfusion and diminished metabolic acidosis, and to its stimulation of liver cells to metabolize lactic acid. Give hydrocortisone sodium succinate (Solu-Cortef®), or equivalent, 0.5-1 Gm. every 4-6 hours I.V. for 24-48 hours. Begin cortisone therapy as soon as septic shock is suspected.

E. Vasodilator Therapy: Isoproterenol should be tried if central venous pressure is initially high or if shock persists after it becomes normal. Administer isoproterenol, 2.5 mg. in 5% dextrose in water, at a rate of 0.5-1 ml./minute. If shock persists after 15 minutes, if urine output remains less than 30 ml./hour, or if central venous pressure is elevated, double the infusion rate. Monitor the vital signs, including continuous observation for excessive tachycardia. Isoproterenol is a beta-adrenergic stimulator which increases cardiac output by its action on myocardial contraction. It produces peripheral vasodilatation. Because of its inotropic effect, an increased incidence of arrhythmia makes its use hazardous if the cardiac rate is greater than 120/minute. Vasoconstrictor drugs are rarely indicated in septic shock.

F. Disseminated Intravascular Coagulation (DIC): This may occur in septic shock. When blood pressure returns to normal and sepsis is controlled, the condition tends to subside without specific therapy. Under these circumstances, consumption of coagulation factors usually ceases and they regenerate rapidly. If coagulation studies confirm the presence of persistent DIC and there are significant hemorrhagic manifestations, heparin should be administered. Give 100 units (1 mg.)/Kg. of body weight I.V. initially and every 4 hours thereafter by continuous I.V. administration. Response to heparin is indicated by improvement of bleeding and a rise within 12 hours of factors V and VIII and fibrinogen. Platelets rise at a slower rate. Discontinue heparin therapy when the cause of DIC has been corrected and coagulation factors have been restored to hemostatic levels.

CARDIOGENIC SHOCK

Cardiogenic shock may be described as a failure of the circulation resulting from an acute decrease of cardiac output (so-called "forward heart failure"). It is typically characterized by severe hypotension, low pulse pressure, oliguria, cold and clammy skin, and dulling of the sensorium. It may be caused by myocardial infarction, cardiac tamponade, severe tachycardia or bradycardia, terminal congestive failure, or massive pulmonary embolism. Cardiogenic shock may be precipitated by trauma, or it may be an intercurrent development in the course of a surgical illness. Recognition of cardiogenic shock is important, since intensive parenteral fluid administration - as for hypovolemic shock - is usually contraindicated.

Treatment consists of relief of pain, administration of oxygen, correction of arrhythmia, relief of tamponade if present, and control of hypotension with vasopressor agents. When vasoconstrictor drugs such as metaraminol (Aramine®) and levarterenol (Levophed®) are used, systolic blood pressure should usually be maintained between 90 and 100 mm. Hg. No attempt should be made to achieve the level of blood pressure before shock, providing that the sensorium is clear and urine output is satisfactory. Ecg., central venous pressure, and other vital signs should be monitored at all times, and the patient should be placed in an intensive care or coronary care unit if one is available. Equipment for D.C. defibrillation of the heart is essential.

Right heart failure is suggested when central venous pressure is above 20 cm. of water, in which case rapid digitalization may be in order. Intravenous digitalization is accomplished by giving digoxin, 0.5 mg. I.V., slowly as an initial dose, followed by 0.25 mg. I.V. every 3 hours until a total dose of 1.5 mg. has been administered.

Isoproterenol may be useful when low cardiac output, hypotension, elevated venous pressure, and peripheral vasoconstriction persist in spite of the above measures. Beneficial effects are due to increased myocardial contractility and decreased peripheral resistance. There is danger of serious cardiac arrhythmia if isoproterenol is continued when the heart rate exceeds 120 (see p. 24).

Significant atrial and ventricular arrhythmias may call for I.V. administration of lidocaine (Xylocaine®) (see p. 72). Various mechanical assistance devices for the failing heart are still in the experimental stage.

ANAPHYLACTIC REACTIONS
(Anaphylactic Shock)

These catastrophic and frequently fatal allergic reactions may occur within seconds or minutes after parenteral administration of animal sera or drugs, including antibiotics. These reactions also may occur rarely after orally administered drugs or foods. Although there is occasionally no history of previous exposure to the foreign substance, anaphylaxis undoubtedly represents induced hypersensitivity by previous injection or ingestion.

Clinical Findings.

Symptoms and signs include apprehension, generalized urticaria or edema, a choking sensation, wheezing, cough, or status asthmaticus. In severe cases there may be hypotension, loss of consciousness, dilatation of pupils, incontinence, and convulsions, with death occurring suddenly. Three syndromes of anaphylaxis may be recognized, based upon the most conspicuous presenting feature: (1) laryngeal edema, (2) bronchospasm, and (3) vascular collapse.

Emergency Treatment. (Act immediately!)

A. Position the patient for comfort and ease of respiration. If he is unconscious, place him in the supine or slightly head-down position.
B. Maintain oxygenation and keep the airway open (see p. 126). If respirations have ceased, give artificial respiration by the

mouth-to-mouth technic (see pp. 8-9); or with mask or endotracheal tube and positive pressure oxygen breathing (see p. 126). If equipment for insertion of an endotracheal tube is not available, tracheostomy may be necessary.

C. Medical Measures: Epinephrine is the drug of choice for emergency use. It may be necessary to supplement it with intravenous antihistaminic drugs or steroids and, in case of intense bronchospasm, with intravenous aminophylline (see below).

1. Epinephrine hydrochloride - (The drug of choice.)
   a. I. M. - 1 ml. of 1:1000 solution I. M., repeat in 5-10 minutes and later p. r. n.
   b. I. V. (for even more rapid effect) - 0.1-0.4 ml. of 1:1000 solution in 10 ml. of saline slowly I. V.
2. Diphenhydramine hydrochloride (Benadryl®), or tripelennamine hydrochloride (Pyribenzamine®), 10-20 mg. (1/6-1/3 gr.) I. V. if response to epinephrine is not prompt and sustained.
3. Hydrocortisone sodium succinate (Solu-Cortef®), 100-250 mg., or prednisolone hemisuccinate (Meticortelone Soluble®), 50-100 mg. I. V. over a period of 30 seconds as adjunct to epinephrine and diphenhydramine. Dosage depends upon the severity of the condition; the drug may be repeated at increasing intervals (1, 3, 6, 10 hours, etc.) as indicated by the patient's clinical condition.
4. Aminophylline injection, 0.25-0.5 Gm. (3 3/4-7 1/2 gr.) in 10-20 ml. saline I. V. slowly for severe bronchospasm. Duration of action is 1-3 hours. May repeat in 3-4 hours.

Prophylaxis.

Avoid using potentially dangerous drugs or sera if possible. Be particularly cautious when administering parenteral medications to patients with a history of allergy or previous reaction to the agent to be injected. Give injections slowly and keep such individuals under close observation for an hour or more thereafter as required.

Always perform a sensitivity test (intradermal or conjunctival) before injecting animal sera or other agents to which a hypersensitivity reaction may occur. When sensitivity is demonstrated by a positive test or is suggested by the history, the patient must be desensitized by the administration of a series of divided doses.

COMA

Coma is loss of consciousness from which the patient cannot be aroused. A patient is considered semicomatose if he can be partially aroused by loud commands or painful stimuli but promptly lapses into unconsciousness again when the stimulus is withdrawn. Coma may be caused by poisoning (e.g., alcohol, barbiturates, narcotics, carbon monoxide), cerebral lesions (e.g., trauma, vascular accidents, tumors, infections, epilepsy), metabolic and constitutional disorders (e.g., diabetes mellitus, hypoglycemia, Addison's disease, uremia, hepatic coma, eclampsia), and by such miscellaneous disorders as toxemia of infection, hypovolemic shock, asphyxia, heat stroke, severe heart failure, and hysteria.

Diagnosis.

The "diagnosis" of coma consists of determining the specific causative factor. This requires a searching history from the patient or his friends or relatives and a complete physical examination with specific attention to the neurologic examination. When the diagnosis is still in doubt, the following examinations may be obtained rapidly and provide leads for further studies if required: urinalysis, CBC; blood glucose, urea, ammonia, electrolytes, and alcohol; analysis of gastric content; and CSF examination, skull x-rays, and blood cultures.

Treatment.

A. Emergency Measures: Recognize and treat life-endangering conditions immediately.
   1. Maintain adequate oxygenation. This is a cardinal principle in all emergency treatment.
      a. Keep the airway clear.
      b. Administer oxygen by nasal catheter, cannula, or mask if oxygenation is poor, as indicated by depressed respirations, cyanosis, or dyspnea.
      c. Use artificial respiration if breathing is failing or has stopped (see p. 10). Endotracheal intubation with mechanical ventilation is required in respiratory failure.
   2. Treat shock.
   3. Hospitalize the patient as soon as possible.

B. General Measures: Observe the patient constantly, record vital signs at regular intervals, and change his position every 30-60 minutes to avoid hypostatic pneumonitis and decubiti. A lateral and slightly head-down position is best for patients likely to vomit. Have a suction machine and an alert attendant near the bedside.

   Maintain fluid, electrolyte, and caloric intake (see pp. 129 and 150). Consider tube feeding if coma lasts more than 2-3 days (see p. 139). Recording the urine output is the best guide to fluid therapy (see p. 152). Catheterize if the bladder is distended or if the patient is unable to void within 8 hours. In critically ill patients and those with urinary retention, an indwelling catheter is advisable for closer observation of urine volume.

   Avoid narcotics, sedatives, and other medications until the diagnosis is established; marked restlessness can then be treated by administration of a parenteral sedative or tranquilizer preparation.

DIAGNOSTIC FEATURES OF SPECIFIC TYPES OF COMA

Nonsurgical causes of coma must be promptly recognized when they occur in surgical patients. Trauma and surgical operations not infrequently aggravate a preexisting metabolic or other derangement and cause rapid deterioration and coma. Medical consultation should be sought immediately.

Acute Alcoholic Intoxication.

Always rule out other causes of coma. **Caution:** Do not overlook head trauma or other injury in the alcoholic patient. Diagnosis is based on a history of drinking, alcoholic breath, flushed face, injected conjunctivas, slow and stertorous respirations, diminished reflexes, and a blood alcohol level above 0.5%. If coma is light, it may alternate with periods of delirium and restlessness.

Narcotic Poisoning.

Even small doses of narcotics may cause respiratory depression and coma in liver insufficiency, myxedema, emphysema, head injuries, and in debilitated or elderly patients. Delayed absorption of toxic amounts may occur if multiple subcut. or I.M. injections are given during a period of vasoconstriction, as in hypovolemic shock.

Diagnostic features include cold, clammy, cyanotic skin; pinpoint pupils, respiratory depression (breathing slow and irregular, sometimes Cheyne-Stokes); and a feeble and often irregular pulse.

Acute toxicity due to an overdose of a self-administered narcotic occurs commonly in some localities. Type and purity of the drug involved are usually difficult to determine, although a companion or acquaintance may know the patient's drug habits. Laboratory tests are of value in determining barbiturate, alcohol, or narcotic levels. The examiner should look for needle tracks along veins in the arms and wrists.

Diabetic Coma.

Coma may be precipitated in a diabetic patient by infection or failure to regulate insulin dosage. Diagnostic features include the following: history of diabetes, gradual onset with blurred vision and thirst, air hunger or Kussmaul breathing, dehydration (soft eyeballs), acetone breath (''fruity'' odor on breath), glycosuria, acetonuria, hyperglycemia, ketonemia, and low plasma bicarbonate.

The objective of treatment is to correct the acidosis by administering large doses of insulin with an abundance of fluid to overcome dehydration. The greatest single factor in reducing mortality is vigorous insulin therapy during the first 2-3 hours. Act promptly when coma is impending or present, and obtain the consultation of an internist.

Diabetic acidosis can be prevented by careful regulation of insulin and caloric intake during surgical illnesses (see p. 76).

Hypoglycemic Shock.

Weakness, hunger, irritability, faintness, tremors, and convulsions or coma. History of diabetes and use of insulin. Blood sugar consistently below 50 mg./100 ml. No sugar in urine.

If the patient is conscious, give sugar, glucose, or sweetened orange juice by mouth. If he is unconscious, give glucose I.V. (preferably 50%).

Uremic Coma.

A history of chronic renal disease may be obtained. The breath is urinous, and there is twitching of the extremities and, frequently, convulsions. Albuminuric retinitis, papilledema, and hypertension are characteristic of severe chronic nephritis. CBC shows anemia, usually normochromic. Urinalysis shows low sp. gr. (about 1.010), albumin, cells, and casts. Blood NPN is usually over 100 mg./100 ml. Creatinine and potassium levels are elevated. Blood bicarbonate and pH are depressed.

BLAST AND CRUSH INJURIES

BLAST INJURY

The blast force from an explosion may be transmitted to the body through air, water, or solid objects on which the patient is standing or resting. Serious internal damage may occur without evidence of surface injury. Victims are most likely to suffer damage or rupture involving the lungs or abdominal viscera. Localizing symptoms and signs are frequently delayed in onset.

Widespread alveolar hemorrhage with dyspnea, frothy hemoptysis, and cyanosis is typical of blast injury to the lungs. Tracheal intubation or tracheostomy may be required to aspirate secretions and administer oxygen (see p. 126). Do not overlook pneumothorax or hemothorax. Mild contusions of the abdominal viscera cause moderate discomfort and occasionally colicky pain which subsides within 48-96 hours. More serious injuries with impending or actual perforation produce signs of peritoneal irritation or shock.

Rupture of the ear drum by blast causes severe pain and often deafness. No local treatment is required. Packs and ear drops are contraindicated.

CRUSH INJURY

Patients who have been crushed and whose limbs have been com-pressed for an hour or more are likely to develop hypovolemic shock due to extravasation of blood and plasma into the injured tissues after the compression is released. If this shock is not treated, the prolonged hypotension often causes kidney damage and acute renal insufficiency. The combination of compression injury, shock, and acute renal failure is known as the "crush syndrome."

Treatment consists of controlling shock (see p. 18) and observing carefully for acute renal insufficiency (see p. 74).

BURNS

Burns are caused by a wide variety of agents, including flame, hot water, steam, electricity, and chemicals. The general principles of treatment are the same in all.

Depth or Degree of Burn.

A. First Degree: Erythema.

B. Second Degree: Erythema with blistering.

C. Third Degree: Destruction of full thickness of skin and frequently of deeper structures also.

Estimate of Extent of Burn.

The amount of body surface burned and the depth of the burn determine the fluid losses. The "rule of nines" is a useful means of estimating the percentage of total body surface involved by second or third degree burns of specific skin ares (see p. 36). The extent of burn is commonly overestimated. Second and third degree burns of over 15-20% of total body surface (10% in children and the elderly) usually cause marked fluid loss which results in burn shock. Burn mortality is markedly influenced by the depth and extent of the burn and the age of the patient. Burns of over 50% of body surface are frequently fatal, especially in children and the older age group.

Special Laboratory Examination.

A. Hematocrit: In severe burns, determine the Hct. repeatedly as a guide to fluid therapy.

B. Blood typing and cross-matching.

Symptoms of Fluid Deficiency in Burns.

Very close attention to clinical signs and symptoms is of great importance, particularly during the first 24 hours after the burn has occurred. Excessive thirst, vomiting, restlessness, disorientation, and mania - together with increase in pulse rate, decrease in BP, collapsed veins, and oliguria - are indications that fluid losses have exceeded the rate of fluid replacement. During this critical early phase the adequacy of treatment is best judged by the urinary output, which should ideally be 30-50 ml./hour. If the rate of urinary excretion is below these suggested volumes, it is important to exclude acute renal insufficiency as a cause of the oliguria before increasing the fluid intake (see p. 74).

Urine volumes greater than 100 ml. /hour indicate that too much fluid has been given, but after 48 hours the urinary output is completely unreliable as a guide to therapy. In part this is due to the release of nitrogenous wastes from the burned tissues, which act as diuretics; in addition, electrolyte deficits may force compensatory elimination of water, as in the developing phase of a low-salt syndrome. Under these conditions, therapy is guided almost exclusively by clinical signs and symptoms, using enough fluid to maintain normal turgor of the unburned skin, fullness of the veins, and moisture of the oral mucosa. The quantities of fluid required to accomplish this may be surprisingly large. However, care must be taken to avoid simple overhydration with edema of the unburned tissues or water intoxication, which may lead to coma or death.

Intravenous Replacement Therapy.

The objective of fluid therapy in acute burns is to maintain adequate tissue perfusion as indicated by blood pressure, pulse, urine output, acid-base balance, and the clinical state of consciousness and hydration of the patient. The volume of fluid required can

ESTIMATION OF BODY SURFACE AREA IN BURNS

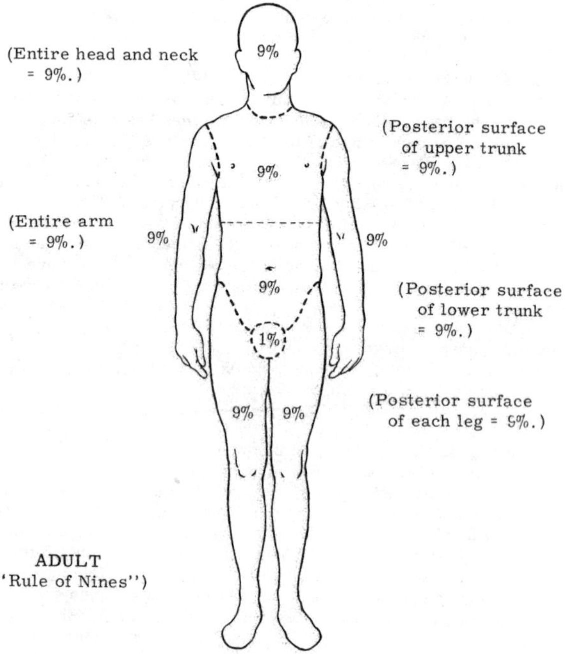

ADULT
("Rule of Nines")

Variations from Adult Distribution in Infants and Children (in %)*

	Newborn	1 yr.	5 yrs.	10 yrs.
Head	19	17	13	11
Both thighs	11	13	16	17
Both lower legs	10	10	11	12
Neck	2			
Anterior trunk	13			
Posterior trunk	13			
Both upper arms	8	These % remain		
Both lower arms	6	constant at all		
Both hands	5	ages.		
Both buttocks	5			
Both feet	7			
Genitals	1			
	100			

*After Berkow.

be calculated initially in a variety of ways provided that the replacement program is adjusted in accordance with the clinical response of the patient. With this principle in mind, the following formula can be used to make a preliminary estimate of fluid needs:

During the first 24 hours after a severe burn, give 1 ml. of plasma and 1 ml. of balanced electrolyte solution (e.g., Lactated Ringer's Injection, U.S.P.) for each 1% of body surface burned and each Kg. of body weight. In addition, adults require 1000-2000 ml. of balanced electrolyte solution to replace insensible loss.

Example: 70 Kg. man with a 40% burn

1. Plasma: $1 \times 70 \times 40$ =	2800 ml.
2. Electrolyte solution: $1 \times 70 \times 40$ =	2800 ml.
3. Insensible loss (electrolyte solution) =	1400 ml.
Total fluids first 24 hours =	7000 ml.

During second 24 hours, give one-half this amount.

If more than 50% of the body surface is burned, calculations should be based on only 50% involvement. In no case should more than 10,000 ml. of fluid be given in the first 24-hour period. In fact, 100 ml./Kg. body weight is usually sufficient as a maximum. Excess fluid in the early postburn period serves to increase the amount of edema formation and exerts little or no effect on blood volume. For this reason, the hematocrit may remain elevated during the first day and fluid intake should not be increased with a view to restoring the hematocrit rapidly to normal.

Experience shows that an electrolyte solution such as lactated Ringer's can usually be substituted for plasma in the above formula in burns of less than 35-40% of body surface.

Acidosis is frequently present and may be corrected by administration of 0.5 mEq. of $NaHCO_3$/Kg. body weight per mEq./L. decrease in plasma bicarbonate. Isotonic $NaHCO_3$ solution containing the calculated mEq. of $NaHCO_3$ required for treatment of the acidosis can be substituted for an equivalent volume of balanced electrolyte solution in the fluid replacement formula. After the first few days, potassium loss is usually marked, making it advisable to give about 100 mEq. potassium ion per day intravenously or by mouth.

Destruction of erythrocytes occurs in deep burns, but blood replacement is rarely required early in the postburn period. Later, 3-5 days after the burn, transfusion of whole blood or packed red cells may be used to correct a reduced red cell mass.

Oral Replacement Therapy.

Fluid and electrolyte replacement by the oral route can frequently be employed, alone or as a supplement to the intravenous route. For oral administration, a solution containing 5.5 Gm./L. of sodium chloride (93 mEq. Na^+/93 mEq. Cl^-) and 4 Gm./L. of sodium bicarbonate (47 mEq. Na^+/47 mEq. HCO_3^-) may be used. This mixture contains 140 mEq./L. of sodium and is usually well tolerated if given slowly as repeated sips.

Guides to Fluid Therapy.

Patients with burns greater than 25% will probably require intravenous therapy - at least initially - because of their tendency to vomit. In such patients an intravenous catheter for infusion and an inlying bladder catheter for bladder drainage should be promptly inserted. Elderly patients and those with extensive burns should have a catheter inserted via the subclavian or internal jugular vein into the superior vena cava for determination of central venous pressure. Fluid therapy and bladder drainage should be instituted before care of the burn wound is begun.

The objectives of fluid administration are to maintain plasma volume, urinary output, and blood pressure at satisfactory levels. Initially, lactated Ringer's injection is administered rapidly during the first two hours until a urinary output of 30-50 ml. per hour is established. Plasma may then be administered simultaneously with the electrolyte solution, the rate being determined by the volume of fluid required to maintain the urinary output. Central venous pressure is monitored to avoid circulatory overloading, especially in elderly patients or when there is pre-existing cardiovascular disease.

When urinary output lags below the optimum of 30-50 ml. per hour, the rate of administration of the electrolyte solution may be doubled and the urinary response noted. Alternatively, one liter of plasma may be administered in 30 minutes as test of renal function. Hypotension as a cause of the oliguria must be ruled out; plasma must be administered rapidly if hypotension occurs or is suspected. If urinary output remains low in spite of satisfactory venous and arterial pressure and a presumably adequate fluid intake, it may be helpful to give mannitol as described for the treatment of oliguria in hypovolemic shock (see p. 19). If no increase in urine output occurs in response to fluid loading and mannitol administration, it is probable that renal insufficiency exists. Under these circumstances, determination of urine osmolality and sodium content may be of diagnostic value. Low osmolality suggests renal failure and high osmolality suggests a need for additional fluid replacement. Urinary sodium above 40 mEq./L. suggests failure to reabsorb sodium due to renal insufficiency. Urinary sodium below 20 mEq./L. indicates adequate tubular reabsorption of sodium and the probable need for additional fluid.

The hematocrit rises in severe burns and may reach 60-65%. Adequate fluid therapy will control the rising hematocrit, but it is unnecessary and unwise to push fluids during the first 24-48 hours with the primary objective of lowering the hematocrit. It will come down spontaneously as edema fluid is returned to the circulation from the burn site. The most important parameters to observe in following the burn patient are the urinary output, the central venous and arterial blood pressures, and the clinical condition. Determination of pH and electrolyte values on blood and urine will serve as a guide to the adjustment of the electrolyte composition of the intravenous fluids. In respiratory tract burns, arterial pH, pCO_2, and pO_2 aid in early detection and management of respiratory insufficiency.

EARLY CARE OF THE BURN WOUND

First Aid.

Immersion of the burned area in cold water for 20-30 minutes immediately after burning, if feasible, will relieve pain and reduce cell damage.

A. **First degree burns require no treatment.**
B. Minor second degree burns may be washed with bland soap and water. Large blebs should be punctured aseptically but not removed. The wound is then covered with sterile petrolatum gauze and a pressure dressing. Change the dressing every 5-8 days. Healing usually takes about 2 weeks.
C. Severe burns should not be washed, greased, powdered, or painted with medication of any kind. Wrap the burned area in clean towels or sheets and transfer the patient to a hospital immediately.

Surgical Measures in Severe Burns.

A. Control pain, which is usually marked, with morphine sulfate, 10-15 mg. (1/6-1/4 gr.) I. V. or I. M., or other narcotic. General anesthesia is unnecessary for the initial cleansing and dressing of severe burns if a narcotic is used and procedures are done gently.
B. Treatment of Burned Area:
   1. **Aseptic technic is essential. Wear cap, mask, sterile gown, and gloves when dressing burns. Sterile linen, instruments, and dressings are required.**
   2. **Cleanse burn and surrounding area with bland or hexachlorophene soap and sterile warm water. Wash gently with gauze sponges. Remove grease or oil with ether or benzene.**
   3. **Debride carefully. Remove only loose and necrotic tissue. Puncture blebs aseptically and leave them in place as protective coverings.**
   4. Closed treatment - Apply petrolatum gauze and a pressure dressing. Place a single layer of petrolatum (or Xeroform®) gauze smoothly over the burn, cover this with soft pads or other absorbent dressings, and secure firmly in place with stockinet or elastic or gauze bandage. Dressings are changed every 2-5 days. The wound surface is debrided and cleansed as indicated at these times.

      A variation of the closed technic is advocated by Monafo and Moyer (Arch. Surg. **91**:200, 1965), who cover the burn with roller bandages of absorbent gauze soaked in 0.5% silver nitrate solution. Catheters may be placed within the dressing for periodic (e.g., every 2 hours) instillation of more solution as required to keep the dressing wet. The dressing is changed daily in bed, and all burns are covered, including those on the hands, face, and genitalia. The antibacterial action of the silver nitrate appears to diminish significantly the surface infection and systemic toxicity which are inevitable in the extensive deep burn. Debridement of slough is accomplished in bed as separation occurs. Fluid and electrolyte derangement, particularly hyponatremia and hypochloremic alkalosis, may result from absorption and excretion across the burn surface. This must be counteracted by appropriate replacement therapy. Although argyria is said not to be a complication of the treatment, this must be finally proved by further experience with the method. Additional disadvantages are that this method causes pain on dressing change, is cumbersome to use, discolors and obscures the wound, and stains linens.

5. Exposure treatment - In this form of treatment, no dressings or medications are applied to the burn after cleansing and debridement. On exposure to air a coagulum of serum seals the burn wound. This is the preferred method of treating burns of the head, neck, genitalia, and perineum. It is also suitable for limited burns on one side of the trunk or extremity. In mass casualities it may be necessary to treat the burns in this manner. The patient is placed on clean sheets. He must be turned frequently when burns encircle the body in order to avoid maceration. If infection occurs beneath the coagulum, it should be removed and warm saline compresses applied to the area.

C. Prevention of Infection: Reliance is placed on thorough cleansing of the burn and on aseptic dressing technics. Prophylactic systemic antibiotics are rarely used. Cultures are obtained from exudates, and specific antibiotics chosen on the basis of sensitivity studies when signs of infection appear.

The outlook for control of burn sepsis in extensive burns has been improved by the incorporation of antibacterial agents in dressings used in closed treatment of burns and by topical application of these agents in the exposure method of treatment (Moncrief, J. A., Surgery 63:862-867, 1968). Silver nitrate has been discussed above. **Mafenide (Sulfamylon®)** - a sulfonamide derivative - reduces surface infection when incorporated in a fine mesh gauze dressing or when applied 1-2 times daily as an 8.5-10% cream to the exposed burn surface. It is easy to apply and remove, is locally nontoxic, and has a wide spectrum of bacterial effectiveness. It has the disadvantage of pain on application and of carbonic anhydrase inhibition on absorption; the latter may result in blocking of the renal buffering mechanism, excessive bicarbonate excretion, impaired ammonia production, and chloride retention. Inhibition of carbonic anhydrase also interferes with CO_2 transport and may result in hyperventilation, decreased serum CO_2, and respiratory alkalosis. Sensitivity leads to the development of rash in about 5% of patients. **Gentamicin** - as 0.1% ointment or, preferably, cream - is an excellent but expensive topical application for burns. It is effective against many strains of pseudomonas as well as some gram-negative bacilli. Since resistant strains of bacteria may develop, topical gentamicin should be restricted to patients with severe burns and these patients isolated to prevent the spread of resistant organisms. The possibility of systemic toxic effects should be kept in mind when treating large burns with a gentamicin preparation. **Silver sulfadiazine,** a promising topical preparation for use in burn therapy, is still an experimental drug and is not yet available for general use.

Early vaccination with a polyvalent pseudomonas vaccine is an experimental and unproved approach to control of burn wound sepsis.

There is suggestive but inconclusive evidence that 1 ml./Kg. of human gamma globulin, administered shortly after a major burn and repeated in 2 days, may result in a reduction of pseudomonas sepsis in certain children.

D. Immunization against tetanus should be given during the first 24 hours in all major burns.

Burns of Specific Anatomic Areas.

A. Respiratory tract burns should be suspected in extensive burns of the head and neck. Inhalation of flame or hot gases produces severe tracheobronchitis and pneumonitis. Obstructive laryngeal edema may develop rapidly, preceded by stridor, copious respiratory tract secretions, dyspnea, and cyanosis. Tracheostomy should be done without delay if there is significant obstruction or retained secretions. Antimicrobial therapy for subsequent respiratory tract infection - which is virtually inevitable - should be based on culture and sensitivity studies of sputum or aspirated tracheal secretions.

B. Head and neck burns are treated by exposure (see above). They are often less deep than suspected initially, and rapid healing is favored by the great vascularity of the region. Early grafting of eyelid burns is important to avoid ectropion and corneal ulceration due to exposure.

C. Hand burns must be carefully cleansed and the fingers dressed individually with petrolatum gauze. Remove rings. Immobilize the entire hand in the position of function by pressure dressings and splints. Soon after the first redressing, which is done 5-8 days after the burn, areas of third degree burn should be excised in a bloodless field (using a pneumatic tourniquet) and a skin graft applied in order to obtain the earliest possible restoration of function. (See also Chapter 17.)

D. Joints should be maintained in optimal position and all third degree involvement grafted early to avoid disabling contractures.

E. Perineum and genitalia burns are left exposed and cleansed with soap and water when they become soiled with feces or urine. An inlying Foley catheter for constant drainage of the bladder may be advisable in genital burns.

LATER CARE OF THE BURN WOUND

Re-dressing and Reevaluation.

Observe strict aseptic technic in all burn dressings. Remove the original burn dressing down to the petrolatum gauze after 5-8 days. The depth and extent of the burn can be accurately determined at this time. Second degree burns require only reapplication of the pressure dressing and should heal in about 2 weeks. Third degree burns require special management.

Treatment of Third Degree Burns.

A. Removal of Slough: The necrotic surface of a third degree burn usually does not separate for many weeks. Significant areas of slough or necrosis should therefore be removed in the operating room under general anesthesia 10-14 days after the burn if the patient's general condition allows. Burns of the face permit more conservative debridement since slough separates rapidly in this region.

B. Skin Grafting: (See Chapter 16.) Early skin grafting (preferably within the first few weeks following the burn) is essential to avoid chronic sepsis, malnutrition, and scar contractures.

Skin grafting should be started as soon after removal of slough as possible. The denuded granulating surface should be firm and bright red, with a minimum of exudate. Compression dressings for 1-2 days may aid in flattening the granulations. Warm saline dressings (changed several times daily) may also be of assistance in the preparation of the burn wound for skin grafting.

Cutaneous homografts and heterografts are effective when applied to the surface of burn wounds, where they serve essentially as dressings. Homograft skin is obtained aseptically from cadavers. These biologic dressings are useful as cover for third degree burns when the eschar has begun to separate and granulations have begun to form. They are changed every 2-4 days until the wound is healed or ready for autografting.

C. Control of Infection: Signs of infection include rising temperature, tachycardia, general toxicity, local pain and tenderness, and increased drainage. Pockets of pus trapped beneath slough must be sought and liberated by debridement. Warm saline dressings (changed several times daily) are applied to infected areas. Cultures are taken and antibiotic chosen by sensitivity studies. Prolonged antibiotic therapy is not necessary if drainage and dressings are adequate. Skin grafts will not survive in the presence of a virulent, invasive infection, but grafting should be done as soon as the infection is under control. A daily tub bath in warm water with hexachlorophene soap may be helpful in cleaning up a chronically septic burn. Bland ointment dressings can be soaked off relatively painlessly in the tub and reapplied after the bath.

Dressings of 0.5% silver nitrate solution and applications of antibacterial creams (as noted above) may aid in control of infection.

General Supportive Measures.

Chronic infection, exudative loss of protein, catabolic response to stress, and anorexia and depression caused by pain and toxemia can produce rapid nutritional depletion in the severely burned patient. The anemia that is often present is usually the result of hemolysis at the time of burning with subsequent inhibition of erythropoiesis by infection. The most effective supportive measures are a high-caloric, high-protein intake at the outset of therapy, vitamin supplementation, and blood transfusions to keep the Hgb. above 12 Gm./100 ml.

The excretion of potassium is high during the acute phase of burns and may remain so for several weeks. In addition, poor food intake at this time frequently prevents adequate potassium in the diet. Beginning on the third or fourth day of treatment, give potassium chloride, 3-4 Gm. (45-60 gr.) orally in fruit juice or broth 3 times a day until a full normal diet is being taken.

OTHER EMERGENCIES

HEAT STROKE
(Sunstroke)

Heat stroke is characterized by fainting, fever, and cessation of sweating due to the failure of the hypothalamic heat-regulating mechanism during exposure to high temperatures. Absence of sweating is an important premonitory sign. Prodromal symptoms include headache, dizziness, nausea, and visual disturbances. Convulsions sometimes occur. The skin is hot, flushed, and dry. The pulse is rapid and weak. Rectal temperatures may be as high as 108-112° F. (42-44° C.). Hydration and salt content of the body are normal. Old people and alcoholics are especially prone to this condition, which may be fatal.

The objective of treatment is to reduce high body temperature by means of ice packs, sponging with cold alcohol, immersion in a cold bath (10° C.), and/or ice water enemas. Massage the skin to maintain peripheral vasodilatation while cooling. Reduce rectal temperature promptly to 102° F. (39° C.). Proceed more slowly thereafter.

HEAT CRAMPS

Heat cramps are painful spasms of the voluntary muscles of the abdomen and extremities due to depletion of body salt by sweating during prolonged exposure to heat. Heavy manual labor in a hot environment may result in the loss of 3-4 L. of sweat (containing 0.2-0.5% sodium chloride) per hour. In addition to cramps, there may be muscle twitchings. The skin is moist and cool, and body temperature is normal or only slightly elevated. Laboratory studies reveal a low serum sodium. Persons working in high temperatures should take an increased amount of salt, either (1) by adding 1 level tsp. of table salt to each quart of water; or (2) by taking one 1 Gm. (15 gr.) sodium chloride tablet with every 1-2 glasses of water.

Remove the victim to a cool place. Cramps will frequently subside on rest alone. Give sodium chloride, 1 Gm. (15 gr.) by mouth every hour with 1-2 glasses of water until 15 doses have been administered. In severe cases, give 1000-2000 ml. of physiologic saline I.V.

COLD INJURY

The fundamental pathologic process in all types of cold injury is the same. Exposure to cold causes arteriolar and capillary spasm, and ischemia and tissue hypoxia produce varying degrees of tissue damage. Because the endothelium of capillaries is damaged, blistering and edema due to plasma leakage are characteristic of severe cold injury. The most serious destruction occurs in the skin and subcutaneous tissues, since cooling is greatest in these superficial structures.

In the great majority of cold injuries the tissues are not actually frozen but suffer from ischemia and thrombosis in the smaller vessels induced by wet cold at temperatures above freezing (e.g., trench foot). True freezing injury (frostbite) does not occur until the skin temperature drops to -4 to $-10°$ C. (25 to 14° F.).

The likelihood of cold injury is increased by immobility, venous stasis, occlusive arterial vascular disease, and previous cold injury.

Prophylaxis. - "Keep warm, keep dry, and keep moving." Wear sufficient windproof and water-repellent clothing; change wet garments and footgear as quickly as possible; and maintain the circulation by frequently exercising the arms, legs, fingers, and toes. Avoid constrictive clothing and shoes and prolonged dependency of feet.

Chilblain (Pernio).

Chilblain is a relatively mild and superficial form of cold injury. It is most common on the dorsum of the hands of outdoor workers. It may also affect the legs, particularly the anterior tibial surface in young women. The acute form is characterized by a transient bluish-red appearance of the skin and mild edema, often associated with itching or burning which is aggravated by warmth. Repeated exposure may cause chronic manifestations: increased swelling, reddish-purple discoloration of the skin, blisters, and hemorrhagic ulcers which heal slowly and leave pigmented scars.

Treatment consists of rewarming the affected area promptly to body temperature. Avoid trauma, rubbing, massage, and excessive heat. Elevate the part if edema is present. Protect from infection by gentle cleansing and aseptic dry dressings over open vesicles and ulcers.

Trench Foot (Immersion Foot) and Frostbite.

Trench foot (which may also affect the hands) results from prolonged exposure to cold at temperatures from just above freezing to 50° F. (10° C.), often in a damp environment and usually in connection with immobilization and dependency of the extremities. Immersion foot is caused by exposure to water at temperatures below 50° F. (10° C.), usually for more than 12 hours. The first symptom is usually an uncomfortable coldness, followed by numbness. Throbbing, aching, or burning and varying degrees of redness, cyanosis, edema, blistering, and skin necrosis occur after rewarming. In severe injuries the tissues become black, dry, and mummified, and later develop a sharp line of demarcation.

Frostbite is due to actual freezing of the tissue fluids after exposure to freezing temperatures. The exposure necessary to produce frostbite varies from a few seconds to several hours, depending upon the temperature of the environment. Local sensations of coldness or stinging pain give way to numbness. The skin becomes pale after severe exposure. A phase of hyperemia may occur after rewarming during which the skin is acutely painful, warm, and red or bluish in color. These changes are followed by varying degrees of edema, blistering, and skin necrosis, depending upon the depth of injury. The phase of hyperemia and local warmth gives way to cyanosis, hyperhidrosis, and coldness; and persistent, burning pain often sets in. Pre-necrotic skin becomes dark brown and finally black. These areas of dry gangrene eventually mummify; 1-2 months are required for separation and epithelization.

A. Immediate Treatment:
   1. Rewarm rapidly by immersion in water at 104-107.5° F. (40-42° C.), with body heat, or by exposure to warm air. Do not expose to an open fire. Maintain general body warmth.
   2. Avoid trauma - All casualities with foot involvement are litter cases. Do not rub or massage the affected part.
   3. Prevent infection - Cleanse the part gently with bland or hexachlorophene soap. Dressings are not necessary if the skin is intact.

B. General Treatment:
   1. Absolute bed rest is required when the feet are involved.
   2. Slight elevation of the part controls edema. Marked elevation diminishes blood flow and is contraindicated.
   3. Expose closed lesions to room air at a temperature of 70-74° F. (21-23° C.).
   4. Rigid asepsis is mandatory in dressing open lesions. Use sterile dry gauze dressings, loosely applied.
   5. Antibiotics - "Prophylactic" antibiotics are contraindicated. Treat invasive infection with specific antibiotics chosen by sensitivity studies on cultures of exudate. If bacteriologic facilities are not available, use penicillin empirically.
   6. Heparin may be of some use in preventing secondary thromboses in surrounding areas if given within 24 hours after thawing and continued for 1 week.
   7. Administer tetanus toxoid or antitoxin.
   8. Regional sympathectomy performed as early as possible after a severe third degree cold injury appears to diminish pain, promote rapid demarcation and healing, conserve tissue, and minimize or eliminate late sequelae.

C. Surgical Treatment: Debride conservatively and advise amputation only when demarcation is definite. Remove superficial necrotic tissue with aseptic precautions, and cover large open areas with skin grafts as early as possible. In general, the tissue loss in cold injury will be less than appeared likely at the outset. Necrosis may be superficial and the underlying skin may heal well spontaneously.

D. Treatment of Sequelae:
   1. Neurologic measures - Late sequelae such as hyperhidrosis, coldness, cyanosis, edema, chronic ulcers, and pain may be palliated by sympathectomy.
   2. Orthopedic measures - Foot pain on weight-bearing should be treated with well-fitted shoes and the use of pads, supports, and other orthopedic devices. Contractures due to fibrosis of muscles pose special orthopedic problems.

ELECTRIC SHOCK

Electric shock produces 4 significant types of reaction, 1 or all of which may occur depending upon the circumstances: (1) Electric burn at the point of contact with the current and in the tissues through which heavy current passes. The skin and adjacent structures are intensely charred to variable depths. (2) Loss of consciousness, which may be momentary or prolonged. With recovery there may be muscle pain, fatigue, headache, and nervous irritability. (3) Respiratory paralysis, which is accompanied by coma and may persist for 6-8 hours if artificial respiration is provided. (4) Ventricular fibrillation. The patient is comatose and pulseless, and no heart sounds can be heard. Respirations cease, and death supervenes within a few minutes unless circulation is restored by cardiac massage (see pp. 12-15).

Alternating current is more dangerous than direct current. With alternating currents of 25-300 cycles, low voltages (below 200) tend to produce ventricular fibrillation; high voltages (over 1000), respiratory failure; intermediate voltages (220-1000), both.

Treatment.

Emergency measures consist of (1) immediate removal of the patient from the electric current; (2) administration of mouth-to-mouth artificial respiration; and (3) treatment of cardiac arrest by external massage and countershock with an external defibrillator (see pp. 10-18). Electric burns are usually third degree and require skin grafting after sufficient time has elapsed for demarcation.

DROWNING

Respiratory obstruction is the primary disturbance in drowning. Spasm of the larynx usually develops, followed by acute oxygen deprivation and respiratory arrest; only a small amount of water may be aspirated. The stomach, however, may be filled with water. The body is cold and the face cyanotic and congested.

Emergency Treatment.

A. Clear the airway. Remove mucus and foreign matter manually from the nose and throat and drain water from the respiratory tract by gravity. Use suction if available. If possible, insert an endotracheal tube and inflate the lungs with oxygen, using an anesthesia bag.

B. Begin mouth-to-mouth artificial respiration immediately (see pp. 8-9) and continue until spontaneous respiration returns or until heart action is stopped and death absolutely certain.

C. If heart action is failing or inaudible, combine mouth-to-mouth breathing with closed chest massage. If ventricular fibrillation is suspected, attempt external defibrillation if equipment is available (see pp. 12-15).

D. Loosen or remove constricting clothing.

E. Keep the patient comfortably warm.

F. In cases of near drowning from salt water, blood studies may indicate the need for plasma infusions to correct hemoconcentration, electrolyte disturbances, or hypovolemia.

CARBON MONOXIDE POISONING

Carbon monoxide is a colorless and odorless gas produced by the incomplete combustion of carbon-containing material; it can therefore be emitted by any flame or combustion device, including gas stoves, coal-burning heaters, and automobiles. Carbon monoxide combines 250 times more readily with hemoglobin than does oxygen. Carbon monoxide and hemoglobin form a stable compound, carboxyhemoglobin, which is incapable of carrying oxygen. Tissue hypoxia results, and if sufficient carbon monoxide is inhaled it may produce unconsciousness and death in a few minutes.

Manifestations include headache, faintness, dizziness, tinnitus, vomiting, cherry-red skin and mucous membranes, loss of memory, collapse, and coma. When the patient's blood is boiled or shaken with 1-2 volumes of normal sodium hydroxide, normal blood becomes black or brown-black but blood containing high levels of carboxyhemoglobin remains red.

Emergency treatment consists of removing the patient to fresh air and keeping him warm and at rest. Give 100% oxygen by mask for 1 hour. If respirations are depressed, give 5% CO_2 in oxygen to stimulate breathing. Positive pressure breathing of 100% oxygen will reduce the blood carboxyhemoglobin below the danger level. Respiratory failure is treated by mouth-to-mouth breathing (see p. 8) with positive pressure oxygen administration by mask or endotracheal tube as soon as possible if resuscitation is difficult. If BP is markedly depressed, use a vasopressor drug.

SNAKE BITE

The venom of poisonous snakes may be neurotoxic or hemotoxic. There are 4 types of poisonous snakes found in the U.S.A.: rattlesnake (several species), copperhead, cottonmouth moccasin, and coral snake. (About 15% of adults bitten by rattlesnakes will die.) It is important to determine whether a bite is by a poisonous snake: Poisonous snakes have fangs within the mouth; nonpoisonous snakes do not. Bites from poisonous snakes are characterized by 2 puncture wounds where the fangs enter the skin; nonpoisonous snakes leave semicircular rows of tooth marks. The manifestations of poisonous snake bite are severe and persistent local pain, redness, and swelling followed rapidly by nausea, vomiting, and collapse; nonpoisonous snake bite causes little pain or other symptoms. Hemotoxic venoms cause hemolysis, local hemorrhage, and bleeding from the mucous membranes. Neurotoxins tend to cause respiratory failure.

Treatment.

A. Emergency Measures: Prompt treatment is of paramount importance.
   1. Immobilization and transportation - Keep the patient recumbent and quiet; muscular action tends to spread the venom. Transport the patient by stretcher to a hospital at once. Give barbiturates for restlessness. **Do not give alcohol.**
   2. Tourniquet - Apply a tourniquet proximal to the bite. The tourniquet should be loose enough to permit insertion of a finger between it and the skin. It can be left continuously in place for one hour. Frequent release of the tourniquet permits absorption of the venom.
   3. Cold pack - Application of an ice pack to the area of the

wound will slow absorption of the venom and relieve pain in the site. Packing of an extremity in ice is not advised.

4. Care of the wound - Wash thoroughly with soap and water to remove venom from the skin. Within the first hour after the bite, a physician may wish to prepare the skin with an antiseptic and make longitudinal incisions through the fang marks. Then apply suction by a suction device (or by mouth, if necessary, spitting out the venom and washing out the mouth frequently with water). Up to 10% of the venom can be removed in this manner if tourniquet, incision, and suction are used within the first 30 minutes. If appropriate facilities are available within the first half-hour (or 1½ hours if a tourniquet has been in place), the bite wound can be elliptically excised with a 1-inch margin and to the depth required to remove the venom, which may be down to the fascia or into the muscle.
5. Antivenin - (To be given only by a physician.) Species-specific antivenin should be administered as soon as possible, after testing for sensitivity to horse serum. (Follow printed instructions in the package.) Identification of the snake is important in order to choose the correct antivenin. Polyvalent pit viper antivenin and coral snake antivenin are available from Wyeth Laboratories. The latter is also available from the National Center for Disease Control in Atlanta and from other sources in southeastern U.S.A.

B. General Measures: Respiratory failure is managed by oxygen administration and artificial ventilation (see p. 126). Supportive treatment is provided for shock (see p. 18). Antibiotics have no specific value. Cortisone or substitute in large doses will relieve symptoms temporarily but may not reduce mortality. Do not give corticosteroids if the patient is receiving antiserum. The snake bite wound may produce extensive local tissue necrosis, and the prognosis should be guarded. Fasciotomy may be indicated if severe edema of an extremity produces nerve or vascular compression. (McCollough, N.C., and Gennaro, J.F., Clin. Toxicol. **3**:483-500, 1970; Minton, S.A. Jr., Trauma **11**: 1053-1054, 1971.)

SPIDER BITES AND SCORPION STINGS

The toxin of the less venomous species of spiders and scorpions causes only local pain, redness, and swelling. That of the more venomous species is quite toxic. For example, the bite of the black widow spider (Latrodectus mactans) causes severe systemic symptoms, including generalized muscular pains, abdominal cramps, nausea and vomiting, and collapse. The abdominal muscles may become rigid, in which case the clinical picture resembles that of an acute abdominal emergency. However, the patient with black widow spider bite is extremely restless.

Treat the local wound by application of cold compresses. If symptoms are severe, give specific spider or scorpion antiserum after skin testing. For convulsions or muscle cramps, give calcium gluconate, 10 ml. of 10% solution I.V., and repeat as needed. Additional measures consist of hot baths and control of restlessness with barbiturates.

EYE INJURIES

In severe eye injuries it is important for the nonspecialist to avoid causing further damage by unnecessary manipulation and to refer the patient immediately to an ophthalmologist. An injured eye has no defense against infection, and any local anesthetics, dyes, or other medication used **must be sterile**. Examinations should be made with a well-focussed light and with a magnifying glass or loupe if necessary.

Foreign Bodies.

Superficial metallic corneal or conjunctival foreign bodies are extremely common. Penetrating ocular foreign bodies are rare, and there is almost always a history of striking steel on steel. X-rays are always indicated if an intraocular foreign body is suspected. Intraocular and deeply embedded foreign bodies should be removed by an ophthalmologist; superficial corneal foreign bodies may be safely removed by a general practitioner.

A. Conjunctival Foreign Bodies: The only important conjunctival foreign bodies are those which lodge beneath the upper tarsal conjunctiva and rub on the cornea, causing extreme pain. Foreign bodies on the lower tarsal and palpebral conjunctiva seldom cause pain and are usually washed away by the action of the tears plus blinking.
   1. Evert the lid, if necessary by pressing gently downward across its outer surface with a match or applicator stick while pulling upward on the eyelashes.
   2. Remove free particles with a moist cotton-tipped applicator or by gentle irrigation with warm sterile saline solution.

B. Corneal Foreign Bodies:
   1. Instill 2 drops of sterile 0.5% tetracaine (Pontocaine®) solution or other sterile anesthetic into the conjunctival sac.
   2. Superficial particles may be removed with a moist cotton-tipped applicator.
   3. Embedded particles are removed with a delicate instrument, preferably a special "hockey stick" (actually referred to as a golf club) spud. An antibacterial ointment (e.g., polymyxin B–bacitracin [Polysporin®]) is instilled after the foreign body has been removed.

      Most patients are more comfortable without a patch on the eye after removal of a corneal foreign body. It is essential to see the patient on the next day to be certain that no infection has occurred and that healing is under way.

Corneal Abrasions.

Corneal abrasion is a common injury which must be treated promptly and with great care in order to speed healing and to prevent infection and recurrent corneal erosions.

The history should be taken and visual acuity tested before treatment. A patient with a corneal abrasion complains of severe pain, especially with movement of the lid over the cornea. The surface of the cornea may be examined with a light and loupe. If an abrasion is suspected but cannot be seen, stain the cornea with sterile fluorescein. The area of corneal abrasion will have a deeper green stain than the surrounding cornea.

Instill polymyxin B–bacitracin (Polysporin®) ophthalmic ointment. Apply a tight pressure bandage to prevent movement of the lid and resultant irritation of the abraded corneal area. Bed rest may be necessary. The patient should be observed on the following day to be certain that the cornea is healing. Corneal abrasions heal in 24-72 hours if a pressure bandage is properly applied. In contrast to corneal foreign body wounds, there is little chance of infection. The main dangers are delayed healing and recurrent corneal erosion due to imperfect healing.

Burns of the Eye.

A. Thermal: These are usually associated with face or body burns. If the conjunctivas are involved, adhesions may develop. If the cornea is severely damaged, perforation or infection is apt to occur and an ophthalmologist should be consulted. Dilate the pupil with sterile 5% homatropine solution, instill an antibiotic ointment frequently, relieve pain with cold compresses and systemic analgesics or narcotics, and keep the eyes closed.

B. Ultraviolet: Arc welding may produce a superficial painful keratitis which usually heals without complications within 24-48 hours. Relieve pain by an initial instillation of sterile 0.5% tetracaine (Pontocaine®) solution and subsequently with systemic analgesics or narcotics. Keep the eyes bandaged and apply cold compresses until the initial reaction subsides. In severe cases it may be necessary to instill corticosteroid drops locally to relieve inflammation and associated pain.

C. Chemical: Flush out the conjunctival sac immediately with tap water for several minutes. Neutralizing solutions are unnecessary and may even be harmful. If fluorescein stain after irrigation indicates that corneal damage has occurred, treat as for thermal burn and refer to an ophthalmologist for definitive care.

Contusions of the Eyeball.

If ophthalmoscopic examination shows any evidence of internal hemorrhage or damage to the iris, lens, or retina, specialist care is indicated. Any injury severe enough to produce anterior chamber hemorrhage (e.g., hyphema) may cause secondary hemorrhage and intractable glaucoma.

Lacerations of the Eyeball.

Minor lacerations of the conjunctivas may be left alone or closed by fine silk suturing. Lacerations of the cornea or sclera require specialist care since they may lead to blindness or loss of the globe itself. Emergency and temporizing measures include dilatation of the pupil with sterile 5% homatropine solution, instillation of an ophthalmic antibiotic ointment t.i.d., systemic antibiotics, analgesics or narcotics, and bilateral eye bandages. If the wound is extensive and loss of contents has been great enough to preclude function, enucleation may be indicated. If uveal tissue has been injured and the eye is retained, sympathetic ophthalmia may occur

2 weeks to several years after the initial injury. Fortunately, this dread complication is rare.

COMMON SOFT TISSUE INJURIES

Contusions.

Nonpenetrating blunt trauma produces tissue damage and interstitial hemorrhage, but the superficial soft tissue injury itself is rarely significant. Underlying fracture or damage to an internal organ must be ruled out.

Contusions usually require no treatment. The application of an ice pack within the first few hours may limit interstitial hemorrhage and subsequent ecchymosis.

Hematomas.

A large subcutaneous or intramuscular hematoma occasionally results from contusion. If subsidence is slow, aspiration with a No. 15 or 17 gauge needle may be attempted under local anesthesia but this is usually unsuccessful. Before withdrawing the needle, inject 1500 U.S.P. units of hyaluronidase (Wydase®) and repeat the injection daily or oftener. Incision and evacuation of a hematoma is rarely necessary. Aseptic technic is important when aspirating or evacuating hematomas since they provide ideal conditions for bacterial growth.

Lacerations.

The basic steps in management are debridement, irrigation, and wound closure, usually under local procaine anesthesia. Always examine for damage to nerves and tendons and for the presence of foreign material. Lacerations of the hand and those associated with loss of skin require specialist care.

A. Primary vs. Delayed Wound Closure: Repair of a laceration should be done as soon after injury as possible. The more heavily contused or contaminated the wound, the more important it becomes to treat within a few hours. Certain wounds, however, may occasionally be safely sutured as long as 24 or more hours after injury. This applies to neatly incised lacerations occurring under relatively clean conditions, especially around the head and neck where blood supply is generous and a good cosmetic result is important. Catgut is used in the deeper layers; and fine, nonabsorbable sutures are used in the skin. Heavily contaminated wounds or those considered too old for primary closure should be covered with a single layer of petrolatum gauze and packed lightly open with fluffed gauze; 48-72 hours later the wound should be inspected and loosely closed with sutures or adhesive strips if it appears clean.

B. Antibiotics: Most small or clean lacerations do not require antibiotic therapy. When contamination is marked or when primary closure must be done late, systemic penicillin therapy is justified.

C. Tetanus Prophylaxis: This is advisable if soil contamination is suspected. When in doubt, administer antitoxin or toxoid as indicated.

Penetrating Wounds.

The chief complications of penetrating wounds are (1) perforation of a viscus, (2) introduction of pyogenic or tetanus organisms, and (3) retained foreign body. Treatment must be individualized. Clean puncture wounds and through-and-through missile wounds which cause no serious damage may require only observation. Penetrating injuries which drive clothing or other foreign material into the wound require exploration and debridement. Tetanus prophylaxis is usually indicated.

Foreign Bodies.

Any open wound may contain a foreign body. Attempt removal of a foreign body only after adequate localization by (1) x-rays in 2 or more planes with lead markers on the skin, (2) placing identifying marks on the skin under fluoroscopy, or (3) inserting a needle down to the foreign body under fluoroscopy. Small (less than 1 cm.), deep, inert foreign bodies can usually be left alone and observed by x-ray several months later. A foreign body should be removed if it protrudes through the skin; if it causes pain; if it consists of or is contaminated with dirt, cloth, wood, or other material likely to cause infection or reaction; if the wound is infected or draining; or if it may migrate to or impinge upon important structures. Tetanus prophylaxis should be given as indicated.

HUMAN BITE

Human bites are rare but important because of the virulence of aerobic and anaerobic mouth organisms. Deep penetrating wounds of the knuckles incurred by fighting are especially serious due to frequent involvement of the metacarpophalangeal joint and extensor tendon. When the hand is opened, the proximal glide of the extensor tendon carries infecting organisms proximally into anaerobic sites on the back of the hand. Cellulitis usually appears within 24-72 hours and may extend rapidly. Necrosis, abscess formation, and marked pain and swelling are the typical findings.

Emergency treatment consists of irrigation and debridement, extending the wound as required. Aerobic and anaerobic cultures should be taken and tests made for antibiotic sensitivity. Do not suture the wound, but cover it with petrolatum gauze and a dry dressing and splint the hand and wrist as necessary. Observe for infection, and administer full doses of penicillin pending the results of antibiotic sensitivity tests. Consider tetanus prophylaxis.

If such a wound is seen late, obtain cultures, drain abscesses, place the patient at bed rest with the part elevated, apply hot moist packs, and give penicillin until the antibiotic of choice can be chosen on the basis of sensitivity studies.

ANIMAL BITES

Dog Bites. (See also Rabies, p. 53.)

Penetrating small wounds should be thoroughly irrigated and left open. Lacerations are debrided, irrigated, and sutured according to the usual principles (see p. 51). Tetanus prophylaxis is usually indicated.

Cat Bites and Scratches.

Cat bites are more likely to cause infection than dog bites. Cleanse the area thoroughly with soap and water, apply a dry sterile dressing, splint the part if possible, and observe for infection. Administer penicillin pending antibiotic sensitivity studies. Tetanus prophylaxis is given as indicated.

Cats may also transmit by scratching a condition known as cat-scratch fever, probably of viral origin. At the wound site there is localized cellulitis followed by regional adenopathy, which may suppurate. Encephalitis or pneumonitis may occur rarely. Tetracycline may shorten the course of the disease.

RABIES

Rabies is a viral encephalitis transmitted through the saliva of an infected animal. Humans are usually inoculated by the bite of a rabid dog, but bites of other animals, including the cat, rat, bat, skunk, squirrel, fox, wolf, etc., can transmit the disease. Since the established disease is invariably fatal, early preventive treatment is of paramount importance.

The incubation period varies in humans from 10 days to several months. The onset is with pain and numbness around the site of the wound followed by fever, irritability, malaise, and spasms of the muscles of swallowing. Paralysis and convulsions occur terminally. Absolute quiet and anticonvulsant drug therapy are indicated for established cases.

Prophylaxis.

Do not kill the animal, but confine it under veterinary observation for 10 days. If it becomes rabid, the animal should be sacrificed and its brain cells examined for Negri bodies. If the animal dies of any cause, or if it is inadvertently killed before 10 days have passed, the head should be sent to the nearest public health or other competent laboratory for examination. Consult the local health authorities to determine if any cases of rabies have been reported recently.

Vaccines for immunization of man against rabies have been prepared by many different technics. The vaccines have been of 2 main types: those containing live, attenuated virus and those containing virus that has been inactivated. Duck-embryo vaccine (Lilly) contains an inactivated virus and has been widely used in the U.S.A. Postvaccinal complications of the central nervous system have been reduced but not entirely eliminated by the use of this vaccine.

Antirabies serum and its globulin fractions are of proved effectiveness in preventing rabies. Potent antirabies serum has been produced in horses and other animals. Antirabies serum should be given as promptly as possible after exposure in accordance with the general guidelines given below. Reactions to antirabies horse serum occur with approximately the same frequency as with other sera of animal origin. Sensitivity tests and the usual precautions to avoid an anaphylactic type of reaction should be taken (see p. 30). Rabies immune human gamma globulin may become available.

SPECIFIC SYSTEMIC TREATMENT FOR RABIES*

Nature of Exposure	Status of Biting Animal (Vaccinated or Not)		Recommended Treatment
	At Time of Exposure	10 Day Observation Period	
No lesions (indirect contact)	Rabid	–	None
Licks			
Unabraded skin	Rabid	–	None
Abraded skin, scratches, and unabraded or abraded mucosa	Healthy	Clinical signs of rabies or proved rabid (laboratory)	Start vaccine† at first signs of rabies in biting animal.
	Signs suggestive of rabies	Healthy	Start vaccine† immediately; stop treatment if animal is normal on fifth day after exposure.
	Rabid, escaped, killed, unknown	–	Start vaccine† immediately.
Bites			
Mild exposure	Healthy	Clinical signs of rabies or proved rabid (laboratory)	Start vaccine‡ at first sign of rabies in biting animal.
	Signs suggestive of rabies	Healthy	Start vaccine† immediately; stop treatment if animal is normal on fifth day after exposure.
	Rabid, escaped, killed, unknown	–	Start vaccine†‡ immediately.
	Wild (wolf, jackal, fox, bat, etc.)	–	Serum‡ immediately, followed by vaccine.†
Severe exposure (multiple, or face, head, finger, or neck bites)	Healthy	Clinical signs of rabies or proved rabid (laboratory)	Serum‡ immediately; start vaccine† at first sign of rabies in biting animal.
	Signs suggestive of rabies	Healthy	Serum‡ immediately, followed by vaccine. Vaccine may be stopped if animal is normal on fifth day after exposure.
	Rabid, escaped, killed, unknown Wild (wolf, jackal, pariah dog, fox, bat, etc.)	–	Serum‡ immediately, followed by vaccine†

*From WHO Expert Committee on Rabies, Fifth Report. World Health Organization Technical Report Series No. 321, 1966.

†Practice varies concerning the volume of vaccine per dose and the number of doses given. (See package insert for further details.)

‡In all severe exposures and in all cases of unprovoked wild animal bites, antirabies serum or its globulin fraction together with vaccine should be employed. Because both the serum and the vaccine can cause deleterious reactions, continued therapy in mild exposures is considered optional. As with vaccine alone, it is important to start combined serum and vaccine treatment as early as possible after exposure, but serum should still be used no matter what the time interval. Serum should be given in a single dose (40 I.U./Kg. body weight) and the first dose of vaccine inoculated at the same time. Sensitivity to the serum must be determined before its administration. (See package inserts for further details.)

A. Local Treatment of Wounds Involving Possible Exposure to Rabies:*

1. Recommended in all exposures -
   a. First-aid treatment - Immediate washing and flushing with soap and water, detergent, or water alone (recommended procedure in all bite wounds including those unrelated to possible exposure to rabies).
   b. Treatment by or under direction of a physician -
      (1) Adequate cleansing of the wound.
      (2) Thorough treatment with 20% soap solution and/or application of a quaternary ammonium compound or other substance (70% ethanol, tincture of thimerosal, tincture of iodine) of proved lethal effect on the rabies virus. (See WHO reference for details.) Where soap has been used to clean wounds, all traces of it should be removed before the application of quaternary ammonium compounds because soap neutralizes the activity of such compounds.
      (3) Topical application of antirabies serum or its liquid or powdered globulin preparation (optional).
      (4) Administration, where indicated, of antitetanus procedures and of antibiotics and drugs to control infections other than rabies.
      (5) Suturing of wound is not advised.
2. Additional local treatment for severe exposures only -
   a. Topical application of antirabies serum or its liquid or powdered globulin preparation.
   b. Infiltration of antirabies serum around the wound.

B. Specific Systemic Treatment: See table on p. 54.

*This and the section on Specific Systemic Treatment are slightly modified from WHO Expert Committee on Rabies, Fifth Report. World Health Organization Technical Report Series No. 321, 1966.

2...

Preoperative & Postoperative Care

GENERAL CONSIDERATIONS IN MANAGEMENT

PREOPERATIVE EVALUATION

The basic work-up for surgery is also a general health examination and should include a complete history and physical examination, urinalysis, complete blood count (CBC), serology, chest x-ray, and, in patients over 50, an Ecg. and stool test for occult blood. For the older age group, a BUN and postprandial blood sugar are often advisable as screening measures. It may be appropriate to order a chemical screening battery of 12 or more tests, including calcium, inorganic phosphorus, glucose, BUN, uric acid, cholesterol, total protein, albumin, total bilirubin, alkaline phosphatase, LDH, and SGOT. A Papanicolaou smear for cytologic study should be obtained from the vagina or cervix of all women over 30. When blood transfusion is anticipated, blood typing and cross-matching should be ordered. Open wounds and infections usually require bacteriologic investigation.

In addition to the foregoing more or less routine studies, all significant complaints and physical findings should be adequately evaluated by appropriate special tests, examinations, and consultations. Bleeding tendencies, medications currently being taken, and allergies to antibiotics and other agents should be carefully noted. Psychiatric consultation is advisable in patients with a history of significant mental disorder which may be exacerbated by surgery and in patients whose complaints may have a psychoneurotic or psychophysiologic basis.

The preoperative work-up should be sufficiently comprehensive to disclose occult conditions as well as establish the diagnosis and determine the risk of surgery for the presenting illness. Recording of peripheral pulses is frequently overlooked. Pelvic and rectal examinations should always be performed unless contraindicated by age, marital status, or other valid reasons. Sigmoidoscopy may provide valuable information and can often be done on the initial visit.

Surgical intervention, particularly in a major operation, subjects the patient to the risk of infection, hemorrhage, and metabolic imbalance as well as to complications from existing conditions which may be latent or well-tolerated until exacerbated by the stress of surgery. Preoperative preparation is directed toward the identification and, as far as possible, correction of disorders which will increase the risk of operation. Among the conditions requiring preoperative correction are shock, hypovolemia, anemia, electrolyte imbalance, respiratory infection, cardiac decompensation, diabetic acidosis, renal insufficiency, and hyperthermia. In emergency surgery, time is limited but is usually sufficient to permit significant progress to be made in the preparation of the patient, particularly with respect to correction of hyponatremia and fluid and electrolyte imbalance. In elective surgery, meticulous preparation is possible and, indeed, mandatory in order to minimize morbidity and mortality. The usual preoperative routines are described in the following sections. Conditions and diseases that commonly affect operative risk are subsequently discussed.

CONSULTATIONS

The opinion of a qualified consultant should be obtained (1) when it may be of benefit to the patient, (2) when requested by the patient or his family, or (3) when it may be of medicolegal importance. The physician should take the initiative in arranging consultation when the treatment proposed is controversial or exceptionally risky, when dangerous complications occur, or when he senses that the patient or his family is unduly apprehensive about the plan of management or the course of events. Preoperative consultation with cardiac or other medical or surgical specialists is important if the patient's abnormal findings fall within their fields of competence. If it is possible that the consultant will be called upon for advice in connection with a postoperative complication or development, it is beneficial for him to become acquainted with the patient and his condition preoperatively.

Anesthesia consultation is always requested prior to major surgery if an anesthesiologist is available. In poor risk patients this consultation should be requested several days in advance of operation if possible. The patient's prospects for smooth and uncomplicated anesthesia are greatly improved by the anesthesiologist's preoperative evaluation and advice. Respiratory, cardiovascular, and other complications related to anesthesia are forestalled or minimized when the anesthesiologist has an opportunity to adapt the anesthesia to the patient's special circumstances.

When an anesthesiologist is available for preoperative consultation, he usually writes the orders for premedication, for the withholding of oral intake, and for other measures which relate directly to the anesthesia. When an anesthesiologist is not available, preanesthetic orders are written by the surgeon in accordance with the principles discussed in Chapter 3.

INFORMING THE PATIENT

Surgery is a disturbing prospect for the patient and his family. Their psychologic preparation and reassurance should begin during their initial meeting with the surgeon. Appropriate explanation of the nature and purpose of preoperative studies and treatment establishes confidence. When all pertinent information has been gathered, it is the surgeon's responsibility to describe to the patient (and, usually, to his next of kin) the planned procedure, its risks, and its possible consequences in understandable terms. Similarly, prompt interpretation of pertinent postoperative findings and prospects to the patient and his family contributes to rapport and to intelligent cooperation during the recovery period.

OPERATIVE PERMIT

The patient or his legal guardian must sign a permit in advance that authorizes major or minor operations or exploratory or therapeutic procedures (e.g., thoracentesis, lumbar puncture, sigmoidoscopy). The nature, risk, and probable result of the operation or procedure must be made clear to the patient or to a legally responsible relative or guardian so that the signed permit indicates "informed consent." A signed consent is ordinarily valid **only** for the specific operation or procedure for which it was obtained.

Therapeutic abortions and operations which adversely affect the sexual or childbearing functions should usually be undertaken only with the concurrence in writing of the marital partner. It may not be required in a particular state or jurisdiction that the husband give his consent, but it is generally desirable that he be informed of and, if possible, agree to the proposed procedure and its effects.

Emergency lifesaving operations or procedures may have to be done without a permit. In such cases, obtain adequate consultation and inform the director of the hospital in advance, if possible, of the situation.

Legal and institutional requirements vary regarding permits. It is essential that the physician know and follow local specifications.

PREOPERATIVE NOTE

When the diagnostic work-up and the preoperative evaluation have been completed, all details should be reviewed and a "preoperative note" written in the chart. The note summarizes the pertinent findings and decisions and gives the indications for the operation proposed. This constitutes a final check on the adequacy of the analysis of the patient's problem and his requirements for treatment. The note is usually written on the day before operation.

PREOPERATIVE ORDERS

On the day before surgery, orders are written which assure completion before operation of the final steps in the preparation of the patient. These orders usually include the following:

A. Skin Preparation: Designate the specific region to be prepared by shaving, cleansing, or other procedure.

B. Diet: Omit solid foods for 12 hours and fluids for 8 hours preoperatively. Special orders must be written for diabetics and for infants and children.

C. Enema: Enemas need not be given routinely. Patients with well-regulated bowel habits do not require a preoperative enema except in the instances of (1) operations, chiefly abdominal, likely to be followed by paralytic ileus and delayed bowel function, and (2) operations on the colon, rectum, and anus.

Constipated patients and those scheduled for the above types of operations, should be given a flushing enema 8-12 hours preoperatively with 500-1500 ml. of warm tap water or, preferably, physiologic saline or with 120-150 ml. of hypertonic sodium phosphate solution (conveniently available in a commercial kit, e.g., Travad® Enema, Fleet® Enema). Tap water enemas are contraindicated in congenital megacolon because of the danger of excessive water absorption. When thorough cleansing of the bowel is not essential, satisfactory evacuation on the evening before operation can usually be accomplished by use of a 10 mg. bisacodyl rectal suppository (Dulcolax®). Hypertonic sodium phosphate enema or bisacodyl rectal suppository is also effective in the rapid preparation of the colon and rectum for sigmoidoscopy.

D. Bedtime and Preanesthetic Medication: If the anesthesia is to be given by a physician anesthesiologist, he will usually examine the patient and write the premedication order. If not, follow the guidelines in Chapter 3.

E. Special Orders: In addition to the above more or less routine preoperative orders required for most major operative procedures, additional special orders related to the type and severity of the operation should be written. Examples of these are:

1. Blood transfusion - If blood transfusions may be needed during or after operation, have the patient typed and arrange for a sufficient number of units to be cross-matched and available prior to operation.
2. Nasogastric tube - A nasogastric tube on suction is usually advisable after operations on the gastrointestinal tract to prevent distention due to paralytic ileus. If the patient has gastrointestinal obstruction with possible gastric residue, a nasogastric tube is passed preoperatively and the stomach aspirated or placed on continuous suction to reduce the possibility of regurgitation and aspiration during induction of anesthesia. If an emergency operation is to be undertaken on a patient who has eaten within the past 8-12 hours, lavage of the stomach with a large-bore Ewald tube followed by insertion of a nasogastric tube should be considered. When there is no indication for nasogastric intubation prior to surgery and the patient is to be under general anesthesia, the anesthesiologist can pass the tube into the stomach after the patient is asleep.
3. Bladder catheter - If urinary retention is anticipated or if there is a need for hourly monitoring of urinary output postoperatively, a Foley catheter can be inserted for constant bladder drainage. If bladder distention interferes with exposure in the pelvis (e.g., during abdominoperineal resection), a catheter should be placed preoperatively. Catheterization can be done on the nursing unit just before the patient leaves for the operating room, or it can be done after the patient has been anesthetized.
4. Venous or arterial catheter - Operations associated with marked blood loss call for placement of one or two 14- or 16-gauge intravenous plastic catheters preoperatively for rapid administration of blood, fluid, or medication. Percutaneous insertion is usually possible; if not, a cutdown

should be done to expose a vein, usually the antecubital vein. Central venous pressure monitoring may be required for assessment of the circulation during certain procedures (e.g., complicated cardiovascular and pulmonary operations). For central venous pressure determination, a catheter should be passed into the superior vena cava via the subclavian or internal jugular vein. Arterial catheterization or cannulation, usually of the radial or brachial artery, is done primarily for monitoring blood pressure and obtaining blood gas measurements during and after operation in selected patients in whom repeated, accurate measurement of these parameters is essential. Usually, central venous and arterial catheterization can be deferred until the patient is anesthetized.

5. Continuing medications - Certain patients will be receiving continuing medications whose dosage or route of administration should be altered as the result of operation. Insulin and cortisone are examples of hormone preparations requiring special preoperative orders. Such agents as digitalis, other cardiac drugs, and antibiotics may require a shift to the parenteral route of administration and altered dosage in the immediately preoperative period and during operation. Foresight in the adjustment of medication orders will minimize the possibility of underdosage or overdosage of potent and essential drugs.
6. Prophylactic antibiotics - See Chapter 6.
7. Miscellaneous - Complex operations may require additional preparation.

POSTOPERATIVE ORDERS

Postsurgical patients should be accompanied by a physician or other qualified attendant while en route to the recovery room, intensive care unit, or general nursing unit. Detailed written orders should be sent with each postoperative patient, and the nurse receiving the patient should be given a verbal report of his condition. The postoperative orders should provide for appropriate observation and treatment. In the case of the patient requiring intensive care, these may include many of the procedures listed above under the parameters to be monitored. As a guide to the preparation of an inclusive set of postoperative orders, each of the following categories should be considered.

A. Special Observations:

1. Vital signs - BP, pulse, and respiration should be recorded at regular intervals after all major operations (e.g., every 15-30 minutes until stable, then hourly). A significant drop in BP should be reported to the surgeon immediately (specify the level to be reported).
2. Continuous monitoring of Ecg. - This is indicated in many critically ill patients. Other parameters to be monitored continuously depend upon the patient's needs and the equipment available.
3. Central venous pressure - Central venous pressure monitoring requires percutaneous placement of an inlying catheter

in the superior vena cava or right atrium via the internal jugular or subclavian vein. Record central venous pressure at stated intervals in patients with shock, borderline cardiac or respiratory status, large fluid volume replacement, or oliguria.

4. Specific observations - Orders should be given as indicated to observe closely for such developments as cardiac arrhythmias, respiratory distress, wound bleeding or drainage, impaired circulation in an extremity (e.g., distal to a cast or vascular procedure), or other possible developments.

B. Position in Bed: Designate specifically the position desired (e.g., flat or on side, sitting, or foot of bed elevated).

C. Mobilization: Prescribe bed rest, standing to void, up in chair, or ambulation. While recovering from general anesthesia, the patient should be turned from side to side every 30 minutes until he is conscious and then hourly for the first 8-12 hours. Require active position change and active motion of feet and legs every 1-2 hours while the patient is awake until he is ambulatory. To minimize the possibility of embolism, order elastic stockings for legs in elderly patients or when ambulation is delayed.

D. Respiratory Care: Hyperventilation, coughing, tracheal suction, and inhalation therapy should be ordered as required. Percutaneous placement of a small catheter in the trachea may be needed for injection of saline or water to stimulate cough.

E. Oxygen Therapy: See p. 126.

F. Intake and Output: Order either nothing by mouth or a specific diet. Record the fluid intake and output for as long after surgery as required for control of fluid balance. Prescribe the parenteral fluids to be administered during the first 24 hours. Continuous catheter drainage of the bladder may be required to follow urine output closely in suspected renal impairment due to shock or other cause. If the patient is on catheter drainage, specify intervals for measurement of urine volume and specific gravity (e.g., hourly).

G. Voiding: Place an order for notification of the surgeon if the patient is unable to pass urine within a specified period (usually 6-8 hours) after operation.

H. Body Weight: Patients with fluid balance problems should be weighed daily.

I. Drainage Tubes: If a nasogastric or intestinal tube is in place, it should be connected to suction and irrigated every 1-2 hours with 15-30 ml. of saline. Urethral, chest, biliary, and other drainage catheters call for specific orders.

J. Medications: A narcotic for pain relief is usually required. Other drugs frequently used include sedatives, antibiotics, and antiemetic drugs. Always resume essential preoperative medications (e.g., digitalis, insulin, cortisone).

K. Special Laboratory Examinations: During the first 24 hours it may be necessary to obtain Hct., CBC, urinalysis, blood chemistries, blood pH, pO_2, pCO_2, and portable x-rays.

GENERAL CONDITIONS AFFECTING OPERATIVE RISK

The Pediatric Patient.

Infants and young children have a relatively low tolerance for infection, trauma, blood loss, and nutritional and fluid disturbances. The management of these disorders in infants and children differs somewhat from their treatment in adults, and the margin of safety is narrower. Because specialized knowledge and experience are required to treat infants and children, pediatric consultation is advisable.

As a result of the limited fluid and electrolyte resources of the infant and small child, dehydration and acid-base imbalance tend to develop rapidly, especially when fluid intake reduction is accompanied by unusual gastrointestinal losses from vomiting, diarrhea, or pooling of secretions in obstructed bowel. Dehydration is indicated by decreased skin turgor, recession of eyes, flatness or concavity of fontanelles, and low urine output. The status of acid-base balance requires determination of serum Na, Cl, K, and CO_2 and, in severe cases, pH, pO_2, and pCO_2 on arterial blood. Metabolic alkalosis is usually associated with a lesion causing vomiting. Respiratory alkalosis is most often the result of artificial ventilation, while respiratory acidosis is rarely a problem in children. Risk of surgery is substantially increased when undertaken before correction of fluid and electrolyte disturbances.

Another common occurrence in the acutely ill pediatric patient is high fever. Children with high temperatures are poor operative risks since they are prone to develop marked tachycardia, convulsions, or cardiovascular collapse. Rectal temperature should be reduced to less than 102° F. (38.9° C.) preoperatively by sponging the patient with tepid water or alcohol, fanning, ice bags, rehydration, and antibiotic therapy as indicated.

The newborn infant may be deficient in vitamin K and have a bleeding tendency caused by hypoprothrombinemia. Water-soluble vitamin K (Aqua-Mephyton® or Hykinone®), 2 mg. I.M. once, is sufficient; repeated administration may be dangerous since large doses to infants, particularly the prematurely born, may cause hemolytic anemia, hyperbilirubinemia, hepatomegaly, and even death. Vitamin C and other vitamins are important in the preoperative management of depleted children (see Chapter 4).

The Elderly Patient.

Operative risk should be judged on the basis of physiologic rather than chronologic age. Do not deny the elderly patient a needed operation because of his age alone. The hazard of the average major operation for the patient over 60 is increased only slightly provided there is no cardiovascular, renal, or other serious systemic disease. Assume that every patient over 60, even in the absence of symptoms and physical signs, has generalized arteriosclerosis and potential limitation of myocardial and renal reserve. Accordingly, the preoperative evaluation should be comprehensive (see above). Occult cancer is not infrequent in this age group; therefore, investigate suggestive gastrointestinal and other complaints, even though they might be minor.

Administer intravenous fluids with care so that the circulation in the elderly is not overloaded. Monitoring of intake, output, body weight, serum electrolytes, and central venous pressure is an important means of evaluating the cardiorenal response and tolerance in this age group.

Regarding medications, aged patients generally require smaller doses of strong narcotics and are frequently depressed by routine doses. Codeine is usually well tolerated. Barbiturates often cause restlessness, mental confusion, and uncooperative behavior; sedative and hypnotic drugs should be used cautiously. Preanesthetic medications should be limited to atropine or scopolamine in the debilitated elderly patient, and anesthetic agents should be administered in minimal amounts.

The Obese Patient.

Obese surgical patients have a greater than normal tendency to serious concomitant disease and a higher incidence of postoperative wound and thromboembolic complications. Also, obesity usually increases the technical difficulty of surgery and anesthesia. For these reasons, it may at times be advisable to delay elective surgery until the patient loses weight by appropriate dietary measures.

The Pregnant Patient.

Elective major surgery should be avoided during pregnancy. Normal, uncomplicated pregnancy is not debilitating, however, and does not significantly alter operative risk except as it may interfere with the diagnosis of abdominal disorders and increase the technical problems of abdominal surgery. Abortion is not a serious hazard after operation unless peritoneal sepsis or other serious complication occurs. During the first trimester, congenital anomalies may be induced in the developing fetus by hypoxia. It is preferable to avoid surgical intervention during this period; if surgery does become necessary, the greatest precautions must be taken to prevent hypoxia and hypotension. The second trimester is usually the optimum time for operative procedures.

Roentgenograms may be needed in connection with the diagnostic work-up and preoperative evaluation of the pregnent surgical patient. Diagnostic radiologic examinations of the lower abdomen and pelvis should be avoided during pregnancy, if possible, especially during the first 6 weeks of gestation. The fetus is particularly susceptible to irradiation effects during this period, which is also the period when pregnancy is likely to be overlooked. Although there is no conclusive evidence that exposure to diagnostic radiation during pregnancy produces a malformed baby, there is statistical evidence that mothers of leukemic children had a higher incidence of abdominal radiologic studies during pregnancy. It is also probable that the relatively small amount of irradiation to the fetus which results from multiple abdominal roentgenograms may slightly increase the risk of cancer in later life. Therefore, radiologic studies involving exposure to the abdomen and pelvis should be ordered in pregnant women only when essential to management. Precautions should include (1) a minimal number of films, (2) minimal exposure to the patient per film, and (3) irradiation of the minimal area of fetus and mother. Generally speaking, fluoroscopy of the abdomen during pregnancy is undesirable.

The Compromised or Altered Host.

A patient may be considered a ''compromised or altered host'' if the capacity of his systems and tissues to respond normally to infection and trauma has been significantly reduced or changed by some disease or agent. Obviously, preoperative recognition and special evaluation of these patients is important.

A. Increased Susceptibility to Infection: Certain drugs may reduce the patient's resistance to infection by interfering with host defense mechanisms. Corticosteroids, immunosuppressive agents, cytotoxic drugs, and prolonged antibiotic therapy are associated with an increased incidence of invasion by fungi and other organisms not commonly encountered in infections. A combination of irradiation and corticosteroid therapy is found experimentally to produce lethal fungal infections. It is possible that the synergistic combination of irradiation, corticosteroids, and serious underlying disease may set the stage for clinical fungal infection. A high rate of wound, pulmonary, and other infections is seen in renal failure, presumably due to decreased host resistance. Granulocytopenia and diseases which may produce immunologic deficiency (e.g., lymphomas, leukemias, and hypogammaglobulinemia) are frequently associated with septic complications. The uncontrolled diabetic is also observed clinically to be more susceptible to infection (see p. 76).

B. Delayed Wound Healing: This problem can be anticipated in certain categories of patients whose tissue repair process may be compromised. Many factors have been alleged to influence wound healing; however, only a few are of possible clinical significance - protein depletion, ascorbic acid deficiency, marked dehydration or edema, and severe anemia.

It has been shown experimentally that hypovolemia, vasoconstriction, increased blood viscosity, and increased intravascular aggregation and erythrostasis due to remote trauma will interfere with wound healing, probably by reducing oxygen tension and diffusion within the wound.

In animal studies, large doses of corticosteroid depress wound healing. This effect is apparently increased by mild starvation and protein depletion. Humans appear to react similarly to corticosteroid excess and it is therefore reasonable to assume that wounds in patients who have received appreciable doses of corticosteroid preoperatively should be closed with special care to prevent disruption and managed postoperatively as though healing will be delayed.

Surgical intervention may be required with a patient receiving cancer chemotherapy with cytotoxic drugs. These drugs usually interfere with cell proliferation and would theoretically tend to decrease the tensile strength of the surgical wound. Although experimental evidence for this assumption is equivocal, it is wise to manage wounds in patients on cytotoxic drugs as though healing will be slower than normal.

Decreased tensile strength and slow healing are sometimes observed clinically in such debilitated patients as those with advanced cancer, renal failure, gastrointestinal fistulas, and chronic infection. Protein and other nutritional deficiencies are doubtless the chief cause of the sluggish wound repair.

Preoperative assessment and correction of nutritional depletion may serve to minimize troublesome wound complications in such cases.

Systemic factors are, on the whole, only infrequently the cause of delayed wound healing. This is because the healing wound receives high priority in the body economy of even the aged or depleted patient for the protein, catalysts, and other resources that are required for collagen synthesis and deposition. This knowledge serves to emphasize the paramount importance of adhering strictly to basic surgical principles in the creation, closure, and care of wounds.

Decreased vascularity and other local changes occur after a few weeks or months in tissues which have been heavily irradiated. That they are potential deterrents to wound healing is a point which should be kept in mind in planning surgical incisions in patients who have been irradiated. Radiation therapy at levels of 3000 R and above is injurious to the skin, connective tissue, and vascular tissue. Chronic changes include scarring, damage to fibroblasts and collagen, and degenerative changes with subsequent hyalinization in the walls of blood vessels. Capillary budding in granulation tissue and collagen formation are inhibited when these changes are well established so that surgical wounds in heavily irradiated tissues may heal slowly or may break down in the presence of infection. When therapeutic doses of radiation are used as a surgical adjunct, it is generally agreed that there is an optimum delay period to minimize wound complications. This optimum period is from 2-12 weeks after completion of the radiation therapy. In general, technical problems in correctly timed operations for cancer are not increased by low-dose adjunctive radiotherapy (2000-4000 R). With radiation dosage in the therapeutic range (5000-6000 R), increased wound complications can be expected, although these can be minimized by careful surgical technic and proper timing.

Allergies and Sensitivities.

The surgical patient who is being evaluated and prepared for a major operation is about to face a formidable series of stresses, in the course of which he will probably receive a variety of potent medications. Drug allergies, sensitivities, incompatibilities, and adverse drug effects which may be precipitated by surgery must be foreseen and, if possible, prevented. A history of skin or other untoward reaction or sickness after injection, oral administration, or other use of any of the following substances should be noted so that they may be avoided: (1) penicillin or other antibiotic, (2) morphine, codeine, meperidine, or other narcotics, (3) procaine or other anesthetics, (4) aspirin, Empirin® Compound, or other pain remedies, (5) barbiturates, (6) sulfonamides and sulfones, (7) tetanus antitoxin or other sera, and (8) iodine, thimerosal (Merthiolate®), or other germicide. Untoward reactions to any other medication, to any foods (e.g., egg, milk, chocolate), and to adhesive tape should also be noted. Personal history or strong familial history of asthma, hay fever, or other allergic disorders should alert the surgeon to possible hypersensitivity to drugs.

Current Medications.

Drugs currently taken by the patient should be considered for continuation, discontinuation, or dosage adjustment. Medications such as digitalis, insulin, and cortisone must usually be maintained and their dosage carefully regulated during the operative and postoperative periods. Prolonged use of such corticosteroids as cortisone (even though discontinued 1 month or more preoperatively) may be associated with hypofunction of the adrenal cortex, which impairs the physiologic responses to the stress of anesthesia and surgery. Such a patient should receive cortisone immediately before, during, and after surgery. Anticoagulant drugs comprise an example of a medication to be strictly monitored or eliminated preoperatively.

The anesthesiologist is concerned with the long-term preoperative use of CNS depressants (e.g., barbiturates, opiates, alcohol), which may be associated with increased tolerance for anesthetic drugs, and with tranquilizers (e.g., phenothiazine derivatives such as chlorpromazine) and antihypertensive agents (e.g., rauwolfia derivatives such as reserpine), which may be associated with hypotension in response to anesthesia.

NONSURGICAL DISEASES AFFECTING OPERATIVE RISK

HEART DISEASE

Cardiac conditions severe enough to decrease the capacity of the heart to respond to stress can increase operative risk. Myocardial failure, ischemia, or serious arrhythmia may be precipitated by operation or its complications in patients who have minimal or absent cardiac symptoms under normal conditions. Cardiovascular function may be adversely affected by such common sequelae of surgery as apprehension, severe pain, fluid and electrolyte imbalance, infection, hypoxemia, hypercapnia, hypovolemia, decreased peripheral resistance, hypotension, tachycardia, bradycardia, and arrhythmia. The cardiac patient therefore requires careful preoperative evaluation and close observation during and after operation. A cardiologist should be consulted if a significant cardiac condition is present preoperatively or if it develops in the postoperative period.

Cardiac conditions most commonly associated with increased surgical risk are as follows: (1) cardiac failure or limited myocardial reserve, (2) coronary heart disease with a history of myocardial infarction or angina pectoris, (3) major arrhythmia (fibrillation, flutter, or block), (4) hypertension associated with coronary heart disease, cardiac failure, or renal insufficiency, (5) valvular heart disease, and (6) congenital heart disease.

Preoperative Evaluation.

A. History and Physical Examination: The most common symptoms of heart disease are dyspnea, fatigue, chest pain, and palpitation. Signs include cardiac enlargement, murmurs, hypertension, arrhythmias, and such evidence of cardiac failure as distention of neck veins, dependent edema, rales, liver enlargement, and ascites. A past history of angina pectoris, myocardial infarction, Stokes-Adams attacks, stroke, cerebral ischemic attacks, intermittent claudication, or previous treatment for heart disease or hypertension should alert the surgeon to the possibility of a cardiac abnormality requiring special study.

Conditions that contraindicate elective surgery because of increased risk are a recent occurrence of angina pectoris, a crescendo change in the pattern of angina pectoris in recent weeks or months, preinfarction angina, acute myocardial infarction, severe aortic stenosis, and a high degree of atrioventricular block.

B. Special Examinations: If symptoms, signs, or past history are suggestive of heart disease, the following examinations may be helpful in further clarifying the diagnosis and the functional state of the heart.

1. Electrocardiography - The Ecg. is useful diagnostically and as a baseline for evaluating subsequent changes in the myocardium and conduction system. It may provide evidence of arrhythmia, myocardial hypertrophy or strain, coronary artery disease, digitalis effect, or electrolyte disturbance. The Ecg. has its limitations, however: Some patients with known previous myocardial infarction or, more importantly, with preinfarction angina may have a normal Ecg., while, in other patients, grossly abnormal changes may be due to an old infarct that has healed and is therefore of lesser significance.

   In general, a stable abnormality in the Ecg., in the absence of cardiac failure or angina pectoris, indicates that the operative risk is probably only slightly increased. A patient with a healed myocardial infarction has an added mortality factor of about 3-5%.
2. Chest x-ray - This should be checked for abnormalities in the size and shape of cardiac and vascular contours and for evidence of valvular calcifications and pulmonary vascular congestion.
3. Central venous pressure - This should be determined when congestive failure is suspected (normal range: 6-12 cm. of water). If central venous pressure is elevated, determination of right ventricular end-diastolic pressure is useful.
4. Cardiac catheterization and angiography - These examinations are rarely required except in preparation for cardiac surgery. However, if a patient with serious congenital or coronary heart disease is under consideration for elective surgery, it may be necessary to complete one or both of these studies in order to decide whether corrective cardiac surgery should take precedence.
5. Exercise tolerance tests - Rarely, an exercise Ecg. test may be warranted if the diagnosis of coronary heart disease is seriously in doubt. Do not do an exercise test unless the resting Ecg. is normal, the patient has had no digitalis for 3 weeks, and the onset of pain of an anginal type is not of recent origin. A simple but adequate exercise tolerance test is to have the patient walk up 3 flights of stairs. If he

can accomplish this without precipitating angina or stopping because of dyspnea, he probably does not have a significant deficit in cardiopulmonary function.

Preoperative Preparation.

Before surgery, the cardiac patient should have the best possible cardiac status. Special attention should be paid to correction of electrolyte imbalance, fluid excess, and anemia (with packed red cells rather than whole blood). Alert all those concerned with the patient's care during and after the operation to the importance of avoiding hypotension, hypoxia, excessive sodium, fluid, and blood administration, and undue pain or excitement. These stresses may precipitate the major cardiac complications: failure, myocardial infarction, or serious arrhythmia.

A. Cardiac Failure: Cardiac failure should be treated adequately before surgery. It is desirable to have the patient stabilized for at least one month preoperatively, with special care to avoid digitalis toxicity and potassium depletion from diuretics. If the patient is well-controlled for a month, digitalis and diuretics can be avoided for a few days before surgery. In the presence of such signs as dyspnea when walking on level ground, orthopnea or nocturnal dyspnea, gallop rhythm, increased venous pressure, and rales, risk of surgery is significantly increased and the operation should be delayed if possible. Patients with mild cardiac failure whose symptoms and signs are controlled with digitalis and diuretics have only a slightly increased surgical risk, provided that they are able to perform ordinary activities without symptoms. It is probably unwise to use digitalis in patients with cardiac hypertrophy who do not have heart failure, since there is no clinical evidence that digitalis is of benefit under these circumstances and there is the hazard of digitalis toxicity. If the presence of cardiac failure is questionable, a preoperative period of bed rest and a restricted sodium diet may be adequate treatment.

B. Coronary Heart Disease: Many surgical patients, most of whom are in the older age group, have either occult or symptomatic coronary heart disease. A history of previous myocardial infarction or angina is frequently obtained and its implication must be assessed. Important danger signals, indicating markedly increased surgical risk, are (1) crescendo in the character of the anginal pain, (2) pain at rest, and (3) the possibility of preinfarction angina or actual recent myocardial infarction. Under these circumstances, elective surgery should be deferred.

When emergency surgery must be done in spite of recent myocardial infarction, the mortality rate has been 30-50%. Surgery that is important but not urgent should be delayed at least 3 weeks if possible following myocardial infarction. Elective surgery should be postponed 6 months. If at least 6 months have elapsed following a myocardial infarction, if the coronary artery disease is presumed stable as evidenced by no change in pattern of pain or in the serial Ecg., if there are no signs of cardiac failure, and if the indications for surgery are definite, operation can be undertaken.

C. Arrhythmias: Atrial premature beats occur with equal frequency in normal and diseased hearts and are not by themselves a sufficient basis for a diagnosis of heart disease. They can usually be abolished by speeding the heart rate by any method. Similarly, occasional ventricular premature beats generally have no definite significance; they may respond to treatment with phenobarbital. When ventricular premature beats are frequent and arise from multiple foci, when they occur with rapid ventricular rates or in runs, or when they appear during digitalis administration, they may be an indication of severe myocardial disease or digitalis toxicity and thus may require preoperative study and treatment. Partial (second degree) or complete (third degree) heart block indicates organic heart disease. The patient should be monitored; prior to a surgical procedure, it may be advisable to insert a transvenous electrode catheter into the right ventricle and have a pacemaker available in case ventricular standstill occurs.

D. Hypertension: Moderate hypertension alone does not affect the surgical risk significantly unless renal or cardiac complications are present. Patients with uncomplicated chronic hypertension, even with left ventricular hypertrophy and an abnormal Ecg., tolerate surgery well if there is no evidence of coronary heart disease or cardiac failure and if renal function is normal. Unless the diastolic pressure is above 110-115 mm. Hg, it is best to decrease or stop antihypertensive drugs for one week prior to surgery. If thiazides have been used, be certain that the body potassium level is normal. Catechol depletion following reserpine, methyldopa, and guanethidine can be managed satisfactorily if the anesthesiologist is forewarned and is prepared to give vasopressors if hypotension occurs.

E. Valvular Heart Disease: Acquired valvular conditions that affect operative risk adversely are severe aortic stenosis and tight mitral stenosis. An aortic systolic murmur without significant valvular disease or important left ventricular hypertrophy does not increase the mortality rate. Mitral insufficiency is usually well-tolerated, but tight mitral stenosis may result in pulmonary edema, especially if the patient has sinus rhythm and if there is abrupt fibrillation during surgery. Severe coronary ostial involvement from syphilitic aortitis considerably increases the hazard of operation.

F. Congenital Heart Disease: Uncomplicated ventricular or atrial septal defect does not usually increase surgical risk. Coarctation of the aorta and patent ductus arteriosus should usually be repaired before elective surgery. Patients with tetralogy of Fallot are poor surgical risks because of polycythemia and the probability of contraction of the infundibulum and decreased cardiac output; corrective surgery should be considered before major elective surgery. Pulmonic stenosis, if mild, does not contraindicate elective surgery, but severe pulmonic stenosis does; it should probably be corrected before elective surgery because of the danger of acute right heart failure or a reversed shunt through a patent foramen ovale or atrial septal defect. Pulmonary hypertension with Eisenmenger's syndrome significantly increases mortality and is a contraindication to surgery unless the need is urgent.

Treatment of Cardiac Complications.

A. Treatment of Acute Pulmonary Edema (Acute Congestive Failure): Acute pulmonary edema is a grave emergency. **Act immediately.** It is most likely to occur postoperatively and is often precipitated by stress, transfusion of too much blood, or excess administration of sodium-containing fluids intravenously. Myocardial infarction or an attack of atrial fibrillation with a rapid ventricular rate may be the precipitating factor.
   1. Position - Place the patient in a sitting position in bed or in a chair in order to decrease venous return to the heart.
   2. Morphine sulfate, 10-15 mg. (1/6-1/4 gr.) I. V. or I. M. every 2-4 hours, depresses pulmonary reflexes, relieves anxiety, and induces sleep.
   3. Give oxygen in high concentrations, preferably by mask. Positive pressure breathing for short periods may be of value.
   4. Reduction of blood volume is accomplished in 1 of 2 ways:
      a. By application of rubber tourniquets or BP cuffs to 3 extremities with sufficient pressure to obstruct venous but not arterial flow. Rotate the tourniquets every 10-15 minutes by placing a tourniquet on the fourth extremity and releasing one of the others.
      b. By venesection of 300-700 ml. of blood in successive bleedings.
   5. Rapid digitalization - This is of great value. Extreme care is necessary in giving digitalis I.V. to a previously digitalized patient (see Appendix).
   6. Aminophylline, 0.25-0.5 Gm. (4-7 1/2 gr.) slowly I.V., may be helpful. A rectal suppository, 0.5 Gm., or rectal instillation of 0.5 Gm. in 30 ml. of tap water may be effective if the I.V. route is not feasible.
   7. Rapid diuresis may be useful in some circumstances. This may be accomplished with ethacrynic acid (Edecrin®), 25-100 mg. orally or 25-50 mg. I.V., or furosemide (Lasix®), 40-80 mg. orally or I.V.

B. Treatment of Congestive Failure: Symptoms and signs include dyspnea, orthopnea, rales at lung bases, venous and hepatic engorgement, dependent edema, prolonged circulation time, and increased venous pressure.
   1. Eliminate or control precipitating factors such as stress, sepsis, anemia, excess sodium administration, arrhythmias, and thyrotoxicosis.
   2. Rest in bed or chair with appropriate sedation decreases the work required of the heart.
   3. The diet should be bland, low-residue, and low in sodium (less than 0.6 Gm. of sodium or 1.5 Gm. of sodium chloride). With sodium restriction, fluids may be allowed ad lib.
   4. Digitalis (see above).
   5. Diuretics (see above and Appendix).
   6. The patient will lose weight and dyspnea will subside as improvement occurs. Activity can then be resumed gradually within appropriate limits.

C. Treatment of Acute Myocardial Infarction: Prolonged, usually severe precordial or substernal pain, sometimes radiating to the neck or upper extremities, is typical, but these symptoms may be masked by anesthesia or narcotics. Infarction is often associated with shock, congestive failure, and arrhythmias. Other manifestations include fever, leukocytosis, and elevation of sedimentation rate and the serum levels of glutamic-oxaloacetic transaminase (SGOT), lactic dehydrogenase (LDH), and creatine phosphokinase (CPK). There are characteristic Ecg. changes (which may be delayed). During the acute stage, the patient's Ecg., pulse, and possibly the venous and arterial pressures should be continuously monitored in a coronary care or equivalent unit.

1. Rest - Complete bed rest for 1-4 weeks is advocated, with gradual resumption of activity as tolerated. Use sedatives as required.
2. Relief of pain - Give morphine sulfate, 10-15 mg. (1/6-1/4 gr.) subcut., I.M., or slowly I.V., or choose an alternative narcotic.
3. Oxygen therapy is usually necessary.
4. Shock - If cardiac shock is present, treat with an inotropic drug, such as isoproterenol (Isuprel®), and with cautious digitalization. Vasopressor drugs such as metaraminol (Aramine®) or levarterenol (Levophed®) are thought by some clinicians to be helpful, but inotropic drugs are usually more helpful.
5. Digitalis and drugs to control arrhythmia are prescribed for specific indications.

D. Treatment of Cardiac Arrhythmias: The treatment of the major arrhythmias is a complex problem calling for the close collaboration of the internist and surgeon. However, the surgeon may be required to give emergency treatment or initiate treatment until the services of an internist can be obtained. The final diagnosis of the type of arrhythmia present is made from the Ecg.

1. Atrial fibrillation - Rapid atrial fibrillation decreases the efficiency of the heart and may lead to congestive failure. Emergency treatment consists of slowing the rate by adequate digitalization. Conversion to normal sinus rhythm by quinidine or D.C. countershock can be considered later.
2. Atrial flutter - Rapid atrial flutter may lead to congestive failure. Digitalization will slow the rate, either by increasing the degree of block or by converting the flutter to sinus rhythm or atrial fibrillation. The final conversion is best supervised by one familiar with the treatment of this condition. D.C. countershock may be the treatment of choice.
3. Paroxysmal supraventricular tachycardia - Paroxysmal atrial tachycardia is the most common paroxysmal tachycardia. Other types are paroxysmal nodal tachycardia and a group of tachycardias in which the source of the ectopic focus cannot be determined. Supraventricular tachycardias often occur in patients with otherwise normal hearts. In the absence of heart disease, serious effects are rare. Remedies that are more dangerous than the disease should be avoided. Rule out digitalis toxicity as a cause of the tachycardia. Vagus stimulation (carotid sinus pressure, gagging, Valsalva's maneuver) should be tried initially. If mechanical measures fail, drugs should be used. Sedation alone may be sufficient. There is no unanimity regarding the most

effective cardiac medication, but the following may be tried: (1) Digitalis orally or, if no digitalis has been given in the preceding 2 weeks. I.V. (see Appendix). (2) Vasopressor agents (see p. 24). (3) Procainamide hydrochloride (see below). Continuous Ecg. or monitoring of heart rate and monitoring of BP are essential. (4) Propranolol (Inderal®), 10-30 mg. t.i.d. before meals and at bedtime, or 1 mg. I.V. slowly, and with continuous clinical and Ecg. monitoring, until therapeutic effect begins. If necessary (and there have been no untoward effects), a second dose of 1 mg. may be given in 2-5 minutes. Atropine, 0.5-1 mg., should be given I.V. if excessive bradycardia occurs. **Caution:** Propranolol should be given I.V. only if other measures fail and the clinical situation warrants the risk. Rarely, cardioversion by D.C. countershock may be required if the patient's condition deteriorates in spite of the above measures.

4. Ventricular paroxysmal tachycardia - This arrhythmia is usually associated with myocardial damage, especially myocardial infarction. Digitalis toxicity may cause this arrhythmia.
   a. Lidocaine (Xylocaine®) - This is the drug of choice for emergency treatment because of its short duration of action and infrequent hypotensive effect. Give 50-100 mg. I.V. as a bolus and repeat the injection if the initial bolus is not effective. If the arrhythmia recurs, an I.V. infusion of 50 mg./hour (1 Gm. diluted to 1 L. in 5% glucose solution) may be given or the I.V. injection repeated twice at 20-minute intervals. If lidocaine is without effect, cardioversion by D.C. countershock is preferred to additional pharmacologic methods of treatment in all but the mildest cases (see below).
   b. Quinidine -
      (1) Oral - Quinidine sulfate, 0.4 Gm. (6 gr.) orally every 2 hours for 3 doses, if the attack is well tolerated and the patient is not in shock (otherwise, give parenterally). If the attack continues and quinidine toxicity does not appear, increase the dose to 0.6 Gm. (9 gr.) orally every 2 hours for 3 doses. This usually terminates the attack. If it does not, give the drug I.M. or use procainamide.
      (2) I.M. - Quinidine gluconate, 0.8 Gm. (12 gr.), or 0.5 Gm. (7 1/2 gr.) of quinidine base, may be given I.M. and repeated every 2 hours for 2-3 doses.
   c. Procainamide (Pronestyl®) - This drug causes hypotension; BP must be observed frequently during its use.
      (1) Oral - Procainamide hydrochloride (Pronestyl®), 0.5-1.5 Gm. (7 1/2-22 1/2 gr.) orally every 4-6 hours.
      (2) I.M. - 0.5-1 Gm. (7 1/2-15 gr.) may be given I.M. and repeated in 4 hours.
      (3) I.V. - 1 Gm. (15 gr.) ampul in 10 ml. diluent given slowly at a rate of 50-100 mg. (3/4-1 1/2 gr.) per minute to a total of 1 Gm. (15 gr.) with continuous BP determinations and, if possible, Ecg. control. Discontinue drug as soon as conversion takes place.
   d. Propranolol (Inderal®) may be tried if the above drugs fail.

e. Give a vasopressor drug for shock. **Note**: Digitalis must be used cautiously in this disorder, and only in patients with cardiac failure in whom other drugs have failed to restore sinus rhythm.

f. Electrical cardioversion - Conversion to normal sinus rhythm by depolarization of the entire heart with a D.C. shock is an important method of therapy in arrhythmias. Initial energy settings of 25 watt-seconds are employed for atrial flutter and supraventricular tachycardias, and 50 watt-seconds for atrial fibrillation and ventricular tachycardia. If the initial energy is ineffective, sequential increases in energy may be required. General anesthesia is not necessary. Amnesia is induced with sodium methohexital (Brevital® Sodium), 25-75 mg. I.V., or diazepam (Valium®), 5-20 mg. I.V.

5. Ventricular fibrillation produces cardiac arrest and requires cardiopulmonary resuscitation and electric shock defibrillation (see pp. 10-18).

Prognosis.

Generalizations about the cardiac patient's prognosis for survival of surgery are difficult. Large series of cardiac patients have shown an average mortality of only 3% after major abdominal and thoracic surgery. Certain cardiac conditions, however, are associated with an inherently greater surgical risk. Coronary heart disease is the commonest of these encountered in practice. In general, surgical mortality for major procedures is doubled by congestive failure or angina with mild exertion. Risk is further increased in the presence of serious arrhythmia or a history of myocardial infarction within 6 months. Angina at rest quadruples the risk and recent myocardial infarction raises the risk to a practically prohibitive level.

RESPIRATORY TRACT DISEASE

Operative morbidity and risk are affected adversely by acute or chronic respiratory tract diseases.

Acute Conditions.

Acute respiratory tract infection (coryza, pharyngitis, tonsillitis, laryngitis, bronchitis, or pneumonitis) is a contraindication to elective surgery because it is associated with an increased postoperative incidence of atelectasis and pneumonitis. The patient should be completely recovered for 1-2 weeks before operation. If emergency operation must be undertaken in the presence of acute respiratory tract infection, avoid inhalation anesthesia if possible, employ prophylactic measures for atelectasis postoperatively (see p. 85), and administer antibiotics if the infection is marked or progressive. Penicillin is usually given until the antibiotic sensitivity reports on throat or sputum cultures can be obtained.

Chronic Conditions.

A. Chronic Bronchopulmonary Infection: Chronic bronchitis, bronchiectasis, emphysema, asthma, pulmonary fibrosis, and tuberculosis are among the commonest disorders associated with bronchial or pulmonary infection in surgical patients. Many of these patients are elderly, and smoking is often an aggravating factor. Any patient with a history of having smoked over 20 cigarettes a day for 10 years can be assumed to have a chronic bronchopulmonary disorder. Heavy smokers should abstain for at least 2 weeks before elective major surgery.

Respiratory reserve may be diminished, but is usually adequate. The major hazard is excessive bronchial secretions, with a marked tendency to postoperative atelectasis and pneumonitis.

Preoperative and postoperative management is discussed under Atelectasis (see p. 81).

B. Diminished Pulmonary Reserve: With the exception of thoracic procedures, pulmonary insufficiency is rarely severe enough to contraindicate necessary surgery. Diminished reserve is caused by a wide variety of disorders, particularly those mentioned above as being associated with bronchopulmonary infection. When the clinical examination shows that pulmonary function is significantly reduced, special tests should be performed (see Chapter 6). Preoperatively, respiratory function can often be improved by treatment of infection and bronchospasm. Atelectasis and hypoxia are the chief dangers postoperatively. Acutely diminished pulmonary function after operation or injury may occasionally require tracheal intubation and mechanical ventilation as lifesaving measures.

RENAL DISEASE

Chronic impairment of renal function may be fully compensated and asymptomatic under normal conditions, but renal insufficiency may develop under the adverse conditions of surgical illness. About 700 ml. /day of urine are normally required for the excretion of nitrogenous wastes. In patients with damaged kidneys, considerably larger volumes of urine (1500 ml. or more) may be necessary as a result of the kidneys' inability to concentrate urine. Such patients will develop uremia if they become dehydrated or if the nitrogen load is increased, e.g., in fever and as a catabolic response to trauma or infection. Metabolic acidosis is a common additional complication (see p. 157).

The following types of renal disease are most frequently responsible for diminished reserve in surgical patients: chronic glomerulonephritis, chronic pyelonephritis, toxic nephritis, amyloid renal disease, obstructive uropathy, and acute renal failure.

Before major operations it is often advisable to evaluate kidney function by 1 or more special examinations if any of the following is present: (1) a history of renal disease, (2) age over 60, (3) diabetes mellitus, (4) hypertension, (5) abnormal urinalysis (proteinuria, casts, low or fixed sp. gr.), or (6) oliguria or polyuria not caused by variations in fluid intake. The following special examinations are frequently of value in addition to the routine urinalysis: BUN, creatinine, PSP, a clearance test (urea or creatinine), plasma electrolyte determinations, and intravenous urogram.

Principles of Management.

A. Preoperative Care:
  1. Evaluate renal function carefully.
  2. Correct electrolyte imbalance (see p. 150).
  3. Correct nitrogen retention by proper fluid intake and reduction of dietary protein.
  4. Correct anemia and hypovolemia by transfusion of packed red cells or, if necessary, whole blood.
  5. Be alert for the dangerous accumulation of medications excreted by the kidneys.

B. During Operation: The same general rules for operation and anesthesia apply as for patients with heart disease (see p. 66).

C. Postoperative Care:
  1. Record intake and output accurately.
  2. Maintain electrolyte balance carefully with attention to adequate fluid intake and output (see Chapter 5).
  3. Weigh patient daily.
  4. Determine BUN and creatinine postoperatively as indicated.

D. Treatment of Complications:
  1. Acute renal failure (see p. 171).
  2. Urinary tract infection and obstruction (see Chapter 14).
  3. Uremia - **Nitrogen retention in surgical patients is usually reversible when precipitating factors such as dehydration and urinary obstruction are corrected. Diagnosis and treatment of these should be prompt. In the management of uremia,** acidosis and other electrolyte derangements are more important than the elevation of the BUN.
     a. Diet - Restrict protein to 0.5 Gm. /Kg./day plus the amount lost in the urine. The diet should include adequate calories, and sodium should usually not be restricted.
     b. Fluids - Unless the patient is anuric, fluid intake should be sufficient to maintain adequate urine volume, which may be quite high because of a large solute load (e.g., sodium and urea) excreted by a reduced number of nephrons. Intake should be great enough to maintain renal function without excessive diuresis or edema. Water restriction may be hazardous.
     c. Electrolytes - Correct imbalance cautiously (see p. 150). Serum sodium and calcium concentrations may be low and potassium increased. Retention of phosphate, sulfate, chloride, and organic acids, plus the loss of sodium, may result in a decrease of plasma bicarbonate concentration and of pH. Sodium supplements may be needed to replace losses due to failure of the kidneys to provide NH_4^+ and H^+ for sodium conservation. A mixture of NaCl and $NaHCO_3$ in equal parts, 1-2 Gm. 2-3 times daily with meals, may be required, in addition to the sodium in the diet. Potassium intake may have to be restricted or, more rarely, supplemented. If severe hyperkalemia is present, active measures to remove potassium may be necessary, such as cation exchange resins or dialysis (see p. 172). Frequent measurement of electrolytes will usually be essential for proper management of imbalances.
     d. Anemia - Correct by transfusions of whole blood or

packed red cells if severe. Iron is usually ineffective.

e. Medications -

(1) Aluminum hydroxide gel, 30 ml. q.i.d. orally, causes precipitation of soluble phosphates in the bowel and aids in reducing hyperphosphatemia. This helps to elevate serum calcium and prevent tetany.

(2) Calcium gluconate, 10%, 10 ml. I.V. p.r.n., is useful to prevent or treat tetany. (**Note**: Calcium gluconate should be used cautiously or not at all in digitalized patients.) Calcium lactate, 4 Gm. 2-3 times daily by mouth, may also be satisfactory for this purpose.

Extrarenal Azotemia.

Extrarenal azotemia is the abnormal accumulation of nitrogenous waste products in the presence of normal or potentially normal renal function. The most common cause is inadequate glomerular filtration secondary to decreased effective circulating blood volume, as occurs in shock and dehydration. BUN, NPN, and blood creatinine are elevated. After massive gastrointestinal bleeding, extrarenal azotemia may occur as a result of protein digestion and absorption plus decreased circulating blood volume. Under these circumstances the blood creatinine level is not elevated.

Since no renal disease is present, treatment is aimed at improving circulating blood volume (transfusion), electrolyte balance, and urinary output (increased fluid intake).

DIABETES MELLITUS

Well-controlled diabetes probably does not increase operative risk. However, the diabetic patient is physiologically older than his chronologic age and tends to develop atherosclerosis early; the possibility of cardiac, renal, and cerebral complications is therefore greater. The uncontrolled diabetic is also more susceptible to infection, which in turn aggravates his metabolic disorder. For this reason the diabetic patient must be protected from even minor infections and must receive prompt antibiotic treatment when infections do occur. Furthermore, diabetes is frequently put out of control by the very conditions so often associated with surgical illness: excitement and stress, anesthesia; fluid, electrolyte, and nutritional derangements; and inflammation. Early diagnosis and therapy are therefore essential to minimize these disturbances. The collaboration of an internist in the management of the diabetes is advisable.

Simple and rapid testing of urine glucose may be accomplished with Clinitest®, Clinistix®, and Tes-Tape®. These proprietary preparations require no heating and only a few drops of urine.

Elective Surgery.

A. Preoperative Care:

1. Diet - If diabetes is moderate or severe, admit patient several days before surgery. Discontinue oral and long-acting insulins and bring diabetes under optimum control with crystalline zinc insulin. Ketosis should be absent before operation.

In a well-regulated diabetic, continue the diet and insulin to which the patient is accustomed. If the patient is not on an adequate diet, he should be placed on a diabetic diet and insulin dosage given q.i.d. (a.c. and h.s.) according to the urine reactions listed in the table above. A diet suitable for a normally active 70 Kg. patient should consist of 1750 Cal.: 175 Gm. (700 Cal.) carbohydrate, 105 Gm. (420 Cal.) protein, and 70 Gm. (630 Cal.) fat.

2. Urinalysis - In every diabetic surgical patient, examine for sugar and ketone bodies before each meal and at bedtime or every 4 hours to evaluate the status of the disease. If catheterized, diabetic patients are very susceptible to urinary tract infections. The procedure should be avoided if possible.
3. Blood chemistry - Fasting blood sugar should be determined on one or 2 occasions before operation. Blood level of sodium, potassium, chloride, bicarbonate, and BUN should be measured as a baseline.
4. If infection is present, insulin therapy will often fail to eliminate glycosuria; control of infection is frequently necessary before carbohydrate tolerance will improve.
5. If diabetes is newly discovered or out of control on admission, consult an internist for assistance in regulating it.

Action of Insulin*

Product	Action		
	Onset	Maximum	Total Duration
Short-acting Insulins			
Regular, I.V.	Immediate	1 hr.	....
Regular, subcut.	1/2 hr.	3 hrs.	7 hrs.
Crystalline Zinc (CZI)	1/2 hr.	3 hrs.	7 hrs.
Intermediate Insulins			
NPH	3 hrs.	8-9 hrs.	16-17 hrs.
Globin	3 hrs.		16-17 hrs.
Long-acting Insulins			
Protamine Zinc (PZI)	10 hrs.	18 hrs.	24-36 hrs.
Newer Insulins			
Semi-lente	3-4 hrs.	7 hrs.	9-10 hrs.
Ultra-lente	8-9 hrs.	16-19 hrs.	24-48-96 hrs.
Lente® (30% semi and 70% ultra)	3 hrs.	8-9 hrs.	18-24 hrs.

*Adapted from Read and Baer.

Tests for Urine Glucose

Color of Benedict's Test Solution	% Glucose	Amount of Regular Insulin Needed
Blue to cloudy green = 0	–	0
Greenish-yellow = +	< 5%	0
Yellow = ++	0.5-1%	5 units
Orange = +++	1-2%	10 units
Red = ++++	> 2%	15 units

6. Ketonuria and acidosis must be corrected prior to elective operations.

B. Day of Operation:
1. Assign the patient an early position on the operating schedule.
2. Omit modified insulin on the day of operation (and usually for several days thereafter). Perform urinalyses every 4 hours and administer regular insulin according to the color reaction (see above).
3. Continue regular oral intake up to 12 hours before surgery.
4. Patients with mild diabetes may usually be fasted preoperatively for 8-12 hours, just as is done for patients without diabetes. Patients with more severe diabetes should be given 1 L. of 5% glucose in water or saline (to which is added 25 units of regular insulin) before surgery.
5. Give fluids, electrolytes, and glucose on the day of operation according to the requirements of the operative procedure and the patient's condition.
6. When prolonged procedures are contemplated or when the patient is unable for other reasons to void at regular in-intervals, insert an inlying catheter. **Note:** Catheterization may produce urinary tract infection and for this reason should not be done unless definitely required. Use all appropriate means to elicit spontaneous urination.

C. Postoperative Care:
1. Continue urinalyses at intervals of 4 hours and administer regular insulin according to the color reaction until the patient's accustomed diet and insulin regimen can be resumed.
2. Provide at least 150 Gm. of carbohydrate daily, either orally or by vein.
3. Do not attempt to keep the urine completely free of sugar during the first day or 2 postoperatively. Control of blood sugar within the normal range is not necessary or desirable during the operative or immediate postoperative period. Mild hyperglycemia is not hazardous and hypoglycemia is to be avoided.

Emergency Surgery.

A. Treatment of Diabetic Acidosis Preoperatively: These patients frequently have ketonuria. If acidosis is also present (as indicated by ketonuria, red reduction for sugar in urine, and blood bicarbonate below 27 mEq. /L.), treatment is urgently required along the following lines:
1. Urinalysis - Examine urine hourly for sugar and ketone bodies. (Insert an inlying catheter only if absolutely necessary.) The urine should contain some sugar at all times during intensive treatment with insulin to avoid a hypoglycemic reaction.
2. Blood chemistry - Draw blood for blood glucose, bicarbonate, sodium, potassium, and chloride. In acidosis, in addition to the losses caused by the surgical condition, there is usually acute loss of water, sodium, chloride, bicarbonate, and potassium.
3. Insulin therapy - Intensive insulin therapy is indicated. Give 50-100 units of regular insulin I.V. and a similar

amount subcut. unless the patient is in shock, in which case only the intravenous route should be used. Repeat 50-75 units subcut. every 1-2 hours until there is a rapid diminution in urinary and/or blood sugar; then give insulin intravenously in glucose and saline as described below. The average amount of insulin required in the first 3 hours in the treatment of severe diabetic acidosis with coma was 200-225 units at the Joslin Clinic.

4. Fluids and electrolytes - Begin an infusion of physiologic saline at the outset of treatment and restore water and electrolyte balance. If blood bicarbonate is low, give sodium bicarbonate or sodium lactate by vein in calculated amounts (see p. 169). Marked potassium deficit is usually present and, when a urine output of 40-50 ml./hour has been established, requires correction with potassium (preferably as the phosphate), 20-30 mEq./L. of intravenous fluid.
5. Glucose - As soon as urinary sugar has fallen to the point where an olive or green reduction is shown on Benedict's test, change intravenous fluids to 5% glucose in saline to which is added 0.5-1 unit of insulin/Gm. of glucose (25-50 units of insulin/L.) and 20 mEq. /L. potassium phosphate. The urine should contain sugar at all times to avoid hypoglycemic reactions. Continue this infusion slowly (60-70 drops/minute) throughout the surgical procedure. This will supply glucose on which the insulin can act in overcoming the acidosis.
6. Timing of operation - Unless surgical intervention (e.g., drainage of an abscess) is essential to management of the acidosis, delay operation until acidosis is controlled.
7. Postoperatively - Continue slow infusion of 5% glucose in saline or water with insulin until ketonuria has disappeared. Administer additional insulin subcut. every 1-2 hours as required to maintain slight glycosuria. Insulin dosage is based on the color of the reduction in hourly urinalyses (see p. 77). As soon as possible, shift to oral intake and give insulin every 4 hours in amounts depending upon the color reaction on urinalysis.

B. Emergency Operation for Trauma: Injured diabetic patients under insulin treatment may develop a severe hypoglycemic reaction because of failure to eat. Determine blood and urine glucose levels. If laboratory findings, history, or physical examination suggest the possibility of an insulin reaction (weakness, faintness, hunger, tremor, convulsions, or hypoglycemia), give sweetened orange juice or candy by mouth or 5% glucose in water or saline by vein. Administer 5% glucose in water or saline at 60-70 drops/minute I.V. throughout the operation. One unit of insulin per 2 Gm. of glucose may be added to this infusion. Test urine every 1-4 hours and administer regular insulin accordingly. When surgery has been completed, follow as after elective surgery.

Anesthesia. (See Chapter 3.)

With the aid of insulin practically any type of anesthetic may be used, but some are better than others. The following principles should be kept in mind:

A. Premedication: Keep this to a minimum. Avoid depressing the patient with narcotics unless they are definitely made necessary by severe pain. Obtain mild sedation with a barbiturate; in the older diabetic patient, use only atropine.
B. Anesthetic Agents: The anesthetist should be experienced in the problems of surgical anesthesia in diabetic patients.
   1. Local or regional procaine anesthesia is the method of choice if suitable.
   2. Spinal anesthesia is next in order of preference.
   3. General anesthesia - Ether is the least desirable of these agents since it impairs the formation of glycogen and tends to increase the severity of the diabetes. Avoidance of hypoxia is essential.

POSTOPERATIVE COMPLICATIONS

OPERATIVE WOUND COMPLICATIONS

Abdominal Wound Disruption.

An incidence of wound rupture of up to 3% in laparotomies has been reported, but the frequency can be kept well under 1%. Vertical abdominal wounds are slightly more vulnerable to dehiscence than transverse wounds. Disruption may occur as late as a month postoperatively, but is commonest between the fourth and twelfth days.

A. Predisposing Factors: The major cause is poor surgical technic in wound closure. Malnutrition, vitamin C deficiency, hypoproteinemia, anemia, obesity, drains, postoperative cough, vomiting, distention, premature removal of sutures, infection, and all disorders which put an undue strain on the wound may predispose to wound disruption.
B. Sudden serosanguineous drainage from the wound is practically pathognomonic of wound rupture. Occasionally the patient is conscious of a tearing sensation as the suture line gives way during coughing or straining. Rarely, a loop of bowel or the omentum will prolapse through the wound. There is little pain or reaction unless extensive evisceration takes place.
C. Prophylaxis: Predisposing conditions should be corrected or prevented as far as possible. Drains and colostomies should be brought out through separate stab wounds when feasible. Clean wounds should be closed in layers, preferably with interrupted nonabsorbable sutures, approximating fascial structures under proper tension. In addition, retention sutures should be placed through all layers of the abdominal wall if wound closure is precarious, or if postoperative stress on the wound or delayed healing is expected. Retention sutures may be tied over special plastic suture bridges if the wound must be left open or if infection is anticipated.
D. Treatment:
   1. Minimal disruption - Using aseptic technic, hold the wound edges together with strips of adhesive tape, apply a sterile dressing and an abdominal binder, maintain bed rest,

relieve abdominal distention with nasogastric suction as required, and treat the systemic condition. This procedure is applicable only when the sole evidence for dehiscence is slight serosanguineous drainage without apparent separation of the fascial layers. Frequently the extent of disruption of deeper layers is far greater than suspected and exploration of the wound with a sterile instrument will disclose separation of fascia and peritoneum. In that case, treat as a major disruption.

2. Major disruption - Resuture the entire wound with through-and-through wire, nylon, or silk sutures. General anesthesia with adequate relaxation is highly desirable. Primary healing usually takes place.

E. Prognosis: Mortality after wound dehiscence is about 10% and is due primarily to the patient's underlying disease. The incidence of hernia following through-and-through closure of disrupted wounds is also about 10%.

Wound Infection.

Postoperative wound infection is usually obvious within the first week after operation, but its appearance may be delayed, especially if antibiotics are given. Infection most commonly occurs in the fat and subcutaneous tissues. The development of fever 4-7 days postoperatively is frequently due to wound infection. Treatment consists of early drainage and appropriate anti-infective therapy.

PULMONARY COMPLICATIONS

Atelectasis.

Obstruction of a bronchus or bronchiole with resultant collapse of a portion of the lung occurs after 10-20% of major operations and is the most frequent complication of thoracic surgery. Involvement of multiple, small patchy areas is most common, but massive atelectasis of an entire lobe or lung may occur. Onset usually occurs within the first few days postoperatively, and is almost invariably associated with pneumonitis in the collapsed area.

A. Predisposing Factors:

1. Preoperative - Atelectasis is 4 times as frequent in patients over 60, and twice as frequent in males. The rate of occurrence is higher when the patient is 30% or more above ideal weight. Chronic bronchitis, bronchiectasis, asthma, and smoking predispose to increased secretions and a higher incidence of atelectasis and pneumonitis postoperatively. For similar reasons, acute respiratory infection definitely increases the incidence and severity of pulmonary complications.
2. Operative - Hypoventilation, accumulation of bronchial secretions, aspiration of gastric contents, and prolonged immobilization during operation set the stage for the development of atelectasis postoperatively.
3. Postoperative - Inadequate ventilation, failure to change position, and failure to remove tracheobronchial secretions

by cough or aspiration are the most important factors. Depressant doses of narcotics, abdominal distention, wound pain, and general debility are aggravating conditions.

B. Diagnosis: Higher than anticipated fever in the first few days after operation is frequently the earliest sign of atelectasis. Temperature may rise suddenly, reaching 102° F. (38.9° C.) or more. Cough and sputum may not be present at the onset, but usually develop within 1-2 days. Diminished breath sounds and bronchial breathing with scattered moist rales are heard over the area of collapse if sufficiently large. When a major portion of the lung is atelectatic, the mediastinal structures shift to that side and deviation of the trachea may be apparent at the jugular notch. Dyspnea, cyanosis, and prostration indicate extensive atelectasis and pneumonitis.

C. Treatment: Examine the chest of postoperative patients once or twice daily during the first week after surgery. Act promptly on the earliest signs of atelectasis since this disorder is often quickly reversible if treated immediately. Obtain a chest x-ray and sputum culture at the beginning of treatment in severe cases.

Vigorous coughing, deep breathing, and change of position at intervals of 30 minutes to several hours are the most important preventive and therapeutic measures. Early ambulation is also of value.

1. Voluntary coughing - Insist on a short period of hyperventilation and forceful coughing every hour. Close supervision and encouragement are essential. Cough and cooperation will be improved by administration of a narcotic to relieve wound pain and apprehension. The expectoration of thick, yellowish, tenacious plugs of sputum often brings improvement.
2. Tracheal aspiration - If voluntary coughing is inadequate, aspirate the trachea as often as required to clear secretions. Tracheal catheterization is best accomplished with the patient in a sitting position and the tongue held forward by an assistant. A 16-20 F. catheter (connected to suction with a "Y" tube so that suction may be interrupted) is then passed through the nostril into the pharynx. The patient is then instructed to take a few deep breaths, and the catheter is advanced quickly into the trachea during inspiration. Paroxysmal cough and loss of voice indicate that the catheter is in correct position. The catheter is then moved up and down the trachea for aspiration. Suction is interrupted as necessary to allow the patient to rest and breathe.
3. Transtracheal catheter - Transtracheal insertion through the cricothyroid membrane of a small inlying (I.V. type) plastic catheter (such as a standard No. 14 Intracath [Bard]) will permit repeated injection of a few ml. of saline or distilled water into the trachea to stimulate cough and assist mobilization of secretions in the patient unable to clear his airway because of diminished cough and tenacious sputum.
4. Bronchoscopic aspiration - This may occasionally be necessary at the conclusion of an operation to remove foreign material or plugs of mucus from the bronchi and when catheter aspiration of the trachea is unsuccessful postoperatively.

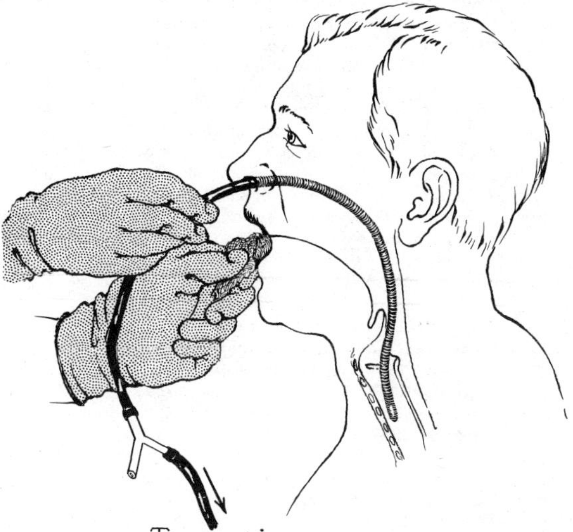

Technic of Tracheal Aspiration

5. Tracheal intubation - In debilitated patients unable to raise secretions, respiratory insufficiency may become an added problem. In such cases, tracheal intubation by the oral or nasal route may be necessary to permit frequent suctioning of secretions and mechanical assistance to ventilation. Rarely a tracheostomy may be required for this purpose.
6. Intermittent positive pressure breathing (IPPB) - This type of breathing for 3-5 minutes every hour is an aid in the prevention and treatment of atelectasis. Oxygen or air may be used and should be humidified by nebulization of water or saline. A bronchodilator is most effectively administered by the IPPB apparatus.
7. Humidification - Inhalation of warm, moist air is soothing, and helps to mobilize tracheobronchial secretions, chiefly by improving ciliary activity. When oxygen is administered, it should be humidified by passage through a heated, thermostatically controlled nebulizer. Alternatively, "cold" mist for humidification can be provided by an ultrasonic nebulizer. Either distilled water or normal saline can be used for humidification by these methods. A positive pressure breathing apparatus should have a humidifier in the circuit.
8. Aerosol therapy - A nebulizer which will produce fluid particles smaller than 8-10 μ in diameter is required. Continuous aerosol therapy with water or saline is accomplished

by placing the nebulizer in the oxygen or air line to the patient. Intermittent therapy can be administered with a hand nebulizer or, more effectively, with an IPPB apparatus such as the Bennett or Bird respirator. The following agents may be used in aerosol therapy:

a. Water or saline - Nebulization of water or physiologic saline solution is more satisfactory than steam inhalations and should be used when oxygen or air is administered by nasal catheter, face mask, or tracheal tube.

b. Surface tension lowering agents - Detergents or "wetting" agents such as tyloxapol (Alevaire®) and sodium ethasulfate (Tergemist®) have been recommended on the theory that they lower the viscosity of the sputum. Double-blind studies show them to be no more effective than saline as an aerosol.

c. Mucolytic agents - Acetylcysteine (Mucomyst®) is used to lyse secretions prior to their aspiration. It may be necessary to dilute the 20% solution with equal parts of normal saline. Copious secretions may be produced. This type of medication is rarely indicated in the postoperative patient.

d. Antibiotics - Inhalation of antibiotics is not advisable because the patient may become sensitized to the drug. Use systemic antibiotics if anti-infective therapy is necessary.

e. Bronchodilator drugs - These are indicated when bronchospasm contributes to cough and respiratory distress, as in asthmatic bronchitis, which may be exacerbated by surgical illness. An aminophylline rectal suppository (0.5 Gm.) every 6-12 hours may be of value when prolonged bronchodilator effect is desired (see p. 70).

One of the following may be administered by nebulization:

(1) Isoproterenol hydrochloride inhalation (Isuprel®, Aludrine®), usually 3-7 inhalations of 1:100 solution or 5-15 inhalations of 1:200 solution with hand nebulizer; with oxygen aerosolization, give no more than 0.3 ml. of 1:100 solution or 0.5 ml. of 1:200 solution in a 15-20 minute period. Repeat every 4 hours p.r.n. or more often in severe cases. Simultaneous use of epinephrine is contraindicated.

(2) Epinephrine inhalation, 0.5-1 ml. of a 1:100 aqueous solution by inhalation every 2-4 hours. Use cautiously in hypertensive and elderly patients.

9. Carbon dioxide and oxygen - Inhalation of a mixture of 5% carbon dioxide and 95% oxygen at a rate of 5-7 L./minute by means of a mask or nasal catheter for 10-15 minutes 3-4 times daily tends to improve depth of respiration and has some bronchodilator effect. Alternatively, pure CO_2 may be blown gently over the patient's nose and mouth while he inhales deeply. When this has stimulated 6-7 deep inhalations, the flow is discontinued. These actions make cough more effective, clear out secretions, and thus relieve chronic coughing. This regimen may be particularly useful in prevention or treatment of postoperative atelectasis.

10. Antibiotics - Pneumonitis should be treated with penicillin

or cephalothin (Keflin®) (see Chapter 6) until sputum culture and sensitivity studies are available.

11. Expectorants - These are sometimes prescribed but have little or no practical value.
12. General measures - Treat all contributory conditions, such as abdominal distention (see p. 90). Change the patient's position hourly and encourage early ambulation. Respiratory exchange and coughing are most efficient in the semi-sitting position.

D. Prophylaxis:
   1. Preoperative measures -
      a. Never perform elective surgery in the presence of an acute respiratory tract infection.
      b. Treat chronic respiratory disorders such as bronchitis, bronchiectasis, and asthma in order to reduce infection and sputum volume and to improve ventilatory capacity.
         (1) The patient should stop smoking.
         (2) Give aerosol therapy with a bronchodilator drug 4 times daily by IPPB.
         (3) Tetracycline, one specific antibiotic based on sensitivity study of sputum culture, is usually effective in reducing excessive sputum production in bronchiectasis or chronic bronchitis. Postural drainage may also be useful.
         (4) Repeated pulmonary function tests may be helpful in evaluating effectiveness of treatment.
         (5) Instruction in breathing and coughing exercises preoperatively ensures better postoperative cooperation.
   2. During operation - Expert anesthesia management is the most important feature.
   3. Postoperative measures -
      a. Postoperative orders should include instructions for turning, hyperventilating, and coughing.
      b. If chronic respiratory tract disease was present preoperatively, institute IPPB and aerosol therapy postoperatively as for established atelectasis.

Respiratory Insufficiency.

Subclinical respiratory insufficiency is common after major operations, especially thoracic or abdominal procedures, as the result of hypoventilation or accumulated secretions. Patients with chronic lung disease or general debility or who have had extensive operations are particularly susceptible. Dyspnea or cyanosis may or may not be present. Restlessness or coma may occur. Respiratory insufficiency should be suspected when conditions favor its occurrence, and measures should be taken at once to assure oxygenation, adequate ventilation, and the removal of secretions (see p. 82). When hypoxia is a possibility, administer humidified oxygen at 6-10 L./min. by nasal catheter or face mask. Depressing doses of narcotics should be avoided, but relief of severe pain is necessary if the patient is to breathe deeply and cough. Recovery from mild postoperative respiratory insufficiency is usually progressive and without incident. When response to empirical measures is inadequate or when severe pulmonary failure is imminent due to the patient's general condition, the following additional measures should be considered.

A. Diagnostic Tests: Measurement of arterial pO_2, pCO_2, and pH are of great value in establishing the nature and extent of respiratory derangement and in determining the effects of treatment. A portable chest film is usually indicated.

B. Artificial Ventilation: Continuous positive pressure breathing with either a pressure-limited (Bennett, Bird) or volume-limited (Emerson, Engstrom, Morch) machine may be life-saving. Assisted or controlled ventilation via a tracheal tube is often essential for oxygenation, CO_2 excretion, and pH control. The patient is also relieved of the work of breathing, which may be an intolerable burden in the critically ill. Tracheal intubation may be via the nose or mouth if artificial ventilation is expected to last only 4 or 5 days; for longer periods, a tracheostomy should be considered. Frequent tracheal aspiration will be required and should be done aseptically. Pulmonary sepsis is a threat. Antibiotic therapy is indicated, based on endotracheal cultures every few days. Control of the respiratory rhythm by the machine does not require a sedative or relaxant if there is slight hyperventilation.

Following cardiac operations and other procedures likely to be associated with respiratory insufficiency in the immediate postoperative period, the anesthesiologist often leaves the endotracheal tube in place. Artificial ventilation is then continued for 24-48 hours, until arterial blood gas determination shows that ventilatory assistance is no longer required.

Pneumonitis and Bronchial Pneumonia.

These pulmonary infections are usually secondary to atelectasis and respond to treatment for that condition. When they occur independently, the principal treatment is with an antibiotic drug chosen on the basis of sputum culture and sensitivity studies. After specimens have been obtained, an antibiotic may be chosen empirically until reports of these tests are available.

Pulmonary Embolism and Infarction.

This complication is so common in older, bedridden, early postpartum, or postoperative patients - especially after extensive surgery on the abdomen, pelvis, and hips - that any sudden appearance of pulmonary or cardiac symptoms in such patients should at once suggest this diagnosis. Other predisposing factors include obesity, cardiac disease, and general debility.

Pulmonary emboli occur following 0.1-0.2% of operations, but the overall incidence of pulmonary embolism is much higher and ranges from 5-15% in general autopsy series. About 80% of emboli arise from thromboses in the deep veins of the legs, and about 10% arise from the pelvic and prostatic veins. The remaining 10% arise from the right heart and are associated with cardiac failure, myocardial infarction, atrial fibrillation, cardiac myopathies, and bacterial endocarditis involving the tricuspid or pulmonic valve. Probably only about 10% of pulmonary emboli are recognized clinically; the remainder either do not produce significant symptoms or are misdiagnosed as atelectasis, pneumonitis, congestive failure, or some other cardiac or pulmonary condition.

Although the most common origin of embolism is due to thrombosis in the leg veins, embolism frequently precedes the clinical appearance of thrombophlebitis by 1-3 days. In about 40% of cases, no evidence of thrombophlebitis will ever be found. Pulmonary emboli are usually not fatal, and their transient effects may go unnoticed. It is important to realize that 85% of patients with fatal pulmonary embolism have such prior warning signs as minor emboli or symptomatic venous disease. Therefore, prompt recognition and treatment of pulmonary emboli and thrombophlebitis of the legs are essential.

A. Diagnosis: Pulmonary embolism may occur at any time in the course of a complicated illness but is most likely to occur late in the postoperative course, on the seventh to tenth postoperative day. Early diagnosis depends upon a high index of suspicion. Differential diagnosis includes myocardial infarction, acute pneumonia, atelectasis, pneumothorax, and obscure cardiac and pulmonary cause of chest pain and dyspnea.

1. Symptoms and signs - The cardinal symptom of a small pulmonary embolus is a sudden onset of pleuritic pain, occasionally associated with blood streaks in the sputum. This is due to the development of a pulmonary infarct in the periphery of the lung, accompanied by parenchymal hemorrhage and pleural inflammation. Friction rub, cough, and localized signs of pulmonary consolidation may or may not occur. Frequently, there is an associated rise in respiratory and pulse rates disproportionate to the rise in temperature.

   The manifestations of a larger embolus include various combinations of (1) sudden dyspnea, (2) precordial or substernal oppressive pain, occasionally with radiation to shoulders and neck, (3) tachycardia, (4) accentuation of pulmonic second sound with pulmonary hypertension and right heart failure, (5) hypotension or shock, (6) cyanosis, (7) anxiety, (8) restlessness, and (9) syncope or convulsions.

   If a major pulmonary artery is obstructed, sudden death may result from acute cor pulmonale. Alternatively, recurrent pulmonary embolism may be overlooked because of the absence of characteristic clinical features; it may occasionally culminate in progressive pulmonary arterial obstruction, pulmonary hypertension, and chronic cor pulmonale.

2. Laboratory findings - Moderate leukocytosis (up to 15,000 WBC) occurs in 70% of cases. Elevated bilirubin level is frequent and is related to heart failure rather than to hemorrhage in the lung. Elevated LDH and normal SGOT is seen in about one-half of patients; both enzymes are elevated in about one-fourth and are normal in the remainder.

3. Electrocardiography - Changes in the Ecg. occur in only about one-fourth of patients. Arrhythmias account for about 80% of these changes. The following abnormalities consistent with right heart strain or dilatation are usually considered to be characteristic but are seen in only about 5% of patients with proved pulmonary embolus: Standard leads show a deep S in lead I, prominent Q with inverted T in lead III, tall P in lead II (occasionally) and right axis deviation; precordial leads show inverted T waves in V_{1-4}, transient and incomplete right bundle branch block, prominent R waves over right precordium, and displacement of transitional zone to the left ("clockwise rotation").

4. Chest x-ray - Chest x-ray may show no abnormality, or changes may be delayed 24-48 hours. In about 15% of patients, pulmonary density occurs which is sometimes (but not always) in the periphery of the lung and roughly in the shape of a triangle, with its base at the lung surface. Other possible findings include enlargement of the main pulmonary artery, small pleural effusion, and elevated diaphragm. Embolism involves the lower lobes in 75% of cases, more often on the right than on the left.
5. Pulmonary scan - Scanning the lung fields for radioactivity after intravenous injection of radioiodinated, macroaggregated human albumin is a simple and valuable diagnostic procedure which characteristically reveals negative defects in the lung areas distal to pulmonary artery obstruction. This is a particularly useful screening technic when the chest x-ray reveals no lesions. The scan essentially demonstrates diminished blood flow in the lung. Change similar to that of pulmonary embolus can be produced by atelectasis, pneumonia, and neoplasm; however, the clinical picture is usually sufficiently distinct in these conditions to permit differentiation from pulmonary embolus.
6. Angiography - Pulmonary angiography should always be done before embolectomy is undertaken. It is the most reliable procedure for confirming the diagnosis and determining the location and extent of large emboli. It is performed on selected patients in whom definitive diagnosis is essential. Pressures taken in the right heart and pulmonary artery in conjunction with catheterization for angiography will aid in evaluating the degree of right heart failure secondary to pulmonary artery obstruction. Angiography should be preceded by a pulmonary scan; if the scan is negative, massive pulmonary embolus can be virtually ruled out and angiography may be avoided.
7. Blood gases - When dyspnea is present, arterial pH, pO_2, and pCO_2 are obtained to assess the degree of respiratory insufficiency and the need for oxygen or assisted respiration.

B. Treatment: For mild symptoms, anticoagulants and bed rest are usually adequate treatment. For severe symptoms indicating the occurrence of a major embolus, the following measures are to be considered:
1. Oxygen - Give oxygen in high concentration, preferably by mask, to relieve hypoxia and dyspnea. This also helps prevent cardiopulmonary failure.
2. Anticoagulants - If there is no contraindication to anticoagulation, give heparin, 10,000 units I.V. every 4 hours for 6 doses, either by continuous infusion or intermittently through an indwelling catheter. If continuous infusion is used, give an initial loading dose of 10,000 units. Beginning with the second day, regulate the continuous infusion so that the Lee-White clotting time is maintained between 30-45 minutes. For intermittent injections, the clotting time should be maintained at this level about one hour before the next dose. Heparin therapy should be continued for 7-10 days before oral anticoagulation with a coumarin drug is introduced; this should then be continued for 6 weeks to 6 months, depending upon circumstances.

Intensive heparin therapy carries a significant risk of bleeding. If this occurs, heparin in the circulation can be immediately neutralized by I.V. injection of protamine sulfate.

3. Narcotics - For severe pain, give meperidine hydrochloride (Demerol®), 50-100 mg. subcut. or I.V., or morphine sulfate, 8-15 mg. subcut. or I.V. Avoid these agents in presence of shock. Only the I.V. route should be used in the heparinized patient.
4. Vasopressors - Treat shock, if present, with metaraminol bitartrate (Aramine®), 15-100 mg., or levarterenol bitartrate (Levophed®), 2 mg. in 500 ml. of 5% dextrose solution. Adjust the rate of infusion to maintain systolic pressure at about 90 mm. Hg. Also monitor central venous pressure, Ecg., arterial blood gases, and urine output.
5. Vena cava interruption - Ligation or plication of the vena cava should be considered when pulmonary emboli occur during anticoagulant therapy or when anticoagulants are contraindicated. However, a minor episode of embolism during the first few days of heparinization does not necessarily mean failure of anticoagulant therapy. Vena cava interruption is not indicated unless there is a recurrence of major embolization or unless the emboli are septic.
6. Pulmonary embolectomy - This procedure is indicated in critically ill patients with angiographic evidence of massive embolism and with persistent hypotension in spite of appropriate supportive measures. It may also be considered for patients who have survived a massive embolus which continues to block the pulmonary artery, producing pulmonary hypertension and progressive cor pulmonale. Pulmonary embolectomy requires cardiopulmonary bypass; an experienced cardiac surgical team is essential. The operation may be lifesaving, but the mortality rate is high due to the serious condition of the patients.

C. Prophylaxis: The prophylaxis of pulmonary embolism depends upon the prevention and treatment of thrombophlebitis (see Chapter 15).

Fat Embolism.

Embolization involving fat globules may occur following extensive crushing injuries to soft tissues and bones or following extensive surgery on bone or fatty tissue. Liquid fat from ruptured fat cells is forced into the circulation, where it forms a myriad of fat globules as a result of surface tension. These globules diffusely embolize the small pulmonary capillaries. The clinical picture is variable, but pulmonary manifestations generally consist of dyspnea, tachypnea, and cyanosis; these develop suddenly on the first or second day following injury or operation. The findings are frequently suggestive of disseminated bronchopneumonia.

In addition to the pulmonary involvement, many of the fat emboli escape through pulmonary capillaries or pulmonary arteriovenous shunts into the systemic circulation, where they occlude and damage peripheral capillaries. This is most strikingly observed in the brain, skin, and kidneys and accounts for the development of additional clinical signs within 1-2 days after injury or operation.

These include (1) neurologic changes such as restlessness, delirium, twitchings, convulsions, and coma, (2) petechiae over the upper trunk and in conjunctivas and retina, and (3) the escape of fat globules through renal glomeruli into the urine, unassociated with significant impairment of renal function.

Diagnosis is usually made by finding fat globules in sputum, urine, and retinal arteries and by observing petechiae over the upper trunk and in the axillas.

Treatment is nonspecific. Administration of oxygen is beneficial if hypoxia is present. Heparin has been recommended because of its lipemia-clearing action but may be contraindicated in the presence of recent extensive soft tissue and bone injury. Most patients recover on symptomatic therapy.

DEEP THROMBOPHLEBITIS

(See Chapter 15.)

ABDOMINAL COMPLICATIONS

Acute Gastric Dilatation.

Acute gastric dilatation is caused by a reflex inhibition of the stomach. It occurs most commonly early in the postoperative period after major surgery or severe trauma.

A. Diagnosis: Repeated regurgitation of small quantities of thin, dark, brownish-green or black fluid with a foul (but not fecal) odor is characteristic. Copious vomiting is rarely seen. Several liters of fluid may accumulate in the stomach so that the patient becomes hypovolemic and hypochloremic. The appearance may be that of shock, and failure to relieve distention promptly at this stage may be fatal. Diagnosis is confirmed by observing the distended, tympanitic stomach in the epigastrium or by upright abdominal x-ray.

B. Treatment: Pass a nasogastric tube and aspirate the stomach immediately if gastric dilatation is suspected. Relief is usually dramatic. Correct electrolyte and fluid imbalance. Continue nasogastric suction and parenteral alimentation until gastric emptying resumes.

Subphrenic Abscess and Intrahepatic Abscess.

Subphrenic abscess is secondary to intra-abdominal sepsis and occurs most frequently after a perforated appendix or peptic ulcer. The right subphrenic space is the commonest site. Subphrenic abscess is a serious complication, and the mortality in various series ranges from 20 to 50%.

Intrahepatic abscess is less common. It also is usually secondary to intra-abdominal sepsis and has essentially the same clinical findings as subphrenic abscess. If amebic abscess of the liver is present, the therapy is different from that of pyogenic liver abscess. (See Chapter 12.)

A. Diagnosis: There is almost invariably a history of intra-abdominal operation or sepsis. Fever and leukocytosis of unexplained origin should arouse suspicion of a subphrenic or hepatic abscess in such a patient. Localizing symptoms and signs are usually slow to appear and may be further delayed by antibiotic therapy.

1. Symptoms and signs - Pain, tenderness, and occasionally edema of the skin develop in the lower thoracic region overlying the abscess. Pain may be referred to the top of the shoulder due to diaphragmatic irritation. There may be signs of fluid or basilar atelectasis and limitation of diaphragmatic motion on the side of the lesion. Pleural effusion may be present. The liver may be displaced downward and may appear to be enlarged. Septic fever and leukocytosis will be present. Rupture of the abscess into the pleural cavity usually results in massive pyopneumothorax with dyspnea and marked toxemia. Rupture into the bronchial tree results in a lung abscess with copious expectoration of pus.
2. X-ray findings - Diaphragmatic motion on the side of the lesion is usually limited or absent. Elevation or upward bulging of the diaphragm and a small pleural effusion are often noted. A fluid level in an abscess cavity is pathognomonic but is not always present.
3. Radioactive scintiscan - Simultaneous radioisotope scanning of the liver and lung may demonstrate a defect between the base of the lung and the dome of the liver on the right. Liver scan may delineate an intrahepatic abscess.
4. Angiography - Search for an intrahepatic abscess may be aided by a hepatic arteriogram, which, if positive, will indicate the size and location of the lesion.

B. Treatment: Surgical drainage is mandatory when a collection of pus is present. The extraperitoneal, extrapleural posterior approach with rib resection was formerly used almost exclusively for drainage of subphrenic abscess, but the anterior approach through a subcostal incision is also satisfactory and provides better exposure for anterior collections. Essentially, the approach to subphrenic abscess is dictated by anatomic location. Abscesses posterior to the right coronary ligament can be drained through the bed of the twelfth rib if low, or, if high, through the bed of the tenth or even eighth rib. Care should be taken to obliterate the costophrenic sinus in order to prevent pleural contamination. An anterior subcostal extraperitoneal or transperitoneal approach is most appropriate for subphrenic abscess anterior to the right coronary ligament or for abscess in the right lobe of the liver. Exploration of the subphrenic space on the basis of suspicion of abscess may be necessary and is justifiable to avoid the serious complications which follow diaphragmatic perforation. Broad-spectrum antibiotic therapy is employed as an adjunct and may abort the process in the early stage of subphrenic infection before abscess formation.

C. Prophylaxis: Early recognition and prompt surgical treatment of predisposing lesions, such as appendicitis and perforated peptic ulcer, and intensive antibiotic therapy of all forms of intra-abdominal sepsis have, in recent years, greatly reduced the incidence of subphrenic abscess.

Paralytic Ileus.

See p. 417.

Peritonitis.

See p. 403.

Pancreatitis.

See p. 477.

URINARY TRACT COMPLICATIONS*

Acute Postoperative Retention.

A. Etiology: Inability to void after operation is most often due to (1) reflex spasm of the sphincters, caused by pain or anxiety; (2) paralysis of the detrusor mechanism, caused by operations within the pelvis; (3) vesical neck obstruction by an enlarged prostate; and (4) narcotic or parasympatholytic drugs. The incidence of acute postoperative retention is highest following rectal, perineal, and abdominal surgery.

B. Diagnosis: Failure to pass urine postoperatively may be simply the result of inadequate fluid intake with oliguria. More rarely the cause will be acute renal failure. If the patient is unable to void in spite of an urgent desire to do so, or if his bladder is palpable above the pubis, he probably has acute retention. A deeply sedated patient may be unaware of a distended bladder postoperatively. **NOTE:** Because an overdistended bladder becomes atonic, in which case prolonged catheter drainage will probably be required, no patient should be allowed to go more than 8 hours postoperatively without an evaluation of his inability to void.

C. Treatment: Catheterization is followed by cystitis in about 20% of cases. Therefore, try simpler measures first.

1. Relieve acute pain and anxiety by a narcotic or sedative and reassurance.
2. Have the patient sit on a commode or stand to void. Warm the bed pan if one must be used.
3. Turn on a water faucet to encourage urination.
4. Give bethanechol chloride injection (Urecholine®), 2.5 mg. (1/24 gr.) subcut., followed in one-half hour by 5 mg. (1/12 gr.) subcut. if there have been no untoward side effects and spontaneous urination has not occurred. This drug should never be given in the presence of organic obstruction of the urinary or gastrointestinal tract; whenever increased peristalsis might prove harmful; or in asthma or thyrotoxicosis. Mild side effects such as abdominal cramps, flushing, and sweating occur occasionally even with small doses.
5. Catheterization - Catheterize when other measures fail and before marked bladder distention (over 500 ml.) occurs. Repeat catheterization every 8-12 hours if necessary. In some instances it will be necessary to insert a Foley catheter and leave the patient on constant bladder drainage until he is ambulatory or for a few days. Patients who are unable to void postoperatively because of an enlarged prostate may

---

*Urinary infection, see Chapter 14; acute renal failure and uremia, see p. 74.

require prostatectomy before they can regain their power to urinate spontaneously.

If urinary tract infection follows catheterization, obtain a urine culture and treat on the basis of antibiotic sensitivity studies. Continue antibiotic therapy until the catheter has been removed. If the urinary tract infection is not readily controlled after removal of the catheter, investigate for underlying urinary tract disease.

D. Prophylaxis: Examine preoperatively for prostatic hypertrophy, cystocele, and other disorders likely to cause postoperative retention. When such defects are found they should be corrected before operation if possible; otherwise the patient should be watched carefully so that overdistention of the bladder postoperatively can be prevented. Excessive use of narcotic or parasympatholytic drugs should be avoided, especially in the presence of bladder neck obstruction. A Foley catheter should be inserted preoperatively on all patients scheduled for extensive pelvic operations, and bladder drainage should be continued after surgery until the patient is fully ambulatory.

ACUTE PAROTITIS

Acute parotitis as a complication of surgery is now rare because of the declining incidence of such predisposing disorders as dental sepsis and postoperative dehydration. It is most likely to occur in a debilitated, febrile, dehydrated, elderly patient with poor oral hygiene, or in patients on diuretic therapy or anticholinergic drugs.

Swelling and tenderness appear in the parotid gland at the angle of the jaw, accompanied by trismus, systemic toxicity, tachycardia, leukocytosis, and fever sometimes rising to 104°F. (40°C.). Bilateral involvement can occur. Pus may sometimes be expressed from a swollen, inflamed Stensen's duct. Abscesses may form within the gland, but fluctuation is late because of the deep location and trapping by fibrous septa and tense capsule.

X-ray treatment is effective in aborting the process if carried out immediately after onset. Established parotitis will usually respond to penicillin, local hot packs, mouth care, and restoration of fluid balance. When abscesses develop, drainage is required; incisions must be made parallel to the facial nerve to avoid injuring it.

Preoperative correction of dental sepsis and good postoperative oral hygiene and adequate fluid intake are effective preventive measures.

COMPLICATIONS OF BLOOD COAGULATION

Mechanism of Hemostasis.

The mechanism of hemostasis is a complex process involving vasoconstriction, platelet adhesion and aggregation, initial formation of platelet plugs in small vessels, and eventual development of a fibrin clot. The coagulation system is usually activated initially by exposure of subendothelial connective tissue at the cut ends of blood vessels which provide sites to which platelets adhere. The

Numerical System for Naming Blood Clotting Factors*

Factor†	
I	Fibrinogen
II	Prothrombin
III	Thromboplastin
IV	Calcium
V	Proaccelerin, labile factor, accelerator globulin
VII	Proconvertin, SPCA, stable factor
VIII	Antihemophilic factor (AHF), antihemophilic factor A, antihemophilic globulin (AHG)
IX	Plasma thromboplastic component (PTC), Christmas factor, antihemophilic factor B
X	Stuart-Prower factor
XI	Plasma thromboplastin antecedent (PTA), antihemophilic factor C
XII	Hageman factor, glass factor
XIII	Fibrin-stabilizing factor, Laki-Lorand factor

*Reproduced, with permission, from Ganong: Review of Medical Physiology, 6th ed. Lange, 1973.

†It is no longer felt that factor VI is a separate entity, and it has been dropped from the list.

Disease States Due to Deficiency of the Various Clotting Factors*

Deficiency of Factor	Clinical Syndrome	Cause
I	Afibrinogenemia	Depletion during toxic pregnancy with premature separation of placenta; also congenital (rare)
II	Hypoprothrombinemia (hemorrhagic tendency in liver disease)	Decreased hepatic synthesis, usually secondary to vitamin K deficiency
V	Parahemophilia	Congenital
VII	Hypoconvertinemia	Congenital
VIII	Hemophilia A (classical hemophilia)	Congenital defect due to abnormal gene on X chromosome; disease is therefore inherited as x-linked characteristic
IX	Hemophilia B (Christmas disease)	Congenital
X	Stuart-Prower factor deficiency	Congenital
XI	PTA deficiency	Congenital
XII	Hageman trait	Congenital

*Reproduced, with permission, from Ganong: Review of Medical Physiology, 6th ed. Lange, 1973.

Summary of Reaction Involved in Hemostasis

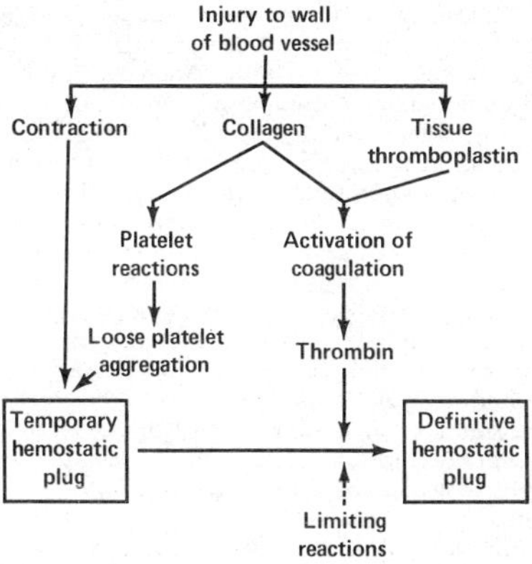

Diagrammatic Summary of the Clotting Mechanism

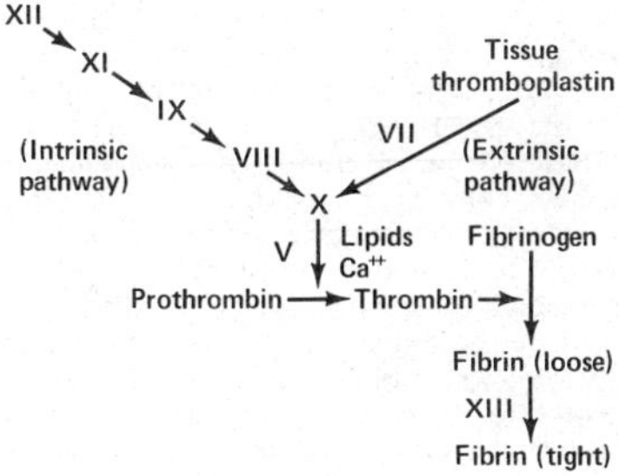

The Fibrinolytic System

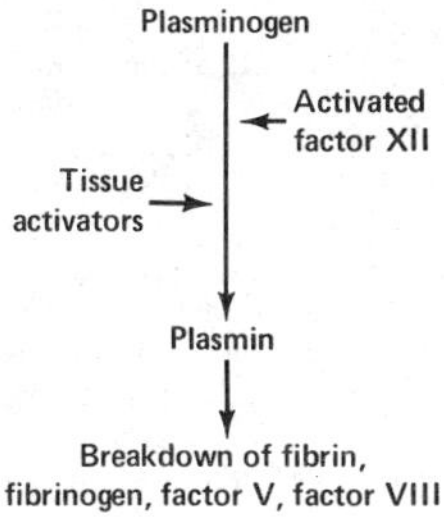

(Drawings on this page modified and reproduced, with permission, from Deykin: Thrombogenesis. New England J. Med. 276:622, 1967.)

initial stimulus for platelet adhesiveness is probably related to contact with connective tissue or collagen as a result of disruption of the vascular endothelium. Aggregating platelets release a number of compounds, including epinephrine, 5-hydroxytryptamine (serotonin), adenosine diphosphate, platelet phospholipid, and thrombosthenin (a factor promoting clot retraction). These products of platelets cause further vasoconstriction and aggregation of platelets leading to formation of platelet plugs sufficient to stop blood flow temporarily in small, constricted vessels and to provide "primary hemostasis."

Simultaneously, exposure of plasma to connective tissue activates a number of plasma enzymes or clotting factors which participate in a series of reactions culminating in the generation of complete thromboplastin, and the conversion sequentially of prothrombin to thrombin and of fibrinogen to fibrin. Fibrin strands reinforce the friable platelet aggregates and plugs to produce a resilient composite clot which provides "secondary hemostasis" of sufficient resistance to withstand arteriolar pressure when vasoconstriction relaxes (see p. 95, top).

The clotting factors in the plasma produce complete thromboplastin by 2 different pathways, designated as **intrinsic** and **extrinsic** (see p. 95, center). The intrinsic pathway operates within the vasculature to form complete thromboplastin by the interaction of factors V, VIII, IX, X, XI, and XII plus platelet phospholipid and calcium. The extrinsic pathway generates a complete thromboplastin by a combination of tissue factor (an incomplete thromboplastin), calcium, and factors V, VII, and X. Tables showing the numerical system for the clotting factors and disease states due to deficiency of various clotting factors are given on p. 94.

Complete thromboplastin from either the intrinsic or extrinsic system acts in the presence of calcium to convert prothrombin to thrombin. Thrombin then converts fibrinogen to fibrin, which is rendered insoluble by the action of factor XIII (fibrin-stabilizing factor), and the fibrin clot retracts under the influence of thrombosthenin, a factor released by platelets. Thrombin accelerates both platelet aggregation and the activation of plasma clotting factors; thus, a small amount of thrombin serves to increase the rate of the coagulation process.

Finally, initiation of coagulation leads to the activation of the **fibrinolytic system,** which is capable of dissolving fibrin clots (see p. 95, bottom). Circulating plasminogen is a plasma globulin which may be converted to **plasmin,** an active fibrinolysin, by a variety of tissue activators. This conversion usually occurs within the fibrin clot, since potent inhibitors of plasmin and plasminogen activator are normally present in the plasma. Activation of plasminogen to plasmin is a normal feature of hemostasis and is a natural defense against pathologic deposition of fibrin. However, fibrinolysis may also occur rarely as a pathologic process resulting in severe bleeding. Under these circumstances, plasmin not only dissolves fibrin clots but also digests fibrinogen and other clotting factors such as V and VIII. The breakdown products of fibrin and fibrinogen are powerful anticoagulants which block the polymerization of fibrin and impede the aggregation of platelets. The net effect of this sequence of events is a marked hemorrhagic diathesis.

Diagnosis of Bleeding and Coagulation Disorders.

Bleeding and coagulation disorders are usually discovered because of (1) a history of abnormal bleeding or a predisposing condition, such as liver disease; or (2) the unexpected occurrence of excessive hemorrhage at operation or after trauma. It is essential in surgical practice to recognize the presence or the possibility of a clotting defect before surgical intervention so that diagnostic and corrective measures can be carried out. Inadequate hemostasis is the commonest cause of postoperative bleeding. Rule out this possibility before assuming that a hemorrhagic disorder is present.

A. Screening Measures: The most important clues to the existence of a clotting disorder are found in the history. Bleeding due to a congenital deficiency of clotting factor will frequently, but not invariably, occur spontaneously into such deep tissues as joints, muscles, and viscera. Hematomas, hemarthroses, or large ecchymoses at the site of trauma suggest hemophilia. Onset of bleeding problems in adult life does not rule out a congenital clotting factor defect. Vascular and platelet abnormalities usually present with spontaneous bleeding from wounds or with hemorrhage into the skin and mucous membranes rather than deep tissues. Purpuric spots suggest a capillary or platelet defect; they are not typical of hemophilia. Every patient should be questioned preoperatively regarding the following conditions, any of which may be associated with a coagulation dyscrasia:
   1. Personal or family history of abnormal bleeding, bruising, or purpura.
   2. Unusual hemorrhage in connection with operation or dental extraction.
   3. Liver disease.
   4. Ingestion of drugs capable of depressing prothrombin, e.g., salicylates and intestinal antiseptics (neomycin, succinylsulfathiazole, etc.).

B. Laboratory Studies: Routine bleeding and clotting times are of little value in detecting occult clotting defects and are not recommended. Preoperative assessment of the number of circulating platelets by examination of a stained blood smear is a simple and useful procedure. A platelet count is not necessary for this gross evaluation. When a coagulation disorder is suspected, chief reliance should be placed on the patient's history and on thorough laboratory investigation. Consultation with a hematologist is desirable in suspicious cases to assist in selection and interpretation of appropriate laboratory tests; these may include bleeding time, clotting time, platelet count, prothrombin time, partial thromboplastin time (PTT), thrombin time and measurement of fibrinogen, fibrinolysis, and circulating anticoagulants. All clinically important bleeding disorders, except factor XIII deficiency, will be disclosed by one or more of these tests. Some screening tests useful in the evaluation of acute bleeding are listed in the table on p. 98. Additional and more specialized clotting studies may be required to identify the specific deficiency involved.

Conditions Associated With Abnormal Bleeding.

A. Congenital Defects: The major clinical syndromes due to congenital clotting factor deficiency are listed in the table on p. 94.

Screening Tests in Acute Bleeding

Condition	Platelet Count	Prothrombin Time	Thrombin Time	Fibrinogen	Fibrinolysis
Congenital clotting factor deficiency	Normal	Normal	Normal	Normal	Normal
Disseminated intravascular coagulation	Low	Increased	Increased	Low	Absent or present
Primary fibrinolysis	Normal	Normal or increased	Normal or increased	Normal or low	Present
Massive transfusion (dilution)	Low	Normal or increased	Normal	Normal	Absent
Heparin effect	Normal	Normal or increased	Increased	Normal	Normal

Definitive diagnosis is made by a combination of the above laboratory tests with special additional studies as required. Clinical manifestations of these disorders are variable. Since clotting factors act to reinforce the initial platelet plugs, the absence of these factors may result in the dissolution of the plugs, with delayed bleeding hours or days after operation or trauma.

Surgery in the presence of a serious coagulation deficiency (e.g., hemophilia) can be hazardous and complicated. The deficient clotting factor should be identified in advance whenever possible and replaced before, during, and after surgery. Planning of therapy in cooperation with a hematology consultant is essential. In emergency situations, when the exact nature of the deficiency is unknown, treatment is by fresh whole blood or plasma or by fresh frozen plasma. Stored plasma is deficient in factors V and VIII. In known classical hemophiliacs (factor VIII deficiency), concentrated factor VIII in the form of cryoprecipitate or glycine-precipitated preparation is used.

Congenital abnormalities of the platelets are rare in comparison with acquired platelet disorders (see p. 99). Thrombasthenia (Glanzmann's disease) is an autosomal recessive defect in which the platelet count is normal. Bleeding time is prolonged, clot retraction is absent or decreased, and platelets do not aggregate with ADP, epinephrine, or other agents. Plasma coagulation is normal but platelet clumping is completely absent. Primary familial platelet–ADP release dysfunction is a milder disorder than thrombasthenia, but symptoms are similar. These uncommon conditions may be associated with easy bruising, skin purpura after minor trauma, dependent petechiae, and mucocutaneous bleeding; some patients have abnormal bleeding after surgery. In severe forms the bleeding time is prolonged, but in mild cases the diagnosis can only be made by specialized tests of platelet function. Unexplained, slight bleeding tendency may be due to a mild form of congenital platelet disorder. All of these patients should avoid the use of aspirin. Treatment is by transfusion of fresh, viable platelets.

B. Acquired Deficiencies:

1. Anticoagulant effects of drugs - Heparin and derivatives of coumarin (oral anticoagulants) result in decreased clotting. Heparin inhibits coagulation by preventing the interaction of thrombin with fibrinogen and by impairing the activation of factor IX. The clotting time is prolonged. Heparin is destroyed in the stomach, must be given parenterally, and is neutralized by protamine, 1 mg. for each 100 units of heparin (approximately). Oral anticoagulants inhibit the synthesis of vitamin K-dependent clotting factors (factors VII, IX, X, and prothrombin [factor II]) by the liver. The prothrombin time is prolonged and, if liver function is not impaired, is reversible by vitamin K. The anticoagulant effects of heparin and coumarin derivatives should be evaluated by appropriate tests and controlled before operation.

   A number of drugs may cause a bleeding tendency by inhibiting the "release reaction" and the aggregation of platelets. Aspirin is most frequently involved. One gram a day will produce an effect lasting 4-6 days. As a result, the drug is now occasionally used therapeutically as an anticoagulant. Aspirin is a possible cause of unexplained diffuse wound bleeding. Agents with a similar effect on platelets include antihistamines, indomethicin, phenylbutazone, chlorpromazine, and many tranquilizers.

2. Thrombocytopenia - Decreased number and function of platelets may be caused by many conditions, including idiopathic thrombocytopenic purpura (autoimmunization), leukemia, marrow metastases, lupus erythematosus, cytotoxic agents (cancer chemotherapy), and allergy to such drugs as quinidine, thiazides, sulfonamides, etc. The danger of a hemorrhagic complication is related to the level of the platelet count. Undue bleeding at operation is unlikely if the platelet count exceeds 60,000-100,000/cu. mm. Platelet counts less than 20,000-30,000/cu.mm. may be associated with spontaneous bleeding, and intracranial hemorrhage is a major hazard when the platelet count is less than 10,000/cu. mm. Bleeding due to thrombocytopenia, or elective surgery on a thrombocytopenic patient (platelet count less than 100,000/ cu. mm.), is an indication for transfusion of fresh, viable platelets. Compatibility tests are not necessary but platelets from a donor of the same blood type as the patient (or from a type O donor in emergency) may be given. Platelet concentrates are available in 30 ml. volumes and contain three-fourths of the platelets found in a unit of fresh blood. Two units of platelet concentrate will raise the platelet count by approximately 15,000/cu. mm. one hour after infusion in an average-sized adult; 8 units are usually considered the minimum effective dose. In idiopathic thrombocytopenic purpura, platelets are generally administered during operation just after removal of the spleen.

3. Functional platelet defects - Dextran with an average molecular weight of 70,000 - and, to a lesser extent, dextran with

an average molecular weight of 40,000 - may cause a functional platelet defect with prolonged bleeding time and clinically significant bleeding tendency in patients who receive more than 1.5 Gm./Kg. Uremia may cause a qualitative defect in platelet function and the danger of hemorrhage is roughly correlated with the degree of azotemia. Dialysis and transplantation have been observed to reverse the defect.

4. Massive transfusions - Bank blood is deficient in platelets and in plasma factors V and VIII because of the lability of these components. Deficient clotting factors are normally replaced rapidly from body stores, but platelets decrease during massive transfusion of stored blood. Rapid transfusions of 8-10 pints may drop the platelet count to less than 100,000/cu. mm., and a rapidly transfused volume of 7-8 liters is likely to cause a significant prolongation of bleeding time and a tendency to increased bleeding. Deficiency of factors V and VIII and dilutional thrombocytopenia can be minimized by giving one unit of fresh blood for each 4-5 units of stored blood. Fresh frozen plasma (which contains factors V and VIII) and platelet concentrates can also be administered if circumstances warrant.

5. Coagulopathy in hepatic and biliary disease - All clotting factors whose source is known are synthesized in the liver. In the presence of portal hypertension and splenomegaly, thrombocytopenia due to hypersplenism may develop. Failure of a damaged liver to remove activators of plasminogen may result in fibrinolysis while the breakdown products of fibrinolysis act as anticoagulants and serve to impair platelet aggregation. Thus, liver failure due to cirrhosis, infectious hepatitis, drug toxicity, or other causes tends to produce a complicated coagulation defect. The treatment of choice is probably fresh frozen plasma or a concentrated preparation of vitamin K-dependent clotting factors (factors II, VII, IX, X) such as Konyne®. There is the risk of hepatitis with either plasma or the concentrate. Platelet concentrates may have a transient effect on thrombocytopenia.

   Vitamin K, which is required for synthesis of factors II, VII, IX, and X, is a fat-soluble vitamin. It is ingested in the diet and is produced by intestinal bacteria. Biliary tract obstruction, biliary fistula, and sterilization of the intestinal tract by broad-spectrum antibiotics result in deficiency of clotting factors as indicated by prolonged prothrombin time (decreased plasma concentration of prothrombin). Bleeding tendency can be expected when the plasma concentration of prothrombin drops below 20% of normal. Administer vitamin K preoperatively and restore prothrombin to an approximately normal level. When liver function is poor, there may be little or no response to vitamin K. For vitamin K preparations and dosage, see Appendix.

6. Disseminated intravascular coagulation - Disseminated intravascular coagulation (DIC), also termed consumption coagulopathy, is a bleeding disorder characterized by (1) diffuse bleeding from wounds, skin, and mucous membranes, (2) poor, small clot, (3) reduced platelets on smear and count, and (4) low concentrations of fibrinogen, prothrombin,

and factors V and VIII. The decreased clotting components are only those consumed in the process of coagulation. DIC is most frequently precipitated by certain obstetric complications (e.g., abruptio placentae, retained dead fetus, amniotic fluid embolism, septic abortion), some types of surgery (e.g., pulmonary, brain, or prostate surgery; open-heart operations on cardiopulmonary bypass), shock, infections (e.g., gram-negative sepsis, meningococcemia, malaria), malignant diseases (e.g., carcinomatosis), hemolytic anemia, snake bite, drug therapy (e.g., ristocetin), and a number of other conditions, including blood dyscrasias. DIC is presumably caused by the entrance into the blood stream of materials which induce widespread intravascular coagulation and platelet aggregation.

The combination of diffuse bleeding from many sites at surgery and from needle punctures - associated with a poor, small clot, reduced platelets on smear, and a prolonged prothrombin time - is very suggestive of DIC. The diagnosis depends essentially upon demonstration of a deficiency of labile clotting factors and of platelets. Platelet counts usually vary from 30,000-120,000/cu.mm. Prothrombin (PT) is usually less than 40% and may be less than 10%. Screening tests for fibrinogen usually indicate values of less than 100 mg./100 ml. (normal: 200-600 Gm./ml.). The activated partial thromboplastin time (PTT) is prolonged to as much as 100 seconds (normal: < 47 seconds). The bleeding time is usually prolonged when platelets are below 70,000/cu. mm. Factors V and VIII are markedly decreased. The fibrinolytic system is often active in DIC, making differentiation from primary fibrinolysis difficult. Low platelet count and very low level of fibrinogen are the most useful features in distinguishing DIC from primary fibrinolysis, which is a much rarer condition requiring very different management (see below).

Treat the underlying disorder (e.g., shock, sepsis) if possible. Heparin may stop the pathologic clotting and thus block the consumption of hemostatic elements. In adults, the usual dose of heparin is 100 U.S.P. units/Kg. every 4-6 hours I.V.; in children, the dosage is 50 units/Kg. every 4 hours after an initial dose of 100 units/Kg. If the diagnosis of DIC is correct and therapy is effective, fibrinogen levels, PT, and PTT should rise within 24 hours, and platelet count within a few days. Whole blood may be necessary to combat shock. Human fibrinogen in doses of 4-6 Gm. may be given I.V. if fibrinogen deficiency is severe but there is considerable risk of hepatitis. Platelet concentrates may be used in marked thrombocytopenia.

7. Primary fibrinolysis - When excessive fibrinolysis occurs, it is usually in association with disseminated intravascular clotting. Some authorities believe that hyperfibrinolysis can exist as an isolated phenomenon. It has been reported following cardiac resuscitation and in severe postprostatectomy bleeding. In primary fibrinolysis, circulating plasmin should be demonstrable by clot lysis time, euglobin lysis time, or fibrin plate. Plasmin, produced by the activation of plasmino-

gen, leads to the dissolution of fibrin clots and digests fibrin, fibrinogen, and other clotting factors (see p. 95, bottom). The breakdown of fibrin and fibrinogen produces polypeptides with anticoagulant activity which block the polymerization of fibrin and the aggregation of platelets. This sequence of events may result in a severe hemorrhagic diathesis.

If fibrinolysis can be identified as the primary cause of bleeding, and if DIC is considered to be highly unlikely on the basis of laboratory findings (including normal platelet count and fibrinogen level), it may be justified to treat with an antifibrinolytic agent such as aminocaproic acid (Amicar®, EACA). The suggested oral and intravenous dose is 5 Gm. initially followed by 1.25 Gm./hour. This agent is a synthetic compound related to lysine. It acts as a competitive antagonist to activators of plasminogen and thus prevents the generation of plasmin. Primary fibrinolysis is doubtless extremely rare. The usual situation is one in which fibrinolysis and DIC are both present and cannot be differentiated. Under these circumstances, the patient should be treated first with heparin; then, if hyperfibrinolysis is found to contribute to continued hemorrhage, it may be advisable to use EACA.

Emergency Treatment of Abnormal Bleeding.

Abnormal bleeding at operation or in the postoperative period is a rare but potentially dangerous complication. Among the most frequent of the causes which must be considered are liver disease (hypoprothrombinemia), hemolytic transfusion reaction, massive transfusion of citrated blood or dextran, fibrinogen-fibrinolysin disorders (disseminated intravascular coagulation), and hemophilia. Always rule out inadequate hemostasis.

A. Diagnosis: Establish the diagnosis at once, if possible, so that specific treatment may be given. Obtain blood for coagulation studies (see p. 95, bottom). An immediate report should be available on hematocrit, CBC, platelet count, coagulation time, bleeding time, and prothrombin time. When transfusions have been given, verify the accuracy of the cross-match if in doubt. Emergency consultation with a hematologist is advisable in all obscure cases.

B. Treatment: Specific diagnosis often cannot be made promptly. If bleeding is serious, it is then necessary to try one or more of the following measures empirically:

1. Fresh blood or plasma - Administer 500 ml. or more of blood or plasma drawn within 6 hours in siliconized or plastic containers. Blood processed in this manner contains platelets. There are no platelets in plasma unless it has been specially prepared as "platelet-rich" plasma. Fresh plasma (or blood) provides prothrombin, fibrinogen, antihemophilic globulin, factor V, and other factors which may be deficient in the patient's own blood.
2. Platelets - Thrombocytopenia below 60,000-100,000/cu. mm. may be associated with continued bleeding. Give 8 units of platelet concentrate and repeat platelet count after one hour.

3. Vitamin K - If prothrombin time is long, give phytonadione (vitamin K_1, Mephyton®), 50-100 mg. (3/4-1½ gr.) I.V. slowly (no faster than 10 mg./minute). This agent is of specific value in hypoprothrombinemia.
4. Corticosteroids - If the platelet count is low or if a drug reaction is suspected, give hydrocortisone sodium succinate (Solu-Cortef®), 100 mg. I.V.
5. Calcium - Depletion of calcium as a result of massive transfusion of citrated blood is a very unlikely cause of abnormal bleeding. If hypocalcemia is suspected, administer 1 Gm. (15 gr.) of calcium chloride or calcium gluconate (10 ml. of 10% solution) I.V. slowly after every 2000 ml. of blood.
6. Fibrinogen - Prompt intensive therapy may be necessary in fibrinogen-fibrinolysin disorders. These are conditions which may occur in carcinomatosis, in a variety of acute stress conditions, and in complications of pregnancy. When fibrinolysis is the cause of bleeding, the patient's clot will usually lyse completely within a few hours at 98.6° F. (37° C.). Fibrinogen (human; Parenogen®) is specific treatment for hypofibrinogenemia, but the risk of hepatitis is considerable. Give a 1-2% solution in water for injection I.V., the dosage depending upon initial fibrinogen level and the response of the patient. Two to 6 Gm. may be needed. If fibrinogen is not available, use fresh plasma or whole blood.
7. Antihemophilic concentrate is specific therapy for bleeding due to hemophilia.

NONSPECIFIC SYMPTOMS

FEVER

Reduction of Fever by Nonspecific Means.

Of primary importance in the control of fever is the removal of the primary cause whenever possible. In general, body temperature above 105° F. (40.6° C.) rectally persisting more than a few hours should be reduced by nonspecific methods if fever is the chief cause of distress or is associated with cerebral symptoms and if it can be reduced without complications.

A. Surface Applications:
   1. Ice or cold water - Cold sponges or baths and the application of ice caps produce surface cooling and make the patient more comfortable. Ice water enemas may occasionally be useful when surface cooling fails.
   2. Alcohol, 70% - Sponging of the trunk and extremities results in cooling by evaporation of the alcohol.
   3. The refrigerated blanket is the most effective means of maintaining temperature at normal or subnormal level for prolonged periods.

B. Antipyretic Drugs: (See Appendix.) These drugs have both an antipyretic and an analgesic effect. They act on the heat-regulating mechanism of the CNS to cause a greater dissipation of body heat through cutaneous vasodilatation. They may obscure the clinical picture or cause undesirable side-effects, especially diaphoresis, nausea and vomiting, or, less commonly, skin eruptions, hematologic changes, and cardiovascular depression.

NAUSEA AND VOMITING

Relief of nausea and vomiting is essential to the patient's comfort and to the prevention of fluid imbalance. The underlying cause should be treated promptly if possible. A wide variety of drugs, including morphine, may produce nausea and vomiting as a side effect. Symptomatic measures include bed rest, withholding of oral intake, and administration of an antiemetic or sedative drug. If gastric retention or dilatation is suspected, aspiration by nasogastric tube is indicated.

HICCUP (SINGULTUS)

Although hiccup is usually self-limited (disappearing within a few minutes to an hour), it can be sufficiently persistent and exhausting to endanger life in a debilitated patient. It may be produced by any condition which irritates the afferent or efferent phrenic nerve pathways. The etiology is therefore quite varied: CNS, cardiopulmonary, or gastrointestinal disorders, renal failure, infectious diseases, etc. Treatment should be directed at the cause when possible, but therapy must frequently be symptomatic.

Treatment.

A. General Measures: Breath-holding, drinking a large glass of water, or gastric lavage with a warm 1% solution of sodium bicarbonate may be effective. Rebreathing into a paper bag or administration of 10-15% CO_2 by face mask induces hyperventilation and may interrupt the reflex. Inhalation of amyl nitrite from a broken ampul will occasionally terminate the attack after a few breaths. Tranquilizing drugs such as chlorpromazine hydrochloride (Thorazine®) or other phenothiazine preparation are worthy of trial in prolonged hiccup. Barbiturate sedation may also be tried.

B. Surgical Measures: Phrenic nerve interruption by procaine block or by crushing may be considered when hiccup is intractable and life-threatening in spite of conservative measures. Only one leaf of the diaphragm may be affected and this should be checked by fluoroscopy.

CONSTIPATION

Constipation is a common postoperative complaint. Resumption of normal bowel habits is encouraged by early ambulation, bathroom privileges, discontinuance of narcotics, and normal oral intake.

Treatment.

A. Laxatives: A mild laxative (e.g., liquid petrolatum, milk of magnesia, methylcellulose, or dioctyl sodium sulfosuccinate) is frequently helpful in the postoperative period but should usually be withheld until peristalsis has returned and oral intake begun. Contraindications to laxatives include peritoneal or bowel inflammation, paralytic ileus, and mechanical intestinal obstruction.

B. Enemas: Enemas should be used only as temporary measures to combat induced constipation and fecal impaction; to cleanse the bowel for diagnostic studies and surgery; and to aid in the restoration of normal bowel habits.
   1. Warm tap water (nonirritating), 500-1500 ml. (1-3 pints). Contraindicated in congenital megacolon because of the danger of excessive water absorption. Use a saline enema instead.
   2. Saline enema (nonirritating), 500-1500 ml. (1-3 pints) of warm physiologic saline.
   3. Soapsuds (S.S.) enema (irritating), 500-1500 ml. White toilet soap is stirred into warm tap water until it is opalescent.
   4. Hypertonic phosphate enema (irritating) consists of saturated solution of sodium phosphate. Commercially available disposable enema kits containing 4-5 oz. of this solution are very convenient (Travad® Enema, Clyserol®, and Fleet® Enema).
   5. Oil Retention Enema: 180 ml. of mineral oil or, preferably, cottonseed oil is introduced to soften impacted feces or in the management of acutely painful rectal lesions. Overnight retention of the oil followed by an S.S. or hypertonic phosphate enema in the morning is often advantageous.

C. Fecal Impaction: When severe constipation or scanty, intermittent diarrhea develops in a bedridden or sedentary patient, fecal impaction should be suspected and a rectal examination performed. Elderly and debilitated patients and those taking narcotics are most susceptible. Fecal impaction is prevented by the judicious use of anticonstipation measures, including laxatives and enemas. Treatment consists of an oil retention enema followed by a cleansing enema. Manual removal of the impaction is frequently necessary.

DECUBITUS ULCER
(Pressure Sore; Bedsore)

Decubitus ulcers are caused by sustained pressure on the skin, usually over bony prominences such as the sacrum, ischium, trochanter, and heel. They occur quite commonly in bedridden patients who are weak, aged, malnourished, or paralyzed and who are receiving poor nursing care. Soiling of the bed by incontinence of stools or urine frequently leads to skin irritation. Unrelieved pressure of only a few hours may be sufficient to produce a decubitus ulcer in a susceptible individual. Decubiti characteristically begin as a small area of redness and tenderness which soon breaks down to form an indolent ulcer unless protected from further pressure. In neglected cases, large defects in skin and soft tissues may result from the combined effects of pressure, infection, and poor healing power. Osteomyelitis of underlying bone may occur.

Treatment.

A. General Measures: Relieve pressure by frequent change of position and protection of the involved area, if necessary, by pillows, pads, and rubber rings. Bed clothing and skin must be kept clean and dry. Correction of malnutrition and anemia and control of infection are often essential to healing.

B. Local Measures: Decubitus ulcers should be kept clean, well-drained, debrided, and either exposed or covered with dry sterile dressings. Topical applications have little value. Invasive local infection is treated by drainage, saline compresses, and systemic antibiotics as indicated.

C. Surgical Treatment: Surgical treatment in large, resistant lesions consists of complete debridement, including removal of any bony prominences or sequestra, and closure of the wound by a local rotation flap. This will provide an adequate pad over the bone and avoids suture lines over the critical area of pressure. The donor area may frequently be closed by direct approximation, but a split-skin graft may be required.

Prophylaxis.

The most important elements in prevention are good nursing care, early mobilization, and good nutrition. Bedridden patients should be inspected frequently for areas of skin damage which might progress to ulceration. Prevent soiling by incontinence. An alternating pressure or foam rubber mattress is useful. Special washable spongy pads under pressure points are protective.

3...

Anesthesia

Anesthetic agents and technics are usually employed to facilitate surgical procedures. In the form of "nerve blocks" they may also be used for diagnostic and therapeutic purposes.

The conduct of a safe anesthetic procedure begins with the preoperative visit to the patient's bedside and ends after the patient has completely recovered from the anesthetic and any postanesthetic complications.

Anesthetic management thus includes: (1) Evaluation and preparation of the patient; (2) familiarity with the action of the drugs to be used; (3) ability to use the recommended technics; (4) ability to administer supportive measures as necessary, e.g., maintenance of adequate pulmonary ventilation; and (4) care of the patient in the postanesthetic period.

EVALUATION OF THE PATIENT

Except in emergencies, patients should be examined by the anesthetist on the day before the proposed procedure. A thorough review of the history, physical examination, and laboratory findings is essential to ensure proper preparation of the patient, to aid in the selection of the agent and type of anesthetic procedure, to anticipate complications, and to suggest postanesthetic care.

History.

In taking the preanesthetic history special emphasis should be placed on the cardiorespiratory system. Question the patient about the following:

A. History of Previous Anesthesia: Agents and methods which have caused difficulties or complications can be avoided or safeguards taken.

B. History of Drugs Used by the Patient: The following groups are of importance.

1. CNS depressants - Barbiturates, opiates, and alcohol may alter a patient's tolerance to anesthetic drugs.
2. "Tranquilizing drugs" - Preoperative use of these drugs reduces the required dosage of general anesthetics. The 3 important groups are as follows:
   a. Dicarbamates (meprobamate, etc.) - These have little effect on the conduct of anesthesia.
   b. Rauwolfia derivatives (reserpine, etc.) - Prolonged use of these drugs may lead to epinephrine depletion, but this does not occur with the usual clinical doses.
   c. Phenothiazine derivatives (chlorpromazine, etc.) - Use of these drugs predisposes to hypotension during anesthesia.

3. Corticosteroids - Prolonged use of cortisone (even though discontinued 1 month or more prior to anesthesia) leads to hypofunction of the adrenal cortex, which impairs the physiologic responses to the stress of anesthesia and surgery. Such a patient should receive cortisone immediately before, during, and after surgery.
4. Any drugs which may have to be continued during anesthesia or which may have a bearing on prognosis and complications (e.g., insulin, nitroglycerin, digitalis).

C. History of Allergies: Asthma and drug sensitivities play an important role in the choice of agents used.

D. Presence of Food in Stomach: Note the interval since food was last taken. Pain and anxiety may delay the emptying time of the stomach. Regurgitation and aspiration are frequent and serious complications of general anesthesia.

Physical Examination.

The preanesthetic physical examination should be complete; special emphasis should be placed on the following:

A. Mental and emotional status.

B. Cardiac status (e.g., decompensation, cyanosis, edema).

C. Status of the respiratory system, with particular reference to (1) obstruction of the airway; (2) conditions which may lead to obstruction of the airway (foreign bodies, such as dentures); and (3) other disorders which may hinder gas exchange, such as pneumothorax, emphysema, poliomyelitis, and abdominal distention.

D. Physical deformities or abnormalities which complicate or contraindicate specific technics. For example, the patient should be examined for spinal or sacral deformities if spinal or caudal anesthesia is contemplated, and ankylosis and other mandibular and oral pathology may render tracheal intubation difficult.

Special Studies.

The minimum preanesthetic laboratory evaluation of a patient scheduled for surgical anesthesia should include a complete urinalysis and Hgb. or Hct. Individual cases may require chest x-rays, blood volume and serum electrolyte determinations, arterial blood gas values, electrocardiograms, and other laboratory tests aimed at the diagnosis or evaluation of disorders which must be treated before anesthesia can proceed safely.

PREPARATION OF THE PATIENT FOR ANESTHESIA

Medical Preparation.

The patient scheduled for surgical anesthesia should be in the best physical condition possible within the limits of medical treatment and the urgency of the surgery. The following conditions must be treated prior to anesthesia in all except extreme emergencies: (1) shock, (2) anemia, (3) hypovolemia, (4) electrolyte imbalance, (5) cardiac decompensation, (6) diabetic acidosis, and (7) acute inflammation of the respiratory system.

The stomach must be allowed to empty itself or must be emptied by gastric tube or induced vomiting.

Patency of the airway must be assured. Tracheostomy made necessary by severe upper respiratory obstruction should be performed under local anesthesia; general anesthesia must not be induced until the tracheostomy has been done.

Psychologic Preparation.

The anesthetist must gain the patient's confidence and make every effort to allay his fears. A personal relationship should be established. The calm, reassured patient is more easily anesthetized.

Pharmacologic Preparation.

The patient should arrive at the operating room in a drowsy but cooperative state and with minimal respiratory depression.

A. Purposes of Preanesthetic Medication: To ensure a good night's rest before surgery, to diminish fear and anxiety and to produce a mild euphoria, to decrease metabolism and anesthetic requirements, to produce amnesia, to decrease secretions in the mouth and respiratory tract, to decrease autonomic reflexes (e.g., cardiac irregularities), to counteract toxic manifestations of local anesthetics, and to minimize postanesthetic nausea and vomiting.

B. Drugs Used for Preanesthetic Medication: (The tables below and on p. 110 list the commonly used preanesthetic drugs and their recommended dosages.)

Common Drugs and Average Doses of Drugs for Premedication (Adults)*

Drug	Dosage	Route and Time
Barbiturates		
Pentobarbital (Nembutal®)	50-200 mg. (3/4-3 gr.)	Give orally 1 1/2-2 hours before induction; or I. M. 30 minutes before induction; or I. V. 15 minutes before induction.
Secobarbital (Seconal®)	50-200 mg. (3/4-3 gr.)	
Amobarbital (Amytal®)	50-200 mg. (3/4-3 gr.)	
Narcotics		
Morphine sulfate	5-15 mg. (1/12-1/4 gr.)	Give subcut. 1 hour before induction; or I.M. 45 minutes before induction; or I.V. 15 minutes before induction.
Meperidine (Demerol®)	50-150 mg. (3/4-2 1/2 gr.)	
Alphaprodine (Nisentil®)	30-60 mg. (1/2-1 gr.)	
Belladonna Alkaloids		
Atropine	0.2-0.6 mg. (1/300-1/100 gr.)	Give subcut. with the narcotic before induction.
Scopolamine	0.2-0.6 mg. (1/300-1/100 gr.)	

*Dosage of barbiturates and narcotics should be reduced when premedication includes tranquilizers.

PEDIATRIC PREMEDICATION* / COMPARABLE DOSES OF NARCOTICS

Age	Average Weight (lb.)	Pentobarbital (Nembutal®) or Secobarbital (Seconal®) mg. (gr.)	Atropine or Scopolamine mg. (gr.)	Morphine mg. (gr.)	Meperidine (Demerol®) mg. (gr.)	Alphaprodine (Nisentil®) mg. (gr.)
Newborn	7	-	0.1 (1/600)	-	-	-
6 months	16	30 (1/2)	0.2 (1/300)	-	-	-
1 year	21	50 (3/4)	0.2 (1/300)	1 (1/60)	10 (1/6)	4 (1/15)
2 years	27	60 (1)	0.3 (1/200)	1.5 (1/40)	20 (1/3)	8 (1/8)
4 years	35	90 (1 1/2)	0.3 (1/200)	3 (1/20)	30 (1/2)	12 (1/5)
6 years	45	100 (1 1/2)	0.4 (1/150)	4 (1/15)	40 (2/3)	15 (1/4)
8 years	55	120 (2)	0.4 (1/150)	5 (1/12)	50 (3/4)	20 (1/3)
10 years	65	150 (2 1/2)	0.4 (1/150)	6 (1/10)	60 (1)	25 (3/8)
12 years	85	150 (2 1/2)	0.6 (1/100)	8 (1/8)	80 (1 1/4)	30 (1/2)

The above dosage scale is for well developed patients of average weight. Reductions must be made for underweight or poorly developed patients. No barbiturate is given to patients under 6 months of age; no narcotic to patients under 1 year of age. Barbiturates are given rectally at least 90 minutes before operation. Dissolve barbiturate in 10 ml. of water and inject rectally. Morphine and atropine are given subcut. 45 minutes before operation.

*Modified and reproduced, with permission, from R.M. Smith, Anesthesia for Infants and Children. Mosby, 1959.

1. Barbiturates - For general sedation, relief of anxiety, hypnosis, and for protection against local anesthetic reactions.
2. Narcotics - For analgesia, euphoria, and general sedation.
3. Belladonna derivatives (scopolamine, atropine) for drying secretions and other vagolytic effects. Scopolamine also produces sedation and amnesia.
4. Tranquilizers - Major tranquilizers such as chlorpromazine or other phenothiazines may be used. They produce drowsiness, are antiemetic, and their vascular effects facilitate hypotension and hypothermia. Chlorpromazine (Thorazine®) may be given orally (25-50 mg.) or I. M. (25 mg.) in place of or in addition to a barbiturate or other sedative. Promethazine (Phenergan®) or promazine (Sparine®) may also be used in the same dosages. Innovar® - a combination of a narcotic (fentanyl) and a tranquilizer (droperidol) - can be a useful premedication for balanced anesthesia.

C. Individualization of Drugs and Dosages:
1. Age - Infants and children can be premedicated according to the table on p. 110. The very aged require little or no premedication.
2. Physical and mental condition - These may increase or greatly diminish the suggested doses.
3. Anesthetic agent - See the table below for examples.

Selection of Premedication for Various Anesthetic Agents*

Anesthetic Agent	Barbiturates	Narcotic	Atropine or Scopolamine
Ether	++	+	+++
Cyclopropane	++	+	++
Thiopental with N_2O	++	+++	++
Halothane	++	+	++
Fluroxene	++	+	+++
Methoxyflurane	++	+	++
Regional Anesthesia			
Low dosage (subarachnoid)	++	++	+
Large dosage (epidural, nerve block, infiltration, etc.)	+++	++	+

+ None or reduced dosage. ++ Desirable. +++ Indicated.
*For selection of drugs in infants and children, see p. 110.

FACTORS INFLUENCING THE SELECTION OF ANESTHETIC AGENTS AND TECHNICS

All of the factors outlined below must be taken into consideration in deciding what type of anesthesia will be used. With few exceptions (e.g., inability to use ether in open chest surgery with cautery), no single factor excludes the consideration of the others.

Patient Factors.

A. Patient's preferences and prejudices.
B. Patient's condition.

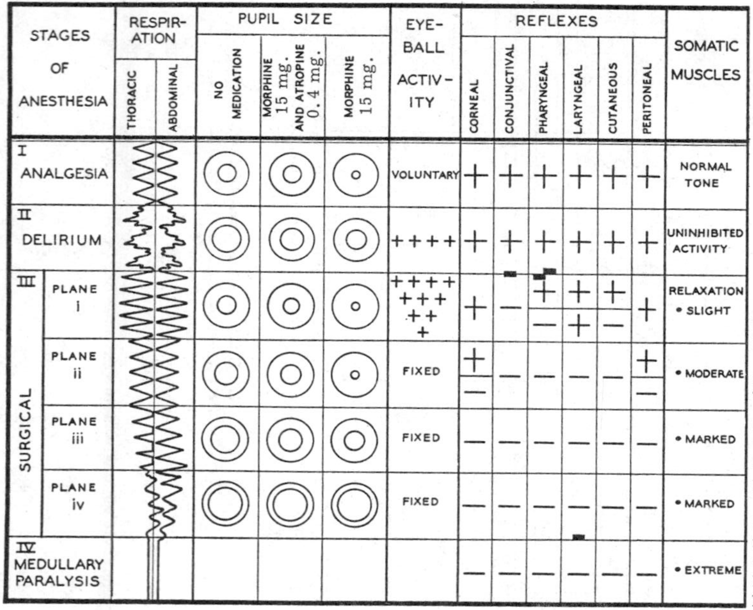
STAGES OF ANESTHESIA
RESPIRATION
THORACIC
ABDOMINAL
PUPIL SIZE
NO MEDICATION
MORPHINE 15 mg. AND ATROPINE 0.4 mg.
MORPHINE 15 mg.
EYEBALL ACTIVITY
REFLEXES
CORNEAL
CONJUNCTIVAL
PHARYNGEAL
LARYNGEAL
CUTANEOUS
PERITONEAL
SOMATIC MUSCLES
I ANALGESIA
II DELIRIUM
III SURGICAL
PLANE i
PLANE ii
PLANE iii
PLANE iv
IV MEDULLARY PARALYSIS
VOLUNTARY
FIXED
FIXED
FIXED
NORMAL TONE
UNINHIBITED ACTIVITY
RELAXATION
• SLIGHT
• MODERATE
• MARKED
• MARKED
• EXTREME

STAGES AND PLANES OF ANESTHESIA

The 4 small black rectangles represent zones, as follows:

1. Conjunctival column - Disappearance and reappearance of lid reflex.
2. Pharyngeal column - Appearance of swallowing (upper border of plane i) and of vomiting (lower border of Stage II).
3. Laryngeal column - Disappearance of carinal reflex.

The large plus and minus signs refer to the presence or absence of the indicated reflex.

Respiration Column:

Thoracic and abdominal inspiration is shown moving away from the mid-line; expiration, toward the mid-line. Regularity, rate, and depth are shown for each stage and plane, in comparison with the normal.

(Modified and reproduced, with permission, from Goodman and Gilman, The Pharmacological Basis of Therapeutics, 2nd Ed., Macmillan, 1955, as modified from Guedel, Inhalation Anesthesia, Macmillan, 1951.)

Surgical Requirements.

A. Speed and skill of the surgeon; individual skill and experience of the anesthetist with the agents and equipment at his disposal.
B. Site of surgery and position of patient.
C. Use of electrocautery.
D. Need for muscle relaxation.
E. Open chest.

TYPES OF GENERAL ANESTHESIA

General anesthesia is a state of drug-induced CNS depression characterized by (1) analgesia and amnesia, (2) unconsciousness, and (3) loss of reflexes and muscle tone. Drugs producing this state must cause no permanent tissue change; must be reversible in action by excretion or destruction; and must have minimal side-effects on other tissues.

Different methods of administration all serve the same purpose, i.e., to introduce the agent into the blood stream for transport to the CNS. The route of administration (inhalation, gastrointestinal absorption, or injection into veins or tissues) depends upon the physical properties of the agent.

Inhalation Anesthesia. (See table on pp. 114-115.)

Inhalation anesthesia is used to administer gases (cyclopropane, nitrous oxide, and ethylene) and volatile liquids (ethers, chloroform, trichloroethylene, halothane, ethyl chloride).

A. Technics:
   1. Open drop - This is the simplest and oldest method and requires the least equipment. A volatile liquid (ethers, chloroform) is administered drop by drop onto the gauze or cloth covering of a wire frame mask applied over the mouth and nose. The inhaled concentration is controlled by the rate of drip. Induction is accomplished with a slow rate of drip, and the rate is increased to the patient's tolerance. When the desired depth of anesthesia is reached, the rate of administration is slowed to stabilize the physical signs of that depth.
   2. Insufflation - This method consists of blowing anesthetic vapors or gases into the mouth, pharynx, or trachea. Some type of apparatus or anesthesia machine is required for metering gas flows and vaporizing volatile agents. Insufflation has its greatest usefulness in operations for which a mask cannot be used (e.g., tonsillectomy).
   3. Nonrebreathing - As the term indicates, nonrebreathing anesthesia supplies a continuous fresh quantity of anesthetic agent with adequate oxygen through an apparatus which evacuates each exhalation to the atmosphere. Leigh valves and Ayre's T pieces are examples of these apparatus.
   4. Partial and total rebreathing - These methods require anesthesia machines and are named according to the amount of exhalation the patient is required to rebreathe. A means of absorbing the exhaled CO_2 must be provided in all instances except where the rebreathing is minimal.

INHALATION AGENTS USED FOR GENERAL ANESTHESIA

	Diethyl Ether $(C_2H_5)_2O$	Chloroform $CHCl_3$	(Divinyl Ether (Vinethene®) $(C_2H_3)_2O$	Methoxyflurane (Penthrane®) $CHCl_2CF_2OCH_3$	Trichloroethylene (Trimar®) C_2HCl_3
Concentration in Inspired Mixture For:					
Analgesia	<1%	0.25-0.75%	0.2%		0.5-1.5%
Anesthesia	3.5-4.5%	0.75-1.65%	2-4%	0.2-0.8%	5-7.5%
Respiratory Arrest	6.7-8%	2%	10-12%		
Use With Soda Lime	Yes.	Yes.	Yes.	Yes.	**Dangerous.**
Depth and Use	Any depth required for surgery.	Rarely used. Light anesthesia.	Light anesthesia for short procedures.	Light to moderate anesthesia.	Analgesia only.
Cardiac Effects: Arrhythmias	Occasional.	Frequent.	Occasional.	Sinus bradycardia.	Frequent
Myocardium	Depressed.	Markedly depressed.	Depressed.	Depressed; hypotension.	Depressed.
Use with epinephrine or norepinephrine	Yes.	**Dangerous.**	Yes.	Heart sensitized to pressor amines.	**Dangerous.**
Respiratory Effects					
Irritating to respiratory passages	Yes.	Not in recommended concentrations.	Yes.	No.	No.
Secretions	Increased.	Slightly increased.	Increased.	Not increased.	Slightly increased.
Respiration	Stimulated, then depressed.	Depressed. Circulation may fail before respiration.	Stimulated, then depressed.	Depressed.	Tachypnea with increasing depth.
Liver Toxicity	Depression of function.	Marked.	Prolonged anesthesia causes central necrosis. Less toxic than chloroform.	None reported.	Yes.
Renal Toxicity				Nephrotoxic.	
Muscle Relaxation	Excellent.	Excellent.	Not used for relaxation.	Good.	Poor.
Explosive	Yes.	No.	Yes.	No.	Not in anesthetic concentrations.
Recovery	Slow. Nausea and vomiting frequent.	More rapid than ether. Nausea and vomiting common.	Rapid. Nausea and vomiting uncommon.	Slow. Nausea and vomiting less than ether.	Rapid. Nausea and vomiting less than with ether.

	Halothane (Fluothane®) $CF_3CHBrCl$	Nitrous Oxide* N_2O	Ethylene* C_2H_4	Cyclopropane C_3H_6	Fluroxene (Fluoromar®) $CF_3-CH_2-O-CH=CH_2$
Concentration in Inspired Mixture For:					
Analgesia	< 0.5%	20-40%	20-25%	3-5%	1.5-2%
Anesthesia	0.4-1.6%	85-90%	80-90%	5-23%	2.4-7%
Respiratory Arrest				23-40%	
Use with Soda Lime	Yes.	Yes.	Yes.	Yes.	Yes.
Depth and Use	Light to moderate depth anesthesia.	1st plane anesthesia.	1st plane anesthesia.	Moderate depth.	Light to moderate depth.
Cardiac Effects					
Arrhythmias	Infrequent; bradycardia.	Rare.	Rare.	Frequent.	Infrequent; bradycardia.
Myocardium	Depressed; hypotension.	Slight depression.	Slight depression.	Moderate depression.	Slight to moderate depression.
Use with epinephrine or norepinephrine	Heart sensitized to pressor amines.	Yes.	Yes.	**Dangerous.** May produce ventricular fibrillation.	Yes.
Respiratory Effects					
Irritating to respiratory passages	No.	No.	No.	Nonirritating with < 50%.	Slight.
Secretions	Not increased.	Not increased.	Not increased.	Minimal.	Slight.
Respiration	Depressed; tachypnea.	Normal.	Normal.	Depressed.	Tachypnea with increasing depth.
Liver Toxicity	†Hepatoxic?	No.	No effect.	Not significantly depressed.	None specific.
Muscle Relaxation	Good.	No relaxation.	Poor.	Good.	Fair.
Explosive	No.	No, but supports combustion.	Yes.	Yes.	Flammable above 4%.
Recovery	Moderately rapid. Nausea and vomiting infrequent.	Rapid. Nausea and vomiting uncommon.	Rapid. Nausea and vomiting less than with ether.	Rapid. Nausea and vomiting frequent.	Rapid. Nausea and vomiting moderately frequent.

*Should not be administered with less than 20% oxygen. The real danger in their use is from hypoxia and not from the gases themselves.
†Not clearly established whether this effect is due to sensitization or direct toxicity.

B. Anesthesia Machines: Anesthesia machines make possible:
  1. The use of anesthetic gases and oxygen supplied in compressed form in tanks.
  2. Accurate metering of these gases.
  3. The vaporization of volatile liquids.
  4. The absorption of CO_2.
  5. The conservation of expensive agents.
  6. Artificial respiration (by using the reservoir bag as a bellows for inflation of the lungs).

Intravenous Anesthesia.

A. Commonly Used Agents:
  1. Barbiturates - Thiopental (Pentothal®) or thiamylal (Surital®) is administered slowly in 2.5% solution until loss of consciousness occurs. Dosage is limited by respiratory depression. Increments may be added as needed.
  2. Narcotics.

B. Advantages: Ease of administration with a rapid and pleasant induction.

C. Disadvantages: Lack of control after administration. The duration of action depends upon the destruction or renal excretion of the agent.

Rectal Anesthesia.

A. Commonly Used Agents: Barbiturates, tribromoethanol (Avertin®).

B. Advantages: Ease of administration with pleasant induction when the intravenous approach is impractical (children, obese patients).

C. Disadvantages: Same as for intravenous anesthesia; in addition, the rate of absorption is slow and the amount of anesthetic which can be absorbed in this way is difficult to predict.

Balanced Anesthesia.

In balanced anesthesia several agents are administered by 1 or more of the above methods. Each agent is used for its most desirable properties, and none is given in toxic amounts. By variations in the dose of different agents the anesthetic is made to suit the surgical requirement. A typical example is the combination of (1) an intravenous barbiturate for induction, (2) nitrous oxide by inhalation for maintenance of light anesthesia, (3) supplementation of nitrous oxide with an intravenous narcotic or potent inhalation agent (e.g., halothane), and (4) muscle relaxants to diminish or abolish muscle tone.

Dissociative Anesthesia.

Ketamine (Ketaject®, Ketalar®), a nonbarbiturate general anesthetic administered either intravenously or intramuscularly, rapidly produces somatic analgesia and anesthesia without respiratory depression or loss of motor tone. The patient appears to be in a catatonic trance. Circulation is well maintained, and blood pressure may be elevated. The duration of action is brief (5-15 minutes). Repeated injections may be administered. This agent is useful when inhalation or the intravenous route is not easily available (e.g., severe burn cases) and when respiratory depression might be particularly hazardous. Unpleasant postanesthetic hallucinations are the principal disadvantage.

Muscle Relaxants.

Curare and allied drugs are discussed in the Appendix. These agents act peripherally at the myoneural junction to diminish or abolish the action of the skeletal muscle. In sufficient doses they paralyze all voluntary muscles, including those of respiration. **Caution:** Succinylcholine administered intravenously to infants may produce bradycardia and sinus arrest. Curare and allied drugs must never be used unless the means for effective artificial respiration (preferably with oxygen) are available. Following the administration of these agents, the patient must be observed until the return of muscular strength demonstrates a reserve well beyond the minimum requirements for ventilation and maintenance of the airway.

MANAGEMENT OF GENERAL ANESTHESIA

Regulation of Depth of Anesthesia.

By ''depth of anesthesia'' is meant the degree of depression produced by the anesthetic agent. Increasing doses of anesthetic agents progressively depress physiologic functions such as respiration, cardiac action, muscle tone, and reflexes. Changes in these functions are the signs of anesthesia. Different agents depress these functions in a different order and to different degrees. For example, at the same level of respiratory depression, the muscle relaxant and circulatory effects of ether, chloroform, cyclopropane, and halothane are very different. The clinical signs at various stages and planes of ether anesthesia were classically described by Guedel (see p. 112). All of these signs are useful in monitoring a patient's response to any agent, but there significance in determining the depth of anesthesia will vary with the agent. By observing these signs one strives to provide satisfactory surgical conditions with minimal depression of those functions which are vital.

Care of the Unconscious Patient.

The nervous system depression produced during anesthesia permits painless surgery but deprives the patient of important protective reflexes and homeostatic responses which maintain the efficiency of the cardiorespiratory functions. The anesthetist must correct or compensate for these undesirable effects. The most serious are those which interfere with the adequate oxygen supply to the tissues, i.e., hypoxia. Prevention of hypoxia during anesthesia is the most important task of the anesthetist.

Hypoxia During Anesthesia.

Hypoxia during anesthesia may be due to inadequate pulmonary ventilation (with reference to its volume, its inspired oxygen tension, and its distribution) or to circulatory deficiencies. The diagnosis should be established by arterial blood gas determinations.

A. Inadequate Pulmonary Ventilation:
   1. Signs -
      a. Early - Cyanosis and tachycardia.
      b. Late - Bradycardia, failing circulation, dilated pupils, and cardiac arrest.

2. Etiology -
   a. Insufficient oxygen tension in the inspired gases.
   b. Insufficient total pulmonary ventilation due to (1) central depression by narcotics or anesthetics; (2) weakness or paralysis of respiratory muscles caused by muscle relaxants or deep anesthesia; or (3) obstruction of the air passages.
   c. Maldistribution of the inspired gases due to obstruction of selected air passages, or due to atelectasis which may involve a lung, a lobe, or be patchy. This permits some venous blood to shunt through the lung.

      Note: Obstruction is the most frequent of all causes of hypoxia during general anesthesia. It is detected by noticing the signs of obstruction: (1) noisy respiration; (2) increased muscular effort during inspiration; (3) indrawing of the soft tissues of the thorax, such as the suprasternal notch, the supraclavicular fossae, and the intercostal spaces; and (4) a diminished gas movement for the effort involved. The volume can be assessed by observation of the rebreathing bag of the anesthesia machine or by listening with the ear close to the patient's mouth.

      Obstruction of the airway may occur anywhere along the tract from the nose and lips to the pleurae (pneumothorax). Any narrowing or occlusion of the air passages or impediments to expansion of the lungs constitutes a form of obstruction. Hundreds of causes have been reported, including foreign bodies, inflammatory disorders, and neoplasms. The 3 most common causes of obstruction are as follows:

      (1) Relaxation of the mandibular and lingual muscles, so that the tongue blocks the pharynx.
      (2) Laryngospasm - This consists of the reflex closure of the glottis when stimulated during light anesthesia. Thiopental, which does not suppress the laryngeal reflex, predisposes to a severe and obstinate type of laryngospasm.
      (3) Vomitus in the throat or trachea.
3. Treatment -
   a. Low inspired oxygen tension - Increase oxygen concentration.
   b. Respiratory depression - Lighten anesthesia and assist respirations.
   c. Muscle weakness or paralysis - Assist or control respirations until muscle power returns.
   d. Obstruction of respiratory passages -
      (1) Relaxation of mandibular and lingual muscles - This is treated by pulling the mandible forward, inserting an oropharyngeal airway, or both. The airway must reach behind the tongue and not push the tongue farther back.
      (2) Laryngospasm - Removal of the stimulus, deepening the anesthetic level if possible, or the use of some form of positive pressure to assist respiration, may relieve the spasm. Succinylcholine, 10-20 mg. (1/6-1/3 gr.) I.V. or I.M., may be resorted to if other methods fail.

(3) Vomiting - This is best treated prophylactically by emptying the stomach before general anesthesia. Aspirated vomitus must be suctioned out. Bronchoscopy is sometimes necessary. Cortisone therapy may be of value.

(4) Tracheal intubation (see below) must be resorted to if treatment by the above measures is not successful.

B. Circulatory Deficiencies:

1. Signs - Falling BP, weak pulse, ashen gray color, altered central venous pressure (normal: 4-14 cm. H_2O).
2. Etiology -
   a. Diminished cardiac output brought on by -
      (1) Myocardial depression by diseased myocardium, arrhythmias, anesthetic drugs (e.g., halothane) or by hypoxia. Suggested by rising central venous pressure.
      (2) Poor venous return caused by incorrect posture, loss of peripheral venous tone, increased intrathoracic pressure, manipulation of major vessels during surgery, etc.
   b. Diminished circulating blood volume relative to capacity of vascular bed (e.g., hemorrhage, peripheral vasodilatation). Central venous pressure low.
   c. Diminished peripheral arteriolar resistance, most often caused by the depressant actions of many anesthetic drugs on the sympathetic nervous system.
3. Treatment -
   a. Reduction in depth of anesthesia. Be certain that oxygenation is adequate.
   b. Replacement of blood volume.
   c. Change of position (Trendelenburg) to aid venous return.
   d. Vasopressor drugs - Ephedrine or other vasopressor drugs should be used as adjuncts to other methods of treatment as indicated.
   e. Digitalis for myocardial failure. Lidocaine for reduction of cardiac irritability.

Tracheal Intubation.

Obstruction of the upper respiratory passages may best be treated or prevented by inserting an endotracheal tube. This is done by visualizing the larynx with a laryngoscope and inserting the tube into the trachea. Muscle relaxant drugs or deep anesthesia may be used to facilitate nontraumatic intubation. The tube should not reach the carina (teeth to carina in adults is 24-26 cm.), and must be narrow enough to enter the glottis with ease.

Intubation is indicated (1) in upper respiratory obstruction, (2) to remove the anesthetic mask from the vicinity of the surgical field, (3) to facilitate controlled respiration (e.g., open chest operations), and (4) prophylactically, when emergency intubation would be difficult during surgery (e.g., when the face-down position is necessary).

REGIONAL ANESTHESIA
(Local Anesthesia)

Regional anesthesia is used to render a selected part of the body insensitive to pain and, if necessary, incapable of muscular

DRUGS USED FOR LOCAL ANESTHESIA

	Cocaine	Procaine (Neocaine®, Novocaine®)	Tetracaine (Pontocaine®)	Lidocaine (Xylocaine®)	Dibucaine (Nupercaine®)	Mepivacaine (Carbocaine®)
Potency*	3	1	10	1.5-2	15	1.5-2
Toxicity*	4	1	10	1-1.5	10-15	1-1.5
Stability	Cannot be autoclaved	Stable	Stable	Stable	Stable	Stable
Recommended Concentration for Anesthesia:						
Caudal-epidural	Do not use	2%	0.2%	1.2-2%	Not commonly used	1-2%
Nerve blocks	Do not use	1-2%	0.1-0.2%	1-2%	Not commonly used	1-2%
Infiltration	Do not use	0.25-0.5%	0.05-0.1%	0.5%	Not commonly used	0.5%
Topical						
Eye	2-10%	Not effective	0.5%	0.5%	0.1%	Not established; probably same as lidocaine
Nose and throat	4-10%	Not effective	2%	4%	0.5-2%	
Urethra	Absorption rapid	Not effective	Too toxic	4%	0.05-0.2%	
Onset of Action	Immediate	5-15 minutes	10-20 minutes	5-10 minutes	8-15 minutes	5-20 minutes
Duration of Action	30-60 minutes	45-60 minutes	1 1/2-3 hours	1-2 hours	2-3 hours	1 1/4-3 hours
Total Maximum Dose†	100-200 mg.	1 Gm.	50-100 mg.	500 mg.	35 mg.	500 mg.
Spinal Anesthesia:						
Recommended Conc.	Do not use	3-5%	0.3-0.5%	Not commonly used	0.06%‡ / 0.25%§	Not commonly used
Dose Range		50-200 mg.	5-20 mg.		4-13 mg.‡ / 2.5-7.5 mg.§	
Onset of Action		3-5 minutes	5-10 minutes		7-15 minutes	
Duration of Action		45-60 minutes	1 1/2-2 hours		2 1/2-3 hours	

*Potency and toxicity relative to procaine = 1.

†Maximum dose administered at one time.

‡Hypobaric.

§Hyperbaric.

1. Duration of anesthesia can be prolonged by using epinephrine or phenylephrine (Neo-Synephrine®).
   (a) For epidural and nerve blocks, use epinephrine with resultant concentration of 1:200,000.
   (b) For spinal anesthesia use epinephrine, 0.1-0.3 mg., or phenylephrine (Neo-Synephrine®), 2-4 mg.
2. AUTOCLAVE all drugs used for epidural or spinal anesthesia. DO NOT COLD STERILIZE.
3. Solutions for spinal anesthesia are made hyperbaric by using 10% dextrose as the diluent.

action; the patient retains consciousness. Regional anesthesia is achieved by blocking the conduction of nerve impulses from and to a well-defined area. The interruption of the nerve impulses may be done anywhere along the length of the peripheral nerves from their motor or sensory endings to their entry into the CNS in the spinal canal or skull.

Agents Used in Regional Anesthesia.

Drugs used for regional anesthesia must have a limited duration of action and must not cause permanent damage to the nerves blocked or to other tissues. Their therapeutic dose must be well below the toxic dose.

The table on p. 120 lists the local anesthetic drugs commonly employed together with their uses, individual properties, dosages, and toxic amounts.

Toxic Manifestations of Local Anesthetics.

Local tissue toxicity is rare.

Systemic reactions are more common than local reactions and may affect the CNS or the cardiovascular system, or may be of an allergic nature. Reactions occur when toxic concentrations are absorbed from the site of topical application or injection. The factors which favor such concentrations are (1) accidental intravascular injections and (2) rate of absorption. Rate of absorption is increased by large total dose or by vascularity at the site of injection (reduced by the addition of epinephrine to the anesthetic).

A. CNS Reactions: Twitches and tremors, first seen about the mouth and eyes, progress to convulsions which so impair the coordination of respiratory efforts that severe hypoxia ensues. The prognosis depends upon the severity and duration of hypoxia and the physical condition of the patient. Varying degrees of permanent brain damage may occur, or the patient may die in convulsions.

   The hypoxia caused by convulsions is prevented or corrected by adequate pulmonary ventilation, preferably with oxygen. Intravenous barbiturates, by their central effect, or intravenous muscle relaxants, by their peripheral effect, may be used to control convulsions. Oxygenation is more important and takes precedence. **Caution:** Small doses (100 mg. of thiopental, pentobarbital, or amobarbital) are adequate and more should not be given; large doses may synergize with postconvulsive depression and lead to severe central respiratory depression.

B. Cardiovascular Reactions: Tachycardia, palpitation, and anxiety are more likely to be caused by the epinephrine which is added to the local anesthetic.

   Anaphylactic shock (see p. 30) is a rare complication of regional anesthesia and requires vigorous antishock measures. The sudden cardiovascular collapse with absent BP and pulse and ashy pallor may require cardiac massage (see Cardiac Arrest, p. 10).

C. Allergic manifestations in susceptible individuals include the usual variety of skin manifestations and bronchospasm. Treatment is with epinephrine or antihistamines.

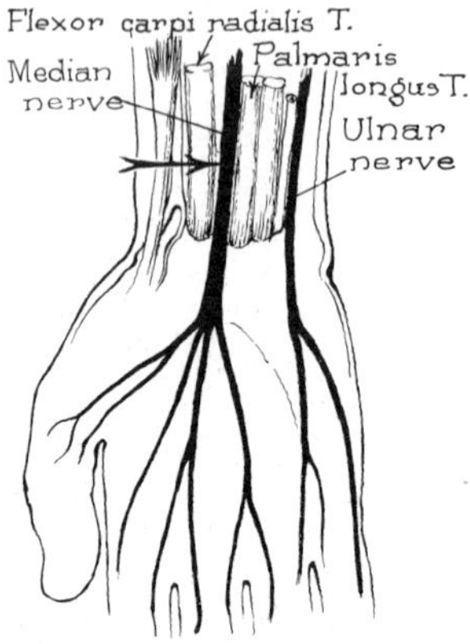

Median Nerve Block at Wrist

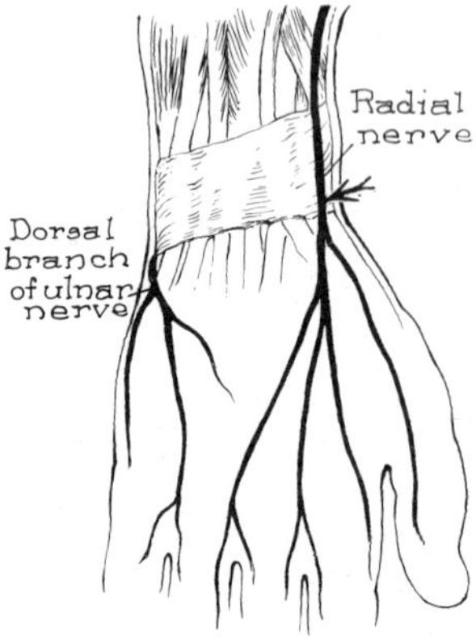

Radial Nerve Block at Wrist

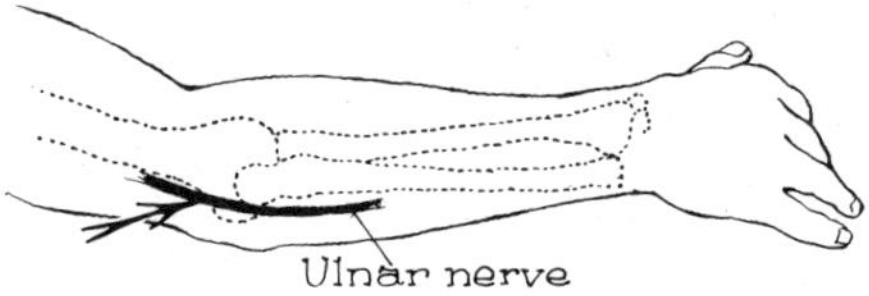

Ulnar Nerve Block at Elbow

Brachial Plexus Block in Axilla

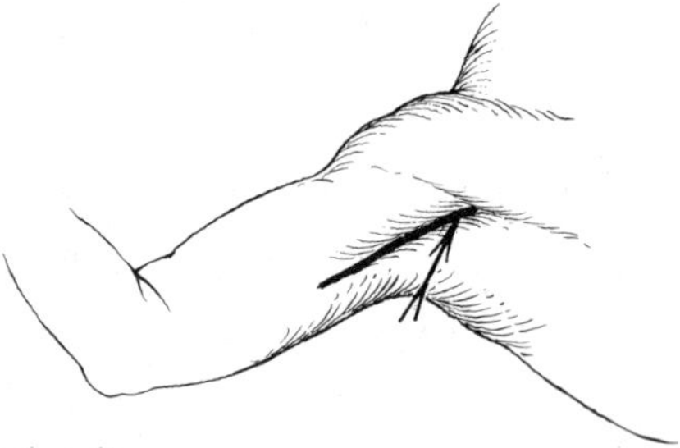

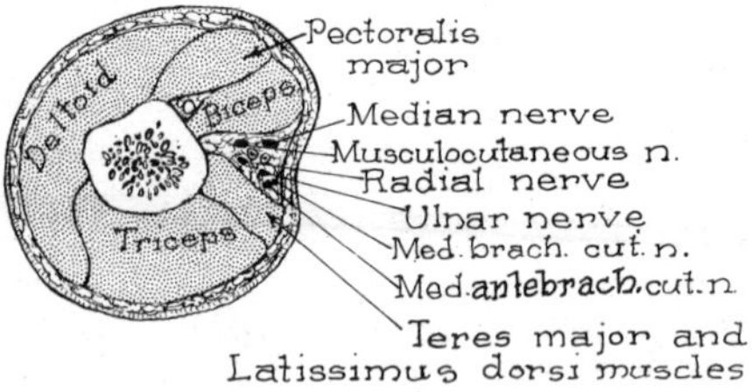

Cross-section of Arm at Level of Brachial Plexus

(Heavy arrows show point of injection of anesthetic agent.)

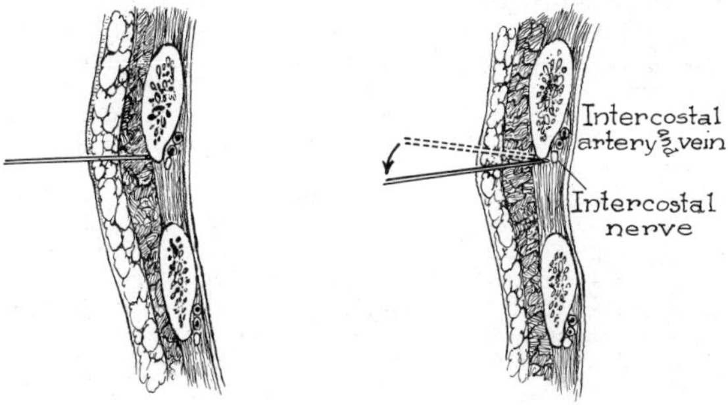

Intercostal Nerve Block. Left: Needle locating lower edge of rib. Right: Needle under edge of rib for injection of anesthetic agent.

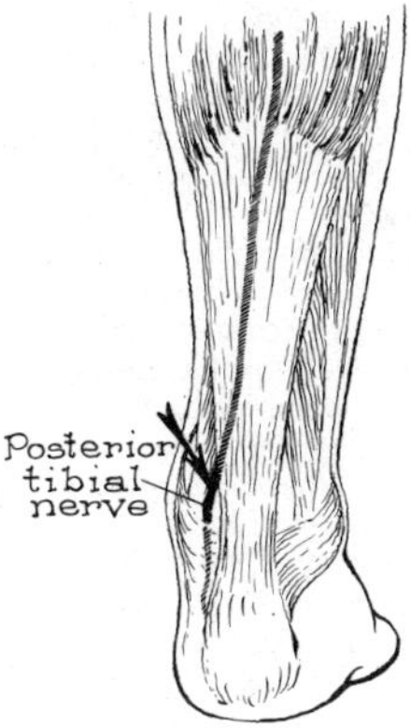

Posterior Tibial Nerve Block at Ankle

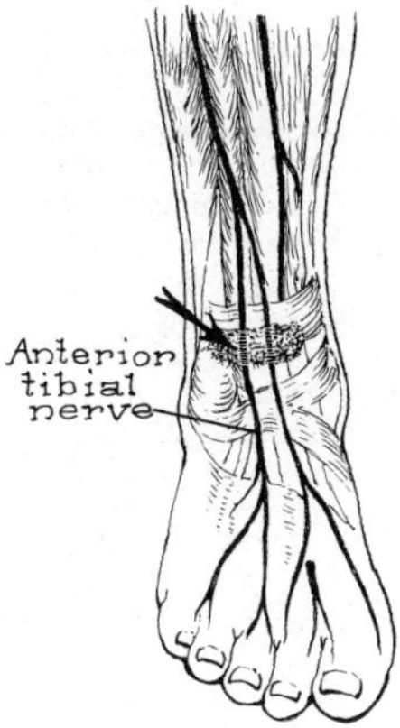

Anterior Tibial Nerve Block at Ankle

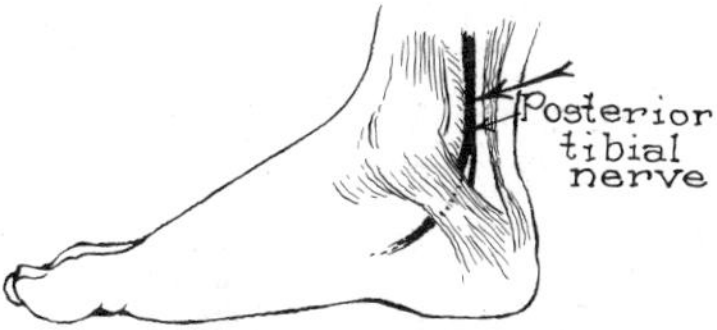

Posterior Tibial Nerve Block at Ankle. Side view.

(Heavy arrows show point of injection of anesthetic agent.)

Technics of Regional Anesthesia.

Surgical asepsis must be maintained. Do not inject into an infected area. Always aspirate before injecting to avoid intravascular injection.

A. Topical: Application of readily absorbed local anesthetic agents (cocaine, tetracaine) on mucous surfaces. Examples:
   1. Eye - 2-10% cocaine.
   2. Pharynx and trachea for bronchoscopy - 4% cocaine, 1-2% tetracaine (Pontocaine®), or 2-4% lidocaine (Xylocaine®).
   3. Urethral for cystoscopy - Females: Cocaine, 10%, on cotton swab. Males: Lidocaine (Xylocaine®), 1%, 10 ml.

B. Infiltration: Injection of local anesthetic into tissues, e.g., into the fracture site for Colles' fracture, around a laceration to be sutured, around donor areas before taking skin grafts, etc.

C. Field Block: Injection of local anesthetic into tissues surrounding the area to be made insensitive without infiltrating the area itself, e.g., for excision of sebaceous cysts or lipomas and for herniorrhaphies.

D. Nerve Blocks: Injection of anesthetic agent to permeate nerves at some point proximal to the area to be anesthetized. Almost every peripheral nerve in the body may be blocked if the anatomy of the region is known. In many cases, eliciting paresthesia with the injecting needle helps locate the nerve to be blocked. The illustrations on pp. 122-123 show some common nerve blocks useful in outpatient practice.

E. Intravenous Block: Fifty to 100 ml of 0.5% lidocaine may be injected into the vein of a limb drained of blood by an elastic bandage and kept avascular by a pneumatic cuff inflated to a pressure above systolic. Complete anesthesia of the limb is achieved below the cuff and lasts until the cuff is deflated. Reactions to the lidocaine may occur on deflation of the cuff.

F. Spinal Anesthesia: In spinal anesthesia the spinal nerves are blocked between their emergence from the cord and their exit from the spinal canal through the intervertebral foramens. This may be done in the subarachnoid space by injecting a local anesthetic agent into the CSF or into the epidural space at any level of the vertebral column, including the sacral hiatus. The table on p. 120 gives the doses of drugs used for spinal anesthesia.
   1. Types of spinal anesthesia -
      a. Subarachnoid spinal anesthesia - Sterile technic is used; ampuls must be autoclaved, not kept in alcohol or other disinfectants. With the patient in either the lateral decubitus or sitting position, lumbar puncture is done at any level between the second and fifth lumbar vertebrae. When a free flow of CSF is obtained, the anesthetic is injected into the subarachnoid space. This blocks all spinal nerves below the site of injection as well as those above the site of injection which are reached by the anesthetic solution in its upward spread. This upward spread can be controlled by limiting the volume and concentration of the injection and by judicious use of posture and the curves of the spinal canal to "float" or "sink" an anesthetic solution which is heavier (hyperbaric) or lighter (hypobaric) than the CSF. Dilution by the CSF also limits

the effective spread. After 20 minutes the solution is "fixed" and further spread is unlikely.

A "high spinal" (reaching the upper thoracic nerves) is obtained by injecting a large volume of a hypobaric solution with the patient sitting or with a hyperbaric solution with the patient placed in 5-10° degrees of Trendelenburg.

Duration of subarachnoid spinal anesthesia depends upon the agent selected:

Procaine	-	30-75 minutes
Tetracaine (Pontocaine®)	-	1-2 hours
Dibucaine (Nupercaine®)	-	2-3 hours

Increased dosages increase the duration of anesthesia only slightly. The addition of 0.2-0.4 ml. of 1:1000 epinephrine or 3 mg. of phenylephrine (Neo-Synephrine®) increases the duration of anesthetic effect 30-50%.

b. Epidural spinal anesthesia - A needle is introduced into the epidural space, either in the lumbar area or into the sacral canal, through the sacral hiatus. In the lumbar area the space is recognized by advancing the needle in the same manner as for a lumbar puncture, but stopping when resistance to injection is no longer felt even though no CSF can be aspirated. A test dose of local anesthetic sufficient to achieve subarachnoid spinal anesthesia (e.g., 5 ml. of 1% lidocaine) but insufficient for epidural anesthesia proves in 5 minutes that the subarachnoid space has not been entered. The anesthetic dose is then given either by single injection or through a plastic catheter advanced through the needle for continuous epidural anesthesia. (**Caution:** Catheters should never be withdrawn through the needle for fear of cutting the catheter in the spinal canal.)

The concentrations used and the rates of onset of the block are the same as in peripheral blocks of large nerves. Lidocaine (Xylocaine®), 1-2%, tetracaine (Pontocaine®), 0.1-0.2%, or mepivacaine (Carbocaine®), 1-2%, may be used. Since the epidural space extends from the foramen magnum to the sacral hiatus, the area anesthetized is limited only by the spread of the injected solution and is subject to considerable individual variation. The dangers of toxicity must be borne in mind because the total dose required may be quite large.

(1) Caudal approach - 20 ml. for sacral nerves for perineal surgery; 30-35 ml. for lumbar and lower thoracic nerves.
(2) Lumbar approach - 20-25 ml. for lower abdominal surgery; 25-30 ml. for upper abdominal surgery.
(3) Repeat doses by catheter require half the initial dose.

2. Comparison of subarachnoid and epidural block -
   a. Advantages of subarachnoid block -
      (1) Technically easier.
      (2) Rapid onset.
      (3) Small drug doses with less chance of toxic reactions.

b. Advantages of epidural block -
(1) Fewer postoperative complications, such as spinal headaches.
(2) Less patient prejudice against this technic.

3. Effects of spinal anesthesia -
a. Analgesia over distribution of the spinal nerves anesthetized.
b. Paralysis of muscles innervated by the spinal nerves anesthetized. If the anesthetic reaches the level of the fourth cervical segment in sufficient concentration, all respiratory muscles are paralyzed and respiration ceases.
c. Sympathetic paralysis (thoracolumbar outflow from T1 to L2) causes the following:
(1) Loss of vasomotor tone in the affected area, with peripheral vasodilatation, diminished vascular resistance, and loss of ability to control blood distribution. This impairment leads to a fall in BP which is particularly severe in hypertensive and in hypovolemic states.
(2) Active intestinal peristalsis.
(3) Warmth and dryness of skin, which is easily distinguished from the damp pallor seen in shock.

4. General management of patients during spinal anesthesia -
a. Prevent hypoxia by the administration of oxygen or assisted respiration.
b. Support circulation by -
(1) Positioning patient to promote venous return.
(2) Use of vasopressors (see Appendix). When high spinal anesthesia is planned, an intravenous infusion should be started before the spinal anesthetic for easy administration of vasopressors. Vasopressors may be given prophylactically before the spinal.

5. Sequelae of spinal anesthesia -
a. "Spinal headache" - Occurs during the first week after subarachnoid block and may last several days. Treatment consists of keeping the patient flat in bed for the first 24 hours to diminish CSF loss at the site of the puncture of the dura. Severe cases may require injection of saline into the epidural space. The incidence is 1-15% depending on the age of the patient (low in the elderly) and the size of the needle used for lumbar puncture.
b. Nerve injuries and transverse myelitis may cause transient or permanent disabilities ranging from minor paresthesias to paraplegia. These sequelae are rare, but their tragic impact gives them notoriety out of proportion to their frequency. They may be due to contaminants, drug sensitivities, or excessive dosages. Cases have been reported following epidural as well as subarachnoid spinal anesthesia.

OXYGEN THERAPY

Oxygen therapy consists of increasing the oxygen concentration of inspired air. At sea level the normal 21% oxygen concentration constitutes 159 mm. Hg (partial pressure) of the total 760 mm. Hg atmospheric pressure. Dead space, water vapor, CO_2 diffusing from the blood, and oxygen diffusing into the blood unite to reduce the alveolar oxygen to the 100 mm. Hg partial pressure normally found in the alveoli. This alveolar oxygen pressure is sufficient to saturate hemoglobin with oxygen, but may be reduced by (1) diminished oxygen partial pressure in the inspired air (e.g., high altitudes), or (2) diminished pulmonary ventilation as seen in respiratory depression or obstruction.

The objective of oxygen therapy is to raise the alveolar oxygen partial pressure and arterial oxygen saturation to normal. Values are best determined by blood gas analysis of arterial blood samples. If ventilation is inadequate it is a temporary life-saving measure, but it must not be used as a substitute for measures necessary to return pulmonary ventilation to normal (i.e., clearing the airway, etc.).

Signs and symptoms of hypoxia in the conscious patient include tachycardia, restlessness, mental confusion, and air hunger in the early stages; and cyanosis, bradycardia, and loss of consciousness when the hypoxia becomes severe.

Methods of Administration.

All methods require a source of oxygen (usually tanks of compressed oxygen), reducing valves, and flow meters.

A. Oropharyngeal Catheter: By this method the oxygen is administered through a catheter introduced through the nose and advanced until the tip can be seen below the uvula. Flows of 6-8 L. of humidified oxygen raise the oxygen in the inspired air to 35-40%.

B. Oxygen Mask: A wide variety of rubber and plastic masks with and without rebreathing bags, or valves to offer positive pressure on expiration, are available. They permit higher oxygen concentrations.

C. Oxygen Tents: In these the patient is not encumbered by masks or catheters. High concentrations are possible, but without expert adjustment and supervision oxygen administration by tent may be most inefficient and useless.

D. Mechanical Ventilators: These assist or control pulmonary ventilation by increasing the airway pressure intermittently and are important adjuncts to oxygen therapy. Their management requires personnel trained in their use.

POSTANESTHESIA CARE

Anesthesia does not terminate with closure of the incision; its termination depends upon the elimination of the anesthetic agent by pulmonary or renal excretion or by metabolic destruction. The duration of the period required for recovery from the effects of the anesthetic varies with the agents and technics used (regional anesthesia not excepted). During this time the protective reflexes and homeostatic responses which control vital respiratory and circulatory functions return gradually. The anesthetist must continue to provide the same care as during surgery until the patient is conscious and his vital signs have stabilized. Above all, **the patient must not be left unattended.** Respiration, circulation, and state of reactivity must be monitored at frequent intervals.

The serious hazards peculiar to the postanesthetic period are respiratory and circulatory collapse.

Respiration.

HYPOXIA IS ONE OF THE MOST FREQUENT CAUSES OF POSTOPERATIVE RESTLESSNESS.

Respiratory depression may be due to the prolonged effect of the agents used during surgery or may be caused by postoperative pain medication. Increasing respiratory depression may occur as the painful stimuli of surgery subside. Respiratory obstruction may be due to undrained secretions, tight dressings or casts, etc. Hematomas, pneumothorax, and atelectasis must be kept in mind.

Treatment is by removal of all impediments to respiration, oxygen therapy, and assisted respiration if necessary.

Circulation.

Postoperative hypotension may be caused by drug depression, blood loss, sudden elimination of excess CO_2, and hypoxia. Two or more of these factors are usually involved.

Treatment consists of placing the patient in the shock position (elevate foot of bed), oxygen therapy, fluid replacement, and (rarely) the use of vasopressor drugs. Monitoring of central venous pressure assists in the management of postanesthetic hypotension.

4 . . .
Nutrition

Energy for physiologic processes is provided in the metabolism of carbohydrate, fat, and protein. The daily requirement for energy (the daily caloric need) is the sum of the so-called basal energy demand (the energy required merely to maintain life) plus that required for additional activity. Extra energy is needed also during periods of growth, pregnancy, or convalescence. Accelerated metabolism, as in hyperthyroidism or during fever, also increases the energy demand. For example, in fever there is an increase of approximately 12% of the basal caloric requirement per degree centigrade (8% per degree Fahrenheit) rise in temperature over normal.

The total caloric requirements of healthy persons of both sexes and various ages is given in the table on pp. 130-131. These intakes provide for average activity. However, caloric requirements in pathologic states (even at bed rest) increase sometimes to very high levels, as indicated below.

Daily Caloric Requirements in Adult Patients

Afebrile, minor injury or illness, at bed rest	2000 Cal.
Severe injury or illness	2500-4000 Cal.
Previously depleted	3500 Cal.
Severe chills, fever	5000 Cal.

PROTEIN NUTRITION

Protein is not replaceable by any other food and is therefore absolutely necessary in all diets. The recommended daily intakes of protein for healthy individuals are shown in the table on p. 88. However, the quantity of protein required by various surgical patients is highly variable, ranging from 80 Gm. /day to a high of 200-300 Gm. /day or more in severe burns. At least 100 Gm. of protein should be given daily to sick or injured persons.

The metabolism of protein is profoundly affected by the stress incurred in such pathologic states as infections, injuries, major surgery, and burns. For a variable period after the onset of stress, patients undergo a period of obligatory negative nitrogen balance. Prolonged bed rest will also induce a negative nitrogen balance. It is difficult or impossible to avoid this apparently physiologic catabolic response to stress even after greatly increased intakes of protein and calories have been provided.

Depletion of body protein is associated with prolonged convalescence, poor healing of wounds, more frequent and more severe postoperative complications, increased susceptibility to infection, anemia, edema, impaired gastrointestinal motility, and skeletal muscle weakness.

RECOMMENDED DAILY DIETARY ALLOWANCES, REVISED 1968[1]

	Age Years[2] From-To	Weight Kg.	Weight (lb.)	Height cm.	Height (in.)	K Calories	Protein Gm.	Fat Soluble Vitamins: Vitamin A Activity I. U.	Vitamin D I. U.	Vitamin E Activity I. U.	Water Soluble Vitamins: Ascorbic Acid mg.	Folacin[3]
Infants	0-1/6	4	9	55	22	Kg. × 120	Kg. × 2.2[4]	1500	400	5	35	0.05
	1/6-1/2	7	15	63	25	Kg. × 110	Kg. × 2.0[4]	1500	400	5	35	0.05
	1/2-1	9	20	72	28	Kg. × 100	Kg. × 1.8[4]	1500	400	5	35	0.1
Children	1-2	12	26	81	32	1100	25	2000	400	10	40	0.1
	2-3	14	31	91	36	1250	25	2000	400	10	40	0.2
	3-4	16	35	100	39	1400	30	2500	400	10	40	0.2
	4-6	19	42	110	43	1600	30	2500	400	10	40	0.2
	6-8	23	51	121	48	2000	35	3500	400	15	40	0.2
	8-10	28	62	131	52	2200	40	3500	400	15	40	0.3
Males	10-12	35	77	140	55	2500	45	4500	400	20	40	0.4
	12-14	43	95	151	59	2700	50	5000	400	20	45	0.4
	14-18	59	130	170	67	3000	60	5000	400	25	55	0.4
	18-22	67	147	175	69	2800	60	5000	400	30	60	0.4
	22-35	70	154	175	69	2800	65	5000	---	30	60	0.4
	35-55	70	154	173	68	2600	65	5000	---	30	60	0.4
	55-75+	70	154	171	67	2400	65	5000	---	30	60	0.4
Females	10-12	35	77	142	56	2250	50	4500	400	20	40	0.4
	12-14	44	97	154	61	2300	50	5000	400	20	45	0.4
	14-16	52	114	157	62	2400	55	5000	400	25	50	0.4
	16-18	54	119	160	63	2300	55	5000	400	25	50	0.4
	18-22	58	128	163	64	2000	55	5000	400	25	55	0.4
	22-35	58	128	163	64	2000	55	5000	---	25	55	0.4
	35-55	58	128	160	63	1850	55	5000	---	25	55	0.4
	55-75+	58	128	157	62	1700	55	5000	---	25	55	0.4
Pregnancy						+200	65	6000	400	30	60	0.8
Lactation						+1000	75	8000	400	30	60	0.5

[1] Intended to cover individual variations among most normal persons in the U. S. A. The recommended allowances can be attained with a variety of common foods, providing other nutrients for which human requirements have been less well defined.

[2] Entries for age range 22-35 represent 22-year requirements; others represent the midpoint of the specified age periods.

[3] Refers to dietary sources as determined by Lactobacillus casei assay. Pure forms may be effective in doses less than 1/4 of the RDA.

[4] Assumes protein equivalent to human milk. For proteins not 100 percent utilized factors should be increased proportionately.

RECOMMENDED DAILY DIETARY ALLOWANCES, REVISED 1968, Cont'd.

	Age Years[2]	Water Soluble Vitamins					Minerals				
	From-To	Niacin Equiv.[6] mg.	Riboflavin mg.	Thiamine mg.	Vitamin B_6 mg.	Vitamin B_{12} μg.	Calcium Gm.	Phosphorus Gm.	Iodine μg.	Iron mg.	Magnesium mg.
Infants	0-1/6	5	0.4	0.2	0.2	1.0	0.4	0.2	25	6	40
	1/6-1/2	7	0.5	0.4	0.3	1.5	0.5	0.4	40	10	60
	1/2-1	8	0.6	0.5	0.4	2.0	0.6	0.5	45	15	70
Children	1-2	8	0.6	0.6	0.5	2.0	0.7	0.7	55	15	100
	2-3	8	0.7	0.6	0.6	2.5	0.8	0.8	60	15	150
	3-4	9	0.8	0.7	0.7	3	0.8	0.8	70	10	200
	4-6	11	0.9	0.8	0.9	4	0.8	0.8	80	10	200
	6-8	13	1.1	1.0	1.0	4	0.9	0.9	100	10	250
	8-10	15	1.2	1.1	1.2	5	1.0	1.0	110	10	250
Males	10-12	17	1.3	1.3	1.4	5	1.2	1.2	125	10	300
	12-14	18	1.4	1.4	1.6	5	1.4	1.4	135	18	350
	14-18	20	1.5	1.5	1.8	5	1.4	1.4	150	18	400
	18-22	18	1.6	1.4	2.0	5	0.8	0.8	140	10	400
	22-35	18	1.7	1.4	2.0	5	0.8	0.8	140	10	350
	35-55	17	1.7	1.3	2.0	5	0.8	0.8	125	10	350
	55-75+	14	1.7	1.2	2.0	6	0.8	0.8	110	10	350
Females	10-12	15	1.3	1.1	1.4	5	1.2	1.2	110	18	300
	12-14	15	1.4	1.2	1.6	5	1.3	1.3	115	18	350
	14-16	16	1.4	1.2	1.8	5	1.3	1.3	120	18	350
	16-18	15	1.5	1.2	2.0	5	1.3	1.3	115	18	350
	18-22	13	1.5	1.0	2.0	5	0.8	0.8	100	18	350
	22-35	13	1.5	1.0	2.0	5	0.8	0.8	100	18	300
	35-55	12	1.5	0.9	2.0	5	0.8	0.8	90	18	300
	55-75+	10	1.5	0.9	2.0	6	0.8	0.8	80	10	300
Pregnancy		15	1.8	+0.1	2.5	8	+0.4	+0.4	125	18	450
Lactation		20	2.0	+0.5	2.5	6	+0.5	+0.5	150	18	450

[5] Entries for age range 22-35 represent 22-year requirements; others represent the midpoint of the specified age periods.

[6] Niacin equivalents include dietary sources of the vitamin itself plus 1 mg. equivalent for each 60 mg. of dietary tryptophan.

The efficiency with which administered protein is utilized for tissue repair depends upon an adequate intake of calories from non-protein nutrients. In the postoperative period an intake of as much as 0.5 Gm. of nitrogen (1 Gm. of nitrogen = 6.25 Gm. protein) and 45 Calories/Kg. may be necessary to restore positive nitrogen balance in a nutritionally depleted patient.

CARBOHYDRATES AND FATS IN NUTRITION

In the usual well-balanced diet about 50-60% of the total calories may be derived from carbohydrates and 20-30% from fats. Necessary increases in caloric intake are usually achieved by increasing the fat content of the diet.

The presence of carbohydrate is essential to permit the efficient utilization of fats without the development of ketosis. At least 5 Gm. of carbohydrate/100 Calories of the total diet are required for this purpose. Surgical patients maintained exclusively on intravenous fluids will probably obtain much of their required energy from their own reserve stores of fat because of the difficulty of providing adequate nutrition when only the parenteral route is available to supply nutrient substances. Under these circumstances an intake of as little as 100 Gm. of carbohydrate (2000 ml. of 5% dextrose) is adequate to prevent ketosis.

VITAMINS

The vitamin requirements of healthy persons are given in the table on pp. 130-131. Normal persons on an adequate diet can secure all of the required vitamins from natural foods. However, in disease states in which digestion or assimilation is impaired or where the requirements are increased, vitamin supplementation is necessary.

The recommended **therapeutic daily doses** of the most important vitamins are as follows:

Thiamin (B_1)	5-10 mg.
Riboflavin (B_2)	5-10 mg.
Niacinamide	100 mg.
Calcium pantothenate	20 mg.
Pyridoxine (B_6)	3 mg.
Folic acid (folacin)	1.5 mg.
Vitamin B_{12}	4 μg.
Ascorbic acid (vitamin C)	500 mg.

For short-term vitamin supplementation only thiamin, riboflavin, niacinamide, and ascorbic acid need be given. If prolonged intravenous alimentation is required or if an adequate intake of vitamins cannot be obtained from the diet, all of the above vitamins should be given in the doses listed.

When vitamins are added to solutions to be given intravenously, large losses are likely to occur into the urine. For this reason intramuscular or subcutaneous injection is preferred if the oral route cannot be used.

Deficiencies of fat-soluble vitamins (vitamins A, D, and K) will occur if fat digestion or absorption is impaired, as in obstructive jaundice, biliary fistula, pancreatic disease, or in any disease state which extensively involves the gastrointestinal tract. For the surgical patient a deficiency of vitamin K (almost exclusively an effect of malabsorption) is the most significant. Because this fat-soluble vitamin is essential to the production of prothrombin by the liver, its lack in the body causes hypoprothrombinemia and thus disrupts normal coagulation mechanisms. Preoperative administration of vitamin K by injection is indicated in such cases to raise the prothrombin level to at least 60-70% of normal. The usual daily dose is 2-5 mg. of menadione sodium bisulfite injection (Hykinone®), I.V. or I.M. Failure of prompt response to these conservative doses constitutes evidence of severe hepatic damage, and this must be taken into account in assessing the hemorrhagic risks of surgery.

PARENTERAL NUTRITION

Patients who cannot take food orally must be nourished intravenously. By this method it is possible for a limited period to give most of the essential nutrients required for adequate although not ideal nutrition.

Carbohydrates.

The principal problem in parenteral nutrition is to provide sufficient calories. Under the usual circumstances dextrose is relied upon to provide all of the exogenous calories. However, because 1 L. of 5% dextrose (glucose) provides only 200 Calories (1 Gm. dextrose = 4 Calories) and because 3 L./day I.V. is probably an average maximum intake for an adult patient, 5% dextrose solution can provide only about 600 Calories/day. When it is recalled that 2000 Calories/day is the minimum requirement for a bed patient, it becomes obvious that a caloric deficit must often occur when the usual parenteral regimen is employed.

More concentrated solutions of dextrose may be used in an effort to provide more calories, but these solutions are hypertonic and lead to phlebitis. Furthermore, there are limits to the rate at which dextrose can be given intravenously without causing glycosuria, which is wasteful of calories and contributes to dehydration via the polyuria and electrolyte diuresis with which glycosuria is always associated. In general, dextrose should not be given intravenously at rates exceeding 0.5-0.75 Gm. (approximately 10-15 ml. of a 5% solution)/Kg./hour, although somewhat slower rates are to be preferred.

It follows that the higher the concentration of intravenous dextrose solution, the more slowly it must be given. In many clinical situations where the oral route is not available, additional required calories may be given in this way. Examples are when parenteral nutrition must be maintained over a prolonged period or when maximum protein-sparing action is essential, as in the case of patients with acute renal insufficiency who can be given only very small quantities of fluid (see p. 150). In these instances, hypertonic (25-50%) solutions of dextrose are used. Phlebitis can be minimized by administering hypertonic solutions very slowly through a small polyethylene catheter advanced through an arm or leg vein as far as possible into a large vessel.

Fructose has been recommended as a substitute for dextrose in intravenous nutrition because it disappears from the blood faster than dextrose and thus can be administered more rapidly and is less readily lost into the urine. In most situations, however, these advantages do not seem to be sufficiently impressive to recommend its general use as a substitute for dextrose. The caloric contributions of the two sugars are the same.

Ethyl Alcohol.

Ethyl alcohol may be added to dextrose solutions as an additional source of calories. It is metabolized to provide 5.6 Calories/ml. or 7 Calories/Gm. However, alcohol should not be given intravenously in concentrations much exceeding 5% (50 ml. 95% alcohol/L.), which means that only an additional 280 Calories/L. can be administered in this way.

Patients receiving alcohol-containing solutions intravenously must be carefully attended, and the possibility of undesirable reactions with other drugs that are being used must also be considered.

Fat.

From a nutritional standpoint, the most satisfactory concentrated source of calories is fat. Unfortunately, an emulsion of fat suitable for intravenous administration is not presently available in the United States although such an emulsion is available in other countries. This product, designated commercially as Intralipid®, is a 20% soy bean emulsion.

Protein.

When only the parenteral route can be used, the most efficient way to provide nutrients for synthesis of protein is by the administration of amino acid mixtures prepared by enzymatic or acid hydrolysis of casein or fibrin.* The principal disadvantage to the use of intravenous amino acid preparations is that adequate amounts of "protein-sparing" calories from carbohydrates and fat must be administered simultaneously. There is evidence that as much as 53-60 Calories/Kg. may be necessary to attain nitrogen balance when amino acids are used as the sole source of nitrogen, even by mouth, as compared to 35 Calories/Kg. when equivalent amounts of nitrogen are given as whole protein. However, if an adequate caloric intake can be provided, amino acid mixtures are very satisfactory as a source of nitrogen for protein synthesis.

Intravenously administered amino acids are not lost into the urine in any significant quantity.

Most patients tolerate these mixtures well if too rapid administration is avoided. An optimal rate of administration is approximately 300 ml./hour of a 5% solution. It may be assumed that 1 L.

---

*Although plasma or purified protein fractions of the plasma, such as albumin, can be given intravenously, these substances are metabolized slowly and in a manner which is nutritionally uneconomical. Consequently, these substances should not be used for nutritional purposes alone.

of a 5% amino acid solution contributes the equivalent of about 35 Gm. of protein to the diet. Most amino acid preparations contain also 5% dextrose. It is desirable to give the amino acids simultaneously with dextrose.

Sample Regimen.

The following regimen is cited as an example of what is required in parenteral feeding to supply only a modest daily intake of protein and calories at less than an optimal level. The total infusion time required is about 10 hours.

1000 ml.	10% dextrose and 5% ethyl alcohol	- 680 Calories
2000 ml.	5% dextrose - 5% amino acids	- 680 Calories

Totals - 3000 ml. fluid
1380 Calories
70 Gm. protein equivalent

Prolonged Total Parenteral Nutrition.

In the foregoing discussion the problems associated with attempts to nourish adequately a patient who cannot be given nutrients except by the intravenous route were emphasized. Massive catabolism of body protein presents a particularly difficult problem. During the period immediately after severe trauma, the extensive protein catabolic response to stress appears not to be substantially affected by large infusions of carbohydrate; as a result, administration of amino acids does not seem to restore positive nitrogen balance or even to compensate for the protein nitrogen losses.

Nevertheless, it has been shown that the intravenous infusion of a fat-free amino acid and glucose solution could under some circumstances support normal nutritional needs. For example, in a study of 30 patients with chronic complicated gastrointestinal disease nourished exclusively by the intravenous route for 10-200 days, positive nitrogen balance was achieved in all, and this was associated with healing of wounds, closure of fistulas, gain in weight, and increased strength and activity. Caloric intakes up to 3300 Calories/day and nitrogen intakes of 16-25 Gm./day were achieved. The average positive nitrogen balance was 4 Gm./day.

The method used for total parenteral (intravenous) nutrition is based on the infusion of glucose for calories and a protein hydrolysate as a source of nitrogen to provide for synthesis of protein. The hypertonic basal solution can be prepared in the hospital pharmacy by mixing routinely available solutions of glucose and 5% protein (fibrin) hydrolysates.

Preparation of the solution for hyperalimentation is as follows: One liter of solution providing approximately 1000 Calories and 6 Gm. of nitrogen (equivalent to approximately 35 Gm. protein) is prepared by combining 860 ml. of 5% fibrin hydrolysate (Aminosol®) in 5% glucose with 165 Gm. of Dextrose, U.S.P. (anhydrous). Sterilization must be accomplished by the use of an 0.22 μ membrane (Millprose) since such a hypertonic glucose solution would suffer intense caramelization (browning [Maillard] reaction) if autoclaved. This is the stock solution to which additional nutrients can be added. There are approximately 8 mEq. Na^+, 14 mEq. K^+ and traces of other mineral elements such as chloride, phosphate, magnesium, and calcium in the protein hydrolysate added. These values may vary slightly depending on the type of protein hydrolysate used (e.g., fibrin or casein digests).

An alternative method for preparing the basic stock solution consists of discarding 250 ml. from a 1 L. bottle of 5% protein hydrolysate in 5% glucose and then - using strict aseptic precautions - adding 350 ml. of 50% glucose. The resultant 1100 ml. of solution provides approximately 5.25 Gm. of nitrogen (equivalent to 25 Gm. as protein), 212 Gm. of glucose, 7 mEq. Na^+, and 13 mEq. K^+ when fibrin hydrolysate is used. The caloric value is slightly less than 1 Calorie/ml.

Unless contraindicated, 50 mEq. NaCl and 40 mEq. KCl, using concentrated solutions of the electrolyte, should be added per liter of solution prepared by either procedure. Fortification with vitamins is most conveniently accomplished by addition of 10 ml. of a commercially available multivitamin preparation* of fat- and water-soluble vitamins to only one bottle of the daily infusate.

Magnesium (4-8 mEq./day) may also be provided as magnesium sulfate. Vitamins B_{12} and K and folic acid may be necessary during prolonged intravenous alimentation. These may be given intramuscularly. If plasma analyses so suggest, calcium gluconate and potassium acid phosphate (KH_2PO_4) may also be supplied as necessary. Unless there has been a pre-existing iron deficiency or extensive hemorrhage (or both), iron may not be required. Transfusions of whole blood will supply iron as will intramuscular injection of iron-dextran complex as necessary. The trace mineral elements such as zinc, copper, manganese, cobalt, and iodine may be added if total nutrition by intravenous injection is prolonged beyond 1 month. Alternatively, 1 unit of plasma twice weekly will serve also as a source of trace elements.

The table on p. 137 summarizes the average nutrient composition of 2500 to 3000 ml. of the solution prepared as described above, for hyperalimentation in adults. Solutions intended for use in children requiring long-term nutrition exclusively by the intravenous route are prepared as for adults with only minor modifications.

Administration of the solution described below requires continuous infusion over the 24-hour day. The injection is made into a large vessel such as the superior vena cava, preferably using an indwelling catheter threaded carefully and with aseptic technic into the vessel by way of the subclavian vein. For newborn infants or those weighing less than 10 lb., the superior vena cava may be reached via the jugular vein. Initially, only the normal amounts of fluid are given (2500 ml./day in adults; 125 ml./Kg. in infants); the volume infused is then slowly increased over a period of several days as tolerated, with careful attention to avoidance of overhydration. Alternate-day measurement of plasma electrolytes and weekly measurement of BUN and glucose should serve as monitors of the safety of the infusion. Testing for urine glucose, collected at 6-hour intervals during the infusion, is also recommended.

The rate of glucose utilization is between 0.5 Gm./Kg./hour in adults and 1.2 Gm./Kg./hour in infants, the average being 0.9 Gm./

---

*M.V.I.®, U.S. Vitamin Corporation.

Average Composition of Adult Nutrient Solution

Water	2500-3000 ml.
Protein hydrolysate (amino acids)	100-130 Gm.
Nitrogen	12-18 Gm.
Carbohydrate (dextrose)	525-625 Gm.
Calories	2500-3000
Sodium	125-150 mEq.
Potassium	75-120 mEq.
Magnesium	4-8 mEq.
Vitamin A	5000-10,000 U. S. P. units
Vitamin D	500-1000 U. S. P. units
Vitamin E	2.5-5 I. U.
Vitamin C	250-500 mg.
Thiamine	25-50 mg.
Riboflavin	5-10 mg.
Pyridoxine	7.5-15 mg.
Niacin	50-100 mg.
Pantothenic acid	12.5-25 mg.

Calcium and phosphorus are added to the solution if indicated.

Iron is added to the solution, or given intramuscularly in depot form as iron-dextran complex, or given as blood transfusion, if indicated.

Vitamin B_{12}, vitamin K, and folic acid are given intramuscularly or added for intravenous administration, as indicated.

Trace elements such as zinc, copper, manganese, cobalt, and iodine are added only after total intravenous therapy exceeds one month. Alternatively, 1 unit of plasma twice a week will provide required amounts of trace elements.

Kg./hour in an adult. These are the rates for normal individuals; in seriously ill patients, infusion rates may need to be lower, and periodic adjustment in rate of administration of the nutrient solution may be required.

Giving glucose intravenously at a rate which permits less than 2% excretion of glucose in the urine avoids the danger of osmotic diuresis, with resulting dehydration and electrolyte imbalance. The normal pancreas will increase its output of insulin in response to the continuing infusion of glucose. If a diabetic patient is being treated, appropriate doses of insulin may be given subcutaneously every 6 hours, or the total dose may be added to the intravenous fluid. Indeed, 5-25 units of crystalline insulin per 1000 Calories may be added routinely to the nutrient solution to improve utilization of glucose and promote nitrogen retention in elderly patients with evidence of some degree of intolerance to glucose or in patients with severe nutritional depletion.

Potassium is usually required in patients receiving hyperalimentation in larger than maintenance amounts. Forty mEq. of KCl per liter of infusate is a minimum dose; more is required (with careful attention to the prevention of hyperkalemia) if there are substantial gastrointestinal fluid losses or extensive burns. Although 50 mEq. of sodium per 1000 Calories is a satisfactory intake in these patients, reduction of intake or even total elimination of sodium may be necessary in clinical states which predispose to retention of sodium.

Significant hypoalbuminemia or anemia may require initial administration of albumin or whole blood.

COMPLICATIONS OF HYPERALIMENTATION

Septicemia.

The problem of septicemia developing during intravenous hyperalimentation must be kept in mind. Solutions to be used for parenteral alimentation are nutritionally very favorable to the growth of infectious organisms. Several reports emphasize infection as a dangerous complication of hyperalimentation. The infectious agents include not only bacteria but - even more commonly - fungi such as Candida albicans. The incidence of septicemia is related both to the duration of hyperalimentation and to the time elapsing between changes of an indwelling catheter. At present, there does not appear to be any absolutely safe method to prevent these infections, particularly when the pathogen is a fungus. Every effort must be made to maintain aseptic conditions when giving parenteral alimentation. The use of external arteriovenous shunts for injection of the nutritional solution may be preferred to direct catheterization of a vein.

Metabolic Hazards.

In addition to the hazards of infection, there are reports of a peculiar metabolic disturbance associated with intravenous hyperalimentation. Silvis & Paragas observed 3 severely malnourished patients who were given intravenously the hyperalimentation solution described above. Although the patients appeared to be doing well for the first few days after the infusion was begun, between the fourth and seventh days each developed muscular weakness and paresthesias; 2 progressed to convulsions and coma, and one died in coma after 5 days. The most significant and characteristic finding was a profound decline in serum phosphate to mean levels of less than 0.3 mg./100 ml. None of the patients showed evidences of hyperosmolarity, uremia, or ketoacidosis.

In experimental studies with animal models (dogs or rats), effects similar to those observed with the patients were produced by intravenous hyperalimentation. The effects were particularly severe in previously starved animals as compared with those entering the experiment without a prior period of undernutrition. Attempts to correct the significantly low serum phosphate levels by including phosphate in the infusions did not prevent the syndrome. Balance studies on one dog indicated that the fall in phosphate was not attributable to negative phosphate balance since the amount of phosphate excreted fell far short of accounting for the fall in serum phosphate. It was concluded that an extravascular shift of phosphate had occurred.

In any case, it seems certain from these studies that a depression of central nervous system activity can occur in humans as a result of intravenous hyperalimentation and that the syndrome can be reproduced in experimental animals, although the causes of these occasionally fatal symptoms have not yet been elucidated. A possibly important clue is the observation in the rat experiments that the animals most susceptible to this fatal syndrome were those having a chronic and continuing weight loss at the time hyperalimentation was instituted. Both the animals totally fasted for a week and those allowed to stabilize at a constant albeit subnormal weight - i. e., who have had an opportunity to adjust to the suboptimal intake of calories - were relatively resistant to the development of the full-blown fatal syndrome. Obviously, the metabolic circumstances in the patients who may be selected for intravenous hyperalimentation resemble those of the chronically malnourished rats. Further studies may better define all of the abnormal metabolic parameters that predispose to the development of this serious complication of intravenous hyperalimentation.

Glycolysis in red blood cells differs somewhat from the classic Embden-Meyerhof (E-M) pathway as it occurs in other tissues by the ability of the erythrocyte to form significant quantities of 2, 3-diphosphoglycerate (2, 3-DPG) from 1, 3-diphosphoglycerate (1, 3-DPG), which is the usual major product of the oxidation of glyceraldehyde-3-phosphate in the E-M glycolytic pathway. The formation of 2, 3-DPG from 1, 3-DPG is catalyzed by phosphoglycerate 2, 3-mutase.

An important function of 2, 3-DPG in red cells is its ability to enhance the dissociability of oxyhemoglobin by decreasing the tendency of oxygen to bind to hemoglobin, an effect similar to that of CO_2 (the so-called Bohr effect) or of a decline in intracellular pH. Thus, the P-50 for oxyhemoglobin (i. e., the oxygen tension at which hemoglobin is 50% saturated with oxygen) is lowered. This is often referred to as a shift of the oxyhemoglobin dissociation curve "to the right." An important physiologic function of red cell 2, 3-DPG, therefore, is to improve the delivery of oxygen to the tissues, particularly in circumstances where low oxygen tension prevails. Hypophosphatemia reduces the red cell 2, 3-DPG content and thus may be considered as impairing oxygenation of the tissues. This is certainly a serious additional hazard in hypotension, ischemia, reduction of circulating red cell mass as in anemia, or after extensive hemorrhage uncorrected by adequate transfusions. While an increase in the amount of phosphate infused is said not to affect the CNS depression described above as being occasionally associated with severe hypophosphatemia, it will nonetheless prevent a fall in erythrocyte 2, 3-DPG.

TUBE FEEDING

Feeding by nasogastric tube is occasionally necessary to prevent serious malnutrition, e.g., in severe anoxia, coma, obstructive lesions of the esophagus, fractures of the jaw, and after severe burns.

When liquid formulas are used, very small polyethylene nasogastric tubes (e.g., K-30) which may be left in place for many days are suitable. These tubes may even be used for supplemental feedings in patients who can ingest some of their meals in the usual manner (such as burned patients who may be unable to eat adequate quantities of protein).

In preparing formulas for tube feeding it will probably be necessary to avoid the use of simple sugars, such as dextrose, and too much fat, such as cream, since both tend to cause diarrhea in tube-fed patients. The preferred source of carbohydrate is a dextrinized starch, such as Dexin® or Dextri-Maltose®. A simple formula for feeding by gastric tube is as follows:

Homogenized milk	2200 ml.
Half-and-half (cream and milk)	600 ml.
Eggs	6
Dextri-Maltose®	7 Tbsp.

(In a total volume of 3000 ml. this mixture contains 120 Gm. protein and 3000 Calories.)

Homogenized milk alone is often the simplest substance to use at the beginning of a tube feeding regimen. It contains 3.5 Gm. of protein and about 70 Calories/100 ml. During the first few days after an operation, the initial rate of feeding should not exceed 50 ml./hour. Thereafter the rate may be increased gradually in accordance with the patient's tolerance until a maximum of 150-200 ml. every 2 hours is reached, usually about 1 week later. If, at this time, the patient is tolerating the feedings well, the homogenized milk may be fortified with 50 Gm. of a powdered protein hydrolysate and 30 Gm. of Dextri-Maltose® or Dexin®. If this is well tolerated, the carbohydrate may be gradually increased over a three-day period to 60 Gm./L. This final formula contributes 160 Gm. of protein and about 2500 Calories in 2400 ml. Vitamins may be added to the formula, using a concentrated solution similar in composition to that given on p. 132.

The formulas and rates of administration described above may also be used for jejunostomy feedings.

A more concentrated tube feeding mixture can be used with the aid of a pump to maintain the flow of the mixture. A sample formula which utilizes commercially available puréed infant foods is as follows:

	Protein (Gm.)	Calories
3 1/2 oz. strained beef	14.6	103
4 1/2 oz. beets	1.5	51
3 raw eggs	18.0	225
Homogenized milk (640 ml.)	23.3	466
Totals	57.4	845

Other meats and vegetables can be used to vary the formula.

Use of Medium-Chain Triglycerides.

Fat introduced into the tube feeding formula, while valuable as a concentrated source of additional calories, is often difficult for patients to digest and absorb and tends to favor fermentative activity within the bowel, leading to diarrhea, a complication that severely limits the usefulness of a tubal nutrient. However, triglycerides containing fatty acids of medium-chain length (C_6 to C_{10}) have proved to be useful clinically since the short-chain fatty acids formed after digestion of a medium-chain triglyceride can be readily digested and absorbed. Furthermore, they are transported as free fatty acids - rather than as chylomicrons - directly to the liver via the portal venous blood. Indeed, there is evidence that medium-chain triglycerides can be absorbed with no intestinal intraluminal hydrolysis whatever.

Using medium-chain triglycerides in a tubal nutrient formula, greater absorption of fat is possible in the presence of shortened lengths of small intestine or where there is an abnormally rapid transit time. It can also be expected that, with the use of medium-chain triglycerides, there will be an advantageous reduction in the bulk of the stools as well as a minimization of the foul quality of steatorrheic stools.

The dose of medium-chain triglycerides, like all tubal nutrients, must be adjusted to the tolerance of the patient. These lipid materials occur as oily liquids and are usually given in that form. Flavored preparations are available, although their content of lactose may limit their tolerance in patients with a shortened small intestine.

A major use for formulas fortified with medium-chain triglycerides is in patients with short bowel syndromes or internal or external fistulas. The benefit to be expected from the use of medium-chain triglycerides is illustrated by the patient with total colectomy and ileostomy who after 70 Gm. of ordinary triglyceride retained only 27% of ingested fat, whereas 54% was retained using medium-chain triglyceride.

Elemental Diets.

The commercial availability of amino acid preparations, usually as powdered hydrolysates of natural proteins but occasionally as mixtures of synthetic amino acids, has made it possible to construct "elemental diets" made up of amino acids as a source of protein with the addition of sugars, minerals, and vitamins. Such an elemental mixture contains no fats, proteins, or higher peptides which require digestion preliminary to absorption. These dietary mixtures are of particular usefulness in nutritional balance studies. Stimulation of exogenous secretion by the pancreas is much reduced by the absence of lipid. There is also a diminution of enteric secretion. This reduces drainage from fistulas, and the absence of residue obviously reduces the volume of stools.

However, these elemental diets have the disadvantage of being quite hypertonic. Consequently, this diet should be given to patients very gradually, and care should be taken that adequate water is also provided, particularly when normal thirst mechanisms are impaired. Although nitrogen is provided for protein synthesis from the constituent amino acids, the amounts may be inadequate when the metabolic demands are excessive, as after extensive trauma or stress or when there are large external losses of protein.

These elemental dietary mixtures are difficult to administer for prolonged periods unless given by tube because of their unpalatability. Nevertheless, they may be very useful adjuncts to the therapy of chronic pancreatic disease or severe ulcerative colitis. While the disadvantages of prolonged intravenous infusions are avoided, some gastrointestinal function is obviously required.

Precautions in Tube Feedings.

1. If given rapidly by gravity drip or by injection into the gastric tube, the formula should first be warmed to body temperature.

2. Do not give over 200 ml. at a time.
3. Use special care to prevent aspiration in unconscious patients.
4. Supply sufficient water in addition to the formula to permit excretion of nitrogenous end products. This is particularly important if the formula is high in protein.
5. When stopping or starting a feeding, or whenever the question of gastric retention arises, aspirate the gastric tube and wash it out with water.
6. Avoid constipation and fecal impaction in debilitated patients, if necessary by introducing 30 ml. of milk of magnesia into the tube.

THE NORMAL DIET

Parenteral and tube feedings should be discontinued as soon as possible in favor of a full normal diet taken by mouth. Foods should be palatable and attractively prepared as a stimulus to appetite. The physician should not overlook his responsibilities in this matter since a properly compounded nutritional prescription can be just as important to his patient's welfare as the drugs he may order.

The daily diet for the convalescent adult patient should contain 3000-3500 Calories and 100-150 Gm. of protein. It is not sufficient merely to place these nutrients on a tray within the patient's reach; care must be taken to make certain that the entire nutritional prescription is actually consumed.

It is often difficult for surgical patients to eat large amounts of high-protein foods such as muscle meats. Intermittent feedings may have to be given, but must be carefully spaced so as not to spoil the patient's appetite for regular meals. Fruit juices and broths are of little value as supplementary nutrients because they contribute practically nothing toward remedying protein and caloric deficits, the major dietary faults in need of correction; in fact, these liquid supplements may actually dull the appetite and thus indirectly impair nutrition.

A simple but useful supplementary drink may be prepared by stirring 50 Gm. of skimmed milk powder into 200 ml. of water. This supplies 17 Gm. of protein and 26 Gm. of carbohydrate, more than is available in 1 pint of milk but in only half the volume. Six glasses will supply over 100 Gm. of protein of excellent nutritional quality. Other valuable protein supplements are ice cream, cottage cheese, and eggs.

The "Basic" Foods.

As a guide to the formulation of an adequate diet, various foods have been arranged into 4 "basic" groups each of which makes a major contribution to the diet. To maintain an adequate diet, some foods from each of the 4 groups should be taken each day as follows:

1. Milk group -
   a. Children - Three or more 8 oz. glasses. (Smaller servings for some children under age 9.)
   b. Teenagers - Four or more glasses.
   c. Adults - Two or more glasses.
   d. Cheese, ice cream, and other foods derived from milk can supply part of the milk requirement.

2. Meat group - Two or more servings of meats, fish, poultry, eggs, or cheese, with dry beans, peas, and nuts as alternatives.
3. Vegetable and fruit group - Four or more servings. Include dark-green or yellow vegetables; citrus fruits or tomatoes.
4. Bread and cereal group - Four or more servings. (One serving = 1 slice enriched or whole grain bread, 3/4 cup enriched or whole grain dry cereal, 1/2 cup enriched or whole grain cooked cereal.)

The basic diet outlined above will provide approximately 1200 Calories. Additional calories may be derived from other foods as desired, or by increasing the quantity of servings of the listed foods.

SPECIAL DIETS FOR SURGICAL PATIENTS

Surgical diets are listed below according to the purpose for which each is designed. Therapeutic diets are modifications of the Regular or House Diet devised to meet the unusual demands imposed by the illness under treatment. The increased nutritional requirements created by many surgical conditions must be kept in mind. Inadequate diets should be used for only the briefest possible time, and vitamin supplements should be prescribed with them. When the oral intake is insufficient, parenteral supplementation should be considered.

Difficulty with mastication may prevent ingestion of the prescribed diet and must be considered in edentulous patients or those with oral neoplasms. A "mechanical" or puréed regular diet will be nutritionally complete.

Types of Surgical Diets

Diet	Indications
Regular or house	Normal maintenance.
High-protein, high-caloric, high-vitamin	Malnutrition; increased nutritional requirements.
Liquids without milk Liquids with milk Surgical soft	Depressed or disturbed gastrointestinal function, e.g., postoperatively.
Postgastrectomy	After gastric resection or gastroenterostomy.
Peptic ulcer regimens	Peptic ulcer.
Low-fat	Biliary tract disease.
Minimal residue	Colon preparation, rectal surgery, colitis.
Low-sodium	Cardiac disease, e.g., congestive failure; edema.
Gastric tube feeding	Comatose, uncooperative, malnourished, or severely anorexic patients; markedly increased nutritional demands, e.g., burns; gastrostomy.
Jejunostomy feeding	Jejunostomy.

High-Protein, High-Calorie, High-Vitamin Diet.

This diet is prescribed for malnourished patients or those with increased requirements, as in hyperthyroidism, febrile illness, and surgical convalescence. At least 3000-3500 Calories and 100-150 Gm. of protein should be provided.

Composition: All the basic foods with increased amounts of meat, liver, fish, poultry, eggs, milk, cheese, whole grain cereals, carrots, green vegetables, citrus fruits, and butter or margarine. Recipes and drinks may be fortified with such protein sources as skimmed milk powder.

Liquid Diet Without Milk.

Liquid and soft diets are suitable after injury or surgery when the function of the gastrointestinal tract is impaired. Under these circumstances the transition to a regular diet must be made in gradual stages when anorexia, nausea, vomiting, and paralytic ileus subside. The absence of distention, the return of peristalsis, and the passage of flatus are indications that the diet may be advanced.

Composition: Cereal gruel made with water, clear broth, bouillon, tea, coffee, plain gelatin, sugar, strained fruit juice, and carbonated beverages.

Liquid Diet With Milk.

Composition: Broth, bouillon, cereal gruel made with milk, strained creamed soups lightly seasoned, tomato juice, strained fruit juice, lemonade, sherbet, ice cream, plain gelatin, junket, all milk and cream beverages, cocoa, ginger-ale, carbonated beverages, coffee, tea.

Surgical Soft Diet.

This diet is transitional between the liquid and regular diets. The basic foods are included in each day's menu, but only those are selected which are lowest in cellulose and connective tissue. All foods are bland, smooth, and easily digested; stimulating factors (acids, extractives, concentrated carbohydrates, and condiments) are kept to a minimum. When served in 3 meals with 3 between-meal feedings, the surgical soft diet qualifies as a ''six-meal bland diet'' suitable for patients with peptic ulcer, gastritis, hiatus hernia, and after gastric resection.

Composition: Lean meat, fish, poultry, eggs, milk, mild cheese, potatoes; cooked, tender, or purėed vegetables and fruits; refined cereals and breads, custards, puddings, gelatin desserts, ice cream, plain cake, cream, butter, margarine, salt, and sugar in moderation.

Restrictions: Fried foods, meat soups and gravies, raw or coarse vegetables and fruits, whole grain cereals or bread, spices, highly seasoned foods, rich desserts and pastries, coffee, tea, carbonated and alcoholic beverages.

Postgastrectomy Diet.

It is likely that postgastrectomy patients will be maintained exclusively by parenteral feeding for at least the first 3 postoperative days or until bowel sounds return. When oral feeding can be instituted, it is important to increase gradually the quantity of small, frequent, bland, low-residue feedings. Undue distention of the stomach must be avoided. Feedings should be reduced or omitted if nausea, vomiting, or a marked sense of gastric fullness occurs.

A diet which serves for postgastrectomy patients is exemplified below:

A. Foods Which May Be Used:

Soups	Broth; cream soups made with purе́ed vegetables listed below.
Meat and meat substitutes	Beef: tender roast, steak, or ground. Lamb: tender chop, roast, or ground. Fowl: chicken, turkey. Fish: white fish, salmon. Eggs: soft cooked or poached.
Starches	White bread or toast, soy bread, soda crackers, melba toast. Refined cereals: cornmeal, cream of rice, cream of wheat, cornflakes, puffed rice, rice krispies. Macaroni, noodles, potato, rice, spaghetti - buttered or creamed.
Vegetables	Cooked artichoke, asparagus tips. Cooked and purе́ed beets, carrots, chard, peas, potato, spinach, squash, string beans.
Fruits	Ripe banana. Purе́ed cooked fruits; applesauce, apricots, peaches, pears, prunes.
Desserts	Plain cake, plain cookies, plain gelatin desserts, ice cream without fruit or nuts, milk puddings, purе́ed fruit whip. No chocolate.
Beverages	Coffee, tea, milk if tolerated.
Miscellaneous	Butter or margarine, cream, jelly, salt, sugar.

B. Foods Which May Not Be Used:

Soups	All except those listed above.
Meat and meat substitutes	Very rare meat. All except those allowed. Avoid dried, smoked, and spiced fish, fowl, and meat. No pork.
Starches	Whole grain breads and cereals; hot breads.
Vegetables, fruits, desserts	All except those allowed.
Beverages	Alcoholic beverages, carbonated beverages, cocoa, fruit juice.

Miscellaneous Dried and highly seasoned foods and sauces; condiments and spices, gravy, nuts, chocolate, cocoa.

Low-Fat Diet.

The basic foods are included in each day's menu, but those of low fat content are selected. Fat intake should be reduced to 30-50 Gm./day. The energy requirements are made up by increasing the protein and carbohydrate intake. Because of the reduced fat intake and the associated restrictions in fat-soluble vitamins, fruits and vegetables high in vitamin A should be served daily.

Composition: Lean meat, fish, poultry, skimmed milk or buttermilk, cottage cheese, cereal products, bread, vegetables, fruits (except those listed below), gelatin desserts, sherbet, puddings without cream, sugars, jellies.

Restrictions: Pork, ham, bacon, fatty cuts of meat, cream, cabbage family, onions, turnips, cucumbers, radishes, green peppers, dried beans and peas, melons, raw apples, butter, margarine, mayonnaise, oil, nuts, chocolate, fried foods, pastries, and highly seasoned foods.

Minimal Residue Diet.

This diet is planned to leave only a small residue after digestion. It is useful during preoperative and postoperative periods when it is desirable to reduce the fecal residue to prevent bowel movements for several days (as after rectal surgery). This diet is inadequate and should be used as briefly as possible. The surgical soft diet is also low in residue and can be made even more so by the omission of milk. It should be prescribed when a less restrictive regimen is satisfactory.

Composition: Eggs (soft-cooked, poached, or hard-cooked), meats (tender beef, veal, liver, fowl, oysters, sweetbreads), cereals (farina made with water, rice, rice-products), soda crackers, zweibach, arrowroot wafers, desserts (jello, arrowroot cookies, gelatin flavored with coffee or carbonated beverages), clear broths, bouillon, carbonated beverages, tea, coffee, butter, sugar, pure sugar candies, and jelly.

Restrictions: All foods not listed.

Low-Sodium Diet.

The low-sodium diet is used in those conditions associated with generalized edema, with or without ascites, secondary to chronic heart failure or hepatic insufficiency. In the preparation of such patients for surgery and during the postoperative period, sodium restriction may be indicated.

Restrictions:

1. Ham, bacon, bacon fat, salt pork, corned beef or pork, luncheon meats, canned meats, fish, or poultry.
2. Prepared cereals with salt, "quick-cooking" cereals, breads leavened with baking powder or baking soda.
3. Prepared foods or prepared desserts except as allowed.
4. Regular canned vegetables, dried fruits (except sun-dried), commercial salad dressings, ketchup.
5. Salted nuts, salted popcorn, potato chips.

6. Salt, garlic salt, onion salt, celery salt, baking powder, baking soda, and monosodium glutamate.
7. Sauerkraut, olives, pickles, relishes, chard, spinach.
8. To avoid distention - Cabbage family, onions, turnips, peppers, dried beans, cucumbers, raw apples, melons.

A diet containing no more than 500 mg. sodium per day may be summarized as follows. If low-sodium milk is substituted, the diet qualifies as a 250 mg. sodium diet.

A. Foods Which May Be Used:

1. **Soups** - Homemade vegetable soup, creamed soups prepared with milk allowance and purée of one of the vegetables allowed.
2. **Meat and meat substitutes** - 5 oz. daily (cooked weight) divided into one portion of 2 oz. and a second portion of 3 oz. of fresh meat (beef, lamb, veal, liver, rabbit), fresh fish (salmon, halibut, cod), or poultry (duck, chicken, turkey), 1 egg daily.

   Substitutes for 1 oz. of meat:

   1/4 cup dietetic pack tuna or salmon (canned without salt).
   1/4 cup washed cottage cheese.
   1 oz. dietetic low-sodium cheddar cheese.
   2 Tbsp. low-sodium peanut butter.
3. **Breads and cereals** - Homemade or commercial low-sodium bread as desired.

   Most cooked cereals if cooked in unsalted water.

   Exception: "Quick" Cream of Wheat. "Regular" and "Instant" Cream of Wheat are permitted.

   Three prepared dry cereals are low in sodium: puffed wheat, puffed rice, and shredded wheat.

   Noodles, spaghetti, macaroni, and rice.
4. **Vegetables** - Potato daily: baked, boiled in the jacket, mashed, or scalloped with a part of the milk allowance. Sweet potatoes and yams may also be used.
   Fresh or frozen (except lima beans, mixed vegetables, peas) or dietetic pack (canned without salt) artichoke, asparagus, carrots, lettuce, mushrooms, peas, pumpkin, romaine, string or wax beans, squash (summer, winter, zucchini), tomatoes. The following vegetables may be used only if well tolerated: broccoli, Brussels sprouts, cabbage, cauliflower, cucumbers, dried beans and peas, green pepper, radishes, onions, rutabagas, turnips.
5. **Fruit and fruit juices** - All fruits and fruit juices - fresh, canned, or frozen - are permitted. If not well tolerated, raw apples and melons should be avoided. Cooked apples are usually tolerated, so that applesauce or baked apples may be used. Citrus fruit or juice such as orange, grapefruit, or dietetic pack tomato juice should be included each day.
6. **Desserts** - Homemade cake or cookies prepared with sodium-free baking powder; homemade fruit pie from which salt has been omitted; gelatin prepared with plain gelatin, fruit juices, and sugar; puddings prepared with cornstarch, rice, or tapioca and a part of the milk allowance.

7. **Beverages** - Coffee, tea, coffee substitute; 2 cups of whole or skimmed milk per day.
8. **Miscellaneous** - Sweet butter, unsalted margarine, sugar, pepper, jelly, jam, syrup, spices, herbs, flour, cornstarch, tapioca, salad oil, vinegar, unsalted nuts, unsalted popcorn, vanilla and other extracts for flavoring, dry mustard, fresh garlic, garlic powder, garlic purée, 2 oz. cream (half and half).

B. Foods Which May Not Be Used:

1. **Soups** - Ordinary canned soups, dehydrated soup mixes, bouillon cubes.
2. **Meat and meat substitutes** - Corned beef, corned pork, dried beef, canned meat, fish and poultry unless canned without salt, ham, bacon, salt pork, pork sausage, cold cuts, shellfish, frozen fish fillets, frozen fish sticks, frozen precooked meals and entrée, kidney, brains, and cheese of all kinds except washed cottage cheese and low-sodium cheddar.
3. **Breads and cereals** - All commercial baked products, including bread, rolls, muffins, biscuits, pie, cake, cookies, coffee cake, sweet rolls, doughnuts.

   Pancakes, waffles, biscuits, cornbread, muffins, and similar products even if prepared without salt unless special sodium-free baking powder has been used. "Self-rising" flours, pancake mixes, cookie and coffee cake mixes, pie crust mix.

   Crackers of all kinds including those not salted "on the outside."

   Prepared dry cereals other than those specifically allowed.
4. **Vegetables** - All vegetables and vegetable juices which are commercially canned unless they have been canned without salt and the label so states. If the label does not state whether salt has or has not been added, assume that salt has been added.

   Frozen peas, frozen lima beans, and mixtures of frozen vegetables containing one or the other.

   Sauerkraut, spinach, beets, beet greens, dandelion greens, chard.
5. **Desserts** - Pudding mixes, pie fillings, gelatin mix, ice cream, iced milk, sherbet, commercially prepared desserts of any kind, most commercial candy.
6. **Fats** - Salted butter or margarine, peanut and other nut butters, bacon grease, commercial mayonnaise, commercial salad dressing of all kinds unless label specifically states that the dressing has been made without salt and is low in sodium.
7. **Beverages** - Milk in excess of 1 pint per day, buttermilk, prepared chocolate drinks and mixes.
8. **Miscellaneous** - Salt, baking powder, baking soda.

   Salted nuts, salted popcorn, potato chips, pretzels.

   Ketchup, prepared mustard, steak sauces, Worcestershire sauce, soy sauce, prepared horseradish, chili sauce, pickles, olives, pickle relish.

   Garlic salt, onion salt, celery salt, monosodium glutamate (Accent®, Zest®), salted meat tenderizers.

   Gravy and meat sauces.

Note: With the advent of effective medication designed to control sodium retention, there has been a tendency to permit patients who require a low-sodium regimen to consume a diet which is somewhat less restrictive in its sodium content. As a guide to the modifications in the diet which are required for daily intakes for varying amounts of sodium, the accompanying table is useful. A daily intake of 2400-4500 mg. of sodium is considered mild in its restriction; a limit of 1000 mg. as moderate; 500 mg. as strict; and 250 mg. as extreme. Most outpatients to be placed on a restricted sodium intake may be maintained on mild sodium restriction with the aid of appropriate medication. Strict restriction of sodium is difficult for outpatients to maintain, and the extreme restriction to a sodium intake of 250 mg. daily is practical only under hospital conditions.

Daily Allowance of Certain Foods According to Requirement for Sodium Restriction

Food Substance	2400-4500 mg. Sodium	1000 mg. Sodium	500 mg. Sodium	250 mg. Sodium
Milk	1 pint	1 pint	1 pint	Low-sodium ad lib.
Egg	1	1	1	1
Salt-free meat, fish, poultry	Ad lib.	6 oz.	5 oz.	5 oz.
Bread	Ad lib.	2 slices plus low-sodium bread ad lib.	Low-sodium bread ad lib.	Low-sodium bread ad lib.
Butter, margarine, mayonnaise	Ad lib.	2 tsp. sweet ad lib.	Sweet ad lib.	Sweet ad lib.
Cream	Ad lib.	2 oz.	2 oz.	2 oz.
Vegetables	Ad lib.	Low-sodium ad lib.	Low-sodium ad lib.	Low-sodium ad lib.
Fruits and juices	Ad lib.	Ad lib.	Ad lib.	Ad lib.
Desserts	One serving: cake, gelatin, ice cream, pie, pudding, sherbet.	Special low-sodium only.	Special low-sodium only.	Special low-sodium only.
Cereals and starches	Ad lib.	Low-sodium only.	Low-sodium only.	Low-sodium only.

5...

Fluid & Electrolyte Therapy

WATER METABOLISM

BODY WATER AND ITS DISTRIBUTION

The total body water comprises 40-65% of total body weight (avg., 55% for adult men and 47% for adult women). The body water is distributed throughout 2 main compartments: the extracellular compartment (plasma and interstitial fluid), which contains about one-fourth of the total body water; and the intracellular compartment, which contains about three-fourths of the total body water.

Distribution of Body Water in the Male

Fluid Compartment	Per Cent of Body Weight	ml. of Water in a 154 lb. (70 Kg.) Man
Extracellular water		
Plasma	4-5 %	3,200
Interstitial fluid	11-12%	7,300
Intracellular water	40-45%	31,500

The considerable variation in percentage of body weight which is water is due mainly to the effect of body composition on the water content of the tissues. The higher the fat content of a given subject, the smaller the percentage of his body weight which is water. If a correction for the fat content of the body is made, the total body water in various subjects is relatively constant when expressed as a percentage of the so-called lean body mass, i.e., the sum of the fat-free tissue. Consideration should be given to this fact when calculating fluid requirements on the basis of body weight in order to avoid excess administration of water to obese patients.

NORMAL WATER LOSSES AND WATER REQUIREMENTS

Water is lost from the body by 4 routes: from the skin, as sensible and insensible perspiration; from the lungs, as water vapor in the expired air; from the kidneys, as urine; and from the intestines, with the feces. In the absence of visible perspiration, the total losses from the skin and the lungs are generally referred to as the "insensible loss." In adults, this loss is considered to be 0.5 ml./Kg./hour (12 ml./Kg./day), i.e., approximately 800 ml./day for the average adult. In children, the insensible loss is somewhat higher when estimated on the basis of body weight, varying from 1.3 ml./Kg./hour in infants to 0.6 ml./Kg./hour in the older child.

The normal daily water losses and water allowances are summarized in the following table:

Daily Water Losses and Water Requirements for Normal Individuals Who Are Not Working or Sweating

	Losses				Requirements	
	Urine (ml.)	Stool (ml.)	Insensible (ml.)	Total (ml.)	ml./ person	ml./ Kg.
Infant (2-10 Kg.)	200-500	25-40	75-300 (1.3 ml./ Kg./hr.)	300-840	330-1000	165-100
Child (10-40 Kg.)	500-800	40-100	300-600	840-1500	1000-1800	100-45
Adolescent or Adult (60 Kg.)	800-1000	100	600-1000 (0.5 ml./ Kg./hr.)	1500-2100	1800-2500	45-30

ADDITIONAL WATER REQUIREMENTS IN DISEASE

Insensible losses may rise much higher than normal postoperatively or in febrile or debilitated states. The quantity of fluid lost from the surface of the body may also be very large in the extensively burned patient.

In high environmental temperatures or when visible sweating occurs for any reason, additional water must also be provided to replace the additional losses of sensible perspiration. It is difficult to estimate these losses accurately. During moderate sweating the fluid lost is about 300-500 ml./day, but in cases where extreme sweating occurs the losses may exceed 2000-3000 ml./day.

Water loss from the gastrointestinal tract is negligible under normal circumstances. However, this route of loss may assume great importance in patients with prolonged diarrhea or vomiting, in cases where nasogastric suction is in use, or where there is drainage from fistulas or an ileostomy.

In kidney disease in which the ability to form a concentrated urine may be impaired, such as chronic nephritis, nephrosclerosis, or pyelonephritis, it may be necessary to provide additional fluid. This is illustrated in the table below, which relates the daily volume of urine necessary for removal of metabolic wastes to the concentrating power of the kidney expressed in terms of the sp. gr. of the urine. On a regular diet, 50-60 Gm. of metabolic wastes must be excreted daily (approximately 1.5-2 Gm./100 Calories metabolized). This may be reduced to 30-35 Gm./day by decreasing the protein intake. From the table it is evident that a patient on a normal diet who is unable to form a urine more concentrated than sp. gr. 1.010-1.014 must be given enough fluid to permit a daily urine output of as much as 2100 ml. if uremia is to be avoided.

Relation Between Urine Volume Necessary to Remove Metabolic Wastes and Concentrating Power of Kidney (Expressed as Sp. Gr. of the Urine)

Sp. Gr. of Urine	Urine Volume	
	35 Gm. Load of Metabolic Wastes	50 Gm. Load of Metabolic Wastes
1.032-1.029	500	700
1.028-1.025	600	850
1.024-1.020	700	1000
1.019-1.015	850	1200
1.014-1.010	1200	2100

ESTIMATION OF WATER LOSSES

An accurate record of the quantity and source of the fluid lost by all routes is of utmost importance for proper replacement therapy. This ordinarily includes measurement of daily urinary excretion and of any fluid recovered from the gastrointestinal tract. It is often difficult to obtain an accurate measurement of total fluid losses when a major category of loss is from perspiration, from exudation (as in burns), from diarrhea, or when fluid is lost into dressings. In such circumstances, daily weighing of the patient is of great value. In many hospitals special bedside scales are available for patients who cannot be weighed on the usual scales.

Patients maintained on parenteral fluids (and seriously ill patients generally) cannot be expected to gain weight unless they are overhydrated. Properly hydrated adult patients should normally lose 0.5-1 lb./day until adequate nutrition can be established during convalescence. If rapid losses in weight occur, the patient must be presumed to be dehydrated. The table below shows the approximate relationship between the extent of a rapidly occurring weight loss and the degree of dehydration.

Relation of Acute Weight Loss to Degree of Dehydration

Weight Loss Expressed as % of Normal (or Preoperative) Body Weight	Degree of Dehydration
Loss of 4% body weight	Mild
Loss of 6% body weight	Moderate
Loss of 8% body weight	Severe

Because such rapidly occurring weight losses are due mainly to loss of fluid, the extent of the loss may be used to estimate the amount of fluid to be replaced. Each Kg. of weight loss is assumed to be equivalent to 1 L. of fluid.

An exception to the foregoing remarks concerning the relationship between acute weight loss and dehydration must be made in the case of receding edema or a diuresis after administration of diuretic agents.

FLUID REQUIREMENTS IN THE IMMEDIATE POSTOPERATIVE PERIOD

During the immediate postoperative period the posterior pituitary and the adrenal cortex, in responding to the stress of the operation, cause excessive retention of water (increased antidiuretic effect) and sodium. Urinary output then becomes a poor guide to the need for fluid; in fact, oliguria at this time may be considered a normal physiologic response, particularly after severe stress and/or trauma. Additional fluid given under these circumstances in an effort to increase the urinary output will not only be ineffective but may actually result in serious overhydration. It is therefore recommended that during the first postoperative day conservative amounts of water (e.g., up to 1500 ml./day for an adult) and no electrolyte be given unless significant gastrointestinal losses have occurred, in which case small amounts (50-75 mEq.) of sodium salts may be given. As noted above, patients can be expected to lose 0.5-1 lb./day during the first few days after surgery. The absence of a weight loss or a gain in weight is strong presumptive evidence for overhydration.

INTERNAL LOSSES OF FLUID AND ELECTROLYTE

The extracellular fluid space may be depleted of both fluid and electrolyte by losses into fluid spaces newly created by a disease process. Examples are the accumulation of fluid in the edema of burns; in an area of infection, as within a serous cavity; or in the intestine during ileus. The fluid and electrolyte thus lost results in what may be termed "internal dehydration." Unless prompt and adequate replacement of these losses is made, the effect on the circulating plasma volume will be just as serious as if the losses had been external.

These fluids will be reabsorbed later unless they have been removed (as by suction in a case of ileus), and the replacement of fluid and electrolyte must be reduced to compensate for this. In the case of a burn, resolution of fluid pooled outside the circulation usually begins after 48-72 hours, whereas a longer period is required in the case of infection or trauma.

ELECTROLYTE METABOLISM

ELECTROLYTE COMPOSITION OF BODY FLUIDS

The table on p. 154 lists the concentrations of the various inorganic salts (electrolytes) in the plasma and in the cells. It will be noted that the electrolyte composition of intracellular fluid differs from that of the plasma in that potassium (rather than sodium) is the principal cation, and phosphate (rather than chloride) is the principal anion. The amount of protein within the cell is also considerably larger than that in its extracellular environment.

Normal Electrolyte Composition of Body Fluids

	Atomic or Radicular Weight	mEq. Wt. (mg.)	Extracellular Fluid (Plasma) mEq./L. (Avg.)	Extracellular Fluid (Plasma) mEq./L. (Range)	Extracellular Fluid (Plasma) mg./100 ml.	Intracellular Fluid (Muscle) mEq./L. (Avg.)
Cations						
Na^+	23	23	143	135-147	310-340	13
K^+	39	39	5	4.6-5.6	18-22	140
Ca^{++}	40	20	5	4.5-5.5	9-11	Trace
Mg^{++}	24	12	2	1.5-3.0	1.8-3.6	45
Total			155			198
Anions						
Cl^-	35	35	103	100-112	350-390	3
(As NaCl)	(58)	(58)			(590-660)	
HCO_3^-*	-	-	27	25-30	56-65†	10
$HPO_4^=$ (as P)‡	31	17.2	2	1.8-2.3	3-4	100
SO_4 (as S)	32	16	1			20
Org. Acids§	-	-	6			Trace
Protein§	-	-	16			65
Total			155			198

*HCO_3^- is measured as CO_2 content and frequently reported in Vol.% (ml./100 ml. plasma). To convert Vol.% of CO_2 to mEq./L. HCO_3^-, divide Vol.% by 2.24.

†Vol.%.

‡The inorganic phosphorus in the serum exists as a buffer mixture in which approximately 80% is in the form of $HPO_4^=$ and 20% as $H_2PO_4^-$. For this reason the mEq. weight is usually calculated by dividing the atomic weight of phosphorus by 1.8. Thus, the mEq. weight for phosphorus in the serum is taken as 31/1.8 = 17.2.

§The organic acids and the proteins are expressed in terms of their combining power with cations. For protein, the cation equivalence in mEq. is calculated by multiplying the number of grams of total protein/100 ml. by 2.43.

The chemical reactivity of the various electrolytes in the body fluids cannot be evaluated when their concentrations are given only in accordance with their weights in a given volume (e.g., mg./100 ml.) any more than the work performance (horsepower) of an electric motor can be expressed merely in terms of its weight. In order to convert electrolyte concentrations to a common unit which expresses the individual contribution of each to the total chemical reactivity of all, it is necessary to express their concentrations in mEq./unit of volume.

The mEq. weight of an element is simply its atomic weight divided by its valence (number of electric changes carried by the element). In the above table the mEq. weights of the electrolytes of the body fluids are listed. To convert a concentration of an electrolyte from mg./100 ml. to mEq./L., the formula shown below is used:

$$\frac{\text{mg./100 ml.} \times 10}{\text{mEq. weight}} = \text{mEq./L.}$$

For example, if the concentration of plasma sodium is reported as 322 mg./100 ml., the equivalent concentration is 140 mEq./L.:

$$\frac{322 \times 10}{23} = 140 \text{ mEq./L.}$$

COMPOSITION OF GASTROINTESTINAL SECRETIONS AND SWEAT

The volume and composition of gastrointestinal secretions and sweat are shown in the table below. It will be noted that large quantities of fluid and electrolyte are normally secreted into the gastrointestinal tract but that almost all are subsequently reabsorbed (mainly in the colon), as evidenced by the normal minimal losses of fluid and electrolyte in the feces. When reabsorption is impaired, as may occur during vomiting, diarrhea, obstruction, or a fistulous process such as a biliary or pancreatic fistula, or when fluid is removed by nasogastric suction or is lost in a recent ileostomy, depletion of fluid and electrolyte can occur rapidly. **Note:** In surgical patients such gastrointestinal losses are the principal causes of severe dehydration and electrolyte depletion.

Other disorders in which disturbances of fluid and electrolyte metabolism are prominent include diabetes mellitus, congestive heart failure, hepatic cirrhosis, Addison's disease, kidney disease, extensive burns, and shock.

Volume and Composition of Gastrointestinal Secretions and Sweat*

Fluid	Avg. Volume (ml./24 hr.)	Electrolyte Concentrations (mEq./L.)			
		Na^+	K^+	Cl^-	HCO_3^-
Blood plasma†		135-150	3.6-5.5	100-105	24.6-28.8
Gastric juice	2500	31-90	4.3-12	52-124	0
Bile	700-1000	134-156	3.9-6.3	83-110	38
Pancreatic juice	>1000	113-153	2.6-7.4	54-95	110
Small bowel (Miller-Abbott suction)	3000	72-120	3.5-6.8	69-127	30
Ileostomy					
Recent	100-4000	112-142	4.5-14	93-122	30
Adapted	100-500	50	3	20	15-30
Cecostomy	100-3000	48-116	11.1-28.3	35-70	15
Feces	100	<10	<10	<15	<15
Sweat	500-4000	30-70	0-5	30-70	0

*After J.S. Lockwood and H.T. Randall, Bull. New York Acad. Med. **25**:228, 1949; and H.T. Randall, S. Clin. North America **32**:3, 1952.

†Blood plasma included for purposes of comparison.

mEq. /L.	Normal	Respiratory Acidosis and Alkalosis				Metabolic Acidosis and Alkalosis			
		Acidosis	Compensation	Alkalosis	Compensation	Acidosis	Compensation	Alkalosis	Compensation
$H.HCO_3$	1.35	> 1.35	> 1.35	< 1.35	< 1.35	1.35	< 1.35	1.35	> 1.35
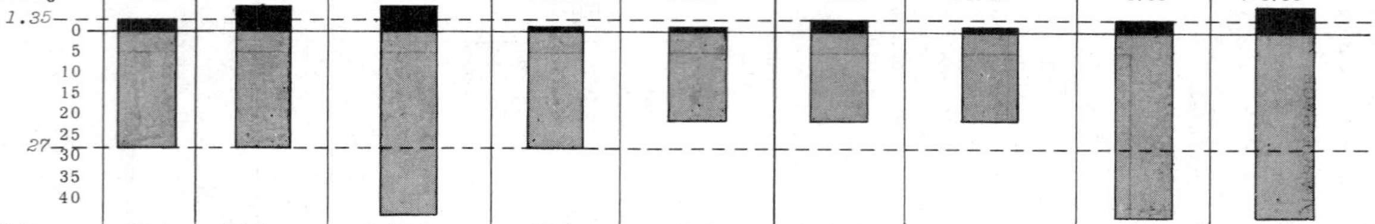									
$B.HCO_3$	27.0	27.0	> 27.0	27.0	< 27.0	< 27.0	< 27.0	> 27.0	> 27.0
Serum pCO_2		Increased	Increased	Decreased	Decreased		Decreased		Increased
$B.HCO_3$ / $H.HCO_3$	20/1	< 20/1	20/1	> 20/1	20/1	< 20/1	20/1	> 20/1	20/1
pH	7.4	< 7.35	7.4	> 7.45	7.4	< 7.35	7.4	> 7.45	7.4
Mechanism		Acidosis is due to retention of CO_2 resulting from improper ventilation. Compensation occurs with saving of fixed base by renal synthesis of NH_4.		Alkalosis due to excessive blowing off of CO_2. Compensation occurs by renal excretion of fixed base.		Acidosis results from loss of fixed base and/or accumulation of organic or fixed acids. Compensation occurs by the blowing off of CO_2 if respiratory mechanism is normal.		Due usually to excessive K^+ loss, loss of acid, or, rarely, alkali ingestion. Compensation occurs by CO_2 retention.	
Diseases or Causes		Any disease interfering with proper respiration: pneumonia, emphysema, congestive failure, asthma, poorly functioning respirator.		Hyperventilation, voluntary, psychological, or overuse of resp. aids (e.g., respirator). Liver failure.		Renal loss (failure), diabetic acidosis, loss of base from GI tract, other causes.		Urinary K^+ loss without replacement, gastric vomiting, or, rarely, alkali ingestion.	
Treatment		Treat underlying disease and attempt to improve ventilation. Base is rarely used. Correction will result when disease resolves or is corrected and excess CO_2 is "blown off."		Hold breath, rebreathe into paper bag, breathe 5% CO_2-O_2, remove cause. Correction will occur, fixed base will return to normal by body's retention of base.		Remove excessive anions and replace fixed base by the use of fluids and electrolytes (if diminished). Correction of HCO_3^- results from respiratory retention of CO_2.		Replace K^+ deficit (large doses of K^+ are often necessary) and any Na^+ deficit indicated by using Cl^- salt. May use NH_4Cl but with caution.	

ACID-BASE BALANCE

The laboratory detection of disturbances of acid-base balance is best accomplished by measurement of the pH of the arterial blood and of the total CO_2 in the plasma (plasma CO_2 content). Carbonic acid (H_2CO_3) and bicarbonate (HCO_3^-) (as well as small amounts of physically dissolved CO_2, which need not be considered) constitute the measured total CO_2 of the plasma. When the pH of the blood is normal (pH 7.4), it may be assumed that 1 part of H_2CO_3 is present for each 20 parts of HCO_3^-. As long as this ratio is maintained, the pH of the blood remains normal.

RESPIRATORY ACIDOSIS AND ALKALOSIS

The content of H_2CO_3 in the blood is under the control of the respiratory system because of the effect of respiratory elimination of CO_2 on the following reaction:

$$CO_2 + H_2O \rightleftharpoons H_2CO_3$$

Disturbances in acid-base balance which are due to alterations in content of H_2CO_3 in the blood are said to be respiratory in origin. Thus, respiratory acidosis will occur if CO_2 and consequently H_2CO_3 accumulate in the blood. Examples are pneumonia, emphysema, congestive failure, asthma, and inadequate ventilation during anesthesia and in the postanesthetic period. Depression of the respiratory center, as by overdosage of morphine or other respiratory depressants, may also be a cause of respiratory acidosis.

Compensation for respiratory acidosis occurs by an increase in plasma bicarbonate to restore the normal 1:20 ratio between carbonic acid and bicarbonate at which the blood pH is normal. The total CO_2 is therefore elevated in compensated respiratory acidosis.

Respiratory alkalosis will occur when the rate of elimination of CO_2 is excessive so that blood H_2CO_3 is reduced. This may be brought about by voluntary or forced hyperventilation. Examples are hysterical hyperventilation, CNS disease affecting the respiratory system, the early stages of salicylate poisoning, the hyperpnea occurring at high altitudes, or injudicious use of respirators. Respiratory alkalosis may also occur in patients in hepatic coma.

In respiratory alkalosis compensation occurs by a decrease in plasma bicarbonate; the total CO_2 is therefore decreased in compensated respiratory alkalosis.

These changes are illustrated in the chart on p. 156.

METABOLIC ACIDOSIS AND ALKALOSIS

Disturbances in acid-base balance which are due to alterations in content of bicarbonate in the blood are said to be metabolic in origin. A deficit of bicarbonate will produce a metabolic acidosis; an excess of bicarbonate, a metabolic alkalosis. Compensation occurs by adjustments of the H_2CO_3 concentration - in the first instance by elimination of CO_2 (hyperventilation) and in the latter instance by retention of CO_2 (depressed respirations). The total CO_2 content of the plasma will be lower than normal in metabolic acidosis and higher than normal in metabolic alkalosis. These changes are illustrated in the chart on p. 156.

Metabolic acidosis is the most common type of acidosis. It occurs in uncontrolled diabetes with ketosis, in some cases of vomiting (when the fluids lost are not acid), in renal disease, or after poisoning by an acid salt. In surgical patients, metabolic acidosis most frequently occurs after excessive loss of intestinal fluids, particularly from the lower small intestine and colon (diarrhea and colitis), or after losses of pancreatic and biliary secretions. This is readily understandable in view of the high bicarbonate concentrations of these fluids (see table on p. 114). Increased respirations (hyperpnea) are an important sign of uncompensated metabolic acidosis.

Metabolic alkalosis. - A simple alkali excess can be produced by the chronic ingestion of large quantities of alkali, as might occur in patients under treatment for peptic ulcer; but perhaps the most common type of metabolic alkalosis is that which occurs as a consequence of high intestinal obstruction (as in pyloric stenosis), after prolonged vomiting, or after the excessive removal of gastric secretions containing hydrochloric acid (as in nasogastric suction). A chloride deficit develops because of the loss of secretions which are low in sodium but high in chloride (e.g., hydrochloric acid). The chloride ions are then replaced by bicarbonate. The resultant electrolyte disturbance is thus aptly termed "hypochloremic alkalosis." Almost invariably in surgical patients, hypochloremic alkalosis is accompanied by potassium deficiency, and the alkalosis is enhanced and persists as long as the potassium deficit remains. It is for this reason that the treatment of hypochloremic alkalosis is accomplished mainly by the provision of relatively large quantities of potassium (see p. 162).

Hypochloremic alkalosis may also occur in Cushing's disease and during administration of corticotropin or cortisone.

METABOLISM OF SODIUM

IMPORTANCE OF SODIUM IN WATER BALANCE

The maintenance of both the volume and the distribution of fluids in the body is almost entirely a function of the inorganic electrolytes, principally salts of sodium and potassium. For this reason the sum of the sodium and potassium concentrations in the body best defines the status of the total body water. However, in the extracellular fluid, salts of sodium are the most important in regulating the volume of this fluid because sodium salts constitute the great majority of the extracellular electrolyte. For this reason changes in total body sodium or its distribution in the body are immediately reflected by changes in body water. A sodium-depleted patient must necessarily become dehydrated, and such a patient cannot be rehydrated unless the sodium deficit is simultaneously corrected. Conversely, retention of sodium or its administration in excess is usually associated with overhydration, often detectable by the appearance of excess extracellular fluid (i.e., edema).

The effect of excess sodium in producing and maintaining edema is enhanced in the presence of hypoproteinemic states (particularly hypoalbuminemia). Hypoproteinemia commonly occurs in chronic disease (e.g., cirrhosis), in malnourished patients (who may come to surgery in a semi-starved condition), and in patients for whom adequate nutrition must be unduly postponed postoperatively.

Mobilization of excess body sodium and restriction of sodium intake is essential to reduce the overhydration of edematous patients. This may be accomplished by the use of diuretic agents, which increase elimination of sodium salts in the urine; in severely hypoproteinemic patients, it may also be useful to administer salt-poor albumin to aid in mobilizing edema fluid.

INTERPRETATION OF THE SERUM SODIUM

Measurement of the serum sodium is frequently employed in an effort to ascertain the status of a patient with regard to sodium and thus to investigate an important phase of water balance as well as acid-base balance. However, such a measurement does not necessarily reflect total body sodium because the amount of water in the body affects the **concentration** of many substances in the plasma, including the plasma electrolytes. Serum sodium determinations should thus be interpreted (in the light of the clinical circumstances) as a reflection of the **relationship** between sodium and water. The insight thus gained into the sodium status of the patient can be used in determining the need for (1) administering or withholding sodium, in cases where the serum sodium is low or normal; (2) administering more sodium than water (hypertonic solutions); or (3) rigidly restricting sodium and rapidly administering sodium-free fluids, as in hypernatremic states.

The relationship of serum sodium concentration to total body sodium in various clinical states is summarized on p. 160. It will be noted that a serum sodium may be low in the presence of high, normal, or low total body sodium. Similar variations are possible with a normal or high serum sodium. It is therefore important to correlate measurements of serum sodium with pertinent clinical observations as a proper guide to fluid and electrolyte therapy.

As already noted, edema is a sign of an increase in body water. In edematous states, regardless of the apparent concentration of sodium in the serum, it can be concluded that the total body sodium is actually increased. Electrolyte therapy to raise the serum sodium is not indicated.

Low serum sodium in the presence of a normal total body sodium, which is a sign of excess water intake, is a feature of so-called "dilutional hyponatremia." If excessive amounts of water are given rapidly, water intoxication will occur.* These syndromes are observed in surgical patients given excessive amounts

---

*A useful diagnostic aid in the dilutional states is the measurement of Hgb. and PCV on the same sample of blood. A normal Hgb. appears to be low, whereas the PCV will appear to be high. The Hgb.

[Note cont'd. on p. 161.]

RELATIONSHIP OF SERUM SODIUM TO TOTAL BODY SODIUM IN VARIOUS CLINICAL STATES

Serum Sodium	Total Body Sodium	Clinical States	Fluid and Electrolyte Therapy
Low (hyponatremia) < 130 mEq. /L.	High	Edematous states (e.g., nephrosis, cirrhosis, cardiac disease). May also occur after severe burns and in the immediate post-operative period.	Not indicated to raise serum sodium.
	Normal	Patients on low sodium intake retaining water as a metabolic response to trauma or surgery, particularly if given excess water (dilution syndrome; water intoxication). May also occur in cirrhotic patients after paracentesis.	Mild: Restrict fluids. Severe: Hypertonic (3-6%) sodium chloride solution may be needed.
	Low	Addison's disease; salt-wasting nephritis; gastrointestinal fluid and electrolyte losses; prolonged sweating with free access to water; perhaps in prolonged use of diuretic agents and on salt-free diets.	Isotonic sodium chloride solution.
Normal 135-145 mEq. /L.	High	Renal, cardiac, or hepatic disease; also carcinoma involving pleural or peritoneal cavities. Caused by renal retention of water and salt in the same osmotic ratio.	
	Low	In the early stages of rapid salt depletion from gastrointestinal losses, renal excretion of a dilute urine preserves osmolarity of body fluids. A similar situation prevails in diabetic acidosis.	
High (hypernatremia) > 150 mEq. /L.	High	Excess administration of sodium salts.	Water by mouth or dextrose and water I.V. Withhold electrolytes.
	Normal	Simple dehydration due to deprivation of water; diabetes insipidus (congenital, or acquired, as in the diuretic phase of acute renal insufficiency or after cerebral trauma).	
	Low	Prolonged sweating without access to water.	Hypotonic sodium chloride solution.

of electrolyte-free fluids, particularly in the immediate postoperative period when water requirements are reduced because of the retention of fluid which normally occurs as a result of stress (see p. 153).

In mild dilutional hyponatremia, restriction of fluid may be all that is required to return the serum sodium to normal. If signs of acute water intoxication are apparent, hypertonic (3-6%) solutions of sodium chloride may be needed.

The therapy of hyponatremic states with low total body sodium usually requires both salt and water because the patient is both salt-depleted and dehydrated. Isotonic saline solutions are therefore used for replacement therapy of these patients.

The patient with a high serum sodium is usually water depleted, so that water by mouth (or dextrose and water by vein) is indicated to return the serum sodium to normal. Electrolyte must be withheld, particularly in cases where the cause of the hypernatremia is excess administration of salt.

METABOLISM OF POTASSIUM

Potassium is the chief cation of the intracellular fluid. Like sodium in the extracellular fluid, it influences acid-base balance and the retention of water. Because potassium is almost entirely an intracellular component, the levels of potassium in the serum may not accurately reflect the true potassium status of the patient. As with sodium, the significance of serum potassium levels must be interpreted by correlation with clinical observations.

High levels of potassium in the serum (hyperkalemia) are not indicative of an excess of total body potassium but rather of excessive loss from the cell accompanied by some degree of failure of the kidney to excrete potassium, as in renal failure, advanced dehydration, or shock. Hyperkalemia may also occur if potassium is administered at an excessive rate, usually by the intravenous route.

The clinical manifestations of hyperkalemia are chiefly cardiac and CNS depression. Cardiac signs include bradycardia and poor heart sounds, followed by peripheral vascular collapse and, ultimately, cardiac arrest. Ecg. changes are characteristic, and include elevated T waves, widening of the QRS complex, progressive lengthening of the P-R interval, and, finally, disappearance of the P wave. Other symptoms commonly associated with elevated extracellular potassium include mental confusion; weakness, numbness, tingling, and flaccid paralysis of the extremities; and weakness of the respiratory muscles.

A low serum potassium (hypokalemia) is almost inevitably an indication of true potassium depletion, but it must be emphasized that an intracellular deficit of potassium may coexist with normal serum levels.

Potassium deficiencies develop readily during the postoperative period when solutions which do not contain potassium are given intravenously for more than a few days. This occurs because these

---

reflects dilution of the blood; the PCV the swelling of the red cells because of excess accumulation of intracellular water.

patients are in negative nitrogen and caloric balance, so that increased quantities of potassium are lost from the cells and then excreted into the urine. Furthermore, all of the gastrointestinal fluids contain considerable quantities of potassium; removal of these fluids in nasogastric suction, losses from a fistulous process, or diarrhea - all enhance potassium depletion.

Alkalosis favors potassium depletion principally by increasing its excretion into the urine. The adrenocortical hormones, particularly aldosterone, also increase excretion of potassium. Thus the adrenocortical response to severe stress (as after surgery, trauma, or severe burns) further contributes to potassium loss.

Certain of the diuretic drugs, such as acetazolamide (Diamox®) or chlorothiazide (Diuril®), increase potassium excretion. Patients who come to surgery after treatment with adrenocortical steroids or diuretic drugs or who have been malnourished and in negative nitrogen balance for some time must be considered to have a chronic potassium depletion. Such patients may develop severe signs of potassium deficiency very early in the postoperative period.

The persistence of alkalosis after adequate replacement of sodium chloride and water is a strong indication of an underlying potassium deficiency. Other symptoms of a potassium deficit are muscle weakness, irritability, and paralysis. Tachycardia and dilatation of the heart with gallop rhythm are also noted. Characteristic Ecg. changes in hypokalemia are, first, a flattened T wave; later, inverted T waves with a sagging ST segment and atrioventricular block; and finally cardiac arrest.

Because of the occasional unreliability of the serum potassium levels, the Ecg. is of great diagnostic value in that it assesses the cellular status of this element.

Correlation of the Serum Potassium Concentration and the Electrocardiogram (Providing there is no parallel change in Na and Ca)*

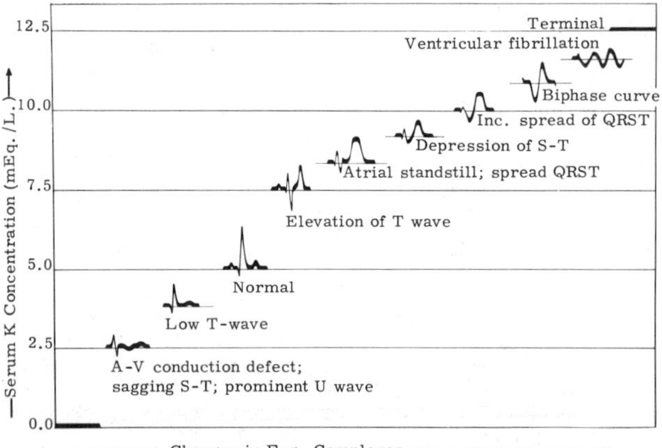

*From Krupp, Sweet, Jawetz, Biglieri, and Roe: Physician's Handbook, 17th Ed. Lange, 1973.

BLOOD AND PLASMA VOLUME

A surgical patient may readily develop a reduction in blood volume because of dehydration, losses of blood and plasma, or chronic undernutrition. Patients who come to surgery with a decreased blood volume are more susceptible to the hypotension which may be induced by anesthetic drugs, or to vascular collapse and shock after even a minimal operative loss of blood. It is therefore important to anticipate this possibility in such patients by a preoperative determination of the blood volume and to correct blood volume deficits before surgery. Because of the wide range of "normal" values for plasma volume (30-65 ml./Kg.) which have been reported, it may also be of value to obtain a measurement of plasma and blood volume preoperatively as a baseline reference for each patient. Such information will be particularly useful if extraordinary losses of blood or plasma require frequent transfusions in the postoperative period. Blood and plasma volume determinations are more useful than measuring simply the PCV or Hct. as a means of assessing the adequacy of replacement of blood or plasma.

MEASUREMENT OF PLASMA AND BLOOD VOLUME

The simplest method of measuring plasma volume is by the use of the blue dye T-1824 (Evans blue). However, the entire blood volume must then be calculated from the Hct. This may not be entirely reliable because the Hct. of the peripheral blood does not necessarily reflect that of the entire blood supply, particularly in pathologic states. For this reason isotopic technics which depend on direct labeling of the red cells are preferred if available. Plasma volume may also be measured by the use of isotopically labeled (I^{131}) human serum albumin. This technic seems to have no particular advantage over the T-1824 method except when repeated determinations at frequent intervals are required.

USE OF BLOOD TRANSFUSIONS

Surgical patients are often found to be anemic, frequently as a result of chronic blood loss. This anemia must be corrected as soon as practicable. In patients who are protein-deficient as well as anemic, the regeneration of Hgb. takes precedence over that of other proteins; consequently, it cannot be expected that the serum proteins will rise until the Hgb. concentration of the blood has first been brought to normal.

Blood transfusions are required to correct anemia only when the loss of blood is acute and/or further bleeding at a rapid rate may be expected. In anemia due to chronic blood loss, iron deficiency is the predominant defect that must be corrected.

Iron deficiency anemia in patients who have sustained chronic losses of blood is of the hypochromic microcytic type. RBC, Hgb., and Hct. determinations are usually sufficient to make a diagnosis of iron deficiency anemia in a patient with a history of chronic blood loss. In these circumstances adequate treatment with iron is all that is required to correct the anemia. Blood transfusions are not required unless the rate of bleeding is very rapid, immediate surgery is required, or the anemia is in itself more dangerous to the patient than the dangers of transfusion.

Normal persons can probably replace blood at a rate of at least 1000 ml./week when sufficient iron is made available; thus in most patients a blood loss of 500-1000 ml./week can be sustained, and some increase in Hgb. can still occur if adequate amounts of iron are supplied. Iron therapy may have to be continued for 3-5 weeks before the Hgb. levels return to normal. Iron must be given by a parenteral route if the patient cannot tolerate iron salts given orally or if absorption of iron from the intestine is inadequate, as is the case after resection of the stomach or in widespread disease of the small intestine.

In treatment of an iron deficiency anemia, Ferrous Sulfate, U.S.P., may be given in a dose of 200 mg. (3 gr.) orally t.i.d. If oral therapy is not possible, a form of iron which can be administered parenterally should be used. The total amount of iron to be given parenterally is determined by providing 1 Gm. to replenish iron stores plus that represented by the Hgb. deficit. If Hgb. is normal (100%), the total body Hgb. contains 3 Gm. of iron. An iron-deficient patient with a Hgb. of 50% would therefore require 1.5 Gm. to provide for the synthesis of Hgb. to a normal level and 1 Gm. to replenish iron stores (total of 2.5 Gm.). Because of the danger of overdosage when iron is given parenterally, it is important to give only that amount of iron which is required to correct the existing iron deficiency.

POSTOPERATIVE MAINTENANCE

POSTOPERATIVE BLOOD AND PLASMA

Prevention of shock due to excessive blood or plasma loss is of first priority. A 30% reduction in the normal circulating blood volume threatens shock, and even a more moderate blood loss may lead to shock if it occurs rapidly or if it occurs in a patient whose blood volume is already low.

Properly cross-matched whole blood is the preferred replacement fluid in most instances of threatened or actual shock or in the presence of excessive hemorrhage. When whole blood is not available, blood plasma or a plasma expander, such as dextran, may be used instead. In the treatment of shock characterized by a high PCV (as in the early phase of severe burns), these latter substances may be preferred until the PCV begins to fall.

POSTOPERATIVE WATER

An accurate record of the quantity and routes of fluid loss is essential to proper replacement therapy. On the basis of such a record, fluids (dextrose and water or dextrose and saline solution) are given to replace the measured losses of the preceding 24-hour period (12 hours for infants) together with additional fluid to compensate the insensible losses.

POSTOPERATIVE ELECTROLYTES

Sodium chloride is given in an amount of 6 Gm./L. of fluid lost by the gastrointestinal route during the preceding 24 hours. This may be administered as "half-normal" (0.45%) sodium chloride or as a "normal" (0.9%) solution in 5 or 10% dextrose. An additional 4.5 Gm. of sodium chloride may be given to compensate losses via urine and sweat. As a rule, all of the fluids prescribed for a patient need not contain electrolytes because a major segment of the 24-hour fluid losses (the insensible perspiration) does not contain electrolytes.

Exceptions to the foregoing are discussed on pp. 150-153.

Potassium should be added to the intravenous regimen when a patient must be maintained on intravenous fluids for more than 2 days. If there has been a preoperative potassium deficiency, potassium should be given postoperatively as soon as practicable. Potassium should ordinarily not be given intravenously if the urinary output is less than 400 ml. in a 24-hour period.

Forty to 50 mEq./day (approximately 4 Gm. KCl) is a satisfactory maintenance dose of potassium for adults if there are no fluid losses from the gastrointestinal tract. Additional amounts of potassium must be given to replace gastrointestinal losses. Approximately 20-25 mEq. of potassium should be given per day for each liter of gastrointestinal fluid which has been lost during the previous day. However, a total of more than 100 mEq. of potassium is seldom required during a single 24-hour period.

Sodium lactate (or sodium bicarbonate) solutions may be required instead of sodium chloride in replacement of fluid losses which predispose to acidosis (see table on p. 155). A useful guide for replacement of gastrointestinal losses is outlined below. This table* relates the proportions of the various fluids to use in replacement of gastrointestinal losses to the source of the loss.

Source of Loss	Dextrose in Water	Dextrose in Saline	M/6 Sodium Lactate
Gastric			
Average	33%	67%	
Low acidity	67%	33%	
Small intestine	20%	70%	10%
Ileostomy	10%	75%	15%
Bile		67%	33%
Pancreas		50%	50%

*Modified from Randall (S. Clin. North America **32**:3, 1952).

PARENTERAL SOLUTIONS
(See table on p. 167.)

Sodium chloride solution is the most commonly employed electrolyte solution. Although so-called "normal" (actually isotonic, 0.85-0.9%) sodium chloride is the most commonly used concentration, there is now a tendency to prefer "half-normal" (hypotonic, 0.45%) solutions with a view to administering the electrolyte over a longer period of time in order to promote better utilization.* It must be emphasized that the total amount of salt required must still be provided regardless of the concentration of sodium chloride in the solutions given.

Hypertonic saline solution (3-6% solutions of sodium chloride) is required in the treatment of acute water intoxication (see p. 161). It may also be given initially (followed by normal saline) in acute sodium depletion.

Sodium lactate is approximately isotonic in a 1/6 molar (M/6) concentration. It is used to repair acidotic states. However, in order to be effective as an alkalinizing agent the lactate radical must be metabolized to bicarbonate; in severe acidosis, or in pathologic states where hepatic function is depressed (as may occur in prolonged hypotension or in shock), sodium bicarbonate may therefore be preferred. This is available in ampuls containing 3.75 Gm. (45 mEq.) in a 50 ml. volume. It is to be added to dextrose and water in the quantity required to provide the calculated need (see p. 169).

Lactated Ringer's injection resembles plasma in its electrolyte concentration. It differs from Ringer's injection by its content of lactate (bicarbonate precursor). The small amounts of potassium and calcium in these solutions are of insignificant value in therapy. The only advantage of lactated Ringer's injection over sodium chloride solutions is in the maintenance of patients who may develop acidosis. The so-called **"balanced electrolyte" solutions** which have recently come into use are somewhat more useful for this purpose because of their higher content of bicarbonate precursors (lactate, citrate, or acetate). Their content of potassium, however, may not be adequate. It is important to emphasize that balanced electrolyte solutions or lactated Ringer's injection should not be used in patients with alkalosis. These solutions are therefore not indicated to replace losses from the stomach or upper small intestine.

Darrow's solution is especially useful for replacement therapy in patients with acidosis and potassium deficiency. Thus it is particularly indicated for deficit therapy of diarrhea, especially in infants and children, and as a replacement fluid in the treatment of diabetic coma.

Ammonium chloride solutions should be used only for the initial treatment of very severe metabolic alkalosis. In most instances increased amounts of potassium chloride together with sodium chloride will satisfactorily correct metabolic alkalosis. Ammonium-containing solutions may be toxic, particularly in the presence of depressed liver function. They should be given slowly and with

---

*The electrolyte-containing solutions are usually made up in at least 5% dextrose solution (isotonic) rather than in water. For this reason all of these solutions are actually hypertonic to varying degrees.

careful attention to development of the neurologic signs of ammonium intoxication.

Calcium gluconate may be required to treat tetany which accompanies uncompensated alkalosis or hypocalcemic states. The usual dose is 10 ml. of a 10% solution I.V., which may be repeated hourly as required for control of symptoms. In alkalosis, correction of the alkalotic state will promptly correct the tetany because the syndrome is in this instance actually attributable to the elevated blood pH rather than to an absolute calcium deficit.

A summary of the various electrolyte repair solutions described above is given in the table below. The solutions described in the table are the standard formulas generally available. However, it is a simple matter to prepare other types of electrolyte repair or maintenance solutions of varying constitution to suit special needs. This is conveniently accomplished by the addition (to 5 or 10% of dextrose in water) of electrolytes prepared in concentrated form in 20 or 40 ml. vials. Many manufacturers supply solutions of potassium chloride containing 20 or 40 mEq. of potassium in a 20 ml. vial; 50 mEq. NaCl in 20 ml. or 100 mEq. in 40 ml.; 50 mEq. of sodium lactate in 20 ml. or 100 mEq. in 40 ml., etc. By the use of these concentrates one can "tailor" solutions for more precise therapeutic purposes than can be served by the fixed formulations usually available. An example of the value of tailored solutions would be their use in the type of electrolyte therapy recommended in the table on p. 165. These special solutions are also of value in the treatment of patients with acute or chronic renal insufficiency, where the day-to-day needs for electrolytes may be highly variable.

Composition of Electrolyte Repair Solutions (in mEq./L.)

	Na^+	K^+	Ca^{++}	Cl^-	HCO_3^-*
Normal saline (0.85% NaCl)	145			145	
Half-normal saline (0.45% NaCl)	77			77	
Hypertonic saline (3% NaCl)	513			513	
1/6 Molar (M/6) sodium lactate	167				167
Lactated Ringer's Injection, U.S.P.	130	4	3	109	28
Ringer's Injection, U.S.P.	147	4	4	155	
Darrow's solution (KNL)	122	35		104	53
Balanced electrolyte solution†	140	10	5	103	55
Ammonium chloride (0.9%)‡				170	
Calcium gluconate (10%)			446		

*As bicarbonate or its precursors (such as lactate, citrate, or acetate).

†Contains also 3 mEq./L. of Mg^{++}.

‡Contains also 170 mEq./L. of NH_4^+.

CALCULATIONS USED FOR REPLACEMENT THERAPY OF ELECTROLYTE DEFICITS

Although some idea of the quantity of electrolyte required to correct an electrolyte deficit is helpful, it must be emphasized that no method of calculation is so completely trustworthy that it can be recommended as a rigid prescription for replacement therapy. Clinical and biochemical response must be used as the primary guide; mathematical calculations are of value only as a preliminary basis for planning fluid and electrolyte therapy.

Sodium Chloride Deficit.

Total body water is used as the basis for calculation of sodium deficits because sodium is directly concerned with the movement of water in and out of cells; in order to correct deficits it may be necessary to supply sufficient osmotic activity to mobilize or retain large quantities of fluid. For the purpose of sodium replacement, 50% of body weight is taken to represent the clinical average of total body water.

Example A:

1. A 70 Kg. patient with a history of excessive sodium and chloride losses which have not been adequately replaced is found to have a serum sodium of 120 mEq./L.
2. The deficit of sodium, based on a normal of 140 mEq./L., is 140 − 120 = 20 mEq./L.
3. Total body water (50% of 70 Kg.) = 35 L.
4. Sodium deficit (20 × 35) = 700 mEq.
5. One L. of 0.9% sodium chloride contains approximately 150 mEq.
6. The total quantity of 0.9% NaCl theoretically required = 700 ÷ 150 = about 4.7 L. (4700 ml.).
7. Give **one-half** (2500 ml.) the calculated dose in 12-24 hours; if biochemical and clinical signs warrant, the remainder can be given in the next 24-48 hours. Remember that deficit therapy must be given in addition to the required maintenance therapy.

Example B: Assume that the patient in Example A has the same low value of serum sodium but that hyponatremia is not due to sodium chloride losses but to excessive water intake (dilutional hyponatremia; water intoxication; see p. 161). If the symptoms are mild, complete restriction of fluid until the serum sodium returns to normal may be all that is needed. However, in severe states of water intoxication, hypertonic solutions of sodium chloride are required. The solutions usually employed range in concentration from 3-6% NaCl. While hypertonic solutions are being used, rigidly restrict fluid intake only as necessary for administration of the hypertonic solution. The degree to which water must be restricted governs the choice of solution, i.e., 3% up to 6%. A 6% solution of NaCl contains approximately 1 mEq. of sodium/ml. Thus, if a 6% solution is used, the volume of solution to be used equals the quantity of sodium required. In

Example A, 700 ml. of a 6% solution would theoretically be required. Again it is to be emphasized that only one-half of the calculated dose would be given in the first 12 hours. After that the patient should be sufficiently improved to permit recalculation of his needs on the basis of another electrolyte determination.

Bicarbonate Deficit.

Use only the extracellular fluid space for calculation of the amount of alkali required. This will probably suggest a dose that is too low for complete correction; but the calculated dose, when given over a 24-hour period, should be adequate for the immediate emergency. A reappraisal of the biochemical and clinical status of the patient can then be made and additional therapy provided to restore the plasma bicarbonate to a normal level.

Example:

1. A 70 Kg. patient with a plasma bicarbonate of 15 mEq./L.
2. Normal plasma bicarbonate = 26 mEq./L.
3. Deficit = 26 − 15 = 11 mEq./L.
4. Extracellular fluid (20% of 70 Kg.) = 14 L.
5. Theoretical bicarbonate deficit = 11 × 14 = 154 mEq.
6. Administer 1 L. (166 mEq.) of M/6 sodium lactate in addition to maintenance therapy to make an initial correction of this bicarbonate deficit.

FLUID THERAPY IN CHILDREN

In children, a larger proportion of the total body water (50% of body weight) is in the extracellular space than is the case in adults (20% of body weight). Furthermore, the average daily output of fluid in an infant is equal to about one-half the extracellular fluid volume, whereas in the adult the output is only about one-seventh the extracellular volume. Because of this rapid turnover of fluid, the infant is able to tolerate only very short periods of negative fluid balance before severe dehydration results. The renal regulation of electrolyte and acid-base balance is also less efficient in the infant than in the older child or adult.

ESTIMATION OF FLUID AND ELECTROLYTE REQUIREMENTS FOR MAINTENANCE IN CHILDREN

The fluid and electrolyte needs of infants and children vary with the age of the child. It is therefore usual to express these requirements on the basis of body weight.

Average requirements for water, electrolyte, and carbohydrate in infants and children are as follows (see also the table on p. 151):

	Water (ml./Kg.)	Sodium (mEq./Kg.)	Potassium (mEq./Kg.)	Dextrose (Gm./Kg.)
Premature	50	1.5	1.5	2
Newborn	40	0.5	0.5	2
4-10 Kg.	120-140	1.8-1.5	1.8-1.5	5
10-20 Kg.	100-80	1.5-1.3	1.5-1.3	4
20-40 Kg.	80-60	1.3-1.0	1.3-1.0	3

Except in premature infants, a solution containing 15 mEq./L. each of sodium, potassium, chloride, and bicarbonate (or bicarbonate precursor, as lactate) is convenient to provide the maintenance requirements listed above. To 900 ml. of 5% dextrose in water, add 90 ml. M/6 sodium lactate (or 16.7 ml. of 7.9% sodium bicarbonate) and 7.5 ml. of 14.9% potassium chloride. The solution may be administered in a quantity determined by the maintenance water requirement shown above. It is desirable that the required fluids and electrolytes be given slowly over the greater part of the 24-hour period for which they are calculated.

The maintenance requirements listed above may be reduced in the immediate postoperative period or in edematous states. They may be increased if activity exceeds quiet bed rest and in conditions characterized by salt loss, such as adrenal insufficiency or salt-losing nephritis, as well as in hyperventilation, fever, and excessive sweating. In fever, increase the requirements 8% per degree Fahrenheit or 12% per degree centigrade. The precautions against administration of potassium in the presence of a reduced urinary output must also be observed; if preoperative potassium deficiency has been corrected, it is not necessary to give potassium until the second postoperative day.

CORRECTION OF FLUID AND ELECTROLYTE DEFICITS

When water and salt **deficits** have been incurred it is necessary to give fluid and electrolyte **in addition** to that required for maintenance. The usual deficits which may be incurred in severe dehydration (after acute loss of 12-15% body weight and with clinically evident signs of dehydration) are shown below.

	Water (ml./Kg.)	Sodium (mEq./Kg.)	Chloride (mEq./Kg.)	Potassium (mEq./Kg.)
Diarrhea	100-150	8-12	7-10	8-14
Pyloric stenosis	150-200	12-17	15-19	10-14
Diabetic acidosis	100-150	6-12	5-9	4-7

In mild dehydration (approximately 5% loss in body weight), reduce the above intakes proportionately.

If extrarenal losses persist it is necessary to continue to give fluid and electrolyte in addition to maintenance requirements. The nature of the electrolyte losses by way of the gastrointestinal tract may be recalled by reference to the table on p. 155. A frequent cause of fluid and electrolyte losses in infants is by way of diarrheal stools. With severe diarrhea the fluid loss approximates 50-70 ml./Kg./day; in less severe cases, 20-40 ml./Kg./day. The electrolyte losses are (in severe cases):

Sodium	3-6 mEq./Kg./day
Potassium	3-5 mEq./Kg./day
Chloride	2-4 mEq./Kg./day

FLUID AND ELECTROLYTE THERAPY IN ACUTE RENAL INSUFFICIENCY

In the oliguria of acute renal insufficiency which may occur as a result of trauma, shock, transfusion reactions, or tissue insult from various causes (so-called lower nephron nephrosis, lower nephron syndrome, etc.) it is important to restrict fluid and electrolyte intake to the minimum requirement. For this reason this syndrome must be diagnosed promptly so that excess administration of fluid and electrolyte - which may easily produce generalized edema and death from respiratory and cardiac failure - can be avoided.

Except for the first few hours after operation, acute renal insufficiency should be suspected in any patient previously well hydrated who exhibits (1) oliguria (less than 400 ml. of urine/day*) in the presence of a normal BP; and (2) urine of low sp. gr. (1.008-1.014).

The fluid intake of the oliguric patient must be strictly limited to that lost by all routes. Ordinarily this will total no more than 500-800 ml./day (12 ml./Kg. for insensible losses plus the output in the urine for the previous 24 hours less 250 ml. produced endogenously as metabolic water of oxidation). If visible perspiration occurs or if there are gastrointestinal losses, as in the presence of diarrhea, vomiting, or gastric suction, these fluid losses must also be replaced. Unless the oliguric patient loses about 0.5-1 lb. of body weight/day he is probably being overhydrated.

Because of tissue breakdown, potassium is liberated in increased quantities. Since potassium cannot under these circumstances be excreted, it may rise to toxic levels in the blood. The accumulation of potassium in the extracellular fluid is perhaps the most serious complication of oliguria. In an attempt to spare tissue breakdown and thus minimize the mobilization of potassium and nitrogenous waste products such as urea, hypertonic (25-50%) solutions of dextrose are used. These must be given slowly with a view to maintaining elevated levels of the blood sugar throughout the 24 hour period. The addition of insulin to hypertonic dextrose solutions aids in the storage of glycogen in the tissues, and this process tends to shift potassium from the extracellular fluid. For this purpose 1 unit of regular insulin may be added for each 2 Gm. of dextrose administered (50 units in 500 ml. of 20% dextrose).

*It is not usual for absolute anuria to occur in these patients. If this does occur, obstructive uropathy should be strongly suspected.

The accumulation of phosphate in the oliguric patient leads to a depression in the blood calcium, which enhances the cardiac toxicity of the elevated serum potassium. Calcium is therefore administered in doses of 50-100 ml. of 10% calcium gluconate added to 500 ml. of the hypertonic dextrose solutions to antagonize the elevation in potassium.

It is obvious with the very restricted electrolyte and fluid intake permitted these patients that complete correction of electrolyte and acid-base imbalance is not possible. However, normal saline and/or M/6 sodium lactate may be used in conservative amounts (250-400 ml./day).

Potassium intoxication may be treated by the use of a sulfonated polystyrene resin in the sodium cycle such as Kayexalate®. The resin may be given by mouth every 4-6 hours, the average dose being 15 Gm. suspended in a minimal amount of fluid. When the resin is being administered orally, a mild laxative should also be given to guard against intestinal impaction. The dose range and duration of therapy vary widely depending on the status of the serum potassium and the Ecg. Frequently the oral route cannot be used because of nausea and vomiting. In such cases the resin can be given every 4 hours by rectum as a retention enema. It is desirable that the resin be retained for about 3 hours and then washed out. This resin is more effective in removing potassium than those previously used for this purpose. Consequently, the effect of therapy with resin on the electrolyte changes in the patient must be carefully appraised at regular intervals.

When urine flow is restored, renal tubular function is still poor, so that disorders of fluid and electrolyte regulation are to be expected. During this so-called "diuretic" phase very careful attention to and the prompt replacement of electrolyte losses is of utmost importance until recovery of renal tubular function is assured.

In severe cases of acute renal insufficiency not amenable to the conservative therapy described above, extracorporeal dialysis may be required. The Travenol coil kidney is of great value in such cases. If this is not available, intermittent peritoneal lavage may be indicated. A simplified procedure and the indications for the use of this technic have been described by Doolan et al. (Am. J. Med. **26**:831, 1959). Where it is applicable, peritoneal lavage can be attempted in any hospital because it requires no special equipment or dialyzing solutions that are not readily available.

ROUTES OF PARENTERAL FLUID ADMINISTRATION

VENOCLYSIS

Solutions containing glucose, electrolytes, or amino acids, as well as fat emulsions, and whole blood or plasma fractions, may all be administered intravenously. Fluids which are isotonic and of a neutral pH are tolerated best. Pure water must never be given intravenously because it will cause hemolysis. When electrolyte-free solutions are required in therapy, solutions of 5-10% dextrose in water are used. Solutions of sugars which are more hypertonic than that of a 10% glucose solution produce phlebitis and obliteration of veins when administered for other than a very short period. If hypertonic solutions are necessary, as may be the case in patients who require an increased caloric intake in a small volume (such as in acute renal insufficiency; see p. 74), the infusions should be made through a polyethylene cannula threaded high into a large vein with a free flow of blood (see below).

Sites for Venoclysis.

The veins of the forearm and of the back of the hand are preferred. Infusions into the antecubital vein have the disadvantage of requiring prolonged extension of the elbow. The long saphenous vein in the leg and its tributaries on the dorsum of the foot are convenient, but occasionally a deep femoral phlebitis results. Femoral vein puncture about 3 cm. below the inguinal ligament, using the femoral artery (which lies just lateral to the vein) as a landmark, may be necessary in emergencies when safer and more superficial veins are temporarily inaccessible. The scalp veins of infants can be punctured with a No. 24-21 gauge needle. The superior longitudinal sinus should not be used.

Venous Cut-down.

When prolonged, continuous infusion is needed, when venipuncture is difficult, when a secure infusion is essential, when rapid infusion is important, or when emergency situations combine these indications, it is advisable to ''cut down'' on a vein in order to tie a cannula or polyethylene tube in place. The distal saphenous vein, lying just anteromedial to the medial malleolus of the tibia, is first choice. When repeated cut-downs are necessary, this vein (which has a fairly predictable course) may be exposed and cannulated at successively higher levels between the ankle and groin. Alternatively, the median cubital or the basilic vein of the antecubital region (there are many variations of venous anatomy here) or any other sizable superficial vein may be chosen.

Rate of Administration.

Isotonic and hypotonic solutions may usually be given intravenously at a rate of 250-500 ml./hour. When glucose is present in the infusion, the rate of administration should not exceed 0.5-0.75 Gm. of glucose/Kg. body weight/hour to avoid glycosuria and diuresis (e.g., in a 70 Kg. patient, 1000 ml. of 5% glucose solution should take at least 90-120 minutes to administer). Potassium should usually not be administered faster than 20 mEq./hour.

HYPODERMOCLYSIS

This procedure consists of the subcutaneous administration of isotonic fluid, usually by gravity flow from a reservoir. In surgical patients, the chief indication for hypodermoclysis is inability to find a vein for venoclysis. In small infants this occurs frequently; in adults it occurs very rarely.

Only fluids which are approximately isotonic should be given subcutaneously. Glucose, 2.5%, in 0.45% saline is a satisfactory solution, or physiologic saline or Ringer's injection may be given. Glucose, 5% in water, is acceptable but causes more local reaction and is definitely contraindicated in debilitated elderly patients.

In adults the subcutaneous tissues of the anterior or lateral aspect of the mid thigh are preferred. In small infants, fluid can also be injected subcutaneously in the upper back, axillas, and lower abdomen, using a 20-50 ml. syringe and No. 20 gauge needle.

In infants, up to 50 ml. can be injected into each of several sites at 1 time to a total volume of up to 30-40 ml./Kg. body weight. In adults, 750 ml. can be injected into each thigh at 1 time at a rate of 250-500 ml./hour for each thigh. The practical maximum which can be absorbed in 1 day is 3000-4000 ml. Hyaluronidase (250 viscosity units/500-1000 ml. of fluid) will increase the absorption rate about 12 times if it is injected into the tubing at the beginning of the clysis, or into the solution. Hyaluronidase is contraindicated with solutions containing large amounts of potassium, as it may produce excessively rapid absorption. Two ml. of 1% procaine added to each 1500 ml. of solution lessens the discomfort of the clysis.

Precautions.

A. Never give concentrations of glucose greater than 5% to any patient, as sloughing of tissues may occur.
B. Avoid over-distention of tissues because it will cause avascularity and necrosis. Whenever the skin over a subcutaneous clysis becomes blanched, discontinue the clysis temporarily or select another site.
C. Rigid aseptic technic is necessary to avoid cellulitis and abscess formation.

6 . . .

Surgical Infections *

ANTIMICROBIAL THERAPY OF SURGICAL INFECTIONS

Principles of Therapy.

A. Identify the infecting organism and choose an antimicrobial drug on the basis of sensitivity studies whenever possible. Once bacteriologic specimens are obtained it is justifiable, when necessary, to start therapy on the basis of clinical judgment, although the choice of drug may have to be reconsidered when laboratory investigation is complete. Because of the possibility of acquired resistance or change in the bacterial flora, culture and sensitivity studies should be repeated at intervals (e.g., weekly) if infection continues.

B. Treat clinically significant infections only. Minor or superficial infections are best treated with conservative local measures. Indiscriminate use of antimicrobial agents may lead to toxic reactions, drug sensitization, the emergence of resistant strains of bacteria, and disturbances in the mechanisms of host resistance.

C. Give adequate doses of an effective drug and discontinue administration as soon as possible. In most surgical infections, response will be apparent within 5 days if the drug and dosage are properly chosen and if there are no undrained foci of infection. The dosages usually employed are listed in the following pages. Pediatric dosages are listed on pp. 176-177.

D. Use combinations of antimicrobial agents only when required (1) to treat mixed infections, (2) to prevent emergence of resistant mutants (as in antituberculosis therapy), or (3) to obtain additive or synergistic effects in overwhelming infections (e.g., enterococcal sepsis).

E. Do not substitute chemotherapy for definitive surgical measures such as the drainage of abscesses.

F. Avoid "prophylactic" antibacterial therapy to prevent infection in clean wounds except for definite indications (see below).

G. Avoid topical administration of absorbable systemic drugs (especially penicillin and sulfonamides). Such "sensitizing" applications may form the basis of a severe hypersensitivity reaction upon later systemic use. Irrigation of operative wounds with antibiotics probably does not reduce the incidence of wound infection.

---

*The section on antimicrobial drugs is contributed by Ernest Jawetz, PhD, MD.

PEDIATRIC DOSAGES OF ANTIBIOTIC AND CHEMOTHERAPEUTIC AGENTS

(NOTE: Premature infants and newborns should receive one-half of lower dose of parenteral medication.)

Drug	Oral	Intramuscular	Intravenous	Intrapleural Intra-articular Intraperitoneal
Aminosalicylic acid	0.5-2 Gm. 4 times daily		0.5-2 Gm. 4 times daily (30 mg./ml.)	
Bacitracin	2000 units/Kg./day in 4 doses (not absorbed)	600-1200 units/Kg./day in 2 doses.	200-250 units/Kg./day (premature, newborn)	1000 units/ml.
Cephalothin	Not absorbed	40-80 mg./Kg./day in 4 doses (deeply I. M.)	Same as I. M.	
Chloramphenicol*	50-100 mg./Kg./day in 4 doses	100-150 mg./Kg./day in 4 doses†	Same as I. M.	5 mg./ml.
Colistin	5 mg./Kg./day in 3 doses (not absorbed)	2-5 mg./Kg./day in divided doses		
Erythromycin	30-40 mg./Kg./day in 4 doses		40-50 mg./Kg./day in 4 doses	1 mg./ml.
Gentamicin	5-10 mg./Kg./day in 4 doses	3-5 mg./Kg./day in divided doses every 6-8 hours	Same as I.M., but experience is limited	
Isoniazid	15-20 mg./Kg./day in 2-4 doses	10 mg./Kg./day in 2 doses		
Neomycin, kanamycin	100 mg./Kg./day in 4 doses (not absorbed)	10-15 mg./Kg./ lay in 4 doses		2 mg./ml.
Nitrofurantoin	5 mg./Kg./day in 4 doses		6 mg./Kg./day in 2 doses	
Novobiocin	20-45 mg./Kg./day in 4 doses	15-40 mg./Kg./day in 2 doses		
Penicillins				
Ampicillin	50-200 mg./Kg./day in 4 doses	Same as oral		

Benzathine penicillin G	300,000 units 4 times daily	600,000 or 1,200,000 units as single injection		
Cloxacillin	<20 Kg., 50-100 mg./Kg./day. >20 Kg., same as adult.			
Methicillin		100-300 mg./Kg./day in 4 doses. (Total: 6-8 Gm./day.)	Same as I. M.	
Nafcillin	25 mg./Kg./day in 4 doses	25 mg./Kg. 1-2 times daily	Same as I. M.	
Oxacillin	<20 Kg., 50-100 mg./Kg./day. >20 Kg. 500 mg. every 4-6 hours. (Total: 3-6 Gm./day.)			
Penicillin G, V	100,000-400,000 units 4 times daily (penicillin G, buffered, or penicillin V p.c.)	20,000-50,000 units/Kg./day in 4-6 doses	20,000-100,000 units/Kg./day in 4 doses	10,000-20,000 units/ml.
Phenoxymethyl penicillin, phenethicillin	0.5-2 million units 4 times daily			
Procaine penicillin G		0.6-1.2 million units/injection		
Polymyxin B	10-20 mg./Kg./day in 4-6 doses (not absorbed).	2.5 mg./Kg./day in 4-6 doses		1 mg./ml.
Streptomycin	40 mg./Kg./day in 4 doses	20-40 mg./Kg./day in 2 doses		50 mg./ml.
Sulfisoxazole‡	120 mg./Kg./day in 4 doses		120 mg./Kg./day in 4 doses	
Tetracyclines	20-40 mg./Kg./day in 4 doses with water	12 mg./Kg./day in 2 doses	12 mg./Kg./day in 2 doses	5 mg./ml.

*Should be administered with extreme caution to premature infants.
†Premature infants: 25 mg./Kg./day in 2-4 doses.
‡Initial dose should be twice subsequent dose.

Drug Resistance.

An infectious organism may be naturally resistant to a given drug, may acquire resistance as a result of prior exposure, or may acquire resistance as a result of prior exposure to a similar drug (cross-resistance). Drug-resistant organisms arise by mutation and are selectively favored in the antimicrobial environment.

The emergence of resistant organisms can be reduced by the application of the following empiric rules.

A. Adequate Dosage: High tissue levels of drug inhibit both the original population and certain of the mutants.
B. Combined Therapy: If 2 drugs which do not give cross-resistance are administered simultaneously, each drug might delay the emergence of mutants resistant to the other.

Antibiotic Sensitivity Testing.

Sensitivity tests should be done whenever there is any doubt regarding the drug of choice.

A. Disk Test: This is a rapid test performed by noting the zone of inhibition of bacterial growth around small paper disks saturated with various antibiotics and placed on the surface of the culture plate. The zone size for a given drug can be compared with a standard for that drug to give a semiquantitative estimate of the relative susceptibility of organisms. This test does not always correlate with the clinical response, but it is generally true that drugs failing to give a zone of inhibition are not likely to be useful against the organism.
B. Serum Assay: The surgeon may establish whether the proper drug is administered in an adequate dose by assay of serum or urine. Body fluid from the patient under treatment is mixed in the laboratory with a dilution of the culture obtained from the patient prior to treatment. Diluted ($>$1:5) serum should inhibit or kill the organisms.

Side-Effects.

The undesirable side-effects of antimicrobial therapy fall into 3 general categories: (1) sensitivity reactions (fever, rash, anaphylactic reactions, etc.); (2) toxicity (suppression of renal function, deafness, etc.); and (3) superinfection with nonsusceptible organisms (candidiasis, enterocolitis, etc.).

Prior to administration of an antibiotic, sensitivity to that drug or to a chemically related agent should be reulted out by means of the patient's history. The potential allergic and toxic effects of the chosen antibiotic should be thoroughly understood. The patient's reaction should be monitored by observation and by appropriate laboratory tests.

When side reactions occur, the antimicrobial drug should usually be discontinued at once and another drug effective against the offending organism substituted. If necessary for the control of the infection, an antimicrobial drug may be continued when side effects are minimal and not potentially dangerous (e.g., nausea, eosinophilia). For example, patients who are hypersensitive to penicillin may be given full doses of corticosteroids and penicillin therapy continued when this is absolutely necessary.

Absolute indications for discontinuing the offending drug include bone marrow suppression, hepatitis, exfoliative dermatitis, progressive renal insufficiency, and ototoxicity. Proteinuria is a relative contraindication to continuing the drug, depending upon the need for it. Serious superinfection requires discontinuance of the drug and treatment with an agent effective against it.

Selection of Antibiotics.

When possible, antibiotics are selected on the basis of culture and sensitivity studies (see p. 178). It is frequently necessary, however, to prescribe an antibiotic or combination of antibiotics without a bacteriologic diagnosis, e.g., in peritonitis, cholangitis, cellulitis, and suspected septicemia. Under these circumstances, agents must be chosen empirically. The following are the commonest organisms encountered in surgical infections and the antimicrobial agents to which they are usually sensitive.

A. Gram-Positive Cocci:

1. Hemolytic streptococci - Group A β-hemolytic streptococci are a common cause of upper respiratory infections, cellulitis, and lymphangitis and are occasionally involved in pneumonia, meningitis, peritonitis, and bacteremia. Infections with this organism are usually characterized by sudden onset and rapid progression. Group D β-hemolytic streptococci (Streptococcus faecalis) inhabit the alimentary tract and usually are of low-grade pathogenicity. They are commonly involved in infections of the biliary and urinary tracts, peritoneum, and operative wounds. They are most often associated in peritoneal infections with gram-negative intestinal organisms. α-Hemolytic streptococci (Streptococcus viridans) frequently cause subacute bacterial endocarditis.

   Penicillin G is the drug of choice in hemolytic streptococcal infections. Cephalothin may be used in patients with penicillin allergy, but cross-sensitivity may rarely occur. In that case, erythromycin or lincomycin may be tried. None of these drugs is as effective as penicillin G.

2. Staphylococci - The hemolytic Staphylococcus aureus is the most important organism of this group from the surgical point of view. Diseases caused by it range from limited lesions such as boils and localized cellulitis to more extensive infections such as spreading cellulitis, abscesses, wound infection, pneumonia, osteomyelitis, enterocolitis, peritonitis, and bacteremia. The commonest cause of infection in clean surgical wounds is Staphylococcus aureus, which is often resident on the skin or in the nasopharynx or alimentary tract of patients or hospital personnel. Penicillinase-producing strains of this organism are common. Because of this possibility, selection of antibiotic in severe staphylococcal infections should be based on sensitivity tests. Penicillinase-resistant penicillins (methicillin, nafcillin, dicloxacillin) are an empiric choice.

   For nonpenicillinase-producing staphylococci, the antibiotics of choice are the same as for hemolytic streptococci. When penicillin allergy exists, alternatives are cephalothin, lincomycin, and erythromycin. Vancomycin is rapidly bactericidal but has nephrotoxic and ototoxic potential.

B. Gram-Positive Bacilli: The most important of these from the surgical point of view are Bacillus anthracis, Clostridium tetani, and Clostridium welchii (see pp. 207-210). Penicillin is the drug of choice in infections caused by these bacilli. Tetracycline is the preferred alternate in clostridial infections.

C. Gram-Negative Bacilli: Of chief surgical importance are the coliform organisms, generally of low pathogenicity and found normally in the alimentary tract. Prominent among these are Escherichia coli, Aerobacter aerogenes, Proteus vulgaris, P. mirabilis, P. morganii, and Pseudomonas aeruginosa. They are often involved in "mixed infections" consisting of gram-positive cocci and gram-negative bacilli, as after perforation of the bowel. Gram-negative bacteremia may occur, usually in association with burns, intra-abdominal sepsis, or urinary tract infections, or as superinfection during antibiotic treatment. Because many of these organisms form potent endotoxins, bacteremia may be associated with profound prostration ("gram-negative sepsis") or septic shock demanding intensive supportive and antimicrobial therapy (see p. 27).

When a severe "mixed infection" is suspected, a combination of 2 or more drugs is advisable. Give penicillin (as an agent against gram-positive cocci and rods) plus a second drug such as an aminoglycoside (against the coliform group). If there is no clinical improvement after 48 hours, ampicillin may be added as a third drug or substituted for the second drug. These antibiotics are usually effective in infections of mixed type involving coliform bacilli. If the response is poor, chloramphenicol or polymyxin B may be considered.

In recent years, infection with gram-negative bacilli has become an increasingly important cause of morbidity and mortality. Accurate bacteriologic diagnosis and sensitivity studies are mandatory for the most successful management of these complicated infections, which often occur in elderly and debilitated patients. On the other hand, intensive empirical management, particularly of mixed intraperitoneal sepsis, frequently permits the normal defense mechanism to contain the infection provided that necessary surgical procedures are also done.

Preventive Antibiotics.

The prevention of surgical wound infection by the **postoperative** administration of antibiotics has proved unsuccessful. Many studies have shown that the rate of wound infection is not diminished by the postoperative use of these agents, and in some series the incidence of infection has actually been higher in the treated patients. Indiscriminate postoperative use of antibiotics is not only worthless in the prevention of wound sepsis but is also hazardous because it favors the development in the hospital environment of virulent strains of bacteria resistant to those antibiotics chosen for frequent postoperative administration.

When antibiotics are selectively administered just before and during operation, however, therapeutic serum and tissue levels are present during operation so that the blood and serum coagulum which forms in the fresh wound contains bacteriostatic or bactericidal concentrations of antibiotic. Since postoperative infection is almost invariably the result of either exogenous (e.g., patient's skin, hands of operating team) or endogenous (e.g., an open viscus) contamination of the wound during surgery, the presence of antibiotic in the wound coagulum tends to inhibit bacterial growth from the very outset.

A. Indications: Preoperative administration of preventive antibiotics is not necessary or desirable in the great majority of surgical patients, but there are circumstances in which the danger of wound infection is sufficient to warrant this procedure. The parenteral injection of antibiotic may be considered preoperatively under the following circumstances:
   1. When the consequences of wound infection will be grave, such as in open heart surgery, transplant operations, vascular, neurosurgical, and very extensive operations, and in procedures involving implantation of prosthetic materials.
   2. When the patient's condition is thought to increase the risk of serious wound sepsis, e.g., steroid and immunosuppressive therapy, blood disorders, infection elsewhere, obesity, old age.
   3. When wound contamination during operation is expected, as in certain procedures involving (a) opening of the respiratory, gastrointestinal, or genitourinary tract, or (b) an internal focus of sepsis such as ruptured appendix, peritonitis, or empyema.
   4. In contaminated traumatic and other obviously dirty wounds.

B. Prophylactic Regimens: Various preventive antibiotic regimens have been tried. When the potential bacterial contaminants are known, the preoperative antibiotics should be chosen accordingly. Parenteral antibiotics may be started the night before or on the morning of operation. A simple and apparently equally useful method is to begin an intravenous infusion containing antibiotics immediately before operation, continue the infusion during surgery, and maintain the patient on parenteral antibiotics for several days postoperatively. The drug regimen of choice varies from year to year. It should be emphasized that the preventive administration of antibiotics continues to be under study and that the indications and results are still not finally established. Either of the following 2 alternative prophylactic antibiotic programs will provide broad-spectrum coverage.
   1. For control of infection associated with elective operations on the stomach, small intestine, and small bowel, give cephaloridine (Keflordin®), 1 Gm. I.M. on call to the operating room and at 5 and 12 hours thereafter. Alternatively, give cephaloridine, 1 Gm. I.V. upon induction of anesthesia and I.V. or I.M. at 5 and 12 hours thereafter. Polk and Lopez-Mayor (Surgery 66:97, 1969) found - in a double-blind, prospective study - that this short 3-Gm. regimen was effective in reducing postoperative wound and intra-abdominal infection rates and that it was not associated with toxicity, emergence of resistant organisms, or masking of later postoperative infections. Ferguson (S. Clin. North America 51:49, 1971) has used cephalothin (Keflin®), 4 Gm. I.V. every 24 hours, starting just before operation and continuing for no more than 2-5 days if nc signs of infection appear.
   2. Various combinations of antibiotics have been proposed in order to achieve a broad spectrum of preventive coverage - for example, in cardiac surgical patients. The following is an example of such a regimen. It includes 3 drugs (penicillin G, methicillin, and kanamycin), which are to be started the

day before surgery and usually continued for 2-5 days thereafter:

a. Penicillin G, 4-6 million units/day I.V. or I.M (1 million units every 4-6 hours). Penicillin G is the drug of choice against nonpenicillinase-producing staphylococci, group A hemolytic streptococci, and the clostridia.
b. Methicillin, 4 Gm./day I.V. or I.M. (1 Gm. every 6 hours). Methicillin is the prototype of the semisynthetic penicillins. These are resistant to penicillinase, an enzyme produced by certain strains of staphylococci and gram-negative bacilli, which destroys penicillin by hydrolysis before it can injure the microorganism. High serum concentrations of methicillin are required for effective treatment. Other penicillinase-resistant penicillins that may be used instead of methicillin and at the same dosage, I.M. or I.V., are nafcillin and oxacillin. Unlike methicillin, which is not effective when given by mouth, these drugs are suitable for oral administration at the dosage level of 50-100 mg./Kg./day in 4 divided doses.
c. Kanamycin, 15 mg./Kg./day I.M. (daily dose may be given in 2-4 divided doses every 6-12 hours). The total daily dose is not to exceed 1.5 Gm., regardless of body weight. Kanamycin, one of the aminoglycoside antibiotics akin to streptomycin, is bactericidal for many gram-positive cocci (except enterococci) and gram-negative bacteria, including some strains of proteus. Pseudomonas and serratia are often resistant to kanamycin. When pseudomonas is a possible invader, substitute gentamicin, 3 mg./Kg./day I.M. in 3 equal doses every 8 hours, for kanamycin. Both kanamycin and gentamicin may cause eighth nerve damage and kidney damage; they should be avoided or used with caution in patients with renal disease.

PENICILLINS

All penicillins share a common chemical nucleus (aminopenicillanic acid) and a common mode of antibacterial action - the inhibition of cell wall mucopeptide (peptidoglycan) synthesis. The penicillins can be arranged according to several major criteria:

(1) Susceptibility to destruction by penicillinase (i.e., hydrolysis by the β-lactamase of bacteria).
(2) Susceptibility to destruction by acid pH (i.e., relative stability to gastric acid).
(3) Relative efficacy against gram-positive versus gram-negative bacteria.

Antimicrobial Activity.

All penicillins specifically inhibit the synthesis of rigid bacterial cell walls which contain a complex mucopeptide. Most penicillins are much more active against gram-positive than against gram-negative bacteria, probably because of chemical differences in cell wall structure. Penicillins are inactive against bacteria which are not multiplying and thus not forming new cell walls ("persisters").

One million units of penicillin G equal 0.6 Gm. Other penicillins are prescribed in grams. A blood serum level of 0.01-1 μg./

ml. penicillin G or ampicillin is lethal for a majority of susceptible microorganisms; methicillin and isoxazolyl penicillins are 1/5-1/50 as active.

Resistance.

Resistance to penicillins falls into 4 different categories:

(1) Certain bacteria (e. g., some staphylococci, gram-negative bacteria) produce enzymes (penicillinases, β-lactamases) which destroy penicillin G, ampicillin, and other penicillins. Clinical penicillin resistance of staphylococci falls largely into this category.

(2) Certain bacteria (e. g., coliform organisms) produce an enzyme (amidase) which can split off the side chain from the penicillin nucleus and thus destroy biologic activity.

(3) Certain bacteria are resistant to some penicillins although they do not produce enzymes destroying the drug. Clinical methicillin resistance falls into this category.

(4) Metabolically inactive organisms which make no new cell wall mucopeptide are temporarily resistant to penicillins. They can act as "persisters" and perpetuate infection during and after penicillin treatment. L-forms are in this category.

Indications, Dosages, and Routes of Administration.

The penicillins are by far the most effective and the most widely used antimicrobial drugs. All oral penicillins must be given away from meal times.

A. Penicillin G: This is the drug of choice for infections caused by gonococci, pneumococci, streptococci, meningococci, non-β-lactamase-producing staphylococci, Treponema pallidum and many other spirochetes, Bacillus anthracis and other gram-positive rods, clostridia, listeria, and bacteroides.

1. Intramuscular or intravenous - Most of the above-mentioned infections respond to aqueous penicillin G in daily doses of 0.6-5 million units (0.36-3 Gm.) administered by intermittent I.M. injection every 4-6 hours. Much larger amounts (6-120 Gm. daily) can be given by continuous I.V. infusion in serious or complicated infections due to these organisms. Sites for such intravenous administration are subject to thrombophlebitis and superinfection and must be rotated every 2 days and kept scrupulously aseptic. In enterococcus endocarditis, kanamycin, streptomycin, or gentamicin is given simultaneously with large doses of a penicillin.
2. Oral - Buffered penicillin G (or penicillin V) is indicated only in minor infections (e.g., of the respiratory tract or its associated structures) in daily doses of 1-4 Gm. (1.6-6.4 million units). About one-fifth of the oral dose is absorbed, but oral administration is subject to so many variables that it should not be relied upon in seriously ill patients.
3. Intrathecal - With high serum levels of penicillin, adequate concentrations reach the central nervous system and cerebrospinal fluid for the treatment of meningitis. Therefore, and because of the danger of injection into the subdural space of more than 10,000 units of penicillin G (which can give rise to convulsions), intrathecal injection has been virtually abandoned.

4. Topical - Penicillins have been applied to skin, wounds, and mucous membranes by compress, ointment, and aerosol. These applications are highly sensitizing and rarely warranted. Rarely, solutions of penicillin (e.g., 100,000 units/ml.) are instilled into joint or pleural space infected with susceptible organisms.

B. Benzathine Penicillin G: This penicillin is a salt of very low water solubility. It is injected I.M. to establish a depot which yields low but prolonged drug levels. A single injection of 2.4 million units I.M. is satisfactory for treatment of beta-hemolytic streptococcal pharyngitis and perhaps for early syphilis. An injection of 1.2-2.4 million units I.M. every 3-4 weeks provides satisfactory prophylaxis for rheumatics against reinfection with group A streptococci. There is no indication for using this drug by mouth. Procaine penicillin G is another repository form for maintaining drug levels for up to 24 hours; for highly susceptible infections, 300-600 thousand units I.M. are usually given once daily.

C. Ampicillin, Carbenicillin: These drugs differ from penicillin G in having greater activity against gram-negative bacteria, but, like penicillin G, they are destroyed by penicillinases.

Ampicillin is the drug of current choice for bacterial meningitis in small children, especially meningitis due to Haemophilus influenzae; 150 mg./Kg./day are injected I.V. Ampicillin can be given orally in divided doses, 3-6 Gm. daily, to treat urinary tract infections with coliform bacteria, enterococci, or Proteus mirabilis. It is ineffective against enterobacter and pseudomonas. In salmonella infections, ampicillin, 6-12 Gm. daily orally, can be effective in suppressing clinical disease (second choice to chloramphenicol in acute typhoid or paratyphoid) and may eliminate salmonellae from some chronic carriers. Ampicillin is somewhat more effective than penicillin G against enterococci and may be used in such infections in combination with kanamycin or streptomycin. Hetacillin is converted in vivo to ampicillin and should not be used. Carbenicillin is relatively active against proteus and pseudomonas.

D. Penicillinase-Resistant Penicillins: Methicillin, oxacillin, cloxacillin, dicloxacillin, nafcillin, and others are relatively resistant to destruction by β-lactamase. The only indication for the use of these drugs is infection by β-lactamase-producing staphylococci.

1. Oral - Oxacillin, cloxacillin, dicloxacillin (the isoxazolylpenicillins), or nafcillin may be given in doses of 0.25-0.5 Gm. every 4-6 hours in mild or localized staphylococcal infections (50-100 mg./Kg./day for children). Food must not be given in proximity to these doses because it will seriously interfere with absorption.
2. Intravenous - For serious systemic staphylococcal infections, methicillin, 8-16 Gm., or nafcillin, 6-12 Gm., is administered I.V., usually by injecting 1-2 Gm. during 20-30 minutes every 2 hours into a continuous infusion of 5% dextrose in water or physiologic salt solution. The dose for children is methicillin, 100-300 mg./Kg./day, or nafcillin, 50-100 mg./Kg./day.

Adverse Effects.

The penicillins undoubtedly possess less direct toxicity than any other antibiotics. Most of the serious side-effects are due to hypersensitivity.

A. Allergy: All penicillins are cross-sensitizing and cross-reacting. Any preparation containing penicillin may induce sensitization, including foods or cosmetics. In general, sensitization occurs in direct proportion to the duration and total dose of penicillin received in the past. The responsible antigenic determinants appear to be degradation products of penicillins, particularly penicilloic acid and products of alkaline hydrolysis bound to host protein. Skin tests with penicilloyl-polylysine, with alkaline hydrolysis products, and with undegraded penicillin will identify many hypersensitive individuals. Among positive reactors to skin tests, the incidence of subsequent penicillin reactions is high. Although many persons develop antibodies to antigenic determinants of penicillin, the presence of such antibodies does not appear to be correlated with allergic reactivity (except rare hemolytic anemia), and serologic tests have little predictive value. A history of a penicillin reaction in the past is not reliable; however, in such cases the drug should be administered with caution.

   Allergic reactions may occur as typical anaphylactic shock, typical serum sickness type reactions (urticaria, fever, joint swelling, angioneurotic edema, intense pruritus, and respiratory embarrassment occurring 7-12 days after exposure), and a variety of skin rashes, oral lesions, fever, nephritis, eosinophilia, hemolytic anemia, other hematologic disturbances, and vasculitis. LE cells are sometimes found. The incidence of hypersensitivity to penicillin is estimated to be 5-10% among adults in the U. S. A., but is negligible in small children.

   Individuals known to be hypersensitive to penicillin can at times tolerate the drug during corticosteroid administration. "Desensitization" with gradually increasing doses of penicillin is also occasionally attempted but is not without hazard.

B. Toxicity: The toxic effects of penicillin G are due to the direct irritation caused by I.M. or I.V. injection of exceedingly high concentrations (e.g., 1 Gm./ml.). Such concentrations may cause local pain, induration, thrombophlebitis, or degeneration of an accidentally injected nerve. All penicillins are irritating to the central nervous system. There is little indication for intrathecal administration at present. In rare cases, a patient receiving more than 50 Gm. of penicillin G daily parenterally has exhibited signs of cerebrocortical irritation, presumably as a result of the passage of unusually large amounts of penicillin into the central nervous system. With doses of this magnitude, direct cation toxicity (Na^+, K^+) can also occur. Potassium penicillin G contains 1.7 mEq. of K^+ per million units (2.8 mEq./Gm.), and potassium may accumulate in the presence of renal failure.

   Large doses of penicillins given orally may lead to gastrointestinal upset, particularly nausea and diarrhea. Oral therapy may also be accompanied by luxuriant overgrowth of staphylococci, pseudomonas, proteus, or yeasts, which may occasionally cause enteritis. Superinfections in other organ systems may occur with penicillins as with any antibiotic therapy.

Methicillin and isoxazolyl-penicillins have occasionally caused granulocytopenia, especially in children.

CEPHALOSPORINS

Cephalosporins are a group of compounds closely related to the penicillins. The mode of action is the same as that of penicillins, there is some (limited) cross-allergenicity, and they are resistant to destruction by β-lactamase.

Antimicrobial Activity.

Cephalosporins, like penicillins, inhibit the synthesis of bacterial cell wall mucopeptide. They are resistant to destruction by β-lactamase, but they can be hydrolyzed by a cephalosporinase produced by certain microorganisms. The cephalosporins are bactericidal in vitro in concentrations of 1-20 μg./ml. against most gram-positive microorganisms, except Streptococcus faecalis, and in concentrations of 5-30 μg./ml. against many gram-negative bacteria, except pseudomonas, herellea, proteus, and enterobacter. There is at least partial cross-resistance between cephalosporins and β-lactamase-resistant penicillins. Thus, methicillin-resistant staphylococci are also resistant to cephalosporins.

Indications, Dosages, and Routes of Administration.

A. Oral: Cephaloglycine, 0.5 Gm. 4 times daily orally, yields urine concentrations of 50-500 μg./ml. - sufficient for treatment of urinary tract infections due to coliform organisms. Cephalexin, 0.5 Gm. 4 times daily orally (50 mg./Kg./day), can be given in urinary or respiratory tract infections due to susceptible organisms.

B. Intravenous: Cephalothin (Keflin®), 8-16 Gm. daily (for children, 50-100 mg./Kg./day) by continuous drip, gives serum concentrations of 5-20 μg./ml. This is adequate for the treatment of gram-negative bacteremia or staphylococcal sepsis, or as a substitute for penicillin in serious infections caused by susceptible organisms in persons allergic to penicillin (although some cross-hypersensitivity exists). Cephaloridine (Keflordin®, Loridine®), 4 Gm. daily I.V. (for children, up to 100 mg./Kg./day), gives serum levels of 10-25 μg./ml. It is used for the same indications.

C. Intramuscular: Cephaloridine, 0.5-1 Gm. I.M. every 6 hours, is used for the same indications as above in less severely ill patients. Cephalothin is too painful when injected intramuscularly.

Adverse Effects.

A. Allergy: Cephalosporins are sensitizing and a variety of hypersensitivity reactions occurs, including anaphylaxis, fever, skin rashes, granulocytopenia, and hemolytic anemia. Cross-allergy also exists with penicillins and can produce the same hypersensitivity reactions. Perhaps 10-30% of penicillin-allergic persons are also hypersensitive to cephalosporins.

B. Toxicity: Local pain after intramuscular injection, thrombophlebitis after intravenous injection. Cephaloridine can cause renal damage with tubular necrosis and uremia.

ERYTHROMYCIN GROUP
(Macrolides)

The erythromycins are a group of closely related compounds. Erythromycins inhibit protein synthesis and are active against gram-positive organisms (especially pneumococci, streptococci, staphylococci, and corynebacteria) in concentrations of 0.02-2 μg./ml. Neisseriae and mycoplasmas are also susceptible. Activity is enhanced at alkaline pH. Resistant mutants occur in most microbial populations and tend to emerge during prolonged treatment. There is complete cross-resistance among all members of the erythromycin group. Absorption varies greatly. Basic erythromycins are destroyed by gastric acid. Stearates are somewhat resistant. The propionyl ester of erythromycin (erythromycin estolate) and the triacetyl ester of oleandomycin are among the best absorbed oral preparations. Oral doses of 2 Gm./day result in blood levels of up to 2 μg./ml., and there is wide distribution of the drug in all tissues except the central nervous system. Erythromycins are excreted largely in bile; only 5% of the dose is excreted into the urine.

Erythromycins are the drugs of choice in corynebacterial infections (diphtheroid sepsis, erythrasma) and in mycoplasmal pneumonia. They are most useful as substitutes for penicillin in persons with streptococcal and pneumococcal infections who are allergic to penicillin.

For oral administration, give erythromycin stearate, erythromycin estolate, or troleandomycin, 0.5 Gm. every 6 hours (for children, 40 mg./Kg./day). For intravenous administration, give erythromycin lactobionate or gluceptate, 0.5 Gm. every 12 hours.

Such adverse effects as nausea, vomiting, and diarrhea may occur after oral intake. Erythromycin estolate or troleandomycin can produce acute cholestatic hepatitis (fever, jaundice, impaired liver function). Most patients recover completely. Upon readministration, the hepatitis promptly recurs. It is probably a hypersensitivity reaction.

TETRACYCLINE GROUP

The tetracyclines constitute a large group of drugs with common basic chemical structures, antimicrobial activity, and pharmacologic properties. Microorganisms resistant to this group show complete cross-resistance to all tetracyclines.

Antimicrobial Activity.

Tetracyclines are inhibitors of protein synthesis and are bacteriostatic for many gram-positive and gram-negative bacteria, including anaerobes, and are strongly inhibitory for the growth of mycoplasmas, rickettsiae, chlamydiae (psittacosis-LGV-trachoma agents), and some protozoa (e.g., amebas). Equal concentrations of all tetracyclines in blood or tissue have approximately equal antimicrobial activity. Such differences in activity as may be claimed for individual tetracycline drugs are of no practical importance. However, there are great differences in the susceptibility of different strains of a given species of microorganism, and laboratory tests are therefore important. Because of the emergence of resistant strains, tetracyclines have lost some of their former usefulness. Proteus and pseudomonas are regularly resistant; among coliform bacteria, pneumococci, and streptococci, resistant strains are increasingly common.

Indications, Dosages, and Routes of Administration.

At present, tetracyclines are the drugs of choice in cholera, mycoplasmal pneumonia, infections with chlamydiae (psittacosis-LGV-trachoma), and infections with some rickettsiae. They may be used in various bacterial infections provided the organism is susceptible, and in amebiasis.

A. Oral: Tetracycline hydrochloride, oxytetracycline, and chlortetracycline are dispensed in 250 mg. capsules. Give 0.25-0.5 Gm. orally every 6 hours (for children, 20-40 mg./Kg./day). In acne vulgaris, 0.25 Gm. once or twice daily for many months is prescribed by dermatologists.

Demeclocycline and methacycline are slowly excreted. Give 0.15-0.3 Gm. orally every 6 hours (12-20 mg./Kg./day for children). Doxycycline is available in capsules of 50 or 100 mg. Give 100 mg. every 12 hours on the first day, then 100 mg./day.

B. Intramuscular or Intravenous: Several tetracyclines are formulated for I.M. or I.V. injection. Give 0.1-0.5 Gm. every 6-12 hours in individuals unable to take oral medication (for children, 10-15 mg./Kg./day).

C. Topical: Topical tetracycline, 1% in ointments, can be applied to conjunctival infections.

Adverse Effects.

A. Allergy: Hypersensitivity reactions with fever or skin rashes are uncommon.

B. Gastrointestinal Side-Effects: Gastrointestinal side-effects, especially diarrhea, nausea, and anorexia, are common. These can be diminished by reducing the dose or by administering tetracyclines with food or carboxymethylcellulose, but sometimes they force discontinuance of the drug. After a few days of oral use, the gut flora is modified so that drug-resistant bacteria and yeasts become prominent. This may cause functional gut disturbances, anal pruritus, and even enterocolitis with shock and death.

C. Bones and Teeth: Tetracyclines are bound to calcium deposited in growing bones and teeth, causing fluorescence, discoloration, enamel dysplasia, deformity, or growth inhibition. Therefore, tetracyclines should not be given to pregnant women or small children.

D. Liver Damage: Tetracyclines can impair hepatic function or even cause liver necrosis, particularly during pregnancy, in the presence of preexisting liver damage, or with doses of more than 3 Gm. I.V.

E. Kidney Damage: Outdated tetracycline preparations have been implicated in renal tubular acidosis and other forms of renal damage.

F. Other: Tetracyclines, principally demeclocycline, may induce photosensitization, especially in blonds. Intravenous injection may cause thrombophlebitis, and intramuscular injection may induce local inflammation with pain.

CHLORAMPHENICOL

Chloramphenicol is a synthetic drug which inhibits the growth of many bacteria and rickettsiae in concentrations of 0.5-10 μg./ml. There is no cross-resistance with other drugs.

Because of its potential toxicity, chloramphenicol is at present a possible drug of choice only in the following cases: (1) symptomatic salmonella infection, e.g., typhoid fever; (2) Haemophilus influenzae meningitis, laryngotracheitis, or pneumonia that does not respond to ampicillin; (3) occasional gram-negative bacteremia; (4) severe rickettsial infection; and (5) meningococcal infection in patients hypersensitive to penicillin. It is occasionally used topically in ophthalmology.

In serious systemic infection, the dose is 0.5 Gm. orally every 4-6 hours (for children, 30-50 mg./Kg./day) for 7-21 days. Similar amounts are given intravenously.

Nausea, vomiting, and diarrhea occur infrequently. The most serious adverse effects pertain to the hematopoietic system. Adults taking chloramphenicol in excess of 50 mg./Kg./day regularly exhibit disturbances in red cell maturation after 1-2 weeks of blood levels above 25 μg./ml. There is anemia, rise in serum iron concentration, reticulocytopenia, and the appearance of vacuolated nucleated red cells in the bone marrow. These changes regress when the drug is stopped and are not related to the rare aplastic anemia.

Serious aplastic anemia is a rare consequence of chloramphenicol administration and represents a specific, probably genetically determined individual defect. It is seen more frequently with either prolonged or repeated use. It tends to be irreversible and fatal. Fatal aplastic anemia occurs 13 times more frequently after the use of chloramphenicol than as a spontaneous occurrence. Hypoplastic anemia may be followed by the development of leukemia.

Chloramphenicol is specifically toxic for newborns, producing the highly fatal "gray syndrome" with vomiting, flaccidity, hypothermia, and collapse. Chloramphenicol should only rarely be used in infants, and the dose must be limited to less than 50 mg./Kg./day in full-term infants and less than 30 mg./Kg./day in prematurely born infants.

AMINOGLYCOSIDES

Aminoglycosides are a group of drugs with similar chemical, antimicrobial, pharmacologic, ototoxic, and nephrotoxic characteristics. Important members are streptomycin, neomycin, kanamycin, and gentamicin.

1. STREPTOMYCINS

Streptomycin is a product of Streptomyces griseus. Dihydrostreptomycin was derived from it by chemical reduction, but it is no longer used because of serious ototoxicity. Streptomycin can be bactericidal for gram-positive and gram-negative bacteria and for Mycobacterium tuberculosis. Its antituberculosis activity is described below.

In all bacterial strains there are mutants which are 10-1000 times more resistant to streptomycin than the remainder of the microbial population. These are selected out rapidly in the presence of streptomycin. Treatment with streptomycin for 4-5 days thus results either in eradication of the infecting agent or the emergence of resistant infection which is intractable by the drug. For this reason, streptomycin is usually employed in combination with another drug to delay the emergence of resistance. Streptomycin may enhance the bactericidal action of penicillins, particularly against Streptococcus faecalis. Activity is enhanced at alkaline pH.

Indications and Dosages.

The principal indications for streptomycin at present are (1) serious active tuberculosis, (2) plague, tularemia, or occasional gram-negative sepsis, (3) acute brucellosis (used in conjunction with tetracycline), (4) bacterial endocarditis caused by Streptococcus faecalis or S. viridans (used in conjunction with penicillin), and (5) rare acute urinary tract infections caused by susceptible organisms.

The dose in the nontuberculous infections is 0.5-1 Gm. I.M. every 6-12 hours (for children, 20-40 mg./Kg./day), depending on severity of the disease.

Adverse Effects.

Allergic reactions, including skin rashes and fever, may occur upon prolonged contact with streptomycin, e.g., in personnel preparing solutions. The principal side-effects are nephrotoxicity and ototoxicity. Renal damage with nitrogen retention occurs mainly after prolonged high doses or in persons with preexisting impairment of renal function. Damage to the eighth nerve manifests itself mainly by tinnitus, vertigo, ataxia, loss of balance, and occasionally loss of hearing. Chronic vestibular dysfunction is most common after prolonged use of streptomycin. Streptomycin, 2-3 Gm./day for 4 weeks, has been used to purposely damage semicircular canal function in the treatment of Ménière's disease.

Streptomycin should not be used concurrently with other aminoglycosides, and great caution is necessary in persons with impaired renal function.

2. KANAMYCIN
(Kantrex®)

Kanamycin is the most prominent aminoglycoside for systemic use in gram-negative sepsis. Kanamycin is bactericidal for many gram-positive (except enterococci) and gram-negative bacteria in concentrations of 1-10 μg./ml. Activity is enhanced at alkaline pH. Some strains of proteus are susceptible, but pseudomonas and serratia are often resistant. In susceptible bacterial populations, resistant mutants are rare. Kanamycin exhibits complete cross-resistance with neomycin but not with gentamicin.

Indications and Dosages.

The principal indication for systemic kanamycin is bacteremia caused by gram-negative enteric organisms or, occasionally, serious urinary tract infection with enterobacter, proteus, or other "difficult" organisms. The I.M. dose is 0.5 Gm. every 6-12 hours (15 mg./Kg./day). In renal failure the dose is reduced and the interval between injections is prolonged.

Adverse Effects.

Like all aminoglycosides, kanamycin is ototoxic and nephrotoxic. Kanamycin is probably less toxic than neomycin. Proteinuria and nitrogen retention occur commonly during treatment. This must be monitored and the dose or frequency of injection adjusted when creatinine clearance falls. In general, these nephrotoxic effects are reversible upon discontinuance of the drug. The auditory portion of the eighth nerve can be selectively and irreversibly damaged by kanamycin. The development of deafness is proportionate to the level of drug and the duration of its administration, but it can occur unpredictably even after a short course of treatment. Loss of perception of high frequencies in audiograms may be a warning sign. Ototoxicity is a particular risk in patients with impaired kidney function. The sudden absorption of large amounts of kanamycin (or any other aminoglycoside) can lead to respiratory arrest. This has occurred after the instillation of 3-5 Gm. of kanamycin (or neomycin) into the peritoneal cavity following bowel surgery. Neostigmine is a specific antidote.

3. NEOMYCIN

Neomycin is analogous in all pharmacologic and antibacterial characteristics to kanamycin. However, it is believed at present to be somewhat more toxic when given parenterally and is therefore used mainly for topical application and for oral administration.

After oral intake, only a minute portion of neomycin is absorbed. Most of the drug remains in the gut lumen and alters intestinal flora. For preoperative reduction of the gut flora, give neomycin, 1 Gm. orally every 4-6 hours for 2-3 days before surgery. In hepatic coma, ammonia intoxication can be reduced by suppressing the coliform flora of the gut with neomycin, 1 Gm. orally every 6-8 hours, and limiting the protein intake. Oral neomycin, 50-100 mg./Kg./day, is effective against enteropathic Escherichia coli. To control surface infections of the skin (pyoderma), ointments containing neomycin, 1-5 mg./Gm., are applied several times daily. Solutions containing 10 mg./ml. of neomycin can be instilled (up to a total of 0.5 Gm./day) into infected joints, pleura, or tissue spaces. Paromomycin (Humatin®), a close relative of neomycin, is given in a dosage of 1 Gm. orally every 6 hours for the treatment of intestinal amebiasis.

All topically administered forms of neomycin may produce sensitization. Hypersensitivity reactions occur particularly in the eye and skin after repeated use of neomycin ointments. Topical or oral neomycin rarely produces systemic toxicity. However, oral neomycin alters the intestinal flora and thus predisposes to superinfection. Staphylococcal enterocolitis, occasionally fatal, has followed the use of neomycin for preoperative "bowel sterilization."

4. GENTAMICIN
(Garamycin®)

Gentamicin is an aminoglycoside antibiotic which shares many properties with kanamycin but differs in its antimicrobial activity. In concentrations of 0.5-5 μg./ml., gentamicin is bactericidal not only for staphylococci and coliform organisms but also for many strains of pseudomonas, proteus, and serratia. Gentamicin is not significantly absorbed after oral intake.

Gentamicin is used in severe infections caused by gram-negative bacteria which are likely to be resistant to other, less toxic drugs. Included are sepsis, infected burns, pneumonia and other serious infections due to coliform organisms, klebsiella-enterobacter, proteus, pseudomonas, and serratia. The dosage is 2-3 mg./Kg./day I.M. in 3 equal doses for 7-10 days. In life-threatening infections, 5-7 mg./Kg./day have been given. In urinary tract infections caused by these organisms, 0.8-1.2 mg./Kg./day is given I.M. for 10 days or longer.

For infected burns or skin lesions, creams containing 0.1% gentamicin are used.

Renal function must be monitored by repeated creatinine clearance tests, although nephrotoxicity is said to be infrequent with recommended doses and in the absence of preexisting renal damage. About 2-3% of patients develop vestibular dysfunction (perhaps because of destruction of hair cells), and occasional cases of loss of hearing have been reported.

POLYMYXINS

The polymyxins are a group of basic polypeptides bactericidal for most gram-negative bacteria except proteus and especially useful against pseudomonas. Only 2 drugs are used: polymyxin B sulfate and colistin (polymyxin E) methanesulfonate.

Indications, Dosages, and Routes of Administration.

Polymyxins are indicated in serious infections due to pseudomonas and other gram-negative bacteria which are resistant to other antimicrobial drugs.

A. Intramuscular: The injection of polymyxin B is painful. Therefore, colistimethate, which contains a local anesthetic and is more rapidly excreted in the urine, is given I.M., 2.5 mg./Kg./day, for urinary tract infection.

B. Intravenous: In pseudomonas sepsis, polymyxin B sulfate, 2.5 mg./Kg./day, is injected by continuous I.V. infusion.

C. Intrathecal: In pseudomonas meningitis, give polymyxin B sulfate, 2-10 mg. once daily for 2-3 days, and then every other day for 2-3 weeks. (Colistimethate must not be given intrathecally.)

D. Topical: Solutions of polymyxin B sulfate, 1 mg./ml., can be applied to infected surfaces, injected into joint spaces, intrapleurally or subconjunctivally, or inhaled as aerosols. Ointments containing 0.5 mg./Gm. polymyxin B sulfate in a mixture with neomycin or bacitracin are often applied to infected skin lesions. Solutions containing polymyxin B, 20 mg./L., and neomycin, 40 mg./L., can be used for continuous irrigation of the bladder with an indwelling catheter and a closed drainage system.

Adverse Effects.

The toxicities of polymyxin B and colistimethate are similar. With the usual blood levels there are paresthesias, dizziness, flushing, and incoordination. These disappear when the drug has been excreted. With unusually high levels, respiratory arrest and paralysis can occur. Depending upon the dose, all polymyxins are nephrotoxic, producing tubular injury. Proteinuria, hematuria, and cylindruria tend to be reversible, but nitrogen retention may force reduction in dose or discontinuance of the drug. In individuals with preexisting renal insufficiency, kidney function must be monitored (preferably by creatinine clearance) and the dose reduced or the interval between injections increased.

ANTITUBERCULOSIS DRUGS

Singular problems exist in the treatment of tuberculosis and other mycobacterial infections. They tend to be exceedingly chronic but may give rise to hyperacute lethal complications. The organisms are frequently intracellular, have long periods of metabolic inactivity, and tend to develop resistance to any one drug. Combined drug therapy is often employed to delay the emergence of this resistance. "First line" drugs, often employed together in tuberculous meningitis, miliary dissemination, or severe pulmonary disease, are streptomycin, isoniazid, ethambutol, and aminosalicylic acid. A series of "second line" drugs will be mentioned only briefly.

1. STREPTOMYCIN

The general pharmacologic features and toxicity of streptomycin are described above. Streptomycin, 1-10 μg./ml., is inhibitory and bactericidal for most tubercle bacilli; whereas most "atypical" mycobacteria are resistant. All large populations of tubercle bacilli contain some streptomycin-resistant mutants, which tend to emerge during prolonged treatment with streptomycin alone and result in "treatment resistance" within 2-4 months. Therefore streptomycin is usually employed in combination with another antituberculosis drug. Streptomycin penetrates poorly into cells and exerts its action mainly on extracellular tubercle bacilli.

For combination therapy in tuberculous meningitis, miliary dissemination, and severe organ tuberculosis, streptomycin is given I.M., 1 Gm. daily (30 mg./Kg./day for children) for weeks or months. This is followed by streptomycin, 1 Gm. I.M. 2-3 times a week for months or years. In tuberculous meningitis, intrathecal injections (1-2 mg./Kg./day) are sometimes given in addition.

The vestibular dysfunction resulting from prolonged streptomycin treatment results in inability to maintain equilibrium. However, some compensation usually occurs so that patients can function fairly well.

2. ISONIAZID (INH)

Isoniazid is the most active antituberculosis drug. INH inhibits most tubercle bacilli in a concentration of 0.2 μg./ml. or less. However, most "atypical" mycobacteria are resistant. In susceptible large populations of Mycobacterium tuberculosis, INH-resistant mutants occur. Their emergence is delayed in the presence of a second drug. There is no cross-resistance between INH, streptomycin, PAS, or ethambutol.

INH is the most widely used drug in tuberculosis. In active, clinically manifest disease, it is given in conjunction with streptomycin and PAS or ethambutol. The initial dose is 8-10 mg./Kg./day orally (up to 20 mg./Kg./day in small children); later, the dosage is reduced to 5-7 mg./Kg./day.

Children (or young adults) converting from a tuberculin-negative to tuberculin-positive skin test may be given 10 mg./Kg./day (maximum: 300 mg./day) for 1 year as prophylaxis against the 5-15% risk of meningitis or miliary dissemination. For this "prophylaxis," INH is given as the sole drug.

Toxic reactions to INH include insomnia, restlessness, dysuria, hyperreflexia, and even convulsions and psychotic episodes. Many of these are attributable to a relative pyridoxine deficiency and peripheral neuritis and can be prevented by the administration of pyridoxine, 100 mg./day.

3. RIFAMPIN
(Rifadin®, Rimactane®)

Rifampin may be used in combination with ethambutol or INH. It is also active against various bacteria and chlamydiae. Its toxic effects seem only minor. Give 0.45-0.9 Gm./day orally.

4. ETHAMBUTOL

Ethambutol (Myambutol®), a synthetic drug, is well absorbed from the gut. About 20% is excreted in feces and 50% in urine. The drug is widely distributed through the body, including the cerebrospinal fluid, which makes it useful in treatment of meningitis.

Ethambutol, 15 mg./Kg., is given orally as a single daily dose, usually in combination with INH, to prevent the rapid emergence of ethambutol-resistant mycobacteria. The most common side-effects are visual disturbances with daily doses of 25 mg./Kg. or more; these tend to regress when the drug is stopped.

5. ALTERNATIVE DRUGS IN TUBERCULOSIS TREATMENT

The drugs listed alphabetically below are usually considered only in cases of drug resistance (clinical or laboratory) to "first line" drugs and when expert guidance is available to deal with toxic side-effects.

Aminosalicylic acid (PAS), closely related to *p*-aminobenzoic acid, inhibits most tubercle bacilli in concentrations of 1-5 μg./ml.

but has no effect on other bacteria. Resistant Mycobacterium tuberculosis emerges rapidly unless another antituberculosis drug is present.

Common side-effects include anorexia, nausea, diarrhea, and epigastric pain. These may be diminished by taking PAS with meals and with antacids, but peptic ulceration may occur. Sodium PAS may be given parenterally. Hypersensitivity reactions include fever, skin rashes, granulocytopenia, lymphadenopathy, and arthralgias.

Capreomycin, 0.5-1.5 Gm./day I.M., can perhaps substitute for streptomycin in combined therapy. It is not commercially available. It is nephrotoxic and ototoxic.

Cycloserine (Seromycin®), 0.5-1 Gm./day orally, has been used alone or with INH. It can induce a variety of CNS dysfunctions and psychotic reactions. In smaller doses (15-20 mg./Kg./day) it has been used in urinary tract infections.

Ethionamide (Trecator®), 0.5-1 Gm./day orally, has been used in combination therapy but produces marked gastric irritation.

Pyrazinamide (PZA, Aldinamide®), 2-3 Gm./day orally, has been used in combination therapy but may produce serious liver damage.

Viomycin (Vinactane®, Viocin®), 2 Gm. I.M. every 3 days, can occasionally substitute for streptomycin in combination therapy. It is nephrotoxic and ototoxic.

SULFONAMIDES AND SULFONES

More than 150 different sulfonamides have been used at some time, the modifications being designed principally to achieve greater antibacterial activity, a wider antibacterial spectrum, greater solubility, or more prolonged action.

Indications.

Because of their low cost and their relative efficacy in some common bacterial infections, sulfonamides are still used widely in many parts of the world. However, the increasing emergence of sulfonamide resistance (e.g., among streptococci, meningococci, and shigellae) and the higher efficacy of other antimicrobial drugs have drastically curtailed the number of specific indications for sulfonamides as drugs of choice. The present indications for the use of these drugs can be summarized as follows:

(1) First (previously untreated) infection of the urinary tract: Many coliform organisms, which are the most common causes of urinary infections, are still susceptible to sulfonamides.

(2) Chlamydial infections of the trachoma–inclusion conjunctivitis–LGV group: Sulfonamides are often as effective as tetracyclines in suppressing clinical activity, and they may be curative in acute infections. However, they often fail to eradicate chronic infection.

(3) Parasitic and fungal diseases: In combination with pyrimethamine, sulfonamides are used in toxoplasmosis. In combination with trimethoprim, sulfonamides are sometimes effective in falciparum malaria or urinary tract infections. Alone or in combination with cycloserine, sulfonamides may be active in nocardiosis.

(4) Bacterial infections: In underdeveloped parts of the world, sulfonamides, because of their availability and low cost, may still be useful for the treatment of pneumococcal or staphylococcal infections; bacterial sinusitis, bronchitis, or otitis media; bacillary (shigella) dysentery; and meningococcal infections. In most developed countries, however, sulfonamides are not the drugs of choice for any of these conditions, and sulfonamide resistance of the respective etiologic organisms is widespread.

(5) Leprosy: Certain sulfones are the drugs of choice in leprosy.

Antimicrobial Activity.

The action of sulfonamides is bacteriostatic and is reversible upon removal of the drug or in the presence of an excess of *p*-aminobenzoic acid (PABA). Susceptible microorganisms require extracellular PABA in order to synthesize folic acid, an essential step in the formation of purines. Sulfonamides are structural analogues of PABA, can enter into the reaction in place of PABA competing for the enzyme involved, and can form nonfunctional analogues of folic acid. As a result, further growth of the microorganisms is inhibited. Animal cells and some sulfonamide-resistant microorganisms are unable to synthesize folic acid from PABA but depend on exogenous sources of preformed folic acid. Other microorganisms may be sulfonamide-resistant because they produce a large excess of PABA.

Dosages and Routes of Administration.

A. Topical: The application of sulfonamides to skin, wounds, or mucous membranes is undesirable because of the high risk of allergic sensitization or reaction and the low antimicrobial activity. Exceptions are the application of sodium sulfacetamide solution (30%) or ointment (10%) to the conjunctivas or mafenide acetate (Sulfamylon®) to burned surfaces.

B. Oral: For systemic disease, the soluble, rapidly excreted sulfonamides (e.g., sulfadiazine, sulfisoxazole) are given in an initial dose of 2-4 Gm. (40 mg./Kg.) followed by a maintenance dose of 0.5-1 Gm. (20 mg./Kg.) every 4-6 hours. Trisulfapyrimidines U.S.P. may be given in the same total doses. Urine must be kept alkaline.

For urinary tract infections (first attack, not previously treated), trisulfapyrimidines, sulfisoxazole, or another sulfonamide with equally high solubility in urine are given in the same (or somewhat lower) doses as shown above. Following one course of sulfonamides, resistant organisms usually prevail. Simultaneous administration of a sulfonamide, 2 Gm./day orally, and trimethoprim, 400 mg./day orally may be more effective in urinary, respiratory, or enteric tract infections than sulfonamide alone.

Salicylazosulfapyridine, 6 Gm./day, has been given in ulcerative colitis, but there is little evidence of its efficacy.

"Long-acting" and "intermediate-acting" sulfonamides (e.g., sulfamethoxypyridazine, sulfadimethoxine, sulfamethoxazole) can be used in doses of 0.5-1 Gm./day (10 mg./Kg.) for prolonged maintenance therapy (e.g., trachoma) or for the treatment of minor infections. These drugs have a significantly higher rate of toxic effects than the "short-acting" sulfonamides.

C. Intravenous: Sodium sulfadiazine and other sodium salts can be injected intravenously in 0.5% concentration in 5% dextrose in water, physiologic salt solution, or other diluent in a total dose of 6-8 Gm./day (120 mg./Kg./day). This is reserved for comatose individuals or those unable to take oral medication.

Adverse Effects.

Sulfonamides produce a wide variety of side-effects - due partly to hypersensitivity, partly to direct toxicity - which must be considered whenever unexplained symptoms or signs occur in a patient who may have received these drugs. Except in the mildest reactions, fluids should be forced, and - if symptoms and signs progressively increase - the drugs should be discontinued. Precautions to prevent complications (below) are important.

A. Systemic Side-Effects: Fever, skin rashes, urticaria, nausea, vomiting, or diarrhea; stomatitis, conjunctivitis, arthritis, exfoliative dermatitis; hematopoietic disturbances, including thrombocytopenia, hemolytic (in G-6-PD deficiency) or aplastic anemia, granulocytopenia, leukemoid reactions; hepatitis, polyarteritis nodosa, vasculitis, Stevens-Johnson syndrome; psychosis; and many others.

B. Urinary Tract Disturbances: Sulfonamides may precipitate in urine, especially in neutral or acid pH, producing hematuria, crystalluria, or even obstruction. They have also been implicated in various types of nephritis and nephrosis.

Precautions in the Use of Sulfonamides.

(1) There is cross-allergenicity among all sulfonamides. Obtain a history of past administration or reaction. Observe for possible allergic responses.

(2) Keep the urine volume above 1500 ml./day by forcing fluids. Check urine pH; it should be 7.5 or higher. Give alkali by mouth (sodium bicarbonate or equivalent, 5-15 Gm./day). Examine fresh urine for crystals and red cells every 2-4 days.

(3) Check hemoglobin, white blood cell count, and differential count every 3-5 days to detect possible disturbances early.

SULFONES USED IN THE TREATMENT OF LEPROSY

Several drugs closely related to the sulfonamides have been used effectively in the long-term treatment of leprosy. The clinical manifestations of both lepromatous and tuberculoid leprosy can often be suppressed by treatment extending over several years.

The sulfones may cause any of the side-effects listed above for sulfonamides. Anorexia, nausea, and vomiting are common. Hemolysis or methemoglobinemia may occur.

Diaminodiphenylsulfone (DDS, dapsone, Avlosulfon®) is the most widely used and least expensive drug. It is given orally, beginning with a dosage of 25 mg. twice weekly and gradually increasing to 100 mg. 3-4 times weekly and eventually to 300 mg. twice weekly.

Sulfoxone sodium (Diasone®) is given orally in corresponding dosage.

Solapsone (Sulphetrone®), a complex substituted derivative of DDS, is given initially in a dosage of 0.5 Gm. 3 times daily orally. The dose is then gradually increased until a total daily dose of 6-10 Gm. is reached.

Other classes of drugs are used uncommonly. An ethyl mercaptan (Ditophal®) may be applied to the skin. Thiosemicarbazones (e.g., amithiozone, Tibione®) permit the rapid emergence of resistance if used alone. Therefore, if administered, they are given with a sulfone.

SPECIALIZED DRUGS AGAINST GRAM-POSITIVE BACTERIA

1. BACITRACIN

This polypeptide antibiotic is selectively active against gram-positive bacteria, including penicillinase-producing staphylococci, in concentrations of 0.1-20 units/ml. Bacitracin is very little absorbed from gut, skin, wounds, or mucous membranes. Topical application results in local effects without significant toxicity. Bacitracin, 500 units/ Gm. in ointment base, is often combined with polymyxin or neomycin for the suppression of mixed bacterial flora in surface lesions. Systemic administration of bacitracin has been abandoned because of its severe nephrotoxicity.

2. LINCOMYCIN (Lincocin®) AND CLINDAMYCIN (Cleocin®)

These drugs resemble erythromycin and are active against gram-positive organisms (except enterococci) in concentrations of 0.5-5 μg./ml. Lincomycin, 0.5 Gm. orally every 6 hours (30-60 mg./Kg./day for children), or clindamycin, 0.15-0.3 Gm. orally every 6 hours, yields serum concentrations of 2-5 μg./ml. The drugs are widely distributed in tissues. Excretion is through bile and urine. Lincomycin, 0.6 Gm., can also be injected I.M. or I.V. every 8-12 hours. The drugs appear to be an alternative to erythromycin as a substitute for penicillin. Success in bone infections and against bacteroides has been reported.

Common side-effects are diarrhea and nausea. Clindamycin may have a lower incidence of gastrointestinal side-effects than lincomycin. Impaired liver function and neutropenia have been noted. If 3-4 Gm. are given rapidly intravenously, cardiorespiratory arrest may occur.

3. NOVOBIOCIN

Many gram-positive cocci are inhibited by novobiocin, 1-5 μg./ ml., but resistant variants tend to emerge during treatment. Novobiocin, 0.5 Gm orally every 6 hours, yields serum concentrations of 2-5 μg./ml. It is widely distributed in tissues and excreted in urine and feces. It can also be given I.M. or I.V. In the past, a possible indication for novobiocin was infection caused by penicillinase-producing staphylococci. However, many better drugs are now available, so that no clear indication for novobiocin exists.

Skin rashes, drug fever, and granulocytopenia are common side-effects.

4. VANCOMYCIN
(Vinactane®, Vancocin®)

This drug is bactericidal for most gram-positive organisms, particularly staphylococci and enterococci, in concentrations of 0.5-10 μg./ml. Resistant mutants are rare, and there is no cross-resistance with other antimicrobial drugs. Vancomycin is not absorbed from the gut. It is given orally (3-4 Gm./day) only for the treatment of staphylococcal enterocolitis. For systemic effect the drug must be administered I.V. After I.V. injection of 0.5 Gm. over a period of 20 minutes, blood levels of 10 μg./ml. are maintained for 1-2 hours. Vancomycin is largely excreted into the urine. In the presence of renal insufficiency, marked accumulation may occur and have toxic consequences.

The only indications for vancomycin are serious staphylococcal infection or enterococcal endocarditis intractable with penicillins. Vancomycin, 0.5 Gm., is injected I.V. over a 20-minute period every 6-8 hours (for children, 20-40 mg./Kg./day). It can also be given by continuous intravenous infusion.

Vancomycin is intensely irritating to tissues. Intramuscular injection or extravasation from intravenous injection sites is very painful. Chills, fever, and thrombophlebitis commonly follow intravenous injection. The drug is both nephrotoxic and ototoxic, and renal function must be monitored.

URINARY ANTISEPTICS

These drugs exert antimicrobial activity in the urine but have little or no systemic antibacterial effect. Their usefulness is limited to urinary tract infections.

1. NITROFURANTOIN
(Furadantin®)

Nitrofurantoin is bacteriostatic and bactericidal for both gram-positive and gram-negative bacteria in concentrations of 10-500 μg./ml. The activity of nitrofurantoin is greatly enhanced at pH 6.5 or lower.

Nitrofurantoin is rapidly absorbed from the gut. The drug is bound so completely to serum protein that no antibacterial effect occurs in the blood. Nitrofurantoin has no systemic antibacterial activity. In kidney tubules, the drug is separated from carrier protein and excreted in urine where concentrations may be 200-400 μg./ml.

DRUG SELECTIONS, 1973-1974*

Suspected or Proved Etiologic Agent	Drug(s) of First Choice	Alternative Drug(s)
Gram-negative cocci		
Gonococcus	Penicillin (1), ampicillin	Tetracycline (2), erythromycin (3)
Meningococcus	Penicillin (1)	Chloramphenicol
Gram-positive cocci		
Pneumococcus	Penicillin (1)	Erythromycin, lincomycin
Streptococcus, hemolytic groups A, B, C	Penicillin (1)	Erythromycin, lincomycin
Streptococcus viridans	Penicillin (1)	Cephalosporin (4), vancomycin
Staphylococcus, non-penicillinase-producing	Penicillin (1)	Cephalosporin, vancomycin, lincomycin
Staphylococcus, penicillinase-producing	Penicillinase-resistant penicillin (5)	Cephalosporin, vancomycin, lincomycin
Streptococcus faecalis (enterococcus)	Ampicillin plus streptomycin or kanamycin	Penicillin plus kanamycin or gentamicin
Gram-negative rods		
Enterobacter (Aerobacter)	Kanamycin or gentamicin	Tetracycline, chloramphenicol, polymyxin
Bacteroides	Clindamycin	Ampicillin, chloramphenicol
Brucella	Tetracycline plus streptomycin	Streptomycin plus sulfonamide (6)
Escherichia		
E. coli sepsis	Kanamycin, gentamicin	Cephalothin, ampicillin
E. coli UT infection (first attack)	Sulfonamide (7)	Ampicillin, cephalexin
Haemophilus (meningitis, respiratory infections)	Ampicillin	Chloramphenicol
Klebsiella	Cephalosporin or kanamycin	Gentamicin, chloramphenicol
Mima-Herellea	Kanamycin	Tetracycline, gentamicin
Pasteurella (plague, tularemia)	Streptomycin plus tetracycline	Sulfonamide (6)
Proteus		
P. mirabilis	Penicillin or ampicillin	Kanamycin, gentamicin
P. vulgaris and other species	Kanamycin or carbenicillin	Chloramphenicol, gentamicin
Pseudomonas		
Ps. aeruginosa	Polymyxin or gentamicin	Carbenicillin
Ps. pseudomallei (melioidosis)	Chloramphenicol	Rifampin, tetracycline
Ps. mallei (glanders)	Streptomycin plus tetracycline	
Salmonella	Chloramphenicol	Ampicillin
Serratia	Gentamicin	Kanamycin
Shigella	Ampicillin	Tetracycline, kanamycin
Vibrio (cholera)	Tetracycline	Chloramphenicol
Gram-positive rods		
Actinomyces	Penicillin (1)	Tetracycline, sulfonamide
Bacillus (eg, anthrax)	Penicillin (1)	Erythromycin
Clostridium (eg, gas gangrene, tetanus)	Penicillin (1)	Tetracycline, erythromycin
Corynebacterium	Erythromycin	Penicillin, cephalosporin
Listeria	Ampicillin plus aminoglycosides	Tetracycline

DRUG SELECTIONS, 1973-1974* (cont'd.)

Suspected or Proved Etiologic Agent	Drug(s) of First Choice	Alternative Drug(s)
Acid-fast rods		
Mycobacterium tuberculosis	INH plus rifampin/ ethambutol	Other antituberculosis drugs
Mycobacterium leprae	Dapsone or sulfoxone	Other sulfones
Nocardia	Sulfonamide (6)	Tetracycline, cycloserine
Spirochetes		
Borrelia (relapsing fever)	Tetracycline	Penicillin
Leptospira	Penicillin	Tetracycline
Treponema (syphilis, yaws)	Penicillin	Erythromycin, tetracycline
Mycoplasma	Tetracycline	Erythromycin
Psittacosis–LGV–trachoma agents (chlamydiae)	Tetracycline, sulfonamide (6)	Erythromycin, chloramphenicol
Rickettsiae	Tetracycline	Chloramphenicol

*Reproduced, with permission, from Krupp and Chatton (editors): Current Diagnosis & Treatment 1973. Lange, 1973.

(1) Penicillin G is preferred for parenteral injection; penicillin G (buffered) or penicillin V for oral administration. Only highly sensitive microorganisms should be treated with oral penicillin.

(2) All tetracyclines have the same activity against microorganisms and all have comparable therapeutic activity and toxicity. Dosage is determined by the rates of absorption and excretion of different preparations.

(3) Erythromycin estolate and troleandomycin are the best absorbed oral forms.

(4) Cephalothin and cephaloridine are the best accepted cephalosporins at present.

(5) Parenteral methicillin, nafcillin, or oxacillin. Oral dicloxacillin or other isoxazolylpenicillin.

(6) Trisulfapyrimidines have the advantage of greater solubility in urine over sulfadiazine for oral administration; sodium sulfadiazine is suitable for intravenous injection in severely ill persons.

(7) For previously untreated urinary tract infection, a highly soluble sulfonamide such as sulfisoxazole or trisulfapyrimidines is the first choice.

(8) Either or both.

The average daily dose in urinary tract infections is 100 mg. orally 4 times daily (for children, 5-10 mg./Kg./day), taken with food. If oral medication is not feasible, nitrofurantoin can be given by continuous I.V. infusion, 180-360 mg./day.

Oral nitrofurantoin often causes nausea and vomiting. Hemolytic anemia occurs in G-6-PD deficiency. Hypersensitivity may produce skin rashes and pulmonary infiltration.

2. NALIDIXIC ACID (NegGram®)

This synthetic urinary antiseptic inhibits many gram-negative bacteria in concentrations of 1-50 μg./ml. but has no effect on pseudomonas. In susceptible bacterial populations, resistant mutants emerge fairly rapidly.

Nalidixic acid is readily absorbed from the gut. In the blood, virtually all drug is firmly bound to protein. Thus, there is no systemic antibacterial action. About 20% of the absorbed drug is excreted in the urine in active form to give urine levels of 10-150 μg./ml.

The dose in urinary tract infections is 1 Gm. orally 4 times daily (for children, 55 mg./Kg./day). Adverse reactions include nausea, vomiting, skin rashes, drowsiness, visual disturbances, and, rarely, convulsions.

3. METHENAMINE MANDELATE AND METHENAMINE HIPPURATE

These are salts of methenamine and mandelic acid or hippuric acid. The action of the drug depends on the liberation of formaldehyde and of acid in the urine. The urinary pH must be below 5.5, and sulfonamides must not be given at the same time. The drug inhibits a variety of different microorganisms except those (e.g., proteus) which liberate ammonia from urea and produce strongly alkaline urine. The dosage is 2-6 Gm. orally daily.

4. ACIDIFYING AGENTS

Urine with a pH below 5.5 tends to be antibacterial. Many substances can acidify urine and thus produce antibacterial activity. Ammonium chloride, methionine, and mandelic acid are sometimes used. The dose has to be established for each patient by testing the urine for acid pH with test paper at frequent intervals.

SYSTEMICALLY ACTIVE DRUGS IN URINARY TRACT INFECTIONS

Many antimicrobial drugs are excreted in the urine in very high concentration. For this reason, low and relatively nontoxic amounts of aminoglycosides, polymyxins, and cycloserine (see Antituberculosis Drugs) can produce effective urine levels. Many penicillins and cephalosporins can reach very high urine levels and can thus be effective in urinary tract infections.

ANTIFUNGAL DRUGS

Most antibacterial substances have no effect on pathogenic fungi. Only a few drugs are known to be therapeutically useful in mycotic infections. Penicillins and sulfonamides are used to treat actinomycosis; sulfonamides and cycloserine have been employed in nocardiosis.

1. AMPHOTERICIN B (Fungizone®)

Amphotericin B, 0.1 μg./ml., inhibits in vitro several organisms producing systemic mycotic disease in man, including histoplasma, cryptococcus, coccidioides, candida, blastomyces, sporotrichum, and others. Amphotericin B, 100 Gm. I.V., results in average blood and tissue levels of 1-2 μg./ml., and thus can be used for treatment of these systemic fungal infections. Intrathecal administration is necessary for the treatment of meningitis.

Amphotericin B solutions, 0.1 mg./ml. in 5% dextrose in water, are given I.V. by slow infusion. The initial dose is 1-5 mg./day, increasing daily by 5 mg. increments until a final dosage of 1-5 mg./Kg./day is reached. This is usually continued for many weeks. In fungal meningitis, amphotericin B, 0.5 mg., is injected intrathecally 3 times weekly; continuous treatment (many weeks) with an Ommaya reservoir is sometimes employed.

The intravenous administration of amphotericin B usually produces chills, fever, vomiting, and headache. Tolerance may be enhanced by temporary lowering of the dose or administration of corticosteroids. Therapeutically active amounts of amphotericin B commonly impair kidney and liver function and produce anemia. Electrolyte disturbances, shock, and a variety of neurologic symptoms also occur.

2. GRISEOFULVIN
(Fulvicin®, Grifulvin®)

Griseofulvin is an antibiotic that can inhibit the growth of some dermatophytes but has no effect on bacteria or on the fungi that cause deep mycoses. Absorption of microsized griseofulvin, 1 Gm./day, gives blood levels of 0.5-1.5 μg./ml. The absorbed drug has an affinity for skin and is deposited there, bound to keratin. Thus, it makes keratin resistant to fungal growth and the new growth of hair or nails is first freed of infection. As keratinized structures are shed, they are replaced by uninfected ones. The bulk of ingested griseofulvin is excreted in the feces. Topical application of griseofulvin has little effect.

Oral doses of 0.5-1 Gm./day (for children, 15 mg./Kg./day) must be given for 6 weeks if only the skin is involved and for 3-6 months or longer if the hair and nails are involved. Griseofulvin is most successful in severe dermatophytosis, particularly if caused by trichophyton or microsporon.

Side-effects include headache, nausea, diarrhea, photosensitivity, fever, skin rashes, and disturbances of nervous and hematopoietic systems. Griseofulvin increases the breakdown of coumarin anticoagulants.

3. NYSTATIN
(Mycostatin®)

Nystatin inhibits Candida species upon direct contact. The drug is not absorbed from mucous membranes or gut. Nystatin in ointments, suspensions, etc. can be applied to buccal or vaginal mucous membranes to suppress a local candida infection. After oral intake of nystatin, candida in the gut is suppressed while the drug is excreted in feces. However, there is no good indication for the use of nystatin orally because increase in gut candida is rarely associated with disease.

4. FLUCYTOSINE
(Ancobon®)

Flucytosine, 3-8 Gm. daily orally, has been used in amphotericin-resistant yeast meningitis or sepsis. It can produce bone marrow depression and loss of hair.

ANTIVIRAL CHEMOTHERAPY

Several compounds are now available which can influence viral replication and the development of viral disease.

Amantadine hydrochloride (Symmetrel®), 200 mg. orally daily for 2-3 days before and 6-7 days after influenza A infection, reduces the incidence and severity of symptoms. The most marked untoward effects are insomnia, dizziness, and ataxia.

Idoxuridine (Herplex®, Stoxil®), 0.1% solution or 0.5% ointment, can be applied topically every 2 hours to acute dendritic herpetic keratitis to enhance healing. It is also used, in conjunction with corticosteroids, for stromal disciform lesions of the cornea to reduce the chance of acute epithelial herpes. It may have some toxic effects on the cornea and should probably not be used for more than 2-3 weeks. Intravenous injection of idoxuridine, 100-400 mg./day for 5 days, has been proposed for herpetic encephalitis. Cytarabine, 0.3-2 mg./Kg. as a single daily dose I.V., is an alternate drug in disseminated herpes or varicella.

Methisazone (Marboran®) can inhibit the growth of smallpox virus in man if administered to exposed persons within 1-2 days after exposure. Methisazone, 2-4 Gm. daily orally (for children, 100 mg./Kg./day), gives striking protection against the development of clinical smallpox and permits an asymptomatic, immunizing infection. Methisazone can also inhibit the growth of vaccinia virus and is used for the treatment of complications of smallpox vaccination (e.g., progressive vaccinia). The most pronounced toxic effect is profuse vomiting.

SPECIFIC TYPES OF SURGICAL INFECTIONS

FURUNCLE

A furuncle or boil is an abscess of a sweat gland or hair follicle, usually caused by Staphylococcus aureus. Treatment consists of hot packs and, if necessary, incision and drainage when the process has localized. Squeezing or incision before localization is to be avoided. Antibiotics are rarely indicated. Furuncles are usually self-limited and of minor significance except when multiple (furunculosis) or when they occur on the face. Rule out diabetes by urinalysis in every case of multiple or recurrent furuncles.

Furunculosis.

Predisposing factors include low resistance to infection, as in uncontrolled diabetes or debilitation; high virulence of the invading staphylococcus; poor body hygiene; and folliculitis. Treatment consists first of controlling diabetes or other systemic or local predisposing conditions. Have the patient bathe all over once or twice daily with soap containing hexachlorophene. Use aseptic dressing technic on draining furuncles to avoid contaminating surrounding skin. Administration of an antibiotic chosen by sensitivity studies may help reduce the surrounding inflammation.

Furuncles of the Face.

Infections in the mastoid and occipital areas and on the face above the level of the mouth may produce septic phlebitis of the emissary veins with extension into the cavernous sinus. Furuncles in these regions are therefore dangerous and must not be squeezed or incised. They should be allowed to localize under treatment by rest and hot packs. Drainage can then be encouraged by gentle manipulation. Antibiotics chosen by sensitivity tests are frequently advisable.

CARBUNCLE

Carbuncle is a staphylococcal infection of the skin and subcutaneous tissues which resembles a cluster of partially confluent furuncles. There is considerable surrounding brawny induration, and localization tends to proceed slowly. The back of the neck is a common site. Fever, malaise, and prostration may occur. Carbuncles are more common in diabetic patients, and diabetes should be ruled out in every case. These lesions can be quite extensive locally, and may endanger life in debilitated or diabetic patients.

Treatment.

A. Antibiotic therapy will frequently help localize the process or reduce the extent of surgery required.
B. General supportive measures include application of hot moist packs to the lesion, control of diabetes if present, rest, and symptomatic treatment of malaise and pain.
C. Incision and drainage or excision of the area is necessary for patients who fail to respond to antibiotics and supportive measures.

CELLULITIS, LYMPHANGITIS, AND LYMPHADENITIS

These common, nonsuppurative infections of the subcutaneous tissues may be caused by aerobic or anaerobic bacteria. The usual sequence of events is the development of an area of spreading infection and cellulitis, generally at the site of an infected wound. Involvement of the lymphatic channels is indicated by the red streaks on the skin extending proximally to draining nodes - which are usually, by this time, tender and enlarged. Rarely the nodes will suppurate and form abscesses requiring drainage. General measures for this group of infections include rest or splinting, elevation, hot packs, drainage of the entry wound if necessary, and symptomatic treatment of the systemic reaction, which usually consists of moderate fever and malaise. Antibiotic therapy is indicated when cellulitis is extensive or rapidly progressive, and should always be instituted when lymphangitis or lymphadenitis appears. Penicillin should be given when cultures for sensitivity studies cannot be obtained since the hemolytic streptococcus is frequently the cause.

The hemolytic streptococcus is also responsible for the following 2 severe types of cellulitis:

A. Erysipelas: This form of cellulitis is characterized by a marked erythematous blush of the skin in and around the area of infection. Elderly or debilitated patients are more susceptible. Penicillin is specific. General measures are as outlined in the preceding paragraph.

B. Hemolytic Streptococcus Gangrene: This is a rare and intense form of streptococcal cellulitis which progresses to necrosis of the skin and subcutaneous tissues. It is most likely to occur if the blood supply to the part is diminished, as in peripheral vascular disease of an extremity. Gangrene may be prevented if the virulent nature of the infection is recognized early, when it begins to involve the fascial planes. The fascia should then be opened widely to allow free drainage. Large doses of penicillin and general measures as above are recommended.

PILONIDAL SINUS

Pilonidal sinus or cyst is caused by the penetration of hair into the subcutaneous tissues as a result of trauma. The hair acts as a foreign body and nidus for the development of infection. The commonest location is in the midline of the back over the sacrococcygeal junction, but the lesion may also occur on the hands or in the umbilicus. The majority of patients are hirsute males in their late teens or early twenties. The first symptom is either an acute abscess or a chronic draining sinus. Sinus tracts may ramify to form several openings on either side of the midline. When a sinus opening is near the anus it may be confused with fistula in ano.

Treatment.

Treatment of the acute abscess is by incision and drainage, usually under local anesthesia. If the infected cavity or "cyst" is small and superficial, unroofing the abscess and packing it open, followed by a sitz bath daily, may result in complete healing. As a rule, however, a chronic draining sinus persists which must be surgically extirpated by excision and primary closure or, preferably, by an "open" technic such as marsupialization. Marsupialization can frequently be done under local anesthesia in the outpatient clinic with minimum morbidity. The procedure consists of opening the sinus and all of its ramifications over a grooved director or hemostat. The sinus tract is then completely exteriorized by circumcising the overhanging skin edges. Finally, the intact skin edge is sutured to the edge of the sinus tract and a pressure dressing applied. There is little postoperative pain. The pressure dressing is removed on the second postoperative day. Sutures are removed in 7-9 days and daily sitz baths are then begun. The wound is inspected every 5-7 days and wiped out carefully to prevent bridging-over. Healing time depends upon the size of the defect, but is usually 3-6 weeks. Daily dressings are applied by the patient, who is entirely ambulatory throughout the treatment. The recurrence rate with this method is 5-10%.

PROGRESSIVE BACTERIAL SYNERGISTIC GANGRENE

This is a mixed and synergistic infection with a microaerophilic nonhemolytic streptococcus (derived from the patient's intestinal tract) and hemolytic, coagulase-positive Staphylococcus aureus. Most cases involve the abdominal wall. The lesion may develop following drainage of a peritoneal abscess or an empyema, wound infection, or infection around an ileostomy or colostomy.

The principal symptom is excruciating pain and tenderness in the infected area. The lesion consists of progressive superficial ulceration and a narrow circle of gangrenous skin surrounded by a margin of erythema. The diagnosis is suggested by the course and appearance of the infection, which may progress to involve large areas of the abdominal wall, flank, and neighboring regions. Careful bacteriologic methods are required to identify the microaerophilic streptococcus which grows in the advancing margin of the ulcer.

Treatment.

Appropriate antibiotic therapy is indicated, usually following cultures and sensitivity studies. Penicillins and aminoglycosides are sometimes effective. If chemotherapy is not effective it may be necessary to excise the region completely (including the erythematous margin). Sterilized medicinal grade zinc peroxide, freshly prepared by suspension in distilled water to make a thin, creamy paste, is then applied once or twice daily to the wound and sealed over with vaseline gauze in order to prevent recurrence of infection. Skin grafting is required after the infection has been controlled.

ANTHRAX

Anthrax is an acute infectious disease of domesticated animals (cattle, horses, sheep, swine) which may be transmitted to man either directly or by contact with hides or hair. The characteristic lesion in humans is a "malignant pustule" resembling a carbuncle but distinguished by a central necrotic eschar surrounded by violaceous, bullous cellulitis. The diagnosis is made by identifying the gram-positive anthrax bacilli in the serum from 1 of the blebs. Treatment is with large doses of penicillin. Surgical intervention is not necessary for the acute process.

TETANUS

Tetanus is a nervous system intoxication caused by the toxin of Clostridium tetani. The organism most often infects puncture wounds or injuries associated with devitalized tissue (anaerobiosis), such as compound fractures, but even trivial wounds may be infected.

Clinical Findings.

The incubation period is usually 7-14 days, but symptoms can appear as early as 24 hours or as long as 8 months after injury. The first symptom may be pain and tingling at the site of the con-

taminated wound. Tetany may be limited to the injured extremity, or local spasm may be the first sign of the disease. More frequently, however, the earliest evidence of nervous system irritation is trismus ("lockjaw") followed by spasms which gradually progress to involve the rest of the body. Dysphagia, opisthotonos, a rigid but nontender abdomen, spasms of the facial muscles (risus sardonicus), and laryngeal spasm are classical manifestations. Trivial stimuli such as bright illumination or jarring the bed may elicit gross spasms or convulsions. Neonatal tetanus, caused by unclean management of the umbilical cord, is relatively common in underdeveloped parts of the world.

Death is most frequently caused by asphyxia from prolonged spasm of the respiratory muscles. Pneumonia is also a common cause of death.

The diagnosis of tetanus must be based on the clinical picture, since the organism is difficult or impossible to recover.

Prophylaxis.

A. Active Immunization: It is strongly advised that all persons be actively immunized with alum-precipitated tetanus toxoid (APT). Give 2 injections of 0.5 ml. I. M., 4-8 weeks apart, and a third injection approximately 12 months after the second. Fluid tetanus toxoid, 0.5 ml. I. M. or subcut., is given as a booster dose at the time of injury. Adequate responses to booster doses are obtained many years after a previous dose. However, to maintain maximum protection against tetanus from obscure or trivial injuries, a booster dose of 0.5 ml. I.M. of toxoid every 6-10 years is desirable. When an unimmunized person receives an injury for which tetanus prophylaxis is indicated, begin active immunization by injection of toxoid at another site at the same time that tetanus antitoxin is given.

B. Passive Immunization: For patients not actively immunized, give human Tetanus Immune Globulin, U. S. P., 250 units I. M., following wounds potentially contaminated with tetanus bacilli. Patients with dirty puncture wounds, compound fractures, major burns, and severe wounds of any type should receive the immune globulin and active immunization should be begun. When in doubt, immunize. Human tetanus immune globulin can be given without sensitivity testing and causes no allergic reactions. If it is not available, give equine or bovine tetanus antitoxin, 3000 units I. M. (6000 units if wound is heavily contaminated or severe), after sensitivity test is performed and proves negative. If the sensitivity test is positive, do not give equine or bovine antitoxin. Desensitization procedures may be dangerous, and the antitoxin will be valueless because of rapid destruction by antibodies. For such patients, rely on good wound care and prophylactic antibiotic therapy (penicillin or oxytetracycline). Give human tetanus immune globulin if possible.

C. Wound Care: Adequate debridement and delayed closure of wounds which are heavily contaminated and traumatized remove the conditions which favor the growth of tetanus bacilli. Penicillin or tetracycline prophylactically is also of value.

D. Tetanus is a particular risk in "skin-popping" heroin addicts. They should be fully immunized.

Treatment.

Tetanus is a true emergency. Intensive treatment should be started as soon as the earliest signs are noted. Ideally, the patient should be under the combined care of an internist, a surgeon, and an anesthesiologist.

A. Neutralization of Toxin: Toxin which has already entered and damaged the patient's cells is termed "fixed toxin," and cannot be reached by antitoxin. Circulating toxin must be neutralized with massive doses of antitoxin. Use human tetanus immune globulin if available. If not, use equine or bovine antitoxin after preliminary skin testing. Do not give bovine or equine antitoxin if sensitivity tests are positive.
   1. Systemic serotherapy - Give human tetanus immune globulin, 3000-6000 units, if available. Otherwise give equine or bovine tetanus antitoxin (TAT), 50,000 units I. V. and 50,000 units I. M. Stat., followed by daily injections of 5000 units I. M. until the disease is under control. In critically ill patients it may be advisable to give up to 1 million units I. V. in 24 hours. Intraspinal injection is contraindicated.
   2. Local serotherapy - Inject 250-500 units of tetanus immune globulin into the tissues at multiple sites around the wound 1 hour or more before surgical treatment. If not available, use 10,000 units of TAT for injection around the wound site.

B. Surgery: Locally excise (or incise) and debride the suspected wound under local procaine or intravenous thiopental (Pentothal®) anesthesia when feasible. Withhold surgery until at least 1 hour after systemic serotherapy. The wound should be left open, and may be packed with zinc peroxide paste.

C. Control of Muscle Spasms: The patient should be placed in a dark, quiet room and should be spared all unnecessary noise, movement, and excitement. Muscle spasms and most convulsions can be controlled with chlorpromazine (Thorazine®), 50-100 mg. 4 times daily, combined with a sedative (amobarbital, phenobarbital, or meprobromate). Other anticonvulsant regimens which have been advised are: (1) Tribromoethanol (Avertin®), 15-25 mg./Kg. rectally every 1-4 hours p. r. n. (2) Amobarbital sodium (Amytal Sodium®), 5 mg./Kg. I. M. p. r. n. (3) Paraldehyde, 4-8 ml. (1-2 dr.) I. V. (2-5% solution), may be combined with barbiturates.

D. General Measures:
   1. Nursing care must be expert and constant.
   2. Fluid balance and nutrition (see p. 150) must be maintained by parenteral or nasogastric tube feeding.
   3. Tracheostomy (see p. 251) - A tracheostomy set should be at the patient's bedside. If respiratory arrest occurs or if excessive mucus blocks the airway, tracheostomy may be lifesaving. Tracheostomy should probably be performed on every severe case.
   4. Artificial respiration - Use of a mechanical respirator may be required for days or weeks.
   5. Antimicrobial agents are not effective against tetanus toxin, but penicillin (or oxytetracycline) is useful in treating pulmonary, urinary, or pyogenic wound infections and in preventing multiplication of clostridia. The preferred antibiotic management during tetanus is aqueous penicillin G,

12 million units daily in divided doses I.M. or by intravenous drip.

6. Hyperbaric oxygen treatment may be of value in the management of tetanus. It is reported to delay or arrest progression of the condition and to reduce the severity of muscle spasms. Response is not as predictable and dramatic as in gas gangrene.

Prognosis.

The prognosis varies with the facilities available for treatment. The mortality rate in large series is 25-35%. The longer the incubation period, the better the outlook. If the incubation period is less than 7-10 days, the mortality rate will be almost twice as high as with longer incubation periods.

GAS GANGRENE

Gas gangrene, caused by Clostridium perfringens (welchii) and other toxigenic anaerobic clostridia, is an occasional complication of extensively traumatized and soil-contaminated wounds.

Clinical Findings.

The diagnosis is made primarily on clinical grounds. Do not wait for bacteriologic studies before starting therapy. Smears for Gram staining and fluid and tissue for aerobic and anaerobic culture should be obtained. Keep in mind that clostridial organisms may be noninvasive contaminants of wounds and that other organisms such as E. coli may produce gas in wounds and tissues.

The onset is generally abrupt, 1-4 days after injury, although the first symptoms may appear as early as 6 hours after injury. Wound pain is the earliest symptom, followed soon by a rapid, feeble pulse, pallor, prostration, and, frequently, septic shock. Varying degrees of fever and leukocytosis are reported. Anemia usually appears rapidly as a result of extensive hemolysis. The wound becomes swollen and exudes a dirty brown, watery, sometimes malodorous discharge. Exposed muscle is usually discolored, edematous, and nonviable. Gross crepitation around the wound (caused by gas in the tissues) occurs sooner or later in most cases, and the gas can be demonstrated by x-ray before it becomes palpable. Spread of the infection along fascial planes and muscle bellies is rapid, and toxicity becomes overwhelming, sometimes within a few hours. Results may be further improved by hyperbaric oxygen therapy.

Prophylaxis.

A. Debridement must be adequate to remove devitalized tissue; heavily traumatized and contaminated wounds should be left open.
B. Antibiotic therapy with penicillin or tetracycline for contaminated wounds.
C. Antitoxin is of no value in prophylaxis.

Treatment.

Gas gangrene is a surgical emergency. Begin therapy immediately.

A. Antibiotics: Large doses of penicillin inhibit growth of vegetative forms of clostridia. Give 20-40 million units of aqueous penicillin G daily by continuous intravenous drip as the preferred treatment. The following are also effective: tetracycline, 4 Gm. daily; chloramphenicol, 3 Gm. daily; or cephalothin, 6 Gm. daily I.V.

B. Antitoxin: The value of antitoxins is doubtful. After appropriate skin tests and desensitization as necessary, give pentavalent gas gangrene antitoxin I.V. prior to surgery. The dose is 2-4 vials (about 20,000 units/vial).

C. Operative Treatment: General anesthesia, rapid and wide removal of affected tissue, and, frequently, excision of entire muscle bellies are necessary. The fascial planes and muscle sheaths must be freely incised to promote drainage. Pack the wounds loosely to keep them open, and splint extremities as required. The most important aspect of treatment is radical surgical debridement.

D. General Supportive Measures: Combat septic shock (see p. 27), anemia, and fluid and electrolyte abnormalities.

E. Avoid cross infection of other patients by strict isolation procedures in the operating room and on the nursing unit.

F. Hyperbaric Oxygen Therapy: This is probably helpful in the treatment of gas gangrene and may be attempted whenever possible (see Appendix).

Prognosis.

Gas gangrene can be an extremely fulminant disease, fatal within a few hours. However, it can also be very gradual, and it responds well to surgical care. It must be differentiated from other conditions which it may resemble and which require less aggressive management.

ACTINOMYCOSIS

Actinomycosis is a chronic suppurative and granulomatous process caused by infection with Actinomyces israelii (A. bovis), a relatively common saprophytic resident of the mouth and the respiratory and gastrointestinal tracts. Invasion occurs through a break in the mucous membranes caused by infection or trauma. The 3 regions most commonly involved are the cervicofacial area (60%), the thorax (20%), and the abdomen (20%).

Clinical Findings.

There is usually a precipitating trauma or infection (e.g., dental extraction, lung abscess, appendicitis, or gastrointestinal perforation), followed by an indolent, burrowing network of sinuses and abscesses which tends to cross tissue planes indiscriminately and reach the body surface. Around the sinuses there is firm induration, and the overlying skin becomes brawny and dusky red. The granulation tissue is vascular, and drainage varies from serous to purulent. The systemic reaction is at first minimal, but as the infection becomes extensive the condition of the patient deteriorates from the effects of chronic sepsis. Pyogenic or intestinal organisms are invariably present also (mixed infection).

The diagnosis is made by finding "sulfur granules" in the

drainage or curettings from sinuses and abscesses. These are tiny yellowish masses composed of a central dense network of mycelial filaments which project radially and are usually enveloped by eosin-staining hyaline clubs. The granules are often difficult to find, and the diagnosis of actinomycosis is thus not easy to establish. Repeated smears and anaerobic cultures should be made and biopsy material obtained for pathologic examination.

Treatment.

A. Medical Measures: Perform sensitivity tests on culture material. Penicillin is the drug of choice for Actinomyces israelii. Dosage should be 10-20 million units of penicillin G I.M. daily for 4-6 weeks. Treatment should be continued for weeks after the clinical manifestations have disappeared in order to prevent relapse. Tetracycline may be of value if the organism is resistant to penicillin. Concomitant use of sulfadiazine or an aminoglycoside with penicillin may be advisable depending upon the nature of the mixed infection as determined by culture and sensitivity studies.

B. Surgical Treatment: Radical drainage and excisional procedures are no longer necessary since the antibiotics have come into wide use. Sinuses and abscesses should be conservatively incised and drained as required by the mixed infection and as an adjunct to intensive and prolonged chemotherapy. In rare cases (e.g., tubo-ovarian actinomycotic abscess), resection of the infected focus may be advisable.

BLASTOMYCOSIS

North American blastomycosis, caused by Blastomyces dermatitidis, is characterized by chronic ulcerating lesions of the skin, resembling boils with multiple draining sinuses; and pulmonary lesions which may simulate tuberculosis. Hematogenous spread may follow pulmonary infection, and further abscesses may then develop in bone, brain, or subcutaneous tissues.

The etiologic agent in South American blastomycosis is Blastomyces brasiliensis, which causes primary papillomatous granulomas of the buccal mucosa. Involvement of the skin, lymphatic tissues, and viscera also occurs. The diagnosis of either variety depends upon microscopic recognition of the fungus in tissues and exudates, followed by its isolation in culture. Complement fixation antibody titer is useful for prognosis.

The drug of choice in treatment of blastomycosis is hydroxystilbamidine (Lockwood et al.: Ann. Int. Med. **57**:553, 1962). Amphotericin B (Fungizone®) is also effective, but is more toxic. Surgical procedures may be successful for removal of cutaneous lesions, persistent cavities, or other localized pulmonary lesions.

HISTOPLASMOSIS

(See p. 311.)

COCCIDIOIDOMYCOSIS

(See p. 312.)

HOSPITAL INFECTIONS

Hospital cross-infection with hemolytic, coagulase-positive Staphylococcus aureus and with gram-negative enteric organisms is always a potential problem. Strains endemic in hospitals are often resistant to many antimicrobial drugs as a consequence of the widespread use of these agents. Relaxation of aseptic precautions in the operating theater and wards and an unwarranted reliance on "prophylactic" antibiotics contribute to the development of resistant strains. The result may be a significant increase in the incidence of hospital-acquired wound infection, pneumonitis, and septicemia, the latter 2 complications especially affecting infants, the aged, and the debilitated.

Although the pyogenic cocci are the major offenders, it is important to recognize that the enteric gram-negative bacteria (particularly the coliform and proteus group and Pseudomonas aeruginosa) are increasingly prominent in hospital-acquired infections.

Preventive Measures.

A. Hospital Administration:
1. The surgical infection control program should be coordinated closely with that of other services through a Hospital Infection Committee set up to promulgate and enforce regulations.
2. All significant infections should be reported immediately. A clean wound infection rate of more than 1-2% is excessive and indicates a need for more effective control measures. The wound infection rate should be continuously observed on the surgical services.

B. Cultures:
1. Obtain culture and antibiotic sensitivity studies on wounds, ulcerations, and significant infections of all types.
2. Phage-typing of staphylococci and detailed identification of other organisms may be useful in studying epidemics.

C. Isolation:
1. Isolate every patient with a significant source of communicable bacteria.
2. Isolate every case of suspected communicable infection until the diagnosis has been ruled out.
3. Isolate every patient in whom cross-infection will be serious.

D. Aseptic Technic:
1. Operating room - The operating room should be considered an isolation zone which may be entered only by persons wearing clean operating room attire (which may not be worn elsewhere).
2. Ward procedures - All open wounds should be aseptically dressed to protect them from cross-infection and to prevent heavy contamination of the environment. Eliminate dressing carts containing supplies and equipment for multiple bedside dressings.
3. Hand washing, preferably with hexachlorophene soap, before and after each contact with a patient is a simple but important routine measure in control of infection.

E. Nursing and Housekeeping:
1. Bedding must be laundered, and mattresses, furniture, and

cubicles cleaned with a general utility antiseptic (see p. 216) after a patient is discharged.
2. Housekeeping procedures throughout the hospital must be thorough. Wet mopping and cleaning are required in order to prevent accumulation or raising of dust.

F. Antibiotics:
1. Prophylactic use of antibiotics should be minimized.
2. When possible, antibiotic therapy should be based on sensitivity studies.
3. Antibiotics should be given in adequate doses and discontinued as soon as possible.

G. Epidemiology:
1. Personnel with active staphylococcal infections should be excluded from patient contact until they have recovered. Personnel carrying staphylococci in their nasal passages or gastrointestinal tracts must observe personal hygiene, but need not be removed from duty unless they prove to be a focus of infection. The advisability of treatment of the carrier is uncertain since the carrier state is frequently transient or recurrent in spite of treatment.
2. Every significant infection acquired in the hospital should be investigated to determine its origin and spread, possible contacts and carriers, and whether improper technics may have been responsible.

STERILIZATION, ASEPSIS, AND ANTISEPSIS

The protection of the surgical patient from infection is a primary consideration throughout the preoperative, operative, and postoperative phases of care. The factor of host resistance that influences the individual patient's susceptibility to infection has been discussed elsewhere. The incidence and severity of infection, particularly wound sepsis, are related also to the bacteriologic status of the hospital environment and to the care with which basic principles of asepsis, antisepsis, and surgical technic are implemented. The entire hospital environment must be protected from undue bacterial contamination in order to avoid colonization and cross-infection of surgical patients with virulent strains of bacteria which will invade surgical wounds in the operating room in spite of aseptic precautions taken during surgery. Prevention of wound infection therefore involves both application of general concepts and technics of antisepsis and asepsis in the hospital at large, and the use of specific procedures in preparation for operation.

Sterilization.

The only completely reliable methods of sterilization in wide current use are by steam under pressure (autoclaving), by dry heat, and by ethylene oxide gas.

A. Autoclaving: Saturated steam at a pressure of 750 mm. Hg (14.5 lb./sq. inch above atmospheric pressure) at a temperature of 120° C. (248° F.) destroys all vegetative bacteria and most resistant dry spores in 13 minutes. Additional time (usually a total of 30 minutes) must be allowed for the penetration of heat and moisture into the centers of packages. Sterilization time is markedly shortened by the high-vacuum or high-pressure autoclaves now widely used.

B. Dry Heat: Exposure to continuous dry heat at 170° C. (338° F.) for 1 hour will sterilize articles which would be spoiled by moist heat or which are more conveniently kept dry. If grease or oil is present on instruments, safe sterilization calls for 4 hours of exposure at 160° C. (320° F.).

C. Gas Sterilization: Liquid and gaseous ethylene oxide as a sterilizing agent will destroy bacteria, viruses, molds, pathogenic fungi, and spores. It is also flammable and toxic, and will cause severe burns if it comes in contact with the skin. Gas sterilization with ethylene oxide is an excellent method for sterilization of most heat-sensitive materials, including telescopic instruments, plastic and rubber goods, sharp and delicate instruments, and miscellaneous items such as electric cords and sealed ampuls. It has largely replaced soaking in antiseptics as a means of sterilizing materials that cannot withstand autoclaving. Care must be exercised in selecting items for gas sterilization because chemical interaction may occur with ethylene oxide or the agent with which it is mixed. For example, some acrylic plastic materials, polystyrene, certain lensed instruments, and pharmaceuticals may be damaged by ethylene oxide. Gas sterilization is normally carried out in a pressure vessel (gas autoclave) at slightly elevated pressure and temperature. It requires one hour and 45 minutes for sterilization in a gas autoclave utilizing a mixture of 12% ethylene oxide and 88% dichlorodifluoromethane (Freon 12®) at a temperature of 55° C. (131° F.) and a pressure of 410 mm. Hg (8 lb./sq. inch above atmospheric pressure). Following sterilization, a variable period of time is required for dissipation of the gas from the materials sterilized. Solid metal or glass items such as knives, drills, and thermometers may be used immediately following sterilization. Lensed instruments and packs including cloth, paper, rubber, and other porous items must usually be kept on the shelf exposed to air for 24-48 hours before use. Certain types of materials or complex instruments, such as a cardiac pacemaker, may require 7 days of exposure to air before use.

D. Boiling: Instruments should be boiled only if autoclaving, dry heat, or gas sterilization is not available. The minimum period for sterilization in boiling water is 30 minutes at altitudes less than 300 meters. At higher altitudes, the period of sterilization must be increased. The addition of alkali to the sterilizer increases bactericidal efficiency by raising pH so that sterilization time can safely be decreased to 15 minutes.

E. Soaking in Antiseptics: Sterilization by soaking is rarely indicated and should never be relied upon if steam autoclaving, dry heat, or gas sterilization is suitable and available. Under some circumstances, it may be necessary or more convenient to sterilize lensed or delicate cutting instruments by soaking in a liquid germicide. A wide variety of such germicides is available. The liquid disinfectant of current choice for lensed instruments and certain other critical items which should be sterile when used is glutaraldehyde in 2% aqueous alkaline concentration (Cidex®). This solution is bactericidal and virucidal in 10 minutes and sporicidal within 3 hours.

Antiseptics.

Antiseptics are chemical agents which kill bacteria or arrest their growth; they may or may not be sporicidal. Antiseptics should not be used in wounds since their toxicity to host cells far outweighs the possible advantages of their antibacterial effect. Many new and more versatile antiseptics have been developed in recent years. The most promising of these are discussed below.

A. Antiseptics for General Utility Purposes: Soap solution is one of the best all-purpose cleansing agents, but it is a weak antiseptic. A number of basic chemicals, more bactericidal than soap, are now in general use in hospitals and offices for cleaning floors, furniture, and operating room equipment and for soaking contaminated utensils and materials. The most valuable of these germicidal chemicals are (1) synthetic phenolics, (2) polybrominated salicylanilides, (3) iodophors, (4) alcohols, and (5) quaternary ammonium compounds. An increasing number of institutions are using the synthetic phenolics and polybrominated salicylanilides (PBS) as general purpose disinfectants because of their effectiveness under actual working conditions. These agents retain high potency in the presence of organic matter and are notable for their excellent residual activities on surfaces. This is probably a reflection of their inherent stability, their compatibility with ionic and alkaline agents, and their marked resistance to deactivation by organic matter. Synthetic phenolics and PBS compounds are compatible with soaps, detergents, and numerous other anionic and alkaline agents broadly used in hospitals. Iodophors and quaternary ammonium compounds tend to be rapidly diminished in activity by anionic or alkaline materials and are subject to a certain degree of volatilization. Glutaraldehyde preparations have the germicidal qualities of formaldehyde without the toxic and irritating properties.

1. Phenol compounds - Phenol (carbolic acid) is one of the most potent bactericidal chemicals available, but it is too caustic for safe use. The same is true to a lesser degree of cresol (Lysol®). These have been superseded by synthetic phenolic germicides such as Lamar SP-63®, Vestal Vasphene®, and Western Polyphene®. They kill gram-positive and gram-negative bacteria (including tubercle bacilli) and fungi. Surfaces properly treated with these compounds have demonstrated antibacterial properties for periods of 10-14 days. However, residual antibacterial activity should not be relied upon as a substitute for adequate routine cleaning and disinfection.
2. Polybrominated salicylanilide (PBS) - This is the newest class of antibacterial chemical. The antimicrobial spectrum and residual surface action are similar to those of the phenolics. When PBS preparations are used in laundries, textiles take on a self-sanitizing antibacterial finish. A disadvantage of PBS preparations is the white powdery film which remains on metal and other surfaces when the cleaning solution dries. PBS is the essential ingredient in Lamar L-300®.

3. Iodophors - These are chemicals in which iodine is combined with a detergent (Wescodyne®, Surgidine®) or with polyvinylpyrrolidone (Betadine®, Isodine®). The toxicity of the iodine is practically eliminated, but surface and skin disinfection is efficient.
4. Alcohols - Seventy percent ethyl alcohol is a powerful germicide. Isopropyl alcohol should be used as 70-90%. Neither of these alcohols is effective against spores.
5. Quaternary ammonium compounds - These are less effective than phenol, iodine, and alcohol and are inactivated by soap and adsorbed by fibers. Benzalkonium chloride is the prototype.
6. Formaldehyde and glutaraldehyde - Aqueous solutions of formaldehyde are known as formalin, which, when purchased commercially, is approximately 40% formaldehyde in water. The high-level germicidal activity of formaldehyde is increased by adding alcohol; a combination of 8% formaldehyde (20% formalin) in 70% alcohol is rapidly bactericidal and is sporicidal within 3 hours. Irritating fumes and tissue toxicity limit the usefulness of formaldehyde preparations. Glutaraldehyde is chemically related to formaldehyde, but it has a low tissue toxicity and does not have an irritating odor. Glutaraldehyde in 2% aqueous alkaline concentration (Cidex®) is approximately equivalent to 8% formaldehyde in alcohol. Glutaraldehyde is a good chemical sterilizing agent for soaking of instruments, cleaning of anesthesia equipment, and decontamination of operating room items such as basins, bottles, tubing, rubber goods, etc. after exposure to septic fields.
7. Other chemicals - Hypochlorites, chloramine, mercury salts, and solutions of azo dyes have been largely replaced by more reliable compounds.

B. Skin Antiseptics: The most important applications of skin antisepsis are the hand scrub of the operating team and the preparation of the operative field. Hexachlorophene is widely used in skin disinfection, usually in combination with a detergent (e.g., pHiso-Hex®) or with liquid or bar soap (e.g., Septisol®, Gamophen®, Dial®). Daily use of hexachlorophene produces a sustained lowering of the bacterial count on the skin. Sporadic or one-time use of hexachlorophene in soap or other preparation has no special value. Alcohol dissolves hexachlorophene and should not be applied if a prolonged surface effect is desired.

1. Hand scrub routine - Always scrub for 10 minutes except when changing gloves and gown aseptically between clean cases; in these circumstances, scrub for 5 minutes.
   a. Wash hands and forearms thoroughly with soap or a hexachlorophene preparation.
   b. Clean fingernails.
   c. Scrub for 5 minutes with a sterile brush or sponge, covering the entire surface of the hands and forearms repeatedly with soap or a hexachlorophene preparation.
   d. Scrub for another 5 minutes with a second sterile brush or sponge (a total of 10 minutes by the clock). Dry with sterile towel.
   e. Wash with 70% ethyl alcohol for 1 minute while rubbing the skin surface with a gauze sponge and allow to dry.

This optional step in the scrub routine will improve its effectiveness. Omit alcohol rinse if hexachlorophene preparation is used regularly for prolonged effect.

2. Preparation of the operative field -
   a. On the day before operation - Initial preparation of the skin is usually done the afternoon or evening before operation. Designate the specific area to be prepared in the preoperative orders. The area should be washed with soap and water, making sure that it is grossly quite clean. A shower or tub bath is satisfactory. The type of soap used makes little difference. Soap is a weak antiseptic and it is useful because of its nonirritating detergent action, especially when washing is combined with mechanical friction.

      Shaving is usually but not always required as part of the ward preparation. Shaving may be omitted where no hairs are present, as on the abdomen of a child. Where coarse hairs are present, shaving is necessary. Shaving must be skillfully done with a new blade and adequate soap lather. Slight nicks and scratches of the skin may be followed in a few hours by an abnormal increase in bacterial flora of the skin. For this reason, it is sometimes preferred (e.g., by neurosurgeons) to have the patient shaved just prior to surgery. It is not necessary to apply antiseptics such as alcohol or other germicides to the skin or to cover the prepared area with a sterile dressing.

      For elective operations involving areas with high levels of resident bacteria (e.g., hands, feet) or likely to be irritated by strong antiseptics (e.g., face, genitalia), preoperative degerming of the skin can be improved by repeated use of hexachlorophene soap or solution. Instruct the patient to wash the area several times daily for 3-5 days before operation exclusively with a soap or solution containing hexachlorophene.
   b. In the operating room - Use aseptic technic and prepare the operative field as follows:
      (1) Wash for 10 minutes with gauze and detergent or with soap solution. Wipe off with 70% ethyl alcohol and dry with a sterile towel or gauze. (This step may be omitted without change in the wound sepsis rate if preoperative preparation has been meticulous.)
      (2) Apply an antiseptic in one of the following ways: (a) Apply 70% ethyl alcohol to the skin with a gauze swab for 3 minutes and allow to dry before draping. Several applications of tinted tincture of benzalkonium (1:1000) may be alternated with applications of 70% ethyl alcohol for the same effect. (b) Apply 1-2% iodine in 70% (by weight) ethyl alcohol and remove with 70% ethyl alcohol. Repeat once. Iodine is one of the most efficient skin antiseptics available, but it occasionally causes skin reactions. Avoid streaming of iodine outside of operative field. Do not use iodine on the perineum, genitalia, or face; on irritated or delicate skin (e.g., small children); or when the patient gives a history of iodine sensitivity. In practice, careful skin preparation with

tincture of iodine is highly effective and safe. One percent iodine solution in 70% ethyl alcohol is an inexpensive all-purpose skin preparation. It has the same iodine concentration as the iodophors and is nonirritating unless there is a problem of sensitivity. (c) Apply an iodophor tincture to the skin. (d) For especially sensitive areas (perineum, around the eyes, etc.), apply aqueous iodophor solution repeatedly; or apply 1:1000 aqueous benzalkonium solution (first swabbing the area with water to remove any residual soap).

7 . . .

Pediatric Surgery

SPECIAL CONSIDERATIONS IN PEDIATRIC MANAGEMENT

Infants and young children have a relatively low tolerance to infection, trauma, blood loss, and nutritional and fluid disturbances. The management of these disorders in infants and children differs somewhat from their treatment in adults, and the margin of safety is narrower. Because specialized knowledge and experience are required to treat infants and children, the specialty of pediatric surgery has come into being. Certain unique aspects of surgical care in infants and young children deserve emphasis.

Fluid and Electrolyte Management.
Parenteral fluids must be adjusted to the size of the patient. Maintenance fluid and electrolyte requirements may be calculated according to body weight:

Weight	Water Requirements ml./Kg.	Na^+ mEq./Kg.	K^+ mEq./Kg.
< 10 Kg.	120	1-1.5	1-1.5
10-20 Kg.	100	1.5-2	1.5-2
20-30 Kg.	90	1-1.5	1-1.5
30-40 Kg.	80	1-1.5	1-1.5
> 40 Kg.	70	0.5-1	0.5-1

The physiologic limits of water replacement are 30 ml./Kg. above or below these mean daily requirements. The maintenance electrolyte requirements may be given by using solutions such as 5% dextrose and 0.2% saline or by mixing 5% dextrose and Ringer's lactate, 2 parts, and 5% dextrose and water, 1 part. Potassium chloride should be added to a concentration of 20 mEq./L.

Higher than maintenance requirements should be given when there is visible perspiration or abnormally high environmental temperature, fever, hyperventilation, and chronic renal insufficiency.

Previously existing deficits from external fluid losses such as vomiting, diarrhea, and third space losses into the bowel lumen, peritoneal cavity, or large wounds require rapid blood volume expansion. When a severely contracted blood volume exists, Ringer's lactate or 5% albumin solution (or both) should be given rapidly in a volume of 10-20 ml./Kg. Rehydration may then be continued with 5% dextrose and 0.45% saline until the clinical status of the baby is improved. Placement of a catheter in the right atrium by a cutdown in the external jugular vein or brachial vein will allow monitoring of central venous pressure. Methods for evaluating the response to therapy include assessment of weight, skin turgor, mucous membrane moisture, pulse and central venous pressure response, skin perfusion, urine output and specific gravity, serum and urine osmolarity, hemoglobin, hematocrit, and serum electrolyte changes.

Continuing losses such as gastrointestinal secretions, chest tube or bile drainage, and "third space" losses require replacement along with maintenance requirements. Gastric secretion is replaced by using 5% dextrose and 0.45% saline solution to which 20 mEq./L. of potassium has been added. Small bowel and "third space" losses should be replaced with lactated Ringer's injection.

The fluid requirements should be reassessed continuously and the prescribed orders should be rewritten at intervals of not more than 8 hours.

Intravenous Alimentation.

Prolonged starvation should be treated by intravenous alimentation. This requires the use of concentrated solutions which thrombose peripheral blood vessels, and it is necessary to place a catheter into the superior vena cava or right atrium where a large blood flow will dilute the solution immediately. A cutdown is required over the external jugular, anterior facial, internal jugular, or brachial veins. This should be performed with strict aseptic technic under general anesthesia. The catheter should be of inert material such as Silastic® or polyvinyl tubing. The tubing should be sutured to the skin to prevent accidental dislodgement. The cutdown site dressing should be changed daily and cleansed with an iodine solution. A bacterial filter in line with the intravenous tubing may minimize the risk of infection.

The intravenous alimentation solution is made up by mixing equal amounts of 10% protein hydrolysate and 50% glucose solutions (Hyprotigen®). The electrolyte composition of the protein hydrolysate solution must be recognized, and the desired additional maintenance requirements should be added. A stock solution (Hyprotigen®) consists of:

Water	1000 ml.
Glucose	20%
Protein	5%
Sodium	25 mEq.
Potassium	18 mEq.
Chloride	18 mEq.
Phosphate	25 mEq.
Magnesium	2 mEq.
Calcium	5 mEq.

Multivitamins are added to this solution. M.V.I.®, 2.5 ml./L., provides:

Vitamin A	2500 units
Vitamin D	250 units
Vitamin E	1.25 units
Thiamine (B_1)	12.5 mg.
Riboflavin (B_2)	2.5 mg.
Niacinamide	25.0 mg.
Pyridoxine (B_6)	3.75 mg.
Pantothenic acid	1.0 mg.
Ascorbic acid (C)	20.0 mg.

Added to the above (per liter):

Folic acid	2.5 mg.
Vitamin B_{12}	10 μg.
Vitamin K	0.5 mg.
Iron	5.0 mg.

Trace elements may be supplied by using a stock solution with the following composition in each 10 ml.:

Copper sulfate · 5 H_2O	25.5 mg.
Cobalt chloride · 6 H_2O	16.1 mg.
Manganese chloride · 4 H_2O	48.3 mg.
Zinc sulfate · 7 H_2O	59.4 mg.
Potassium iodide	6.5 mg.
Glycine	25.0 mg.

To each liter of alimentation solution, 0.33 ml. of the above trace element stock solution is added.

This solution must be given at a constant rate of infusion to prevent wide fluctuations of blood glucose and amino acid concentrations. This requires the use of an infusion pump. Complications include clotting or accidental dislodgement of the catheter, requiring replacement in a new site; sepsis, particularly due to Candida; thromboembolism, acidosis, hyperammonemia, and secondary liver damage; and sudden hypoglycemia following abrupt cessation of the infusion. When properly given, a normal growth rate can be maintained in infants by this technic.

DISORDERS OF THE HEAD, NECK, RESPIRATORY TRACT, AND MEDIASTINUM

BRANCHIOGENIC CYSTS AND FISTULAS

During the first month of fetal life, the primitive neck develops 4 external branchial clefts. Each cleft overlies outpocketings of the foregut, the pharyngeal pouches, so that the external cleft is separated from the internal pouch by only a membrane. The ridges between the clefts, or branchial arches, ultimately form portions of the face and neck. The first arch becomes the upper lip, cheek, maxilla, mandible, submaxillary gland, tragus, and helix. The second branchial arch forms the antitragus, antihelix, and the lesser horn of the hyoid bone. The third arch gives rise to the greater horn of the hyoid bone and the skin of the mid neck.

Clinical Findings.

A persistent first branchial cleft may present as a cyst or fistula in front of or below the ear, or below the margin of the mandible. The tract commonly extends to the external auditory canal near the facial nerve.

A second branchial cleft remnant may be a cyst or fistula located along the anterior border of the sternocleidomastoid muscle. The tract extends between the internal and external carotid arteries, coursing above the hypoglossal nerve to the tonsillar fossa (see p. 224). The cyst or fistula is lined by squamous or columnar epithelium and is surrounded by lymphoid follicles. Branchiogenic fistulas and cysts are bilateral in approximately 10% of cases.

A cyst produces localized painless swelling unless secondary infection has occurred, in which case erythema and tenderness are present. If a fistula opens into the pharynx, a sour taste may be noted.

A fistula produces mucoid material or crusting from a pinpoint skin opening over the middle or lower third of the sternocleidomastoid muscle. Milking the tract from above downward may produce mucoid material at the orifice of the fistula. If the fistula becomes secondarily infected, symptoms of inflammation are present.

Treatment.

Surgical excision through a transverse incision is the treatment of choice. If the tract is long, it may be necessary to place a second or third transverse incision above the first for ease of dissection.

THYROGLOSSAL DUCT CYSTS AND SINUSES

Thyroglossal duct cysts and sinuses may develop from cell rests at any point along the migratory path of the thyroid gland. If the cyst suppurates and drains externally, a fistula will result. The cysts contain mucoid material and are lined by squamous or columnar epithelium. Mucous glands occur in 60% of tracts. Scattered islands of thyroid follicles may be present. Sinuses pass a variable distance upward toward the foramen cecum at the base of the tongue. Multiple tracts are frequent.

Clinical Findings.

Thyroglossal duct cysts may be asymptomatic, may be large enough to cause symptoms by pressing on adjacent structures, or, if infected, may be tender and have a discharge. They are found in the midline of the neck anywhere from the submental region to the suprasternal notch, but are most commonly located at the level of the hyoid bone. They vary in size from a barely palpable nodule to a mass 3-4 cm. in diameter. Motion of the cyst during protrusion of the tongue is characteristic.

Thyroglossal duct fistulas usually develop after a thyroglossal duct abscess has been incised and drained. A deeply placed cord of dense tissue passing upward in the neck with attachment to the hyoid bone suggests the diagnosis.

Differential Diagnosis.

Dermoid cysts may also occur in the midline. Ectopic thyroid tissue is clinically difficult to distinguish from a cyst. The distinction can be made by radioactive scintiscans.

Treatment.

Cysts and sinuses should be removed because they are apt to become infected. The tracts must be completely removed, including the central portion of the hyoid bone and a block of tissue to the base of the tongue (see p. 224). Infected cysts must be drained,

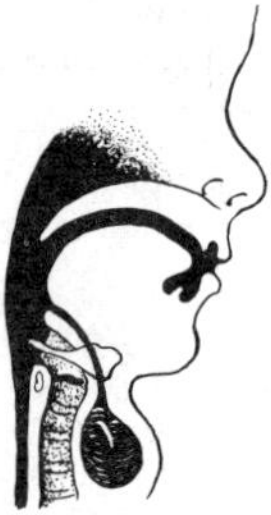

Thyroglossal duct cyst

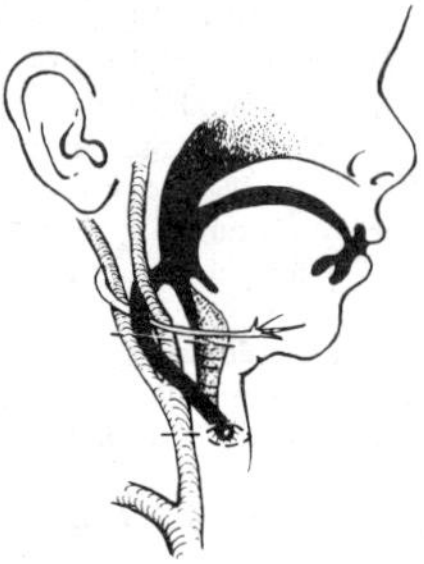

Branchial cleft fistula

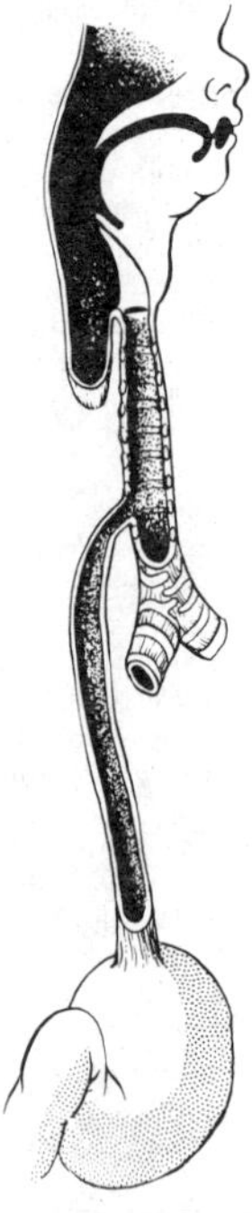

Esophageal
atresia

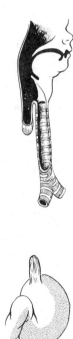

Esophageal
atresia
without
fistula

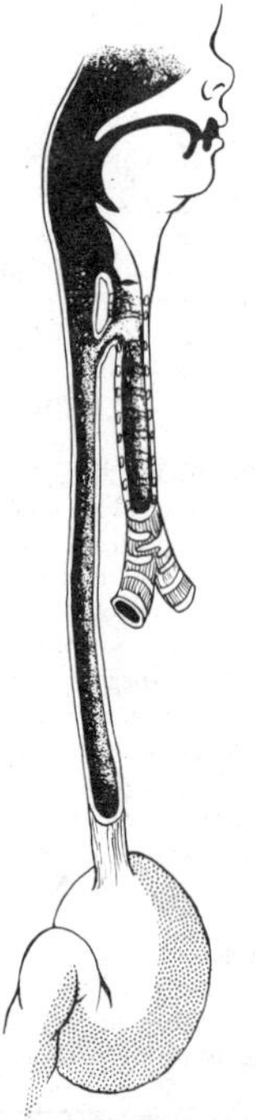

H-type
tracheoesophageal
atresia

and definitive removal should be delayed until the inflammation has subsided. A sinus or cyst will recur if a branch of the original sinus is overlooked at the first operation.

CERVICAL LYMPHADENOPATHY

Pyogenic Lymphadenitis.

Acute inflammation of cervical lymph nodes in the submandibular and anterior cervical triangles usually develops after a respiratory infection. These enlarged nodes ordinarily subside within several weeks. Occasionally, a streptococcal or staphylococcal abscess develops in the nodes and incision and drainage are necessary.

Granulomatous Lymphadenitis.

Typical or atypical tuberculosis lymphadenitis develops slowly and may suppurate. The diagnosis is established by appropriate skin tests. These nodes should be excised rather than drained to prevent a chronically draining sinus.

Lymphatic Tumors (Lymphosarcoma and Hodgkin's Disease).

Lymphomatous nodes are usually located in the posterior as well as the anterior cervical triangle. These nodes may be solitary, but they are usually multiple, rubbery-hard, matted together, and painless.

Metastatic cervical nodes in children are usually due to primary thyroid carcinoma or neuroblastoma.

SURGICAL RESPIRATORY EMERGENCIES IN THE NEWBORN

Certain aspects of respiration peculiar to infants must be appreciated:

(1) Babies are obligate nasal breathers. Mouth breathing is an acquired habit which may not be learned for days or weeks.

(2) Infants breathe primarily by diaphragmatic movement. The accessory and intercostal muscles contribute little to ventilation in the newborn.

(3) An infant's response to hypoxia is an increase in respiratory rate before an increase in volume. Normal tidal volume is 15-20 ml.

(4) Infants have a flaccid chest wall and mediastinum. Paradoxical motion and increased work in breathing occur with any degree of respiratory distress.

(5) Infants have a small, flaccid airway. The tracheal cartilages are readily compressed by slight external pressure. The subglottic area is the narrowest part of the upper airway, measuring about 14 sq. mm. If mucosal edema of 1 mm. occurs, it will reduce the subglottic area to 5 sq. mm.

(6) Air swallowing develops rapidly during respiratory distress which produces abdominal distention and impaired diaphragmatic excursion.

(7) During ventilatory assistance, transpulmonary pressure must be less than 30 cm. of water to prevent alveolar rupture.

Symptoms and Signs.

Symptoms and signs suggestive of respiratory distress in the newborn include the following:

(1) Respiratory rate greater than 40/min.
(2) Retraction of the chest wall or stridor.
(3) Cyanosis.
(4) Increased salivation.
(5) Episodes of choking.
(6) Episodes of apnea.

Differential Diagnosis of Surgical Respiratory Emergencies.

The diagnosis must be established as soon as possible. Causes of airway obstruction above the thoracic inlet can be identified by physical examination, by attempting to pass a tube through the nasopharynx and esophagus, or by direct laryngoscopy. Intrathoracic lesions must be diagnosed by chest x-ray examination.

Surgically treatable causes are choanal atresia, Pierre Robin syndrome; congenital laryngeal obstructions due to webs, cysts, or tumors; tumors of the neck and mediastinum, esophageal anomalies, diaphragmatic eventration or hernia, vascular rings, congenital lobar emphysema, pulmonary parenchymal anomalies, pneumothorax, and pneumomediastinum.

CHOANAL ATRESIA

Complete obstruction at the posterior nares due to choanal atresia may be unilateral and relatively asymptomatic. When it is bilateral, severe respiratory distress is manifest by marked chest wall retractions on inspiration and a normal cry.

Clinical Findings.

There is arching of the head and neck in an effort to breathe, and the baby is unable to eat. The diagnosis is confirmed by inability to pass a tube through the nares to the pharynx. With the baby in a supine position, radiopaque material may be instilled into the nares and lateral x-rays of the head taken to outline the obstruction.

Treatment.

The emergency treatment of choanal atresia consists of maintaining an oral airway by placing a nipple, with the tip cut off, in the mouth. The membranous (10%) or bony (90%) occlusion may then be perforated by direct transpalatal excision, or it may be punctured and enlarged by using a Hegar's dilator. The newly created opening must be stented with plastic tubing for 5 weeks to prevent stricture.

PIERRE ROBIN SYNDROME

Pierre Robin syndrome is characterized by micrognathia, glossoptosis, and cleft palate.

Clinical Findings.

The small lower jaw allows the tongue to fall back and occlude the laryngeal airway.

Treatment.

Most infants should be kept in the prone position during care and feeding, and a nasogastric or gastrostomy tube may be necessary. If conservative measures fail, tracheostomy is indicated. The tongue may be sutured forward to the lower jaw, but this frequently breaks down. In time the lower jaw develops normally. These infants eventually learn how to keep the tongue from occluding the airway.

CONGENITAL LARYNGEAL OBSTRUCTIONS

Laryngeal obstructions may be due to intraluminal webs or cysts or to extraluminal tumors such as hemangiomas, cystic hygromas, large congenital goiters, or thyroglossal cysts.

Clinical Findings.

These infants have stridor and chest wall retraction. When the vocal cords are involved the cry is hoarse or aphonic. Examination of the neck and direct laryngoscopy will usually identify the cause.

Treatment.

An airway must be established by placing an endotracheal tube through the larynx or by tracheostomy. Webs and cysts as well as extraluminal tumors must be excised.

ESOPHAGEAL ANOMALIES

Classification. (See p. 224.)

There are 6 types of esophageal anomaly:

A. Esophageal atresia with a blind proximal esophageal pouch, no tracheo-esophageal fistula, and rudimentary distal esophagus, usually a long distance from the proximal end. This accounts for 10% of esophageal anomalies.

B. Esophageal atresia in which the proximal pouch has a fistula between the trachea and esophagus. The blind end of the distal esophageal segment is usually adjacent to the carina. This anomaly accounts for 0.3% of cases.

C. Esophageal atresia in which there is a blind proximal pouch and the distal esophageal end communicates with the trachea as a tracheo-esophageal fistula. This anomaly accounts for 85% of cases.

D. Esophageal atresia in which both the proximal and distal esophageal segments communicate with the trachea. This accounts for 0.5% of cases.

E. No esophageal atresia but an H type tracheo-esophageal fistula. This accounts for 4-5% of esophageal anomalies.

F. Congenital esophageal stenosis usually consists of a membranous occlusion between the middle and distal thirds of the esophagus.

Clinical Findings.

A. Symptoms and Signs: The infant appears to have excessive salivation because of inability to swallow. There are repeated episodes of cyanosis, coughing, and gagging. Attempts to feed these babies results in choking and regurgitation. Pneumonia is common because of aspiration and reflux of gastric contents through the tracheo-esophageal fistula. When there is a fistula to the distal esophagus, abdominal distention is common because air is forced into the bowel during crying and fretting.

B. X-ray Findings: A nasogastric tube passed through the nose will not traverse the expected esophageal length. If 1 ml. of propyliodine (Dionosil®) or barium is injected into the tube, followed by air, it will outline the blind pouch on an A-P and lateral chest x-ray. The presence or absence of air in the stomach will indicate whether a distal esophageal fistula is present. The most reliable method of proving an H-type fistula is by cine-esophagography.

Treatment.

Aspiration pneumonia must be treated before surgical treatment is begun. A sump suction catheter should be placed in the infant's upper esophageal pouch and connected to continuous suction. The head of the bed should be elevated. The infant should be placed in a humidified incubator and should be turned from side to side every hour and stimulated to cry and cough. Antibiotic therapy should be given, e.g., ampicillin, 50 mg./Kg. every 6 hours I.M., and kanamycin, 7 mg./Kg. every 12 hours I.M. Infants that are fully mature and without severe anomalies should have a gastrostomy and an extrapleural thoracotomy for division of tracheo-esophageal fistula and primary esophageal anastomosis. The operation should be staged for premature babies, for infants with associated severe anomalies, or for babies with a short upper esophageal segment. The first stage consists of a gastrostomy and transpleural division of the tracheo-esophageal fistula. A sump suction catheter is maintained in the upper esophageal pouch, and the baby is fed by gastrostomy until he has become strong enough to tolerate the second stage procedure. A short upper pouch can be elongated with a 22-24 F. Hurst bougie over a period of 2-3 weeks. The second stage procedure consists of an extrapleural thoracotomy and anastomosis of the 2 esophageal segments.

The infant with esophageal atresia and no tracheo-esophageal fistula requires a cervical esophagostomy and gastrostomy. He is fed through the gastrostomy tube until he weighs 20-25 pounds, at which time a colon interposition is used to establish continuity between the cervical esophagus and the stomach.

In infants with an H-type tracheo-esophageal fistula, the fistula is located above the thoracic inlet in two-thirds of cases. These fistulas may be divided through a left transverse cervical incision. Intrathoracic fistulas may be divided by an extrapleural right thoracotomy. A gastrostomy is commonly employed for feeding until the esophageal closure is healed.

DIAPHRAGMATIC EVENTRATION AND POSTEROLATERAL (BOCHDALEK) DIAPHRAGMATIC HERNIA

Eventration of the diaphragm may be a congenital defect in which the diaphragm consists of a thin membrane lacking tendon and muscle, or it may be acquired by injury to the brachial plexus during birth, and is usually associated with Erb's palsy. The phrenic nerve may be injured during thoracotomy, producing diaphragmatic paralysis.

Posterolateral (Bochdalek) diaphragmatic hernia is a congenital defect in the posterior and lateral portion of the diaphragm caused by failure of the septum transversum to fuse with the pleuroperitoneal folds during the eighth week of fetal life. The defect occurs on the left side 3-5 times more frequently than on the right side, possibly because the right diaphragm is protected by the liver. During fetal development, the intestinal contents are pushed into the pleural cavity by abdominal muscle tone (see p. 230). Varying degrees of pulmonary hypoplasia result, depending on the size of the defect and the amount of intestinal content compressing the lungs.

Clinical Findings.

The onset and severity of symptoms are dependent upon the degree of pulmonary hypoplasia and the amount of lung compressed by the bowel. These infants have markedly labored respiration and cyanosis. The heart sounds are displaced, and there is apparent dextrocardia with left-sided hernias. The ipsilateral chest is flat to percussion and has diminished breath sounds. The abdomen is characteristically scaphoid. The diagnosis is confirmed by chest x-ray showing the bowel, spleen, and portions of the liver within the thorax. The lungs, mediastinum, and trachea are displaced to the opposite chest.

Treatment.

A nasogastric tube should be placed in the stomach to prevent distention of the bowel with air. For severely distressed infants, an endotracheal tube should be placed in the airway and ventilation assisted with transpulmonary pressure less than 25 cm. water. A catheter should be placed in the distal aorta via the umbilical artery, and the blood gas and pH levels should be monitored. Metabolic acidosis due to hypoxia should be corrected with sodium bicarbonate.

Infants with eventration may develop severe respiratory distress, and they may require a thoracotomy and plication of the diaphragm to prevent paradoxical motion of the diaphragm and mediastinum.

For infants with a posterolateral diaphragmatic hernia, an abdominal incision is preferred. The bowel is reduced from the pleural space and a hernia sac lining the pleural space should be looked for and excised. A chest tube should be placed in the pleural space and connected to water-seal without suction. The diaphragmatic defect is closed. Forced expansion of the lung must not be attempted to prevent rupture of alveoli. A gastrostomy is beneficial. A large ventral hernia should be created by closing the skin, but not the fascia, to accommodate the intestine in the small abdominal cavity.

VASCULAR RINGS

The genesis of vascular rings may be understood if the embryo is considered to have 2 aortic arches, each with a carotid and sub-

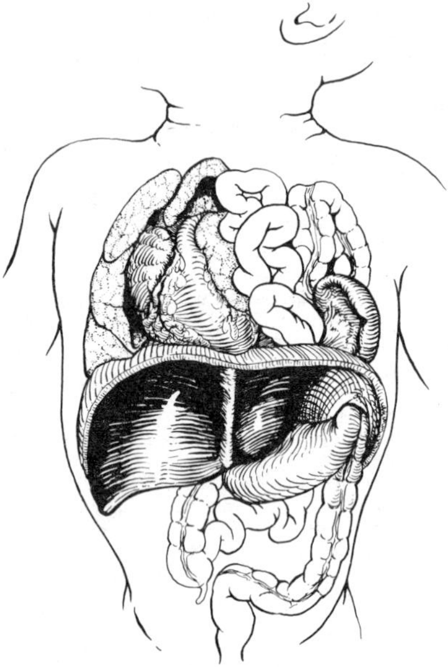

Congenital diaphragmatic hernia

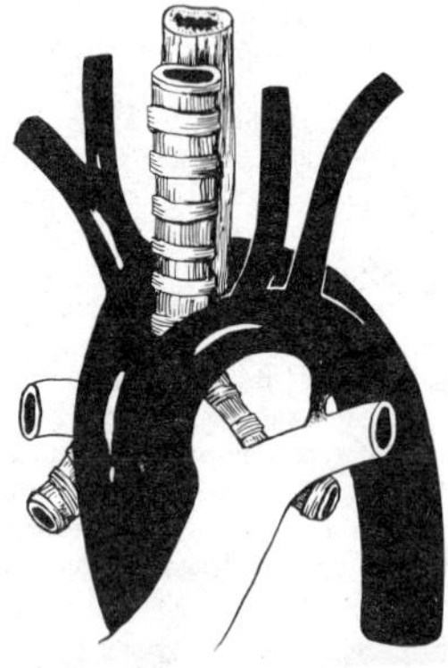

Double aortic arch

clavian artery and a ductus arteriosus. In the normal development of the aortic arch, the distal portion of the right arch is obliterated. There are 5 main types of vascular rings: (1) persistence of both arches gives rise to double aortic arch (see p. 230); (2) obliteration of the left distal arch generates right aortic arch and persistent left ligamentum arteriosum; (3) obliteration of the right arch between the right carotid and subclavian arteries results in anomalous origin of the right subclavian artery; (4) incorporation of the right proximal arch into the left arch produces anomalous origin of the innominate artery; and (5) incorporation of the left proximal arch into the right arch gives rise to an anomalous origin of the right common carotid artery. Each of these anomalies may compress and encircle the trachea and esophagus, producing respiratory distress and swallowing symptoms of obstruction.

Clinical Findings.

These infants have a characteristic inspiratory and expiratory wheeze, stridor, or crow. The head is held in an opisthotonic position to prevent compression of the trachea. If the head is forcibly flexed, the stridor is increased and apnea may be produced. There may be hesitation on swallowing with episodes of choking - so called "dysphagia lusoria." Chest x-rays may show compression of the trachea. A-P and lateral esophagograms show indentation of the esophagus at the level of T-3 and T-4. When there is no esophageal indentation, a tracheogram may be necessary to demonstrate tracheal compression due to an anomalous origin of the innominate or left common carotid artery. An arteriogram is almost never needed. Esophagoscopy and bronchoscopy may be helpful in assessing the degree and level of compression.

Treatment.

The aortic arch anomaly must be completely dissected and visualized through a left thoracotomy. The smallest component of a double aortic arch must be divided. An anomalous right subclavian artery is divided at its origin. The anomalous innominate or left carotid arteries are pulled forward by placing sutures between their adventitia and the sternum. The accompanying fibrous bands and sheaths constricting the trachea and esophagus must also be divided. Occasionally, symptoms persist postoperatively because of deformed tracheal cartilage rings which require tracheostomy or nasotracheal intubation for a period of time.

CONGENITAL LOBAR EMPHYSEMA

Emphysema may be due to deficiency in the involved bronchial cartilage, partial obstruction by a redundant or edematous membrane, or compression of the bronchus by an anomalous pulmonary vessel. This almost always involves the upper lobes or middle lobe. The emphysematous lobe becomes progressively enlarged, compresses the normal lung, and displaces the mediastinum to the opposite side. These infants have wheezing, dyspnea, and cyanosis. The chest is hyperresonant and the breath sounds are decreased over the involved lobe. The diagnosis is established by chest x-ray showing the overdistended lobe and compression of the normal lung. The mediastinum may be displaced and the emphysematous lobe may herniate into the opposite chest.

Treatment.

Occasionally, bronchoscopy and aspiration of mucus are curative. In severely distressed infants, immediate thoracotomy is usually required, and the abnormal lobe must be resected. Relatively asymptomatic patients should be followed closely and may require no treatment.

PULMONARY CYSTS AND CONGENITAL CYSTIC ADENOMATOID MALFORMATION

Lung cysts may be congenital or acquired. They may become large enough to be confused with lobar emphysema or pneumothorax and produce symptoms of severe pulmonary insufficiency. In cystic adenomatoid malformation, usually only one lobe is involved by cysts containing proliferating respiratory epithelium but no cartilage and bronchioles.

The involved lobe should be removed to relieve the symptoms of respiratory insufficiency and to prevent pulmonary suppuration.

MEDIASTINAL TUMORS

Respiratory distress may develop due to displacement of the lungs or compression of the airways from masses involving the anterior, middle, or posterior mediastinum. Examples of such masses are as follows:

(1) Anterior mediastinum: Thymoma, teratoma, lymphangioma, intrathoracic goiter.

(2) Middle mediastinum: Pathogenic lymph node enlargement (lymphoma, etc.), aneurysm.

(3) Posterior mediastinum: Neurogenic tumor (neuroblastoma), gastrointestinal duplication (neurenteric cyst), bronchogenic cyst, achalasia or hiatus hernia, mediastinal meningocele.

SPONTANEOUS ALVEOLAR RUPTURE

Rupture of an alveolus may occur spontaneously or may be caused by excessive intratracheal pressure during resuscitation. Initially, the air dissects along the bronchovascular planes, producing pulmonary interstitial emphysema. Further dissection of the air may produce pneumomediastinum or pneumothorax. Mediastinal air does not readily dissect into the tissues of the neck and may markedly compress the trachea. An incision above the clavicles may be necessary to release the mediastinal air. Pneumothorax requires chest tube suction.

INTESTINAL OBSTRUCTION AND PROBLEMS IN THE NEONATAL PERIOD

The cardinal signs and symptoms of intestinal obstruction are (1) polyhydramnios in the mother, (2) vomiting, (3) abdominal distention, and (4) failure to pass meconium. Polyhydramnios is related to the level of obstruction, occurring in approximately 45% of women who have infants with duodenal atresia and 15% of those who have infants with ileal atresia. When a tube is routinely passed into the stomach of a newborn, a residual greater than 40 ml. is diagnostic of obstruction. Vomiting occurs early in upper intestinal obstruction, and it is bile-stained if the obstruction is distal to the ampulla of Vater. Abdominal distention is related to the level of obstruction, being most marked for distal obstructions. Meconium is passed in 30-50% of newborn infants with intestinal obstruction, but the failure to pass meconium within the first 24 hours is distinctly abnormal. Approximately one-fourth of infants with congenital intestinal obstructions weigh less than $5^1/2$ pounds.

Causes of neonatal intestinal obstruction include intestinal atresia or stenosis, annular pancreas, malrotation with peritoneal bands or volvulus, meconium ileus, Hirschsprung's disease, and meconium plug syndrome.

CONGENITAL DUODENAL OBSTRUCTION

Duodenal atresia and stenosis and annular pancreas are frequently associated with other anomalies, and 30% of these patients have Down's syndrome. In 25% of the patients with duodenal atresia, the obstruction is proximal to the ampulla of Vater.

Clinical Findings.

Abdominal x-rays show gastric and duodenal distention (double-bubble sign) when obstruction of the duodenum is almost complete. Total absence of gas distal to the duodenum indicates atresia rather than stenosis. Barium enema (in saline) identifies the presence or absence of malrotation of the colon. The colon is usually very narrow (microcolon).

Treatment.

A nasogastric tube should be placed and continuous suction applied. Dehydration should be treated preoperatively. Duodenal atresia, stenosis, and annular pancreas should be treated by a retrocolic, side-to-side duodenojejunostomy. A right upper quadrant transverse incision is used. The overdistended proximal duodenum frequently fails to function well for many days, and a gastrostomy is helpful for decompression and to check gastric residual during graded feedings.

MALROTATION OF THE MIDGUT

During the 10th week of fetal development the small bowel and colon undergo counterclockwise rotation and fixation to the posterior peritoneum. If bowel rotation fails to occur, intestinal obstruction may be produced by 2 mechanisms. First, when the cecum is arrested in the upper abdomen, filmy or dense adhesive bands from the right abdomen to the cecum may obstruct the duodenum and other portions of the small bowel. Second, the failure in fixation of the mesentery produces a "universal mesentery" based on the superior mesenteric vessels. Volvulus of the intestine, always following clockwise torsion of the bowel and mesentery, will also obstruct the duodenum. The mesenteric blood supply may become embarrassed and produce infarction of the entire small and proximal large bowel.

Clinical Findings.
Mesenteric bands usually produce symptoms of duodenal obstruction early in infancy. The abdomen is not distended, and abdominal x-rays show little gas in the small bowel. In contrast, when volvulus occurs, the bowel is usually distended. Bloody stools are a late sign of bowel infarction. A barium enema confirms the abnormal position of the colon and cecum.

Treatment.
The adhesive bands are divided through an upper abdominal transverse incision. When a volvulus is present, the torsion is reduced by counterclockwise rotation of the gut. The duodenum is mobilized and placed in the right lower quadrant, and, following appendectomy, the cecum is placed in the left lower quadrant. Suturing the mesentery to the posterior peritoneum may prevent subsequent volvulus. Frankly necrotic bowel should be resected and continuity established either by primary anastomosis or by Mikulicz enterostomy. After reduction of the volvulus, intestine with questionable viability should be left alone and the abdomen reexplored 24 hours later to confirm the viability of the bowel. Hyperbaric oxygen treatment may be beneficial for infants with severely ischemic bowel.

JEJUNAL, ILEAL, AND COLONIC ATRESIA OR STENOSIS

Small intestinal and colonic atresias probably follow a vascular accident in utero such as volvulus, intussusception, or gangrenous obstruction. Following aseptic necrosis and resorption of the segment of bowel, the atresia may be a membranous occlusion, may produce 2 blind ends connected by a cord, or there may be a complete separation of the bowel ends. Multiple atresias occur in 10% of cases. Infarction of long lengths of bowel in utero results in abnormally short intestine. The markedly distended proximal bowel frequently functions abnormally and produces a functional obstruction after repair of the atresia.

Clinical Findings.
The vomiting, distended infant should have abdominal roentgenograms. Air is sufficient contrast to outline the presence of obstruction, and barium by mouth is not indicated. The colon cannot be distinguished from the small bowel in the newborn. Therefore, a barium enema (in saline) will demarcate the colon and determine the presence of colonic obstruction or malrotation. The colon is usually small in caliber (microcolon) because it has been unused, but it is not abnormal. The onset and severity of symptoms from intestinal stenosis is dependent upon the degree of lumen narrowing.

Treatment.
A transverse upper abdominal incision is used for jejunal atresia, and a transverse infra-umbilical incision is employed for ileal

or colonic atresia. The bulbously dilated proximal blind end of the bowel should be resected. End-to-oblique anastomosis is preferred. A gastrostomy is valuable because prolonged postoperative functional obstruction of the dilated proximal bowel frequently occurs.

MECONIUM ILEUS

About 15-20% of infants born with cystic fibrosis will have meconium ileus. Cystic fibrosis is an inherited disease transmitted by an autosomal recessive trait. The disease affects all the exocrine glands. The secretion from the mucous glands is abnormally viscid and produces varying degrees of obstruction of the bronchi and the pancreatic and bile ducts. Obstruction of the distal small bowel in utero occurs because of the abnormal viscosity of intestinal mucus and not because of pancreatic enzyme deficiency.

Clinical Findings.
Enormous abdominal distention may produce dystocia at birth. Dilated intestinal loops are palpable, and plain abdominal x-rays show dilated loops of bowel of varying diameter. Air-fluid levels are not prominent because of delayed layering of the viscous fluid. Small "soap" bubbles of gas can be seen in the meconium-filled bowel. Calcification in the abdomen may be seen. About 50% of cases are complicated by volvulus and atresia, with or without perforation of the bowel, and meconium peritonitis. The sodium and chloride content of sweat and fingernails is abnormally high.

Treatment.
A nasogastric tube should be placed into the stomach and connected to suction. Under fluoroscopic control, enemas containing methylglucamine diatrizoate (Gastrografin®), which is hygroscopic, or acetylcysteine (Mucomyst®), which is mucolytic, may effectively unplug the meconium in uncomplicated cases. Most patients require a right lower quadrant transverse incision and Mikulicz resection of the most dilated portion of the ileum. The proximal and distal bowel loops may then be irrigated with acetylcysteine. Subsequently, the Mikulicz enterostomy is closed.

HIRSCHSPRUNG'S DISEASE

The congenital absence of myenteric ganglion cells, extending for a varying distance from the anus, produces functional obstruction of the colon. The normally ganglionic bowel becomes markedly dilated and hypertrophic. The transition zone between aganglionic and ganglionated bowel involves the rectosigmoid in 75% of cases. The entire colon may be lacking ganglion cells in 10% of cases.

Clinical Findings.
Invariably, constipation begins at birth and may be obstinate enough to cause intestinal obstruction in the neonatal period. Paradoxically, symptoms of abdominal distention and diarrhea in infancy are due to Hirschsprung's disease until proved otherwise. Rectal examination may reveal a tight and narrow anus and rectum. The

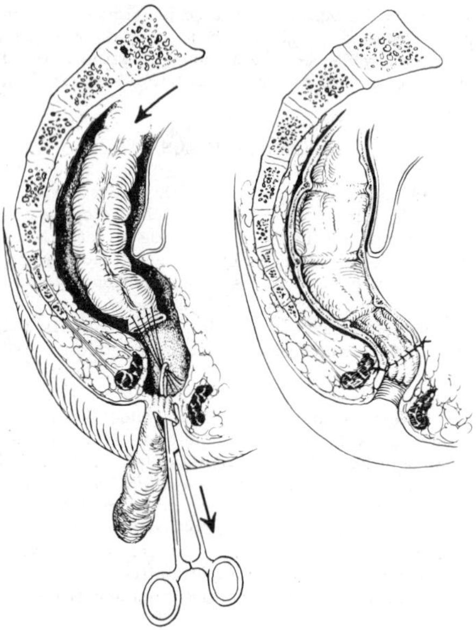

Swenson abdominoperineal pull-through

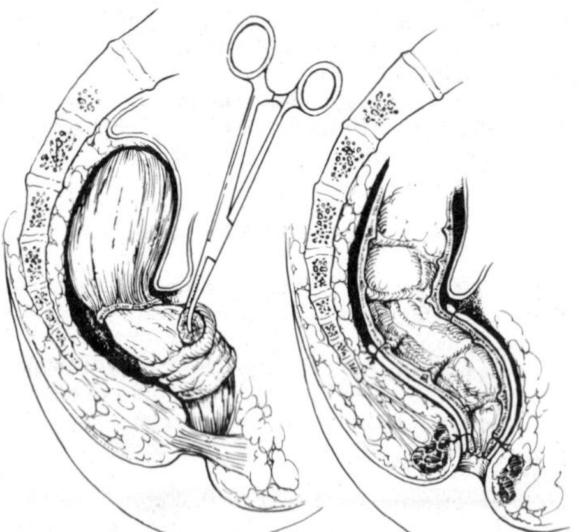

Soave endorectal pull-through

diagnosis is suspected by barium enema (in saline) showing a normal or small caliber distal intestine and dilatation of the bowel above the transitional zone. No effort should be made to evacuate the contents of the colon before barium enema, so that the transition zone will be retained. The infant is usually unable to evacuate the barium during the next 24 hours. Rectal biopsy, including a full thickness of the rectal wall and measuring at least 2×1.5 cm., is required to confirm the absence of ganglion cells.

Enterocolitis is a serious and often fatal complication before the first year of life.

Treatment.

Conservative measures to evacuate the colon are inadequate. Therefore, for infants less than 1 year old, colostomy should be performed at the transition zone (established by biopsy) in an area of ganglionated bowel. When the child weighs more than 20 pounds, a choice of 3 abdominoperineal pull-through procedures is available. In the Swenson procedure (see p. 236), the overly dilated and aganglionic colon and rectum are excised to a point 1.5 cm. anteriorly and 0.5 cm. posteriorly from the dentate line. In the Duhamel (see p. 238) and Soave (see p. 236) procedures, the overly dilated and aganglionic bowel is removed down to the rectum at the level of pelvic peritoneal reflection. In the Duhamel operation, the proximal bowel is brought between the sacrum and rectum and sutured end-to-side to the rectum above the dentate line. The intervening spur of rectum and bowel is crushed to form a side-to-side anastomosis. The Soave operation consists of dissecting the mucosa out of the residual rectal stump, pulling the proximal bowel through, and suturing it to the rectal muscular sleeve.

MECONIUM PLUG SYNDROME

Unusually thick meconium may block the colon at varying distances from the rectum in newborn infants. Many of these infants pass some meconium after birth, but obstruction persists, producing abdominal distention and vomiting which mimics other causes of obstruction. Rectal examination and barium enema are usually curative following evacuation of the plug. These patients must be examined regularly, since some actually have Hirschsprung's disease or cystic fibrosis.

ANORECTAL ANOMALIES

Two important types of anorectal malformations must be distinguished depending on whether the distal rectum extends through the levator ani (puborectalis) muscle: the low type of imperforate anus or ectopic anus and the high type of imperforate anus or anorectal agenesis (see p. 239).

The low type of imperforate anus may be diagnosed by the presence of an ectopic (and usually stenotic) anal orifice anterior to the normal position. In the male, a fistulous tract may extend along the perineal raphe; more rarely, the fistula is higher and enters the bulbous urethra. In the female, the ectopic orifice may be in the perineum, vestibule, or lower vagina.

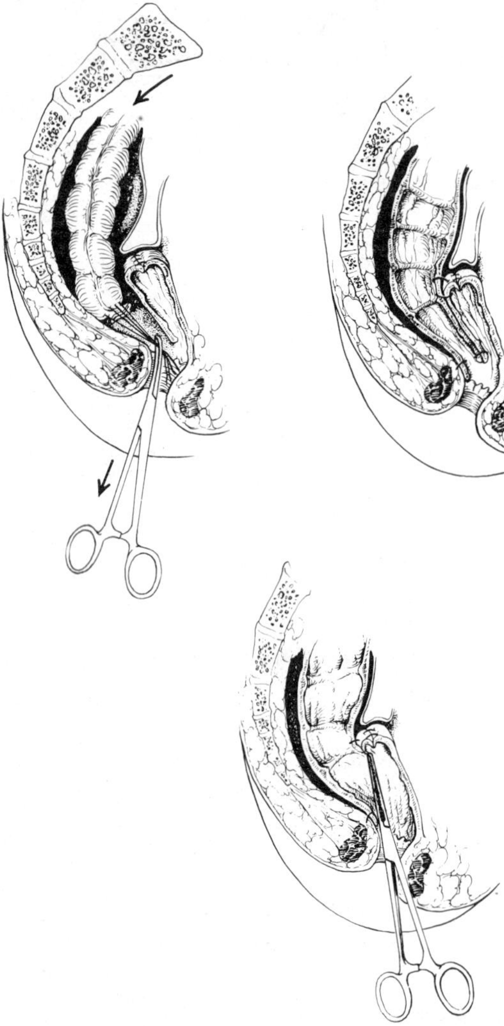

Duhamel abdominoperineal pull-through

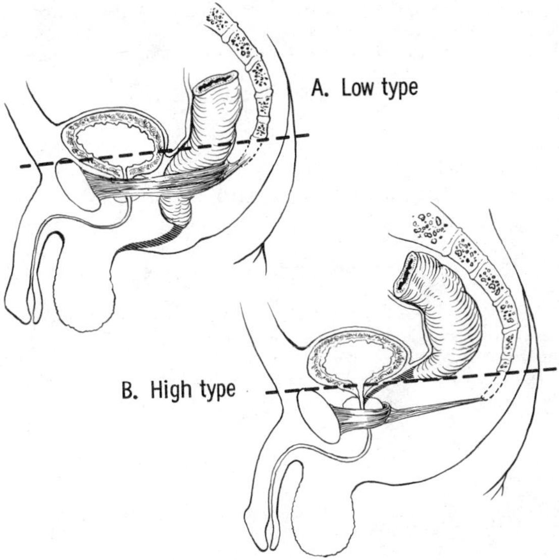

Imperforate anus

In anorectal agenesis, the distal rectum and anus fail to develop. In the female, there is usually a fistula to the upper vagina or, rarely, to the bladder. In the male, there is usually a fistula to the urethra or bladder.

Clinical Findings.

If a communication between the bowel and perineum cannot be seen, a lateral upside down x-ray of the infant pelvis may be helpful. This should be taken several hours after birth to allow time for swallowed gas to travel to the distal end of the rectum. The baby should be held upside down for several minutes, and the x-ray should be centered over the greater trochanter. X-ray studies of the spine often reveal vertebral anomalies. Intravenous urograms and voiding cystourethrograms must be done because of the frequency of associated urinary malformations, particularly with anorectal agenesis.

Treatment.

If the bowel gas shadow extends below the ischial spine, the malformation is a low anomaly and can usually be surgically repaired from a perineal approach with a good prognosis for continence. Bowel gas that does not extend below the ischium - or gas seen in the bladder - indicates anorectal agenesis. This malformation requires a right transverse colostomy in the newborn period. When the infant grows to 20 pounds, the anorectal agenesis should be repaired by abdominoperineal operation in which the distal colon is brought anterior to the puborectalis muscle and is sutured to the perineum. In this anomaly, the external anal sphincter is inadequate and the internal sphincter is absent. Therefore, continence is dependent upon a functional puborectalis muscle.

GASTROINTESTINAL PROBLEMS PECULIAR TO OLDER INFANTS AND CHILDREN

HYPERTROPHIC PYLORIC STENOSIS

Progressive hypertrophy of the circular muscle of the pylorus produces narrowing and obstruction of the pyloric canal. The cause is unknown. There is a familial tendency, and males - particularly first-born males - predominate over females 4:1.

This disorder must be differentiated from feeding problems, hiatus hernia, pylorospasm, chalasia, intracranial lesions, uremia, adrenal insufficiency, duodenal stenosis, and malrotation of the bowel.

Clinical Findings.

The symptoms are nonbilious projectile vomiting, failure to gain weight or weight loss, dehydration, and diminished number of stools. The onset of symptoms may occur shortly after birth but is usually delayed until 2-3 weeks after birth. Prominent gastric waves may be seen traversing from the left costal margin across the upper abdomen. A pyloric "tumor" or "olive" 1-2 cm. in size is palpable in the upper abdomen in more than 95% of the cases. This latter finding is diagnostic, and x-ray studies to show the pyloric "string sign" are rarely indicated.

Treatment.

A Fredet-Ramstedt pyloromyotomy through a right upper quadrant muscle-splitting incision is curative. This is an elective operation that should be performed only after dehydration and metabolic alkalosis have been treated. Postoperatively, feeding may begin within 6 hours, starting with 1 oz. of 10% dextrose solution every 2 hours, and then be advanced to increasing amounts of formula every 3-4 hours. There should be no mortality in the treatment of this disease. Complications such as duodenal mucosal perforation, intra-abdominal bleeding, and aspiration of vomitus must be carefully watched for in the immediate postoperative period.

INTUSSUSCEPTION

Telescoping of a segment of bowel (intussusceptum) into the adjacent segment (intussuscipiens) produces intestinal obstruction, and it may result in gangrene of the intussusceptum. The terminal ileum is usually telescoped into the right colon, producing ileocolic intussusception but ileo-ileal, ileo-ileocolic, jejuno-jejunal, and colo-colic intussusceptions also occur. In 95% of infants and children the cause is unknown, but this disorder may be related to adenovirus infection. The most frequent occurrence is in midsummer and midwinter. The peak age is in infants 5-9 months old; 65% are less than 1 year old; and 80% are less than 2 years old. Causes such as Meckel's diverticulum, polyps, intramural hematoma (Henoch-Schönlein purpura), and hypertrophic Peyer's patches are reported with increasing frequency in children older than 1 year.

Clinical Findings.

The typical patient is a healthy, robust child who has sudden onset of crying and doubles up his knees on the abdomen because of pain. The ratio of males to females is 3:2. The pain is intermittent, lasts for about 1 minute, and is followed by intervals of apparent well-being. Reflex vomiting is a frequent early sign and results from bowel obstruction later in the course. Blood and mucus in the rectum produce a "currant jelly" stool. In small infants, colicky pain may not be apparent; these babies become withdrawn, and the most prominent symptom is vomiting. Pallor and sweating during colic are frequent. A mass is usually palpable along the distribution of the colon. A hollow right lower quadrant (Dance's sign) may be noted. Occasionally the intussusception is palpable on rectal examination. The blood count usually shows a polymorphonuclear leukocytosis and hemoconcentration.

Treatment.

Hypovolemia and dehydration must be corrected. The patient is sedated, and barium enema is then performed with a surgeon present. The enema bag must not be raised to more than 30 inches above the patient, and under fluoroscopic control the barium enema may distend the intussuscipiens and reduce the intussusceptum in 65-70% of cases. If enema reduction cannot be accomplished, the patient is anesthetized and the abdomen is explored through a right lower quadrant transverse incision. The intussusception is then reduced by gentle, retrograde compression of the intussuscipiens and not by traction on the proximal bowel. Intestinal resection is indicated if the bowel cannot be reduced or if the bowel is gangrenous. Mikulicz resection may be necessary in critically ill patients. Resection of a Meckel's diverticulum, polypectomy, and incidental appendectomy may be performed. Intussusception recurs in 1-2% of cases.

OMPHALOMESENTERIC DUCT ANOMALIES

When the entire duct remains intact it is called an **omphalomesenteric fistula**. When the duct is obliterated at the intestinal end, but communicates with the umbilicus at the distal end, it is called an **umbilical sinus**. When the epithelial tract persists but both ends are occluded, an **umbilical cyst** or intra-abdominal **enterocystoma** may develop. The entire tract may be obliterated, but it may form a band between the ileum and the umbilicus.

The most common remnant of an omphalomesenteric duct is a Meckel's diverticulum, which occurs in 1-3% of the population. Meckel's diverticulum may be lined in part or totally by small intestinal, colonic, or gastric mucosa, and it may contain aberrant pancreatic tissue. In contrast to duplications and pseudo-diverticula, it is located on the antimesenteric border of the ileum 10-90 cm. from the ileocecal valve.

Clinical Findings.

Omphalomesenteric remnants may produce symptoms of continuous mucus discharge at the umbilicus, umbilical mass, or abscess. Intestinal obstruction may develop from a persistent band occluding the bowel lumen, or by volvulus of the intestine about the band.

Meckel's diverticulum is most commonly symptomatic of painless, sudden, severe intestinal hemorrhage due to peptic ulceration of the adjacent bowel. The hemorrhage usually occurs in infants less than 2 years old. Peptic ulceration may lead to perforation and generalized peritonitis.

Meckel's diverticulum with a narrow lumen may become occluded and result in diverticulitis, similar to phlegmonous appendicitis. A Meckel's diverticulum may also become inverted into the bowel lumen and act as a leading edge for an intussusception.

Treatment.

Umbilical fistulas, sinuses, and cysts should be excised to prevent the development of infection. Meckel's diverticulum should be considered the source of peritonitis or massive gastrointestinal bleeding when some other cause cannot be identified. Usually the omphalomesenteric remnant can be excised and the communication with the ileum oversewn. Resection of the small intestine is occasionally required.

MALIGNANT TUMORS IN CHILDHOOD

NEUROBLASTOMA

Of all childhood neoplasms, neuroblastoma is second only to leukemia and brain tumors in frequency. Two-thirds of cases occur within the first 5 years of life. This tumor is of neural crest origin and may originate anywhere along the distribution of the sympathetic chain. The tumor is of retroperitoneal origin in 65% of cases, and 40% of the tumors arise from the adrenal gland. The tumor originates in the posterior mediastinum in 15% and is of cervical and sacral origin in 5% of cases. The site of primary origin may not be determined in 10% of cases.

The biologic behavior of neuroblastoma is frequently different in infants under 1 year old than in older children. The tumor is more frequently localized in infants, but distant metastases have developed in more than 70% of older children at first diagnosis. In infants, distant metastases are commonly confined to the liver and subcutaneous tissues, whereas in older children bone and lymph node metastases are most common.

Clinical Findings.

The symptoms in infants are an isolated tumor, hepatomegaly, or subcutaneous nodules. Older children may also have an isolated tender mass, but they also frequently have pain in the bones and joints and associated malaise, fever, vomiting, and anemia, which may mimic infection or rheumatic fever. Hypertension occurs in less than 20% of patients. Abdominal neuroblastoma may be distinguished from other tumors by the hard, irregular surface of the tumor and tendency to cross the midline. X-rays show a soft tissue mass displacing surrounding structures, and calcification is present in 45% of the tumors. For retroperitoneal tumors, an intravenous pyelogram shows displacement or compression of the adjacent kidney without distortion of the renal calyces. Approximately 70% of the neuroblastomas produce norepinephrine and its precursor metabolites. The breakdown products of excess norepinephrine production, most commonly vanillylmandelic acid (VMA) and homovanillic acid (HVA), should be measured in urine specimens at intervals so that the clinical course of the patient can be followed.

Treatment.

A localized neuroblastoma should be excised and the local area of the tumor bed should be irradiated. An unresectable primary tumor and its metastases should be treated by irradiation therapy. Chemotherapeutic agents such as cyclophosphamide (Cytoxan®) and vincristine (Oncovin®) produce tumor regression, which is sometimes permanent in infants but usually only temporary in older children. The two-year "cure" rate in infants with distant metastases is 45%. Cure in older children is much less frequent.

WILMS'S TUMOR

This tumor arises within the capsule of the kidney and consists of a variety of epithelial and sarcomatous cell types such as abortive tubules and glomeruli, smooth and skeletal muscle fibers, spindle cells, cartilage, and bone. Hence the tumor is also called nephroblastoma, embryoma, carcinosarcoma, or mixed tumor of the kidney. Eighty per cent of patients are under 4 years old. Bilateral tumors occur in 5-10% of cases. Metastases most commonly occur in the liver and lungs.

Clinical Findings.

A large, firm, smooth, lateral abdominal mass is always palpable. An intravenous urogram shows distortion of the calyces and kidney silhouette. Very rarely there is nonfunction of the kidney, in which case the mass must be distinguished from hydronephrosis. Cystoscopy, retrograde urograms, and renal arteriograms are unnecessary.

Treatment.

The preferred treatment is immediate nephrectomy and excision of all the surrounding tissues within Gerota's fascia, followed by irradiation therapy to the tumor bed. Very large tumors should be treated with irradiation therapy preoperatively to reduce the size of the tumor; nephrectomy should then be performed. The nephrectomy is accomplished through an abdominal incision in which the renal artery and vein are divided before any other dissection is performed. Dactinomycin (Cosmegen®) should be given intravenously (10-15 μg./Kg./day), intraoperatively, and for 4-7 days postoperatively, and it should be repeated every 3 months for 2 years. Patients with distant metastases are curable. Solitary liver and lung metastases should be resected. Multiple metastases should be treated with irradiation therapy in conjunction with dactinomycin. The cure rate is more than 85% when this tumor is treated in pediatric oncology centers.

TERATOMAS

Teratomas are congenital tumors derived from pluri-potential embryonic cells. They are located in the midline or paramedian parts of the body. Teratomas consist of cells representing the 3 germ layers such as neural tissue, dermal epithelial elements and teeth, intestinal and respiratory epithelium, chorio-epithelioma, and mesenchymal tissue such as smooth and striated muscle, connective tissue, fat, cartilage, and bone. There are benign and malignant types of teratomas. Metastases may represent one cellular element but usually consist of most of the cellular types present in the primary lesion. Sites of origin in order of frequency are the ovaries, testes, anterior mediastinum, presacral and coccygeal regions, and retroperitoneum. Most ovarian teratomas are benign "dermoid" tumors. Most testicular teratomas are malignant, and the incidence of malignancy is higher than the normal population in undescended testes and in pseudohermaphrodites. Most of the mediastinal, retroperitoneal, and coccygeal teratomas are benign. These tumors should be excised because of their malignant potential and the symptoms produced by their size.

RHABDOMYOSARCOMAS

The histologic varieties of rhabdomyosarcomas are the embryonal cell, the alveolar cell, and the pleomorphic types. Sarcoma botryoides is a variant of the embryonal type which is characterized by grape-like masses located in areas of mucosal-lined cavities such as the bladder, vagina, bile ducts, middle ear, and sinuses. The embryonal type of tumor occurs primarily in infants and children and arises from the urogenital tract, and skeletal muscles of the head and neck, the extremities, and the trunk. The alveolar cell type occurs in adolescents and young adults and arises from skeletal muscles in the trunk and extremities. The pleomorphic type develops mainly in adults. Metastases spread to regional lymph nodes and to the lungs and liver. Treatment requires radical excision. Irradiation therapy and dactinomycin are effective in supplementing surgical excision and for palliation of disseminated tumor.

CYSTIC HYGROMA AND LYMPHANGIOMA

These tumors of lymph vessels occur at the junction of large lymphatic trunks such as the neck, axilla, and groin. Cystic hygromas contain large cysts with a well-defined capsule. Lymphangiomas consist of microcystic lymph masses and characteristically invade surrounding structures without respect for tissue planes. Whether these tumors are true neoplasms or whether they represent malformations of the lymphatic system is controversial. Indications for treatment are cosmetic deformity, functional impairment, and prevention of repeated lymphangitis. These lesions do not respond to drugs or injection of sclerosing agents, and they are radioresistant. Excision is the only method of treatment. Every effort should be made to spare normal structures, particularly nerves.

NEONATAL JAUNDICE

The numerous medical causes of jaundice in the newborn include giant cell hepatitis, cytomegalic inclusion disease, herpes simplex, toxoplasmosis, rubella, syphilis, and galactosemia. Surgically treatable causes of jaundice are biliary atresia and choledochal cyst (see below). During the first months of life, liver function studies cannot identify these various conditions. Microcephaly, choreoretinitis, intracranial calcification, and cytomegalic inclusion bodies in the cells of urinary sediment suggest toxoplasmosis or cytomegalic inclusion disease. Excretion in the stools of more than 10% of an intravenous dose of radioactive rose bengal rules out biliary atresia but not choledochal cyst. Needle biopsy of the liver is diagnostic in 60% of cases. Surgical exploration, cholangiography, and open liver biopsy establish the diagnosis in more than 90% of cases. However, this procedure may enhance the development of progressive cirrhosis in patients with neonatal hepatitis. Since severe grades of cirrhosis in surgically correctable cases of jaundice do not develop before the third month, and since the jaundice of neonatal hepatitis subsides before the third month in half of cases, surgical exploration is advocated at the age of 3 months.

BILIARY ATRESIA

The cause of biliary atresia is unknown, but it is probably acquired after birth. Surgical correction requires a ductal structure at the hilum of the liver which drains a normal intrahepatic biliary tree. Although a hilar ductal structure may be found in 10-20% of cases, only 5% of these drain a normal intrahepatic biliary tree. The bile duct may be anastomosed to the duodenum, but recurrent cholangitis is frequent. A Roux-en-Y choledochojejunostomy or hepatic duct jejunostomy may be preferable.

Uncorrectable biliary atresia may be extrahepatic or intrahepatic. In extrahepatic atresia, both the major extrahepatic and intrahepatic ducts are obliterated, but numerous proliferating cholangioles and varying grades of cirrhosis may be seen on liver biopsy. The average life span of these infants is 19 months. Intrahepatic biliary atresia is characterized by a total absence of intrahepatic ducts with few cholangioles and little cirrhosis. These patients may live for 3-5 years.

CHOLEDOCHAL CYST

The 3 types of choledochal cysts are cystic dilatation of the common bile duct, diverticulum of the common bile duct, and choledochocele. These cysts commonly have thick, fibrous walls which lack an epithelial lining. The onset of symptoms is usually between the age of 3 months and adulthood. Females are affected 4 times as frequently as males. The symptoms are the triad of jaundice, pain, and abdominal mass.

Treatment consists of choledochocystoduodenostomy or Roux-en-Y cystojejunostomy.

ABDOMINAL WALL DEFECTS

INGUINAL HERNIA AND HYDROCELE

Autopsy studies have shown that the processus vaginalis remains patent in more than 80% of newborn infants. With increasing age, the incidence of a patent processus diminishes; at 2 years, 40-50% are open, and in adult autopsy specimens 25% are open. Actual indirect inguinal hernia develops in 1-4% of children; 45% occur in the first year of life.

Clinical Findings.

The diagnosis of a hernia in infancy and childhood can be made only by the demonstration of an inguinal bulge originating from the internal ring. Commonly, the bulge cannot be elicited at will, and signs such as a large external ring, "silk glove" sign, and thickening of the cord are not dependable. Under these circumstances, a reliable history alone may be sufficient. Hernias are found on the right side in 60% of cases; on the left side in 25%; and bilaterally in 15%. Bilateral hernias are more frequent in premature infants. The processus may be obliterated at any location proximal to the testes or labium. When the bowel herniates into the scrotum, it is referred to as a complete indirect inguinal hernia; when it extends to a level proximal to the testes in the male or external ring in the female, it is an incomplete inguinal hernia. Direct inguinal and femoral hernias are very rare in infancy and childhood.

Incarcerated inguinal hernia accounts for approximately 10% of childhood hernias, and the greatest incidence is in young infants. In 45% of females with incarcerated hernia, the contents of the sac consist of various combinations of ovary, tube, and uterus. These structures are usually a sliding component of the sac.

Hydroceles almost always represent peritoneal fluid trapped in a patent processus vaginalis; hence, they are commonly called communicating hydroceles. Hydrocele is characteristically an oblong, nontender, soft mass that transilluminates with light. The sudden appearance of fluid confined to the testicular area may represent a noncommunicating hydrocele secondary to torsion of the testes or testicular appendage, or epididymo-orchitis. Rectal examination and palpation of the peritoneal side of the internal ring may distinguish an incarcerated hernia from a hydrocele or other inguino-scrotal mass.

Treatment.

If expert anesthesia is available, an inguinal hernia in infancy and childhood should be repaired soon after diagnosis. In premature infants under constant surveillance in the hospital, hernia repair may be deferred until the baby is strong enough to be discharged home. Ordinarily, high ligation and excision of the hernia sac at the internal ring is all that is required. When there is a large internal ring, it may be necessary to narrow the internal ring with sutures placed in the transversalis fascia, but use of abdominal muscles for the repair is unnecessary.

An incarcerated hernia in an infant can usually be reduced initially before operation. This is accomplished by sedation with meperidine (Demerol®), 1 mg./lb., and secobarbital, 1 mg./lb., and by elevating the foot of the bed to keep the abdominal pressure from being exerted on the inguinal area. When the infant is well sedated, the hernia may be reduced by gentle pressure over the internal ring in a manner that milks the bowel into the abdominal cavity. During this time, nasogastric suction and intravenous fluids are used as required for bowel distention and fluid and electrolyte losses. If the bowel is not reduced after a few hours, operation is required. If the hernia is reduced, operative repair should be delayed for 24 hours to reduce the edema in the tissues. Bloody stools and marked edema or red discoloration of the skin around the groin suggest strangulated hernia, and reduction of the bowel should not be attempted. Emergency repair of incarcerated inguinal hernia is technically difficult because the edematous tissues are friable and tear readily. Gangrenous intestine should be resected, but black, hemorrhagic discoloration of the testis or ovary does not require excision of the gonad.

UMBILICAL HERNIA

A fascial defect at the umbilicus is frequent in the newborn, particularly in premature infants. The incidence is higher in Negroes. In most children, the umbilical ring progressively diminishes in size and eventually closes. Protrusion of bowel through this defect rarely results in incarceration. Because of these 2 factors, surgical repair is not indicated unless the intestine becomes incarcerated or unless the fascial defect is greater than 1.5 cm. in diameter after the age of 3 years.

OMPHALOCELE

Omphalocele occurs once in every 10,000 births. It is a defect in the peri-umbilical abdominal wall in which the celomic cavity is covered only by peritoneum and amnion. The omphalocele may contain small and large bowel, liver, stomach, spleen, pancreas, and bladder. This defect results from an arrest in mesoblastic infiltration of the ventral body wall. When this mesoblastic arrest takes place in the eighth to tenth week of fetal development, a small defect occurs in which the cord is at the apex of the sac; this is called a **fetal** type of omphalocele, or hernia into the cord. If arrest in mesoblastic infiltration occurs during the third week of fetal development, a large abdominal wall defect is formed and the umbilical cord is located at the edge of the omphalocele. This is called the **embryonic** type of omphalocele. Extensive failure in mesoblastic formation farther craniad causes diaphragmatic hernia and sternal defects with ectopia cordis. The abdominal musculature is usually well developed, but occasionally the "prune belly" syndrome with absence of abdominal muscles may occur. Caudally, when mesoblastic infiltration within the infra-umbilical cloacal membrane fails to develop, exstrophy of the bladder occurs and is usually associated with arrest in the formation of the urorectal septum. This produces an imperforate anus with atresia of the entire large bowel. The ileum terminates between the 2 bladder halves, producing a defect called **exstrophy of the cloaca.** Malrotation of the midgut is commonly associated with omphalocele. Associated major anomalies involving the central nervous, cardiovascular, and skeletal systems are frequent. More than half of these babies are born prematurely.

Treatment.

The conservative treatment of omphalocele consists of painting the amniotic sac with 2% merbromin (Mercurochrome®) every 3 hours in order to form a sterile eschar which becomes vascularized beneath the membrane. Over a period of time, contraction of the skin and the abdominal wall will occur and the skin will grow over the granulating portion of the omphalocele. The disadvantages of this technic are the risk of rupture of the omphalocele, the potential for infection and sepsis, and the prolonged period of hospitalization required until the defect has healed. It is indicated only for patients with extremely large defects which might not be covered by a surgical approach, or for infants who are critically ill because of prematurity, pulmonary complications, or severe associated malformations.

The fetal type of omphalocele, with a small abdominal defect, can be treated by excising the omphalocele sac and by reapproximating the abdominal wall muscles and skin edges. The surgical treatment of the embryonic omphalocele consists of undermining the skin edges in the plane between the subcutaneous fat and the abdominal fascia well around to the back, inguinal area, and costal margin. The skin edges can then be approximated in the midline to cover the abdominal wall defect. There should be no attempt to approximate the abdominal wall muscles in the large embryonic type of omphalocele. The hazards of attempted primary closure of the abdominal wall muscles with large omphaloceles include compression of the inferior vena cava with cardiac arrest from impaired venous return, respiratory insufficiency due to impaired diaphragmatic excursion, vascular insufficiency and infarction of the bowel, and wound breakdown. Because of the frequency of malrotation and potential duodenal obstruction, excision of the omphalocele sac is advised to allow exploration of the abdominal cavity and correction of the existing defects. Gastrostomy is a valuable adjunct in the treatment of this defect. Plastic material such as Marlex® or Silastic®-coated cloth may be sutured to the edges of the abdominal wall defect to prevent a large ventral hernia and lateral displacement of abdominal muscles. Later, the midportion of the skin and underlying plastic material can be removed in stages as the abdominal capacity increases, and the abdominal muscles can then be reapproximated.

GASTROSCHISIS

This rare abdominal wall defect differs from omphalocele because it is characterized by a full-thickness defect in the ventral abdominal wall lateral to and usually to the right of a normal insertion of the umbilical cord. No remnants of a covering amnion are found, and there may be a bridge of skin between the defect and the cord. The small and large bowel are herniated through to the abdominal wall defect, and, having been bathed in the amniotic fluid, have a very thick, shaggy membrane covering the bowel wall. The loops of intestine are usually matted together, and the length of intestine appears to be abnormally short. Since the bowel has not been contained intra-abdominally, the abdominal cavity fails to enlarge and cannot accommodate the protuberant bowel. Over 70% of these infants are premature. Malrotation of the intestine is almost always present, and other associated anomalies are frequent.

Treatment.

A tube may be formed from Silastic®-covered nylon mesh to encompass the bowel, and the tube is sutured to the abdominal wall defect. When this tube is suspended from the top of an isolette, the intestines will progressively fall into the expanding abdominal cavity. The fibro-gelatinous pseudomembrane surrounding the matted loops of bowel will resorb. Once the bowel is reduced, the Silastic® tube may be removed and the abdominal wall layers may be reapproximated. A gastrostomy should be performed for gastrointestinal decompression during the period of ileus, which may be prolonged.

When material is not available to use the above technic, a midline incision is performed from the xiphoid to the symphysis. The skin between the subcutaneous fat and the fascia of the abdominal wall should be undermined laterally from the costal margin to the groin. Marlex® or Silastic®-coated cloth may be sutured to the edges of the abdominal muscles on each side so as to produce a large ventral hernia, and the skin edges should be closed over this. After the baby has thrived well, the large ventral hernia can then be repaired in stages by excising the midportion of the skin and underlying prosthetic material and by reapproximating the edges in the midline.

8 . . .

Surgery of the Head & Neck*

TRAUMA TO THE HEAD AND NECK†

EPISTAXIS

The most frequent cause of epistaxis at any age is spontaneous erosion of a superficial mucosal blood vessel situated over the cartilaginous nasal septum (Kiesselbach's area). External trauma to the nose with or without fracture is a frequent cause. Minor trauma such as nose-picking may lead to ulcerations of the nasal septum and subsequent hemorrhage. Less common causes are neoplasms of the nasal chamber or paranasal sinuses, and spontaneous rupture of a branch of the ethmoidal or sphenopalatine arteries or of vessels within the meatuses.

Acute infectious diseases of childhood, hypertension, arteriosclerosis, cardiac disease, and blood dyscrasias and coagulation defects may be associated with epistaxis.

Treatment.

A. Specific Measures: Treat the underlying disease; give transfusions as necessary if blood loss is excessive.

B. Local Measures: Have the patient sit up and forward to prevent swallowing and aspiration of blood.

1. Anterior epistaxis -
   a. Pressure over the area (pinching the nose) for 5 minutes is usually sufficient to stop bleeding. This may be combined with packing the bleeding nostril with cotton moistened with saline solution or 1:1000 epinephrine solution.
   b. After active bleeding has ceased (or if pressure fails to stop the bleeding), a cotton pledget soaked with 2% lidocaine (Xylocaine®) is applied to the bleeding area and the ruptured vessel is cauterized with a chromic acid or silver nitrate bead or an electrocautery needle. Chromic acid must be neutralized immediately with saline solution. After 24 hours, zinc oxide ointment is applied to relieve crusting. Repeat cauterization may be necessary.
   c. If the source of bleeding is not accessible to cauterization (beneath the middle or inferior turbinates, behind septal spurs, or high in the vault), the nasal chambers must

---

*Congenital anomalies of the head and neck are discussed in Chapter 7, Pediatric Surgery.

†The principles of treatment of soft tissue injuries are discussed in Chapter 1, Trauma and Emergencies. Other fractures are discussed in Chapter 19, Orthopedic Surgery.

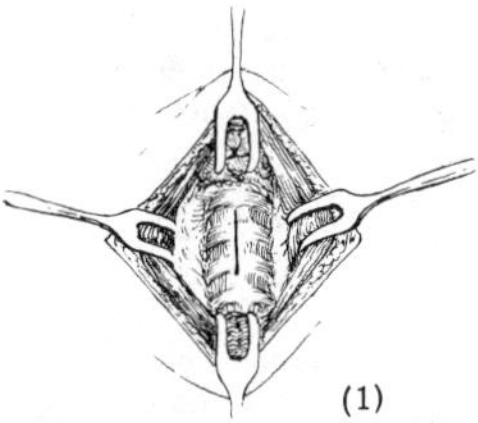

(1)

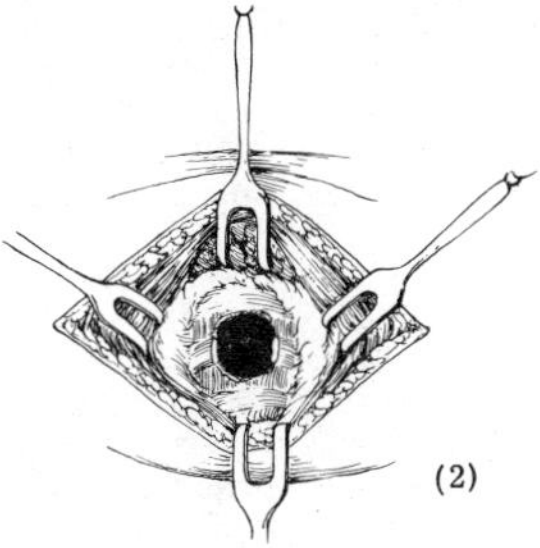

(2)

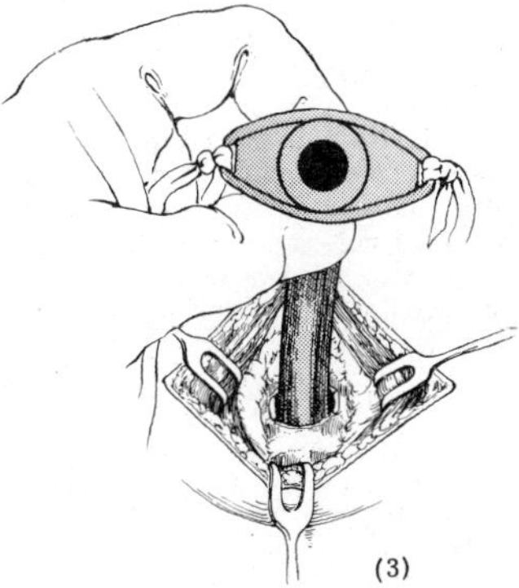

(3)

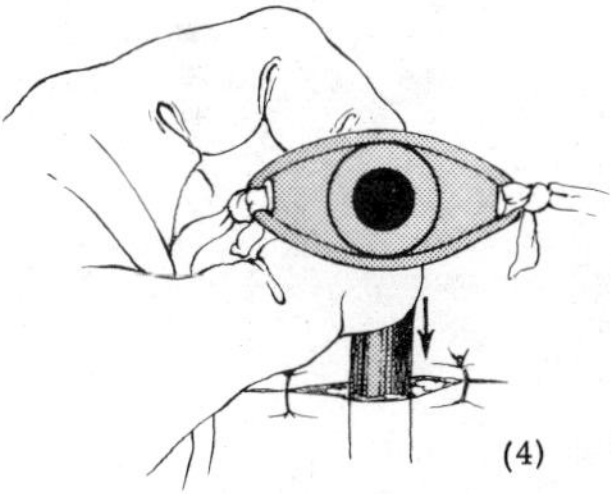

(4)

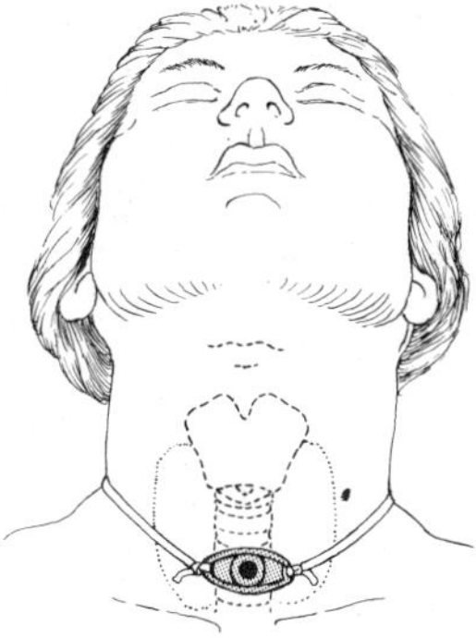

(5)

Technic of Tracheostomy.

(1) Surgical approach in children. Third and fourth tracheal rings split in midline. No cartilage removed.

(2) Surgical approach in adults. Anterior section of third tracheal ring removed.

(3) Insertion of tracheostomy tube.

(4) Loose suturing of both ends of wound.

(5) Tube tied in place.

be anesthetized topically and packed with half-inch selvedged gauze impregnated in cod liver oil or petrolatum. The packing is placed in layers, starting either in the vault or on the floor of the nasal chamber. Anchor the pack by means of a string taped to the face. It is safe to leave the nasal packing in place for as long as 7 days provided the patient is given adequate antibiotic medication to help prevent suppurative otitis media and sinusitis.

2. Posterior epistaxis - In posterior epistaxis it may be necessary to introduce a posterior nasal pack. This is done by sewing 3 strings (braided 0 silk) through and through the center of a rolled 4 × 4 gauze sponge. A soft rubber catheter is passed through the nostril and out through the mouth. Two strings are tied to the catheter and drawn out through the nasal choana posteriorly. The chamber is then packed in layers with selvedged gauze through the anterior nares (see above). The 2 strings are anchored over a gauze bolster at the nares. The third string is shortened and allowed to remain in the pharynx to be used later for removing the pack. The pack should not be left in place more than 5 days. Examine the patient's ears daily for evidence of otitis media. Hemorrhage may recur when the packing is removed or may even continue with the packing in place. If this happens, the pack must usually be changed or reinserted under general anesthesia.
3. If the bleeding persists from a source low in the nasal chamber (middle turbinate or below), external carotid artery ligation in the neck must be considered. In a like situation, the internal maxillary artery may be ligated instead via the maxillary sinus. Uncontrolled bleeding from high in the vault of the nose may have to be controlled by ligation of the anterior ethmoidal artery as it passes from the orbit through the roof of the ethmoidal labyrinth.

FRACTURE OF THE LARYNX

Fracture of the larynx may be caused by direct blunt trauma to the anterior part of the neck. The thyroid cartilages are usually fractured. In more severe injuries, the cricoid cartilage as well as the cartilaginous tracheal rings are crushed. The arytenoid cartilages may be displaced. There are symptoms and signs of laryngeal obstruction. Emphysema of the neck tissues is usually evident.

X-rays of the neck may show gross dislocation of laryngeal structures, narrowing of the airway, and edema and emphysema of the soft tissues. The diagnosis of laryngeal fracture should not depend on x-rays and should be made clinically.

Emergency care is lifesaving. **Establish an airway** with mouth-to-mouth breathing technics. (Establish airway by performing a tracheostomy when feasible. See p. 251.)

Open reduction is the treatment of choice of laryngeal fractures. After the fragments have been reduced, a splint (polyethylene, Silastic®, or tygon tubes) should be placed in the larynx and anchored through the neck tissue with wire or to the tracheotomy cannula with braided silk ligatures. In most cases the splint must be worn for

3-6 weeks before it is removed. **Caution:** Late reduction due to failure to recognize laryngeal fractures early may lead to serious stenosis of the larynx, which may require skin grafting and the use of acrylic splints for many weeks.

INFECTIONS OF THE NECK*

CHRONIC INFLAMMATION OF THE PAROTID GLAND
(Chronic Parotitis, Sialadenitis, Sialectasia, Sialodochitis)

Chronic inflammation of the parotid gland may be secondary to single or multiple calculi or strictures of the duct system, or may occur without apparent cause. There is a recurrent swelling of the gland for months or years which is more pronounced after meals. Chronic enlargement and induration of the gland develops until finally the interlobular ducts become enlarged and sacculated. Thick, tenacious, or purulent secretions may be expressed from Stensen's duct.

X-rays may show calculi. Sialograms often show single or multiple strictures and sacculations of the interlobular duct system.

Dilatations of Stensen's duct, intra-oral removal of stones, and meatotomy of Stensen's papilla are frequently curative in the early stage of the disease. Later, when suppuration, sacculation, and scarring have become extensive, surgical excision of the parotid gland (total parotidectomy) is indicated. The facial nerve must be preserved.

CHRONIC INFLAMMATION OF SUBMAXILLARY GLANDS

Chronic inflammation of the submaxillary gland occurs secondary to calculus or stricture of the duct system. The process continues for years until the gland becomes permanently enlarged by infiltration of lymphocytes and formation of scar tissue.

Probing of the duct with a lacrimal duct probe usually aids in the diagnosis of stricture or stone, or both. X-rays may show stones. Sialography may aid in the diagnosis.

Conservative treatment should be tried early: duct dilatation, removal of stones near the papilla of Wharton's duct, and meatotomy of the duct papilla.

In the advanced case where there is permanent damage to the gland with recurrent pain, suppuration, and scar formation, the gland itself should be removed surgically.

SALIVARY CALCULI

Salivary calculi occur more frequently in the submaxillary duct (Wharton's) than in the ducts of the other salivary glands (parotid

---

*Thyroiditis is discussed on p. 280.

and sublingual). There may be single or multiple calculi or "gravel." The calculi are composed of inorganic salts (primarily calcium and phosphorus), and often have a central core of foreign substance. Calculi vary in size from 1 mm. to several cm.

Symptoms and signs produced by calculi depend upon their size and location. Obstruction of Wharton's duct causes swelling of the submaxillary gland and pain, often after eating. Symptoms and signs of acute inflammation may be most prominent.

Palpation of the calculus or calculi in Wharton's duct in the floor of the mouth is diagnostic. Stones in the hilum of the gland area can usually be felt only with bidigital palpation.

Opaque calculi are readily discernible in the x-ray film.

If symptoms and signs of acute inflammation are present, conservative care should be instituted. When the calculus is near the papilla of Wharton's duct, the papilla may be cut off or slit and the stone evacuated. Some stones in this area may be "milked out" of the duct after dilatation with a lacrimal duct dilator.

The intraoral surgical removal of calculi from Wharton's duct is feasible provided the calculi are not too far posterior in the duct. A probe should be inserted into the duct as a guide for surgical incision. After removing the calculus, the slit duct need not be repaired.

Calculi in the distal third of Wharton's duct and those in the hilum of the gland should not be removed intraorally. The treatment of choice in this instance is to remove the gland and stone by an external surgical approach, ligating the oral stump of the duct. This operation must be performed during remission of an acute inflammatory process.

TUBERCULOSIS OF THE HEAD AND NECK

Cervical Lymph Node Tuberculosis.

Tuberculosis of the cervical lymph nodes may be secondary to a tuberculous focus in the gums or tonsils or may originate in distant sources (e.g., the lungs, by miliary spread). The superior cervical nodes are usually involved first, and the lower nodes of the neck later through lymphatic pathways. The inflammation in the nodes goes through an initial stage of exudation, followed by caseation and liquefaction. Sinuses to the surface may develop, as in scrofula. Pus from the draining sinuses may allow identification of Mycobacterium tuberculosis. In arrested cases x-rays may show calcifications within the cervical lymph nodes.

In early cervical lymph node tuberculosis, the patient should be at bed rest, and measures to promote improvement in general health should be instituted as well as antituberculosis chemotherapy. Observation will usually determine whether the process will resolve or progress. If conservative measures fail, infected nodes should be excised. Antituberculosis chemotherapy should be used as an adjunct to surgical therapy.

Laryngeal Tuberculosis.

Laryngeal tuberculosis follows active pulmonary disease. It must be considered in the differential diagnosis of carcinoma and gummas of the larynx. The diagnosis is usually made by biopsy and microscopic tissue examination. Treatment consists of voice rest and the use of antituberculosis chemotherapy. Tracheostomy has rarely been indicated in recent years.

ACUTE CERVICAL ADENITIS
(With or Without Abscess)

Acute inflammatory adenitis is the most common lesion occurring in the neck both in children and in adults. The anterior or posterior cervical nodes may be involved, depending upon whether the source of inflammation is in the scalp or ear or in the nasal or oral cavity. Cervical lymph gland inflammation is frequently seen with acute or chronic tonsillitis. Symptoms and signs depend upon the virulence of the infection, its location and source, and whether suppuration develops. Many inflammatory processes of the cervical nodes resolve spontaneously when the primary source is eradicated.

In those cases where suppuration and breakdown of lymph nodes occurs, and when fluctuation is evident, incision and drainage are indicated. Superficial abscesses can be entered by sharp incision. The deeper abscesses must be entered by blunt dissection after the skin and platysmus muscle are cleanly incised. If the central mass of the abscessed lymph node is entered and drained (Penrose drain for 3-5 days), resolution usually takes place. Antibiotic therapy is usually indicated as an adjunct to surgery and as an initial treatment also.

INFECTIONS OF THE ORAL CAVITY

PERITONSILLAR ABSCESS

Peritonsillar abscess is a complication of acute tonsillitis. The infection spreads to the potential anatomic peritonsillar space adjacent to the tonsil bed and soft tissues of the palate. Mixed pyogenic organisms (streptococci, staphylococci, and/or pneumococci) are usually obtained upon culture.

The patient complains of sore throat on one side. Pain is severe on swallowing. Trismus is present. Upon inspection there is unilateral swelling which pushes the tonsil toward or across the midline. The swelling extends to the soft palate. The uvula is displaced. Cervical adenitis may be evident. Fluctuation develops between the third and fifth days.

Symptomatic care and antibiotic treatment are indicated early. Incision and drainage of the abscess are indicated after fluctuation develops (3-5 days). Important after-care consists of spreading the abscess cavity walls daily to avoid re-formation of the abscess. Tonsillectomy is usually indicated approximately one month after clearing of the peritonsillar abscess.

LUDWIG'S ANGINA

This is a severe mixed pyogenic infection of the submaxillary and sublingual fascial spaces of the floor of the mouth and upper neck. There is a rapidly spreading, diffuse cellulitis of the submental areas, with limitation of motion of the mandible and tongue. The tongue may be immobilized against the roof of the mouth. The airway may become obstructed. Edema and painful swelling are noted in the submental areas and the floor of the mouth.

Treatment consists of massive doses of antibiotic drugs and supportive measures. If the condition progresses, incision and drainage should be done externally. Local anesthesia must be used to avoid the danger of immediate obstruction of the airway, which may occur if general anesthesia is used. Because of the diffuse nature of the infection, large quantities of free pus are seldom obtained. Incision must be adequate, and the fascial spaces above and below the hyoglossus muscles must be opened by blunt dissection.

Caution: Be prepared to perform a tracheostomy in these patients (see p. 251).

RETROPHARYNGEAL ABSCESS

This pyogenic infection occurs most frequently in infants and children. Suppuration occurs in the areolar tissue spaces between the posterior pharyngeal wall and the prevertebral fascia as a result of suppurative lymphadenitis. The patient may show difficulty in swallowing or breathing, or both, and difficulty in turning his head and neck. Signs of sepsis are present. Examination of the oropharynx will show a swelling of the posterior pharyngeal wall, which may show evidences of fluctuation upon palpation.

Supportive measures (antibiotics, hydration, and proper nourishment) should be instituted. When incision and drainage are required, the patient should be positioned in the deep Trendelenburg position. Adequate lighting and suction are essential, and the physician must be prepared to do a tracheostomy if indicated. General anesthesia is contraindicated because of the danger of laryngeal obstruction and aspiration of pus and blood.

PARAPHARYNGEAL ABSCESS

Parapharyngeal space abscess is a pyogenic infection secondary to acute tonsillitis, peritonsillar abscess, dental infections, or acute pharyngitis. This potential anatomic space lies in close relation to the superior and middle pharyngeal constrictor muscles, the stylopharyngeus and stylohyoideus muscles, and the carotid sheath. This potential space is like an inverted triangle with its base at the base of the skull and its apex at the hyoid (greater cornu). Infection can gravitate along the carotid sheath to the mediastinum. There are symptoms and signs of sepsis with trismus, and bulging of the lateral pharyngeal wall. The veins of the neck and scalp may be distended from jugular vein pressure. In more advanced suppurations of this space, brawny swelling, edema, and redness may develop in the neck below the angle of the mandible.

Supportive measures are indicated early (hydration, antibiotics). Intra-oral incision and drainage are contraindicated. External incision and drainage at the angle of the jaw and upper neck area should be done when pus is sought deep within the neck by blunt dissection.

Caution is required in giving these patients general anesthesia, since the laryngeal airway may be closed off by sudden edema. Local anesthesia should be used for incision and drainage or a tracheostomy performed, after which general anesthesia may be used.

INFECTIONS OF THE EAR AND MASTOID BONE

PERICHONDRITIS AND CHONDRITIS OF THE EAR

Perichondritis of the cartilage of the pinna is important because of the "cauliflower" deformity which may result. Infection is usually due to pyogenic organisms and may follow trauma, surgery, insect bites, or frostbite or may occur spontaneously. If the perichondrium is lifted from the cartilage, necrosis of cartilage may develop. The pinna becomes swollen, reddened, and edematous. Treatment is usually conservative, with supplementary antibiotic therapy. Incision and drainage must be judiciously used and often must be performed in multiple areas.

EXTERNAL OTITIS

External otitis is a common diffuse inflammatory skin infection of the external auditory canal. It is caused by a mixed group of pyogenic organisms (staphylococci, streptococci, proteus organisms) or, less frequently, by fungi. Treatment is conservative, usually in the form of cleansing, Burow's solution compresses (1:12), and systemic antibiotics.

ACUTE SUPPURATIVE OTITIS MEDIA

This disease is most commonly seen in infants and children, but it can occur at any age. Suppuration of the middle ear usually develops following or accompanying disease of the upper respiratory tract.

Pyogenic organisms (beta-hemolytic streptocci, staphylococci, pneumococci, and H. influenzae) are the usual infecting organisms. There are symptoms and signs of inflammation, such as fever, pain, and a serosanguineous or purulent aural discharge if spontaneous rupture has occurred. Examination of the ear shows a reddened, bulging tympanic membrane. There may be exudate in the external auditory canal if the tympanic membrane has ruptured spontaneously. Rarely can the perforation of the tympanic membrane be seen at this stage of the disease. Hearing is impaired.

Acute mastoiditis may occur as a complication.

Systemic antibiotic therapy should be instituted. Penicillin is usually the drug of choice. Paracentesis of the tympanic membrane should be done in most cases.

SEROUS OTITIS MEDIA
(Catarrhal Otitis Media)

Serous otitis media may occur at any age. It is characterized by the presence of serous or mucous discharge in the middle ear cavity. In most cases no organisms can be obtained by culture of the aspirated material from the middle ear. The patient experiences a stuffiness of the ear and a conduction hearing loss. The tympanic membrane is often yellowish and retracted in appearance, whereas the ossicular chain appears chalky. Cancer of the nasopharynx must be ruled out in unilateral instances of serous otitis media.

Local treatment consists of eustachian tube inflations, myringotomy of the drum membrane with aspirations of the middle ear contents, and phenylephrine (Neo-Synephrine®) nose drops (0.25% solution). Systemic antihistamine drug therapy is indicated. Secondary contributing factors must be corrected, e.g., by tonsillectomy and/or adenoidectomy, control of allergic disorders of the respiratory system, and treatment of suppurative sinusitis. The insertion of a plastic tube through the tympanic membrane may be indicated for ventilation of the middle ear. This tube may be left in place for days, months, or years with safety.

CHRONIC OTITIS MEDIA

Chronic inflammatory processes of the middle ear are usually associated with either eustachian tube salpingitis or chronic mastoiditis. They follow acute suppurative otitis media (particularly that associated with acute exanthematous diseases of infancy or childhood). The tympanic membrane is perforated in one of 3 areas: central, marginal, or attic. Hearing is usually impaired.

Contributing factors such as tonsillitis, adenoiditis, sinusitis, and nasal polyps should be corrected. Local treatment is usually in the form of ear drops (alcohol and boric acid, or antibiotic solutions) or powders (iodine, or antibiotics alone or combined with boric acid). Saturated urea solution is an excellent cleansing agent.

If there is evidence of continued suppuration, or if complications occur, radical or modified radical mastoidectomy should be done.

MASTOIDITIS

Acute mastoiditis is a complication of acute suppurative otitis media. Bony necrosis of the mastoid process and breakdown of the bony intercullular structures occurs in the second to third week. When this happens, there is evidence of continued suppuration of the middle ear, mastoid tenderness, signs of sepsis, and x-ray evidence of bone destruction. If suppurative mastoiditis develops in spite of antibiotic therapy, complete mastoidectomy must be done. Acute mastoiditis is rarely seen since chemotherapeutic and antibiotic therapy has become universal in the treatment of acute suppurative otitis media.

Chronic mastoiditis is a complication of chronic suppurative otitis media. If the disease occurs in infancy, the mastoid bone does not develop cellular structures but becomes sclerotic. Infection is usually limited to the antral area. In some cases of marginal and attic perforations of the tympanic membrane, cholesteatomas develop. Cholesteatomas are produced by the ingrowth of squamous epithelium from the skin of the external auditory canal. By their laminated growth, they enlarge and erode adjacent bone.

The use of antibiotic drugs in chronic mastoiditis is usually not helpful in clearing the mastoid infection but may be effective in the treatment of complications. Many cases of chronic otitis media and mastoiditis can be managed by local cleansing of the ear and instillation of antibiotic powders or solutions. In other cases, surgery must be performed. It is the purpose of surgery to cure the disease and maintain or improve hearing. In addition to the classical operations modified and radical mastoidectomies, tympanoplasty procedures have been introduced in the past 20 years.

COMPLICATIONS OF EAR INFECTIONS

Following Acute Suppurative Otitis Media and Mastoiditis.

A. Subperiosteal abscess secondary to acute mastoiditis and suppurative acute otitis media may be encountered.

B. Facial nerve paralysis developing in the first few hours or days after the onset of acute suppurative otitis media is due to edema about the nerve in the bony facial canal. Early conservative treatment is usually indicated (antibiotic therapy, paracentesis, and supportive measures); later, surgical decompression and neurolysis of the nerve sheath may be indicated.

C. Meningitis, abscess (epidural, subdural, and brain), and sigmoid sinus thrombosis are serious complications following suppurative otitis media and mastoiditis. These complications may be masked by use of the antibiotic drugs. Surgical treatment of the mastoid disease and its complications is indicated.

Following Chronic Suppurative Otitis Media.

A. Acute exacerbations of chronic otitis media and mastoiditis may lead to meningitis, epidural and brain abscess, and sigmoid sinus thrombosis. Antibiotic therapy and surgical intervention should be carried out.

B. Facial nerve paralysis is usually the result of direct pressure from cholesteatomas or granulation tissue. Surgical intervention is imperative.

Labyrinthitis.

Acute suppurative labyrinthitis is an infection of the intralabyrinthine structures. It may be secondary to acute suppurative otitis media and mastoiditis, acute exacerbations of chronic suppurative otitis media and mastoiditis, or meningitis unrelated to otitis media and mastoiditis. There is usually complete destruction of labyrinthine function and total deafness. Antibiotic drugs and surgical drainage are indicated.

Chronic labyrinthitis is secondary to erosion of the lateral bony semicircular canal by cholesteatoma. The patient is chronically dizzy. Mastoidectomy and removal of the cholesteatoma is the treatment of choice.

INFECTIONS OF THE PARANASAL SINUSES

The maxillary sinuses are involved in acute suppuration which follows upper respiratory disease, swimming, foreign bodies, neoplasms, abscessed teeth, dental extractions, and nasal allergies. Pyogenic organisms are the etiologic agents. Acute inflammatory processes of the maxillary sinuses are characterized by pain and tenderness over the cheek and teeth. Pus is evident in the nose. The early treatment of acute empyema of the maxillary sinus is conservative, with the use of hot packs, oral antihistaminic drugs, local vasoconstrictors, and control of pain by narcotic drugs if necessary. Antibiotic drugs are indicated, particularly when the patient has fever, tenderness, and pus exuding from the sinus ostium. Antral irrigations should be done later, after the acute process subsides.

Isolated infection of the frontal sinuses is rare. Treatment is usually conservative. The frontal sinus or its nasofrontal ostium should rarely be cannulated. Trephining of the sinus floor may be indicated in acute fulminating infections.

Acute ethmoiditis may cause swelling along the inner canthus of the eye. It occurs most frequently in children and infants. At these ages the ethmoidal sinuses are developed. Treatment in most instances is conservative, with the use of antibiotic drugs; only if fluctuation develops externally should incision and drainage be done.

Chronic suppurative sinus disease occurs principally in adults. Chronic pyogenic infections of single sinuses do occur, but are less common than pansinusitis. The patient has few symptoms except purulent rhinorrhea. Antibiotic drug therapy is usually indicated when the specific pyogenic organism is isolated. Conservative surgery (including irrigations) to promote drainage must be used whenever possible. If conservative treatment fails, more radical sinus surgery (external approach) is permissible.

The following complications of chronic suppurative sinus disease may occur: (1) Osteomyelitis of the facial or skull bones. (2) Meningitis and epidural, subdural, and brain abscess. The treatment of (1) and (2) consists of supportive measures, adequate antibiotic and chemotherapy, and surgery as indicated. (3) Draining orbital fistulas are complications of frontal or ethmoidal chronic suppurative disease. The underlying pathology of the sinus must be eliminated surgically before the fistulous tract can be closed permanently. (4) Oro-antral fistulas occur following tooth extractions, trauma (penetrating wounds, surgical procedures), bone infection, and neoplasms occurring in the area of the maxillary sinus. Chronic suppuration of the sinus frequently is present. The successful surgical treatment of the fistula is dependent for the most part on eradicating the sinus disease successfully. (5) Mucoceles (mucopyoceles) develop most frequently in the anterior ethmoidal sinuses and encroach upon the floor of the frontal sinuses by extension. They result from the blocking of sinus drainage. Proptosis of the orbital contents is common. Surgical excision of the mucocele is necessary for complete cure.

NEOPLASMS OF THE HEAD AND NECK

BENIGN NEOPLASMS OF THE ORAL CAVITY

Warts, Verrucae, and Epithelial Papillomas.

These tumors may be sessile or pedunculated. Microscopically, there is proliferation of the squamous epithelium, which grows into folds; within the stalk there is a small amount of connective tissue and blood vessels. Excision is the treatment of choice either by sharp or electrocautery dissection.

Leukoplakia (Hyperkeratosis).

Leukoplakia appears as whitish plaques on the tongue or palate or on the buccal surfaces of the cheeks, lips, or gingivae, and should be considered premalignant. Patients are often heavy smokers. Microscopically, leukoplakia may be likened to the hyperkeratotic lesions of the skin with the exception that in these locations there are no hair follicles or sweat and sebaceous glands. Malignant changes may occur in the basal cell layers. All suspicious lesions must be adequately biopsied.

Observation is essential to determine changes in growth. Multiple and frequent biopsies may be necessary.

Remove sources of irritation such as ill-fitting dentures, jagged teeth, and tobacco. Excise surgically if healing does not occur following conservative treatment.

Hemangioma and Lymphangioma.

Hemangiomas and lymphangiomas occur on the mucous membranes of any part of the oral cavity and are often noted soon after birth. If they occur within the tongue, "macroglossia" may result. Multiple or single lesions may be present.

Hemangiomas have a purplish color; lymphangiomas are the color of the underlying mucous membrane or paler. Microscopically, these lesions may be capillary or cavernous or mixed. The diagnosis is made by inspection and palpation and not by biopsy.

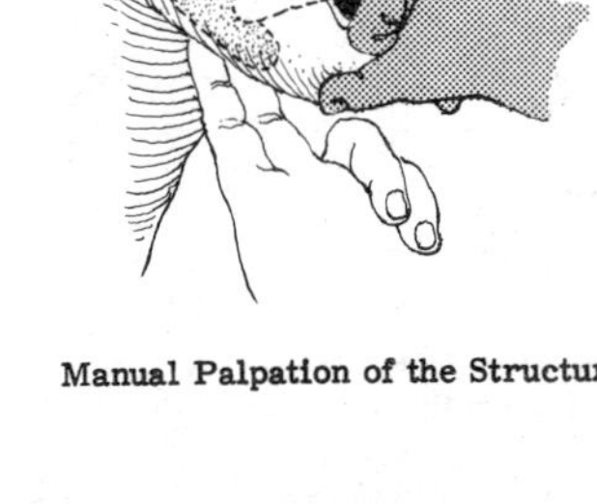

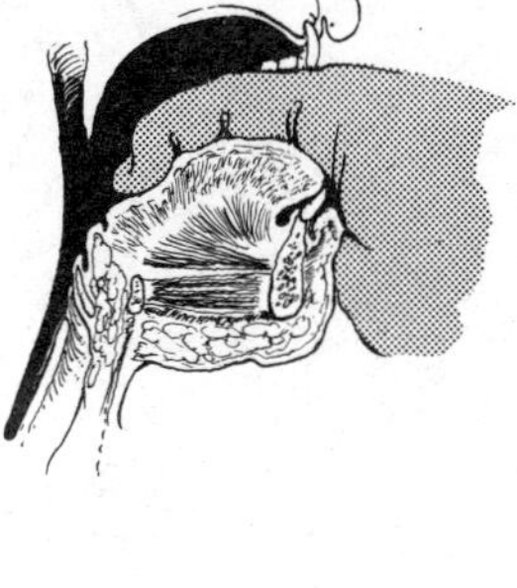

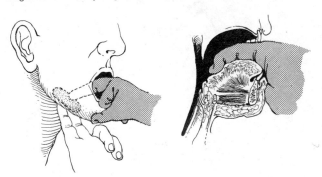

Manual Palpation of the Structures of the Floor of the Mouth

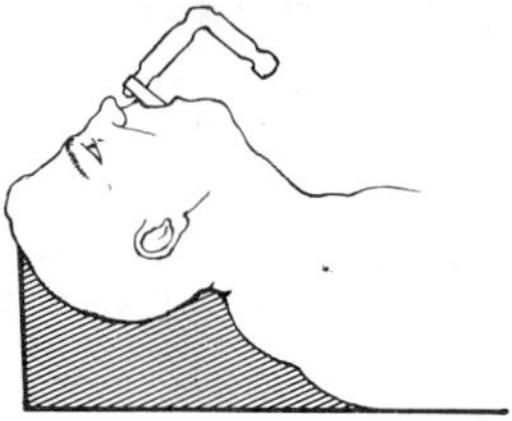

Position of Patient for Direct Laryngoscopy

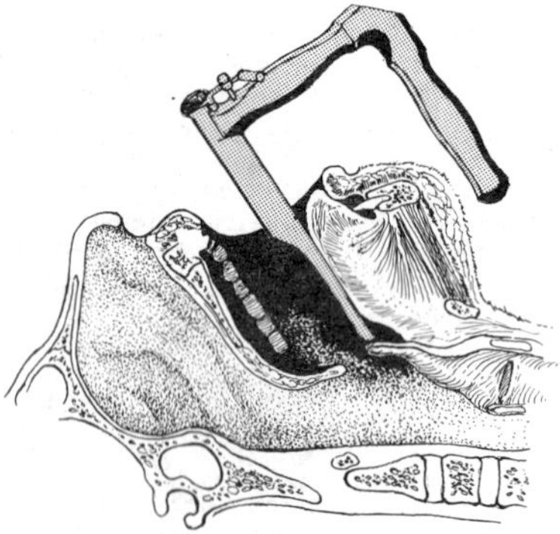

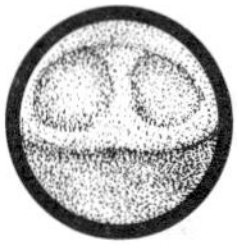

Standard Distal Lighting Laryngoscope Being Introduced. Tip of laryngoscope in vallecula. At right, anterior surface of epiglottis and vallecula as seen with the laryngoscope in the position shown at left.

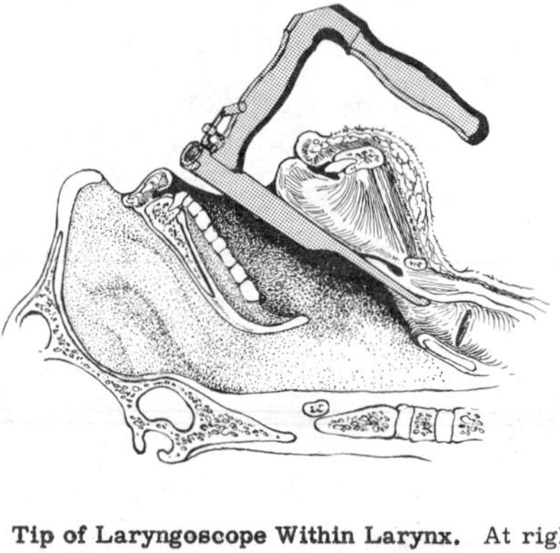

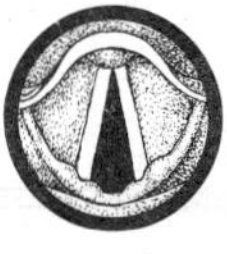

Tip of Laryngoscope Within Larynx. At right, direct view within larynx as seen with the laryngoscope in the position shown at left.

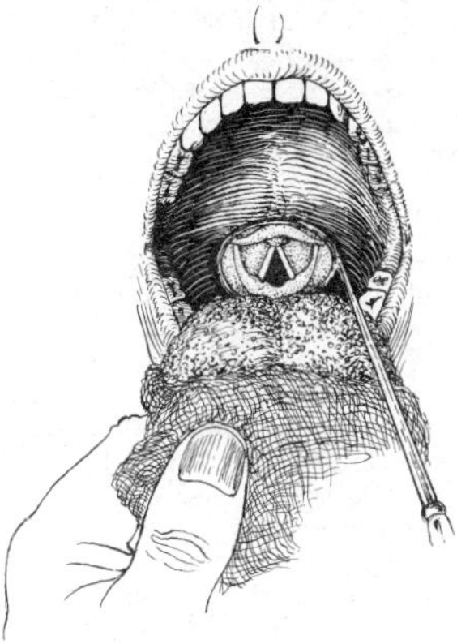

Indirect Mirror Examination of the Larynx and Adjacent Structures

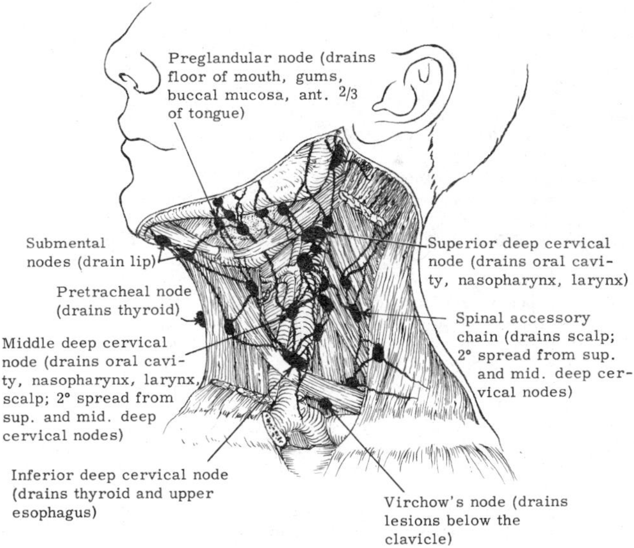

Lymphatic Drainage in the Neck (Left Lateral View)
(Modified after Richards)

Surgical excision, whether by sharp dissection or electrocautery, is the treatment of choice if it can be done safely. Sclerosing agents (sodium morrhuate, urethane, and quinine hydrochloride) may be tried, but excessive amounts of these drugs must not be injected. In some patients, especially those with hemangiomas, the policy of "watchful waiting" should be adhered to since the lesion may disappear.

Median Rhomboid Glossitis.

Median rhomboid glossitis is considered here since it is frequently confused with neoplastic disease. It occurs as a painless, shiny, reddened, raised, firm lesion in the midline of the tongue just in front of the circumvallate papillae. The cause is not known. Microscopic examination shows chronic inflammatory changes of the tissue. No treatment is necessary, and biopsy is not indicated.

Aberrant Salivary Gland Tumors.

Aberrant salivary gland tumors may occur in the cheeks, the palate, or the pharynx. They arise from epithelial salivary gland rests or from epithelial metaplasia of lesser salivary glands. There are usually few or no symptoms. The surface is covered with intact epithelium.

Treatment is by complete surgical excision.

Palatal Exostosis (Torus Palatinus).

An exostosis is frequently seen in the bony palate. It occurs as a painless bony swelling in the midline covered by intact mucosa. Exostoses are usually found on routine examination. No treatment is required unless the process interferes with the wearing of artificial dentures.

MALIGNANT NEOPLASMS OF THE ORAL CAVITY

Squamous Cell Carcinoma.

Squamous cell carcinoma is the most common malignant neoplasm in the oral cavity. (Adenocarcinoma is rare.) It may arise in areas of leukoplakia. On the mucous membrane surfaces it appears as ulcerations with elevated borders. Infiltration and induration may be evident, or the growth may be papillary, or both. The lesions tend to spread by direct extension and through the lymphatic vessels to regional lymph nodes or, less commonly, via the blood stream. Persistent ulcers of the oral cavity should be biopsied promptly.

A. Palate and Gingivae: Squamous cell carcinoma may arise on the hard or soft palate or gingivae. If it originates on the surface of the hard palate, erosion into the nasal cavity or into the maxillary sinus may be evident. Lesions of the soft palate arise on the dorsal or ventral surface or on the uvula. If they arise on the dorsum, early clinical diagnosis can be made only by mirror or nasopharyngoscopic examination of the area. Definitive diagnosis is made by microscopic examination of biopsy specimens. Pain is the most frequent complaint. X-rays should be obtained to rule out bone invasion.

   Small lesions may be excised if they are surrounded by a wide margin of normal tissue. More extensive lesions can be treated with radiation or sharp and electrocautery excision, or both. If bone is invaded, surgical excision is the treatment of choice. Regional neck lymph node metastases should be treated by radical neck dissection only if the primary lesion has been treated successfully.

B. Buccal Mucosa: Squamous cell carcinoma of the buccal mucosa may arise in an area of leukoplakia. Small lesions can be treated by surgical excision or radiation therapy; more extensive lesions may require both. Regional lymph node metastases are treated by surgical excision (block dissection of the neck if the primary lesion is controlled). If there is extensive loss of tissue following treatment, plastic repair in the form of pedicle grafting may have to be carried out.

C. Floor of Mouth: Squamous cell carcinoma arising in the floor of the mouth may involve a portion of the tongue or mandible by direct extension. Because the area contains abundant lymphatic channels, early metastasis to submental, submaxillary, and jugular lymph nodes on either side is the rule. Diagnosis is made by inspection, palpation, and microscopic examination of biopsy specimens. Bimanual palpation is important to determine the extent of infiltration into the tissues of the floor of the mouth. X-rays should be obtained to rule out bone involvement of the mandible.

Small primary lesions can be excised (scalpel or electrodissection) intraorally; some clinicians use radiation therapy also. More extensive lesions require surgical excision by an external approach. If the lesion has involved the periosteum or the bone of the mandible, a section of the mandible must be excised in continuity with the primary growth. A section of the tongue may have to be excised as well. Block dissection of the neck is indicated if the primary lesion is arrested and if resectable nodes are present in the neck, and in patients with extensive primary lesions as a prophylactic measure and in continuity with the primary lesion.

D. Tongue: Squamous cell carcinoma may occur on the body, tip, sides, under-surface, and posterior surface of the tongue. The tongue is rich in lymphatic channels, and these lesions tend to metastasize early. Pain is the most common symptom. Palpation reveals the extent of local infiltration and involvement of the lymph nodes of the neck. The diagnosis is confirmed by microscopic examination of biopsy specimens.

The treatment of squamous cell carcinoma of the tongue depends upon the location of the primary lesion and its potential or actual lymph node extensions. Small cancers of the tip are ideally located for wedge-shaped excision of the tip of the tongue. Cancer of the moveable tongue must be excised widely. Hemiglossectomy - often combined with radical neck dissection - is the treatment of choice. Primary cancer of the posterior third of the tongue has a poor prognosis regardless of treatment. Total glossectomy combined with radical neck dissection and partial mandibulectomy and/or radiation and chemotherapy have been used. Laryngectomy may also be indicated in such a patient.

If neck nodes develop after x-ray therapy to the primary lesion and it is reasonably certain that the primary lesion has been arrested, radical neck dissection should be done.

Intra-oral and external x-ray therapy has been used extensively and successfully in some clinics.

BENIGN NEOPLASMS OF THE LIPS

Hyperkeratosis.

Hyperkeratosis of the upper or lower lip often develops in persons whose occupations keep them out-of-doors. These lesions are considered premalignant. Leukoplakia and hyperkeratosis may be adjacent lesions, the former occurring on the inner surface of the lip and the latter on the vermilion border. Hyperkeratosis may appear as a discrete area, or the whole lip may be involved along its vermilion border. Microscopically, the stratified epithelium becomes thickened and hypertrophied, and excessive keratin layers are formed and shed so that the surface appears cornified and scaly. The rete pegs are elongated, but the basement membrane is intact. Malignant change "in situ" or invasive carcinoma may be evident. Induration as noted by palpation is suggestive of malignant change. Biopsy or biopsy excision (small lesions) should be done for definitive microscopic diagnosis.

In cases showing early hyperkeratosis, the application of protective ointments may be sufficient to promote healing. Slightly larger areas may be treated by electrodesiccation if malignancy has been ruled out by biopsy. Such coagulated areas should be protected by bland oils, ointments, or 2% aqueous gentian violet applications.

When the entire lip is involved, the vermilion surface is excised and the buccal mucosa undermined, advanced, and sutured to cover the defect.

MALIGNANT NEOPLASMS OF THE LIPS

Squamous Cell Carcinoma.

Squamous cell carcinoma of the lips occurs spontaneously in areas of hyperkeratosis (leukoplakia) and in ulcerations. The lower lip is more frequently involved, and the lesion is more common in men than in women. Sunlight appears to be a predisposing factor. The lesion appears as a raised, ulcerated area which cracks and bleeds easily on manipulation. Induration is evident upon palpation. In all lesions the submental areas and neck should be palpated to determine lymph node involvement. Diagnosis is confirmed by microscopic examination of suitable tissue.

Lesions 1.5-2 cm. in diameter which do not infiltrate deeply may be excised by removing a full-thickness wedge or V of the lip. Suprahyoid node dissection is not indicated. External radiation therapy is sometimes used.

Larger lesions require more extensive local excision and often flap rotation and suprahyoid and radical neck dissection as well.

If the primary lesion is controlled and the nodes appear in the neck at a later date, radical neck dissection should be done.

Radiotherapists may be most adept at treating cancer of the lip.

BENIGN NEOPLASMS OF THE NASAL CHAMBERS AND PARANASAL SINUSES

Squamous Papillomas (Inverting Papillomas).

Squamous cell papillomas arise either in the paranasal sinuses or in the nasal chambers. They are benign lesions in the sense that they do not metastasize; however, they erode adjacent structures (soft tissue and bone) by their local growth. Grossly, the papillomas appear irregular on the surface and firm in character, often filling a whole nasal chamber. Histologically, they show squamous epithelium growing in papilliferous cords surrounding a fibrous core. Occasionally, malignancy is diagnosed. Definitive diagnosis is made by microscopic tissue examination. X-rays should be taken to identify the sinuses involved and to determine if bony erosion has occurred.

Complete removal often requires radical surgery, to the point of eradicating the paranasal sinuses and, at times, the orbital contents as well.

Hemangiomas.

Hemangiomas in the nose or paranasal sinuses are diagnosed by a history of epistaxis and the finding of the characteristic bluish tumor. Treatment is usually by radiation therapy in combination with surgical excision.

Osteomas and Ossifying Fibromas.

Osteomas occur characteristically in the maxillary, ethmoid, and frontal sinuses. They usually cause no symptoms unless they grow to excessive size. Many are diagnosed only by routine x-rays. No treatment is indicated unless symptoms are present.

Ossifying fibromas may occur in the maxillary sinus and upper jaw. These benign tumors contain bone as well as fibrous tissue in varying amounts. They grow slowly and may thin adjacent bone by their expansive growth. Symptoms depend on the size of the lesion and involvement of neighboring structures. X-rays are an aid in diagnosis. Treatment is by surgical excision, which must be extensive if the palate or orbital bony structures are involved.

Nasal Polyps.

Nasal polyps are not neoplastic in origin but are considered here because they are often confused with neoplastic lesions. They are associated with allergy and infection or both. Treatment is by surgical removal. All excised tissues, regardless of their gross appearance, should be examined microscopically.

MALIGNANT NEOPLASMS OF THE NASAL CHAMBERS AND PARANASAL SINUSES

Squamous Cell Carcinoma.

Squamous cell carcinoma can develop in the nose or in any of the paranasal sinuses. It occurs most frequently in the maxillary antrum. The sinus mucosa undergoes metaplasia and malignant changes. Microscopic examination of the lesion shows squamous cell carcinoma of varying degrees of differentiation. Symptoms and signs often appear late in the disease and depend upon the extent of the lesion, its speed of growth, the nerves involved, and the presence of infection and bone involvement. All tumors of the nasal chambers or paranasal sinuses which are not obviously benign should be considered carcinoma until proved otherwise. Biopsy and microscopic tissue examination will confirm the diagnosis. Spread is by direct extension to adjacent structures; via lymphatic channels to regional lymph nodes in the pterygomaxillary space, submandibular nodes, and cervical nodes; and, infrequently, via the blood stream.

Radiation therapy followed by radical surgery is the treatment of choice.

If the primary neoplasm is arrested and resectable cervical metastases are present, radical neck dissection should be done.

BENIGN NEOPLASMS OF THE JAW

Adamantinomas (Ameloblastomas).

Adamantinomas occur more frequently in the lower than in the upper jaw. They grow by expansion, causing a swelling intraorally or externally (or both). They arise from the enamel organ epithelium of a tooth. The tumor itself contains cystic spaces which are filled with colloid, mucinous, or clear yellow fluid. Microscopically, the cystic spaces are surrounded by bony trabeculae that contain cuboidal stellate or tall columnar epithelium alone or in combination. Some tumors may be predominantly cellular. They metastasize rarely to distant long bones, lungs, and regional lymph nodes. Symptoms and signs are those of a slowly growing, painless mass in the upper or lower jaw. As the cortex of the jaw is thinned, palpation may elicit a sense of crackling. X-rays aid in the diagnosis if the cystic areas are a prominent feature of the lesion. Biopsy, usually through an intact mucosa or intact skin surface, and microscopic tissue examinations are essential for final diagnosis.

Surgical excision of small lesions of the lower or upper jaw usually present no difficulties. However, large tumors may require extensive resection of the mandible or maxilla and palate. Complete surgical excision of the lesion must be done if local recurrences are to be prevented.

Giant Cell Tumor.

Giant cell tumors of the mandible are not unlike those found elsewhere in the body. Treatment is by surgical excision, which can usually be accomplished without interrupting the continuity of the jaw.

MALIGNANT NEOPLASMS OF THE JAW

Sarcoma is the most common of the rare primary malignant tumors of the jaw. Metastatic tumors may invade the jaw, or the jaw may be involved by direct extension from neighboring neoplasms. X-rays may aid in diagnosis. A diligent search for the primary lesion must be made elsewhere in the body.

BENIGN NEOPLASMS OF THE NASOPHARYNX

Juvenile Fibroma (Juvenile Nasopharyngeal Angiofibroma).
Juvenile fibromas occur most frequently in the adolescent male. They arise in or near the vault of the nasopharynx and may reach considerable size. They are attached to the underlying bony structures by a stalk or by a sessile base. Extensions of the tumor may reach the paranasal sinuses, pterygomaxillary space, and orbit. Histologically, the tumor is composed of vascular connective tissue. The vascularity of individual tumors varies considerably.

These tumors do not metastasize. Nasal obstruction is a prominent symptom. Nasal hemorrhage may occur. The tumor mass may be seen by elevation of the soft palate, indirect mirror examination of the nasopharynx, or by inspection through the nasal chambers. On finger palpation the tumor is firm and smooth. Biopsy should not be attempted unless complete hospital surgical facilities are available. X-rays reveal a soft tissue mass in the nasopharynx, and often show an extension to the maxillary sinus, sphenoid sinuses, pterygomaxillary space, and orbit. Arteriograms also help in determining the size of the tumor.

Surgical removal is the treatment of choice. An attempt is made to evulse the lesion at its base. Hemorrhage may be a serious complication. The external surgical approach is indicated in most cases.

SQUAMOUS CELL CARCINOMA OF THE NASOPHARYNX
(Lympho-epithelioma, Transitional Cell Carcinoma)

Squamous cell carcinoma of the nasopharynx arises in any part of the nasopharynx. Histologically, the cells may be so anaplastic that it is difficult to determine their type. Lymphoid tissue can be abundant in the stroma. Invasion of the base of the skull by direct extension and neck lymph node metastases often occurs early. There are few symptoms and signs until later in the disease, when epistaxis, pain, unilateral serous otitis media, a mass in the neck, and cranial nerve involvement may occur. There is a high incidence of this neoplasm in Orientals. The diagnosis is made by microscopic examination of representative tissue specimens. X-rays are necessary to determine bony involvement of the base of the skull and invasion of the paranasal sinuses.

External x-ray therapy is the treatment of choice not only for the primary disease but for lymph node metastases as well. Radical neck dissection is indicated in some patients.

SQUAMOUS CELL CARCINOMA OF THE TONSILS

Squamous cell carcinoma of the tonsils accounts for about 10% of all intraoral carcinomas. Microscopically, the cell type may vary considerably from the epidermoid to the transitional cell type. The symptoms and signs depend on the size of the lesion, ulceration, infiltration, and secondary infection. Pain may be an outstanding symptom. The exact origin of the primary lesion is often difficult to determine if the process has spread to the tongue, pillars, and soft palate. Diagnosis is confirmed by microscopic examination of representative tissue. Since lymph channels are abundant in this area, neck lymph node involvement occurs early and frequently.

If surgical excision of squamous cell carcinoma arising in the tonsil is attempted, it should be radical. In order to remove the lesion and its regional lymph nodes, radical neck dissection in continuity with excision of the primary lesion must be done. To accomplish this the mandible must be partially resected.

Radiation therapy is regarded as the treatment of choice by some clinicians. Surgery and radiation therapy may be combined.

BENIGN NEOPLASMS OF THE LARYNX AND HYPOPHARYNX

Polyps, papillomas, vocal nodules, and leukoplakia may occur on the vocal cords, producing hoarseness. Diagnosis is made by direct and indirect laryngoscopy and biopsy (often biopsy excision). The lesions are treated by excision except for the vocal nodules, which may be treated by voice training to prevent misuse and overuse of the voice.

MALIGNANT NEOPLASMS OF THE LARYNX AND HYPOPHARYNX

Squamous Cell Carcinoma.

Squamous cell carcinomas represent 99% of all malignant tumors of the larynx. About 60% originate on the true vocal cord; the rest in the laryngeal ventricles, false cords, aryepiglottic folds, epiglottis, and arytenoid and subglottic areas. The sites of primary malignancy in the pharynx are the pyriform sinuses, pharyngeal walls, and postcricoid areas. Histologically, the lesions of the true cord are more differentiated than those of other locations.

Hoarseness is an early symptom of true vocal cord cancer. Laryngeal cancers of other areas are less apt to produce hoarseness, but cause pain and dysphagia. Biopsy (indirect or direct) confirms the diagnosis.

True vocal cord cancer metastasizes late. Cancers arising in other locations metastasize earlier and more frequently because of their anaplastic cell type and the abundant lymph channels in these areas. The lymph nodes involved are along the internal jugular vein; those overlying the thyrohyoid and cricothyroid membranes; and those in the potential anatomic space between the esophagus and trachea. Other routes of spread of laryngeal cancer are by direct extension and, rarely, via the blood stream.

Peroral forceps removal is the treatment of choice in small (2 mm.) true vocal cord cancer. Electrocautery of the base is a further safeguard.

True vocal cord lesions involving the middle third of the cord may be removed by splitting the thyroid cartilage and removing part of the false and the entire true vocal cord (laryngofissure).

More extensive lesions of the true vocal cord require either hemilaryngectomy or wide-field total laryngectomy. True vocal cord lesions require radical neck dissection in continuity with the laryngectomy if nodes are palpable in the neck or if the primary lesion has invaded supraglottic or infraglottic structures. In the latter instances, the node dissection is done as an elective measure.

As a rule those cancers arising in other locations in the larynx or pharynx require wide-field laryngectomy alone (infrequent) or wide-field laryngectomy combined with ipsilateral radical neck dissection. Contralateral neck dissection may be indicated also, but usually at a later date. Prophylactic ipsilateral neck dissection must be done in many cases because of the high incidence of metastatic nodes found on microscopic examination of surgical specimens.

Small cancers of the true vocal cord may also be treated by external x-ray therapy. Larger cancers of the true vocal cord or those arising in other areas carry a less favorable prognosis with this form of therapy.

Surgery combined with preoperative x-ray therapy may be an important form of treatment in certain cases. The surgeon and the radiologist must decide upon the treatment cooperatively.

BENIGN NEOPLASMS OF THE SALIVARY GLANDS

Mixed Tumors.

About 65% of tumors arising in the parotid glands are of the benign mixed cell type. The tumors are encapsulated, but may have finger-like projections which protrude between the lobulations of the gland. Histologically, the tumors are made up of epithelial elements interspersed with fibrous (mesoblastic) tissue. The epithelial elements (alveoli, masses of cells or strands) may predominate in one portion of the tumor, whereas in another the mesoblastic elements may predominate in the form of cartilage, myxomatous connective tissue, and hyalin.

A painless swelling develops in one of the salivary glands. Occasionally these tumors arise in the deep portion of the parotid gland and their main growth is inward, toward the pharynx and palate. Tumors of the submaxillary gland present in the submaxillary triangle area. Although they grow slowly, they may reach several cm. in size. The finding of a discrete, firm, painless mass in these areas suggests the possibility of mixed tumor. Sialograms may show encroachment of the tumor upon the ductal system of the gland. Biopsy should not be done because of the danger of seeding uninvolved tissues.

Treatment of benign mixed tumors of the parotid gland is by wide surgical excision well beyond the tumor capsule, including most of the normal parotid gland.

The facial nerve must be preserved. Before definitive surgery of the tumor is attempted the facial nerve must be identified, either peripherally or at its main trunk. As a rule, the parotid gland lateral to the facial nerve is excised with the superficially placed tumors. Dissection of tumors deep to the facial nerve is much more difficult. Every attempt should be made to perform a total parotidectomy with preservation of the facial nerve. It is imperative also that the capsule of a mixed tumor not be ruptured during removal.

Benign mixed tumors of the submaxillary gland are removed by complete excision of the gland. The mandibular division of the facial nerve must be preserved.

Papillary Cystadenoma Lymphomatosum (Adenolymphoma, Warthin's Tumor).

These tumors usually arise in the inferior pole of the parotid gland. They are composed of lymphocytoid tissues surrounding spaces lined with epithelium (acidophilic cells). They present as benign painless swellings, usually in older patients, and upon palpation appear cystic. Treatment is by surgical excision, taking care to preserve the facial nerve.

MALIGNANT NEOPLASMS OF THE SALIVARY GLANDS

Malignant disease of the salivary glands develops as a firm mass in the substance of the gland affected. Ulceration or infiltration of the skin surface may occur, and adjacent structures such as muscle, other soft tissue, and bone may be invaded by malignant cells. The facial nerve is frequently paralyzed. Definitive diagnosis depends upon microscopic examination of the tumor specimen. Late metastases occur to the lungs, abdominal viscera, bone, and brain.

Squamous cell carcinomas in the salivary glands can be highly malignant. Spread may be rapid, and the prognosis for life is extremely poor.

Adenocarcinomas are not necessarily limited to the salivary glands but may occur in other locations as well, e.g., the oral cavity, nasopharynx, paranasal sinuses, pharynx, and trachea. These tumors are only occasionally rapidly fatal. Metastases to lung, brain, and bone occur late in the course of the disease. In some cell types, the lymph nodes of the neck may be invaded by metastases.

Muco-epidermoid carcinomas are ductal in origin. Their degree of malignancy depends principally upon the type of cell structure which predominates. Highly malignant tumors are composed mainly of mucus-secreting cells; in tumors of low-grade malignancy the epidermoid and intermediate cells predominate.

The treatment of malignancies of the salivary glands should be flexible and individualized. In recent years more and more such cases have been treated by a combination of surgery and x-ray therapy. Frequently, with this combined therapy, the facial nerve can be preserved intact. When feasible, patients with squamous cell carcinomas are so treated. Neck dissections are usually done when nodes are present and only when the primary disease has been arrested by surgery or x-ray therapy or both. If the facial nerve or part of its branches is excised, nerve suture or grafting should be done.

Chemotherapy of Malignancies of the Head and Neck.

The chemotherapeutic agents have not proved satisfactory for malignancies of the head and neck. In most clinics these drugs have been reserved for patients with malignancies which are far advanced and of a hopeless nature. Administration of the drugs has been by arterial infusion or perfusion and by mouth depending upon the location, stage, accessibility, and cell type of the tumor. All of these drugs, whether antimetabolites, alkylating agents, or the newer mycins, must be made more effective before widespread clinical use can be recommended. In some patients combinations of treatment, such as drug therapy in conjunction with surgery or x-ray therapy (or both), may yet prove beneficial. New drugs are being tested, and bio-assays of these materials on animal tumors should continue in the hope of future clinical success.

Local manifestations of constitutional neoplastic disease in the head and neck areas may in some patients respond to systemic drug therapy. Some patients with Hodgkin's disease or other lymphomas fall in this category.

CAROTID BODY TUMOR
(Chemotectoma)

Carotid body tumors arise in the potential anatomic space in the bifurcation of the carotid artery in the nonchromaffin paraganglia. Microscopically the tumors show 2 main types of cellular structure: (1) large cell (alveolar) polyhedral and (2) small cell (peritheliomatous). Vascular tissue may permeate the fibrous tissue stroma so that the whole tumor appears as a dark, blood-red mass.

Clinically, these tumors grow slowly. They may be so vascular that a bruit can be noted by auscultation. Upon palpation they are shown to be fixed to the underlying structures. Carotid body tumors must be considered in the differential diagnosis in all tumor masses of the upper lateral neck. Biopsy is usually contraindicated. Arteriograms may show up-take of dye by the tumor, which helps in diagnosis.

Surgical excision is the treatment of choice. It can usually be done readily if the tumor is not firmly attached to the great vessels. On the other hand, if the tumor is attached to the great vessels, removal may be contraindicated in older patients. The surgeon must assume grave responsibilities in carotid vessel surgery because of its inherent complications.

DISEASES OF THE THYROID

THYROID FUNCTION

The thyroid gland is concerned with iodine metabolism and with synthesis, storage, and secretion of thyroxine (T_4) and triiodothyronine (T_3), which are the principal hormones of the gland. These hormones are synthesized in the thyroid from iodine and tyrosine. They are released from the gland into the blood stream as the need arises by the action of thyroid-stimulating hormone (TSH) from the pituitary. Thyroxine and T_3 in the circulation are both bound to plasma protein, although T_3 adheres to a lesser extent. Circulating thyroxine can be measured as protein-bound iodine (PBI). Thyroid hormone affects cellular oxidative processes throughout the body, and its output is regulated by a feedback mechanism that involves the hypothalamus, the pituitary, and the thyroid. An increase in circulating thyroid hormone inhibits the production of TSH, whereas a decrease stimulates it. Iodine is necessary for thyroid function, although the requirement is minimal (about 20-200 μg./day). Iodine deficiency may arise due to inadequate intake or to ingestion of certain foods and chemical compounds which interfere with the utilization of iodine, or it may arise when the demand for iodine is increased (e.g., during puberty). When iodine deficiency occurs, thyroid hormone production is insufficient and circulating levels are low. This leads to an increase in pituitary TSH output, and hyperplasia of the thyroid results.

Tests of thyroid function are given below.

A. Protein-Bound Iodine (PBI, "Hormonal Iodine"): Normal: 4-8 μg./100 ml. serum.) PBI is elevated in hyperthyroidism and thyroiditis and after administration of iodides, desiccated thyroid, or thyroxine. Inorganic iodides increase levels for up to 3 weeks; organic iodides (e.g., in urograms, cholecystograms) for 6 months or longer; oil-soluble organic iodides (e.g., Lipiodol®) for months or years. Pregnancy and use of Enovid® or similar preparations raise PBI due to increased thyroxine-binding protein. PBI is low in hypothyroidism. It may be falsely low due to mercurial diuretics (low for 3-7 days), urinary loss of protein (e.g., nephrosis), or T_3 (Cytomel®) administration.

B. Butanol-Extractable Iodine (BEI): (Normal: 3-7 μg./100 ml.) BEI roughly parallels PBI. It is not affected by inorganic iodides but is raised by organic iodides.

C. T_4 by Column: (Normal: 3-7.5 μg./100 ml.) This test has largely replaced BEI and is similarly affected by iodides.

D. T_4 CPB-MP or T_4 (D): (Normal: 5.3-14.5 μg./100 ml.) This test measures total thyroxine by competitive protein binding or displacement. It is replacing PBI, BEI, and T_4 by column tests since it is unaffected by exogenous iodides (although it is affected by states of altered thyroxine binding).

E. Radioactive T_3 Uptake of Red Cells or Resin: (Normal [varies with method]: Red cells - males, 12-19%; females, 13-20%. Resin - males, 25-35%; females 24-34%.) Resin uptake is the preferred method. This test is not affected by exogenous organic or inorganic iodides. It is an indirect measure of thyroxine-binding protein and is of value in certain patients (e.g., in pregnancy) when the PBI is falsely high due to increased thyroxine binding while T_3 uptake is low. In general, T_3 uptake test results parallel those of the PBI test.

F. Radioiodine (I^{131}) Uptake of Thyroid Gland: (Normal: 5-35% in 24 hours.) Uptake is increased in thyrotoxicosis, hypofunctioning large goiter, iodine lack, and, at times, chronic thyroiditis. Uptake is low in hypothyroidism and thyroiditis and after administration of iodides (similar to factors raising the PBI), T_4, and antithyroid drugs. A scintigram over the gland outlines areas of increased and decreased activity.

G. Basal Metabolic Rate (BMR): (Normal: ±20%.) This test is rarely used today. It is elevated in hyperthyroidism, polycythemia, leukemia, anemia, congestive heart failure, malignancy, and a number of disorders. It is low (−30% to −60%) in myxedema but is also moderately decreased in chronic debility, starvation, Addison's disease, and a number of other conditions not directly related to the thyroid.

H. Serum Cholesterol: (Normal: 150-280 mg./100 ml.) Cholesterol is usually relatively elevated in hypothyroidism and is occasionally relatively low in thyrotoxicosis. The test is nonspecific and the absolute level is less significant than the change after treatment of the thyroid condition.

I. Serologic Tests: Antibodies against several thyroid constituents may be identified in the sera of patients with various types of thyroiditis (especially Hashimoto's disease); occasionally in nodular goiters and myxedema; and rarely in Graves' disease and thyroid carcinoma.

J. Thyrotropin (TSH) Immunoassay and Response to Thyrotropin-Releasing Factor (TRF): Serum TSH is determined by radioimmunoassay. TSH elevations may occur in subclinical hypothyroidism. A normal TSH rules out primary hypothyroidism. A prolonged and exaggerated rise in TSH after administration of TRF in patients with borderline elevations of TSH may provide further evidence of primary thyroid failure. Patients with hyperthyroidism fail to respond to TRF, and a normal response virtually excludes hyperthyroidism. TSH elevations with nodular goiter usually indicates autoimmune thyroid disease.

ECTOPIC THYROID

The thyroid gland arises embryologically as a midline diverticulum from the pharynx. In normal development it passes downward to its bilobed adult position, but in a rare case it may fail to evolve 2 lobes and is then seen in the neck as a single mass of tissue.

There are no symptoms. A round, smooth, firm, nontender mass is palpable in the midline of the neck below the hyoid bone. The mass is not attached to the skin and moves with swallowing.

Thyroglossal duct cyst is easily mistaken for ectopic thyroid. If there is any question about the diagnosis, a tracer dose of radioiodine will indicate the presence of functioning thyroid tissue.

No treatment is required. Inadvertent excision during surgery for thyroglossal duct cyst may result in hypothyroidism. When ectopic thyroid is encountered during neck surgery for some other disorder, the cosmetic appearance can be improved by dividing the mass in its midline (only if blood vessels enter from both sides) and turning both halves laterally for placement under adjacent muscles (Gross).

NONTOXIC NODULAR GOITER
(Adenomatous Goiter)

The major cause of adenomatous goiter is iodine deficiency, which results in hyperplasia, generalized enlargement of the gland, and, frequently, gross nodule formation. The process is not neoplastic, but when only one nodule is palpable it is usually impossible to distinguish nodular goiter from adenoma or carcinoma except by exploration and biopsy. The overall incidence of carcinoma in multinodular goiter is uncertain, but is probably about 1%. In surgical series, however, the incidence of carcinoma has ranged from 4-30% depending upon the manner in which the patients were selected for operative treatment.

Women are most commonly affected. There are usually no symptoms unless the gland is large enough to produce pressure on the trachea or esophagus. Substernal extension occurs occasionally and appears as a superior mediastinal mass on x-ray. The goiter may have been present for years. Diffuse thyroid enlargement may develop in females during puberty or pregnancy, when iodine requirements normally increase markedly. Hyperthyroidism is the most frequent complication. In addition to evaluation of endocrine status, a radioisotope scan of thyroid is indicated.

It is impractical and unnecessary to advise surgical removal in every case of nodular goiter. The chief indications for surgical removal are (1) hyperthyroidism, (2) pressure symptoms, (3) substernal extension, (4) progressive enlargement, (5) suspicion of malignancy, and (6) cosmetic reasons. The most important question is whether carcinoma is present in a multinodular goiter. Recent onset, rapid growth, hard nodule, fixation, regional node enlargement, and recurrent nerve palsy are suggestive. "Cold" nodules prove to be carcinomatous in about 25% of cases.

Medical measures are of no value in long-standing nodular goiter. In the diffuse type of goiter of recent development (e.g., during puberty or pregnancy), regression may occur following administration of desiccated thyroid, 60-120 mg. (1-2 gr.) daily, and potassium iodide solution (saturated) or strong iodine solution (Lugol's solution), 5 drops daily in one-half glass of water. Continue thyroid and iodine therapy as long as the goiter is regressing; then advise indefinite use of iodized table salt. Endemic goiter is prevented by the use of iodized salt, 1-2 Gm. daily.

HYPERTHYROIDISM

Hyperthyroidism is characterized by excessive secretion of thyroid hormone, probably as a result of autonomous thyroid activity or a nonpituitary thyroid stimulant of unknown nature. Two forms are distinguished: (1) exophthalmic goiter or Graves' disease, and (2) toxic nodular goiter. Rarely, hyperthyroidism may result from an autonomous, hyperfunctioning, solitary ("hot") nodule.

Exophthalmic goiter is usually acute in onset and is associated with diffuse thyroid enlargement. It is 4 times as common in women as in men and typically occurs between puberty and the menopause. Exophthalmos is present in most cases. Exophthalmos is infrequently progressive, and even more rarely unilateral.

Toxic nodular goiter is the result of the development of hyperthyroidism in a preexisting nontoxic nodular goiter. Women in the older age group are usually affected. The onset tends to be insidious, and signs of cardiac insufficiency often dominate the clinical picture to such an extent that the hyperthyroidism is overlooked. Exophthalmos is not present.

Clinical Findings.

A. Symptoms and Signs: Patients with exophthalmic goiter or toxic nodular goiter complain of nervousness, irritability, easy fatigability, increased tolerance to cold, and weight loss in spite of good appetite and food intake. The goiter is diffuse and smooth in Graves' disease and nodular in toxic nodular goiter; other signs in both conditions include a warm moist skin, fine tremors in the hands, restlessness, quick movements, and evidence of weight loss. In Graves' disease there are exophthalmos, stare, and lid lag. A bruit and thrill may be present over the gland. Tachycardia is the most frequent cardiovascular finding in both diseases. Atrial fibrillation and congestive failure are not uncommon in older patients.

B. Laboratory Findings:
  1. PBI values above 8 μg./100 ml. are suggestive of hyperthyroidism.
  2. Radioactive iodine uptake is increased.
  3. Radioactive T_3 uptake of red cells or resin is increased.
  4. The blood cholesterol level may be low.
  5. BMR is usually elevated. A BMR of −5% or below practically excludes hyperthyroidism.

Treatment.

A. Medical Measures.
  1. Radioactive iodine (I^{131} or I^{125}) therapy is the treatment of choice in recurrent thyrotoxicosis after thyroidectomy, and when surgical treatment is refused or is contraindicated. Since irradiation therapy may favor malignant change, it is probably unwise to administer a therapeutic dose of radioactive iodine to patients with a life expectancy of over 25 years except when surgery is unduly hazardous. The incidence of hypothyroidism 5-10 years after radioactive iodine therapy is 25-35%; after subtotal thyroidectomy, 10-15%.
  2. Antithyroid drugs - Thiouracil or thiocyanate preparations may be used as definitive therapy in young patients who refuse surgery, but the course of treatment is prolonged (up to 2 years) and costly and relapses are frequent (about 50%). The major value of antithyroid drugs is in preparation for operation.

B. Surgical Treatment: Subtotal thyroidectomy is the treatment of choice in toxic nodular goiter and in Graves' disease except as noted above. Preoperatively, it is desirable to render the patient euthyroid with an antithyroid drug and iodine. Surgery is not urgent. Preparation should continue until the baseline studies of thyroid function return essentially to normal, signs of toxicity are absent, resting pulse is normal, and weight gain is established. Rest, nutritional support, and mild barbiturate sedation are helpful adjunctive measures. Medical preparation for surgery should be carried out as follows:
  1. Propylthiouracil, 100-200 mg. q.i.d. A larger dose may occasionally be necessary to obtain an adequate response. BMR usually falls at the rate of about 1% per day, so that preparation requires 4-6 weeks. Occasional toxic reactions to propylthiouracil include granulocytopenia, drug fever, and rash. The patient should be examined weekly and a blood count obtained; if the WBC falls below 4500 or if there are fewer than 45% granulocytes, the drug must be discontinued.

     Methimazole (Tapazole®), 10-15 mg. q.i.d., may be used in place of propylthiouracil.
  2. Iodine - Ten to 15 days prior to operation (when the BMR is

+10 to +15%), iodine is given in addition to propylthiouracil. Iodine dosage is 5-10 drops daily of Lugol's solution or saturated solution of potassium iodide. In mild thyrotoxicosis, iodine therapy alone for 10-15 days before operation may be sufficient preparation.

Complications of Hyperthyroidism.

A. Acute Hyperthyroid Crisis (Thyroid Storm): This is usually precipitated by surgery in a patient with severe thyrotoxicosis. Since the advent of antithyroid drugs it is possible to control hyperthyroidism before surgery in most instances. The major features include restlessness, delirium, tachycardia, hyperpyrexia, and vasomotor collapse. The prognosis is grave (mortality over 50%). An "apathetic" type also occurs which is characterized by hypotonia, apathy, and prostration with only mild pyrexia. Treatment is urgent and consists of controlling hyperpyrexia with cold packs or refrigerated blankets and restlessness with sedation. Oxygen and I.V. fluids with glucose, electrolytes, and vitamins are often indicated. Sodium Iodide, U.S.P., 1-2 Gm. (15-30 gr.) I.V. every 12-24 hours, and large doses of an intravenous corticosteroid are advocated. Consider reducing hormone production by giving propylthiouracil, 400 mg. every 8 hours by mouth or nasogastric tube.

B. Severe Exophthalmos: Exophthalmos is the result of edema and later cellular infiltration of the orbital tissues. Removal of the thyroid does not necessarily relieve exophthalmos, and may even aggravate it. In marked exophthalmos there is danger of corneal ulceration, severe limitation of extraocular muscle movement, and blindness. Significant or progressive exophthalmos is an indication for periodic examination with an exophthalmometer. The following treatment measures should be considered:

1. Protection of the eyes with dark glasses during the day and eye shields at night. Ophthalmologic consultation should be obtained. In extreme cases, tarsorrhaphy may be necessary.
2. Thyroid hormone is begun when the BMR or PBI reaches normal during propylthiouracil therapy or after thyroidectomy. Begin with thyroid, 0.1-0.2 Gm. daily, or levothyroxine sodium (Synthroid®), 0.1-0.3 mg. daily. Adjust dosage to maintain PBI at about 7-9 mg./100 ml. This therapy is not invariably effective.
3. Corticosteroids or corticotropin (ACTH) in large doses are reported to be helpful for certain patients.
4. Orbital decompression may rarely be necessary to save the vision if exophthalmos progresses in spite of conservative therapy.

Prognosis.

The results of subtotal thyroidectomy for toxic nodular goiter are generally good, and the incidence of recurrent thyrotoxicosis is low. The recurrence rate following thyroidectomy for Graves' disease is about 10%. Hypothyroidism occurs in about 10% of cases. Operative mortality in experienced hands is as low as 0.25%.

SOLITARY THYROID NODULE

Ten to 20% of solitary thyroid nodules are malignant; the remainder consist chiefly of adenomas and nodular goiter in approximately equal proportion. Unfortunately, there is no certain means of distinguishing benign from malignant nodules. Both are usually asymptomatic incidental findings. The most important diagnostic test is the radioactive scintiscan of the thyroid region after administration of a test dose of radioactive iodine. If the nodule takes up radioactive iodine it is very unlikely to be cancer. "Cold" nodules must be looked upon with suspicion, since about one-fourth of them prove to be carcinomatous.

Single thyroid nodules occur more frequently in women than in men. Neither youth nor long duration rule out cancer, since thyroid malignancy (particularly papillary carcinoma) appears even in the teens and may be present for months or years without discernible change in size. These lesions should therefore be excised completely, usually by lobectomy. From study of an immediate frozen section by an experienced pathologist, it is usually possible to obtain a definitive diagnosis and to decide upon the extent of resection required.

THYROID ADENOMA

Thyroid adenomas are benign, encapsulated, slowly-growing neoplasms which are usually single but may be multiple. Clinically they present as firm, nontender, discrete, ovoid nodules. Adenomas rarely become malignant, but they must be removed because they cannot be differentiated from cancer except on microscopic study. The commonest cell type is the follicular adenoma, which may be difficult to distinguish pathologically from follicular carcinoma since blood vessel invasion and hematogenous metastases can occur in benign-appearing lesions. Papillary adenoma and an atypical type may also occur. Local excision - whether with an adequate margin or by means of lobectomy - is indicated for all true adenomas.

THYROID CARCINOMA

There are 4 general types of thyroid carcinoma: papillary (65%), follicular (25%), medullary (5%), and undifferentiated (5%). An epidermoid type occurs quite rarely. The tumor is firm and nontender, and there are wide variations in rate of growth. Pressure symptoms and recurrent nerve palsy are characteristic of undifferentiated lesions.

Papillary Thyroid Carcinoma.

All ages may be affected, but most patients are under 40. Papillary carcinoma occasionally grows very slowly over a period of 20-30 years, but the assumption that papillary carcinoma can be treated as a benign neoplasm is not warranted. Actually, this is an unpredictable tumor which invades the regional nodes in about 75% of cases and involves the opposite lobe of the gland in about

30%. Treatment should probably consist of total thyroidectomy with dissection if the nodes are positive on frozen section. If nodes are positive on both sides, unilateral neck dissection is carried out at the time of total thyroidectomy. Neck dissection on the opposite side is deferred for a month. Whether sternocleidomastoid muscle is retained depends upon the extent of metastases. The internal jugular on one side is preserved. Total thyroidectomy may result in stimulation of metastases to take up radioactive iodine. This occurs infrequently in papillary tumors. Tumors occur in which there is an admixture of papillary and follicular elements. Metastases can sometimes be inhibited with desiccated thyroid, 0.2 Gm. (3 gr.) daily. The five-year clinical cure rate in papillary carcinoma is about 60%.

Follicular Thyroid Carcinoma.

This type of thyroid cancer usually occurs in patients over 40 years of age. It tends to spread via the blood stream, especially to the bones and lungs, but lymphatic metastases and spread to the opposite lobe are also common. Surgical treatment is the same as for papillary carcinoma. Metastases of follicular cancer may be sufficiently biologically active to permit their localization and palliative treatment with radioactive iodine. The five-year clinical cure rate in follicular carcinoma is about 60%.

Medullary Carcinoma.

This is a solid, hard tumor which may contain amyloid and does not take up radioiodine. The cell of origin is from the final or ultimobranchial cleft. This tumor may be associated with a syndrome of excessive calcitonin secretion, familial in nature, and may be accompanied by pheochromocytoma and hyperplasia or adenoma of the parathyroid glands (Sipple's disease). Metastases occur. Treatment is as outlined for papillary carcinoma.

Undifferentiated Thyroid Carcinoma.

These lesions may be of the small cell, giant cell, or epidermoid variety. They occur after the age of 40 and spread rapidly. Surgical extirpation is often impossible. These tumors do not take up radioiodine, and palliative radiotherapy is the only recourse in nonresectable cases. The five-year survival rate is about 25%.

THYROIDITIS

The various types of thyroiditis are of surgical importance chiefly because they may be confused with thyroid cancer.

Subacute thyroiditis is an inflammatory process, possibly viral in origin, which causes tender enlargement of one or both lobes often accompanied by moderate fever, pain on swallowing, and pain radiating to the ears. Women are affected 6 times as often as men, and the average age at onset is 45 years. The course of the illness is about 10 days. Palliative effects can be obtained with cortisone acetate, 25 mg. q.i.d. orally.

Struma lymphomatosa (Hashimoto's struma) is a disease exclusively of females (average age about 45) characterized by chronic, firm, diffuse, nontender, bilateral enlargement of the thyroid gland. The etiology is uncertain, but an autoimmune reaction may be responsible. Serologic thyroid autoimmune antibody tests may be positive but are nonspecific and may also be positive in goiter, thyroid carcinoma, and occasionally thyrotoxicosis. Biopsy may be required to establish the diagnosis. Hypothyroidism usually develops. In rare cases pressure symptoms may require excision of the isthmus and portions of the lobes. Thyroid therapy is usually indicated.

Riedel's struma is a rare form of thyroiditis in which the gland is fibrotic, hard, adherent, and slightly enlarged, often on one side only. Women are affected twice as often as men, and the average age at onset is about 45. The etiology is not known. Pressure symptoms are the only indication for surgery, but biopsy may be necessary to rule out carcinoma. Myxedema eventually occurs and calls for treatment with thyroid hormone.

COMPLICATIONS OF THYROIDECTOMY

HYPOTHYROIDISM

Postoperative myxedema occurs in about 10% of patients in whom a radical subtotal thyroidectomy is done for Graves' disease. The complication is less common after removal of toxic nodular and other forms of goiter.

Symptoms and signs include weakness, fatigability, intolerance to cold, dry skin, and falling hair (especially the eyebrows), and the face becomes puffy. The BMR is −30% or below, and radioactive iodine uptake is low (about 10% in 24 hours). PBI and T_4 are low. Serum thyrotropin (TSH) levels by radioimmunoassay are high and are of great diagnostic value. Blood cholesterol rises. Patients with hypothyroidism are extremely sensitive to many drugs, such as morphine, and respond poorly to conditions entailing severe stress, such as operations.

Administer desiccated thyroid, 30 mg. (1/2 gr.) daily, increasing by 30 mg. (1/2 gr.) every week until hypothyroidism is controlled. Maintenance dosage is usually 60-130 mg. (1-2 gr.) daily as judged by clinical response and protein-bound iodine or BMR.

In severe myxedema and in the presence of heart disease, begin with small doses, 8-15 mg. (1/8-1/4 gr.) daily, and increase by 15 mg. (1/4 gr.) each week until optimum effect is obtained. Levothyroxine sodium (Synthroid®, Letter®) may be used instead of thyroid, and its action is more predictable.

Sodium liothyronine (Cytomel®) is a rapidly absorbed synthetic drug which produces thyroid effects within 24-48 hours. When a rapid response is desired, it may be used instead of thyroid. Begin with 5 mcg. daily and increase by this amount weekly. Cytomel®, 25 mcg., is equivalent to thyroid, 60 mg. (1 gr.).

HYPOPARATHYROIDISM

Damage to or removal of the parathyroid glands resulting in transient or permanent hypoparathyroidism occurs in about 3% of thyroidectomies. Temporary deficiency of parathyroid hormone (for several months) may develop after excision of a parathyroid adenoma. Primary hypoparathyroidism is extremely rare and usually appears before 16 years of age, though it may persist throughout adult life.

Clinical Findings.

Muscle weakness, irritability, numbness or cramps in the extremities, tetany, carpopedal spasm, laryngeal stridor, and Chvostek's sign are among the characteristic features. Frequently the only clinical evidence of impending tetany is Chvostek's sign. The diagnosis is confirmed by the finding of a low serum calcium and a high or normal serum phosphorus. Symptoms may occur within 2-7 days following surgery, or the disorder may remain latent, causing only vague complaints. If symptoms of hypocalcemia occur on the operative or first postoperative day, the deficiency is probably severe; if they appear on the third, fourth, or fifth day, it is usually mild and transient. Cataracts, convulsive disorders, and mental deterioration are late complications of chronic deficiency.

Treatment.

A. Emergency Treatment of Postoperative Tetany: Give immediately one of the following until tetany subsides: (1) Calcium gluconate injection, 10-30 ml. of 10% solution slowly I.V.; or (2) calcium chloride, 5-10 ml. of 10% solution slowly I.V. Ten to 50 ml. of either solution may be added to 1000 ml. of 5% glucose in water or saline for continuous administration if necessary. Rapid infusion of calcium may cause cardiac arrest in patients receiving digitalis.

   If tetany is otherwise impossible to control, administer 50-100 units of parathyroid hormone I.M. or subcut. 3-5 times daily. Do not use for over 1 week. Parathormone is rarely necessary or used.

B. Maintenance Therapy:
   1. Calcium salts are administered orally as soon as possible. Give calcium lactate or gluconate, 3-4 Gm. (45-60 gr.) 4 times daily.
   2. High-calcium, low-phosphorus diet (omit milk).
   3. Calciferol (Vitamin D_2), 50,000 units 4 times daily if necessary. Vitamin D therapy alone usually reverses all the chemical changes in hypoparathyroidism, but the response is slow and may take 6-12 weeks in the case of chronic hypoparathyroid tetany.
   4. Aluminum hydroxide with magnesium hydroxide or magnesium trisilicate, 15 ml. (or 2 0.5 Gm. tablets) 4 times daily, may be given by mouth to reduce absorption of phosphorus from the intestinal tract if necessary.
   5. If the above measures fail to maintain the blood calcium at a normal level, give dihydrotachysterol (Hytakerol®), 4-10 ml. of oily solution (1.25 mg./ml.) orally daily for 2-4 days, then 1-2 ml. daily for 1-3 weeks. Pure crystalline preparations (e.g., Digratyl®) are available in 0.2 mg. tablets. Dose is 0.8-2.4 mg. daily for several days. Calciferol is just as effective as dihydrotachysterol (though the onset of effect is slower) and is adequate in the great majority of cases. Both dihydrotachysterol and calciferol promote calcium absorp-

tion from the intestine and decrease phosphorus resorption from the kidney tubules.

6. Regulation - Continuing long-term follow-up is essential to prevent serious sequelae. Periodic determination of blood calcium, phosphorus, and proteins is important in management. Treatment of chronic hypoparathyroidism is difficult and costly because a good preparation of parathormone is not available.

RESPIRATORY OBSTRUCTION

Wound hemorrhage, laryngeal edema, tracheal collapse, or bilateral cord palsy may cause airway obstruction in the immediate postoperative period. All thyroidectomy patients should be observed closely for such danger signals as stridor and dyspnea, since severe hypoxia and death may occur shortly after the onset of these symptoms. If significant respiratory distress develops, the wound must be opened immediately and tracheostomy performed (see p. 251). It is preferable to take the patient to the operating room for this procedure, but it may be necessary to do an emergency lifesaving tracheostomy on the ward. The postoperative orders on every thyroidectomy patient should specify that a tracheostomy set be kept at the patient's bedside.

RECURRENT NERVE PALSY

Operative injury of one or both recurrent nerves occurs in about 1% of thyroidectomies. Depending upon the degree of damage, cord palsy may be temporary or permanent. If one nerve is injured, hoarseness is apparent immediately after operation and persists for several months. Hoarseness gradually decreases as the nerve recovers or as laryngeal function compensates for the paralyzed cord.

Bilateral cord palsy is a serious complication usually leading to respiratory obstruction and necessitating tracheostomy immediately after operation. It is advisable to observe cord function by indirect laryngoscopy prior to surgery on the thyroid or parathyroids and to repeat the examination after surgery if hoarseness or stridor develops.

HYPERPARATHYROIDISM

Excessive secretion of parathyroid hormone may be caused by parathyroid adenoma (90%), hyperplasia (10%), or carcinoma (rarely). The result is an increased loss of calcium and phosphorus from the body. Elevated calcium frequently leads to the formation of renal calculi, the commonest complication of hyperparathyroidism. When oral intake of calcium is insufficient to compensate for urinary loss, the bones become decalcified.

Clinical Findings.

A. Symptoms and Signs: Lassitude and fatigability are the earliest symptoms, but are so nonspecific that they rarely suggest the diagnosis. Polydipsia and polyuria may also occur. Hyperparathyroidism is rarely suspected until renal colic or bone pain develops. It is important to consider hyperparathyroidism in all cases of kidney stones. Peptic ulcer and acute pancreatitis may occur with increased frequency in patients with hyperparathyroidism. Some patients are virtually asymptomatic and are accidentally discovered by blood chemistry. About one-half of the cases of hyperparathyroidism are now identified as a result of routine laboratory screening.

B. Laboratory Findings: Serum calcium is elevated, serum phosphorus is low, and urinary excretion of calcium is increased (positive Sulkowitch test). Although there are many other causes of hypercalcemia (e.g., malignancy, immobilization, hyperthyroidism, sarcoid), elevated serum calcium on 3 successive examinations is very suggestive of the diagnosis. Hypercalcemia is often relatively mild; the calcium level is elevated only 0.5-1.5 mg./100 ml. in many cases. Alkaline phosphatase is increased if bone disease is present; a normal level of alkaline phosphatase rules out skeletal involvement. Measure the serum proteins and their electrophoretic patterns in order to evaluate the level of ionized calcium and to exclude myeloma and sarcoidosis by the globin pattern.

Alterations in serum calcium and phosphorus may not be continuously present. Therefore, repeated examination is necessary in suspect cases. Renal damage with uremia, a not uncommon complication, may further confuse the issue by causing a rise in phosphorus and fall in calcium. Tests for determining the renal disposal of phosphorus, such as the evaluation of the maximum tubular reabsorption of phosphate (TRP) during phosphate loading are not infallible and, moreover, are rather cumbersome.

C. X-ray Findings: Decalcification, pathologic fracture, or osteitis fibrosa cystica is found in about 10% of patients. The most important sites to study for bone abnormality are the hands, teeth, and skull. Subperiosteal reabsorption of bone is pathognomonic. Absence of the lamina dura around the teeth is highly suggestive.

Complications.

Renal failure is a common complication of hyperparathyroidism. A significant number of patients die of uremia after successful surgical relief of the hyperparathyroidism. This emphasizes the importance of early diagnosis.

Treatment.

Surgical treatment should be undertaken only after the diagnosis is firmly established on chemical grounds. Localization is best accomplished at operation by an experienced surgeon who is familiar with the normal and unusual locations of the parathyroid glands. Poor surgical technic can result in obscuring the field and in losing the opportunity for proper identification of normal and abnormal glands. Secondary operations are quite difficult. Special preoperative and intraoperative localization technics are unreliable. The thyroid is explored until all of the parathyroids are located. This may also entail exposure of the retrotracheal and retro-esophageal areas and the anterior and posterior mediastinum. All adenomas should be excised. If there is hyperplasia of all 4 parathyroids, 3 should be removed and the fourth subtotally resected. In over 80% of patients there are 4 parathyroid glands, but in about 6% there are 5 and in rare cases only 3 are present. Adenomas are usually single, but in 10% there are 2 and in rare cases 3. In about 5% an adenoma is found in the anterior or posterior mediastinum. Intrathyroid parathyroid adenoma occurs in about 3% of patients with hyperparathyroidism. Hyperparathyroidism disappears rapidly after proper treatment.

Transient hypocalcemic tetany occurs in about 50% of cases, usually 2-4 days after surgery. When generalized decalcification of the skeleton is present and when the serum alkaline phosphatase level is elevated to 10-20 Bodansky units, rapid absorption of calcium by the bone with tetany can be anticipated postoperatively. Treatment is as outlined on p. 282. Several months may be required for the remaining glands to produce sufficient hormone to abolish symptoms.

9 . . .

Surgery of the Pulmonary System

PULMONARY FUNCTION STUDIES

Normal lung function depends upon (1) pulmonary ventilation, (2) diffusion of gases across the alveolar-capillary membrane, and (3) pulmonary blood flow. The simplest and most widely available pulmonary function tests are measurements of ventilation. Specialized studies of lung volume, diffusion, and blood flow are less frequently required for diagnostic purposes.

Pulmonary function tests are of value in assessing operative risk, in the differential diagnosis of pulmonary disease, and as a means of determining response to treatment. In the great majority of cases a satisfactory preoperative estimate of lung function can be made on the basis of history, physical examination, chest x-ray, and fluoroscopy. In borderline cases, function studies provide objective evidence of pulmonary reserve. Certain of these studies, e.g., vital capacity and forced expiratory volume, can be performed in the physician's office by using one of the commercially available spirometer-kymograph units. Such a unit will measure lung and ventilation volumes and the mechanical factors in breathing. These data make possible a satisfactory working diagnosis in the majority of patients with abnormalities of pulmonary function, provided that the physician is well acquainted with pulmonary physiology.

In patients with abnormal ventilation tests or clinical findings suggestive of diminished pulmonary reserve, it may be advisable to do additional ventilation studies as well as measurements of lung volume and blood pH, pCO_2, and pO_2. Analysis of blood gases and pH gives valuable information for the management of certain critically ill patients, particularly after cardiac, pulmonary, and other major procedures which are frequently associated with respiratory failure.

A variety of pulmonary function tests are available in the well equipped cardiopulmonary laboratory, and these may be required to clarify diagnosis and guide therapy in problem cases. A few of the tests most useful to the clinician are summarized in the table on pp. 288-289.

Simple guidelines relating pulmonary function to operative risk are often of more practical value than complex studies. For example, the following preoperative findings are a general indication that the patient will have significant postoperative respiratory difficulty after thoracotomy: inability to climb one flight of stairs without severe dyspnea; hypercapnea at rest; 1-second forced expiratory volume (FEV_1) less than 700 ml., and maximal voluntary ventilation (MVV) less than 50% of predicted normal.

Bronchospirometry consists of inserting a double lumen catheter into the trachea and 1 of the main bronchi so that separate measurement can be made of tidal volume, minute volume, vital capacity, and oxygen consumption in each lung. This is of value in the rare instance when it is desirable to learn whether a patient facing pulmonary surgery will retain adequate pulmonary function after the operation.

Pulmonary function may be diminished by a wide variety of causes, chiefly "obstructive" bronchopulmonary disease and "restrictive" pulmonary disease. Obstructive conditions are those in which there is reduction and prolongation of air flow during expiration due to secretions, mucosal edema or hyperplasia, bronchial spasm, and obliterative bronchiolitis. Predominantly obstructive diseases are bronchial asthma, chronic bronchitis, pulmonary emphysema, mucoviscidosis (cystic fibrosis), coal miners' pneumoconiosis, silicosis, and bronchial obstruction by foreign body, tumor, or infection. Restrictive pulmonary diseases cause an actual reduction in the volume of air-containing tissue and affect principally the volume of air which can be inspired. Mechanisms include replacement of lung tissue by tumor, infiltration, fibrosis, or vascular congestion; filling of alveoli with edema fluid or purulent material (consolidation); restriction of lung expansion by pleural fluid, fibrothorax, or pneumothorax; restriction of chest expansion by kyphoscoliosis, neuromuscular disorders, extreme obesity, spondylitis, or pain; and surgical removal of lung tissues. Obstructive or restrictive conditions, when sufficiently advanced, usually produce the following changes on pulmonary function tests:

Obstructive and Restrictive Pulmonary Diseases

Test	Obstructive Disease	Restrictive Disease
Vital capacity (VC)	Normal or reduced	Always reduced
Forced expiratory volume (FEV)	Always reduced	Normal or reduced
Forced expiratory flow (FEF)	Usually reduced	Normal
Maximal voluntary ventilation (MVV)	Always reduced	Usually reduced

Progressive pulmonary insufficiency is a major contributing cause of death in perhaps a third of patients who survive the immediate effects of severe trauma. A similar proportion of patients dying in the intensive care units of general hospitals die of pulmonary insufficiency. Surgical procedures on patients who are elderly or suffering from chronic lung disease often result in the overtaxing of limited pulmonary reserves. Therefore, pulmonary function testing pre- and postoperatively, often in association with respiratory therapy, is assuming increased importance. (For a detailed discussion of diagnosis and management of respiratory failure after trauma, see Moore, F.D., and others, Post-traumatic Pulmonary Insufficiency. Saunders, 1969.)

DIAGNOSTIC AND THERAPEUTIC PROCEDURES OF VALUE IN THORACIC SURGERY

General Measures in Thoracic Surgical Care.

The immediate objective of management after thoracic surgery

PULMONARY FUNCTION TESTS MOST USEFUL TO THE CLINICIAN*

Test	Clinical Significance	Normal Values
Vital capacity (VC) Maximum volume that can be expelled after a maximum inspiration. No time limit.	Repeated abnormal values (more or less than 20% of predicted) may be significant. Main value is in following course of cardiopulmonary or respiratory disease with serial tests.	Male: VC = [27.63−(0.112 × age in years)] × ht. in cm. Female: VC = [21.78−(0.101 × age in years)] × ht. in cm. (Baldwin, E. de F., & others: Medicine 27: 243, 1948.)
Forced expiratory volume (FEV) "Timed vital capacity." Maximum volume expelled in a timed interval, usually 1 or 3 sec.	A reduced timed volume usually indicates obstructive bronchopulmonary disease. Improvement after a bronchodilator indicates some degree of reversibility.	FEV_1 sec. = 83% of actual VC. FEV_3 sec. = 97% of actual VC.
Maximal expiratory flow rate (MEFR) Measurement of maximal flow rate of a single expelled breath, expressed in L./min.	A reduced flow rate has the same significance as a reduced FEV. The test requires little effort, and several types of small, portable instruments are available. Suitable for screening tests.	Adult male = > 400 L./min. Adult female = > 300 L./min.

Maximal voluntary ventilation (MVV) "Maximal breathing capacity." Maximal volume expelled in 12-15 sec. of forced breathing, expressed in L./min.	Measures essentially the same function as FEV and MEFR. An additional confirmation test of FEV and MEFR. Requires sustained effort and cooperation of patient to a greater degree.	There is a wide variation of normal values depending upon age, size, and sex. The following formulas can be used as a guide for predicted values: Male [86.5−(0.522 × age in years)] × sq. M. body surface. Female [71.3−(0.474 × age in years)] × sq. M. body surface.
When low values are obtained, the above tests should be repeated after administration of a bronchodilator.		
O_2 saturation (arterial) Measure of the % saturation of hemoglobin with O_2.	Hypoxemia which is not apparent clinically can be detected.	Arterial O_2 sat. (%) = 90-100 mm. Hg.
CO_2 tension (arterial)(pCO_2) Plasma bicarbonate (HCO_3^-) pH of arterial blood	Important values in the diagnosis and management of respiratory acidosis due to CO_2 retention. (Now readily measured in arterial blood by the method of Astrup: Clin. Chem. **7**:1-15, 1969.)	pCO_2 40 mm. Hg Plasma HCO_3^- = 24 mEq./L. pH 7.40

*Reproduced, with permission, from Krupp and Chatton (editors), Current Diagnosis & Treatment 1973. Lange, 1973.

or trauma is complete expansion and normal function of the lung without residual air or fluid in the chest. The following measures serve this end:

A. Position and Ambulation:
   1. The patient should be placed in a semi-sitting position as soon as tolerated; this makes breathing and coughing more efficient.
   2. Pneumonectomy patients should lie alternately on the back and on the operated side; if such a patient is placed on his normal side severe respiratory embarrassment may result.
   3. Ambulation should be started as soon as possible (usually on the day following operation). Breathing exercises and other exercises to mobilize the shoulder girdle and thoracic cage should be encouraged throughout the convalescent period.

B. Prevention of Atelectasis:
   1. Deep breathing and repeated vigorous cough at least hourly are essential in the early postoperative period.
   2. Tracheal aspiration is employed as necessary. Bronchoscopy is occasionally useful.
   3. Transtracheal catheterization is useful to stimulate cough if the patient is unable to cough voluntarily. A standard No. 14 catheter (Intracath [Bard]) is inserted percutaneously under local anesthesia into the trachea just below the cricoid cartilage. Injection of 2-3 ml. of saline (or distilled water if necessary for stimulation) through the catheter will excite vigorous coughing.
   4. Positive-pressure breathing with a bronchodilator or saline by aerosol should be used both preoperatively and postoperatively if secretions are marked or bronchospasm is present.
   5. Expectorants are of little value.

C. Pain Relief: The dosage of narcotics given to thoracic patients should be strictly individualized. Pain relief sufficient to make coughing bearable is essential, but depression of respirations and cough reflex must be minimized. Barbiturates can often be used for sedation to reduce the need for narcotics. Blocking of the intercostal nerves with procaine or lidocaine from several spaces above to several spaces below the level of the operative wound or site of chest injury may occasionally be of value.

D. Oxygen Therapy: Pulmonary insufficiency is often present during the first 24-48 hours after chest surgery or severe trauma. Oxygen is usually given routinely after thoracotomy until pulmonary function is adequate. Warm, humidified oxygen prevents drying of the tracheobronchial mucosa and aids in mobilization of secretions, thus helping in the prevention of atelectasis. If hypoxia is suspected - or confirmed by a finding of pO_2 below 85 mm. Hg - humidified oxygen may be delivered at a rate of 10 L./minute by a face tent which will provide about 40% inspired oxygen, which may be adequate; or by a snug mask which will raise inspired oxygen to 60-80%. A nasal catheter or cannula is simpler but provides less humidification; a flow of 100% oxygen at a rate of 5-10 L./minute results in inspired oxygen of 30-40%. A nasal cannula is more comfortable than a catheter and permits oxygen flow of up to 10 L./minute. Flow of oxygen through a nasal catheter should be limited to about 5 L./minute.

E. Assisted or Controlled Ventilation: When pulmonary reserve is markedly diminished, endotracheal intubation and assisted or controlled ventilation may be lifesaving. The preventive value of prolonged controlled or assisted ventilation in selected patients after major surgery or severe trauma is firmly established. Some degree of respiratory failure can be predicted and often forestalled in patients with extensive injuries and operations, particularly if complicated by shock, sepsis, heart disease, obesity, muscular weakness, general debility, or chronic lung disease. The orotracheal tube can be left in place after operation, or a cuffed nasotracheal tube can be substituted for it. Mechanical ventilation, usually volume controlled, can then be continued for 48 hours (and several additional days if necessary) without undue hazard when proper equipment and experienced personnel are available. For example, mechanical ventilation for 24-48 hours after cardiac surgery is common practice and makes it possible to control the ventilatory pattern, lung expansion, and pCO_2; to provide optimum oxygen intake (FI_{O_2}) and oxygenation (pO_2); to remove secretions and prevent atelectasis by endotracheal suction; to reduce the work of breathing; and to facilitate accurate monitoring and control of the major parameters of pulmonary function. In controlled ventilation, the patient's respiratory effort must be eliminated so that the ventilator can completely take over the rhythm and depth of respiration. If sedation is necessary to depress the patient's respiratory drive or to prevent coughing or bucking on the endotracheal tube, small I.V. doses of morphine (2-3 mg.) or meperidine (10-20 mg.) should be given. It may occasionally be necessary to paralyze the patient, preferably with tubocurarine in repeated doses of 5-10 mg. I.V. until the desired effect is obtained.

F. Tracheostomy: Markedly diminished pulmonary reserve which cannot be controlled by endotracheal intubation and controlled ventilation or excessive secretions which cannot be adequately removed by tracheal aspiration may be an indication for tracheostomy. Positive-pressure breathing through a tracheostomy should be instituted promptly when oxygenation is inadequate in spite of other measures.

G. Management of Chest Drainage Tubes: One or more chest tubes for postoperative drainage of fluid and air are usually placed at thoracotomy through the intercostal spaces. (Tubes are rarely used when a pneumonectomy has been performed.) Continuous functioning of these tubes is essential to ensure full lung expansion and obliteration of the pleural space. The tubes must be inspected every few hours, must not be blocked for long periods, and must never be opened to the air. Tubes should be attached at the operating table to waterseal or gentle suction. When there is no pulmonary air leak, waterseal drainage is usually adequate. When an air leak from the lung is present, sufficient suction should be applied to the chest catheter so that bubbles appear in the waterseal bottle on expiration or cough but not on inspiration. The amount of suction usually required is 15-25 cm. of water. Strong suction (up to 40 cm. of water or more) to "pull out" the lung to the chest wall and seal the leak may occasionally be successful. Chest tubes are removed when they have been blocked for 24 hours.

Alveolar air leaks may continue for days and occasionally weeks after segmental resection or lobectomy. These usually seal if tube drainage and suction are maintained. If an undrained air space of significant size persists, a tube should be placed in it for closed drainage. Small, uninfected air pockets usually absorb completely without drainage.

Bronchopleural fistula (an air leak from a bronchus into the pleural space) may or may not be associated with an empyema. The fistula usually opens within the first 1-2 weeks after pulmonary resection. Many will close on prolonged tube drainage; others require open drainage by rib resection. When simpler measures fail, suture of the fistula or thoracoplasty is necessary. Thoracoplasty is usually required for chronic fistula after pneumonectomy or in tuberculosis.

H. Chest Fluid and Empyema: Fluid or blood occasionally accumulates in the chest in spite of tube drainage. Small amounts of uninfected fluid and blood will absorb without incident. Fluid of sufficient volume to be apparent on x-ray should usually be removed as completely as possible by thoracentesis and cultured. If the fluid is infected (empyema), complete evacuation by repeated thoracenteses or by trocar thoracotomy is indicated. Until sensitivity tests can be completed, a systemic antibiotic is administered empirically (see Chapter 6). The antibiotic regimen can be altered as necessary when sensitivity studies are complete.

Complete removal of air and fluid from the chest and full expansion of the lung postoperatively are the most important means of preventing empyema.

Thoracentesis.

A. Preparation of the Patient: The site of the tap is selected by x-ray, fluoroscopy, or physical examination. When there is a large basilar effusion or total hydrothorax, the best site of aspiration is usually the seventh or eighth interspace in the posterior axillary line. The patient is placed in a comfortable sitting position, leaning slightly forward on a padded stand or supported by an attendant. Premedication with a barbiturate or narcotic is optional. The skin of the chest wall is prepared with antiseptic and draped.

B. Technic of the Tap: (Aseptic technic must be used throughout.) The entire thickness of the chest wall, including the parietal pleura, is infiltrated with 5-10 ml. of 1-2% procaine or lidocaine through a No. 22 gauge needle. Thoracentesis is virtually painless if this is properly done. A short-bevel needle (7.5-10 cm. long, 18-13 gauge) is attached by a 3-way stopcock to a 20-50 ml. syringe. With firm, steady pressure the needle is advanced into the pleural space. In order to avoid injury to the intercostal nerve and vessels, pass the needle through the chest wall at the lower margin of the intercostal space (except when making a tap on the anterior chest wall, in which case the needle is passed through the center of the interspace). A clamp may be placed on the needle to steady it at the chest wall. Care is taken during aspiration to prevent air from entering the chest.

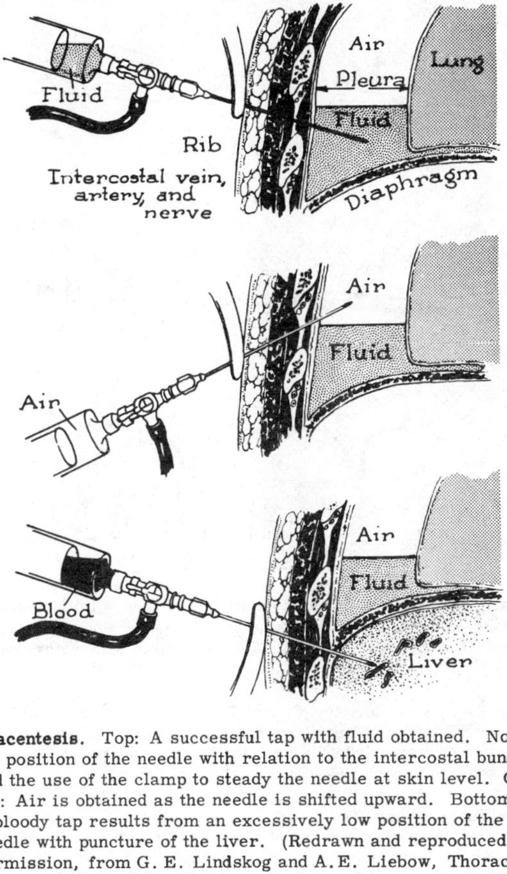

Thoracentesis. Top: A successful tap with fluid obtained. Note the position of the needle with relation to the intercostal bundle, and the use of the clamp to steady the needle at skin level. Center: Air is obtained as the needle is shifted upward. Bottom: A bloody tap results from an excessively low position of the needle with puncture of the liver. (Redrawn and reproduced, with permission, from G. E. Lindskog and A. E. Liebow, Thoracic Surgery and Related Pathology. Appleton-Century-Crofts, 1953.)

C. Volume of Fluid Removed: The amount of fluid removed at one sitting depends upon circumstances. A total of 2000 ml. can often be gradually evacuated at one sitting from a large effusion. If the patient complains of a feeling of tightness in the chest, cough, palpitation, fatigue, faintness, or other untoward symptoms, slow the rate of aspiration or discontinue until another occasion.

D. Laboratory Examination of Pleural Fluid: Laboratory examination of the fluid may include one or more of the following: Total volume, odor, color, turbidity, viscosity, coagulability,

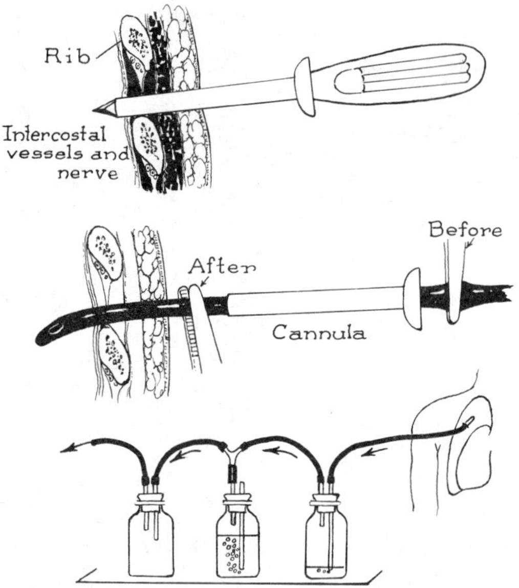

Trocar Thoracotomy. Top: Penetration of trocar into chest. Center: Insertion of flexible catheter through cannula, and removal of cannula. Bottom: Suction bottles with waterseal.

sp. gr.; smear for Gram's and acid-fast stains; total and differential blood cell count; aerobic, anaerobic, and acid-fast cultures; cytologic study for neoplastic cells; histologic study of sediment from a centrifuged specimen.

Trocar Thoracotomy.

Closed drainage of the chest cavity with a catheter is required when thoracentesis is unsatisfactory because of pulmonary air leak or marked viscosity of the pleural fluid. The objective is to place a catheter in the dependent portion of the fluid space when the patient is sitting. If possible, the posterior or midaxillary line is selected (so that the patient will not lie on the tube). An upper anterior interspace is usually chosen for treatment of pneumothorax. The procedure may be done in bed in a critically ill patient. Catheter drainage is usually inadequate when chronic infection has resulted in marked pleural thickening. Under these circumstances, rib resection and open tube drainage of the empyema may be indicated.

Preparation is as for thoracentesis. The chest is tapped with a needle to establish the position of the fluid pocket. After infiltration with 1-2% procaine or lidocaine, a 1 cm. skin incision is made.

A trocar of suitable size is introduced through the chest wall with firm pressure and rotary motion. A flexible catheter of the largest size which will pass through the trocar is passed into the chest. Several extra drainage holes are usually cut in the side of that portion of the catheter which will lie in the chest. The sheath of the trocar is removed and the catheter is secured to the chest wall with a nonabsorbable suture. The catheter is kept clamped during manipulation in order to prevent pneumothorax and is attached immediately to waterseal or suction drainage. If a trocar is not available, the point of a hemostat can be used to dissect a tract through which a catheter can be inserted.

Scalene Node Biopsy.

The anterior scalene and paratracheal nodes may be removed for diagnostic purposes in the investigation of hilar or paratracheal masses, diffuse bilateral lung infiltrates, or palpable nodes. In selected cases of moderate-sized and large peripheral carcinomas of the lung, scalene node biopsy may be of value since a positive node means incurability.

In the absence of enlarged nodes, biopsy is done first on the side of the lesion. Because the lymphatics cross over to the opposite side, bilateral biopsy may be occasionally warranted if ipsilateral nodes are negative.

Wide variation in the reported yield of positive scalene node biopsies is due to differences in selection of cases. When lymph nodes are palpable, the incidence of positive findings will be high. When lymph nodes are not palpable and the above criteria for selection are used, positive nodes will be found in 70-80% of Boeck's sarcoid, 30-50% of hilar masses or diffuse infiltrates, and 5-10% of carcinoma of the lung. Nodes are rarely positive (2-3%) in clinically operable carcinoma of the lung.

Mediastinoscopy.

This procedure is performed by passing a short endoscope into the upper mediastinum through a small transverse incision just above the suprasternal notch under general anesthesia. Biopsy of mediastinal nodes and masses is possible as far down as the carina and upper main-stem bronchi. When nodes are not palpable in the supraclavicular areas, mediastinoscopy offers a better chance of yielding a positive histologic diagnosis than scalene node biopsy in patients with thoracic disease.

Pleural Biopsy.

Percutaneous biopsy of the pleura, using a Vim-Silverman or other type of needle, is helpful in undiagnosed pleural diseases, particularly those due to tuberculosis or malignancy. Pleural effusion must be present unless a special curetting needle is used. The technic is as simple as a thoracentesis, and multiple specimens can be taken. Positive biopsy is reported in 30-70% of cases depending upon the series. Open surgical biopsy of the pleura or pericardium by limited thoracotomy should be considered when pleural or pericardial effusion remains undiagnosed by other means, including needle biopsy.

Bronchoscopy.

Bronchoscopy under local or general anesthesia is an important diagnostic or therapeutic procedure in a wide variety of chest conditions. Bronchoscopy is indicated for diagnosis when it is desirable to visualize a lesion or obtain secretions or tissue for culture or pathologic examination. With the flexible fiberoptic bronchoscope, it is possible to obtain brushings for cytologic examination and even biopsy for histologic study from lobar and segmented bronchi. Excessive secretions which require aspiration and retained foreign body in the bronchial tree are the chief indications for therapeutic bronchoscopy.

Open Lung Biopsy.

Open lung biopsy through a limited thoracotomy is indicated to obtain a wedge of lung tissue for pathology and culture. It is used in selected patients with pulmonary infiltrates requiring definitive diagnosis as a guide to specific treatment (e.g., a patient with lymphoma receiving intensive chemotherapy in whom pulmonary infiltrate may be either a neoplasm or an infection).

CHEST TRAUMA

RIB FRACTURES

Direct violence is the usual cause of rib fractures, but spontaneous fractures, usually of the sixth to ninth ribs, occasionally occur as a result of strenuous coughing. Pathologic fracture in a rib affected by metastatic malignancy or other bone disease is rare.

Pain, sharply localized to the fracture site and aggravated by breathing and other motions of the rib cage, is typical. Limitation of respiratory motion on the injured side is often present. Tenderness and sometimes crepitation are present at the fracture site. Severe injury may be complicated by subcutaneous emphysema, pneumothorax, and hemothorax. Atelectasis and pneumonitis frequently follow rib fracture in elderly persons.

Fractured ribs over the spleen should always raise the question of associated rupture of that organ. Suspicion of rib fracture is an indication for chest x-ray. Special views may be required to show the involved region. Fracture separations at the costochondral junctions do not visualize radiologically.

The pain of uncomplicated rib fracture is best controlled by analgesics or intercostal nerve block. In minor fractures, placement of a wide band of self-retaining web belting around the lower thorax reduces chest motion and pain. A swathe pinned snugly around the lower chest has the same effect but is more difficult to retain in place. Multiple fractures with slight hypermobility of a segment of chest wall are an indication for localized strapping over the mobile segment to control pain and slight paradoxical motion.

Severe thoracic trauma with multiple fractures and flail chest wall require immediate intubation with a cuffed endotracheal tube in order to institute positive-pressure ventilation. Several weeks of controlled respiration may be necessary before the chest wall becomes stabilized. Therefore, tracheostomy is usually done within the first few days and a tracheostomy tube with low pressure cuff is inserted to minimize trauma to the tracheal wall.

Intercostal nerve block, performed as soon after injury as possible, is very useful in severe multiple fractures accompanied by respiratory distress. Five to 10 ml. of 1-2% procaine or lidocaine are injected paravertebrally just beneath the lower margins of the involved ribs and several normal ribs above and below this level. The injection may be repeated as often as necessary.

Rib fractures may lead to atelectasis and serious pulmonary infection in elderly patients. Tracheobronchial secretions in these patients must be removed as often as necessary by coughing and by tracheal aspiration if necessary. Antibiotic therapy is frequently required to control pneumonitis. Depression of cough and respiration by excessive doses of narcotics should be avoided. Strapping of the chest for uncomplicated rib fracture in elderly patients is contraindicated as predisposing to atelectasis.

FRACTURE OF THE STERNUM

Fracture of the sternum is caused by severe direct trauma, as in steering wheel injury. Multiple rib fractures and other injuries are usually also present. Contusion of the heart is not uncommonly present. Severe precordial pain and dyspnea are the chief symptoms. Crepitus and deformity of the sternum may be noted. In most cases the only treatment required is rest in the sitting position, pain relief with narcotics, and intercostal nerve block for associated rib fractures. When there is severe deformity, either closed or open reduction under local anesthesia should be carried out. Hypermobility of the anterior chest wall secondary to multiple fractures can be stabilized by overhead traction. When severe respiratory difficulty cannot be controlled by other measures, positive-pressure breathing through a cuffed tracheostomy tube may be lifesaving. This must be continued for days or weeks until the chest wall is stabilized.

HEMOTHORAX

Bleeding from the lung parenchyma tends to be self-limited. Continued bleeding usually originates in the chest wall, diaphragm, mediastinum, or hilus. Several liters of blood may accumulate in the thorax. In three-fourths of patients the blood remains fluid. In the absence of persistent bleeding, hemothorax can be treated successfully in 80-90% of cases by multiple aspirations or trocar thoracotomy.

Symptoms and signs depend upon the extent of the hemothorax and the associated injuries. If large collections of blood are present, shock and physical signs of chest fluid are seen. Definitive diagnosis is made by x-ray.

Treatment.

A. Emergency Measures: Minor hemothorax not associated with shock or respiratory distress may be treated by thoracentesis. Treatment in massive hemothorax is directed toward immediate replacement of blood loss, and closed drainage by tube thoracotomy to relieve respiratory distress by removing blood and air from the chest. Other general supportive measures are also instituted. If marked hemorrhage continues or recurs (as indicated by reappearance of shock or continued loss of 500 ml. or more of blood every 8 hours through the thoracostomy tube), or if the lung remains collapsed, or if a major collection of blood remains in the chest, thoracotomy is advisable. When hemopneumothorax is present, the early placement of chest tubes by trocar thoracotomy through both the upper anterior and the lower posterolateral chest wall may be necessary to achieve complete evacuation of air and blood and full lung expansion. The intrathoracic condition is monitored by frequent examinations of the chest and by portable sitting chest films.

B. Management of Clotted Hemothorax: Rapid clotting or loculation of hemothorax occasionally prevents satisfactory removal by thoracentesis or tube thoracotomy. When it is estimated that 1-2 L. or more of blood remain in the chest, early thoracotomy should be considered if the patient's general condition is satisfactory. A delay of this procedure will result in the development of an organized hematoma which traps the lung and prevents expansion. There is also added risk of infection when a large quantity of blood remains in the chest.

When a large organizing hemothorax develops because early evacuation of blood is not feasible, the optimum time for evacuation is between the third and fifth week following injury. At this interval, the fibrin peel will separate from the lung with minimal difficulty and the debris can be evacuated from the thorax with relative ease.

TRAUMATIC PNEUMOTHORAX

Pneumothorax may be caused by an open "sucking" wound in the chest wall or, more commonly, an air leak in an injured lung.

Sucking Wounds of the Thorax.

These must be closed immediately with a bulky occlusive dressing held in place by adhesive or a bandage or binder encircling the chest. Vaseline gauze over the wound assists in sealing the leak. Open pneumothorax causes marked to and fro shifting of the mediastinum during respiration ("mediastinal flutter") which must be promptly controlled to prevent respiratory and circulatory failure. Surgical closure of the wound in the chest wall is carried out as soon as the patient's condition permits. Meanwhile, air is evacuated from the chest as described below.

Closed Pneumothorax.

Closed pneumothorax is caused by an air leak from the lung or tracheobronchial tree. It may occur either as a result of a penetrating chest wound or blunt injury.

A. Simple Pneumothorax: Pneumothorax accompanies many blunt and penetrating chest injuries and is often associated with hemothorax. When lung collapse is no more than about 10%, special treatment of the pneumothorax is usually not necessary.

Early and complete expansion of the lung with removal of all air and fluid from the chest is the primary objective of local treatment when a significant pneumothorax is present. Occasionally this can be accomplished by one or more thoracenteses during the first 24-48 hours. If there is lung collapse of more than 25% initially or if pneumothorax recurs after thoracentesis, trocar thoracotomy with placement of a catheter in the upper chest through the second or third interspace anteriorly is indicated. Gentle suction (15-25 cm. of water) is applied for 3-5 days or until blocking of the catheter indicates that expansion is complete and the lung adherent.

B. Tension Pneumothorax: See p. 316.

SUBCUTANEOUS AND MEDIASTINAL EMPHYSEMA

Rib fractures, chest wounds, traumatic rupture of the trachea or a major bronchus, spontaneous pneumothorax, and pulmonary resection are occasionally followed by subcutaneous emphysema. In advanced cases, emphysema extends from head to foot and produces an alarming degree of swelling and crepitation, especially of the head, neck, and scrotum. Air in the tissues causes little harm and, as a rule, requires no treatment.

Attention should be directed toward correction of the underlying cause. Pneumothorax should be controlled by trocar thoracotomy, and irritating, useless cough should be minimized. Major air leaks in the lung or tracheobronchial tree may require surgical repair (see below).

Marked emphysema of the mediastinum will on rare occasions produce sufficient tension to threaten life. If dyspnea, cyanosis, tachycardia, and shock progress in spite of other measures, tracheostomy or cervical mediastinotomy is indicated. Tracheostomy serves to control respirations, remove secretions, and reduce intratracheal pressure during coughing. Mediastinotomy (under local anesthesia) consists of blunt dissection into the superior mediastinum through a transverse incision in the suprasternal notch to permit the egress of air.

TRAUMATIC RUPTURE OF THE TRACHEA OR BRONCHI

Severe crushing or compression trauma to the chest may cause injury to the trachea or major bronchi. Bronchial rupture, usually within 1-2 cm. of the carina, occurs about 4 times as often as tracheal tear. Tracheobronchial injuries are often overlooked.

Symptoms and signs include dyspnea, subcutaneous emphysema, cyanosis, pain, hemoptysis, shock, cough, pneumothorax, extensive atelectasis, and hemothorax. Chest films and bronchoscopy are indicated. The diagnosis may be overlooked until weeks or months after the injury. X-rays then usually show complete atelectasis of the involved portion of lung.

Treatment is by suture of the tear if the patient's other injuries do not contraindicate thoracotomy. Emergency operation is usually required to relieve airway obstruction or to correct uncontrollable air leak, tracheobronchial hemorrhage, or rapidly advancing mediastinal emphysema. Chronic stricture with obstruction due to delayed treatment requires bronchoplastic operation. The distal lung, although collapsed, is often functional when reexpanded; pulmonary resection should therefore be reserved for cases with irreversible damage.

THORACOABDOMINAL WOUNDS

Left-sided wounds are more serious than those on the right because they are more frequently associated with injury to the spleen, stomach, and the splenic flexure; wounds on the right usually involve only the liver and are less likely to cause continuing hemorrhage or massive contamination of the chest and peritoneum. For this reason, suspected penetrating injury to the left diaphragm is an indication for early operation. The principal indication for intervention in right-sided involvement is continued hemorrhage. Blunt, nonpenetrating trauma may cause rupture of the left diaphragm with herniation into the chest. Large herniations cause lung collapse and severe respiratory insufficiency.

The diaphragm may rise as high as the anterior fourth interspace on full expiration, and is thus vulnerable to penetration by injuries of the lower chest. The mechanism of the injury or the trajectory of a missile often indicates that thoracoabdominal injury has probably occurred. Additional information is obtained on physical examination and upright films of the chest and abdomen with a nasogastric tube in place. Films may show that the stomach or bowel is herniated into the chest through a vent in the diaphragm. In some cases, detail in the lower chest is obscured by hemothorax. Administration of barium by mouth or enema may be helpful in identifying intrathoracic herniation after nonpenetrating trauma. Thoracentesis may disclose stomach or colon contents in the chest. Take care not to penetrate a herniated viscus during thoracentesis. The absence of signs of peritoneal irritation does not rule out damage to the abdominal organs.

In left thoracoabdominal injury, treatment is by thoracotomy as soon as the patient's condition permits. Right thoracoabdominal wounds require close observation and supportive measures; intervention is generally reserved for patients with continued bleeding or extensive visceral damage.

TRACHEOBRONCHIAL FOREIGN BODY

Infants, children, and intoxicated, anesthetized, and unconscious individuals are most likely to aspirate foreign bodies. Coughing, choking, and cyanosis may occur immediately after inhalation but often subside for a variable period. Depending upon the size, nature, and site of lodgement of the foreign body, later findings may include cough, wheezing, atelectasis, or pulmonary infection. Unless the foreign body is radiopaque, x-ray evidences are indirect: obstructive emphysema, atelectasis, or pneumonitis. Intermittent findings of this nature, especially in children, are highly suggestive of foreign body. Bronchoscopy and possibly bronchography should be performed. Bronchoscopic removal should be attempted. If successful, inflammatory reactions usually subside promptly; if unsuccessful, thoracotomy and bronchotomy or resection are necessary. Foreign bodies in the tracheobronchial tree should always be removed, since prolonged retention usually leads to bronchiectasis or abscess formation requiring pulmonary resection.

DISEASES OF THE CHEST WALL

PECTUS EXCAVATUM
(Funnel Breast)

Pectus excavatum is a congenital, hereditary malformation characterized by depression of the sternum below the gladiomanubrial junction with symmetric inward bending of the costal cartilages. As the infant develops, kyphoscoliosis may also occur. Severe degrees of funnel breast very rarely embarrass pulmonary and cardiac function. As a rule, the only disturbance is cosmetic. Operative treatment may be indicated for either reason. The preferred operation consists of resection of all the deformed costal cartilages with extensive mobilization of the sternum to allow its elevation to a normal position. Lesser procedures fail. The best results are obtained between the ages of 4 and 8. Successful surgery significantly improves appearance but often will not correct the deformity completely. Placement of a Silastic® implant subcutaneously to fill the defect is currently under trial by plastic surgeons.

CERVICAL RIB AND
THORACIC OUTLET SYNDROME

Supernumerary rib in the cervical region, usually bilateral, is seldom of any clinical significance. When symptoms occur, they frequently involve 1 side only, and are caused by compression of the subclavian artery and a portion of the brachial plexus between the scalenus anticus muscle and the cervical rib. Numbness, tingling, and coldness of the hand and forearm on the involved side are the usual complaints. The most common physical finding is diminution or disappearance of the radial pulse when the patient inspires deeply with his neck extended and his head turned to the affected side (Adson's test). Other signs in the affected extremity may include coolness (occasionally cyanosis), diminished pulse and BP, and atrophic changes of the skin and nails. Vasoconstrictive episodes similar to Raynaud's disease may occur. Poststenotic dilatation of the subclavian artery with aneurysm formation is seen in severe cases. The cervical rib is readily identified by x-ray. Similar symptoms in the absence of a cervical rib constitute the thoracic outlet syndrome (Roos, D. B., Ann. Surg. 173:429-442, 1971).

Mild cases are treated by postural exercises and physical therapy to improve shoulder girdle tone. If these measures fail the scalenus anticus muscle can be divided surgically and the cervical rib or the first rib resected. Minor aneurysmal dilatations of the subclavian artery do not require resection if the proximal constriction is relieved.

DISEASES OF THE PLEURA

ACUTE EMPYEMA

The microorganisms which most frequently cause empyema are the pneumococcus, streptococcus, staphylococcus, and tubercle bacillus. Infections with coliform bacilli, Proteus vulgaris, Friedländer's bacillus, various fungi, and mixed organisms are less common. Invasion of the pleural space occurs in one of the following ways: (1) direct spread from a pneumonic focus, (2) rupture of a pyogenic or tuberculous abscess, (3) contamination as a result of operation or trauma, (4) extension from below the diaphragm, and (5) hematogenous infection.

The principles of treatment in empyema are early evacuation of all fluid and purulent exudate in order to achieve complete lung expansion, and eradication of the infecting organism by adequate drainage, antibiotic therapy, and supportive measures.

Clinical Findings.

The diagnosis of acute empyema is seldom difficult. A predisposing condition is usually apparent. Findings related primarily to the empyema usually consist of chest pain, cough, malaise, fever, and leukocytosis. Large acute effusions may be associated with considerable toxicity and dyspnea. Physical examination discloses signs of pleural fluid; more accurate localization is provided by chest films. If air is seen in the empyema cavity on x-ray, it can be assumed that a bronchopleural fistula has developed. Thoracentesis (see p. 292) is done promptly in order to obtain material for smears, cultures, and antibiotic sensitivity studies.

Treatment.

A. Antibiotic Therapy: Systemic antibiotic therapy based on sensitivity studies is indicated.
B. Thoracentesis: The empyema cavity is evacuated completely by thoracentesis each day until less than 50 ml. can be aspirated on successive days. If the infectious agent is sensitive to a suitable topical antibiotic, intrapleural injections can be given at the conclusion of each aspiration.
C. Trocar Thoracotomy: If the exudate is too thick for complete removal by thoracentesis, or if it is large in volume and requires frequent thoracentesis, a catheter should be introduced into the cavity by trocar thoracotomy in order to establish closed waterseal drainage. Trocar thoracotomy and closed drainage are usually advisable at the outset of treatment if a bronchopleural fistula is present as indicated by pyopneumothorax.

Only closed methods of pleural drainage (e.g., thoracentesis and trocar thoracotomy) should be used until the lung is firmly adherent to the chest wall around the empyema cavity. If open drainage is established before this occurs, total collapse of the lung may result.

Prognosis.

Postpneumonic empyema usually subsides promptly when treatment is begun early. Empyema of other etiology is often more complicated and the prognosis less satisfactory. When closed methods of management fail, treatment must be along the lines described below for chronic empyema (Samson, P.C., Ann. Thoracic Surg. 11:210-221, 1971).

CHRONIC EMPYEMA

As an empyema becomes chronic, the pleura thickens and adheres firmly around the encapsulated exudate. There may be a history of recent acute empyema, or chronic empyema may exist for years in a latent or intermittently symptomatic state.

Empyemas become chronic for the following reasons: (1) delay in diagnosis or inadequate treatment of the acute stage; (2) bronchopleural fistula; (3) specific infection, such as tuberculosis or actinomycosis; (4) retained foreign body, (5) osteomyelitis of a rib, (6) disease of the lung preventing expansion, and (7) underlying malignant neoplasm.

Clinical Findings.

Cough and recurrent fever are usually the principal complaints. When some form of suppurative lung disease is associated with the empyema, the cough is usually productive of frankly purulent and sometimes foul-smelling sputum. Chest pain, clubbing of the fingers, chronic malaise, dyspnea, anorexia, and weight loss may occur. Draining sinuses are occasionally present.

Physical examination discloses signs of chest fluid or thickened pleura. Respiratory excursions are usually limited on the affected side, and there may be contraction of the thoracic cage. These changes are usually readily apparent on x-ray.

Thoracentesis is performed to obtain material for examination of smears and cultures for pyogenic and acid-fast organisms.

Treatment.

A. General Measures: Anemia, malnutrition, and debility due to chronic sepsis should be corrected. Systemic antibiotic therapy is usually indicated as an adjunct to drainage or other local treatment.

B. Specific Measures:

1. Drainage - It is usually impossible to evacuate a chronic empyema cavity adequately by needle aspiration. If the exudate is relatively thin and the pleura not markedly thickened, closed drainage by trocar thoracotomy may be effective (see p. 294).

   Chronic empyema frequently requires open drainage. This is accomplished by resection under local anesthesia of a small segment of rib over the lower portion of the cavity. A generous biopsy of the wall of the empyema cavity should be obtained as it is opened. A large tube is inserted and is shortened gradually as the cavity slowly heals, which may require many weeks or even months. Irrigations are unnecessary if adequate drainage is maintained. The rate of healing may be determined by filling the cavity at weekly intervals with saline.

Large cavities (e.g., postpneumonectomy empyema), especially if associated with bronchopleural fistula, are well managed by the Eloesser flap method of providing continuous open drainage (Panagiotis and others, Ann. Thoracic Surg. 12:69-78, 1971).

A well-drained and stabilized residual cavity - such as a postpneumonectomy empyema space - may occasionally be sterilized and closed after instillation of neomycin, 250 mg./100 ml. of saline solution (Clagett, O. T., S. Clin. North America 53:863-866, 1973).

2. Decortication - Patients in whom infection has been controlled by chemotherapy or drainage may be suitable candidates for decortication, in which thickened pleura is excised in order to permit full expansion of the lung. Expansion is carefully maintained postoperatively by closed tube drainage. Decortication combined with pulmonary resection is the treatment of choice in selected cases of bronchopleural fistula, bronchiectasis, lung abscess, and other disorders in which the underlying lung is severely damaged.

C. Tuberculous Empyema: The management of tuberculous empyema, much less common since the advent of the antituberculosis drugs, is always complex. Bronchopleural fistula and secondary infection are frequently present. The proper timing and selection of therapeutic procedures requires experience and judgment. Consideration must be given to the systemic reaction of the patient, the extent of the tuberculosis, and the response to specific chemotherapy.

Tuberculous empyema (without secondary infection) may respond to general supportive measures, antituberculosis chemotherapy, and closed drainage by repeated thoracentesis or trocar thoracotomy. The trocar thoracotomy is usually placed in the anterior axillary line to reserve the posterolateral chest wall in case thoracoplasty or decortication should become necessary. Closed drainage is always used in order to avoid secondary pyogenic infection.

Mixed infections of the pleura, usually associated with bronchopleural fistula, may occasionally respond to intensive treatment along the same lines combined with penicillin or other antibiotic agent. In these cases, however, thoracoplasty or decortication, with or without resection, is usually required.

NEOPLASMS OF THE PLEURA

Primary tumors of the pleura are very rare and are difficult to distinguish from malignancies arising in the lung, diaphragm, or elsewhere. The most frequent pleural neoplasm is the mesothelioma, which tends to spread diffusely in the pleural space. Mesothelioma is more common in persons with a history of exposure to asbestos (magnesium silicate) dust. It occurs most commonly in men between 40 and 50. The chief complaint is usually pleural pain. Additional symptoms may include malaise, weakness, cough, dyspnea, weight loss, and fever. The physical and radiologic signs are those of pleural fluid and thickening. Plaques of calcium in the pleura are helpful in suggesting the diagnosis of pleural malignancy. Fluid tends to reaccumulate rapidly after thoracenteses. The diagnosis is established by cytologic study of the pleural fluid or by pleural biopsy. Although pleuropneumonectomy has been carried out in some cases, no treatment is curative. Radiotherapy or cancer chemotherapy may have a transient palliative effect.

DISEASES OF THE LUNG

LUNG ABSCESS

The causes of pyogenic lung abscess are (1) necrotizing pneumonia, (2) aspiration of infected material or a foreign body, (3) septic embolus or infection of a pulmonary infarct, (4) bronchial obstruction by tumor, (5) infection of a cyst or bulla, (6) extension of bronchiectasis into the parenchyma, (7) penetrating chest wounds, and (8) transdiaphragmatic extension of infection, e.g., from a subphrenic or amebic abscess. When a lung abscess develops in childhood, suspect a foreign body. In the older age group, consider the possibility of bronchial obstruction by cancer.

Clinical Findings.

A. Symptoms and Signs: A history of a predisposing disorder is usually present. There may be a latent period of several days or weeks during which only malaise and fever are noted. Cough, pleurisy, chills, and fever occur as the process develops. Within a few days the patient may suddenly cough up a large amount of very foul, purulent sputum, usually blood-streaked or frankly bloody. Copious, malodorous sputum associated with the debility of long-standing infection is typical of chronic abscess.

   Signs vary with the size, position, and contents of the cavity and with the local pulmonary reaction. Clubbing of the fingers sometimes develops rapidly.

B. Laboratory Findings: Leukocytosis and anemia are usually consistent with severe infection. Sputum shows infection and may disclose the etiology, e.g., tuberculosis or neoplasm.

C. X-ray Findings: Early films often show only an area of consolidation; cavitation with fluid level and surrounding pneumonitis is seen later. Tomography is useful to reveal the location, extent, and early evidence of cavitation. Bronchography is helpful in chronic cases to delineate local complications such as multiple abscesses and bronchiectasis.

D. Bronchoscopy: Usually indicated to rule out an obstructing bronchial lesion such as carcinoma or foreign body.

Complications.

Complications include brain abscess, massive hemoptysis,

amyloidosis, and pyopneumothorax. Rupture of the abscess into the pleural space may produce tension pneumothorax. There is a sudden onset of pleural pain, dyspnea, and shock. This is a grave surgical emergency requiring immediate closed chest drainage by trocar thoracotomy.

Treatment.

A. Medical Measures:

1. Antibiotics - In acute abscess, treat intensively with an antibiotic in order to minimize lung destruction while sensitivity tests are being done on sputum. Over 75% of acute lung abscesses respond favorably to intensive antibiotic therapy. The response in chronic abscess is less satisfactory, but antibiotics usually reduce the pulmonary infection to a significant degree.
2. Postural drainage.
3. Bronchoscopic aspiration to promote drainage in selected cases.
4. High-protein, high-caloric diet with supplementary vitamins. Correct anemia by transfusions if necessary.

B. Surgical Treatment:

1. Acute abscess - Medical measures should be given a thorough trial before surgery is considered. Evidence of satisfactory progress includes decrease in cough, sputum, fever, and toxicity, and radiologic evidence of diminishing pulmonary infiltration and cavitation. If improvement has not occurred or if progress is arrested after 10-21 days, surgical resection is the treatment of choice. If the condition of the patient makes resection unwise, surgical drainage should be considered. This can be done under local anesthesia. A large tube is inserted into the abscess cavity through the bed of a resected rib. A 2-stage operation is usually required, the first stage consisting of rib resection and packing of the wound to ensure adherence of the lung. Adequate drainage often produces a dramatic clinical response.
2. Chronic abscess - Chronic abscess which is unresponsive to medical management requires resection of the involved segment or lobe. Preoperatively, infection should be vigorously treated by antibiotics, postural drainage, and general supportive therapy. Bronchoscopy should be performed and, in some cases, the bronchial tree in the region of the abscess should be mapped by bronchography. These 2 examinations are done to explore the possibility of foreign body or neoplasm. Neoplasms should be treated as indicated after infection has been controlled sufficiently so that surgery is feasible.

BRONCHIECTASIS

Bronchiectasis is a disorder characterized by tubular or saccular dilatation and chronic infection of the distal bronchial tree. Most clinical cases are probably secondary to focal pneumonitis occurring in childhood during an attack of pertussis, measles, scarlet fever, or other infection. Obstruction of the bronchi by foreign body is an occasional cause. Tuberculosis is frequently associated with bronchiectatic change, but since the lesion commonly is in the upper lobe the bronchial dilatation usually remains asymptomatic. Classical chronic bronchiectasis is a disease largely of the basal segments of the lower lobes, the lingula, and the right middle lobe. Congenital cystic disease of the lung must be considered when saccular dilatation is extensive or present in an unusual location. Kartagener's syndrome or triad consists of situs inversus, pansinusitis, and bronchiectasis. Other congenital lesions rarely associated with bronchiectasis include Fanconi's syndrome, idiopathic kyphoscoliosis, Klippel-Feil syndrome, polydactyly, and congenital heart disease.

Clinical Findings.

A. Symptoms and Signs: There is usually a chronic cough productive of much purulent sputum, more marked on arising in the morning. Recurrent attacks of pulmonary infection, often dating back to childhood, with fever, malaise, and increased cough and sputum, are also characteristic. Sinusitis is occasionally present. Hemoptysis occurs at some time in about half of cases and may be severe.

   Significant bronchiectasis is almost always associated with coarse moist rales over the involved segments. Bronchial breathing and other chest findings are related to the extent of parenchymal involvement. Clubbing occurs in severe cases.

B. Laboratory Findings: Bacteriologic studies of the sputum always reveal mixed infection, usually predominantly streptococci and staphylococci. Antibiotic sensitivity tests should be done. Acid-fast infection should be ruled out by smears and, in questionable cases, by culture. A purified protein derivative (PPD) skin test is indicated.

C. X-ray Findings: Plain films of the chest usually show increased bronchial markings and a variable degree of peribronchial infiltration, but changes may be minimal or absent. Bronchograms should be performed on all suspected cases. The entire bronchial tree must be mapped so that all areas of involvement can be identified. Avoid bronchography during acute episodes of infection and in patients sensitive to iodine. Sinus films should be obtained as indicated.

D. Bronchoscopy should be performed.

Treatment.

A. Medical Measures: Adequate rest, good nutrition, avoidance of respiratory infections, correction of associated conditions such as chronic sinusitis, and postural drainage are the most effective measures. A warm, dry climate is usually beneficial but not curative. Dusty, smoke-filled atmospheres should be avoided. At the onset of a respiratory infection, the patient with bronchiectasis should receive rest, symptomatic treatment, and usually antibiotic therapy to prevent exacerbation of bronchial infection.

   1. Antibiotics - Antibiotic therapy has no lasting effect, but suppresses cough and sputum production for a time. Antibiotics are of greatest value preoperatively, during acute exacerbations in mild cases, or for patients who are not good candidates for operation. Sensitivity studies are indi-

cated. Penicillin G, parenterally or orally, is usually suitable for use in acute exacerbations of bronchitis and pneumonitis pending sensitivity results. For chronic infection, tetracycline, 250 mg. 4 times daily, is often effective in reducing sputum.

2. Aerosol therapy - Saline or a bronchodilator may be administered by aerosol, preferably in conjunction with positive-pressure breathing (see p. 83).

B. Surgical Treatment: Pulmonary resection is indicated in patients who have chronic or recurring symptoms. Fairly extensive areas of involvement can be removed on both sides in properly selected cases.

Preoperative preparation consists of antibiotics, aerosol therapy, and postural drainage for the purpose of minimizing pulmonary infection and decreasing sputum. The daily volume of sputum should be recorded as a guide to progress. It may be of interest to assess improvement by repeated tests of pulmonary function (see p. 215). Operative risk and postoperative complications are materially reduced by careful preparation of patients with bronchopulmonary suppuration.

Postoperatively, excessive secretions are usually troublesome and require attention to coughing, tracheobronchial aspiration, and, occasionally, bronchoscopy.

PULMONARY TUBERCULOSIS

Tuberculosis is a systemic medical disease in which surgical measures occasionally serve as useful adjuncts to other forms of treatment. It is necessary to carry out diagnostic procedures for tuberculosis in surgical patients who have lesions on chest x-rays suspicious of acid-fast infection.

Establishing the Diagnosis of Pulmonary Tuberculosis.

A. Symptoms and Signs: Because early tuberculosis (and even, in some cases, advanced lesions) may be essentially asymptomatic, the routine chest film is an important screening measure prior to major surgery. The characteristic symptoms of cough, weight loss, night sweats, or hemoptysis in established tuberculosis make the diagnosis much less easy to miss. When tubercle bacilli cannot be demonstrated in the sputum, it may be necessary to rely on presumptive evidence of activity such as presence of a cavity, night sweats, blood-streaked sputum, weight loss, easy fatigability, pleurisy with or without effusion, and increased erythrocyte sedimentation rate in a patient with a positive PPD test. In these cases, chest x-rays and sputum examination should be repeated monthly for several months and medical consultation should be obtained.

Note: Elective surgical procedures which are not directed toward the control of the tuberculous lesion should always be deferred until active tuberculosis is excluded or adequately treated.

B. Laboratory Findings:

1. Tuberculin test - For differential diagnosis or screening purposes, administer Intermediate Strength PPD (purified

protein derivative), 0.1 ml. (0.0001 mg.) intradermally on the volar surface of the forearm. Read the test in 48 and 72 hours. The test is positive if induration at the puncture site is 1 cm. in diameter or more. Erythema has no significance. If active tuberculosis is strongly suspected, use First Strength PPD to avoid a severe local reaction. It may occasionally be desirable to use Second Strength PPD if Intermediate Strength PPD gives a negative result in a suspect case. A negative tuberculin test excludes the possibility of tuberculosis in 95% of patients. Old Tuberculin (OT) may be used if PPD is not available.

2. Demonstration of tubercle bacilli - Recovery of tubercle bacilli is the only certain method of establishing the presence of active tuberculosis. This should be attempted by the following methods:
   a. Sputum examination - Simple smears are examined first. If these are negative, 3 or more concentrated 24-hour sputum samples should be studied by direct smear and culture. Culture is more sensitive than smear, but growth of organisms requires 4-6 weeks.
   b. Gastric lavage - If sputum cannot be obtained, or if further study is indicated in spite of negative sputum examinations, 2 or more fasting morning specimens of the gastric contents should be cultured. Stained smears are of no value because of the occurrence of nontuberculous, acid-fast organisms.
   c. Other methods - These include the laryngeal swab or bronchial lavage technics for obtaining culture material. If bronchoscopy is done, introduce 10-15 ml. of normal saline through the bronchoscope and recover by aspiration. This sample can be examined by smear and culture and is also suitable for cytologic study for tumor cells.
3. Antimicrobial sensitivity tests - As a guide to chemotherapy, the cultured acid-fast bacilli should be tested for their sensitivity to the common antituberculosis drugs if facilities are available.

C. X-ray Findings: Full-sized diagnostic chest films will almost always demonstrate a suspicious pulmonary lesion if active tuberculosis is present. Special radiologic studies such as lordotic views and tomograms may be advisable for better delineation of infiltrates and cavities.
D. Bronchoscopy and rarely bronchography may be of value when bronchial disease or bronchiectasis is suspected.
E. Pleural biopsy (see p. 295) is a useful diagnostic procedure when the cause of pleural disease cannot be otherwise determined.

Surgical Measures in Pulmonary Tuberculosis.

Note: Pulmonary tuberculosis is treated most successfully by medical means. Surgical procedures are used with less and less frequency in modern practice.

A. Preoperative Care: Patients with active tuberculous lesions for which surgical treatment is contemplated should have a preoperative period of rest and a course of antituberculosis therapy, preferably with drugs chosen after sensitivity tests.

The time devoted to these measures is usually 3-12 months. In general, it is preferable to delay major thoracic procedures until pulmonary lesions have maximally regressed ("stabilized") as indicated by physical signs and chest films. The systemic reaction should have subsided, as indicated by disappearance of malaise, weakness, and fever, and by the return of the erythrocyte sedimentation rate to normal. Additional signs of improvement include gain in weight, marked decrease in cough and sputum, and disappearance of tubercle bacilli from the sputum.

B. Surgical Treatment: Two types of surgical procedure are used in tuberculosis patients who fail to respond to medical treatment: pulmonary resection and thoracoplasty. The selection of patients, the timing of the operation, and other details of management require the close cooperation of internist and surgeon. Postoperatively, sanitorium care and long-term anti-tuberculosis chemotherapy must be continued as indicated by the general condition of the patient.

1. Pulmonary resection - Patients with active pulmonary lesions should usually receive at least 3-6 months of chemotherapy and supportive care before operation. If the sputum is negative, segmental and subsegmental resections are done to conserve lung tissue when possible. If sputum is positive, lobectomy is associated with fewer tuberculous complications than segmental resection. The following indications for resection are generally accepted.
   a. Localized disease with persistently positive sputum on smear or culture after 3-6 months of adequate chemotherapy.
   b. Open cavity, with or without positive sputum. Thin-walled residual cavities in the presence of negative cultures show a relatively low incidence of relapse on long-term chemotherapy. Nevertheless, resection should be considered in the good risk patient.
   c. Localized nodular disease, especially when a tumor is suspected. It is not necessary to remove multiple small nodular foci; solid lesions representing filled-in cavities, associated with positive sputum or larger than 2 cm. in size, should be resected.
   d. Destroyed lung - Extensive fibrosis, bronchiectasis, and secondary infection are usually present, and pneumonectomy is often required.
   e. Bronchial stenosis - Lung destruction distal to bronchial stenosis may make resection necessary. Bronchoplastic operation to widen a bronchial lumen is indicated if the distal lung is functional and if it is free of active disease.
   f. Thoracoplasty failure - Any of the above conditions may account for the failure of thoracoplasty. Tomography, bronchography, and bronchoscopy may be necessary to determine the extent of residual disease.
2. Thoracoplasty - This operation and its various modifications are now rarely necessary. Indications are as follows:
   a. Chronic cavitary lesions in which resection is not feasible because of the patient's condition and thoracoplasty can be tolerated.

b. Certain cases in which thoracoplasty is used to improve the patient's condition for a later resection.
c. To reduce pleural "dead space" after a large resection and thus minimize over-distention of remaining lung tissue.
d. To close chronic empyema spaces.

Postoperative Tuberculous Complications.

A. Following Pulmonary Resection:
1. Bronchopleural fistula - This is the most frequent serious complication and the commonest cause of postoperative death. Fistula is often followed by the development of tuberculous empyema. The activity of the patient's disease and the type of resection have an important bearing on this complication. In patients with negative sputum preoperatively, the incidence of fistula is about 5%. When sputum is positive, fistulas occur in 10-15% of cases. The highest incidence (15-20%) is noted in patients with positive sputum who have segmental resection. Bronchopleural fistula after pneumonectomy is accompanied by a mortality of about 50%.
2. Postoperative spread - This complication occurs in 5-10% of patients and can be minimized most effectively by preoperative conversion of sputum to negative. Every effort should be made during and after surgery to keep the tracheobronchial tree clear of secretions by aspiration and supervised cough.

B. Following Thoracoplasty: The commonest complication is spread of the disease. In general, thoracoplasty is well tolerated with relatively few complications, considering the fact that most of these patients have advanced disease.

Prognosis.

Operative risk is definitely increased by a positive sputum. The operative mortality for resection is about 3%, with an additional late mortality of around 2%. Relapses or persistent active disease affect a further 10%. The over-all results 5 years after resection are about 85% favorable.

Thoracoplasty mortality is 1-2%, and the long-term satisfactory results are 75-80%. Prognosis is best when the operation results in sputum conversion and cavity closure.

Antituberculosis drug therapy has dramatically reduced the need for surgical treatment in pulmonary tuberculosis and has improved the prognosis in patients who require operation.

HISTOPLASMOSIS

Histoplasmosis is a systemic infection caused by the fungus Histoplasma capsulatum and is usually manifested by a benign transient pneumonia. The organism is world-wide in distribution, but particularly prevalent in central United States, Mexico, Central and South America, northern Europe, and Australia. Histoplasmosis in its chronic form may be associated with nodular pulmonary densities, apical cavities, bronchiectasis, empyema, or pneumothorax. Disseminated histoplasmosis is frequently fatal and fortunately rare.

The diagnosis is based on x-ray findings, serologic and skin tests, and on cultures of sputum, exudates, or tissues. The clinical picture resembles chronic tuberculosis, from which it may be differentiated by positive cultures and skin tests for histoplasmosis and negative cultures and skin tests for tuberculosis. The differentiation is sometimes made difficult by the fact that many patients have both diseases.

Chronic pulmonary lesions such as cavities and large nodules are treated by surgical excision. Amphotericin B (Fungizone®) therapy should be given for several weeks before and after operation.

NOCARDIOSIS

Nocardiosis is caused by a variety of aerobic fungi belonging to the genus Nocardia (e.g., N. asteroides, N. madurae). The infection may resemble actinomycosis or tuberculosis. The diagnosis can only be made by culture of sputum, empyema fluid, blood, or tissue. Distribution is world-wide. The infection usually responds to sulfadiazine in a dosage sufficient to maintain a serum level of about 10 mg./100 ml. (0.5-2 Gm. every 6 hours orally). Sensitivity tests should be used to determine the appropriate antibiotics. Continue drug therapy for 3-4 months after apparent cure. Surgical procedures such as drainage and resection may be required. (Freese, J. W., et al., J. Thoracic Cardiovas. Surg. 46:437, 1963.)

COCCIDIOIDOMYCOSIS

This disease, also known as valley fever, is caused by Coccidioides immitis, which is endemic in certain regions of the Southwest United States, Mexico, and Central and South America, with sporadic cases in Italy and Hawaii. The highly infectious organisms (arthrospores) are carried on wind-borne dust and inhaled. Even very brief exposure may produce the disease, and persons travelling through endemic areas may be infected.

Clinical Findings.

A. Primary Form: About 60% of infections occur without symptoms and are detected only by the conversion of the coccidioidin skin reaction from negative to positive. Clinical manifestations in overt cases usually suggest a respiratory infection and include fever, cough, erythema nodosum, and pleurisy with effusion. Arthralgia is common, and a morbilliform rash may appear 1-2 days after onset of symptoms. X-ray of the lungs during the primary disease, which may last a few weeks, shows patchy soft infiltration; as this clears, residual nodules or thin-walled cavities with little surrounding infiltration may persist. Such cavities may resemble emphysematous blebs or congenital cysts. When marked coccidioidal infection of the cavity is present, the wall may be relatively thick. In the acute stage, the organisms may be found in sputum cultures. The coccidioidin skin test usually becomes positive after 10-14 days and remains positive for years. Precipitating antibodies, as determined by the precipitin test, usually appear in the course of primary infection and tend to disappear with healing. The complement fixation test often shows a low titer in primary infection with a tendency to increase in progressive disease. Complement-fixing antibodies appear later but persist longer. An initial eosinophilia of 15% or higher, with a persistent rising complement-fixation titer, is a bad prognostic sign. A rising complement-fixation titer may indicate dissemination weeks before it is otherwise evident.

B. Chronic or Granulomatous Form: 0.2% of all primary cases progress to the granulomatous stage and may involve the lungs, chest wall, and other structures, including bones and meninges. Diagnosis is made by finding the organisms in infected tissues or discharges. Prognosis was poor in the past but has been improved since the advent of amphotericin B (Fungizone®) therapy.

Treatment.

Surgery is required chiefly in the treatment of the residual pulmonary nodule (coccidioidoma) or cavity left behind by primary coccidioidomycosis. Coccidioidoma usually does not require resection unless it is 2 cm. or more in diameter or unless serial films reveal that the lesion is enlarging. Radiologically, these granulomas appear as coin lesions and may be indistinguishable from carcinoma. They must be resected for diagnostic reasons unless the clinical course, previous chest films, and coccidioidin skin test establish the diagnosis of coccidioidomycosis.

Coccidioidal cavities which persist longer than 1 year should be resected to prevent complications such as secondary infection and hemorrhage. Because wedge and segmental resections may cut across infected tissues and spread the infection, lobectomy is preferred unless the process is well localized.

Encouraging results have been reported with the use of amphotericin B (Fungizone®) in the treatment of coccidioidal disease, particularly the disseminated form. This agent may also prove to be of value in the prevention of spread when infected tissue is traversed in the course of pulmonary resection. It should be given for 3-4 weeks before and after surgery for active or progressive lesions.

ECHINOCOCCUS CYST OF THE LUNG

Echinococcus (hydatid) cyst of the lung is the larval stage of the dog tapeworm, Echinococcus granulosus. Human infection occurs from ingestion of material contaminated with dog feces containing tapeworm eggs, which hatch in the intestine; the larval embryos then penetrate the bowel wall and disseminate via the blood stream. The larvas may come to rest and develop into hydatid cysts in any part of the body, but the liver (70%) and lungs (20%) are most commonly affected.

Hydatid cyst of the lung may be asymptomatic but usually causes cough, minor hemoptysis, sputum, chest pain, and fever by local pressure or by rupture with secondary infection. X-ray shows a sharply defined round or oval density in the lung field. A small crescent of air is sometimes seen between the cyst and the surrounding lung and is pathognomonic. A ruptured, infected cyst has the appearance of a lung abscess. Hydatid cysts are usually solitary, but may be multiple. They usually grow slowly and occasionally reach 15 cm. or more in diameter. They are most commonly confused with neoplasm or lung abscess.

All hydatid cysts should be removed surgically if the patient's general condition permits. The mortality is quite low in uncomplicated cysts. The preoperative diagnosis of hydatid cyst is extremely important because rupture of an unsuspected cyst at operation may result in anaphylactic shock or in spillage of echinococcus scolices onto the pleura or wound with subsequent secondary cyst formation.

PULMONARY ARTERIOVENOUS FISTULA

Pulmonary arteriovenous fistula or aneurysm is a shunt between a pulmonary artery and vein; less frequently, the aneurysm is fed by a bronchial artery or branch from the aorta. This relatively rare anomaly may be hereditary and may be a manifestation of hereditary hemorrhagic telangiectasis (Rendu-Osler-Weber disease), which is transmitted as a simple dominant. Multiple fistulas may be present. When there is a sizable shunt between the pulmonary artery and vein, unoxygenated blood bypasses the pulmonary capillaries in sufficient quantity to produce cyanosis.

Clinical Findings.

Small shunts cause no symptoms and may be discovered on a routine chest film. Fistulas may be progressive; most of them cause no symptoms until adult life. The clinical manifestations of large fistulas include dyspnea, cyanosis, clubbing, hemoptysis, and chest pain. There may be continuous or systolic murmur with or without a thrill over the aneurysm. Epistaxis and telangiectases of the skin and mucous membranes are frequently noted, and nervous aberrations may occur. Paradoxical emboli with hemiplegia and death have been reported.

When arterial oxygen saturation is below normal, polycythemia develops. Diagnosis can often be made from the appearance on x-ray of a rounded, dense shadow connected to the hilum by a broad vascular band. Most lesions occur in the lingula and the middle and lower lobes. They are multiple in 50% of cases. Angiography, including study of both lung fields, is necessary for definitive diagnosis and to detect the presence of fistulas which cannot be visualized on plain films.

Treatment.

If the patient's general health is satisfactory, pulmonary arteriovenous fistulas should be excised (even though asymptomatic), since there is significant danger of progression of the lesion and of such complications as severe hemoptysis or hemothorax. Moreover, there is the threat of paradoxical cerebral emboli or brain abscess.

Surgical excision of the fistula should be accomplished with maximum preservation of pulmonary tissue and care to remove multiple lesions. Persistence or later development of cyanosis or decreased arterial saturation indicates the presence of another aneurysm.

EMPHYSEMATOUS BLEBS AND BULLAE

Air cysts in the lungs usually occur as a local exaggeration of a diffuse emphysematous process. The cause is not known, but bronchial obstruction and advanced age with loss of the elasticity of the alveolar walls may all be contributing factors. Individual alveoli are stretched and interalveolar septa are destroyed, so that the confluence of many alveoli forms cystic spaces.

Emphysematous blebs or bullae cause symptoms (1) by becoming distended with air and compressing the remainder of the lung tissue; (2) by rupturing to cause spontaneous pneumothorax; or, rarely, (3) by causing intramural hemorrhage (which on x-ray is easily mistaken for tumor). Small asymptomatic emphysematous blebs are common incidental findings, especially in the older age group. On x-ray, the bullae appear as translucent areas, usually traversed by fine linear markings. Bronchography may rarely be necessary to determine the presence or absence of bronchiectasis. Scintillation scanning and pulmonary angiography may be helpful in evaluating the status of the lung when excisional surgery is being planned.

Treatment.

Asymptomatic small blebs and bullae usually require no treatment.

A. Medical Measures: When the symptoms are mild or when diminished pulmonary reserve contraindicates surgery, medical treatment is advisable. This may include prevention and early treatment of respiratory infections, avoidance of smoking or inhalation of irritant or allergenic materials, and the use of bronchodilator drugs (see p. 84). Oxygen in appropriate concentration may be required for the relief of dyspnea or hypoxia. Pulmonary function tests (including blood gases) are necessary for evaluation.

B. Surgical Treatment: Large bullae causing significant symptoms or compression of lung tissue should be removed. Lesser surgical procedures than excision are generally reserved for unusual circumstances and poor-risk patients. If a large cyst becomes acutely tense, aspiration with a needle may be lifesaving. Suction drainage by a catheter placed in the cyst cavity with a trocar (Monaldi procedure) may be of value in a severely ill patient.

Prognosis.

The results of excision depend upon the condition of the remainder of the lung. When relatively large areas of normal lung exist and symptoms are due primarily to its compression by giant bullae, excision will usually improve pulmonary function.

SPONTANEOUS PNEUMOTHORAX

Spontaneous pneumothorax is usually caused by the rupture of a small emphysematous bleb.

Clinical Findings.

Spontaneous pneumothorax occurs most frequently in healthy

young adult males. The past history is usually negative, but occasionally there is a history of recurrent pneumothorax. Onset is usually acute and characterized by severe chest pain, cough, and dyspnea. Physical signs are proportional to the extent of pneumothorax and consist of hyperresonance and diminished to absent breath sounds on the involved side. Diagnosis is confirmed by chest film.

Treatment.

A small pneumothorax (less than 25% collapse) will absorb completely within a few weeks unless the air leak in the lung continues. The patient need not be at bed rest during this period, but his activities should be limited. It may be elected to allow the air to absorb spontaneously or to obtain more rapid expansion by aspiration with a needle or small plastic catheter (Intracath), usually through the second interspace anteriorly.

Large pneumothorax (greater than 25% collapse) should be treated by some form of suction drainage of the pleural space in order to expand the lung rapidly and thereby reduce morbidity. A small plastic tube may be introduced into the chest through a needle in the second interspace, or a catheter (e.g., No. 16 F.) may be inserted through a trocar (see p. 294). Constant suction (−25 cm. of water) is applied to the tube or catheter and immediate expansion of the lung will usually occur. Suction is continued until lung expansion is shown on x-ray and the tube or catheter is blocked by the lung. Waterseal drainage is then provided for another 24 hours; at the end of this time, if x-ray shows full expansion, the tube or catheter is removed. The entire process of expansion usually requires only 3-5 days.

Recurrent pneumothorax, either ipsilateral or contralateral, occurs in approximately 20% of cases. If 2 or more episodes have occurred on one side, thoracotomy should be considered in order to excise blebs and create a pleural symphysis, preferably by pleural abrasion. Thoracotomy is also occasionally necessary to control pneumothorax associated with bleeding or persistent air leak.

TENSION PNEUMOTHORAX

Tension pneumothorax occasionally develops as a result of a check-valve type of leak in the lungs. Complete collapse of the lung occurs rapidly, and the mediastinal structures are shifted to the opposite side as intrathoracic tension rises. When positive pressure rises above 15-20 cm. of water, venous return to the heart is impeded and circulatory collapse results unless the tension is relieved immediately. Physical signs include marked dyspnea, cyanosis, shift of the trachea and the apical impulse of the heart to the opposite side, and tympany to percussion and absent breath sounds on the involved side. It may be necessary to begin treatment promptly without waiting for x-rays of the chest.

When tension pneumothorax occurs, a needle should be inserted into the chest through the second or third interspace anteriorly. Air will rush out under pressure and relieve the tension. The needle should then be aspirated with a syringe or connected by a tubing to waterseal drainage until a catheter can be introduced into the chest by trocar thoracotomy (see p. 294). Treatment is the same as for spontaneous pneumothorax. Persistent air leak or recurrent pneumothorax is an indication for thoracotomy.

PRIMARY LUNG CARCINOMA

Bronchogenic carcinoma accounts for about 98% of primary tumors of the lung and is one of the major causes of death from cancer in men. It is 8 times more common in men than in women. Although the peak occurrence is between the ages of 50 and 70, the disease is not rare after 30. The frequency of histologic types in surgical series is approximately as follows: epidermoid, 55%; undifferentiated, 30%; adenocarcinoma, 10%; small (oat) cell carcinoma, 5%; and bronchiolar (alveolar) cell carcinoma, 1%. In autopsy series, undifferentiated carcinoma predominates.

The incidence of primary lung cancer has increased markedly in recent decades as a result of cigarette smoking. Carcinogenic compounds in tobacco smoke are the etiologic agent. The risk of developing lung cancer is much less in pipe or cigar smokers. The risk increases with the duration of smoking and the number of cigarettes smoked per day, and is diminished by discontinuing smoking. In comparison with nonsmokers, males who smoke 10-20 cigarettes a day have an approximately 9- to 10-fold risk of developing lung cancer; heavy smokers (21-40 cigarettes per day) have at least a 20-fold risk. The data for women, though less extensive, point in the same direction. Cigarette smoking is also associated with a higher incidence of chronic pulmonary disease, coronary artery disease, and cancer of the larynx, and with a shortened life expectancy. (Smoking and Health. Report of the Advisory Committee to the Surgeon General. U.S. Department of Health, Education, and Welfare Public Health Service Publication No. 1103 [1964].)

The etiologic relationship between atmospheric pollution in industrial areas and lung cancer is suspected but not proved. Inhalation of radioactive ore in the Schneeburg and Jachymov mines in Czechoslovakia has been shown to be associated with an increased incidence of lung cancer. Inhalation of asbestos dust may also cause carcinoma of the lung.

Clinical Findings.

A. Symptoms and Signs: Early lung carcinoma is asymptomatic and can only be detected by x-ray. Lesions within the parenchyma of the lung may remain silent and will sometimes grow very slowly over a period of several years.

Manifestations of lung cancer are quite varied, depending upon the location and extent of the tumor. The commonest initial complaint is cough, frequently accompanied by a small amount of sputum which may be blood-streaked. Clubbing of the fingers occasionally is present in relatively early lesions.

Obstruction of a small or medium-sized bronchus is quite common, producing a localized wheeze, atelectasis, or obstructive emphysema. Physical signs over such areas may be negligible or may consist chiefly of diminished breath sounds. Acute pneumonitis frequently develops in the partially blocked segments and not infrequently is the earliest clinical evidence of malignancy. For this reason all adults with pneumonitis should have a chest x-ray, and follow-up films should be obtained to prove complete clearing of the process.

Pneumonitis occasionally progresses to abscess formation, or a bulky tumor may break down to form a necrotic cavity. The resulting appearance may be that of a pyogenic lung abscess, and the underlying malignancy may be overlooked unless investigation is complete.

Pleural effusion is a common finding in tumors close to the visceral pleura. The effusion is frequently bloody and may contain cancer cells.

Direct extension beyond the lung may involve (1) the chest wall, causing localized or intercostal nerve pain; (2) the brachial plexus and stellate ganglion in the superior pulmonary sulcus, causing shoulder and arm pain and Horner's syndrome (Pancoast's syndrome); (3) the phrenic nerve, causing paralysis of the diaphragm; or (4) the recurrent laryngeal nerve, usually at the aortic arch on the left, causing cord palsy and hoarseness.

Lymphatic spread is primarily to the hilar and mediastinal nodes, but involvement of the paratracheal and supraclavicular nodes is common. Distant, blood-borne metastases, particularly to the brain, liver, adrenals, and bones, occur frequently in advanced lesions and may occasionally be the first sign of a silent lung primary.

Bronchogenic carcinoma may cause a variety of metabolic disorders, including adrenocortical hyperfunction (Cushing's syndrome) or hypofunction (secondary to adrenal metastases); hypercalcemia (with and without osteolytic metastases) or hypocalcemia; inappropriate secretion of antidiuretic hormone; or carcinoid syndrome. Vascular syndromes such as spontaneous thrombophlebitis (venous thrombosis) or bleeding diathesis due to fibrinogen deficiency may occur. Neuromyopathies such as peripheral neuritis, polymyositis, a myasthenia-like syndrome, and cortical cerebellar and spinocerebellar degenerative myelopathy have been ascribed to lung cancer. When any of the above conditions develop, bronchogenic carcinoma should be considered among the diagnostic possibilities even in the absence of pulmonary symptoms. (Greenberg, E., and others, Am. J. Med. **36**:106, 1964.)

B. Laboratory Findings: Cytologic examination of sputum (Papanicolaou) is positive in 50-75% of patients with lung cancer. The results of sputum examination seldom influence the decision to operate except in a select group of poor-risk patients with questionable lesions in whom a positive diagnosis justifies operation in spite of the hazard. A negative sputum examination is meaningless, and false positives occur.

C. X-ray Findings:

1. Special studies - Determination of the extent and nature of the lesion frequently requires special studies. Tomography is most often helpful. Bronchography is rarely needed to delineate the smaller bronchi. Pulmonary angiography may be of value in deciding the operability of medially placed tumors. Always obtain previous films of the chest for comparison, if they are available.
2. Differentiation of primary from metastatic neoplasm - Primary neoplasms elsewhere in the body, especially the

kidneys, thyroid, testes, and breast, occasionally produce lung metastases indistinguishable from primary lung cancer. An intravenous urogram is advisable in lung tumors to rule out a primary renal tumor if genitourinary tract symptoms or signs are suggestive.

3. The solitary pulmonary nodule - Solitary pulmonary nodules are often incidental findings on chest films. These "coin" lesions are usually asymptomatic, located within the parenchyma, and associated with no distinctive physical or laboratory findings. Calcification is noted in about 50% of benign lesions and about 14% of malignancies. After complete work-up, including a review of previous films, the diagnosis is frequently unsettled. Under these circumstances thoracotomy is indicated, since about 25% of coin lesions prove to be primary lung cancer. The remainder are granulomas (42%), chiefly residuals of histoplasmosis or tuberculosis; hamartomas (8%), metastatic tumors (6%), bronchogenic cysts (4%), or one of a variety of rarer lesions.

D. Bronchoscopy: This examination should be performed on all patients prior to thoracotomy to determine the status of tracheobronchial passages. Biopsy of abnormal tissue and bronchial washings should be submitted for pathologic study. A positive diagnosis can be made by these methods in about 75% of patients. The location of the lesion in the bronchial tree often determines operability. Bronchoscopy can frequently be performed just prior to thoracotomy and under the same anesthesia.

E. Scalene Node Biopsy or Mediastinoscopy: See p. 295.

F. Metastatic Survey: A chemical screening battery - including alkaline phosphatase, LDH, and SGOT - should be obtained on all patients suspected of bronchogenic carcinoma. Elevated enzyme level or any clinical finding suggestive of metastatic disease is a possible indication for radioactive scan of bones and liver and skeletal x-rays (e.g., spine, pelvis, skull).

G. Other Examinations: When pleural fluid is present it should always be examined cytologically before operation. Needle or open biopsy of the pleura occasionally is diagnostic in obscure cases (see p. 295). Needle biopsy of the pulmonary lesion itself is often feasible, but should usually be performed only to obtain a histologic diagnosis in inoperable patients.

Treatment.

Resection is practically the only curative treatment, although a few successes with radiotherapy have been reported.

A. Indications for Thoracotomy: In the absence of evidence of inoperability (see below), all patients with proved or suspected lung cancer should be explored. Because neoplasms often remain stationary in size for many months, failure of the lesion to grow during a short period of observation does not rule out carcinoma.

B. Contraindications to Thoracotomy:
   1. Inadequate pulmonary reserve or poor general health.
   2. Evidence of distant metastases.
   3. Cancer cells in pleural fluid or pleural biopsy. Bloody pleural fluid usually indicates inoperable carcinoma (or tuberculosis).

4. Positive scalene node or mediastinal biopsy. Rarely, the finding of a positive node only along the main stem bronchus at mediastinoscopy may not contraindicate radical pneumonectomy (which includes mediastinal and hilar node excision).
5. Recurrent nerve involvement.
6. Phrenic nerve involvement usually indicates inoperability.
7. Brachial plexus involvement (Pancoast's syndrome) practically always signifies inoperability, although cures have been reported in a few selected cases in whom resection was preceded by radiotherapy.
8. Angiocardiographic evidence of invasion or compression of the main pulmonary artery or vein at the hilus.
9. Unresectable involvement of the chest wall.
10. Bronchoscopic evidence of involvement of the proximal main stem bronchi or trachea.
11. Small (oat) cell carcinoma has been found to metastasize early and to be rarely curable by resection. Some authorities advise radiotherapy instead of resection in such lesions (Coles, D. T., S. Clin. North America 53:769-774, 1973).

C. Palliative Therapy: Roentgen therapy may be of value in the relief of pain, cough, and bronchial obstruction. However, the average survival after x-ray treatment is only about 9 months. If a patient with a small lesion refuses operation or is unsuitable for surgery, intensive supervoltage irradiation offers a faint hope of cure. With the possible exception of superior sulcus tumors, preoperative radiotherapy followed by resection has not been found to increase survival. Postoperative irradiation has had a limited success in selected patients found to be unresectable at thoracotomy, but routine use of postoperative irradiation does not increase survival. Chemotherapy (e.g., cyclophosphamide or other alkylating agents) is occasionally beneficial either alone or combined with radiotherapy.

Prognosis.

Only 8-10% of all patients with carcinoma of the lung survive 5 years. However, asymptomatic patients who are operated on solely on the basis of an abnormal x-ray have a 5-year survival rate of 40-50%. This illustrates the importance of routine chest x-rays. The five-year survival rate for all patients undergoing resection for carcinoma of the lung is about 25%. The prognosis is less favorable if lymph node involvement or blood vessel invasion has occurred. Spidermoid carcinoma is generally considered to have a better prognosis than the other cell types. According to experience at the Mayo Clinic, the 5-year survival rate in squamous cell carcinoma after resection was 37%, in adenocarcinoma 34%, in large cell carcinoma 29%, and in small cell carcinoma 10% (Galofré, M., Surg. Gynec. Obstet. 119:51-61, 1964). Operative mortality is 5-10%.

BRONCHIAL ADENOMA

Bronchial adenoma occasionally invades locally or metastasizes, but its behavior is different from that of bronchogenic carcinoma. Histologically there are 2 characteristic patterns: the carcinoid and cylindroid forms, with transitional and variant types. The carcinoid form resembles carcinoid tumors of the gastrointestinal tract and usually involves one of the major bronchi. Cylindroid adenoma tends to occur near the carina or in the trachea, and typically shows relentless local invasion. Both types of adenoma grow slowly, are more common in women, and tend to occur earlier than bronchogenic carcinoma (mean age 40). Metastases occur in about 15% of cases.

Dry cough, unilateral wheeze, and recurrent hemoptysis are characteristic in the early stage. The average duration of symptoms is over 3 years, and the late changes are due chiefly to bronchial obstruction and pulmonary infection. Findings are often distinguishable from bronchogenic carcinoma only by their chronicity. Most patients show x-ray changes suggesting atelectasis or inflammatory infiltration. Bronchoscopic examination gives the correct diagnosis in less than half of patients.

Bronchoscopic resection is not a reliable method of treatment. Cure usually requires resection of the involved bronchus, adjacent nodes, and damaged lung tissue. Removal of a small adenoma by bronchotomy may occasionally be feasible.

The five-year survival rate after resection is about 80%.

METASTATIC NEOPLASM OF THE LUNG

Metastatic sarcoma and carcinoma of the lung are almost without exception incurable. However, when a slow-growing, solitary pulmonary metastasis appears as the only evidence of persisting disease more than 1 year after the presumed total extirpation of the primary lesion, consideration may be given to local excision of the pulmonary focus. The five-year survival rate in collected series is about 12% for sarcoma and 5% for carcinoma. Many who respond well to surgery do so because they have slow-growing tumors, but in occasional cases a very gratifying long-term result is obtained.

OTHER PULMONARY NEOPLASMS

Hamartomas comprise about 8% of solitary pulmonary nodules. They are usually small, located in the periphery of the lung, and are almost invariably benign (a few malignant hamartomas have been reported). They are 4 times more common in men. Hamartomas are embryologic remnants consisting largely of cartilage containing variable quantities of epithelial, adipose, or muscular tissue. Calcification may be present. These lesions must be excised for diagnostic purposes.

Rare primary pulmonary tumors, including leiomyoma, leiomyosarcoma, and lymphoma, are generally indistinguishable from bronchogenic carcinoma. The diagnosis is usually made only by histologic examination.

Location of Tumors and Cysts in the Mediastinum

Anterior Mediastinum	Superior Mediastinum	Middle Mediastinum	Posterior Mediastinum
Thymoma Thymic cyst Teratoma Goiter Parathyroid adenoma Lymphoma Lipoma Fibroma Lymphangioma Hemangioma Chondroma Rhabdomyo-sarcoma	Goiter Bronchogenic cyst Parathyroid adenoma Myxoma Lymphoma	Bronchogenic cyst Lymphoma Pericardial cyst Plasma cell myeloma	Neurilemmoma Neurofibroma Ganglioneuroma Sympathico-blastoma Fibrosarcoma Lymphoma Goiter Xanthofibroma Gastroenteric cyst Chondroma Myxoma Meningocele Paraganglioma

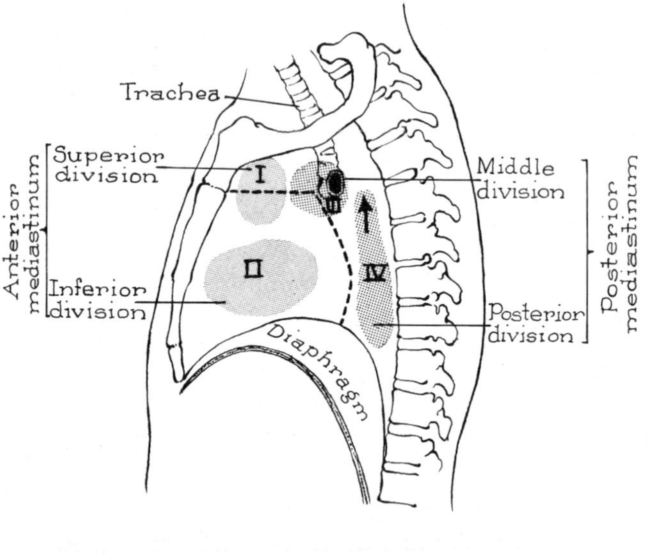

Divisions of the Mediastinum

DISEASES OF THE MEDIASTINUM

TUMORS OF THE MEDIASTINUM

Mediastinal masses consist chiefly of a variety of neoplasms and cysts which tend to occur in characteristic sites (see p. 322). The most frequently encountered tumors are thymomas and teratomas in the anterior mediastinum; lymphomas in the anterior and middle mediastinum; and tumors of the intercostal nerves, sympathetic nerve trunks, and ganglia in the posterior mediastinum. Other conditions which must occasionally be considered in the differential diagnosis of mediastinal masses include cardiovascular abnormalities (especially aneurysm), diaphragmatic hernias, esophageal and pulmonary lesions, granulomas (histoplasmoma, tuberculoma, and sarcoid), hydatid cyst, and metastatic malignancy.

Clinical Findings.

About half of mediastinal tumors are discovered on mass survey or routine chest x-ray, and the majority of these are asymptomatic. Specific symptoms and signs depend upon the size, location, and nature of the tumor. Cough, chest pain, and dyspnea are among the commonest complaints. Physical signs are frequently absent or minimal. The following are of particular interest when present: cervical or generalized lymphadenopathy; venous congestion in the head, neck, and upper extremities (superior vena caval obstruction); hoarseness (recurrent nerve palsy); Horner's syndrome (involvement of the cervical sympathetic nerves); and elevation of the diaphragm (phrenic nerve paralysis). Nerve damage is usually caused by inoperable malignant invasion. When a malignant mediastinal tumor is suspected, a careful search should be made for evidence of primary or metastatic neoplasm outside the mediastinum.

Laboratory examinations include routine chest films, tomography, and, if a vascular lesion is suspected, angiography. Blood and bone marrow studies for blood dyscrasias are indicated if a lymphoma is suspected. Sputum smears, cultures, and cytologic studies may be indicated. Determination by the scanning technic of radioactive iodine uptake by the mediastinal mass is diagnostic in substernal goiter. Scalene or mediastinal node biopsy (see p. 294) may prove valuable, especially if lymphoma or other malignancy is being considered. Extrapleural parasternal mediastinotomy through the second or third intercostal space provides direct access to anterior lesions for biopsy when sternotomy for resection is not indicated. Direct needle biopsy of the mediastinal mass may occasionally be feasible in order to establish the diagnosis in an accessible but obviously inoperable tumor. The response of the mediastinal mass to a course of x-ray therapy is an unreliable diagnostic criterion. Histologic diagnosis is always advisable.

Treatment.

The majority of mediastinal enlargements requires thoracotomy or median sternotomy for positive diagnosis and definitive treatment. In most cases nothing is to be gained by delay of exploration when an operable lesion cannot be ruled out. Even benign, asymptomatic lesions should rarely be treated expectantly. Sooner or later, because of their critical location, they usually cause serious difficulty as a result of pressure, infection, or rupture.

Characteristic Features of the Commonest Mediastinal Tumors.

A. Mediastinal Goiter: This lesion is usually a direct extension of a nontoxic adenomatous goiter in the neck. The usual location of the goiter is the anterior superior mediastinum, but descent into the upper posterior mediastinum does occur.

In 50% of cases the disease is asymptomatic and is detected by routine chest films; in the remainder, symptoms include dyspnea, cough, pain, and dysphagia. The cervical portion of the thyroid is usually, but not always, enlarged and palpable. The substernal thyroid is readily demonstrated by x-ray. Some degree of tracheal (and possibly esophageal) deviation and compression is typically present. The rounded, homogeneous density in the mediastinum is continuous above with the cervical shadow, and on fluoroscopy the mass is usually seen to move upward with swallowing. If functioning thyroid tissue is present in a mediastinal goiter, the diagnosis can be confirmed by administering radioiodine and taking a scan of the area. Superior mediastinal enlargements should be examined by radioisotope scanning unless thyroid origin can be ruled out.

Accurate preoperative diagnosis is especially desirable in superior mediastinal growths since this determines the operative approach. Mediastinal goiters should be approached through the usual thyroidectomy incision except in the rare instance (e.g., posterior mediastinal goiter) where a combined thoracic and cervical approach may be required.

B. Bronchogenic and Gastroenteric Cysts: These cysts represent embryologic remnants or anomalies of the respiratory and alimentary tracts, respectively. Bronchogenic cysts are lined with respiratory epithelium, and may contain smooth muscle and cartilage in the wall. They are most often found in the parahilar or right paratracheal regions. The gastroenteric cysts are usually closely associated with the esophagus or actually intramural, and are lined by squamous, gastric, or intestinal epithelium. They are sometimes referred to as enterogenous cysts or alimentary tract duplications. Those containing gastric epithelium may have acid-secreting cells, and peptic ulceration of the lining sometimes occurs.

Bronchogenic cysts usually become symptomatic only in adult life, if at all, whereas 75% of gastroenteric cysts are diagnosed in the first year of life because of such serious complications as peptic ulceration, perforation into a bronchus or pleural cavity, or hemorrhage. The symptoms of both bronchogenic and gastroenteric cysts depend primarily on their size and location and on the presence or absence of infection. Chest pain, cough, wheezing, and slight dysphagia are the commonest complaints. When the cyst is infected the clinical appearance may resemble lung abscess or empyema. By x-ray, bronchogenic cysts are ovoid, smooth in outline, and homogeneous in density except when a bronchial fistula exists, in which case an air-fluid level can be seen. They are usually located near the midline and, because of their close relation to the trachea, bronchi, and esophagus, may be seen on fluoroscopy to move up and down with respiration or swallowing.

The treatment of bronchogenic and gastroenteric cysts - even if asymptomatic - is surgical removal, provided there is no contraindication to operation.

C. Thymoma: Thymomas are usually composed of lymphocytes and epithelial cells. Since the proportion of these 2 cell types varies in different tumors, the microscopic picture is sometimes difficult to interpret; before diagnosing a tumor as primary in the thymus, one must carefully rule out teratoma, lymphoma, and metastatic tumor. Necrosis, hemorrhage, and cyst formation within thymomas are not uncommon. Cystic change is occasionally so extensive that only a fibrous capsule containing a few remnants of thymic tissue remains (thymic cysts). The histologic differentiation of benign from malignant variants of thymoma is difficult or impossible. About one-fourth of these lesions break through their capsule and invade locally or implant on neighboring surfaces, and in this sense they are "malignant"; lymphogenous or hematogenous metastases are quite rare.

Thymoma occurs in about 15% of patients with myasthenia gravis, and about 75% of patients with thymoma have myasthenia gravis; but removal of the tumor has little or no effect on the myasthenia. Myasthenic symptoms may develop years after a thymoma has been known to be present. In females, especially those under 30 years of age, the removal of a non-neoplastic thymus gland is said to be associated with an increased remission rate in myasthenia gravis.

The average age of patients with thymoma is about 45, and there is no significant difference in sex incidence. The commonest symptoms of thymoma are those of myasthenia gravis. Chest pain occasionally occurs and may indicate invasion of the pleura. Tracheobronchial or superior vena caval obstruction sometimes develops, and hemorrhage into the tumor may produce a rapid onset of pressure symptoms. Roentgenologically, the tumor is usually round or oval and sharply delineated from the surrounding tissues. Its typical location is in the anterior mediastinum, usually anterior to the aortic arch and the base of the heart, but thymomas may be found at lower levels anteriorly or, rarely, posterior to the superior vena cava. Calcification is seen on x-ray in about 25% of tumors and does not rule out local invasion.

Thymomas should be removed since one-fourth of these tumors are locally invasive and it is usually impossible to distinguish these from the noninvasive majority. Myasthenia gravis is the chief cause of operative mortality, and severe grades of this disease may contraindicate surgery. When the tumor is removed completely, recurrence is not likely. Irradiation of thymomas in patients with or without myasthenia gravis only occasionally results in reduction in size of the tumor.

The thymus in neonates and infants is frequently prominent on the chest film. It was formerly thought that infants with larger mediastinal shadows were more susceptible to sudden death. There is no proof of this, and the practice of giving prophylactic roentgen treatment to the thymus gland should be condemned as not only unwarranted but also dangerous. The incidence of carcinoma of the thyroid and of leukemia has been reported to be significantly increased by mediastinal irradiation in infancy.

D. Teratoma: These tumors arise within the anlage of the thymus and consist of tissues derived from 2 or all 3 of the primitive germ layers. About one-third are malignant. Dermoid cyst is a type of benign, unilocular teratoma containing sebaceous material and hair and lined by stratified squamous epithelium and dermal appendages.

Teratomas may occur at any age but are most frequently seen in persons between 20 and 40. About one-third are asymptomatic; the remainder cause cough, chest pain, dyspnea, or other pressure symptoms. In rare cases the tumor ruptures into the esophagus or trachea and the patient vomits or spits up hair. Malignant lesions infiltrate locally, increase rapidly in size, and may produce superior vena caval obstruction, pleural implantation, and distant metastases.

Teratomas are characteristically precordial in location on x-ray, although they may occasionally be found in the posterior mediastinum. They are of homogeneous density, and discrete, round, and smooth in outline unless local invasion has occurred. If the mass is large it may project into either pleural cavity, causing atelectasis, and may even appear to occupy an entire hemithorax. Pleural effusion may be present, especially in malignant teratoma. When the tumor contains bone or teeth, a specific diagnosis can be made. In most cases diagnosis can be established only by exploration.

Treatment is by excision, which is curative in benign lesions. The prognosis of malignant teratoma is very poor; most patients die within 1 year after diagnosis.

E. Lymphoma: This is the most frequent cause of a mediastinal mass. The most common symptoms are cough, pain, dyspnea, wheezing, hoarseness, weight loss, fatigue, and fever. Peripheral lymphadenopathy or splenomegaly may be present. The mediastinal tumor consists of involved lymph nodes, usually in the anterior or middle mediastinum. Bilateral enlargement of the mediastinum is suggestive of lymphoma, but unilateral mass does not preclude the diagnosis. The outlines of the mass on x-ray may appear rounded or lobulated and may be either sharp and clear-cut or indistinct.

Palpable peripheral nodes should be biopsied. If this is not diagnostic (in suspicious cases), the scalene nodes should be removed on one or both sides for histologic examination or mediastinoscopy may be performed (see p. 294). By means of these procedures (as well as blood and bone marrow studies) a positive diagnosis can be made in over half of cases. Exploratory thoracotomy or sternotomy is contraindicated when the diagnosis can be established by other methods since lymphoma is almost invariably a disseminated disease and local manifestations are best managed by x-ray or chemotherapy.

F. Neurogenic Tumors: These are the most frequent primary mediastinal neoplasms. Nearly all neurogenic tumors of the mediastinum arise from the intercostal nerves or the paravertebral sympathetic trunks and are therefore usually found in the posterior mediastinum. Rarely the tumor originates in the neck and extends into the superior mediastinum. Neurilemmoma (schwannoma), a benign neoplasm of the nerve sheath of Schwann, is the most common neurogenic tumor. Many of these neoplasms have been wrongly classified as neurofibromas, which are quite uncommon in the mediastinum. Ganglioneuroma is a rare benign neoplasm of the sympathetic ganglia which may be distinguished by its tendency to reach a very large size and to grow into or out of an intervertebral foramen, producing an "hourglass" tumor which may exert pressure on the spinal cord. The benign neurogenic tumors have malignant counterparts which are fortunately quite rare (malignant schwannoma, malignant ganglioneuroma, sympathicoblastoma).

Neurogenic tumors are usually benign and asymptomatic. The usual complaint is pain referred to the chest, neck, or arm. The diagnosis is usually made on routine x-rays, which characteristically show a round, homogeneous mass with distinct borders in the posterior mediastinum. Occasionally the growth lies behind the heart shadow and is partially obscured on routine exposures. Rib or vertebral erosion may occur, and widening of the intervertebral foramen may be present in the "hourglass" lesions. Calcium can sometimes be visualized. Treatment is by excision.

G. Pericardial Cyst: These cysts probably result from a failure of fusion of 1 or more of the lacunae which merge to form the pericardial sac, but they may represent lymphatic cysts. They are benign, unilocular, and thin-walled; attached to the pericardium, and filled with clear serous fluid. They are usually asymptomatic. Most are discovered on routine chest films, which typically show a smoothly rounded, sharply demarcated tumor of uniform density lying against the pericardium, diaphragm, and chest wall in the right or left anterior cardiophrenic angle. Because of their position they may be confused with diaphragmatic hernia, dermoid cyst, or a pericardial fat pad. Surgical removal of pericardial cysts is indicated because it is not possible to distinguish them from more serious lesions.

H. Granuloma: Granulomatous inflammation of the mediastinal lymph nodes may be caused by histoplasmosis, tuberculosis, coccidioidomycosis, and sarcoidosis. The majority of patients have no symptoms directly related to the enlarged nodes, which are usually located alongside the trachea or hilum and protrude into the thorax as smoothly oval, rounded, or lobulated masses. Calcification may be present. The radiologic appearance is often typical of sarcoidosis, with pulmonary parenchymal involvement and bilateral hilar enlargement. When only unilateral hilar lymphadenopathy is present in sarcoidosis, the diagnosis is difficult. Scalene or mediastinal node biopsy and skin tests for tuberculosis, histoplasmosis, and perhaps coccidioidomycosis should be done. Surgical removal of granulomatous lesions is usually not necessary except for diagnostic purposes when other measures fail. The dense inflammatory reaction around the nodes may make excision difficult.

ACUTE MEDIASTINITIS

Mediastinal infections are chiefly due to perforation of the esophagus by instrumentation or foreign body or to leakage of esophageal suture lines after surgery. Clinical findings usually consist of fever, tachycardia, and prostration. Deep-seated substernal, epigastric, or neck pain is usually present. The superior mediastinum is most frequently involved. Chest films show mediastinal air, widening of the mediastinum, and blurring of the aortic prominence. Pulmonary infiltration and bilateral pleural effusion may occur. A swallow of a soluble contrast medium, e.g., methylglucamine diatrizoate (Gastrografin®) (never barium), should be obtained under fluoroscopy and may show the site of perforation.

Minimal leakage from the esophagus after endoscopy usually responds satisfactorily to intensive antibiotic therapy and restriction of oral intake. Large tears and leaks should be repaired immediately if discovered early; otherwise, drainage is required for abscesses or spreading infection. Cervical esophagotomy, attempt at esophageal repair or resection, and other complex procedures may be required in neglected cases. The mortality rate is high.

10 . . .

Surgery of the Heart & Great Vessels

The orderly evaluation of cardiovascular disease includes the history and physical examination, cardiac x-ray series, Ecg., and cardiac catheterization in most cases. In addition, coexistent disease of the coronary arteries or myocardium requires arteriography or ventriculography for full elucidation.

Despite the sophisticated technics available for preoperative diagnosis, the cardiac surgeon must remain alert at the operating table for unsuspected or misdiagnosed lesions. Exploration at operation provides the opportunity for final diagnosis and plan of management.

In this chapter, the principal surgical aspects of the more common types of congenital and acquired heart disease are discussed.

TRAUMA

Although most traumatic lesions of the heart are due to gunshot or stab wounds, deceleration accidents commonly involve the heart and aorta and should be suspected in all cases of serious injury with or without obvious chest trauma.

PENETRATING INJURY

Almost all persons with direct myocardial perforations due to gunshot wounds die immediately, but a high percentage of patients with stab wounds reach the emergency room alive and salvageable. The most common cause of death in these circumstances is cardiac tamponade secondary to continuing intrapericardial bleeding. Functional sealing of the pericardial laceration occurs rapidly, and the acute accumulation of 150-200 ml. of pericardial blood results in critical limitation of ventricular filling, with decreasing cardiac output and rising venous pressure. The steady accumulation of fluid within the normal pericardium may cause no clinically discernible interference with function until a critical threshold is reached; deterioration is then rapid. Conversely, the removal of seemingly insignificant volumes of fluid from the fully distended pericardium can produce dramatic clinical improvement.

In occasional patients with slow or delayed intrapericardial bleeding, signs of tamponade may develop insidiously after a symptom-free interval. Most patients with significant injury, however, present with some degree of shock. The typical features of acute cardiac tamponade include dyspnea, cool and pale extremities, and weak pulses which may be paradoxical (i.e., become palpably weaker or absent on inspiration, with a measured fall greater than 10 mm. Hg). The small, quiet heart and distant heart sounds often described are not constant findings. The central venous pressure is almost always elevated, although hypovolemia due to severe blood loss may preclude venous engorgement and confuse the clinical picture.

Chest x-rays show fullness of the cardiac silhouette, but total heart size remains normal or minimally increased. If clinical conditions permit, fluoroscopy reveals diminished or absent cardiac pulsations.

The Ecg. is not helpful. Sinus tachycardia is typical, and ST elevation and T wave changes in ventricular injuries are present.

Treatment.

Minimal mortality rates (5-15%) have been obtained by immediate thoracotomy for significant penetrating injuries of the heart. Conservative management can be recommended only in selected cases with minimal blood loss and a stable response to a single pericardiocentesis. As the incidence of delayed hemorrhage and tamponade is high, thoracotomy and definitive repair should be considered from the beginning.

Emergency treatment should include a large-bore venous infusion (preferably a central venous pressure catheter), and blood should be drawn for immediate typing and cross-matching. Saline solution, lactated Ringer's injection, or plasma may be administered until blood is available. Pericardiocentesis should be performed in all cases of diagnosed tamponade.

Technic: This procedure is best performed with the patient semirecumbent or recumbent. The safest site of puncture is between the xiphoid and the left costal margin. (An alternative site is the left fourth intercostal space 3-4 cm. from the sternum.) Preparation of the skin and local anesthesia may be ignored in an acute emergency. A No. 18 or No. 17 gauge, short-beveled needle, 6 inches long, with a 3-way stopcock, is used. (A spinal puncture needle is suitable.) The needle is directed upward at an angle of 35-45° toward the midpoint of the left clavicle. The pericardium is encountered at a variable distance of 3-6 cm. depending upon body build, and a ''pop'' is often felt as the pericardium is entered. A simple safeguard against penetration of the myocardium is to attach the chest lead of the Ecg. to the hub of the needle with an alligator clip connector. Contact with the epicardium produces obvious ST elevation in the Ecg. It must be remembered that inadequate common grounding of the patient and electrical equipment is associated with a small but definite risk of ventricular arrhythmias induced by the leakage of current from the Ecg. machine through the pericardiocentesis needle. After complete aspiration, the needle is withdrawn and reinserted for subsequent pericardiocenteses. A small indwelling plastic catheter inserted into the pericardial space through the needle cannot provide reliable drainage in the presence of active bleeding.

Prognosis.

In cases managed by pericardiocentesis and immediate thoracotomy, survival can be expected in 85-95% of cases. Extensive wounds treated by pericardiocentesis alone are usually fatal. No disability follows recovery from the injury, although rarely a postcardiotomy syndrome or constrictive pericarditis may result.

NONPENETRATING INJURY

A wide variety of myocardial injuries may be produced by blunt chest trauma, today due mostly to automobile accidents. The degree of external thoracic trauma does not necessarily indicate the extent of myocardial damage. These injuries may include rupture or laceration of the cardiac chambers, septa, valves, papillary muscles, and great vessels and traumatic myocardial infarction, but the most common lesion is myocardial contusion with a variable degree of hemorrhagic necrosis (frequently associated with traumatic thrombosis of the left anterior descending coronary artery). Arrhythmias, including ventricular fibrillation and heart block, may occur in the period immediately following injury. Delayed complications include spontaneous perforation, which may involve the ventricular septum (7-10 days), and aneurysm formation (several weeks).

A common iatrogenic cause of cardiac injury is the resuscitation process, which may result in myocardial rupture and laceration of the coronary vessels and ventricles by needles or broken ribs.

Treatment.

Injuries producing acute hemopericardium are treated as outlined above for penetrating injuries. Management of suspected cardiac contusions is conservative (as for myocardial infarction). Digitalis and antiarrhythmic agents should be given only when specifically indicated. The delayed appearance of cardiac tamponade demands immediate investigation with pericardiocentesis, followed by immediate operative exploration if frank hemopericardium is found.

ACUTE AORTIC LESIONS

TRAUMATIC AORTIC RUPTURE

In severe deceleration injuries, rupture of the thoracic aorta is more common than is generally suspected, with an incidence ranging as high as 16%. The most common site of rupture is immediately distal to the origin of the left subclavian artery. Persons with complete rupture die immediately of exsanguination. Incomplete tears, however, involving only intima and media, result in an acute or chronic (delayed) traumatic aortic aneurysm contained by adventitia and pleura.

The diagnosis is strongly suggested by observation of a widened mediastinal silhouette on posteroanterior chest films with loss of definition of the aortic knob. Left hemothorax or pleural effusion is often present. Aortography should be performed immediately in suspected cases.

Treatment.

Diagnosis should be followed by operative repair without delay, since the majority of untreated patients die within weeks. Excision and graft replacement of the involved portion of aorta are performed with cardiopulmonary bypass. Preoperative hypertension should be rigidly controlled, using trimethaphan camphorsulfonate (Arfonad®) if necessary, to minimize the chance of complete rupture prior to operation.

ACUTE AORTIC DISSECTIONS

Except in patients with Marfan's syndrome, acute dissections of the aorta are commonly preceded by a history of uncontrolled hypertension. The resected tissue almost always demonstrates cystic medial necrosis. The most common sites of the presumed origin of the dissection ("intimal tear") are the ascending aorta (60-70%), the descending aorta just distal to the left subclavian artery (20-25%), and the aortic arch (5-10%).

The initial symptoms in almost all cases of acute dissection include sudden and severe deep chest or midscapular back pain. Migrating pain usually accompanies advancing dissection. Syncope or faintness is common, and wide swings in BP occur.

Depending on the site of dissection, inequality of pulses and BP in the upper and lower limbs develops. Dissection of the origins of the renal arteries or celiac axis produces oliguria or abdominal complaints, respectively. Rarely, acute paraplegia is caused by spinal cord infarction. Dissection down to the aortic valve (whether retrograde or originating in the ascending aorta) produces distortion of the valve mechanism, causing aortic insufficiency and a typical murmur. Since aortic valve involvement is often delayed after the onset of the dissection, frequent observation is mandatory. Proximal dissection may also compromise either coronary artery by actual separation of its origin or compression by the intramural hematoma, causing coronary insufficiency or myocardial infarction.

The Ecg. is important in distinguishing this lesion from acute myocardial infarction. In the majority of cases it is normal, but it may show evidence of left ventricular hypertrophy or nonspecific abnormalities.

Mediastinal widening and prominence of the aortic knob are typical findings on plain chest x-rays. Aortography is necessary to establish a definitive diagnosis and should be performed immediately in all suspected cases.

Treatment.

Regardless of the therapy elected (medical or surgical), control of BP is of paramount importance. A systolic pressure below 120 mm. Hg is desirable. Drugs commonly employed include reserpine, 1-2.5 mg. I. M.; guanethidine (Ismelin®), 25-50 mg. orally every 12 hours; and trimethaphan camphorsulfonate (Arfonad®), 1 mg./ml. by I. V. infusion. The latter drug must be administered with caution since sudden and severe hypotension may occur; tachyphylaxis commonly develops after 48 hours. These drugs also depress myocardial contractility, an effect considered important in the limitation of further dissection.

At present, the optimal treatment for acute aortic dissection is controversial. Reports of greatly improved survival with medical therapy based on BP control are considerably more encouraging than the early reported results of surgical treatment alone. However, patients with involvement of the supravalvular aorta remain at high risk. Without operative interruption of the dissection, the vast majority die within days due to intrapericardial rupture. Thus, at the authors' institution, patients with acute dissections of the ascending aorta are always considered for operation, whereas those with dissections limited to the descending aorta may be managed by medical or surgical means with equally good results.

Patients considered for medical management alone include (1) those seen several weeks after the initial event (having survived the period of highest risk); (2) those with diffuse enlargement of the entire descending thoracic aorta; and (3) those with coexistent disease that makes them poor operative risks. Complications such as renal artery involvement do not necessarily contraindicate operation; these lesions are often reversible with restoration of a normal flow pattern.

Operative repair of ascending aortic dissection involves resection of the ascending aorta and graft replacement on full cardiopulmonary bypass. Normal aortic valve configuration can often be restored by removal of the intramural hematoma, and valve replacement is not required. Dissection limited to the descending aorta is treated by excision of a segment of aorta distal to the left subclavian artery (usually the demonstrated site of origin) and graft replacement on partial bypass (femoral vein-femoral artery or left atrial-femoral artery).

Adjunctive therapy to control BP is extremely important throughout all phases of management of acute aortic dissection. Medication should be given as soon as dissection is suspected and continued throughout the postoperative period. Strict antihypertensive control is essential to long-term survival following operative recovery.

Prognosis.

A survival rate of about 80% can be achieved with combined medical and surgical therapy.

DISEASES OF THE PERICARDIUM

ACUTE PERICARDITIS AND TAMPONADE

In the past, the most common recognized cause of surgically significant pericardial disease was tuberculosis; today, viral infection is the presumed cause in the majority of cases. Resected tissue usually presents a histologic picture of acute or chronic nonspecific pericarditis.

An important new cause of both acute and constrictive pericarditis is high-voltage mediastinal irradiation, which may be followed within several months by clinical evidence of pericardial reaction. Acute pericarditis may also be seen following chest trauma, myocardial infarction, or open heart surgery, and occurs in autoimmune disease and uremia. Primary purulent pericarditis is rare. Reviews should be consulted for extensive lists of infrequent causes.

Despite its clinical importance, pericardial disease often goes unrecognized for lack of specific features. Confusion with psychogenic states, primary myocardial disease, and edema syndromes is common. In its primary stages, acute pericarditis is usually associated with fever, vague or localized chest pain, friction rubs, and Ecg. abnormalities. A "flu-like" systemic illness often precedes viral pericarditis. Rapid accumulation of pericardial fluid may result in serious cardiac tamponade; gradual accumulation may cause simple enlargement of the cardiac silhouette ("water bottle heart") on chest x-rays. Frequently, fluid accumulation and clinical deterioration are unpredictable.

The Ecg. shows general ST elevation followed by T wave inversion in the acute stages. With the development of pericardial effusion, Ecg. voltage declines.

Additional aids in the diagnosis of pericardial effusion include radioisotope scans, ultrasound echocardiography, CO_2 contrast studies, and angiocardiography. All are relatively rapid and safe.

Treatment.

The management of acute isolated pericarditis without effusion is conservative. Pericardial effusion producing tamponade demands prompt aspiration or operative intervention since sudden deterioration may develop. Pericardiocentesis is performed as described above for hemopericardium.

Recurrent pericardial effusions or tamponade not easily controlled by a single aspiration are indications for operation. Except in selected cases, the approach should be through a left anterolateral thoracotomy. Most often, the goals of surgical intervention are both diagnostic and therapeutic, and an extensive parietal pericardiectomy is performed. Occasionally, a limited extrapleural incision through the bed of the left fourth costal cartilage is employed for diagnostic purposes or for temporary drainage (pericardial "window").

Prognosis.

The results of elective pericardiectomy for effusion are excellent. Long-term prognosis is chiefly dependent on the type and severity of coexistent myocardial disease.

CONSTRICTIVE PERICARDITIS

An unknown percentage of cases of acute pericarditis progress to a state of cardiac constriction. In occasional patients, a history of acute pericarditis is lacking.

The pathophysiologic features of constrictive pericarditis are related to compromise of ventricular function. Compression of the atria or atrioventricular junctions has not been demonstrated to be significant. The constriction of the ventricles limits diastolic filling, and stroke volume is diminished. Cardiac catheterization demonstrates elevation of intracardiac pressures with equalization of right and left atrial and end-diastolic ventricular pressures. The right ventricular pressure wave shows a prominent early diastolic dip followed by an elevated diastolic plateau.

Clinical manifestations are due to limited cardiac output and systemic congestion. Venous pressure is elevated and typically increases with inspiration (Kussmaul's sign); the neck vein pulsations show early diastolic collapse, corresponding to the right ventricular pressure contour. Hepatomegaly, ascites, and peripheral edema are usually prominent unless diuresis has been vigorous, but pulmonary vascular congestion with associated orthopnea is only occasionally a primary feature. In some patients a secondary syndrome of intestinal lymphangiectasis with malabsorption and immunologic depression may also develop.

Heart size is normal or minimally enlarged upon examination. A palpable early diastolic shock, audible as a third heart sound or pericardial "knock," occurring somewhat earlier than the usual early gallop sound associated with congestive heart failure, is present along the lower left sternal border or near the apex. A paradoxical pulse is present in the peripheral arteries. Although widely considered a misnomer, the term "paradoxical" refers to preservation of the precordial impulse during inspiration while the peripheral pulse weakens.

Ecg. features of chronic constrictive pericarditis include general diminution in size of the QRS complex, ST and T wave changes, and, occasionally, atrial fibrillation. Chest x-rays show a small to minimally increased cardiac silhouette and often foci of calcification in the pericardium. Decreased or absent pulsation of the cardiac border can be observed by fluoroscopy. Left ventriculography demonstrates a small left ventricular cavity with abrupt early diastolic limitation of ventricular filling.

Treatment.

Although digitalis, salt restriction, and diuretics may provide a degree of symptomatic improvement during the early stages of constrictive pericarditis, intractability to medical treatment is a hallmark of this disease. Operative resection of the pericardium provides complete relief in the majority of cases.

Preoperatively, digitalization is recommended to counteract the cardiac dilatation that tends to develop immediately postoperatively. Central venous pressure should be monitored.

The operative approach to complete stripping of the fibrous scar which surrounds the heart should be a left thoracotomy or, with the expectation of severe technical problems, a median sternotomy and cardiopulmonary bypass. Elevation of the epicardial layer is mandatory. Foci of pericardial calcification that extend into the myocardium are more safely left in place as isolated islands. Pericardiectomy should begin over the left ventricle, including the posterior portion, and proceed to the right. Dissection should be especially cautious over the major coronary vessels, atrioventricular grooves, and atria since these structures are easily torn. Complete stripping of the atria and atriocaval junctions is not necessary.

Complications which may occur postoperatively include acute cardiac failure with pulmonary vascular congestion or edema - for which phlebotomy and other routine measures are employed. Excessive early postoperative serous exudation from the denuded cardiac surface occasionally causes a temporary rise in hematocrit.

Prognosis.

Depending on the stage of disease, pericardiectomy can be performed with an operative mortality of 5% or less. Recurrence is uncommon after extensive resections. Limited stripping or creation of a pericardial window for chronic disease is useless.

TUMORS OF THE HEART

Most cardiac tumors are metastatic; primary tumors are comparatively rare. From a therapeutic standpoint, however, primary tumors constitute the more important problem.

Two-thirds of primary tumors are benign, and more than half of these are myxomas. Generally agreed to be true neoplasms, myxomas occur in the left atrium in 75% of cases, usually arising from the atrial septum in the area of the fossa ovalis. Nearly all of the remainder arise in the right side of the septum. Biatrial involvement has been reported.

Malignant cardiac tumors usually originate in the ventricles, more commonly on the right. Because of their mural location, malignant tumors are often far advanced when first diagnosed. Histologically, malignant tumors are sarcomas of variable microscopic type. A serosanguineous pericardial effusion develops in a high percentage of patients with tumors involving the walls of the heart, but is found with both benign and malignant lesions.

Tumors of the heart cause symptoms and signs by virtue of interference with blood flow or ventricular contractions; valvular dysfunction; embolism; and, rarely, arrhythmias. Right-sided lesions usually suggest tricuspid or right ventricular outflow tract anomalies or constrictive pericarditis. Tumors in the left atrium mimic mitral valve disease - either stenosis or insufficiency or a combined lesion.

Features that suggest cardiac tumor include the relatively sudden onset of intractable heart failure, abrupt episodes of syncope, cyanosis, or dyspnea, inconstant or changing murmurs, or strictly position-related symptoms - all in the absence of a history of heart disease. Ultimately, however, a high index of suspicion is necessary for antemortem diagnosis. Many left-sided lesions are still discovered at exploration for mitral disease.

Angiocardiography is the only definitive method of diagnosis and is used to demonstrate the location and extent of the lesion as well as to aid in the differentiation from other conditions.

Treatment.

Benign cardiac tumors usually constitute a pleasant experience for the cardiac surgeon. The pedunculated or sessile myxoma is simply resected at its base. Follow-up studies have shown an excellent prognosis without recurrence.

Cure is not usually possible with malignant tumors. Surgical palliation can be offered for obstructive lesions, and radiotherapy may rarely be effective.

HEART BLOCK

Heart block is a common disease, affecting some 20,000 Americans annually. Before long-term cardiac pacemaking became available, the prognosis was poor, with observed mortality rates as high as 50% within one year of diagnosis.

Heart block is predominantly a disease of the seventh and eighth decades with a higher incidence among men. Most patients pass through a period ranging from a few months to 2 years during which heart block occurs paroxysmally. The intercurrent cardiac rhythm may be normal sinus (often with intermittent first degree heart block), bundle branch block, or second degree block. Following this paroxysmal phase, complete heart block becomes established as the dominant rhythm but is not uncommonly interrupted by occasional episodes of atrioventricular conduction, especially during the early stages. Restoration of atrioventricular conduction after years of established heart block, however, is distinctly rare and remains unexplained.

The manifestations of complete heart block vary considerably and at times inexplicably. The symptomless state is usually associated with a higher idioventricular or nodal rate and probably with better myocardial function (compensatory increase in stroke volume). The majority of patients, however, are symptomatic. Milder symptoms include lightheadedness and exertional dyspnea, and patients with chronic circulatory insufficiency suffer fatigue, shortness of breath, cerebral symptoms, prerenal azotemia, and systemic congestion. The most severe manifestation of heart block is intermittent circulatory arrest due to asystole, or ventricular tachycardia or fibrillation with resultant loss of consciousness. These Adams-Stokes attacks occur without warning, and any single episode may be fatal.

The diagnosis rests on Ecg. findings. If normal sinus rhythm is present at the time of examination, the differential diagnosis of syncope in this elderly age group includes simple syncope, carotid sinus syndrome, cerebrovascular insufficiency, convulsive disorders, and syncope associated with aortic stenosis. Prolonged monitoring may occasionally be necessary to establish the diagnosis.

In addition to complete heart block, there are several less common varieties of bradycardia which are treated similarly. These include severe second degree block, block occurring only with angina, block with atrial fibrillation or flutter, and bradycardia associated with unstable sino-atrial node function ("sick sinus syndrome").

The most common histopathologic finding underlying acquired heart block consists of scattered areas of fibrocalcific degeneration within the conduction system. Major coronary artery lesions are responsible for only a minority of cases. Infiltrative processes or arteritis may infrequently cause permanent heart block in a wide variety of diseases.

In infants with congenital heart block, serious cardiovascular malformations coexist in more than 50%. These include ventricular septal defects, endocardial cushion defects, and transposition abnormalities, especially corrected transposition. In general, the prognosis for children with isolated congenital heart block is more favorable than that for adults with acquired lesions, and in many cases normal activity is possible. Intractable heart failure or recurrent Adams-Stokes attacks, however, are indications for pacemaker insertion despite the greater technical difficulties. In the presence of associated lesions, the prognosis is usually determined by their severity and attendant complications.

Postoperative heart block may follow the repair of congenital defects involving the high ventricular septum or aortic valve replacement. Appreciation of the anatomic relationships of the conduction system has reduced this complication to 1% or less in most centers. Conversion from a temporary postoperative pacemaker to a permanent unit is accomplished in 3-4 weeks if recovery does not occur.

Treatment.

Cardiac pacing is the only definitive treatment for heart block. Although medical therapy is useful for temporary control, prolonged attempts with drug regulation cannot be justified except in cases that respond quickly and completely.

The most effective drug is isoproterenol, which is employed in doses of 5-15 mg. sublingually 3-4 times a day for long-term treatment and as an intravenous infusion containing 2-4 mg./L. for emergencies. Other medical regimens, including anticholinergics, corticosteroids, and kaliuretic agents, are generally ineffective. Drugs that depress cardiac automaticity - e.g., quinidine, procainamide (Pronestyl®), and propranolol (Inderal®) - are contraindicated. Digitalis should be used with caution and only for congestive heart failure.

Temporary pacing is employed (1) for heart block which is expected to be transient, e.g., myocardial infarction, digitalis intoxication, and postoperative heart block; and (2) for temporary control prior to insertion of a permanent unit.

Permanent pacing may be effected with a variety of units that function either synchronously or asynchronously. Synchronous pacemakers offer the physiologic advantage of synchronized atrial and ventricular contractions; a sensing electrode placed on the right atrium monitors atrial depolarization, and the ventricular stimulus is delivered following each P wave after a set delay. The physiologic benefits of synchronized pacing are best suited to the younger patient, whose activity is greater. The disadvantages include the necessity for thoracotomy (systems employing transvenous leads are currently being evaluated) and the lesser reliability associated with increased complexity.

Asynchronous pacing may be delivered on either a fixed rate or demand basis. Because competitive rhythms, due to conducted beats or ventricular extrasystoles, carry a very small but definite risk of pacemaker-induced arrhythmias due to stimulation on or immediately after the peak of the T wave of the preceding extra beat ("vulnerable period stimulation"), demand-type units are now usually employed. These units monitor the intracardiac Ecg. through the pacemaker catheter. Extrasystoles inhibit firing of the pacemaker for a period corresponding to the stimulus-to-stimulus interval of the set rate, and normal sinus rhythm inhibits the pacemaker continuously.

In recent years, the use of the transvenous pacemaker system inserted under local anesthesia has significantly reduced the operative mortality and morbidity associated with thoracotomy and application of epicardial electrodes. Occasional patients (about 5%) defy successful long-term pacing by the transvenous route, and in such cases thoracotomy is mandatory.

The insertion of a transvenous pacemaker should be performed as a major operative procedure. Prophylactic antibiotics are usually employed. Thromboembolism related to the pacemaker catheter has been reported extremely rarely, and anticoagulants are not routinely given.

The most common early postoperative complication is pacing failure, requiring remanipulation of the catheter. Myocardial perforation occurs rarely. Long-term problems include component failure and premature battery exhaustion. Wire breakage has almost been eliminated by the development of better materials. Average battery life is now estimated at $2^1/2$ years.

Recently, atomic power sources (plutonium 238) for electronic pacemakers have been evaluated, both experimentally and clinically. The expected duration of function of such units is 5-10 years.

Prognosis.

The once dismal prognosis for patients with heart block has been greatly improved by pacemaker therapy.

VALVE SURGERY

Valve Substitutes.

The introduction of the caged-ball valve prosthesis in 1960 ushered in an era of remarkable growth in cardiac surgery. The ability to replace diseased valves not amenable to reconstructive procedures led to rapid extension of surgical therapy to thousands of patients whose lesions were otherwise untreatable.

With the widespread application of these new technics has come an appreciation of their inherent limitations. In most patients, pressure gradients at rest can be demonstrated across the prosthetic valve orifice; these increase with exercise. Valve-related thrombosis and embolism constitute a serious problem, occurring in up to 40% of patients with mitral replacement and 25% of patients with aortic replacement in earlier series. Recent valve models incorporating extended cloth covering of nonmoving metal parts are apparently associated with a lower incidence of thromboembolism: less than 5% with aortic replacements and approximately 10% with mitral valves. Anticoagulants exert a slight protective effect. A significant incidence (2-3%) of postoperative endocarditis on prosthetic valves remains a formidable complication. Occasionally, mechanical failure has been caused by physical distortion of the ball in the earlier aortic and even mitral replacements. Finally, traumatic hemolytic syndromes occurring as a result of periprosthetic leaks, tissue ingrowth, or occasionally without known cause may be responsible for serious postoperative morbidity.

These considerations have stimulated intense experimentation in the development of better valve substitutes. Widespread enthusiasm has developed over the use of aortic valve homografts and heterografts in both the aortic and atrioventricular positions. Although freedom from a significant immune response has been demonstrated, the long-term durability of such valves remains in question. Valves subjected to physicochemical trauma such as sterilization and preservation by beta-propiolactone, formaldehyde, or freeze-drying show a significant incidence of delayed tissue failure. Even homografts obtained sterilely and implanted in "fresh" condition may develop late degenerative changes, especially stented valves in the mitral position. Glutaraldehyde-preserved heterograft (porcine) valves are currently under clinical investigation and early reports are encouraging, but their suitability remains unproved. The late results of valves fabricated with autologous fascia lata or pericardium have proved unsatisfactory.

In the mitral or tricuspid position, anatomic relationships necessitate fixation of aortic valve grafts to some kind of supporting prosthetic ring or stent which is then inserted into the annulus. For aortic replacement, tailored homografts may be sewn in directly or may be inserted with a stent as is done with heterografts.

The principal advantage of biologic valve replacement is the virtual absence of thromboembolism. Anticoagulants are unnecessary after aortic substitution but are usually given for several weeks following mitral or tricuspid replacement. Although directly implanted aortic homografts present no central impedance to flow, stented valves are usually associated with small transvalvular pressure gradients. Such valves may impose a lesser risk of postoperative endocarditis. The disadvantages of direct aortic homograft insertion include greater technical difficulty and a high incidence of postoperative diastolic murmurs (15-40%), representing in the majority of cases a trivial hemodynamic insufficiency.

Selection and Preparation of Patients.

With current technics, most patients with primary valvular heart disease are potential candidates for operation regardless of the severity of coexistent myocardial failure. This is not to ignore the fact that advanced heart failure with severe secondary organ dysfunction may carry a poor prognosis with or without operation. There is little or nothing to be gained, however, by reserving surgical intervention until decompensation has become intractable to medical therapy.

For purposes of classification and evaluation, patients with valvular heart disease may be grouped functionally by the following criteria of the New York Heart Association:

- Class I: No limitation of activity.
- Class II: Ordinary activity results in fatigue, dyspnea, or anginal pain.
- Class III: Comfortable at rest, but less than ordinary activity causes symptoms.
- Class IV: Symptoms at rest, increased with any activity.

Following the decision for operation, a variable waiting period is usually necessary. During this interval, it is important that optimal medical therapy be continued. Readmission to the hospital 2 days to a week prior to operation is important in several aspects.

Digitalis and diuretics should be stopped at least 2 days before operation to avoid the apparent precipitation of digitoxic arrhythmias by cardiopulmonary bypass. Patients with a history of severe heart failure and intense diuretic treatment should be given supplemental potassium to replete body stores. If possible, antiarrhythmic drugs should be avoided in the immediate preoperative period. Anticoagulants should be discontinued several days before operation, and vitamin K should be administered if needed to return the prothrombin time toward normal. Persistence of a mild anticoagulant effect, however, is not necessarily a contraindication to operation inasmuch as vitamin K-dependent clotting factors are restored by blood-primed bypass or transfusion. In addition, baseline serum electrolytes, BUN, a hemogram, Ecg., and chest x-rays are obtained.

Although the use of prophylactic antibiotics for open heart surgery remains controversial, it seems unlikely that this issue will be settled by carefully controlled studies. The results of longitudinal studies showing a decrease in the incidence of postoperative endocarditis when antibiotics are employed and the current low incidence of infection preclude any radical change in antibiotic management in the near future. Most centers employ penicillin or a penicillin substitute plus a semisynthetic penicillin resistant to penicillinase as well as another antibiotic active against gram-negative organisms. These are begun 1-2 days prior to operation and continued for several days to a few months postoperatively. During the intraoperative and immediate postoperative periods, intravenous administration to achieve high blood levels is usually employed.

Postoperative Management.

Immediately after operation, several areas of concern simultaneously assume importance. These include respiratory care, hemorrhage, the state of cardiac output, arrhythmias, and renal function. Depending on the preoperative state of the patient and the technical aspects of operation, these problems may demand more or less continuous observation by the physician.

A. Respiratory Care: Respiratory insufficiency of variable degree is common following open heart surgery. Preoperative factors which predispose to respiratory complications include pulmonary hypertension, severe pulmonary congestion or edema, lung disease, chest deformities, cerebrovascular accidents with neurologic residual, extreme age or debilitation, and pulmonary sepsis. Intraoperative complications that lead to postoperative respiratory failure include prolonged cardiopulmonary bypass, acute pulmonary vascular congestion due to left heart distention or pulmonary venous obstruction, overtransfusion, myocardial damage producing left-sided heart failure, and alterations in pulmonary surfactant.

Postoperatively, nearly all patients develop some degree of pulmonary venous admixture due to atelectasis and other factors. The postoperative chest x-rays usually fail to reflect the degree of pulmonary dysfunction indicated by physiologic studies. In the majority of cases, these abnormalities are transient and resolve with the usual measures of vigorous coughing, intermittent positive pressure breathing, and supplemental oxygen. In the remainder, however, some form of respiratory assistance is necessary if serious consequences are to be avoided. In addition to obvious respiratory distress and cyanosis, these patients develop low cardiac output and arrhythmias. Frequent monitoring of arterial blood gases in high-risk patients is recommended.

The management of respiratory insufficiency consists of mechanical assistance for as long as needed and vigorous tracheobronchial toilet. Patients liable to postoperative problems may be ventilated via an endotracheal or nasotracheal tube for 24-72 hours, following which the majority may be extubated to assume spontaneous ventilation with supplemental oxygen. Maintenance of a small and positive end-expiratory pressure during continuous mechanical ventilation may be helpful in minimizing atelectasis. Those patients whose arterial gases during spontaneous respiration show significant desaturation should be ventilated via tracheostomy. Tracheostomy should be performed without delay once its need is established and may be performed at the time of operation after closure of the sternal wound without fear of wound infection.

Although tracheostomy management is not yet fully satisfactory, improvements in tube and cuff design (low-pressure, high-volume cuff) have reduced the incidence of tracheomalacia and consequent late stricture. Tracheal aspiration should be performed gently and sterilely; saline solutions in 5-10 ml. amounts may be used to loosen tenacious secretions. Occlusive cuffs should be deflated at least once every hour to minimize the chances of pressure necrosis.

Weaning from tracheostomy support consists essentially of gradually increasing periods without ventilatory assistance followed by gradually decreasing concentrations of inspired oxygen. Weaning should not be performed abruptly and should be monitored by intermittent blood gas studies.

B. Hemorrhage: Some degree of blood loss is to be expected following open cardiac procedures, and adequate drainage of the pericardial space and chest is essential. What constitutes excessive hemorrhage in any given case is often a matter of experience and individual judgment. Steady and continuous drainage through the chest tubes of more than 100 ml./hour for several hours in the adult, however, usually demands specific investigation.

The great majority of cases of postoperative hemorrhage are due to inadequate surgical hemostasis. In the face of brisk hemorrhage, reoperation should not be delayed while waiting for the determination of coagulation factors and platelet counts. If there is a suspicion of abnormal coagulation, such studies may be obtained simultaneously with reoperation. Procrastination with excessive postoperative hemorrhage is dangerous.

Other causes of hemorrhage include inadequate heparin neutralization, which may be treated with 25-50 mg. incremental doses of protamine, given slowly I. V., controlled if desired by the thrombin time. Thrombocytopenic bleeding is managed with platelet packs or fresh blood. Abnormal fibrinolysis, considered to be an important cause of postoperative bleeding in some patients (especially cyanotic patients), is treated with aminocaproic acid (Amicar®), primarily an inhibitor of plasminogen activation. Hemorrhage associated with generalized depression of clotting factors is treated with fresh whole blood or component products (e.g., Konyne®) as indicated, as well as with vitamin K.

C. Low Cardiac Output: The occurrence of a low cardiac output state (postperfusion low output syndrome) following open heart procedures is always an ominous complication and requires aggressive management. It is a form of postoperative shock and is recognized clinically by the usual signs of hypotension, diminished pulse pressure, cold extremities, oliguria, mental obtundation, and respiratory distress. For practical purposes, the pathogenesis of the low output syndrome may be related to (1) hypovolemia, (2) cardiac tamponade, and (3) factors within the heart itself.

Low output associated with hypovolemia is common and is suggested by low central venous or atrial pressure. Treatment consists of volume expansion with blood. Frequently, despite correction of valvular lesions, blood volume must be restored to preoperative or greater levels to maintain satisfactory cardiac output immediately following operation. Patients with persisting pulmonary hypertension or tricuspid insufficiency often require relatively high venous pressures (e.g., 20-25 cm. saline).

Depressed cardiac output due to cardiac tamponade is suggested by the above signs plus elevated venous pressure and enlargement of the cardiac silhouette and mediastinum on chest x-rays. This complication may occur despite drainage of the pericardium because of the accumulation of clots around the heart. The usual signs of tamponade are indistinct or absent; a paradoxical pulse is impossible to detect reliably with an irregular cardiac rhythm or with positive pressure ventilation. The clinical situation is often precarious, and reexploration should not be delayed.

The contribution of myocardial factors to the postoperative low output syndrome is both complex and incompletely resolved. Although anatomic (incompletely repaired or undetected lesions) or mechanical (obstruction to flow caused by a ball valve prosthesis) problems may be at fault, more frequently no recognizable cause can be defined. These cases presumably relate to injury of the myocardium during cardiopulmonary bypass.

The low cardiac output syndrome is complicated by progressive metabolic acidosis and oliguria. Additional volume loads, digitalis, and vasopressors may temporarily increase the BP but usually do not provide permanent relief. Promising results have been obtained with agents that lower cardiac work while simultaneously increasing myocardial efficiency. Isoproterenol is the drug of choice in patients without excessive tachycardia. Alpha-adrenergic blocking agents, e.g., phenoxybenzamine (Dibenzyline®), or corticosteroids in massive doses are occasionally of value as adjuncts. With peripheral vasodilatation, volume replacement is usually necessary. Meticulous attention to acid-base balance should be maintained and acidosis corrected with bicarbonate. Respiratory support is always necessary. In successful cases, recovery usually occurs within 24 hours, but circulatory support may be required for periods of days.

D. Arrhythmias: Some type of arrhythmia occurs in virtually all patients undergoing open heart procedures. Patients particularly prone to develop serious ventricular arrhythmias include those with advanced myocardial disease or potassium depletion. Postoperative factors responsible for the precipitation of arrhythmias include hypoxia, hypokalemia, alkalosis, myocardial ischemia, and excessive digitalization. Each should be carefully considered before depressant antiarrhythmic drugs are employed.

The management of ventricular arrhythmias depends entirely on the underlying conditions outlined above. Hypoxia should be treated with respiratory assistance, and alkalosis due to hyperventilation should be minimized. Intravenous potassium should be administered unless serum potassium is elevated, and occasional patients may require quite large amounts of potassium to replace urinary loss (up to 300 mEq. daily). Patients with slow sinus or nodal rhythm complicated by ventricular irritability should be treated with isoproterenol infusion or pacing. In most instances, the augmentation of rate alone is sufficient to suppress ventricular foci.

Patients not responding to these measures should receive antiarrhythmic drugs. A continuous infusion of lidocaine (Xylocaine®), 4 mg./ml., is effective and most easily controlled. Procainamide (Pronestyl®) may also be given intravenously, either intermittently or continuously. Propranolol (Inderal®) is occasionally useful, but it is dangerous in the early postoperative period.

Heart block or slow nodal rhythm occurring at the time of operation is managed by temporary pacing instituted on the operating table.

The prompt treatment of ventricular arrhythmias is often crucial to postoperative survival, and there should be no hesitation in the use of countershock once any arrhythmia degenerates into a life-threatening situation.

Atrial arrhythmias occurring postoperatively usually present as flutter or fibrillation, preceded by frequent premature atrial contractions. Paroxysmal atrial tachycardia occurs less commonly, and, if attended by 2:1 block, implies digitalis toxicity. The cardiac rate almost always increases with the onset of these arrhythmias. Digitalis is used to increase the degree of atrioventricular block and is given parenterally (digoxin). Excessive doses should be avoided since sudden toxicity with ventricular fibrillation may occur. Some patients with atrial flutter show a relative resistance to the action of digitalis, and in these it is safer to proceed early with cardioversion. If full doses of digitalis have already been administered, it is reasonable to give a small dose of lidocaine before cardioversion to minimize postconversion ventricular arrhythmias.

The vast majority of patients undergoing isolated aortic valve replacement who develop atrial fibrillation postoperatively will spontaneously revert to sinus rhythm. Those who fail to do so should be cardioverted electively. Many (but not all) patients in whom atrial fibrillation persists following mitral valve operations should be considered for cardioversion. Factors favorable for the maintenance of sinus rhythm after cardioversion include a small left atrium and less than 3 years' duration of atrial fibrillation. Quinidine exerts a stabilizing effect following cardioversion and, if given in full doses, significantly increases the chance of maintaining sinus rhythm. With the availability of present technics, quinidine should never be used as the primary agent in attempted conversion to sinus rhythm.

E. Renal Failure: Acute renal failure secondary to tubular necrosis is currently an infrequent complication of open heart surgery. Its causes include excessive hemolysis or ischemia during prolonged cardiopulmonary bypass, and postoperative hypotension. Patients with depressed renal function preoperatively are significantly more vulnerable.

In some centers, the incidence of renal failure related to bypass has been reduced by the intraoperative use of osmotic diuretics, alpha blocking agents, or fluid loads. The routine use of these methods, however, is not justified where experience has demonstrated technically satisfactory bypass control with a negligible incidence of renal damage, since serious electrolyte imbalance may result from induced diuresis.

The problems of potassium metabolism and acid-base and fluid balance are magnified in the postoperative cardiac patient with borderline myocardial function and renal failure, and recent experience has suggested that dialysis instituted early appreciably improves the survival rate. Rapid shifts in potassium and intravascular volume should be avoided.

Delayed Postoperative Complications.

Two syndromes occurring after cardiac operations - the postcardiotomy syndrome and the postperfusion syndrome - are important from the standpoint of confusion with endocarditis. Both are self-limited and managed conservatively. The former, of unknown cause, develops within days to months following operation and is characterized by fever, fatigue, and pleural pericarditis with chest pain and friction rubs. Treatment with aspirin is usually effective, although in severe cases corticosteroids may be considered. Infrequently, the syndrome recurs one or more times. The principal features of the postperfusion syndrome, occurring 2-6 weeks postoperatively, are fever, splenomegaly, and atypical lymphocytes in the peripheral blood. Rashes and lymphadenopathy may also develop. This complication is probably due to infection by cytomegalovirus.

Endocarditis following prosthetic valve replacement is an extremely serious complication with mortality rates in most series well over 50%. It may be acquired at operation, but usually at some time thereafter. Dental sepsis is a frequent causative factor. The majority of infections are due to staphylococci, with a predominance of penicillin-resistant strains, but a wide variety of organisms has been reported, including gram-negative bacteria, fungi, and yeasts.

Since it is unusual for these patients to present the classic clinical picture of endocarditis, accurate diagnosis depends almost entirely on clinical suspicion followed by thorough blood cultures incorporating technics for the identification of anaerobic bacteria and fungi. Any patient with fever that persists beyond the first postoperative week should be evaluated for endocarditis.

Initial treatment is medical, employing high doses of appropriate antimicrobial agents, but the failure rate is high. For this reason, operative intervention with debridement and replacement of infected valves under antibiotic coverage has been employed with increasing frequency in recent years. Inability to maintain blood stream sterility, disruption of prostheses, repeated emboli, and endocarditis-related congestive heart failure constitute operative indications. Despite theoretic obstacles, many otherwise intractable cases have been apparently cured in this manner.

AORTIC VALVE DISEASE

Calcific aortic stenosis is in most cases probably the result of gradual calcification of a congenitally deformed valve. Noncalcific stenosis in adults nearly always represents rheumatic valvulitis. Aortic insufficiency may result from syphilis (rare), rheumatic valvulitis (most common), endocarditis, congenital deformity (rare except in association with ventricular septal defect), or prolapsing cusps (degenerative). Isolated aortic valve disease is common and constitutes about 40% of valve lesions coming to operation.

Characteristically, cardiac compensation is well maintained with isolated aortic lesions until relatively late in the clinical course. A competent mitral valve and progressive left ventricular hypertrophy protect the pulmonary vascular bed until myocardial failure supervenes. The onset of angina pectoris, syncope, or congestive heart failure initiates a phase of relatively rapid deterioration with expected survivals of approximately 4, 3, and 2 years, respectively.

The clinical findings in isolated aortic stenosis include slow-rising and small arterial pulses, a left ventricular heave, and a systolic thrill and murmur in the second right intercostal space. The aortic component of the second sound is usually diminished or absent, and is frequently followed by a short murmur of aortic insufficiency due to the fixed valve orifice.

Aortic insufficiency is manifested by many signs that reflect the increased left ventricular stroke volume and widened pulse pressure. These include quick-rising and collapsing peripheral pulses, jerking carotid pulses, bobbing of the head, and a prominent left ventricular heave. The aortic component of the second sound may be diminished and initiates a long, high-pitched diminuendo murmur. A systolic flow murmur, transmitted to the neck, and an apical diastolic rumble (Austin Flint murmur) are usually audible.

The Ecg. shows left ventricular hypertrophy in the majority of cases of both aortic stenosis and insufficiency, with ST and T wave changes indicative of a so-called "strain" pattern. Atrioventricular conduction time (P-R interval) is frequently at the upper limits of normal or slightly prolonged, and slight prolongation of the QRS complex (usually an incomplete left bundle branch block pattern) is common. Atrial fibrillation occurs only late in the clinical course and accompanies severe congestive failure. If present earlier, it suggests associated mitral valvular disease.

Chest x-rays in aortic stenosis show a normal-sized or slightly enlarged left ventricle until failure occurs. Poststenotic dilatation of the ascending aorta, best seen on the posteroanterior and left anterior oblique projections, is usually present. Valve calcification is most prominent on the lateral projection. With aortic insufficiency, dilatation of the left ventricle often reaches severe proportions.

In some cases of symptomatic aortic valve disease with typical clinical findings, cardiac catheterization is superfluous. It should be performed, however, in atypical cases, congenital lesions, or cases in which the contribution of coronary disease is uncertain. Coronary artery disease and acquired aortic valve lesions often coexist, and in patients with histories dominated by angina pectoris coronary arteriography should be performed. In the presence of significant stenotic lesions of the major coronary arteries, an aortocoronary vein bypass procedure should be carried out in conjunction with aortic valve replacement. Cardiac catheterization provides little more than an estimate of the degree of heart failure in pure aortic insufficiency. Angiography and ventricular volume studies provide additional data that may be of help in decision-making in some cases.

A valvular gradient in excess of 50 mm. Hg in aortic stenosis is usually indicative of severe stenosis and supports a recommendation for operative repair. It should be remembered, however, that measured gradients are flow-dependent, and heart failure with subnormal cardiac output may produce a gradient considerably less than 50 mm. Hg. Therefore, the calculated aortic valve area is more useful unless significant valvular insufficiency is present.

Areas less than 1 sq. cm. (0.6 sq. cm./sq. meter body surface) indicate severe stenosis and are generally symptomatic. These comments apply also to patients with reduced forward flow due to coexistent mitral lesions.

Treatment.

Debridement of calcified valves and other plastic procedures are employed rarely today. Many types of mechanical prostheses are available, but all possess the drawbacks discussed above.

Aortic valve replacement is performed with operative mortality rates of 5-10% in experienced centers. The operative approach is a median sternotomy which allows access to mitral and tricuspid lesions as well. Many technics are used for myocardial protection during the period of aortic cross-clamping, including right and left coronary artery perfusion, left coronary perfusion alone, and local hypothermia of the heart induced with saline at 4-6° C. The latter technic provides satisfactory myocardial preservation for periods in excess of 2 hours. Coexistent aneurysms of the ascending aorta due to cystic medial necrosis should be replaced by graft simultaneously with valve replacement. Unless treated, these aneurysms commonly dissect and rupture.

Prognosis.

The late results of aortic valve replacement are gratifying in the majority of patients. Angina and syncopal attacks disappear, heart size decreases, and exercise tolerance improves, frequently to normal or nearly normal levels. The late mortality rate appears to be between 5-10% per year for the first 5 postoperative years. Most late deaths are due to persistent coronary artery or myocardial disease, endocarditis, emboli, anticoagulation complications, mechanical valve failure, or unexplained causes (sudden death).

MITRAL VALVE DISEASE

Mitral stenosis is almost always the result of rheumatic valvulitis originating in childhood or adolescence. Congenital mitral stenosis is rare. Mitral insufficiency, due in most cases to rheumatic fever (often as a mixed lesion with stenosis and insufficiency), is also acquired as a complication of coronary artery disease (papillary muscle dysfunction or rupture), endocarditis, or degenerative lesions in the valve tissue (leaflet prolapse, ruptured chordae tendineae).

In contrast to aortic valvular disease, the clinical course with mitral lesions is usually protracted following the onset of symptoms. About 10% of patients with mitral stenosis suffer peripheral emboli (the majority of recognized emboli are cerebral), although the total incidence of left atrial thrombi, including those found at operation, is significantly higher.

Acute severe mitral insufficiency is usually tolerated poorly. Most patients with papillary muscle rupture die within days to weeks.

Clinical findings in patients with pure mitral stenosis and normal sinus rhythm include an accentuated mitral component of the first heart sound and an opening snap followed by a diastolic rumble with presystolic accentuation. A diastolic thrill is frequently palpable at the apex. With the onset of atrial fibrillation, presystolic accentuation of the diastolic murmur is lost. Extensive valve calcification causes loss of the opening snap. Progressive pulmonary hypertension and right ventricular failure cause accentuation of the pulmonic component of the second heart sound which may be followed by a faint murmur of pulmonic insufficiency (Graham Steell murmur), a right ventricular lift, and often a separate murmur of secondary tricuspid insufficiency. A pulsating liver is evidence of severe tricuspid insufficiency.

Mitral insufficiency due to rheumatic damage frequently coexists as a mixed lesion with stenosis. Pure insufficiency causes a full, high-pitched systolic murmur associated with an early diastolic gallop rhythm and left ventricular impulse. Although the murmur typically is transmitted to the left axilla and back, it may radiate to the base of the heart and simulate aortic stenosis if the regurgitant jet is directed toward the root of the aorta.

The Ecg. in isolated mitral disease usually shows a rightward axis and abnormal P waves (left atrial enlargement) or atrial fibrillation. Other signs of right ventricular hypertrophy may be present, and evidence of left ventricular hypertrophy indicates mitral insufficiency, associated aortic valve disease, or systemic hypertension.

Cardiac x-rays reveal features of left atrial enlargement in cases of chronic mitral disease, including posterior displacement of the barium-filled esophagus, elevation of the left main stem bronchus, and a double density or contour at the right border of the heart. The aortic knob is typically normal or small. Mitral insufficiency causes left ventricular enlargement, but, if recently acquired, little or no left atrial dilatation. Additional changes associated with pulmonary hypertension include prominent pulmonary vascular markings with pulmonary venous congestion and evidence of redistribution of blood flow to the upper lobes, and an enlarged pulmonary artery, right ventricle, and right atrium. Valve calcification is often present with rheumatic lesions, but its absence on routine films does not rule it out.

The usual findings at cardiac catheterization include elevated right ventricular, pulmonary artery, and wedge pressures in addition to a diastolic transvalvular mitral pressure gradient. The cardiac output may be normal or low but fails to rise normally with exercise, causing an abnormal increase in mixed arteriovenous oxygen difference. The pulmonary artery wedge pressure, reflecting pulmonary venous pressure, shows high V waves in the presence of mitral insufficiency. Left atrial catheterization, if necessary for pressure measurement or angiocardiography, is best performed by transseptal puncture.

Operative intervention is indicated in those patients whose valve disease causes significant symptoms. The occurrence of emboli alone as a manifestation of the valvular lesion is usually taken as an indication for operation, although this remains controversial.

Treatment.

In many centers, closed mitral commissurotomy is never performed today, and rigorous preoperative evaluation for a closed procedure is superfluous. The risk of intraoperative emboli due to unsuspected left atrial thrombi, the occurrence of significant mitral regurgitation with blind maneuvers, and the better functional result which may attend accurate incision of visualized valves justify routine use of the open approach. Properly performed closed commissurotomy in stringently selected patients, however, may produce excellent results. Ideal patients for this procedure are women under age 40 with pure mitral stenosis, normal sinus rhythm, a small left atrium, and no calcification in the mitral apparatus. Most patients coming to operation fall within functional classes II and III; in these, operative mortality - whether a plastic procedure or valve replacement is performed - is 4-8% in most large series. Class IV disability carries a significantly higher risk, which may exceed 50% in very advanced cases with long-standing myocardial failure and irreversible pulmonary vascular disease.

The type of procedure employed at operation depends entirely on the valvular pathology encountered. Commissurotomy can generally be performed in the earlier stages of rheumatic valvulitis characterized by mild thickening and fibrosis of the leaflets with fusion of the commissures and chordae tendineae. Valve replacement is required, however, when there is progressive damage with calcification of the leaflets and annulus and loss of effective valve substance. Pure mitral insufficiency due to annular dilatation may be approached by annuloplasty, and ruptured chordae may be reattached; however, long-term results are not reliable, and replacement is required in the majority of cases.

Prognosis.

Almost 85% of patients undergoing mitral valve operations are significantly improved postoperatively. The fall in left atrial pressure following operation is accompanied by regression of pulmonary hypertension over periods extending up to a year or more. Poor clinical results not related to complications of mechanical prostheses are usually due to persistent myocardial disease or tricuspid insufficiency. Late mortality rates with valve replacement are approximately 5-12% per year with current technics.

Following mitral commissurotomy, most patients maintain improvement for at least 5-6 years. Unsatisfactory immediate postoperative results are usually due to incomplete relief of stenosis or production of mitral regurgitation. The reported incidence of restenosis varies widely but has ranged from 5-25% at 5 years up to 50% at 10 years postoperatively.

TRICUSPID VALVE DISEASE

Although acquired organic disease of the tricuspid valve is uncommon, secondary dilatation due to chronic right ventricular failure is often seen with advanced mitral lesions. Management depends entirely on evaluation at the time of operation. Lesser degrees of insufficiency do not require manipulation, since valvular competence is usually restored as heart failure recedes postoperatively. Although annuloplasty may be utilized satisfactorily in most instances of moderate or even severe insufficiency, gross insufficiency and stenotic disease usually require valve replacement. Persistent tricuspid insufficiency following mitral valve operations complicates the immediate postoperative course and can account for residual clinical limitations.

MULTIPLE VALVE DISEASE

In recent years, multiple valve replacement has become commonplace, with little increase in operative mortality over that associated with isolated valve replacement in most large series. The least favorable results are obtained in patients in whom triple valve replacement (aortic, mitral, and tricuspid) is necessary, probably because of the severity of myocardial disease encountered in this group. Postoperatively, morbidity rates for replacement of more than one valve are not fully additive, although the incidence of thromboembolism is somewhat increased.

The technical problems encountered at operation are related to the greater length of cardiopulmonary bypass required and the longer period of elective myocardial ischemia. In most instances, this ranges from 1½-2½ hours. The attendant problems of electrolyte imbalance and acid-base disturbance may require more intensive management. Myocardial protection during the prolonged period of aortic cross-clamping can be achieved satisfactorily with local hypothermia of the heart alone, although most centers employ some form of coronary perfusion.

CONGENITAL HEART DISEASE

The importance of congenital heart disease has been appreciated in recent years as methods for palliation or total correction of the majority of these defects have become available. Although the figures of incidence vary considerably, most place the overall incidence between 3 and 8 per 1000 live births. Depending on the criteria for patient selection, wide discrepancies occur in the estimated incidence of individual lesions. Combined statistics, however, show that the commonest lesions are atrial septal defect, ventricular septal defect, tetralogy of Fallot, patent ductus arteriosus, pulmonic stenosis, and coarctation of the aorta. Transposition of the great vessels accounts for the majority of deaths due to congenital heart disease in early infancy.

Complete evaluation of the patient with congenital heart disease, including elucidation of both the functional (cardiac catheterization) and anatomic (angiocardiography) features of the lesion, is the key to an effective surgical approach. In the history and systems review, particular attention should be paid to the chronology of the illness, growth and developmental problems, feeding history, exercise tolerance, respiratory problems, the occurrence of cyanosis or "anoxic spells," and CNS symptoms. Questions regarding both the prenatal history and the occurrence of congenital heart disease in other family members may provide clues to diagnosis.

It should be remembered that although congenital cardiac defects limit life expectancy, many may be found in older people. Corrective operations for symptomatic atrial defects have been performed successfully in persons in the eighth decade.

The selected defects discussed below comprise more than 80% of all those encountered.

ACYANOTIC DEFECTS

1. ATRIAL SEPTAL DEFECT

There are 3 common types of atrial septal defect: ostium secundum, sinus venosus, and ostium primum (a form of endocardial cushion defect). Atrial septal defect is more common in females by a ratio of approximately 2:1.

Cardiac failure in childhood or adolescence due to atrial septal defects of the first 2 types is very unusual. After age 20, the incidence of symptoms rises progressively. In most series, the average survival has been limited to the fifth decade of life. The ostium primum variety, however, frequently causes symptoms during childhood and may cause cardiac failure. The average duration of life is shorter.

The clinical findings in atrial septal defects, in addition to the Ecg. and cardiac x-rays, usually permit diagnosis. The left-to-right shunt causes a systolic flow murmur best heard in the second left intercostal space, and in most cases a diastolic flow murmur arising from the tricuspid valve and heard in the area of the lower sternum. The second heart sound in the pulmonic area is widely split and does not vary with respiration (fixed splitting). Right ventricular dilatation may cause a left-sided chest deformity and a palpable right ventricular lift. Pulmonary hypertension reduces the splitting of the second sound and accentuates the pulmonic component; if severe, it may cause reversal of the interatrial shunt with cyanosis and clubbing. With ostium primum defect, a separate murmur of mitral insufficiency is usually heard at the apex, transmitted to the axilla and back.

Atrial septal defects are characterized on Ecg. by right axis deviation and incomplete right bundle branch block in the secundum and sinus venosus types; the presence of a coronary sinus rhythm strongly suggests a sinus venosus defect or a coexistent left superior vena cava. Left axis deviation with the incomplete right bundle branch block pattern is associated with an endocardial cushion abnormality (ostium primum defect). The typical radiologic features are increased pulmonary vascularity, cardiomegaly with right ventricular and right atrial enlargement, a prominent main pulmonary artery, and a diminutive aortic knob.

The diagnosis is confirmed by cardiac catheterization, which demonstrates an oxygen step-up in the right atrium and allows calculation of the shunt flow.

Treatment.

The surgical treatment of uncomplicated atrial septal defects of the secundum or sinus venosus variety is eminently satisfactory, with operative mortality rates approaching zero. Repair is best performed during childhood. With increasing pulmonary hypertension, the operative risk approaches 25%, and in the presence of a net right-to-left shunt (Eisenmenger reaction) operation is contraindicated. Many secundum defects can be closed primarily, but pericardial or synthetic patches are required in the large circular variety. The high sinus venosus defect with displacement of one or more pulmonary veins into the right atrium is managed easily by patch closure, which simultaneously diverts pulmonary venous drainage into the left atrium. An isolated pulmonary vein draining high into the superior vena cava is best ignored.

In ostium primum defects the associated mitral cleft can usually be obliterated by suturing together the folding edges of the cleft. Complete valve competency, however, is often not restored. Rarely, the interposition of a patch may be necessary to bridge a wide tissue defect. The atrial septal defect is closed by patch, with particular attention to the placement of sutures in the area of the atrioventricular bundle.

Prognosis.

The postoperative response is almost always gratifying, and most patients are restored to normal physical capacity. Those with severe preoperative pulmonary hypertension may be left with residual symptoms.

2. VENTRICULAR SEPTAL DEFECT

The clinical course of patients born with isolated ventricular septal defects is extremely variable, depending upon the size of the defect and the reaction of the pulmonary vasculature to the left-to-right shunt. Patients with small defects and normal pulmonary artery pressure may remain asymptomatic throughout life. Those with larger defects and shunts are vulnerable to the development of pulmonary vascular obstruction and congestive heart failure. These changes usually develop after the first few years of life but may appear during infancy. Infants born with large defects associated with torrential left-to-right shunts frequently develop congestive heart failure and pulmonary complications with an early mortality up to 20%. Spontaneous closure of ventricular septal defects has been well documented, and is estimated to occur in up to 20% of small defects.

A significant risk for patients with ventricular septal defects of all sizes is bacterial endocarditis; this factor may constitute the major indication for operation in patients with small defects.

Clinical findings in patients with small, asymptomatic defects ("maladie de Roger") are limited to a harsh systolic murmur, maximal at the lower left sternal border and associated with an easily palpable thrill. In patients with greater left-to-right shunts, there is an apical diastolic flow murmur due to increased flow across the mitral valve and evidence of biventricular enlargement. The development of pulmonary hypertension causes accentuation of the pulmonic component of the second heart sound with a decrease in inspiratory splitting.

In patients with significant shunts, chest x-rays show increased pulmonary vascularity, prominent pulmonary artery, inconspicuous aortic knob, and cardiomegaly with right and left ventricular enlargement. Left atrial enlargement may be present as well. The Ecg. is usually normal with small defects, but with larger ones demonstrates right ventricular hypertrophy, alone or combined with left ventricular hypertrophy.

Because of the unpredictable course of the pulmonary vascular resistance in patients with significant shunts, operative correction is recommended as soon as feasible. The ideal age is 4-8 years. Repair is contraindicated in patients with severe pulmonary hypertension with predominantly or exclusively right-to-left shunts. Disagreement exists concerning the management of patients with very small shunts (pulmonary to systemic flow ratio less than 1.5). In experienced centers where mortality rates approach zero, operation may be recommended to remove the threat of bacterial endocarditis and the social disadvantages of heart disease.

Treatment.

Operative correction of a ventricular septal defect under direct vision in 1954 marked a milestone in the history of cardiac surgery. The usual approach is through a right ventriculotomy. Technical manipulations are facilitated by elective cardiac arrest with myocardial hypothermia. Only small defects with firm scarred edges should be closed by direct suture; all others require patch closure. Placement of sutures on the right side of the septum away from the posteroinferior edge of the ventricular septal defect is necessary to avoid the main atrioventricular conducting bundle. Right bundle branch block is commonly produced by operation, but is inconsequential.

Prognosis.

In patients without severe preoperative elevation of the pulmonary vascular resistance, operative results are excellent, with mortality rates close to zero. Heart block and residual defects are rare complications. As pulmonary vascular resistance approaches the level of systemic resistance, however, mortality rates rise to 10-20% or higher.

Surgical palliation for infants in intractable congestive heart failure due to large ventricular septal defects can be achieved by simple banding of the pulmonary artery to reduce the left-to-right shunt. Repair of the ventricular septal defect is performed as a second stage procedure, at which time the pulmonary artery is reconstructed.

3. PULMONIC STENOSIS

Isolated pulmonic stenosis with an intact ventricular septum is usually due to valvular obstruction with or without infundibular hypertrophy, but in 10% of cases it may be due to infundibular obstruction alone. While it is clear that severe elevation of right ventricular pressure shortens life expectancy, the natural history of mild stenosis with a right ventricular pressure less than 50 mm. Hg is less well documented.

Clinical limitation is directly related to the degree of obstruction. Symptoms range from florid congestive heart failure with low cardiac output in infants with severe stenosis to mild but progressive limitation appearing in adolescence or early adulthood. Bacterial endocarditis occurring on the abnormal valve remains a significant threat in all patients. Right-to-left shunting through a patent foramen ovale or atrial septal defect produces cyanosis and requires differentiation from other forms of cyanotic disease.

Clinical findings include a right ventricular lift and a systolic thrill and harsh murmur initiated by an early systolic click along the upper left sternal border. The pulmonic component of the second sound is usually diminished.

The Ecg. shows right ventricular and often right atrial hypertrophy.

Radiologic features include diminished pulmonary vascularity, enlarged main pulmonary artery segment (representing poststenotic dilatation), and right ventricular enlargement.

Diagnostic evaluation should include cardiac catheterization or angiocardiography (or both) to rule out associated lesions. Even with these methods, the distinction between infundibular and valvular stenosis may occasionally be unclear.

In symptomatic patients or those with clear Ecg. signs of right ventricular hypertrophy, operation is indicated. In asymptomatic patients, operation is recommended on the basis of catheterization findings; gradients in excess of 50-60 mm. Hg are usually taken as an indication for correction.

Treatment.

In infants with critical valvular stenosis, emergency valvotomy is performed with inflow occlusion with or without hypothermia. No time is available for arterioplastic procedures or resection of infundibular obstruction.

The elective correction of pulmonic stenosis should always be undertaken on cardiopulmonary bypass. The dome-like valvular structure with a central opening is incised along the rudimentary commissures fully to the annulus. Areas of subvalvular obstruction due to muscular hypertrophy or fibrous stricture are resected. Slight pulmonic insufficiency postoperatively is common, but is well tolerated in individuals with normal pulmonary artery pressure.

Prognosis.

The results of surgical treatment are quite satisfactory in nearly all patients. In individuals with very severe preoperative right ventricular hypertension, the reduction of right ventricular systolic and diastolic pressures following operation may be somewhat retarded and slight residual elevation of pressures may persist.

4. AORTIC STENOSIS

Of the 4 types of congenital aortic stenosis, the most common is valvular stenosis with varying degrees of valve deformity, producing in most cases a functionally bicuspid or unicuspid valve mechanism. The second variety is localized subvalvular stenosis, usually due to a fibrous diaphragm-like structure. Less common is left ventricular outflow tract obstruction caused by generalized muscular hypertrophy (idiopathic hypertrophic subaortic stenosis). The least commonly seen lesion is supravalvular stenosis, consisting of localized or diffuse constriction above the valve or diffuse hypoplasia of the ascending aorta. Types 1, 3, and 4 may coexist ("tunnel syndrome"). Although severe aortic stenosis may cause heart failure and death in infancy, most patients pass through childhood without symptoms and are referred for evaluation because of a murmur. Symptoms of later onset include exertional dyspnea and fatigue; syncope and angina (often atypical) are common. The development of frank congestive heart failure suggests the presence of coexistent lesions. Sudden death is an uncommon but dramatic feature of this disease. There is also a significant incidence of bacterial endocarditis.

Physical findings include a systolic thrill and loud murmur at the upper right sternal border, transmitted to the suprasternal notch and carotid arteries. An early ejection click is frequently present in the valvular and fibrous subvalvular types. Mild aortic insufficiency due to severe deformity of the valve is uncommonly present. With subvalvular obstruction, the murmur is usually maximal to the left of the sternum in the third or fourth intercostal space or near the apex. Supravalvular aortic stenosis may occur as part of a syndrome with mental retardation and unusual facial appearance.

The Ecg. is normal in many cases, but with severe stenosis shows evidence of left ventricular hypertrophy. Cardiac x-rays usually show a normal-sized heart and often mild poststenotic dilatation in the localized varieties of obstruction.

Cardiac catheterization and angiocardiography permit definitive diagnosis and should be performed in all cases. Localization of the site of obstruction is usually possible, and contrast studies are extremely helpful in planning the operative approach.

Operation is indicated in symptomatic patients, in patients with advancing left ventricular hypertrophy as evidenced by x-ray or Ecg., and in patients with demonstrated gradients in excess of 50 mm. Hg.

Treatment.

Surgical care is possible in cases of localized supravalvular or subvalvular stenosis. Diffuse subaortic muscular stenosis is more properly considered a myocardial disease, but lasting relief of the obstruction by ventriculomyotomy or resection of obstructing muscle mass (or both) is usually possible. In most cases of valvular stenosis, the valvular deformity is sufficiently severe to preclude restoration of normal function, and operative treatment is palliative. The valve leaflets are usually considerably thickened, and the rudimentary commissures do not permit division all the way back to the annulus without danger of producing significant aortic regurgitation. Although significant reduction in the gradient is achieved, it is thought that the residual deformity predisposes these valves to later calcification and progressive stenosis in adulthood.

Prognosis.

Operative mortality for all types is generally low (5% or less) except in infants submitted to emergency valvotomy under inflow occlusion (20-25%). Postoperative improvement in symptomatic patients occurs in the majority, but the late effects on longevity and valvular calcification are not known.

5. COARCTATION OF THE THORACIC AORTA

Constriction or interruption of the thoracic aorta occurs typically at or just beyond the ligamentum arteriosum ("adult type"). A preductal position ("infantile type") occurs in the minority of cases. Most patients are asymptomatic until early adulthood, but congestive heart failure may develop in infancy, especially if the coarctation is associated with other cardiac anomalies. A bicuspid aortic valve, of varying severity, is a frequently associated lesion.

The hemodynamic consequences of coarctation are systolic hypertension and increased left ventricular work, eventually leading to left ventricular failure. In most cases, only moderate elevation of BP is present until early adulthood, when a progressive increase is seen with advancing age. Early symptoms include exertional dyspnea and fatigue (especially lower extremities).

Physical findings include diminished or absent femoral and lower extremity pulses, with a pulse lag determined by simultaneous palpation of the radial pulse. BP is decreased in the lower extremities and may be unobtainable. The carotid pulses are prominent, and palpation of the latissimus dorsi muscles should reveal collateral vessel pulsations. The absence of detectable collaterals in these muscles suggests atypical location of the coarctation. A systolic murmur is present over the base of the heart and in the back, and multiple bruits of collateral circulation can usually be heard.

The Ecg. shows left ventricular hypertrophy. Important radiologic findings include left ventricular prominence and bony erosions due to enlarged and tortuous collateral vessels. These are most evident along the lower margins of the midthoracic ribs ("rib notching") and the undersurface of the sternum (internal mammary arteries). A "reverse 3" sign in the barium-filled esophagus may be seen in the posteroanterior and left anterior oblique projections due to indentations produced by pre- and poststenotic dilatations of the aorta.

Clinical diagnosis may suffice in many cases. Cardiac catheterization or angiocardiography (or both) is required in infants and in atypical patients.

Treatment.

Operative correction is indicated in childhood before severe symptoms occur. In young patients, operative mortality is almost nil; in older patients, mortality rises to approximately 5%, and in infants operated upon as emergencies it is considerably higher. Increased risk is imposed by cardiac failure, associated anomalies, and the tremendously dilated, thin-walled collaterals found in older adults. Repair consists of excision of the narrowed segment through a left thoracotomy and end-to-end reanastomosis in the majority of instances. In some adults or in cases of elongated stenosis, interposition of a graft is necessary.

Operative complications include hemothorax, cardiac failure (infants), and the "postcoarctectomy syndrome." Features of the latter range from mild abdominal pain to frank bowel infarction associated with fever and leukocytosis within a few days of operation. The cause is not known, but the syndrome is thought to be related to restoration of normal pulsatile flow to the mesenteric circulation, producing widespread hemorrhage and thrombosis. Excised specimens have presented the features of acute arteritis. Occasionally, paradoxical temporary exacerbation of hypertension occurs postoperatively. The threat of cerebrovascular hemorrhage, responsible for 10-15% of medical deaths due to coarctation in reported series, should be kept in mind.

Prognosis.

In general, the results of operation are excellent, and long-term follow-up studies have shown normal hemodynamics in uncomplicated cases. Restenosis is virtually limited to cases corrected during infancy, possibly related to the use of a single continuous suture line that restricts growth at the anastomosis.

6. PATENT DUCTUS ARTERIOSUS

Persistence of the fetal ductus arteriosus was the first type of congenital heart disease to be surgically corrected (1938). Signs and symptoms are dependent upon the magnitude of shunting from the high pressure aorta into the pulmonary vascular bed.

Patients with normal pulmonary vascular resistance are usually asymptomatic, and features of the disease are limited to physical findings. The continuous "machinery" murmur heard maximally in the second left intercostal space and beneath the left clavicle is virtually pathognomonic of this condition. Typically, during infancy, the murmur is limited to systole. Additional findings include bounding peripheral pulses with lowered diastolic pressure, a diastolic flow murmur at the apex (reflecting increased flow across the mitral valve), and a left ventricular impulse. The pulmonic component of the second sound may be accentuated. Radiologic findings caused by the extracardiac left-to-right shunt include an enlarged left atrium and left ventricle and increased pulmonary vascular markings. Calcification of the ductus is a late sign, associated with pulmonary hypertension.

The Ecg. is often normal but may show the pattern of left atrial and left ventricular or combined ventricular hypertrophy.

The development of pulmonary vascular obstruction in patients with significant shunts poses different diagnostic and therapeutic problems. Symptoms are prominent, and congestive heart failure is common. The diastolic component of the previously continuous murmur may be diminished or absent because of the disappearance of a pressure gradient between the aorta and pulmonary artery during diastole. The x-rays and Ecg. show evidence of right ventricular enlargement and hypertrophy.

In addition to its hemodynamic consequences, the left-to-right shunt predisposes patients to bacterial endarteritis, usually occurring at the pulmonary artery end of the ductus. For all these reasons, operation is indicated as soon as feasible after the diagnosis is established.

Cardiac catheterization should be performed in all cases with suspected pulmonary hypertension, in atypical cases, and in adults.

Treatment.

The ductus may be ligated or divided through a left thoracotomy. Because the incidence of recanalization through a ligated ductus is significant, complete division is recommended in most cases. The operative risk varies almost directly with the degree of elevation of pulmonary vascular resistance. In patients with normal pulmonary vasculature, the operative mortality is 1% or less. In the presence of severe pulmonary hypertension and elevated resistance, the mortality rate rises to 20% or more. In occasional patients, severe pulmonary hypertension present at the time of operation will persist and cause death postoperatively due to chronic cor pulmonale. Operation is contraindicated in patients with net right-to-left shunts.

CYANOTIC DEFECTS

1. TETRALOGY OF FALLOT

Two features of the tetralogy of Fallot are important from the surgical point of view: ventricular septal defect and pulmonic stenosis. Ventricular septal defect is usually large and involves the area of the membranous septum close to the crista supraventricularis. In most cases there is infundibular pulmonary stenosis, often combined with valvular stenosis as well. Isolated valvular stenosis with tetralogy of Fallot occurs in 10-20% of cases.

The clinical consequences of the defects involved in tetralogy of

Fallot are determined by the relative resistance to blood flow from the right and left ventricles. During early infancy, a minority of patients are cyanotic; however, by age 2 almost all patients show some degree of arterial desaturation. Exercise tolerance is usually severely limited, and patients characteristically squat to relieve fatigue. Occasional abrupt increases in right ventricular outflow resistance cause hypoxemic spells with or without convulsions or syncope. Evidence of congestive cardiac failure is virtually limited to patients who have undergone shunt procedures with excessive flow.

The physical findings include growth retardation, cyanosis, clubbing of the fingers, and evidence of right ventricular hypertrophy. There is a harsh systolic murmur associated with a thrill along the mid left sternal border, and the pulmonic component of the second heart sound is greatly diminished or inaudible.

Laboratory findings include secondary polycythemia; red cell indices should be determined because of the common finding of relative iron deficiency anemia. The Ecg. shows right axis deviation with a pattern of right ventricular hypertrophy. Chest x-rays reveal the classical boot-shaped heart without cardiomegaly. The pulmonary artery segment is inconspicuous and the pulmonary vascular markings are attenuated unless a previous systemic-pulmonary shunt has been performed. A right-sided aortic arch occurs in approximately 25% of patients.

Findings at cardiac catheterization and angiocardiography, which should be performed in all patients, include elevated (systemic) pressures within the right ventricle and a pressure gradient across the outflow tract or pulmonic valve (or both). Arterial oxygen saturation is decreased, and there is evidence of bidirectional shunting, predominantly right-to-left, through the ventricular septal defect.

Medical complications include severe hypoxic spells, pneumonia, endocarditis, pulmonary hemorrhage or thrombosis, and cerebral embolism, abscess, or thrombosis. In untreated cases, survival is greatly limited.

In children weighing less than approximately 15 Kg., increasingly frequent hypoxic spells constitute indication for a palliative procedure, with definitive correction delayed electively. In patients without severe symptoms - i.e., those with cyanosis only - total correction is best performed electively after age 5, when patient size alone no longer contributes to the operative risk.

Treatment.

Palliative procedures to increase pulmonary blood flow in severely hypoxic infants or small children include anastomosis between (1) the descending aorta and the left pulmonary artery (Potts procedure); (2) the subclavian artery and the right or left pulmonary artery on the side opposite the aortic arch (Blalock-Taussig anastomosis); and (3) the ascending aorta and the right pulmonary artery. Too large an anastomosis with excessive pulmonary blood flow causes postoperative heart failure, usually controllable with digitalis. The results are dramatic, with decreasing cyanosis and improvement in growth.

Total correction of tetralogy of Fallot is fraught with several potential complications which may be avoided by meticulous attention to technic. The ventricular septal defect is best closed by patch with careful attention to suture placement in the area of the atrioventricular conducting bundle. Muscular infundibular obstruction is relieved by division and resection of muscular bands, and a stenotic pulmonary valve is incised along the fused commissures. A hypoplastic pulmonic valve annulus or outflow tract requires patch grafting to avoid residual stenosis. Each of the various systemic to pulmonary artery shunts generates particular technical problems at reoperation. A significant danger is hemorrhage from the area of dissection necessary to take down a previous shunt. An advantage of the ascending aorta to right pulmonary artery shunt is the ease of closure through an aortotomy, and in selected cases a Potts anastomosis may similarly be closed through a left pulmonary arteriotomy. Operation for total correction is greatly facilitated by elective cardioplegia with local hypothermia of the heart. In addition to the still and dry operative field, this technic permits a small right ventriculotomy 1.5-2 cm. in length, which may be maneuvered easily to provide exposure because of the relaxed condition of the myocardium. Pulmonic valvular insufficiency or right bundle branch block resulting from operation is without immediate clinical consequences.

Prognosis.

Although operative mortality has been reduced in recent years, a significant risk of 10% or more persists in most series. The technics for total correction described above, however, have resulted in only 2 deaths in over 100 patients at the authors' institution.

Postoperative improvement may be expected in virtually all cases. Total correction results in normal hemodynamics and clinical status. In occasional instances, elevated right ventricular pressure may resolve slowly.

2. TRANSPOSITION OF THE GREAT VESSELS

Transposition of the great vessels is the commonest congenital defect causing death during early infancy. Fewer than 10% of untreated patients survive beyond the first year.

The isolation of the pulmonary and systemic circuits due to the origin of the aorta from the right (systemic) ventricle and the pulmonary artery from the left (pulmonary) ventricle demands the existence of an additional defect to permit survival. In approximately half of cases, an adequate shunt for intracardiac mixing of the 2 circulations is not present, and closure of the patent ductus creates a critical situation. The remaining cases include an atrial or ventricular septal defect. Pulmonary stenosis is common. The clinical course is determined by the degree of mixing of venous and systemic circuits, either intracardiac or extracardiac, and by the pulmonary blood flow.

Clinically, cyanosis is conspicuous soon after birth. Immediate causes of deterioration are related to congestive heart failure or severe hypoxemia. Respiratory infections are frequent. Physical findings include a nondistinctive systolic murmur, a single second sound, and often a gallop rhythm.

The Ecg. generally shows right axis deviation and right ventricular hypertrophy, with additional features determined by associated lesions. Typical radiologic findings include cardiac enlargement with dominance of the anterior (systemic) ventricle. The base of the heart is narrow. The lung fields usually show increased vascularity, but this is variable depending upon the pulmonary blood flow.

Angiocardiography is required for definitive diagnosis and demonstrates the origin of the aorta anteriorly from the right ventricle. Associated septal defects and patent ductus are defined as well.

A palliative procedure is indicated in virtually all infants.

Treatment.

The operative approach is predicated on the predominant functional lesion present. In most cases, the purpose is to improve cardiac mixing of pulmonary venous and systemic blood. This is accomplished by creation of an atrial septal defect by various technics. Rigid attention to respiratory care and acid-base balance is necessary for survival in these critically ill infants. The presence of an associated ventricular septal defect without pulmonic stenosis requires simultaneous banding of the pulmonary artery to protect the pulmonary vascular bed from systemic BP. In patients with severe desaturation on the basis of inadequate pulmonary blood flow due to left ventricular (pulmonary) outflow tract obstruction, a systemic to pulmonary shunt utilizing the subclavian artery or an ascending aorta to right pulmonary artery anastomosis is required. Operative mortality ranges from 5-10%; most survivors are benefited, and elective total correction may be performed later.

Experience with creation or enlargement of an atrial septal defect by means of a balloon catheter technic (Rashkind procedure) has been encouraging. Although repeated dilatations may be necessary, the shunt produced by this method alone may permit survival until elective total repair or may serve as an important temporizing procedure until operative palliation can be undertaken later, when the operative risk is lower.

Total functional correction of transposition of the great vessels is performed on cardiopulmonary bypass and involves redirection of venous inflow to the appropriate ventricles. The atrial septum is excised, and a rectangular interatrial pericardial or synthetic baffle is sewn into place to conduct blood from the vena cavas through the mitral valve and from the pulmonary veins through the tricuspid valve. Associated defects are repaired simultaneously.

Prognosis.

Accumulating experience with operative correction of this lesion has been associated with lowered operative mortality rates, which presently range from 5-10%. An intact ventricular septum and absence of pulmonic stenosis are favorable factors. Survivors are dramatically improved postoperatively, with essentially normal intracardiac pressures in the few cases studied. Long-term results are not known.

CORONARY ARTERY DISEASE

Coronary artery disease ranks as the most common cause of death in the United States today. Current technics for the surgical treatment of coronary artery disease and its complications include (1) direct myocardial revascularization; (2) indirect myocardial revascularization; (3) resection of ventricular aneurysm; (4) excision of acutely infarcted or chronically ischemic myocardium; and (5) repair of acute complications of myocardial infarction such as ventricular septal perforation or papillary muscle rupture. These will be discussed below.

The ultimate therapy for patients whose disease defies management by any of these methods is cardiac transplantation (see below). All of these areas remain in the stage of exploration and evaluation, and firm conclusions regarding eventual therapeutic value cannot be formed at present.

DIRECT MYOCARDIAL REVASCULARIZATION

The development of successful technics in 1967-1968 for direct myocardial revascularization utilizing aortocoronary autogenous vein bypass grafts produced a quantum advance in the surgical management of coronary artery disease. Such operations are currently the most frequently performed cardiac procedures in the United States.

Approximately 80% of patients with symptomatic coronary disease have lesions which are amenable to bypass - i.e., single or multiple obstructions located sufficiently proximally in the coronary arteries to permit distal vein graft anastomosis. The majority have involvement of 2 or more major vessels. Selective coronary arteriography is essential to preoperative diagnosis and technical planning; lesions associated with a decrease in luminal diameter of 75% or greater are considered hemodynamically significant.

In general, patients with angina pectoris which cannot be controlled at a tolerable level by medical management are considered potential candidates for bypass procedures. Operative indications remain controversial at this time, however, and some centers endorse the application of aortocoronary bypass to all patients with demonstrable significant disease. For many reasons, several patient subpopulations should be distinguished: stable angina (with and without left ventricular dysfunction), crescendo angina, impending myocardial infarction, and acute myocardial infarction (with and without cardiogenic shock). Operative risk and therapeutic outcome differ among these groups, as discussed below.

Preoperative evaluation should include, in addition to selective coronary arteriography and ventriculography, baseline serum enzyme determinations, chest x-rays, and Ecg. close to the time of operation. Profound left ventricular dysfunction - i.e., severe, diffuse left ventricular hypokinesia - is a contraindication to operation. Mild to moderate left ventricular failure, metabolic disorders, hypertension, and smoking are not contraindications to operation but may be expected to significantly affect long-term results.

Technic.

Aortocoronary grafts are best performed on total cardiopulmonary bypass with induced ventricular fibrillation. Segments of the upper saphenous veins are used for bypass unless venous disease is present or previous stripping has been performed. Cephalic veins have been used as substitutes. The distal left internal mammary artery has been utilized for direct anastomosis to the left anterior descending coronary artery in some centers, and early results have been satisfactory.

Distal anastomoses of vein grafts to the coronary arteries are performed in an end-to-side fashion employing microvascular technic. Low power magnification (2-2.5 ×) is helpful. Proximal anastomosis to the ascending aorta should be done separately for each graft. In general, all major coronary arteries with significant lesions should be bypassed, if possible. Manual or gas (CO_2) endarterectomy may be employed for the distally diseased coronary artery, combined with a bypass graft; the early results of such procedures appear to be comparable to those of bypass alone.

Prognosis.

Operative mortality for aortocoronary bypass grafting averages 5% in most centers. Severe disease (e.g., triple vessel involvement) carries a higher operative risk (up to 10-20%). In the presence of acute myocardial infarction or advanced left ventricular failure, mortality rates rise sharply, although salvage of some patients with these complications has been achieved.

Graft patency rates 6-12 months postoperatively range from 75-90%. A comparable percentage of patients are greatly improved or entirely free of angina and are restored to functional class I or II. Absence or regression of symptomatic benefit usually signifies graft occlusion.

Important unanswered questions regarding aortocoronary bypass grafts concern their effects on longevity and on the incidence of recurrence of myocardial infarction.

INDIRECT MYOCARDIAL REVASCULARIZATION

The results of attempted myocardial revascularization by intramyocardial implantation of the distal internal mammary arteries or other arterial source are inferior to those of direct bypass grafts. Implant patency and symptomatic result are unpredictable, and evidence of increased myocardial perfusion is unconvincing. The operative mortality rate with single coronary artery involvement is 2-5%, and is significantly higher with more extensive disease or left ventricular failure. Postoperative complications (infarction, arrhythmias, heart failure) are common. Most centers, including the authors' institution, do not currently perform this operation.

RESECTION OF VENTRICULAR ANEURYSMS

Ventricular aneurysm formation occurs in 10-20% of patients with acute myocardial infarction and accounts for significant long-term disability and mortality in surviving patients. The most common location is in the anterolateral left ventricle near the apex; aneurysms developing posteriorly or involving the septum usually result in early death. The detrimental consequences of ventricular aneurysms stem from interference with myocardial contraction, producing congestive heart failure, and thrombus formation with peripheral embolization. Late rupture of ventricular aneurysms occurs rarely.

Operation is indicated for patients with symptomatic ventricular aneurysms who are at least 3 months past infarction. Earlier intervention is complicated by technical difficulties due to insufficient fibrosis for secure closure of the ventricular incision. Optimal candidates are those with localized aneurysms without gross calcification or diffuse coronary artery disease. Patients with generalized left ventricular dilatation and poor contractility should not be submitted to aneurysmectomy.

Operative repair consists of excision of the aneurysm and removal of mural thrombus on cardiopulmonary bypass. Occasional patients whose aneurysms involve the anterior papillary muscle may require mitral valve replacement as well. Selective coronary arteriography should be performed preoperatively, and significant lesions should be bypassed at the time of aneurysmectomy. Operative mortality rates range from 10-20%. The most common causes of postoperative deaths and morbidity are recurrent myocardial infarction and arrhythmias. In surviving patients, the postoperative results are generally quite satisfactory, and dramatic salvage of some patients in severe intractable congestive heart failure may be achieved.

INFARCTECTOMY

Limited clinical experience with excision of acute myocardial infarcts, combined with direct aortocoronary grafting, has resulted in salvage of some patients, but the operative risk appears high (approximately 50%). Candidates for operation include patients with acute myocardial infarction occurring during or after coronary arteriography (coronary anatomy known) or patients with acute infarction complicated by intractable arrhythmias or cardiogenic shock. In the latter, the necessary preoperative evaluation by coronary arteriography may be possible only with the aid of continuous mechanical circulatory assistance.

REPAIR OF OTHER COMPLICATIONS IN MYOCARDIAL INFARCTION

Acute perforation of the ventricular septum or rupture of a papillary muscle following myocardial infarction is a catastrophic event which leads to rapidly progressive congestive heart failure and death in the majority of untreated patients. Both are diagnosed by sudden deterioration, usually occurring within 2 weeks following myocardial infarction, associated with the abrupt appearance of a precordial murmur. In the case of an acute ventricular septal defect, the murmur is present along the lower left sternal border or midway to the apex; with ruptured papillary muscle, the murmur is maximal at the apex, radiating to the axilla. Prompt diagnosis may permit successful operative repair. Many successful cases of patch closure of acute ventricular septal defects performed as early as 1 week following infarction have now been reported. Repair of mitral lesions necessitates valve replacement. Serious technical complications encountered at operation for fresh lesions relate to friability of the involved myocardium. An elective delay of 2-3 months, if possible, results in higher survival rates. Direct aortocoronary bypass grafting should be performed simultaneously if indicated.

CARDIAC TRANSPLANTATION

The initial clinical trials of cardiac transplantation produced relatively few long-term survivors, with a worldwide 1-year survival rate of 19%. About half of the early postoperative deaths were due to operative complications, reflecting the severity of disease present in these patients, and the remainder were due to graft rejection or complications of immunosuppressive therapy. During the past 2 years, only a few centers, including the authors' institution, have continued to perform cardiac transplants in small numbers. The current results compare favorably with those of renal transplantation from cadaver donors.

Potential candidates for cardiac transplantation usually present with advanced coronary heart disease or idiopathic nonobstructive cardiomyopathy. An increasing number of patients with failed myocardial revascularization procedures have undergone transplantation.

Operative technics used in man are similar in principle to those developed in the laboratory. Two modifications, however, have been imposed by clinical experience. The first involves the usual size disparity between the donor and recipient hearts and necessitates excision of the donor heart by transection of the various venous connections at their junctions with the atria. The left atrium is then opened out by interconnection of the pulmonary vein orifices to increase the available anastomotic circumference. The right atrium is opened by an incision beginning in the inferior vena caval orifice and extending upward into the base of the right atrial appendage. The superior vena cava is simply ligated, thus preserving the integrity of the sinus node.

The lateral left atrial anastomosis is performed first. The atrial septal anastomosis is performed twice, on both the right and left sides, because of the technics for tailoring the donor atria. Following completion of the right atrial suture line, the great vessels are joined and the aorta disoccluded. These technics, combined with local hypothermia of the heart by constant immersion in saline at 4-6° C., have resulted in consistent resuscitation of the graft.

In immediate postoperative management, isoproterenol, cardiac pacing, or digitalis has been used temporarily in most patients. Recipients with severe preoperative pulmonary hypertension and elevated pulmonary vascular resistance require more prolonged and vigorous support.

Clinical experience has confirmed the Ecg. as the most reliable surface-sensed index of cardiac rejection presently available. Most early episodes of rejection occur 5-14 days postoperatively. Preceding the signs of overt heart failure, the Ecg. shows a significant and progressive decrease in voltage. Other abnormalities include right axis deviation, incomplete or complete right bundle branch block, atrial arrhythmias, and first degree heart block. The earliest physical evidence of rejection is usually an early diastolic gallop rhythm. Patient complaints include fatigue and severely reduced exercise tolerance. Measurements made by ultrasound echocardiography demonstrate an increase in total heart size and left ventricular wall thickness with predominant dilatation of the right ventricle during this early period. A striking feature of the cardiac rejection crisis is the rapidity with which patients may progress from this early stage to a point of extremely low cardiac output accompanied by progressive fluid retention and vascular congestion. Chest x-rays show modest enlargement of the cardiac silhouette without prominent pulmonary vascular congestion. Unless effective immunosuppressive therapy is administered, death usually occurs within 48 hours.

Immunosuppressive regimens differ widely among various centers, but essentially include maintenance doses of prednisone and azathioprine in gradually tapering amounts and antilymphocyte or antithymocyte globulin for the first few months postoperatively. Acute rejection, diagnosed by the above parameters, demands immediate and aggressive therapy for reversal. At the authors' institution, this has been achieved in 95% of cases by intermittent intravenous administration of dactinomycin and high doses (1 Gm.) of methylprednisolone. Because of evidence for the participation of intravascular coagulation in the rejecting graft, systemic heparinization has also been employed. Intravenous treatment is given on a daily basis (usually 2-5 days) until initial reversal of the changes described above has occurred. Clinically, complete restoration of myocardial function without residual damage can be achieved.

The complications of immunosuppressive therapy for cardiac rejection are common to organ transplantation in general. Infection, primarily pulmonary, is an ever-present danger. Hepatic and bone marrow toxicity, diabetes mellitus, osteoporosis, myopathy, neuropathy, and psychosis have all been encountered.

Survival rates for the total series of 41 patients at Stanford University are currently 40% at 1 year and 32% at two years after transplantation. A steady increase in postoperative survival by yearly intervals has been observed since 1968. The longest current survivors have now lived more than 3 years after operation.

The clinical and functional status of most long-term survivors is satisfactory. Most ordinary activities are tolerated without difficulty. Cardiac catheterization studies 1 and 2 years postoperatively have shown normal intracardiac pressures at rest, with low normal cardiac outputs. During exercise, cardiac output increases normally in relation to the augmentation of O_2 consumption, although the absolute level remains somewhat low. The mechanisms responsible for increasing output of the transplanted heart during exercise include a gradual elevation in rate, an increased stroke volume via the Frank-Starling mechanism, and enhanced contractility due to circulating catecholamines. Efferent autonomic reinnervation of the donor heart has not been observed in any recipient.

Many recipients who have died in the late postoperative period have shown severe diffuse atherosclerosis of the graft coronary arteries. The cause of this apparently accelerated atherosclerosis is not known at present but may be related to immune injury of the arterial wall in combination with hyperlipidemia, which is exhibited by many recipients. The complications of graft atherosclerosis (arrhythmias, myocardial infarction) have contributed importantly to the majority of deaths after the first postoperative year. Chronic rejection, manifested as proliferation of myointimal cells in the tunica intima of coronary arteries, often coexists with graft atherosclerosis and may be the principal cause of arterial narrowing.

The ultimate value of cardiac transplantation as a therapeutic tool remains to be defined. Current experience demonstrates, however, that long-term survival may be expected in a significant proportion of recipients, and that in successful cases a highly satisfying degree of physical and social rehabilitation may be achieved.

11 . . .

Surgery of the Breast & Soft Tissues

CARCINOMA OF THE FEMALE BREAST

Carcinoma of the breast is among the most common malignant tumors and is a major cause of death in women. The peak incidence is between the ages of 40 and 50, but breast cancer occurs frequently at all ages past 30. The annual incidence of breast carcinoma is about 70 per 100,000, and the mortality rate is about 24 per 100,000. It is estimated that 5% of women develop the disease during their lifetime, and about 20% of deaths from cancer among women are attributable to breast cancer.

A predisposition to breast cancer is inherited; women with a family history of mammary carcinoma, particularly in mothers, sisters, and daughters, are more likely to develop the disease and to be affected at an earlier age. Because mammary dysplasia may possibly be associated with an increased incidence of malignancy, continuous follow-up of patients with this condition is indicated. Women who have never been pregnant are more likely to develop breast cancer than multiparous females. A history of not having nursed a baby and of prolonged lactation (over 2 years) is more common in patients with breast cancer than in controls. There is a greater danger of developing a second primary lesion in the opposite breast, as 7-10% of all breast cancers occur consecutively and 2% concurrently. Inflammation, trauma, and benign neoplasms are not precancerous.

Although the mean duration of life in untreated carcinoma of the breast is about 3 years, the biologic behavior of the disease is highly variable; some untreated patients succumb in 3 months, whereas others survive for 5-30 years. In general, the course of mammary cancer is related to histologic type and grade: well-differentiated tumors tend to progress more slowly. However, the choice of initial treatment is based primarily upon the extent of the disease and not upon the microscopic pattern of the lesion.

It would appear that a significant percentage of women with breast cancer have an abnormal hormonal environment as determined by deviations from normal in excretion of estrogens, androgens, and hydrocorticoids. However, evidence based on hormonal assays is still conflicting, and it is not possible to rely with confidence on such studies to identify individuals with a high risk of developing the disease or likely to respond to hormonal therapy when metastases have occurred.

The relative frequency of carcinoma in various anatomic sites in the breast is as follows: Upper outer quadrant, 45%; lower outer quadrant, 10%; upper inner quadrant, 15%; lower inner quadrant, 5%; central (subareolar of diffuse), 25% (see p. 369, top). Metastasis to regional lymph nodes is the principal mode of spread (see

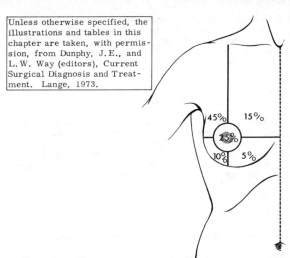

Unless otherwise specified, the illustrations and tables in this chapter are taken, with permission, from Dunphy, J. E., and L. W. Way (editors), Current Surgical Diagnosis and Treatment. Lange, 1973.

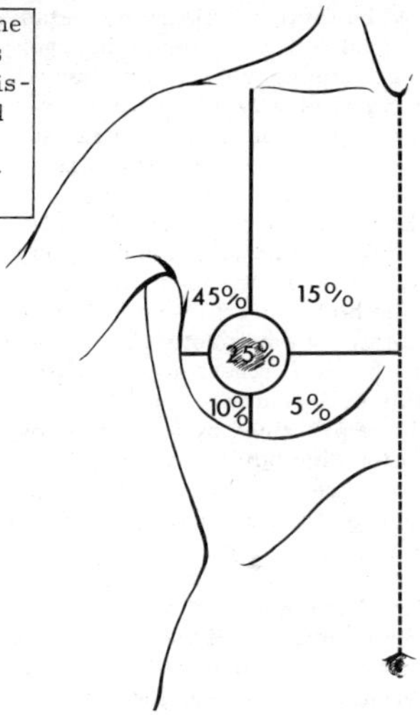

Frequency of Breast Carcinoma at Various Anatomic Sites

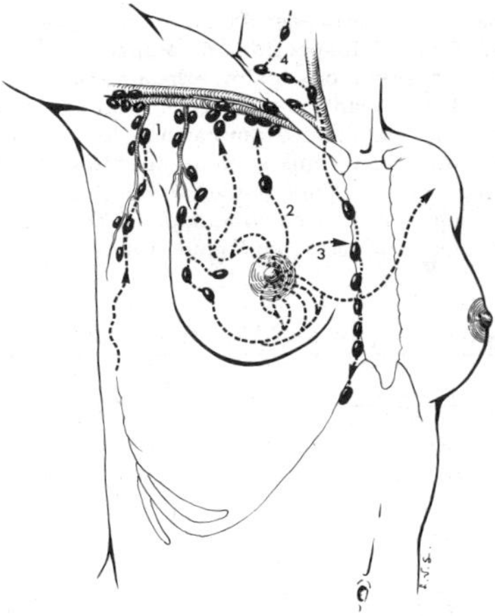

Lymphatic Drainage of the Breast to Regional Node Groups. 1: Main axillary group. 2: Interpectoral node leading to apex of axilla. 3: Internal mammary group. 4: Supraclavicular group. (Modified from Ackerman, L. V., and J. A. Del Regato, Cancer, 3rd ed. Mosby, 1962.)

p. 369, bottom). Axillary metastases are found on microscopic study in 50-60% of patients undergoing radical mastectomy. The internal mammary nodes are invaded in about one-third of patients who have clinically advanced disease of borderline operability. When the tumor is in the central or inner half of the breast and when the axillary nodes have already been invaded, the internal mammary chain is particularly likely to be involved.

Hematogenous spread of breast cancer is common; the bones (especially the pelvis, spine, femur, ribs, skull, and humerus), lungs, and liver are most frequently affected.

The high mortality rate of breast cancer can be most effectively reduced by early detection and adequate surgical treatment. The patient herself is best able to discover the early lesions. Regular monthly self-examination of the breasts after each menstrual period should be practiced by all women over 30. Periodic screening examination, including mammography, is proving effective in detecting early breast cancer. The general availability of such service should significantly reduce the mortality rate from carcinoma of the breast.

Clinical Findings.

A. Symptoms and Signs: The primary complaint in about 80% of patients with breast cancer is a lump (usually painless) in the breast (see table below). Less frequent symptoms are breast pain; erosion, retraction, enlargement, discharge, or itching of the nipple; and redness, generalized hardness, enlargement, or shrinkage of the breast. Rarely, an axillary mass, swelling of the arm, or back pain (from metastases) may be the first symptom.

Examination of the breast should be meticulous, methodical, and gentle. Careful inspection and palpation - with the patient supine, arms at her sides and overhead; and sitting, arms at her sides and overhead - are essential; unless this procedure is followed at all physical examinations, early lesions will be missed and important signs such as dimpling of the skin (see illustration on p. 371) may be overlooked. In some series, 5-10% of cases of breast carcinoma have been discovered during physical examinations performed for other purposes.

Initial Symptoms of Mammary Carcinoma*

Symptom	Percentage of All Cases
Painless breast mass	66
Painful breast mass	11
Nipple discharge	9
Local edema	4
Nipple retraction	3
Nipple crusting	2
Miscellaneous symptoms	5

*Adapted from report of initial symptoms in 774 patients treated for breast cancer at Ellis Fischel State Cancer Hospital, Columbia, Missouri. Reproduced, with permission, from Spratt, J. S., Jr., and W. L. Donegan, Cancer of the Breast. Saunders, 1967.

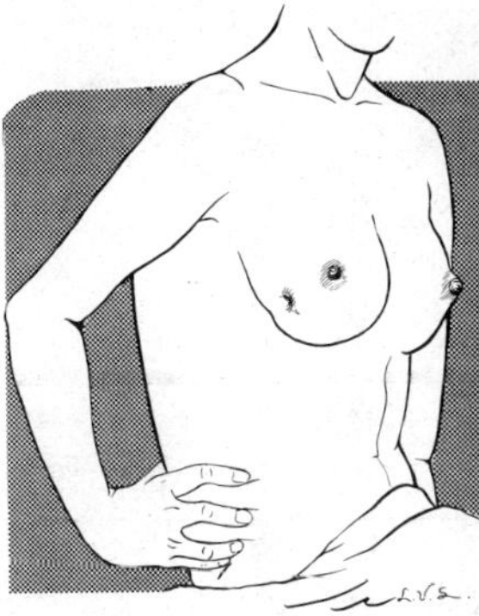

Skin Retraction or Dimpling. This may be accentuated by having the patient press her hand on her hip in order to contract the pectoralis muscles.

A lesion smaller than 1 cm. in diameter may be difficult or impossible for the examiner to feel and yet may be discovered by the patient. She should always be asked to demonstrate the location of the mass; if the physician fails to confirm her suspicions, he should repeat the examination in 1 month. During the premenstrual phase of the cycle, increased innocuous nodularity may suggest neoplasm or may obscure an underlying lesion. If there is any question regarding the nature of an abnormality under these circumstances, the patient should be asked to return after her period.

The location, size, consistency, and other physical features of all lesions should be recorded on a drawing of the breast for future reference.

Breast cancer usually consists of a nontender firm or hard lump with poorly delimited margins (caused by local infiltration). Slight skin or nipple retraction is an important early sign. Minimal assymmetry of the breast may be noted. Very small (1-2 mm.) erosions of the nipple epithelium may be the only manifestation of carcinoma of the Paget type. Watery, serous, or bloody discharge is an infrequent early sign. The following are characteristic of advanced carcinoma: edema, redness, nodularity, or ulceration of the skin; the presence of a large primary tumor; fixation to the chest wall; enlargement, shrinkage, or retraction of the breast; marked axillary lymphadenopathy; and distant metastases.

The axillary and cervical regions must be examined carefully for lymphadenopathy (see p. 372). Involvement of the supraclavicular nodes almost invariably means that distant spread of cancer has already occurred and that attempts at curative surgical treatment are futile. Involvement of the axillary nodes, although an extremely serious prognostic finding, does

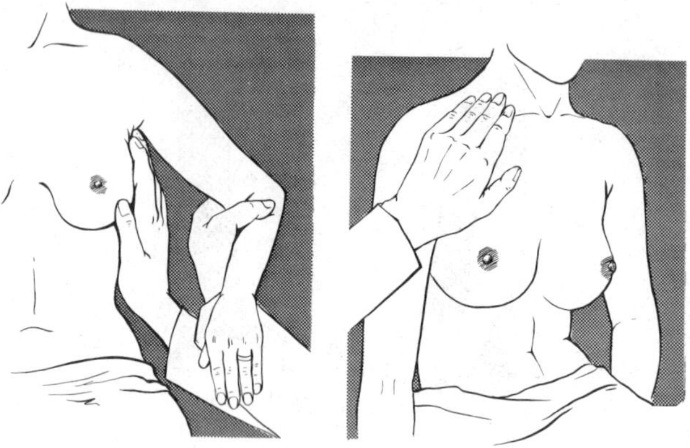

Palpation of Axillary and Supraclavicular
Regions for Enlarged Lymph Nodes

not exclude surgery but does influence the diagnosis and treatment approach. A clinical opinion based on palpation of the axilla should be formed regarding the presence or absence of metastases in the nodes. One or 2 movable, not particularly firm lymph nodes 5 mm. or less in diameter can frequently be palpated in the normal axilla, but firm or hard nodes larger than 5 mm. in diameter must be assumed to contain metastases until proved otherwise. Unfortunately, evaluation of the axillary nodes by palpation is not always accurate. Histologic studies show that microscopic metastases are present in up to 30% of patients considered by the clinician to have "negative nodes." On the other hand, if the clinician thinks that the axillary nodes are involved, he will prove to be correct about 85% of the time. Thus, the examiner is frequently unable to detect early metastatic involvement of the axillary nodes and should recognize his limitations in this regard.

The axillary and internal mammary lymph node chains may be involved independently of each other, or both may be involved. Metastases occur more frequently in axillary than in internal mammary nodes in patients with operable breast cancer. Location in the breast of the primary lesion has relatively little effect on the incidence of axillary lymph node involvement as determined by pathologic examination of the nodes after radical mastectomy. About one-half of the lesions located in any quadrant or centrally in the breast are associated with positive axillary lymph nodes on histologic examination. On the other hand, the incidence of spread to the internal mammary nodes is influenced by the location of the primary tumor. Cancers in the central and medial portions of the breast metastasize to internal mammary nodes more frequently than lateral lesions (see p. 373).

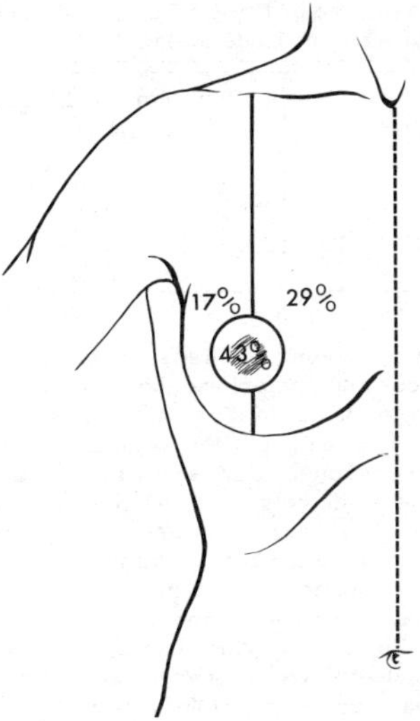

Internal Mammary Node Metastases. The percentage of internal mammary node metastases is shown according to lateral, medial, or subareolar location of the primary tumor. The high percentage of metastases from central tumors is due to the fact that large tumors originating either laterally or medially and extending to the subareolar area are classified as central. (Haagensen, C. D., and others, Ann. Surg. 169:174, 1969.)

The relationship of the size of the primary tumor to the incidence of axillary node metastases is shown in the table on p. 374, top. The influence on location of the axillary nodes to prognosis is shown in the table on p. 374, bottom.

B. Special Clinical Forms of Breast Carcinoma:

1. Paget's carcinoma - The basic lesion is intraductal carcinoma, usually well-differentiated and multicentric in the nipple and breast ducts. The nipple epithelium is infiltrated, but gross nipple changes are often minimal and a tumor mass may not be palpable. The first symptom is often itching or burning of the nipple accompanied by a superficial erosion or ulceration. The diagnosis is readily established by biopsy of the erosion.

   Paget's carcinoma is not common (about 3% of all breast cancers), but it is important because it appears innocuous. It is frequently diagnosed and treated as dermatitis or bacterial infection. This is disastrous, for the lesion metastasizes to regional nodes in up to 60% of cases and should be treated in the same manner as other forms of breast cancer.

Relationship of Size of Breast Tumor to Incidence of Axillary Node Metastases

Size of Primary Tumor	Percentage With Positive Axillary Lymph Nodes
< – 1 cm.	22%
1-1.9 cm.	38%
2-2.9 cm.	41%
3-3.9 cm.	53%
6+	63%

2. **Inflammatory carcinoma - This is the most malignant form of breast cancer and comprises about 3% of all cases. The clinical findings consist of a rapidly growing, sometimes painful mass which enlarges the breast. The overlying skin becomes erythematous, edematous, and warm. The diagnosis should be made only when the redness involves more than one-third of the skin over the breast. The inflammatory changes, often mistaken for an infectious process, are caused by carcinomatous invasion of the subdermal lymphatics with resulting edema and hyperemia. These tumors may be caused by a variety of histologic types. Metastases occur early and widely in all cases, and for this reason inflammatory carcinoma is virtually incurable. Radical mastectomy is not advised. Radiation and hormone therapy are of little value.**

C. Laboratory Findings: Carcinoma localized to the breast and axillary nodes causes no abnormalities detectable by clinical laboratory examinations. Certain tests may be useful as clues to the presence of more widespread disease. A consistently elevated sedimentation rate may be the result of disseminated cancer. Liver metastases may be associated with elevation of alkaline phosphatase. Hypercalcemia is an occasional important finding in advanced malignancy of the breast.

D. X-ray Findings:

1, Metastatic survey - Because of the frequency of metastases to the bones and lungs, preparation for a radical mastectomy should include posteroanterior and lateral chest films. Anteroposterior and lateral views of the lumbar spine and pelvis and a lateral skull x-ray should also be taken preoperatively in all except very early lesions.

Influence of Anatomic Location of Involved Axillary Nodes on Survival in Breast Cancer Treated by Radical Mastectomy

Level	Anatomic Location	Five-Year Survival If Nodes Positive
I	Nodes in low axilla up to the inferior border of the pectoralis minor muscle	65%
II	Nodes posterior to insertion of pectoralis minor muscle	45%
III	Nodes above superior border of pectoralis minor muscle	28%

2. Mammography - A mammogram is a soft tissue radiologic examination of the breast. Xeroradiography is a technical method of mammography that provides especially sharp detail of breast tissues. Mammography is the only reliable means of detecting breast cancer before signs and symptoms appear. Many breast cancers can be diagnosed by mammography as early as 2 years prior to their clinical recognition, and recent reports indicate that certain premalignant conditions of the breast may be identifiable in the future. These developments have led to increased interest in various experimental methods of earlier detection such as thermography, ultrasonography, isotope scanning, and angiography. Wide practical application of certain of these new methods such as thermography may be imminent.

   Indications for mammography include the following: (1) to survey the opposite breast at the time the diagnosis of breast cancer is made and annually thereafter; (2) to complement the annual physical examination of women, particularly those with a family history of breast cancer; (3) as an aid in the evaluation of ill-defined or questionable breast masses; multiple masses; nipple discharge, erosion, or retraction; skin changes; or breast pain; and (4) as an aid in the search for occult primary cancer in women with metastatic disease from an unknown primary.

   Both false-positive and false-negative results are obtained with mammography, but, where mammography is employed proficiently and extensively, the yield of malignant lesions on biopsy remains around 35% - this in spite of the fact that more biopsies are done. The safest course is to biopsy all suspicious masses found on physical examination and, in the absence of a mass, all suspicious lesions demonstrated by mammography.

E. Scanning: Radioisotope scanning of bone is a more sensitive means of identifying bony metastases than skeletal x-rays. Bone scan is indicated when metastases are suspected and x-rays are negative. When x-rays show metastases, bone scan frequently discloses additional lesions. Liver and brain scans are useful when metastatic involvement of these organs is in question.

Differential Diagnosis.

Differential diagnosis depends upon biopsy. The following lesions are most likely to be confused with carcinoma: mammary dysplasia (cystic disease of the breast), adenosis, adenofibroma (in the older patient), intraductal papilloma, and fat necrosis.

With rare exceptions, all breast lumps should be biopsied without delay. Every breast mass in an adult female should be considered malignant until proved otherwise, usually by histologic section. About 30% of lesions thought to be definitely cancer prove to be benign, and about 15% of lesions believed benign are found to be malignant. These findings clearly demonstrate the fallibility of clinical judgment and the necessity for biopsy to settle the issue in most cases.

Biopsy specimens may be obtained by excision of small lesions, removal of a small portion of larger lesions, or by needle. A core of tissue is obtained with a special biopsy needle. Aspiration is not used. There is no evidence that a properly done biopsy procedure causes metastatic spread of cancer. It has not been possible to show by retrospective studies that a delay of a week or so between diagnostic biopsy and definitive treatment of breast cancer has an adverse effect. The preferred approach is incisional or excisional biopsy of the breast mass in the operating room under general or local anesthesia with preparation to proceed immediately with mastectomy if frozen section is positive. However, incisional, excisional, or needle biopsy of the breast mass may be done under local anesthesia on an outpatient or inpatient basis with a view to scheduling definitive surgical or other treatment within a week (see illustration below, left).

Needle biopsy is diagnostic only if positive. A negative needle biopsy should be followed by an open biopsy of the lesion. Needle biopsy is especially useful in making a histologic diagnosis in advanced lesions for which no surgical treatment is planned.

Treatment of breast cancer should never be undertaken without an unequivocal histologic diagnosis. Fortunately, frozen section in this disease is highly reliable. On the rare occasion when diagnosis on frozen section or other type of histologic preparation is questionable, treatment should be deferred pending further tissue examination.

Indications for biopsy of the breast include the following: (1) persistent mass, (2) bloody nipple discharge, (3) eczematoid nipple, and (4) positive mammography. Thermography is an experimental procedure, apparently less reliable than mammography but potentially useful as a screening procedure. In the absence of physical or mammographic findings, positive thermography is a relative indication for biopsy of the suspicious area. Unexplained axillary adenopathy calls for biopsy of the enlarged node after mammography has been done. Random or mirror image biopsy of the contralateral breast is practiced in some centers when the diagnosis of operable

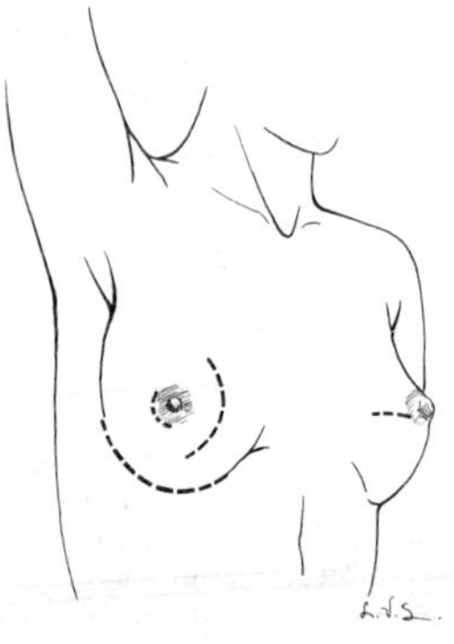

Incisions for Biopsy and for Removal of Benign Tumors

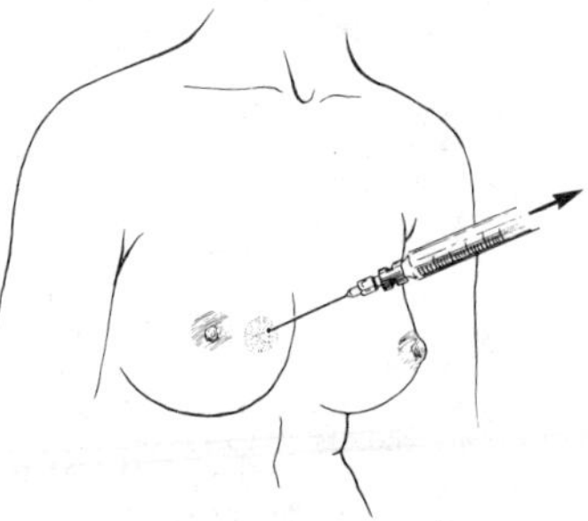

Needle Aspiration of Cyst

breast cancer is established. In patients with a high risk of developing breast cancer, biopsy of the breast for minimal or equivocal change is justified.

In experienced hands, needle aspiration of discrete, spherical lesions of the breast is a useful means of distinguishing the benign cysts of mammary dysplasia from a solid tumor which may be cancer (see illustration on p. 376, right). Turbid greenish or amber fluid is characteristic of a benign cyst, which should disappear completely without residual mass when aspirated. Cytologic examination of the fluid may on rare occasions be of value. Blood-tinged fluid or a persistent mass after aspiration is an indication for biopsy. In any case, patients who develop cysts have an increased risk of developing breast cancer and should be followed regularly. A baseline mammogram should be obtained. When in doubt regarding the diagnosis, biopsy should be performed.

Cytologic examination of nipple discharge is rarely helpful but should be done. Breast biopsy is preferred for bloody or questionable secretions.

In suspected bilateral involvement the preferred biopsy site, provided there are no physical or mammographic indications of a lesion elsewhere, is the upper outer quadrant of the breast since this is the commonest site of the initial lesion. Lobular carcinoma is frequently in situ, and its removal at this stage is generally curative. However, lobular carcinoma in situ may progress to infiltrating lobular carcinoma, the prognosis of which is no better than that of infiltrating ductal carcinoma and actually may be worse.

Treatment.

A. Clinical Staging: Patients with breast cancer can be grouped into stages according to the characteristics of the primary tumor (T), regional lymph nodes (N), and distant metastases (M). Physical, radiologic, and other clinical examinations are used in determining the stage, which is based on all information available before therapy. Staging is useful in evaluating the prognosis and determining the type of treatment indicated. The International Union Against Cancer and the American Joint Committee on Cancer Staging and End Results Reporting have each formulated a standard TNM system to be used by physicians in breast cancer staging. The TNM staging system is summarized in the table on p. 378. The rules for staging of breast cancer as defined by the International and the American systems are given in the table on p. 379.

Both the International and the American staging systems provide sound criteria for the clinical classification of patients with breast cancer. From a practical point of view, it is useful to remember that the International and American systems of staging differ only in detail from this brief definition:

Stage I: The tumor is confined to the breast. There may be early signs of skin involvement such as dimpling or nipple retraction, but there are no signs of axillary or distant metastases.

Stage II: The primary tumor is as in stage I, but there are movable, suspicious nodes in the ipsilateral axilla.

Stage III: The primary tumor is infiltrating the skin or chest wall, or the axillary nodes are matted or fixed.

Stage IV: Distant metastases are present.

TNM System of Staging
(Adopted by the American Joint Committee on Cancer Staging and End Results Reporting.)

		Staging			
		I	II	III	IV
T: Primary Tumor.					
T1 Tumor of 2 cm. or less in its greatest dimension; skin not involved, or involved locally with Paget's disease.	T1	X	X	X	
T2 Tumor over 2 cm. in size or with skin attachment (dimpling of skin) or nipple retraction (in subareolar tumors); no pectoral muscle or chest wall attachment.	T2	or X	or X	or X	Any
T3 Tumor of any size with any of the following: skin infiltration, ulceration, peau d'orange, skin edema, pectoral muscle or chest wall attachment.	T3			or X	
N: Regional Lymph Nodes.					
N0 No clinically palpable axillary lymph nodes (metastasis not suspected).	N0	X		X or	
N1 Clinically palpable axillary lymph nodes that are not fixed (metastasis suspected).	N1		X	X	Any
N2 Clinically palpable ipsilateral axillary or infraclavicular lymph nodes that are fixed to one another or to other structures (metastasis suspected).	N2			or X	
M: Distant Metastasis.					
M0 No distant metastasis.	M0	X	X	X	
M1 Clinical and radiographic evidence of metastasis except those to ipsilateral axillary or infraclavicular lymph nodes.	M1				X

These designations are then combined to define 4 stages which are used for record purposes:

Stage I: T1/N0/M0; T2/N0/M0

Stage II: T1/N1/M0; T2/N1/M0

Stage III: T3/N0/M0; T3/N1/M0; T3/N2/M0; T1/N2/M0; T2/N2/M0; and includes any combination of T1, T2, or T3 with N2 and M0.

Stage IV: Any clinical stage of disease with distant metastasis (M1).

Distribution of breast cancer according to the International and American staging systems is shown in the table on p. 380, top. Five-year survival rates according to the stage of breast cancer are shown in the table on p. 380, bottom.

B. Pathologic Typing: The behavior of breast cancer can be correlated with the histologic appearance of the lesion. Information on the microscopic characteristics of the neoplasm is therefore helpful in deciding on management and in estimating

Clinical Staging of Cancer of the Breast

Stage	International System*	American System†
I	0 No distant metastases. 1 Tumor of 5 cm. or less. 2 Skin fixation absent or incomplete. 3 Nipple may be retracted, or Paget's disease may be present. 4 Pectoral muscle or chest wall fixation absent. 5 No ipsilateral axillary nodes palpable.	0 No distant metastases. 1 Tumor of any size. 2 Skin not involved or involved locally with Paget's disease. 3 Skin attachment (dimpling) or nipple retraction. 4 No pectoral muscle or chest wall attachment. 5 No clinically palpable axillary lymph nodes (no metastases suspected).
II	0-4 As above. 5 Ipsilateral axillary nodes palpable but movable.	0-4 As above. 5 Clinically palpable axillary lymph nodes that are not fixed (metastases suspected).
III	0 As above. 1 Tumor more than 5 cm. in diameter or 2 Skin fixation complete, or skin involvement wide of tumor or 3 Peau d'orange present in tumor area or wide of tumor or 4 Pectoral muscle fixation complete or incomplete, or chest wall fixation or 5 Ipsilateral axillary nodes fixed or 6 Ipsilateral supraclavicular or infraclavicular nodes movable or fixed or 7 Arm edema.	0 As above. 1 Tumor of any size. 2 Skin infiltration or ulceration or 3 Peau d'orange or skin edema or 4 Pectoral muscle or chest wall attachment or 5 Clinically palpable ipsilateral axillary nodes fixed to one another or to other structures (metastases suspected) or 6 Clinically palpable ipsilateral infraclavicular lymph nodes fixed to one another or to other structures (metastases suspected).
IV	Distant metastases, regardless of the condition of the primary tumor and regional lymph nodes.	Clinical, radiographic evidence of metastases except those to ipsilateral axillary or infraclavicular nodes.

*Committee on Clinical Stage Classification and Applied Statistics, Malignant Tumors of the Breast, 1960-1964. International Union Against Cancer, Paris, 1960.

†American Joint Committee on Cancer Staging and End Results Reporting: Clinical Staging System for Cancer of the Breast. American College of Surgeons, 1962.

the prognosis. The pathologist can distinguish 4 types of mammary carcinoma on the basis of cellular differentiation and invasiveness, as shown in the table on p. 381, top.

Type I noninfiltrating neoplasms, particularly those of the intraductal and the lobular in situ variety, are of special inter-

Distribution of Breast Cancer
(According to International and American staging systems.)

Stage	International System	American System
I	42%	48%
II	13%	17%
III	34%	22%
IV	11%	13%
Total	100%	100%

est because of their tendency to occur bilaterally. At the time of initial operation for breast cancer, Urban performed random biopsies of the opposite breast on 73% of 488 patients in his series. When an infiltrating type of carcinoma was present in the primarily involved breast, the overall rate of bilateral cancer was 12% - approximately 8% simultaneous and 4% asynchronous. However, when noninfiltrating cancer was found in the primary breast, the overall rate of bilateral involvement was 20-30% simultaneous and 10% asynchronous. Bilaterality is particularly likely to occur in patients with in situ lobular carcinoma, which should be recognized as a preinvasive form of breast cancer and treated accordingly. Lobular carcinoma may progress in time from an in situ to an infiltrating stage. It may be in situ in one breast and infiltrating in the other. Periods of 1-20 years may elapse between the diagnosis of in situ lobular carcinoma and the development of invasive cancer in the same or opposite breast.

In addition to physical examination and mammography, there is a need to develop ways of diagnosing breast cancer during what may be, especially in type I tumors, a prolonged preclinical or "silent" stage. Biopsy of the opposite "negative" breast at the time of mastectomy for cancer is an approach to the problem of early diagnosis worthy of consideration in patients with lobular and intraductal carcinoma.

In most statistical studies of survival after treatment for carcinoma of the breast, the various pathologic types are not separately identified. As a result, the influence of pathologic type on response to therapy is usually obscured. Those few studies which do correlate clinical stage and pathologic type reveal that stage I lesions less than 5 cm. in size and of pathologic type I or II rarely metastasize beyond the nodes in the lower axilla. Such lesions, therefore, are in a particularly favorable category from the standpoint of such a surgical procedure as modified radical mastectomy.

Five-Year Survival Rates According to Stage of Breast Cancer

Stage	International System	American System
I	80%	75%
II	70%	65%
III	50%	45%
IV	None	None

Classification of Mammary Carcinoma According to the Cellular Growth Pattern

(Kouchoukas and others: Cancer 20:948, 1967.)

Type I: Rarely metastasizing (not invasive)

1. Intraductal or comedocarcinoma without stromal invasion. Paget's disease of the breast may exist if the epithelium of the nipple is involved.
2. Papillary carcinoma confined to the ducts.
3. Lobular carcinoma in situ.

Type II: Rarely metastasizing (always invasive)

1. Well differentiated adenocarcinoma.
2. Medullary carcinoma with lymphocytic infiltration.
3. Pure colloid or mucinous carcinoma.
4. Papillary carcinoma.

Type III: Moderately metastasizing (always invasive)

1. Infiltrating adenocarcinoma.
2. Intraductal carcinoma with stromal invasion.
3. Infiltrating lobular carcinoma.*
4. All tumors not classified as types I, II, or IV.

Type IV: Highly metastasizing (always invasive)

1. Undifferentiated carcinoma having cells without ductal or tubular arrangement.
2. All types of tumors indisputably invading blood vessels.

*Infiltrating lobular carcinoma has been moved from type II to type III because of growing experience with its metastasizing potential.

Relative Frequency of Pathologic Types of Breast Cancer

Type	Characteristics	Percentage of Total Cases
I	Rarely metastasizing (not invasive)	5%
II	Rarely metastasizing (always invasive)	15%
III	Moderately metastasizing (always invasive)	65%
IV	Highly metastasizing (always invasive)	15%

Relationship of Pathologic Type of Breast Cancer to Incidence of Axillary Node Metastases

Type	Percentage With Positive Nodes
I	13%
II	34%
III	58%
IV	57%

Relationship of Pathologic Type of Breast Cancer to Survival

	Five-Year Survival Rate		
	Axillary Nodes		All
Type	Negative	Positive	Cases
I	95%	95%	95%
II	85%	70%	80%
III	80%	50%	60%
IV	80%	40%	55%

C. Curative Treatment: Treatment may be curative or palliative. Curative treatment is advised for clinical stage I and II disease and for selected patients in stage III. Palliative treatment by irradiation, hormones, endocrine ablation, or chemotherapy is recommended for patients in stage IV (distant metastases), for stage III patients unsuitable for curative efforts, and for previously treated patients who develop distant metastases or ineradicable local recurrence.

1. Radical mastectomy - This operation involves en bloc removal of breast, pectoral muscles, and axillary nodes and has been the standard curative procedure for breast cancer since the turn of the century when W.S. Halsted and Willy Meyer independently described their versions of the technic. Experience with radical mastectomy is extensive, and, in properly selected patients, no other form of therapy has produced better results. Radical mastectomy removes the local lesion and the axillary nodes with a wide safety margin of surrounding tissue. Various breast incisions are used depending upon the location of the primary tumor and the preference of the surgeon (see p. 383). If the disease has already spread to the internal mammary or supraclavicular nodes or to more distant sites, radical mastectomy alone will not cure the patient.
2. Extended radical mastectomy - This procedure involves, in addition to standard radical mastectomy, removal of the internal mammary nodes. The extended operation has been recommended by a few surgeons for medially or centrally placed breast lesions and for tumors associated with positive axillary nodes because of the known frequency of internal mammary node metastases under these circumstances. Retrospective clinical comparisons suggest that the 5-year survival and incidence of chest wall recurrence may be slightly better after extended radical mastectomy than after standard radical mastectomy in selected patients, but a controlled prospective clinical trial is required to settle the issue. It does not appear that extended radical mastectomy is significantly more effective than irradiation in preventing recurrence from internal mammary metastases. For this reason, extended radical mastectomy has few advocates at this time.
3. Modified radical mastectomy - This procedure involves complete removal of all breast and subcutaneous tissue (as in standard radical mastectomy) and dissection in continuity of the axillary lymphatic bed up to the level of the coracoid process. The difference between the modified and the stan-

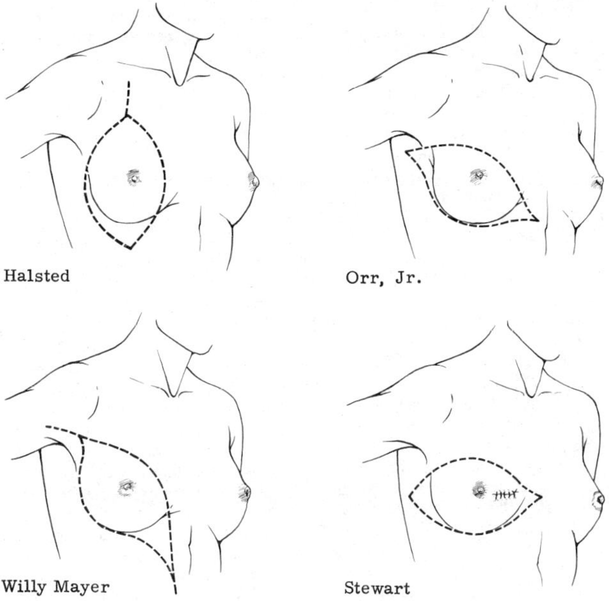

Types of Incisions for Radical Mastectomy

dard radical mastectomy is that the standard operation also removes the pectoralis major and minor muscles and the highest group of axillary nodes just inferior to the clavicle. There is now considerable evidence that morbidity, mortality, survival, and local recurrence rates for standard and modified radical mastectomy are essentially the same for stage I and II breast cancer. Prospective controlled clinical studies will be needed to settle the issue in a definitive manner, but there is already a notable shift in major centers to the use of modified radical mastectomy in patients who, a few years ago, would have been treated by standard radical mastectomy.

4. Simple mastectomy - If the malignancy is confined to the breast without spread to the adjacent muscles or to the regional nodes or beyond (true clinical stage I disease), simple mastectomy (or even wide local excision) should be effective in eradicating the cancer. Clinical experience bears this out in certain cases. The problem is the inability to determine with certainty, prior to their resection and pathologic examination, that the axillary nodes are uninvolved. Reference has already been made to the fact that physical examination is

highly unreliable in detecting axillary metastases. Simple mastectomy must, therefore, be considered an inadequate operation for breast cancer until more is known of the risk associated with leaving axillary metastases until they become clinically evident.

5. Supervoltage irradiation - In recent years, the proved efficacy of supervoltage irradiation in sterilizing the primary lesion and the axillary and internal mammary nodes (Guttman, R. J., Am. J. Roetgenol. **96**:560, 1966; Cancer **20**:1046, 1967) has made radiation therapy with or without simple mastectomy (or wedge resection) an important option for primary treatment of certain breast cancers, particularly those that are locally advanced or when the patient refuses mastectomy. The capability of radical irradiation to destroy or confine metastases in unresected regional nodes has largely eliminated the difference in survival between standard or modified radical mastectomy and simple mastectomy plus irradiation. McWhirtir's policy (since 1941) of treating almost all stages of mammary cancer with simple mastectomy and radical irradiation has been much debated and contested, but the method appears to produce crude survivals at 10 and 15 years equal to those of radical mastectomy for comparable stages of disease (McWhirtir, R., Am. J. Roentgenol. **92**:3, 1964).

D. Choice of Primary Treatment for Breast Cancer: There is evidence that control of mammary cancer confined to the breast and axillary nodes can be achieved by a number of different approaches including standard radical mastectomy, extended radical mastectomy, modified radical mastectomy, simple mastectomy with deferred therapeutic axillary node dissection, and radical irradiation with or without simple mastectomy. The variability in tumor-host relationship from patient to patient and the unpredictability of occult metastases make it difficult to determine with precision the relative merits of current competing forms of treatment without controlled prospective clinical trials.

Relying on evidence now at hand, modified radical mastectomy is recommended as the primary treatment of choice in stage I and II lesions. Results are apparently comparable to those obtained with standard radical mastectomy. Chest wall deformity and problems with shoulder mobility are less with modified radical mastectomy because the pectoral muscles are not removed. The best cosmetic result is achieved when a transverse incision can be used.

Stage III lesions are a borderline group and may or may not be suitable for surgical treatment by either a standard or modified radical mastectomy. Radical surgical treatment is usually contraindicated in stage III lesions with the following characteristics:

(1) Extensive edema involving more than one-third of the skin of the breast.
(2) Satellite nodules on the skin.
(3) Carcinoma of the inflammatory type.
(4) Parasternal tumor nodules.
(5) Edema of the ipsilateral arm.

(6) Palpable ipsilateral infraclavicular lymph nodes (metastases suspected or proved by biopsy).
(7) Two or more of the following grave signs of locally advanced carcinoma:
  (a) Ulceration of the skin.
  (b) Limited edema involving less than one-third of the skin of the breast.
  (c) Fixation of axillary lymph nodes to the skin or the deep structures of the axilla.
  (d) Axillary lymph nodes measuring 2.5 cm. or more in transverse diameter.
  (e) Pectoral muscle or chest wall attachment.

The features listed above are signs of advanced disease and are almost invariably associated with spread to the internal mammary or supraclavicular nodes or other distant sites outside the scope of either standard or modified radical mastectomy. Under these circumstances, operation is not curative and may actually disseminate the disease locally or systemically. Radiotherapy with or without simple mastectomy (or wedge resection) is a more effective approach in these advanced stage III cases.

There remain those stage III lesions which do not exhibit the advanced signs listed above. A modified radical mastectomy may be performed if the primary tumor and the enlarged axillary nodes can clearly be excised with an adequate margin by this procedure. Attachment to the pectoral muscles, high axillary nodes, large primary tumor or nodes, or other technically unfavorable conditions would make standard radical mastectomy the preferred operation.

It is uncertain whether therapeutic abortion significantly improves the prognosis in pregnant patients with cancer which is apparently confined to the breast or to the breast and axillary nodes only. Practice varies widely. It seems reasonable to advise abortion when the child is nonviable. Obviously, the decision must be individualized.

Advice regarding pregnancy must sometimes be given to women who have undergone radical mastectomy or other treatment for cancer of the breast. The weight of the somewhat contradictory evidence is that pregnancy is hazardous and should be avoided or interrupted until the patient has been free of disease for at least 5 years. Thereafter, the presumed stimulating effect of pregnancy on residual cancer is less significant.

E. Radiotherapy as Adjunct to Radical Mastectomy: The purpose of preoperative or postoperative radiotherapy in association with modified or standard radical mastectomy is (1) to reduce the incidence of local recurrence from residual cancer in the operative field, and (2) to sterilize metastatic cancer in the internal mammary and supraclavicular lymph nodes. Patients are therefore selected for radiotherapy on the basis of the likelihood of local recurrence or of the existence of disease in unresected regional nodes. According to these criteria, completely resectable lesions confined to the breast (stage I) do not call for radiotherapy. On the other hand, stage II and stage III patients may be considered for radiotherapy before or after modified or standard radical mastectomy. Only supervoltage irradiation should be advised as adjunctive therapy. Orthovoltage irradiation for this purpose is outmoded.

1. Postoperative radiotherapy - The efficacy of postoperative irradiation in improving survival or recurrence rates has not been decisively demonstrated. However, in view of the proved ability of supervoltage radiotherapy to destroy cancer cells in the breast and regional nodes, postoperative radiotherapy is commonly recommended under the following conditions: (1) if the tumor has been cut through or there is a high likelihood that residual tumor has been left in the operative field; (2) if the tumor is larger than 5 cm. or is located in the central or medial portion of the breast; or (3) if there are metastases to the axillary nodes. Some authorities advise postoperative radiotherapy if one or more axillary nodes are involved; others recommend radiotherapy only if 4 or more nodes are found to contain metastases.

   Radiotherapy is begun as soon after operation as the patient's general condition and state of the wound permit. A tumor dose in the range of 4000-6000 rads (usually 5000 or 5500 rads) is delivered over a period of 4-5 weeks to the internal mammary and supraclavicular and infraclavicular nodal areas. The chest wall is also irradiated only if there is a high probability of chest wall recurrence such as would be the case if the breast lesion was large, cut through, or associated with extensive axillary node involvement. When irradiation is properly managed, delayed wound healing and pulmonary damage are infrequent problems. There is a slight increase in lymphedema of the arm following postoperative radiotherapy.

   In a recent large cooperative study, Fisher and others (Ann. Surg. 172:711-732, 1970) found that although postoperative irradiation slightly reduced the incidence of local recurrence, it did not improve survival.

2. Preoperative radiotherapy - The beneficial results of preoperative radiotherapy are more definite than those of postoperative radiotherapy. Preoperative irradiation reduces the incidence of local recurrence. Fletcher (JAMA 200:140, 1967) demonstrated a 5% local recurrence rate after preoperative radiotherapy, compared to a 16% local recurrence rate following postoperative radiotherapy. Preoperative radiotherapy is possibly also of value in making inoperable patients curable by radical mastectomy, although in such patients the results may not be superior to those obtainable by radiotherapy alone. Indications for preoperative irradiation include the following: (1) primary tumor larger than 5 cm.; (2) limited skin edema or direct skin involvement over tumor; (3) multiple low or midaxillary nodes; or (4) a previous surgical procedure which may have disseminated the tumor locally. A 4000-6000 rad tumor dose is delivered to the axillary, supraclavicular, and internal mammary nodes, and the chest wall and breast are treated tangentially. Radical mastectomy is performed 5-6 weeks after completion of radiotherapy. When cases are properly selected and managed and there is the necessary close cooperation be-

tween radiotherapist and surgeon, there is no significant increase in immediate postsurgical complications as a result of preoperative radiotherapy.

Preoperative Preparation for Radical Mastectomy.

There are 2 objectives of the preoperative work-up: (1) to determine the patient's general condition, with special attention to operative risk; and (2) to search for possible distant metastases.

In patients with no evidence of systemic disease and only a small breast tumor, a complete work-up for metastatic disease is not usually necessary. Only about one in 5 or 6 of such patients is found on breast biopsy to have a malignant tumor. If the local lesion is highly suspicious or if enlarged axillary nodes or other suggestive signs of metastases are present, x-rays should be obtained of the chest (posteroanterior and lateral), skull (anteroposterior and lateral), and lumbar spine and pelvis (anteroposterior). Serum alkaline phosphatase determination and liver scan or needle biopsy are advisable if liver metastases are suspected because of hepatomegaly. Skeletal pain is an indication for films of the painful site, and, if these are negative, bone scans should be considered.

Preoperatively, full discussion with the patient and her next of kin regarding the possible necessity for mastectomy is essential. Because of the controversial nature of the relative benefits of simple, modified radical, or radical mastectomy, many patients wish to discuss the subject in detail and may insist that they wish one or another of the operations. It behooves the surgeon to be patient and understanding, stating his own position as he sees it.

Postoperative Management.

Wound complications following modified or standard radical mastectomy such as marginal slough, fluid collection under the flaps, and infection are minimized by attention during operation to viability of skin flaps and to closure without tension. Suction drainage of the wound by means of catheters placed beneath the skin flaps reduces the collection of blood and serum. Bulky compression dressings are unnecessary.

Active motion of the arm and shoulder on the operated side should be encouraged after the first few days, so that by 10-14 days postoperatively there is a full range of motion. Failure of the patient to cooperate or to make progress may necessitate physical therapy. The Service Committee of the American Cancer Society sponsors a rehabilitation program for postmastectomy patients called Reach for Recovery and will provide useful literature upon request. The patient's morale is improved by early provision of a breast prosthesis held in place by a comfortably fitted brassiere.

Radical mastectomy is well tolerated even by elderly patients. The operative mortality is 1% or less, and the immediate postoperative complications are not usually a serious problem.

Complications of Radical Mastectomy.

A. Local Recurrence: Recurrence of cancer within the operative field following radical mastectomy is due to incomplete removal of tumor or involved nodes, to cutting across infiltrated lymphatics, or to spillage of tumor cells into the wound. The rate of local recurrence correlates with tumor size, the presence and number of involved axillary nodes, the histologic type of tumor, and the presence of skin edema or skin and fascia fixation with the primary. In one series of 704 patients treated with radical mastectomy without ancillary therapy and uniformly followed for at least 5 years, 17% developed local recurrence. When the axillary nodes were not involved at the time of mastectomy, the local recurrence rate was 7%, but the rate was 26% when they were involved. A similar difference in local recurrence rate was noted between small and large tumors. In general, local recurrence rate is a function of the stage of the patient's disease. (Spratt, I. S., Jr., and W. L. Donegan, Cancer of the Breast. Saunders, 1967.)

Chest wall recurrences usually appear within the first 2 years, with a peak incidence in the second year, but may occur as late as 15 or more years after radical mastectomy. Suspect nodules should be biopsied. If the biopsy is positive, disseminated disease must be suspected and a search for metastases made by chest and bone films. Local excision or localized radiotherapy may be feasible if an isolated nodule is present. If lesions are multiple or accompanied by evidence of regional involvement in the internal mammary or supraclavicular nodes, the disease is best managed by comprehensive radiation treatment of the whole chest wall including the parasternal, supraclavicular, and axillary areas. Although local recurrences usually signal the presence of widespread disease, when there is no evidence of metastases beyond the chest wall and regional nodes, radical irradiation for cure should be attempted.

B. Edema of the Arm: Except for local recurrence, the only important late complication of standard radical mastectomy is edema of the arm. Significant edema occurs in 10-30% of cases. When it appears in the early postoperative period, it is usually caused by lymphatic obstruction due to infection in the axilla. Late or secondary edema of the arm may develop years after radical mastectomy as a result of axillary recurrence or of infection in the hand or arm with obliteration of lymphatic channels. After radical mastectomy, the lymphatic drainage of the arm is always compromised and the extremity becomes more than normally susceptible to infection following minor injuries. The patient should be warned of this and treatment instituted promptly if infection occurs. Specific instruction should be given to the patient who has had radical mastectomy to avoid breaks in the skin of the hand and arm on the operated side and to refrain from tasks likely to cause superficial wounds and infections. Injections for inoculation and immunization should not be given in that arm. Well-established chronic edema is managed by elevation and elastic support.

Palliative Treatment.

A. Radiotherapy: Palliative radiotherapy may be advised for locally advanced cancers with distant metastases in order to control ulceration, pain, and other manifestations in the breast and regional nodes. Radical irradiation of the breast and chest wall and axillary, internal mammary, and supraclavicular nodes should be undertaken in an attempt to cure locally advanced and inoperable lesions when there is no evidence of distant metastases. A certain number of patients in this group is cured in spite of extensive breast and regional node involvement.

Palliative irradiation is also of value in the treatment of certain bone or soft tissue metastases to control pain or avoid fracture, particularly when hormonal, endocrine ablation, and chemical therapy are inappropriate or ineffective.

B. Hormone Therapy: When distant metastases have occurred in breast cancer, the patient is incurable; however, disseminated disease may be kept under control or caused to regress for sustained periods by various forms of endocrine therapy, including administration of hormones or ablation of the ovaries, adrenals, or pituitary. About one-third of breast cancer patients will respond to one or more of these endocrine measures. The incidence of hormonal responsiveness is approximately the same in premenopausal women as in postmenopausal women, although the methods of treatment used may be quite different.

The major forms of hormone treatment are estrogen, androgen, and corticosteroid therapy.

1. Estrogen therapy - Estrogens should be reserved for postmenopausal women. The best results of estrogen administration are obtained in women more than 5 years past the menopause. Estrogen is capable of causing exacerbation of tumor growth in 50% of premenopausal women and should not be given to them or to recently postmenopausal women until the vaginal smear ceases to show evidence of estrogenic activity. Tumor remission rates from estrogen (and androgen as well) tend to increase with increasing numbers of years past the menopause.

   Estrogen administered as primary therapy will induce tumor regression in over 30% of postmenopausal patients with advanced breast cancer. Objective evidence of tumor regression is seen most commonly in soft tissue metastases in older patients, and over 40% of this group show remission of tumor growth. Both local soft tissue and visceral lesions show a higher remission rate from estrogen than from androgen therapy. The reverse is true for bone metastases.

   Treatment usually consists of giving diethylstilbestrol (or equivalent), 5 mg. 3 times daily orally, and continued as long as it is beneficial.

   The first evidence of regression of metastatic cancer does not usually appear until about 4 weeks after beginning estrogen therapy, but the trial of estrogen should not be abandoned in less than 2 months except in case of obvious exacerbation or serious side-effects. The average duration of remission is about 16 months, but remissions of soft tissue lesions lasting more than 5 years are occasionally seen. The survival time of women who respond to estrogen therapy is about twice that of nonresponders.

   The most common side-effects are anorexia, nausea, and vomiting. These usually disappear within a few weeks, but when symptoms of toxicity are severe the dosage should be reduced temporarily until tolerance is acquired. Pigmentation of nipples, areolas, and axillary skin, enlargement of the breasts, and sodium and water retention are among the side-effects of estrogen therapy. Uterine bleeding occurs in the majority of postmenopausal patients when estrogen therapy is stopped, and patients should be warned of this possibility to avoid anxiety. Severe bleeding can usually be controlled by administration of testosterone propionate, 100 mg. I.M. daily for 3 or 4 doses.

2. Androgen therapy - Androgen administration causes tumor regression in 10-20% of premenopausal women with advanced breast cancer. However, because of the more frequent and prolonged remission from castration, this procedure is preferred as initial treatment in the premenopausal group. Androgen therapy may sometimes be usefully added to castration in patients under 35 years of age, or in the presence of bone metastases, because of the frequently poor results from castration alone in such patients. Failure of response to castration may be considered an indication for a trial of androgen therapy because of the low likelihood of a favorable response by these patients to adrenalectomy or hypophysectomy. Androgen therapy causes temporary amenorrhea in premenopausal women.

Estrogen therapy is not advisable in recently postmenopausal women until the vaginal smear ceases to show evidence of estrogenic activity because of the danger of exacerbating the disease. A trial of androgen therapy is warranted in this group, but with the expectation of a favorable response in only about 15% of patients.

Since bone metastases are commonly more responsive to androgen than to estrogen therapy, a trial of androgen administration may be advantageous when osseous lesions are present, particularly before adrenalectomy or hypophysectomy is undertaken. About 25% of patients with bone metastases who are more than 5 years past the menopause will respond to androgen therapy. Patients failing to respond can still be subjected to operation if indicated, and surgery will usually have been delayed only about 6 weeks.

Postmenopausal patients who have shown a favorable response to castration or estrogen therapy and have then relapsed may be given a trial of androgen therapy with a 20-30% chance of responding favorably. In patients more than 5 years postmenopausal, bony metastases which have failed to respond to estrogens are more likely to regress on secondary androgen therapy than are soft tissue metastases. Occasionally, androgen administration will cause tumor regression in the completely hypophysectomized patient.

Androgen may be given continuously as long as tumor regression persists. It is probably preferable, however, to administer androgen until the tumor has regressed maximally and then to discontinue administration until reactivation occurs, at which time resumption of androgen therapy will often produce another regression. Intermittent therapy of this kind has the advantage of reducing the tendency to virilization while varying the hormonal environment of the tumor, thereby perhaps postponing the development of autonomy in the tumor.

The androgen preparation most frequently employed is testosterone propionate, 100 mg. I.M. 3 times a week.

However, it is simpler and equally effective to give fluoxymesterone, 20-40 mg. daily orally. An orally administered nonvirilizing androgen, testolactone (Teslac®), is reported to be as effective as testosterone propionate in causing tumor regression. The major reason for interest in this compound is that, since it appears to be relatively inert hormonally, it may have a direct effect on the breast cancer.

About 3 months of androgen therapy are usually required for maximal response. Pain relief may be achieved in up to 80% of patients with osseous metastases. In addition, androgen therapy usually results in a sense of well-being and an increase in energy and weight, particularly in postmenopausal patients. The principal adverse side reactions are increased libido and masculinizing effects, e.g., hirsutism, hoarseness, loss of scalp hair, acne, and ruddy complexion. Virilization occurs in practically all women taking testosterone propionate for longer than 6 months but in only about one-third of patients receiving fluoxymesterone. Fluid retention, anorexia, vomiting, and liver damage are among the rarer side-effects of androgen therapy.

3. Corticosteroids - Corticosteroids are especially valuable in the management of the serious acute symptoms which may result from such conditions as hypercalcemia, brain and lung metastases, and hepatic metastases with jaundice. Corticosteroid therapy is also indicated for patients who are too ill for major endocrine ablation therapy and for those whose tumors do not respond to other endocrine therapy. The combination of systemic corticosteroid and the intracavitary injection of an alkylating agent (see below) may be very effective in controlling pleural effusion due to metastatic breast cancer.

The patient's age and previous response to sex hormone therapy are not correlated with response to corticosteroid therapy, which probably acts through a local effect upon the tumor or the tumor bed. A prior favorable response to adrenocorticosteroids does not guarantee a similar response to adrenalectomy. Objective evidence of tumor regression following corticosteroid administration is less than that following adrenalectomy. Remission on corticosteroid therapy averages about 6 months, whereas that following adrenalectomy is over 12 months.

The subjective response of the seriously ill patient to corticosteroid administration is often striking. Appetite, sense of well-being, and pain from bone or visceral metastases may be markedly improved. However, objective regression of soft tissue lesions occurs in only about 15% of patients. The relief of coma due to brain metastases and dyspnea due to lung metastases is often encouraging but transient. Hypercalcemia is probably improved by specific action on calcium metabolism.

Cortisone acetate, 150 mg. daily orally, or prednisone or prednisolone, 30 mg. daily orally, is an average dose. Twice or 3 times these amounts may be required temporarily for control of severe, acute symptoms. A variety of other corticosteroids has been employed in equivalent dosage with similar results. The dosage of corticosteroids must be reduced slowly if they have been used for prolonged periods because of the adrenocortical atrophy induced.

Adrenocortical hormones may cause numerous undesirable systemic effects and serious complications such as uncontrollable infection, bleeding peptic ulcer, muscle weakness, hypertension, diabetes, edema, and features of Cushing's syndrome.

The best overall tumor remission rate from hormonal therapy in postmenopausal patients can probably be obtained when treatment is individualized. In general, patients with soft tissue and intrathoracic metastases respond best to estrogen therapy. Androgen therapy is usually more effective in patients with bone metastases. Corticosteroid therapy should be considered especially for patients with brain and liver metastases.

C. Therapeutic Endocrine Ablation:

1. Castration - Oophorectomy in premenopausal women with advanced, metastatic, or recurrent breast cancer results in temporary regression in about 35% of cases, with objective improvement lasting an average of about 10 months. Life is definitely prolonged in patients who respond favorably. Patients not responding to castration usually but not always fail to respond favorably to adrenalectomy, hypophysectomy, or specific hormones. Authorities differ on whether castration should be given a trial in all premenopausal women before advising bilateral adrenalectomy or hypophysectomy. Of those patients responding favorably to castration, 40-50% will respond to bilateral adrenalectomy or hypophysectomy. Of those who do not respond to oophorectomy, only 10-15% show tumor regression after one of the major procedures. According to some authorities, simultaneous oophorectomy and adrenalectomy is the palliative treatment of choice in premenopausal women with disseminated breast cancer. Prophylactic castration of all premenopausal women with breast cancer is not of proved value and is not recommended.

   Castration can be performed by bilateral oophorectomy or irradiation. Surgical removal of the ovaries is preferable because it rules out the possibility of residual ovarian function. Therapeutic castration is essentially confined to premenopausal women and is of no value in truly postmenopausal women. Ovarian function may persist for a few years after cessation of menses, and this can be determined by means of the vaginal smear; if evidence of persistent estrogenic activity is found, castration may be beneficial.

2. Adrenalectomy or hypophysectomy - Regression of advanced breast cancer occurs in about 30% of patients after either of these procedures. Patients who respond to castration or to hormone administration are most likely to benefit from removal of the adrenals or pituitary. This information is helpful in the selection of patients for one of these major ablation procedures.

   Adrenalectomy is preferred over hypophysectomy because of its wider availability and greater ease of postoperative endocrine management. The mortality rate of both procedures is in the range of 5%. Transphenoidal implantation (under local anesthesia) of beta ray-emitting yttrium can now be performed with low morbidity and mortality in a few centers, and destruction of the pituitary with great precision by a proton beam is a possible future mode of therapy. Currently, however, adrenalectomy is the procedure of choice in most institutions.

Replacement therapy after adrenalectomy is with oral cortisone acetate, 37.5-50 mg. daily, supplemented in some patients with fludrocortisone acetate, 0.1 mg. orally every other day for its sodium-retaining effect.

The diet following adrenalectomy should include at least 3 Gm. of NaCl daily, which may be achieved by liberal salting of food. Adrenal insufficiency will occur if the maintenance corticosteroid regimen is inadequate or is neglected. Resulting symptoms may include extreme weakness, nausea and vomiting, rapid weight loss, and hypotension. Increased stress calls for increased dosage. Acute crises of adrenal insufficiency require immediate hospitalization and intensive treatment.

In premenopausal women, when oophorectomy alone is followed by a remission and adrenalectomy withheld until progression of the tumor resumes, the overall palliation and length of survival are possibly somewhat better than when adrenals and ovaries are removed at the same operation. Postmenopausal women should be treated by simultaneous oophorectomy and adrenalectomy.

The response of metastatic breast carcinoma to administration of hormones or to ablation of endocrine glands is most likely to be favorable under the following circumstances: (1) slowly growing tumor (e.g., free interval between diagnosis and development of metastases exceeds 24 months), (2) hormone therapy is begun promptly when metastases appear, (3) metastases localized to the soft tissues, bones, and pleuropulmonary region (as opposed to visceral areas such as liver and brain), (4) advanced age, and (5) previous response to hormone therapy or castration. However, favorable responses may occur occasionally when none of these favorable conditions exist.

D. Chemotherapy: Chemotherapy should be considered for palliation in advanced breast cancer when hormone treatment is not successful or when the patient becomes unresponsive to it. Chemotherapy is most likely to be effective in patients who previously responded to hormonal therapy. The most useful chemotherapeutic agent to date is fluorouracil (5-FU), but thiotepa and methotrexate are also of value. These drugs are administered intravenously. Their side-effects include bone marrow depression and nausea and vomiting, which may be so severe as to limit or prevent their use.

Intrapleural injection of methotrexate will frequently control pleural effusion due to metastases. Control of pleural effusion due to metastatic breast cancer is best achieved by trocar thoracotomy to establish closed tube drainage. When the fluid has been practically completely removed, 20 mg. of methotrexate freshly dissolved in 50-100 ml. of diluent are injected through the tube, which is clamped for 2 hours and then reopened to waterseal drainage. The tube is removed in 1-2 days when all the fluid has been evacuated and the lung fully expanded.

E. Hypercalcemia in Advanced Breast Cancer: Hypercalcemia occurs transiently or terminally in about 10% of women with advanced breast cancer. The serum calcium level should be determined periodically in such patients or when suggestive symptoms occur. In the great majority of cases, the cause of elevated serum calcium is not known, but there is a possible relation to (1) immobilization of the patient by progressive invalidism, (2) radiotherapy for osseous metastases, or (3) hormonal therapy. However, hypercalcemia develops in many women without these presumed causes and in the absence of bony metastases or changes in the parathyroid glands. This supports the theory that certain disseminated breast cancers elaborate an osteolytic substance. Some breast tumors have been found to produce parathormone; others elaborate a sterol with vitamin D-like activity.

The symptoms of hypercalcemia are protean, and its course is treacherous. Initial symptoms may include irritability, lethargy, anorexia, nausea, vomiting, nocturia, and dehydration. Many of these symptoms could be attributed to disseminated tumor and hypercalcemia overlooked. Rapid deterioration, anuria, coma, and death may occur unless the hypercalcemia is corrected.

Prevention is important and consists of (1) adequate hydration (at least 2 L. of fluid/day), (2) maintenance of as much physical activity as possible, and (3) a low-calcium diet (avoidance of milk, cheese, ice cream, and vitamin D).

Treatment of hypercalcemia is based on (1) immediate cessation of any hormone therapy, (2) increasing the rate of calcium excretion in the urine by maintaining a fluid intake of 5-6 L./day, and (3) decreasing the mobilization of calcium from the bone by administration of corticosteroids in the form of 20-100 mg. of prednisone (or equivalent) daily. Disodium edetate may be given I.V. For acute, severe, potentially fatal elevations of serum calcium, the intravenous injection of isotonic sodium sulfate may be lifesaving. Major endocrine ablation may be required after the hypercalcemia is controlled or may be necessary (though rarely) as a control measure.

After subsidence of an episode of hypercalcemia, many patients survive for months or years with essentially the same relationship to their disease.

Prevention.

Breast cancer cannot be "prevented," but a diagnosis can be made in an earlier stage provided certain procedures are followed. The most important of these are discussed under Clinical Findings.

Prognosis.

When cancer is confined to the breast, the five-year clinical cure rate by radical mastectomy is 75-90%. When axillary nodes are involved, the rate drops to 40-60%. Operative mortality is about 1%. The most unfavorable anatomic site for breast carcinoma is the medial portion of the inner lower quadrant. Breast cancer is probably more malignant in young than in old women, but the difference is not great. The prognosis of carcinoma of the breast occurring during lactation or pregnancy is generally poor, since over one-fourth are inoperable; but when radical mastectomy is feasible and the axillary nodes are not involved, the over-all five-year clinical cure rate in this group of patients is 60-70%. The presence of axillary metastases in patients who are pregnant or lactating is an extremely poor prognostic sign and the five-year clinical cure rate after radical mastectomy under these conditions is only 5-10%.

Most of the local and distant metastases occur during the first 3 years after radical mastectomy. During this period the patient should be examined every 3-4 months. Thereafter, a follow-up examination is done every 6 months for the life of the patient with special attention to the opposite breast because of the increased risk in such patients of developing a second primary lesion.

CARCINOMA OF THE MALE BREAST

Breast cancer in men is a rare disease; the incidence is only about 1% of that in women. The average age at occurrence is about 60 - somewhat older than the most common presenting age in the female. The prognosis, even in stage I cases, is worse in the male than in the female. Blood-borne metastases are commonly present when the male patient appears for initial treatment. These metastases may be latent and may not become manifest for many years.

As in the female, hormonal influences are probably related to the development of male breast cancer. A high estrogen level (as in liver disease), a shift in the androgen-estrogen ratio, or an abnormal susceptibility of breast tissue to normal estrogen concentrations may be of etiologic significance.

Clinical Findings.

A painless lump, occasionally associated with nipple discharge, retraction, erosion, or ulceration, is the chief complaint. Examination usually shows a hard, ill-defined, nontender mass beneath the nipple or areola. Gynecomastia not uncommonly precedes or accompanies male breast cancer.

There is a high incidence of both breast cancer and gynecomastia in Bantu males, theoretically due to failure of estrogen inactivation by a damaged liver associated with vitamin B deficiency. Breast cancer is staged in the male as in the female patient. Gynecomastia and metastatic cancer from another site (e.g., prostate) must be considered in the differential diagnosis of a breast lesion in the male patient. A biopsy should be performed to settle the issue when in doubt.

Treatment.

Treatment consists of radical mastectomy in operable patients, who should be chosen by the same criteria as for female breast carcinoma. Radiation therapy is also advised as in female patients according to similar indications. Irradiation is the first step in the treatment of localized metastases in the skin, lymph nodes, or skeleton which are causing symptoms.

Since male breast cancer is so frequently a disseminated disease, endocrine therapy is of considerable importance in its management. Castration in advanced breast cancer is the most successful palliative measure and is more beneficial than the same procedure in the female. Objective evidence of regression may be seen in 60-70% of male patients who are castrated (approximately twice the proportion seen in the female). The average duration of tumor growth remission is about 30 months, and life is undoubtedly prolonged. Bone is the most frequent site of metastases from breast cancer in the male (as it is in the female also), and castration relieves bone pain in the vast majority of patients so treated. The longer the interval between mastectomy and recurrence, the longer the tumor growth remission following castration. As in the female, there is no correlation between the histologic type of the tumor and the likelihood of remission following castration. In view of the marked benefits of castration in advanced disease, prophylactic castration has been suggested in stage II male breast cancer, but there is no certainty that this approach is warranted.

Bilateral adrenalectomy (or hypophysectomy) has been proposed as the procedure of choice when tumor has reactivated after castration. Corticosteroid therapy is considered by some to be more efficacious than major endocrine ablation. Male breast cancer is too rare to enable this issue to be decided in a definitive manner at this time. Either approach may be temporarily beneficial. It is probably preferable to reserve corticosteroid therapy for those patients unfit for major endocrine ablation. The recommended dosage of prednisolone or prednisone is 30 mg. daily orally, increased to 100 mg. daily for urgent symptoms. The dosage is reduced to 20 mg. daily when control is established, but it may be necessary to increase the dosage to maintain control over a long period. The side-effects of corticosteroid therapy must be kept in mind.

Estrogen therapy - 5 mg. of diethylstilbestrol 3 times daily orally - may rarely be effective. Androgen therapy may exacerbate bone pain. Castration, bilateral adrenalectomy, and corticosteroids are the main lines of therapy for advanced male breast cancer.

Prognosis.

The absolute 5-year survival of men with breast cancer is about 30%. Following radical mastectomy, the 5-year survival is about 40%. Huggins and Taylor (Arch. Surg. 70:303, 1955) reported a 5-year survival in only 5 of 14 stage I cases of male breast cancer. Palliative therapy is frequently required in this disease because of the frequency of occult metastases and its tendency to present in an advanced stage.

MAMMARY DYSPLASIA

This disorder, also known as chronic cystic disease of the breast, is the most frequent lesion of the breast. It is common in women 30-50 years of age but rare in postmenopausal women, which suggests that it is related to ovarian activity. Estrogenic hormone is considered to be an etiologic factor. The typical pathologic change in the breast is the formation of cysts in the terminal ducts and acini. Cysts may be gross or microscopic. Large cysts are clinically palpable and may be several centimeters or more in diameter.

Sclerosing adenosis is a rare form of mammary dysplasia which may produce a palpable lump and a microscopic picture suggestive of cancer. It also occurs in a diffusely disseminated form consisting of multiple small foci throughout a substantial part of the breast. The microscopic appearance of sclerosing adenosis is varied. Some examples of this lesion show changes quite suggestive of cancer such as marked hyperplasia of ducts. When sclerosing adenosis occurs clinically as a palpable lump in the breast with microscopy suspicious of cancer, the differential diagnosis can be difficult for the pathologist.

Clinical Findings.

Mammary dysplasia may produce an asymptomatic lump in the breast which is discovered by accident, but pain or tenderness often calls attention to the mass. In many cases, discomfort occurs or is increased during the premenstrual phase of the cycle, at which time the cysts tend to enlarge rapidly. Fluctuation in size and rapid appearance or disappearance of a breast tumor are common. Multiple or bilateral masses are not unusual, and many patients will give a history of a transient lump in the breast or cyclic breast pain. Pain, fluctuation in size, and multiplicity of lesions are the features most helpful in differentiation from carcinoma.

Treatment.

Because mammary dysplasia is frequently indistinguishable from carcinoma on the basis of clinical findings, it is advisable to prepare the patient for radical mastectomy and to explore the suspicious lesion in the operating room under general anesthesia with provisions for immediate diagnosis by frozen section. Discrete cysts or small localized areas of cystic disease should be excised when cancer has been ruled out by microscopic examination. Surgery in mammary dysplasia should be conservative, since the primary objective of surgery is to exclude malignancy. Simple mastectomy or extensive removal of breast tissue is rarely, if ever, indicated.

When the diagnosis of mammary dysplasia has been established by biopsy or is practically certain because the history is classical, aspiration of a discrete mass is justifiable. The skin and overlying tissues are anesthetized by infiltration with 1% procaine, and a 20-gauge needle is introduced. If a cyst is present, typical watery fluid (straw-colored, gray, greenish, brown, or black) is easily evacuated and the mass disappears. The patient is reexamined at intervals of 2-4 weeks for 3 months and every 6 months thereafter for life. If no fluid is obtained, if a mass persists after aspiration, or if at any time during follow-up an atypical, persistent lump is noted, biopsy should be performed without delay.

Breast pain associated with generalized mammary dysplasia is best treated by avoidance of trauma and by wearing (day and night) a brassiere which gives good support and protection. Hormone therapy is not advisable because it does not cure the condition and has undesirable side-effects.

Prognosis.

Exacerbations of pain, tenderness, and cyst formation may

occur at any time until the menopause, when the symptoms of mammary dysplasia subside. The patient should be taught to examine her own breasts each month just after menstruation and to inform her physician if a mass appears.

MAMMARY DUCT ECTASIA

This rare disorder is also sometimes called plasma cell mastitis or comedomastitis. It is characterized by dilatation of ducts, inspissation of breast secretion, and inflammation within and around the ducts and in the interstitial tissues. Plasma cells are prominent in the inflammatory reaction, which produces a focal or diffuse area of pain, tenderness, induration, and tumor.

This condition tends to occur in the fifth decade of life. The most likely cause is inspissation of lipid debris within the duct. A sterile ductal inflammation is presumably followed by escape of lipid material into surrounding stroma with resultant more widespread inflammatory reaction. This view of etiology, as opposed to a viral or bacterial cause, is supported by the fact that about one-half of these patients have inverted or cracked nipples or have had difficulty nursing.

Although the lesion is benign and not precancerous, it is easily mistaken for breast carcinoma because of its tendency to cause skin or nipple retraction as a result of skin fixation. Inflammatory enlargement of axillary nodes may occur to heighten the resemblance to carcinoma with metastases. In mammary duct ectasia, however, there is usually a distinguishing history of pain, tenderness, and redness which suggests that the breast induration is due to inflammation. Nevertheless, biopsy will usually be necessary to differentiate mammary duct ectasia from cancer.

FIBROADENOMA OF THE BREAST

This common benign neoplasm occurs most frequently in young women, usually within 20 years after puberty. It is somewhat more frequent and tends to occur at an earlier age in black than in white women. Multiple tumors in one or both breasts are found in 10-15% of patients.

The typical fibroadenoma is a round, firm, discrete, relatively movable, nontender mass 1-5 cm. in diameter. The tumor is usually discovered accidentally. Clinical diagnosis in young patients is usually not difficult. In women over 30, mammary dysplasia and carcinoma must be considered. Fibroadenoma does not normally occur after the menopause, but postmenopausal women may occasionally develop fibroadenoma after administration of estrogenic hormone.

Treatment in all cases is excision and frozen section to determine if the lesion is cancerous.

Cystosarcoma phyllodes is a type of fibroadenoma with cellular stroma which tends to grow rapidly. This tumor may become quite large, and if inadequately excised will recur locally. The lesion is rarely malignant. Treatment is by local excision of the mass with a margin of surrounding breast tissue.

INTRADUCTAL PAPILLOMA AND NIPPLE DISCHARGE

Intraductal papilloma is a rare benign lesion arising from the ducts of the breast. The lesion is usually single and located in the region of the nipple, but multiple papillomas may occur throughout the breast. Papillomas are usually small, soft, and fragile, supported by filamentous fibrous trabeculae. They infrequently become large and may reach 4-5 cm. in diameter. It may be difficult to distinguish intraductal papilloma from cancer on frozen section, and this difficulty increases with the size and complexity of the lesion. Malignant change in intraductal papilloma is very rare. Nipple discharge, which may or may not be bloody, is the commonest complaint associated with papilloma. A mass near the nipple is present in most patients, and pressure at this location usually causes a discharge from the nipple.

In order of decreasing frequency, thc following lesions produce nipple discharge: intraductal papilloma, carcinoma, mammary dysplasia, and ectasia of the ducts. The discharge is usually serous or bloody. When papilloma or cancer is the cause, a tumor can frequently be palpated beneath or close to the areola.

The site of the duct orifice from which the fluid exudes is a guide to the location of the involved duct. Gentle pressure on the breast is made with the fingertip at successive points around the circumference of the areola (see below). A point will be found at which pressure produces discharge. The dilated duct or a small tumor may be palpable here. The involved area should be excised by a meticulous technic that ensurcs rcmoval of the affected duct and breast tissue immediately adjacent to it. If a tumor is present,

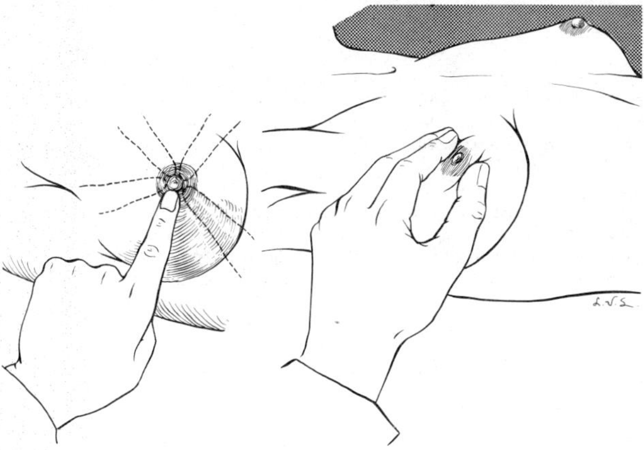

Nipple Discharge. The involved duct can usually be localized by fingertip pressure at successive points around the areola.

it should be biopsied and a frozen section done to determine whether cancer is present. When localization is not possible and no mass is palpable, the patient should be reexamined at intervals of 1-3 months. When unilateral discharge persists, even without definite localization or tumor, exploration must be considered. The alternative is careful, continuous follow-up at intervals of 1-3 months. Mammography should be done. Cytologic examination of nipple discharge for exfoliated cancer cells is occasionally helpful in differential diagnosis.

Although none of the benign lesions causing nipple discharge is precancerous, any of them may coexist with cancer, and it is not possible to distinguish them definitely from malignancy on clinical grounds. Patients with carcinoma almost always have a palpable mass, but in rare instances a nipple discharge may be the only sign. For these reasons, chronic nipple discharge is usually an indication for exploration of the breast.

FAT NECROSIS

Fat necrosis is a rare lesion of the breast but is of clinical importance because it produces a mass, often accompanied by skin or nipple retraction, which is indistinguishable from carcinoma. Trauma is presumed to be the cause, although only about one-half of patients give a history of injury to the breast. Ecchymosis is occasionally seen near the tumor. Tenderness may be present. If untreated, the mass associated with fat necrosis gradually disappears. As a rule, the safest course is to obtain a biopsy. When carcinoma has been ruled out, the area of involvement should be excised.

BREAST ABSCESS

During nursing, an area of redness, tenderness, and induration not infrequently develops in the breast. In the early stages, the infection can often be reversed by discontinuing breast feeding and administering an antibiotic. If the lesion progresses to form a localized mass with increasing signs of infection, an abscess is present and should be drained.

A subareolar abscess may develop in a young or middle-aged woman who is not lactating. These infections tend to recur after incision and drainage unless the area is explored in a quiescent interval with excision of the involved collecting ducts at the base of the nipple.

Except for the subareolar types of abscess, infection in the breast is very rare unless the patient is lactating. Therefore, findings suggestive of abscess in the nonlactating breast require incision and biopsy of any indurated tissue. (See also Mammary Duct Ectasia, above.)

GYNECOMASTIA

Hypertrophy of the male breast may result from a variety of causes. Pubertal hypertrophy is very common during adolescence and is characterized by a tender discoid enlargement 2-3 cm. in diameter beneath the areola with hypertrophy of the breast. The changes are usually bilateral and subside spontaneously within a year in the majority of cases.

Men between 50 and 70 occasionally develop hypertrophy (often unilateral) similar to that occurring at puberty.

Certain organic diseases may be associated with gynecomastia: cirrhosis of the liver, hyperthyroidism, Addison's disease, testicular tumors (especially chorioepithelioma), and adrenocortical tumors.

If there is uncertainty about the diagnosis of the breast lesion, a biopsy should be done to rule out cancer. Otherwise, the treatment of gynecomastia is nonsurgical unless the patient insists on excision for cosmetic reasons. In this case, at least 2 years should be allowed before operation for possible subsidence.

SARCOMA OF THE SOFT TISSUES

Sarcoma of the soft tissues, although rare, is of special importance because adequate initial management will significantly reduce the local recurrence rate. The most prevalent histologic types (in approximate order of incidence) are fibrosarcoma, liposarcoma, rhabdomyosarcoma, myxoma, synovioma, Kaposi's sarcoma, and malignant neurilemmoma. Histogenesis may be difficult to determine, which accounts for the high incidence of "fibrosarcoma," a term applied loosely to many neoplasms for want of a better designation. Sarcoma of the skin (melanoma), lymph nodes (lymphoma), and smooth muscle (leiomyosarcoma) is not included here.

Soft tissue sarcoma involves the extremities, especially the legs, more frequently than the trunk. All age groups are affected, but the highest incidence is between the ages of 30 and 60. In general, these lesions extend locally beyond their visible and palpable margins, tend to metastasize via the blood stream to the lungs, and are radioresistant. The rate of growth and spread is variable.

Principles of Therapy.

A. **The diagnosis of soft tissue masses should be clearly established** without delay by excisional or incisional biopsy. Whenever tissue is removed, microscopic study should be carried out even though the gross appearance is benign.

B. The treatment of soft tissue sarcoma can be properly planned only after the histologic diagnosis is established.

C. **The choice of definitive operative procedure will depend upon the anatomic location of the sarcoma. Enucleation or local excision with narrow margins is inadequate and dangerous. Subcutaneous tumors require wide removal of surrounding tissues, including skin and underlying fascia.** A split-thickness graft is frequently needed. **In deeper lesions, the entire muscle bundles surrounding the neoplasm should usually be removed at points of origin and insertion. During the removal of the sarcoma, the tumor itself must never be exposed, and the site of biopsy or excision should be excised with the tumor. When adequate ablation of the sarcoma is otherwise impossible, amputation is necessary.**

D. **Radiation therapy is reserved for cases unsuitable for surgery.**

12...

Abdominal Surgery

PRINCIPLES OF DIAGNOSIS OF THE ACUTE ABDOMEN

Significance of Acute Abdominal Pain.

Acute, severe abdominal pain must be assumed to be due to a surgical disorder until a definitive diagnosis has been made. Such pain is more likely to be of surgical significance when it occurs in a previously well patient, lasts more than 6 hours, or when signs of peritoneal irritation or shock are present.

Control of Pain.

Narcotics may obscure signs and symptoms of diagnostic value, especially those of peritoneal irritation. If analgesia is essential before the diagnosis can be made, use minimal effective doses and allow the effects to subside at intervals to permit evaluation.

Evaluation of the Patient.

A complete history and physical examination should be done on every patient with an acute abdomen. Special attention should be paid to the mode of onset, localization, and radiation of the pain. The point of maximum tenderness often suggests the diagnosis. It is well to keep in mind, however, that patients who are elderly, acutely ill, or in shock often have less pain, tenderness, and abdominal rigidity than one might expect, and that in obese individuals tenderness and rigidity may be poorly localized. Anorexia, nausea, vomiting, and bowel irregularity are important symptoms.

Laboratory studies which should be done immediately on all patients with an acute abdomen are as follows: (1) Hgb., WBC, and differential count, (2) urinalysis, and (3) stool test for occult blood on a specimen obtained from the rectal glove. Additional examinations are selected as required for differential diagnosis.

When the diagnosis is in doubt, it is advisable to obtain an upright posteroanterior chest film and upright and supine abdominal films. If free air or intestinal obstruction is suspected and the patient is unable to stand, obtain an abdominal film with the patient lying on his side. The upright and lateral decubitus positions should be maintained for about 3 minutes before the x-ray is taken so that free air may collect in the uppermost portions of the abdominal cavity.

Diagnostic abdominal tap is a relatively safe procedure which may be of value in difficult diagnostic problems, particularly after abdominal trauma when there is no clear-cut indication for laparotomy but hemorrhage or perforation of a hollow viscus has not been ruled out. Useful information can be obtained in 50-90% of cases. Both false-negative and false-positive taps occur occasionally. Abdominal distention is not necessarily a contraindication to the procedure. **Technic:** The abdominal wall is infiltrated with 1% procaine, and an 18 gauge, short-bevel spinal needle is carefully introduced into the abdominal cavity. The stylus of the needle is left in place until the peritoneum is entered. The stylus is then removed and the position of the needle repeatedly adjusted as gentle efforts are made to aspirate abdominal fluid. If necessary, a tap can be made in each quadrant of the abdomen. As a rule only a few ml. of fluid will be obtained even though a considerable quantity may be present within the abdomen. The fluid is examined grossly and microscopically. Gram's and Wright's stains are made as indicated. Amylase determination or culture may be advisable.

An alternate - and probably better - method of abdominal tap involves threading a plastic catheter (Intracath) into the abdominal cavity through a needle inserted 2-3 cm. below the umbilicus. When the catheter is in place and the needle is withdrawn, 500 ml. of lactated Ringer's injection is allowed to run into the abdominal cavity over 10-15 minutes. The fluid is then aspirated or siphoned from the abdomen and examined as noted above.

ACUTE PERITONITIS

Localized or generalized peritonitis is the most important complication of a wide variety of acute abdominal disorders. Peritonitis may be caused by infection or chemical irritation. Perforation or necrosis of the gastrointestinal tract is the usual source of infection. Chemical peritonitis occurs in acute pancreatitis and in the early stages of gastroduodenal perforation. Regardless of the etiology, certain typical features are usually present.

Clinical Findings.

A. Systemic Reaction: Malaise, prostration, nausea, vomiting, septic fever, leukocytosis, and electrolyte imbalance are usually seen in proportion to the severity of the process. If infection is not controlled, toxemia is progressive and toxic shock (see p. 27) may develop terminally.

B. Abdominal Signs:

1. Pain and tenderness - Depending upon the extent of involvement, pain and tenderness may be localized or generalized. Abdominal pain on coughing, rebound tenderness referred to the area of peritonitis, and tenderness to light percussion over the inflamed peritoneum are characteristic. Pelvic peritonitis is associated with rectal and vaginal tenderness.
2. Muscle rigidity - The muscles overlying the area of inflammation usually become spastic. When peritonitis is generalized (e.g., after perforation of a peptic ulcer), marked rigidity of the entire abdominal wall may develop immediately. Rigidity is frequently diminished or absent in the late stages of peritonitis, in severe toxemia, and when the abdominal wall is weak, flabby, or obese.
3. Paralytic ileus - Intestinal motility is markedly inhibited by peritoneal inflammation. Diminished to absent peristalsis and progressive abdominal distention are the cardinal signs. Vomiting occurs as a result of pooling of gastrointestinal secretions and gas, 70% of which is swallowed air.

C. X-ray Findings: Abdominal films (see p. 402) show gas and fluid collections in both large and small bowel, usually with generalized rather than localized dilatation. The bowel walls, when thrown into relief by the gas patterns, may appear to be thickened, indicating the presence of edema or peritoneal fluid.

D. Diagnostic Abdominal Tap: Occasionally useful (see p. 402).

Treatment.

The measures employed in peritonitis as outlined below are generally applicable as supportive therapy in most acute abdominal disorders. The objectives are (1) to control infection, (2) to minimize the effects of paralytic ileus, and (3) to correct fluid, electrolyte, and nutritional disorders.

A. Specific Measures: Operative procedures to close perforations, to remove sources of infection such as gangrenous bowel or an inflamed appendix, or to drain abscesses are frequently required. The cause of the peritonitis should always be identified and treated promptly.

B. General Measures: No matter what specific operative procedures are employed, their ultimate success will often depend upon the care with which the following general measures are carried out.

1. Bed rest in the medium Fowler (semi-sitting) position is preferred.
2. Nasogastric suction (see p. 411) is started as soon as peritonitis is suspected. It is important to prevent gastrointestinal distention by the prompt institution of suction, which is continued until peristaltic activity returns and deflation by rectum seems imminent or has begun. The gastric (e.g., Levin) tube is usually adequate. In persistent paralytic ileus, the intestinal tract may be more adequately decompressed by means of a long intestinal tube (e.g., Miller-Abbott), although passage of such a tube into the small bowel is frequently difficult because of poor intestinal motility. In rare cases combined gastric and long intestinal tube suction may be necessary to relieve or prevent distention.
3. Give nothing by mouth. Oral intake can be resumed slowly after nasogastric suction is discontinued.
4. Fluid and electrolyte therapy and parenteral feeding (see Chapter 5).
5. Narcotics and sedatives should be used liberally to ensure comfort and rest.
6. Antibiotic therapy - If infection with mixed intestinal flora is probably present, appropriate antibiotic is chosen empirically in order that treatment may begin at once (see Chapter 6). When cultures are available, antibiotics are chosen according to sensitivity studies.
7. Whole blood or red cell transfusions are used as needed to control anemia.
8. Toxic shock, if it develops, requires intensive treatment (see p. 27).

Complications and Prognosis.

The most frequent sequel of peritonitis is abscess formation in the pelvis (see p. 422), in the subphrenic space (see p. 90), between the leaves of the mesentery, or elsewhere in the abdomen. Antibiotic therapy may mask or delay the appearance of localizing signs of abscess. When fever, leukocytosis, toxemia, or ileus fails to respond to the general measures for peritonitis, a collection of pus should be suspected. This will usually require surgical drainage. Abscess within the liver (see p. 475) and pylephlebitis (see p. 422) are rare complications. Adhesions may cause early or, more frequently, late intestinal obstruction.

If the cause of peritonitis can be corrected, the infection, accompanying ileus, and metabolic derangement can usually be managed successfully.

ABDOMINAL INJURIES

There are 2 general types of abdominal trauma: nonpenetrating and penetrating. The major complications which require surgical intervention are internal bleeding and perforation of a hollow viscus.

NONPENETRATING INJURIES

Clinical Findings.

Blunt injuries are difficult diagnostic problems for the following reasons: (1) They are frequently associated with other serious trauma such as multiple fractures and head injuries with coma. (2) Relatively trivial blows to the abdomen may rupture the bowel or spleen. (3) The absence of an external wound on the abdomen is deceptive. On the other hand, a severe abdominal blow may produce temporary collapse (primary or neurogenic shock), transient paralytic ileus, and a variable degree of abdominal soreness even in the absence of significant visceral damage. There is often a delay in onset of signs when a serious injury exists. For example, evidence of peritonitis may not appear for 8-12 hours or more after rupture of a hollow viscus, and slow or recurrent bleeding may not produce shock until some hours after an injury.

A. Signs of a Ruptured Hollow Viscus: When signs of localized or generalized peritonitis develop within 24 hours following blunt abdominal trauma, perforation of a hollow viscus should be suspected. The usual clinical picture consists of increasing abdominal pain, tenderness, rebound tenderness, muscle spasm, and depression of bowel sounds after a latent period of a few hours following the injury. Tachycardia, fever, and leukocytosis are usually noted. Diagnostic x-rays should be taken as soon after trauma as feasible. Pneumoperitoneum is present in about half of patients with rupture of any portion of the gastrointestinal tract. Diagnostic abdominal tap (see p. 402) may be helpful. Rupture of the duodenum or bladder is a particularly deceptive injury.
   1. Rupture of the duodenum - Retroperitoneal rupture of the duodenum is an insidious and often fatal injury. Signs of generalized peritonitis develop slowly or not at all. Deep

tenderness over the duodenum is the most constant finding. Retroperitoneal air may occasionally be found on x-ray. Fever and leukocytosis occur. The patient may not seem seriously ill for a day or so until fulminating infection becomes manifest. A high index of suspicion is essential in the early diagnosis of this lesion. The serum amylase level may be elevated. Traumatic pancreatitis may be an associated injury.

2. Rupture of the bladder - See Chapter 14.

B. Signs of Ruptured Solid Viscus: The organs most frequently damaged are the kidneys, spleen, and liver, in that order. Hemorrhage is the most important complication.

1. Rupture of the kidney - See Chapter 14.
2. Rupture of the spleen - This is the most common indication for operation after blunt abdominal trauma. Even small tears of the spleen tend to cause continuous or recurrent bleeding. Minor accidents may cause splenic rupture. This is particularly true in children because of the pliability of the overlying rib cage. In adults, splenic injury should always be suspected when there are fractures of the lower ribs on the left side. In certain diseases (e.g., malaria, typhoid, sarcoidosis, and infectious mononucleosis), the spleen is friable and ruptures on minimal trauma or may rarely rupture spontaneously.

   The signs of rupture of the spleen are pain and tenderness in the left upper quadrant, left shoulder pain caused by diaphragmatic irritation (in 75% of cases), and evidence of blood loss. Shock often develops soon after injury, and sufficient blood may collect in the abdomen to cause shifting dullness. Mild generalized peritoneal irritation appears, accompanied by paralytic ileus. The Hct. and Hgb. fall as hemodilution occurs. Moderate leukocytosis is usually present, but the temperature is normal. Diagnostic abdominal tap recovers fresh blood in about 75% of cases, but a negative tap does not rule out intra-abdominal hemorrhage (see p. 402).

   X-rays may occasionally be of value by showing one or more of the following: (1) diffuse haziness in the left upper quadrant, with absent splenic shadow; (2) downward and medial displacement of the stomach and the splenic flexure; (3) elevation and limitation of the left diaphragm; (4) absent left renal and psoas shadows.

   Subcapsular or retroperitoneal rupture of the spleen may occur without bleeding into the free peritoneal cavity and without generalized peritoneal irritation. Pain and tenderness in the left upper quadrant and unexplained anemia may be the only findings. X-rays may show some of the changes mentioned above.

   Delayed rupture of the spleen occurs in one out of 6 cases, with massive hemorrhage beginning usually within 30 days after trauma. The signs are the same as for immediate rupture, but the diagnosis may be missed if a history of trauma is not elicited.
3. Rupture of the liver - More force is required to rupture the liver than the spleen, and bleeding from the liver has a greater tendency to cease spontaneously. The right lobe is

usually involved, and other injuries, such as fractures of overlying ribs and rupture or laceration of the right kidney, are frequently present. The usual signs are pain (accentuated by deep breathing), tenderness, and muscle rigidity in the right upper quadrant, and pain on top of the right shoulder referred from the diaphragm. When significant hemorrhage has occurred, generalized mild peritoneal irritation and shifting dullness due to free blood may be noted. Shock is often present. The Hct. and Hgb. fall as hemodilution occurs and the WBC is elevated. An abdominal tap may be of value (see p. 402).

Treatment.

A. General Measures: A period of observation may be necessary before a diagnosis of serious intra-abdominal injury can be made. Some or all of the following measures are advisable during this interval.
   1. Place the patient at bed rest, record the vital signs (BP, pulse, and respiration) regularly, and observe for increasing abdominal findings or for deterioration of vital signs. Administer narcotics cautiously.
   2. Give nothing by mouth and administer parenteral fluids as required. Nasogastric suction is often indicated. Record the intake and output.
   3. Repeat the WBC, Hgb., and Hct. p.r.n.
   4. Prepare blood for transfusion if internal bleeding is suspected or if operation is imminent.
   5. If bleeding is suspected, repeat the Hct. every 1-2 hours. Signs of actual or impending shock are the most reliable evidence of hemorrhage. If these signs are equivocal and there is a question of significant, continuing blood loss, administer 500 ml. of blood rapidly. If response is prompt and sustained, bleeding is not massive. Failure to respond to two 500 ml. transfusions, or a relapse into shock when they have been completed, indicates continuing major blood loss or fulminating peritonitis due to gastrointestinal perforation. In either case, immediate operation is required.

B. Surgical Treatment: Rupture of a hollow viscus and internal bleeding are absolute indications for laparotomy.

PENETRATING ABDOMINAL WOUNDS

Perforation of a Hollow Viscus.

Any knife, projectile, or other type of wound which could involve the free peritoneal cavity should be assumed to have lacerated a hollow viscus. Immediate operation is indicated in these cases. It is unwise to await the signs of peritonitis, which are often delayed for many hours since leakage may not occur at once. Probing of the wound is not a reliable means of determining the extent of injury. Abdominal x-rays after injection of radiopaque contrast material into the tract of the penetrating wound may, in some instances, indicate whether the abdominal cavity has been entered.

All patients with a perforated hollow viscus should be treated for acute peritonitis (see p. 403). Thoracoabdominal wounds are discussed on p. 300. Injuries of the colon and rectum deserve special comment because they produce the most rapid and serious peritoneal infection. In selected instances lacerations of the colon may be closed primarily, but extensive wounds require resection and proximal colostomy or exteriorization. Penetrating wounds of the buttocks or pelvis frequently perforate the rectum; blood is found on rectal and proctoscopic examination. Such injuries require early and adequate local drainage and sigmoid colostomy.

Laceration of a Solid Viscus.

Intra-abdominal hemorrhage is a common, serious complication of penetrating wounds. The liver, spleen, or kidneys may be torn, or mesenteric or other large abdominal vessels may be cut. Management is as for nonpenetrating trauma with bleeding (see p. 405).

ACUTE MECHANICAL OBSTRUCTION*

The 3 main types of acute intestinal obstruction are **paralytic ileus,** in which the motility of the bowel is diminished or absent (see p. 417); **mechanical obstruction,** in which the lumen of the bowel is actually blocked; and **vascular obstruction,** in which infarction of the bowel and obstructive symptoms are secondary to occlusion of the mesenteric arteries or veins or to acute reduction in blood flow due to other causes (see p. 416). Mechanical obstruction may be simple or due to strangulation obstruction. In **simple obstruction** the blood supply to the bowel is adequate. In **strangulation obstruction** the blood supply is interrupted and gangrene will occur unless the obstruction is relieved. It is always essential to decide whether strangulation may be present, since this is an indication for emergency operation to prevent bowel rupture and peritonitis. The small bowel is the site of mechanical obstruction in about 80% of patients; and the large bowel in about 20%.

Etiology.

A. Small Bowel Obstruction: Approximately one-third of cases are due to incarceration or strangulation of an external hernia. For this reason, the various hernia sites should always be carefully palpated. Adhesions and bands (inflammatory, neoplastic, or congenital) also account for about one-third of cases. Adhesions have markedly increased and hernia decreased as a cause of obstruction in recent years in the United States and Great Britain. Volvulus, intussusception, internal hernia, obturation (e.g., gallstone ileus), and inflammatory or neoplastic stricture of the bowel are less frequent causes of small intestinal obstruction.
B. Large Bowel Obstruction: Neoplasm is the most frequent cause. Volvulus of the sigmoid or cecum is also important, but less common. If strangulated hernia is excluded, cancer of the large bowel is the commonest cause of intestinal obstruction after middle age.

*Obstruction in infants and children is discussed in Chapter 7, Pediatric Surgery.

Clinical Findings.

A. Symptoms:

1. Abdominal pain - Crampy abdominal pain is typical. It is usually mid-abdominal in small bowel obstruction and hypogastric in large bowel lesions. Borborygmus may be loud and coincident with cramps. Continuous abdominal pain, when present, is suggestive of strangulation or peritonitis.
2. Obstipation - Inability to pass stools or more than small amounts of flatus is always noted. In complete obstruction neither feces nor gas will be passed by rectum.
3. Distention - Distention depends upon the accumulation of gas and intestinal secretions proximal to the lesion. In high jejunal obstruction, distention may be minimal or absent.
4. Vomiting - This is usually present from the outset in small bowel obstruction. The higher the obstruction, the more marked the vomiting. In prolonged obstructions at lower levels in the small bowel, fecal vomitus may occur and is pathognomonic. Vomiting is less common and occurs later in large bowel obstruction.

B. Signs: A distended, tympanitic abdomen with hyperactive, rushing peristalsis is typical. Colicky pain coincident with rushes of peristalsis is characteristic when it occurs. Visible peristalsis on the abdominal wall is occasionally present. Late in the course of obstruction or when peritonitis has supervened, peristalsis may be very sluggish or absent. Abdominal tenderness is usually not marked and may be absent in uncomplicated obstruction. Localized tenderness usually develops over a gangrenous segment of bowel. Signs of localized or generalized peritonitis (see p. 403) suggest gangrene or rupture of the bowel wall. Fresh blood may be found in the rectum in intussusception and in carcinoma of the rectum or colon. A sigmoidoscopy is part of the physical examination in every case of colon obstruction. Obstructed patients usually have little or no fever until strangulation or peritonitis occurs.

C. Laboratory Findings:

1. Urinalysis - High sp. gr. and ketonuria, indicating dehydration and metabolic acidosis, are the only common findings.
2. Hct. - Hemoconcentration, caused by dehydration, frequently results in increase in Hct. and Hgb.
3. WBC - Normal or slight elevation is common. A high WBC suggests strangulation obstruction, but gangrenous bowel can be present in the absence of significant leukocytosis.
4. Blood chemistry - Serum sodium, potassium, chloride, and CO_2, and BUN are often deranged and should be determined as an aid to management of fluid imbalance if important losses have occurred.

D. X-ray Findings: Plain abdominal films in the supine and standing positions should be obtained immediately and repeated daily, or oftener if necessary, to follow the course of the illness. A film should be taken in the lateral decubitus position if the patient cannot stand. Normally, the stomach and colon contain a small amount of gas but the small bowel does not visualize. Complete small bowel obstruction is characterized by dilated small bowel, usually with fluid levels. Little or no gas is seen in the colon. In colonic obstruction the large bowel is dilated proximal to the block and may become markedly distended. When the ileocecal valve is incompetent, the small bowel is also dilated.

It is often impossible to differentiate between colonic and small bowel obstruction without a barium enema. A barium enema should be done early in most cases of large bowel obstruction. Care must be taken not to force a large volume of barium past an obstructing lesion. Barium should not be given by mouth in any patient suspected of intestinal obstruction because of the danger of inspissation of barium and aggravation of the obstruction.

Differential Diagnosis.

A. Simple vs. Strangulation Obstruction: This is the most important differential diagnosis to be made since, if strangulation has occurred, emergency operation is required. If the obstruction is simple (i.e., if necrosis of bowel is not present), conservative management is, for the moment, safe. In simple obstruction, the obstruction is often incomplete, so that the patient continues to pass some flatus.

In small bowel involvement, if the obstruction is complete (as indicated by the persistent lack of flatus or stools and by the absence of gas in the colon), it is wise to assume that strangulation may be present. Abdominal tenderness, signs of peritonitis, tachycardia, fever, and marked or rising leukocytosis are also suggestive of strangulation. Additional signs frequently associated with strangulation are (1) the presence of an abdominal, pelvic, or rectal mass; (2) a single, markedly dilated loop on x-ray; (3) blood in the rectum; and (4) the presence of constant, severe abdominal pain. It is important to realize, however, that necrosis may be present in the absence of all definitive signs.

B. Small vs. Large Bowel Obstruction: X-rays are required to make the differential diagnosis, but certain distinctive clinical features are usually present also. Large bowel obstruction is frequently relatively slow in onset and benign in course, without vomiting in spite of considerable distention. Severe cramps, frequent vomiting, and early fluid imbalance are more common in small bowel lesions. A history of previous abdominal surgery or of previous attacks of obstruction favors the diagnosis of small bowel involvement. Elderly patients without such a past history who become obstructed usually have a carcinoma of the large bowel.

C. Mechanical Obstruction vs. Paralytic Ileus: The distinguishing features of paralytic ileus are as follows: (1) There is usually an obvious exciting cause, such as abdominal surgery, acute peritonitis, or trauma to the abdomen or back; (2) the abdomen is silent, and cramps are absent; (3) tenderness may or may not be present, depending upon the underlying cause; (4) on x-ray, gas is distributed throughout the small and large intestines.

The differentiation of paralytic from mechanical obstruction is most difficult in the period immediately following abdominal surgery, when paralytic ileus may be associated with mechanical obstruction caused by adhesions. Under these circumstances, the persistence of abdominal distention, vomiting, and obstipation beyond the expected period of ileus raises the suspicion of a mechanical block and calls for investigation by x-ray and other means.

Treatment.

A. General Measures: Fluid balance must be restored and maintained by the parenteral route. Every patient should be promptly intubated with either a gastric (Levin) or a long intestinal tube and placed on constant suction.

B. Conservative Treatment: This consists of an effort to decompress the bowel and relieve the obstruction by means of intubation with a gastric or long intestinal tube. A trial of intubation as definitive treatment is warranted only when there is no evidence of strangulation. It is most likely to be successful in partial small bowel obstruction caused by adhesions. Conservative management must be vigilant, and immediate surgery is indicated if evidence of strangulation appears or if the patient fails to improve. In general, definitive treatment by intubation should not be attempted in complete large or small bowel obstruction. The 2 types of tubes in common use are the gastric (Levin) and the long intestinal.

1. Use of the gastric tube - Gastric tube suction is specifically indicated in pyloric and duodenal obstruction. Mild degrees of small or large bowel obstruction frequently respond to gastric suction. It may also be used pre- and postoperatively when obstruction is to be treated immediately by operation. A No. 16 tube is passed through the nose into the stomach, placed on constant suction, and irrigated every 1-3 hours with 30 ml. of saline to ensure patency.

2. Use of the long intestinal tube - Partial small bowel obstruction is the primary indication for the long intestinal tube. In partial large bowel obstruction (e.g., due to neoplasm), decompression of the intestinal tract by the long tube may occasionally permit preparation of the colon for a one-stage resection of the obstructing lesion.

   The original long intestinal tube is the Miller-Abbott tube, which has a double lumen, one for suction and one for inflation of the balloon after it passes the pylorus in order to encourage its more rapid propulsion by the peristaltic action of the small bowel. The Harris and Cantor tubes are 2 of the numerous modifications of the Miller-Abbott. They have a single, larger lumen for suction and are thus simpler and somewhat more efficient.

   The most difficult aspect of intestinal intubation is passage of the tube through the pylorus. Four to 6 ml. of mercury are placed in the balloon of long intestinal tubes to aid in positioning within the stomach and also to serve as a bolus when the tube reaches the small bowel. A long, removable metal stylet extending to the tip of the tube can be used to guide the tube through the pylorus. This is often rapidly effective, but the method is more complicated and there is a risk of perforation.

   Technic of intubation:

   a. The well-lubricated tube is passed through the nostril into the stomach, and the gastric contents aspirated.

b. Under fluoroscopic guidance the tip of the tube is passed through the pylorus and into the upper jejunum. This may be difficult or impossible in the obstructed patient. If attempts at passage under fluoroscopy fail or if fluoroscopy is not advisable, elevate the foot of the bed 30 cm. (12 in.) and place the patient on his right side, almost face down, with the tube about 75 cm. (30 in.) past the nares and on suction. With the patient in this position, the tube will often pass the pylorus within a few hours. When bile is aspirated, the tube is probably in the duodenum.

c. When the tip of the tube is in the duodenum, advance the tube 20-25 cm. and place the patient in Fowler's position for one hour to facilitate passage beyond the ligament of Treitz.

d. After the tube reaches the jejunum, advance it 10 cm. (4 in.) an hour. The distal ileum is reached after insertion of about 1.5 meters (5 ft.) of tube if no obstruction is met.

e. The tube is kept on constant suction and irrigated with tap water or saline every hour to keep it open. The progress and effect of the tube is followed by an abdominal film daily or p.r.n.

f. Occasionally the stomach becomes distended when the long tube is in the small bowel. Under these circumstances a gastric tube is passed.

Signs of improvement after intubation are subsidence of pain and distention and decrease in the volume of suction drainage. X-ray shows less dilatation of intestinal loops, and gas can be seen in the colon. The passage of gas and then feces by rectum indicates that the obstruction is relieved.

When improvement has been observed, replace continuous suction by intermittent suction (e.g., 2 hours on and 2 hours off) for 12-24 hours and then gravity drainage for 24 hours while fluids are permitted by mouth. If oral fluids are well tolerated and good bowel function continues, the tube can be removed.

Failure to tolerate oral intake is an indication for resuming suction or for operation.

C. Surgical Treatment: Operation is indicated when strangulation obstruction is present (see p. 410) or when a lesion commonly associated with bowel necrosis is present (hernia, volvulus, intussusception in older children and adults, obturation, and complete obstruction caused by chronic adhesions). Preoperative intubation (see above) and appropriate fluid and electrolyte therapy are always advisable. Failure of the partially obstructed patient to respond adequately to decompression by intubation is an indication for surgical intervention; the partial relief which is usually provided by the tube should not lead to a false sense of security.

Prognosis.

The mortality rate in mechanical obstruction is influenced by many factors, principally age, etiology, the site and duration of obstruction, and, especially, whether or not gangrene has occurred. The very young and the very old tolerate obstruction poorly. In obstruction of the colon the mortality rate is several times higher than in obstruction of the small bowel. The longer the duration of the obstruction, the higher the death rate. When gangrene is present, the over-all mortality rate rises from 10-15% to about 35%. During the past 2 decades the mortality rate from simple obstruction has decreased as a result of improved fluid therapy, emphasis on early operation, and antibiotics. The mortality rate in obstruction due to strangulation has declined very little.

OBSTRUCTION DUE TO EXTERNAL HERNIA

The diagnosis of strangulated hernia (see p. 410) should be considered in every case of intestinal obstruction. The various anatomic sites of hernia and abdominal incisions should be carefully palpated. Femoral hernias are frequently overlooked because they are small and because the physician fails to examine the femoral region. Hernias are often obscured in obese individuals. An irreducible, tender, tense hernia should be assumed to be strangulated, and immediate operation is indicated. Forceful attempts to reduce such a hernia may push a gangrenous loop of bowel into the peritoneal cavity. An attempt to reduce a hernia by gentle manipulation is justifiable if incarceration is recent and painless.

OBSTRUCTION DUE TO VOLVULUS

A volvulus is a twist of a viscus on its mesentery of such a degree as to occlude its blood supply partially or completely. It is most likely to occur where the mesentery of the gastrointestinal tract is long and mobile.

Volvulus of the Stomach.

Volvulus of the stomach is rare and is usually associated with a large para-esophageal hiatus hernia. The stomach may rotate around either its longitudinal or its transverse axis. The major symptoms are severe epigastric or chest pain and vomiting.

Operation is required to reduce the volvulus and repair a hernia if present. It is necessary either to fix the stomach in position or to perform a sleeve resection in order to prevent recurrence.

Volvulus of the Small Intestine.

Volvulus of the midgut due to congenital failure of attachment of the small bowel mesentery occurs in infancy (see p. 233) and, rarely, in adult life. As a rule small bowel volvulus in an adult is secondary to rotation of a loop of bowel around a fixed point such as an adhesion. This is a particularly lethal form of obstruction, since strangulation commonly occurs. Severe and persistent abdominal pain is often present.

Volvulus of the Cecum.

In 10-15% of individuals the cecum is poorly attached to the abdominal wall and is able to rotate on the ascending colon. Cecal volvulus occurs at all ages, but is most common in young adults.

Recurrent attacks may simulate appendicitis. The attack may be acute in onset, or several days of dull pain may precede it. The signs are those of intestinal obstruction. X-rays are diagnostic. The plain film will usually show a large gas bubble in the cecum in the left upper quadrant which may be mistaken for the stomach. The final differentiation is made by immediate barium enema.

Immediate operation is indicated for detorsion and fixation of the cecum or for primary resection and anastomosis. The latter is required if gangrene has occurred.

Volvulus of the Sigmoid Colon.

Sigmoid volvulus is common because the sigmoid is often redundant or may be enlarged by congenital or acquired megacolon. The clinical findings are those of large bowel obstruction. There is frequently a history of previous attacks relieved by enemas. Dilated loops of colon containing gas and fluid are seen on x-ray.

Barium enema confirms the diagnosis by outlining the obstructing twist in the sigmoid. Avoid filling the dilated sigmoid with barium, as this will aggravate the obstruction.

Patients with sigmoid volvulus are often old and debilitated, and the method of treatment must be chosen accordingly. It is frequently possible to decompress the sigmoid with a rectal tube. A sigmoidoscope is inserted to the point of torsion and, if the mucous membrane is of good color, a well-lubricated rectal tube - about 60 cm. (2 ft.) long and size 30 F. - is gently insinuated past the obstruction. Deflation occurs dramatically. The rectal tube is left in place several days and irrigated as necessary to keep it patent. Emergency operation is indicated when decompression is unsuccessful or when strangulation is a possibility. One of 2 types of operation is usually done: (1) simple detorsion of the sigmoid, with drainage of the dilated loop by a rectal tube passed up through the anal canal; or (2) resection of the sigmoid.

When nonoperative decompression by rectal tube is successful in a patient who is a good operative risk, it is possible to prepare the bowel and proceed in a few days with elective resection. Poor-risk patients may be permitted to have 2 or more attacks requiring deflation by rectal tube before resection is advised.

OBSTRUCTION DUE TO ADHESIONS

Thirty to 40% of small bowel obstructions are caused by adhesions secondary to previous surgery, peritonitis, or trauma. Strangulation occurs in 10-20% of cases of obstruction which are caused by long-standing adhesions. Freshly formed adhesions, such as those developing in the early postoperative period, are less frequently associated with bowel necrosis. Adhesions rarely produce colonic obstruction.

Treatment of adhesive obstruction is similar to that for mechanical obstruction (see p. 411). In view of the low incidence of strangulation and the frequently satisfactory response, obstruction caused by early postoperative adhesions is usually given a trial of intubation before surgery is advised.

OBSTRUCTION DUE TO NEOPLASM

Neoplasms of the Small Intestine.

Neoplasm of the small bowel is a relatively rare cause of obstruction. The lesions which occur include carcinoma, lymphoma, leiomyosarcoma, carcinoid, and benign tumors such as adenoma, leiomyoma, and lipoma. Symptoms are often those of chronic or recurrent obstruction. Intussusception of the lesion may precipitate acute obstruction. When intussusception occurs in an adult, a benign or malignant neoplasm should always be suspected as the exciting cause. Treatment is by resection.

Neoplasms of the Colon and Rectum.

Carcinoma is the most frequent cause of large bowel obstruction (see p. 408). The ultimate treatment is by resection. The immediate problem, however, is decompression of the proximal colon when significant obstruction is present. The place of intubation in the management of partial neoplastic obstruction of the colon has already been mentioned (see p. 411). When obstruction is complete and unremitting, surgical decompression of the colon is required prior to resection. Transverse colostomy or cecostomy is employed for severe obstruction located at or distal to the splenic flexure. Tumors which completely obstruct the proximal half of the colon usually require a preliminary cecostomy or side-to-side ileocolostomy. In selected cases, primary resection of the right colon is feasible after intestinal intubation in spite of high-grade obstruction.

Abdominal Carcinomatosis.

Obstruction by peritoneal carcinomatous implants is not uncommon. It can occasionally be palliated temporarily by intubation, limited resection, or entero-enterostomy around the point of obstruction.

MISCELLANEOUS CAUSES OF OBSTRUCTION

Intussusception.

This condition is common in children (see p. 240). In adults it is rare and is usually caused by a benign or malignant tumor of the bowel. Incomplete or intermittent obstruction may be present, and bloody mucus may be found in the rectum. Early operation is required.

Obturation.

Obturation obstruction results when a foreign body is unable to pass through the bowel. Gallstones (gallstone ileus), bezoars, ingested or inserted foreign bodies, worms, and fecal impaction are common causes. All kinds of obturation except fecal impaction most frequently involve the small bowel.

Gallstone ileus is an important syndrome which usually occurs in elderly, obese women, half of whom have a past history of gallbladder disease. A fistula forms between the gallbladder and duodenum for passage of the stone. Intestinal gas which enters through the fistula can almost always be seen in the biliary tree by x-ray if searched for with care. The obstructing gallstone can also be found on x-ray in about half of cases. Treatment is by prompt laparotomy to remove the stone. The cholecystoduodenal fistula should not be disturbed at the operation for obstruction unless the patient's good condition warrants undertaking the added procedure.

Obstruction by worms (usually Ascaris lumbricoides) occurs predominantly in children under 10 years of age. The site of obstruction is most frequently in the lower ileum. Symptoms may be acute or chronic. Diagnosis is made by finding ova in the stools and by thin barium study of the bowel, which may outline the worms. Distention is controlled by intubation, and the worms are removed by vermifuge therapy. Operation is rarely necessary and should be avoided if possible since worms migrate through the suture lines of enterotomies.

Inflammatory Disorders.

The most common inflammatory lesions which cause obstruction are regional enteritis (see p. 437), tuberculosis, and amebiasis. Treatment must be individualized, and operation for acute obstruction is avoided by intubation if possible. In the case of tuberculosis and ameboma, which usually involve the ileocecal region and for which specific drug therapy is available, the differentiation from carcinoma is important but may be difficult.

VASCULAR OBSTRUCTION

The most common causes of vascular obstruction of the bowel are mesenteric artery occlusion and mesenteric vein thrombosis. The relative incidence of the 2 types is probably about the same. Arterial occlusion may be caused by thrombosis of an arteriosclerotic vessel or by embolism. The superior mesenteric artery is involved in most of the cases associated with gangrene. Occlusion of the inferior mesenteric artery (usually asymptomatic) is not uncommon in aneurysm or severe atherosclerosis of the aorta. Mesenteric venous thrombosis may follow appendicitis, strangulation hernia, and abdominal trauma or surgery. It may also occur spontaneously without antecedent cause.

Perhaps a third of the cases of intestinal infarction will be found to have no occlusion of arteries or veins. Most of these patients are elderly and suffering from congestive failure or atrial fibrillation. It is assumed that low cardiac output results in mesenteric vasoconstriction with hypoxia and spasm of the bowel. A vicious cycle is set up leading to progressive diminution of blood supply and, finally, gangrene.

Clinical Findings.

These patients are usually elderly or have cardiovascular disease. In arterial occlusions and in vasospastic infarction the onset is sudden, with severe abdominal pain (may be cramp-like), vomiting, diarrhea, blood in the stools, and shock. In venous thrombosis the onset is frequently more gradual, with relatively mild symptoms and signs until gangrene is marked. The abdomen is tender, peristalsis is diminished or absent, and distention develops gradually. Leukocytosis is variable, but tends to be marked; white counts above 30,000 are not uncommon. Hemoconcentration or hypotension refractory to treatment may also be present. Temperature is at first normal but rises as gangrene and peritonitis progress. The diagnosis may be suggested on x-ray by the appearance of a single loop of distended, thickened bowel and evidence of peritoneal fluid. Recovery of bloody fluid via abdominal tap (see p. 402) indicates the presence of infarcted bowel. Arteriography may be of diagnostic value when indications for immediate operation are in doubt.

Treatment.

These patients should be explored with minimal delay, and resection of gangrenous bowel with end-to-end anastomosis should be performed if possible. Unfortunately, the entire small bowel and right colon are frequently infarcted, in which case resection is usually impossible or fatal. When infarction is due to embolism or localized thrombosis of the superior mesenteric artery, embolectomy or thrombectomy may be feasible and should be attempted. Autogenous vein bypass of the obstructed site may rarely be feasible. Anticoagulants have no place in the preoperative and postoperative treatment of acute mesenteric occlusion.

Postoperative measures after bowel resection should include maintenance of good cardiac output and oxygenation, bowel decompression by nasogastric tube, and broad-spectrum antibiotic therapy. Vasopressors probably aggravate mesenteric vasospasm and are contraindicated.

Prognosis.

The patient is often moribund when first seen. The mortality for mesenteric thrombosis and embolism is 75-100% in reported series. If it is necessary to resect more than 50% of the small bowel because of gangrene, diarrhea and nutritional deficiency may become a chronic problem.

PARALYTIC ILEUS

In paralytic (adynamic) ileus the obstruction is due to inhibition of intestinal motility; there is no organic obstruction. A mild degree of paralytic ileus occurs after every laparotomy, but recovery normally takes place within 2-3 days unless peritonitis develops. Other lesions commonly associated with paralytic ileus are back injuries, fractured vertebrae or ribs, retroperitoneal and intra-abdominal hemorrhage, renal colic, pulmonary lesions such as pneumonia or pneumothorax, torsion of the ovary, testicle, or omentum, CNS diseases, and severe acute infections. Electrolyte imbalance, particularly hypokalemic alkalosis, will cause or aggravate ileus. Distention of the bowel tends to perpetuate ileus.

Clinical Findings.

There is a history of recent operation, injury, or other precipitating condition. Vomiting usually occurs, and obstipation is the rule. Peristalsis is markedly diminished or absent. The abdomen is distended and may or may not be tender, depending upon underlying factors. Plain films of the abdomen show gaseous distention of both colon and small bowel. This observation is helpful in excluding mechanical block in which distention is proximal to the obstruction. When paralytic ileus persists in spite of treatment, suspect sepsis within the abdomen, electrolyte derangement, or an element of mechanical obstruction.

Treatment.

Most cases of ileus are postoperative, mild, and responsive to restriction of oral intake. As the ileus subsides, the diet is liberalized. Supplementary parenteral fluids should be given until oral intake is adequate.

Drugs are rarely of value in improving intestinal motility. The agent of choice for this purpose is bethanechol chloride (Urecholine®), a direct parasympathetic stimulant. The dosage is 10-30 mg. orally or 2.5-5 mg. subcut. 3-4 times daily. The initial parenteral dose should be 2.5 mg. to test the patient's reaction. It should never be administered I.M. or I.V. If distressing side effects of cholinergic stimulation occur (cramps, flushing, sweating, salivation, wheezing, or hypotension), the reaction may be abolished by administration of atropine sulfate, 0.6 mg. subcut. or I.V., which should always be available in a syringe when bethanechol is given by injection. If mechanical obstruction is suspected, bethanechol is contraindicated.

Severe paralytic ileus requires complete restriction of oral intake, parenteral feeding, and gastrointestinal suction with either a gastric or a long intestinal tube (see p. 411). The latter is more effective if it can be passed into the small bowel, but nasogastric suction is usually adequate.

Ileus may rarely be extreme and fail to respond to conservative measures. Marked distention may be a factor in perpetuating the condition. If the patient is deteriorating, abdominal exploration for the following purposes is occasionally necessary: (1) to deflate the gastrointestinal tract by aspiration of the bowel with a catheter passed through a small enterotomy; (2) to maneuver a long intestinal tube through the pylorus into the small bowel; (3) to establish a cecostomy, if necessary; and (4) to rule out mechanical obstruction or intra-abdominal abscess. These procedures serve to relieve distention and prevent its recurrence while the cause of the ileus is being brought under control.

APPENDICITIS

Appendicitis is initiated by obstruction of the appendiceal lumen by a fecalith, inflammation, foreign body, or neoplasm. Obstruction is followed by infection, edema, and frequently infarction of the appendiceal wall. Intraluminal tension develops rapidly and tends to cause early mural necrosis and perforation. All ages are affected, but appendicitis usually occurs in persons between 10 and 30 years of age and is more common in males.

Clinical Findings.

Appendicitis is one of the commonest causes of acute surgical abdomen. The symptoms and signs usually follow a fairly stereotyped pattern, but appendicitis is capable of such protean manifestations that it should be considered in the differential diagnosis of every obscure case of intra-abdominal sepsis and pain.

A. "Classical" Appendicitis:
   1. Symptoms - An attack of appendicitis usually begins with epigastric or periumbilical pain associated with 1-2 episodes of vomiting. Within 2-12 hours the pain shifts to the right lower quadrant, where it persists as a steady soreness which is aggravated by walking or coughing. There is anorexia, moderate malaise, and slight fever. Constipation is usual, but diarrhea occurs occasionally.
   2. Signs - At onset there are no localized abdominal findings. Within a few hours, however, progressive right lower quadrant tenderness can be demonstrated; careful examination will usually identify a single point of maximum tenderness. The patient can often place his finger precisely on this area, especially if asked to accentuate the soreness by coughing. Light percussion over the right lower quadrant is helpful in localizing tenderness. Rebound tenderness and spasm of the overlying abdominal muscles are usually present. Psoas and obturator signs, when positive, are strongly suggestive of appendicitis. Rectal tenderness is common and, in pelvic appendicitis, may be more definite than abdominal tenderness. Peristalsis is diminished or absent. Slight to moderate fever is present.
   3. Laboratory findings - Moderate leukocytosis (10,000-20,000) with an increase in neutrophils is usually present. It is not uncommon to find a few red cells on microscopic examination of the urine, but otherwise the urinalysis is not remarkable.
   4. X-ray findings - There are no characteristic changes on plain films of the abdomen.

B. Factors Which Cause Variations From the "Classical" Clinical Picture:
   1. Anatomic location of appendix - Abdominal findings are most definite when the appendix is in the iliac fossa or superficially located. When the appendix extends over the pelvic brim, the abdominal signs may be minimal, greatest tenderness being elicited on rectal examination. Right lower quadrant tenderness may be poorly localized and slow to develop in retrocecal or retroileal appendicitis. Inflammation of a high-lying lateral appendix may produce maximal tenderness in the flank. Bizarre locations of the appendix may rarely occur in association with a mobile or undescended cecum; in such cases symptoms and signs may be localized in the right upper or the left lower quadrant.
   2. Age -
      a. Infancy and childhood - In infancy appendicitis is relatively rare, but when it occurs the diagnosis is difficult because of the problem of interpretation of history and physical findings. The disease tends to progress rapidly and, when rupture occurs, to result in generalized peritonitis because of poor localizing mechanisms.

b. Old age - Elderly patients frequently have few or no prodromal symptoms. Abdominal findings may be unimpressive, with slight tenderness and negligible muscle guarding until perforation occurs. Fever and leukocytosis may also be minimal or absent. When the white count is not elevated, a shift to the left is significant evidence of inflammation.
c. Obesity - Obesity frequently increases the difficulty of evaluation by delaying the appearance of abdominal signs and by preventing their sharp localization.
d. Pregnancy - Appendicitis occurs occasionally in pregnant women, and the incidence is the same in the 3 trimesters. The symptoms and signs of appendicitis are essentially unchanged, but the diagnosis is usually more difficult because of confusion with the complications of pregnancy. The site of maximal tenderness is usually near McBurney's point - even in the third trimester, when the cecum is displaced upward. Early operation is essential; the somewhat increased mortality rate of appendicitis during pregnancy can be ascribed to delay in treatment. Fetal mortality is about 2-5%. Progesterone administration to prevent abortion is ineffective and may cause female pseudohermaphroditism. A high oxygen intake during anesthesia is mandatory. A muscle-splitting (McBurney type) incision is less likely to cause difficulty during labor.

Differential Diagnosis.

A. Acute gastroenteritis is the disorder most commonly confused with appendicitis. In rare cases it either precedes or is coincident with appendicitis. Vomiting and diarrhea are more common. Fever and WBC may rise sharply and may be out of proportion to abdominal findings. Localization of pain and tenderness is usually indefinite and shifting. Hyperactive peristalsis is characteristic. Gastroenteritis frequently runs an acute course. A period of observation usually serves to clarify the diagnosis.

B. Mesenteric adenitis may cause signs and symptoms identical with appendicitis. Usually, however, there are some clues to the true diagnosis. Mesenteric adenitis is more likely to occur in children or adolescents; respiratory infection is a common antecedent; localization of right lower quadrant tenderness is less precise and constant; and true muscle guarding is infrequent. In spite of a strong suspicion of mesenteric adenitis, it is often safer to advise appendectomy than to risk a complication of appendicitis by procrastination.

C. Meckel's diverticulitis may mimic appendicitis. The localization of tenderness may be more medial, but this is not a reliable diagnostic criterion. Because operation is required in both diseases, the differentiation is not critical. When a preoperative diagnosis of appendicitis proves on exploration to be erroneous, it is essential to examine the terminal 5 feet of the ileum for Meckel's diverticulitis and mesenteric adenitis.

D. Regional enteritis, perforated duodenal ulcer, ureteral colic, acute salpingitis, mittelschmerz, ruptured ectopic pregnancy, and twisted ovarian cyst may at times also be confused with appendicitis.

Treatment.

A. Preoperative Care:
   1. Observation for diagnosis - Within the first 8-12 hours after onset the symptoms and signs of appendicitis are frequently indefinite. Under these circumstances a period of close observation is essential. The patient is placed at bed rest and given nothing by mouth. **Note:** Laxatives should not be prescribed when appendicitis or any form of peritonitis is suspected. Parenteral fluid therapy is begun as indicated. Narcotic medications are avoided if possible, but sedation with barbiturates or tranquilizing agents is not contraindicated. Abdominal and rectal examinations, WBC, and differential are repeated periodically. Abdominal films (see p. 402) and an upright chest film are obtained on all difficult diagnostic problems. In most cases of appendicitis, the diagnosis is clarified by localization of signs to the right lower quadrant within 24 hours after onset of symptoms.
   2. Intubation - Preoperatively, a nasogastric tube is inserted if there is sufficient peritonitis or toxicity to indicate that postoperative ileus may be troublesome. In such patients the stomach is aspirated and lavaged if necessary, and the patient is sent to the operating room with the tube in place.
   3. Antibiotics - In the presence of marked systemic reaction with severe toxicity and high fever, preoperative administration of antibiotics is advisable.

B. Surgical Treatment: In uncomplicated appendicitis, appendectomy is performed as soon as fluid imbalance and other significant systemic disturbances are controlled. Little preparation is usually required. Early, properly conducted surgery has a mortality of a fraction of 1%. Morbidity and mortality in this disease stem primarily from the complications of gangrene and perforation which occur when operation is delayed.

C. Postoperative Care: In uncomplicated appendicitis, postoperative gastric suction is usually not necessary. Ambulation is begun on the first postoperative day. The diet is advanced from clear liquids to soft solids during the second to fifth postoperative days, depending upon the rapidity with which peristalsis and gastrointestinal function return. Parenteral fluid supplements are administered as required. Enemas, except of the small oil retention type, are contraindicated. Mineral oil, milk of magnesia, or a similar mild laxative may be given orally at bedtime daily from about the third day onward if necessary. Antibiotic therapy is advisable for 5-7 days or longer if abdominal fluid at operation was purulent or malodorous, if culture was positive, or if the appendix was gangrenous. Primary wound healing is the rule, and the period of hospitalization is usually one week or less. Normal activity can be resumed in 2-3 weeks after surgery in uncomplicated cases, especially if a McBurney type incision was used.

D. Nonsurgical Treatment: When surgical facilities are not available, treat as for acute peritonitis (see p. 403). On such a regimen acute appendicitis will frequently subside and complications will be minimized.

Complications.

A. Perforation: Appendicitis may subside spontaneously, but it is an unpredictable disease with a marked tendency to progression and perforation. Because perforation rarely occurs within the first 8 hours, diagnostic observation during this period is relatively safe. Signs of perforation include increasing severity of pain and tenderness, and spasm in the right lower quadrant followed by evidence of generalized peritonitis or of a localized abscess. Ileus, fever, malaise, and leukocytosis become more marked. If perforation with abscess formation or generalized peritonitis has already occurred when the patient is first seen, the diagnosis may be quite obscure.

   Treatment of perforated appendicitis is appendectomy unless a well-localized right lower quadrant or pelvic abscess has already walled off the appendix. Supportive measures are as for acute peritonitis (see p. 404).

B. Generalized Peritonitis: This is a common sequel to perforation. Clinical findings and treatment are discussed on p. 403.

C. Appendiceal Abscess: This is one of the possible complications of untreated appendicitis. Malaise, toxicity, fever, and leukocytosis vary from minimal to marked. Examination discloses a tender mass in the right lower quadrant or pelvis. Pelvic abscesses tend to bulge into the rectum or vagina.

   Abscesses usually become noticeable 2-6 days after onset, but antibiotic therapy may delay their appearance. Appendiceal abscess is occasionally the first and only sign of appendicitis and may be confused with neoplasm of the cecum, particularly in the older age group in whom systemic reaction to the infection may be minimal or absent.

   Treatment of early abscess is by intensive combined antibiotic therapy (e.g., penicillin and streptomycin and/or tetracycline). On this regimen, the abscess will frequently resolve. Appendectomy should be performed 6-12 weeks later. A well-established, progressive abscess in the right lower quadrant should be drained without delay. Pelvic abscess requires drainage when it bulges into the rectum or vagina and has become fluctuant.

D. Pylephlebitis: Suppurative thrombophlebitis of the portal system with liver abscesses is a rare complication. It should be suspected when septic fever, chills, hepatomegaly, and jaundice develop after appendiceal perforation. Intensive combined antibiotic therapy is indicated.

E. Other complications include subphrenic abscess (see p. 90) and other foci of intra-abdominal sepsis. Mechanical intestinal obstruction (see p. 408) may be caused by adhesions.

MASSIVE UPPER GASTROINTESTINAL HEMORRHAGE

Massive gastrointestinal hemorrhage is a common emergency. It may be defined as rapid loss of sufficient blood to cause hypovolemic shock. The actual volume of blood loss required to produce shock varies with the size, age, and general condition of the patient and with the rapidity of bleeding. Sudden loss of 20% or more of blood volume (blood volume is approximately 75 ml./Kg. of body weight) produces hypotension, tachycardia, and other signs of shock (see p. 18). For example, a previously well 70 Kg. man who develops shock as a result of gastrointestinal hemorrhage will have lost at least 1000-1500 ml. of blood. The immediate objectives of management are (1) to control shock and (2) to establish a diagnosis on which definitive treatment can be based.

Etiology.

About 75% of cases are due to peptic ulceration of the duodenum or stomach. Esophageal varices and gastritis are each responsible for about 10% of cases. Gastric neoplasm, hiatus hernia, esophagitis, stress ulcer, Mallory-Weiss syndrome, ulcerogenic drugs (e.g., aspirin), and miscellaneous disorders account for about 5%.

Clinical Findings.

There is usually a history of sudden weakness or fainting associated with or followed by tarry stools and/or vomiting of blood. Melena occurs in all patients, and hematemesis in over 50%. Hematemesis is especially common in esophageal varices (90%), gastritis, and gastric ulcer. The patient may or may not be in shock when first seen, but he will at least be pale and weak if major blood loss has occurred.

There is usually no pain, and abdominal findings are not remarkable except when hepatomegaly, splenomegaly, or a mass (neoplasm) is present. There may be a past history of peptic ulcer, cirrhosis, or other predisposing disease, but history often gives no clue to the source of bleeding. About half of all patients will have had at least one previous hemorrhage.

The etiology of bleeding should be established promptly, if possible, since the decision whether to operate or to continue with medical measures often depends upon the diagnosis. The most critical differentiation is between peptic ulcer and esophageal varices, since emergency surgery is frequently indicated and successful in ulcer but less often indicated or successful in varices. Specific diagnosis is of value also because of the difficulties of entering the abdomen in search of an unknown bleeding point.

A history of peptic ulcer, chronic indigestion, or ingestion of antacids favors a diagnosis of peptic ulcer. A history of alcoholism or jaundice favors a diagnosis of liver disease. Jaundice, hepatosplenomegaly, spider angiomas, palmar erythema, and fetor hepaticus are suggestive of liver disease.

The principal diagnostic procedures in the investigation of upper gastrointestinal bleeding, to be carried out after instituting necessary emergency treatment, are as follows:

A. Laboratory Findings: When cirrhosis with bleeding varices cannot be ruled out, the following blood studies should be obtained immediately.
   1. Sulfobromophthalein sodium (BSP) retention test - Normal BSP retention practically excludes cirrhosis severe enough to cause varices. However, because retention (15% or greater) occurs frequently in massive hemorrhage in the

absence of cirrhosis, a positive test is not conclusive evidence of liver disease.

2. Blood ammonia level - Blood ammonia is almost always elevated in cirrhotics with bleeding esophageal varices within 1-2 hours after bleeding begins.
3. Prothrombin time - This test should be performed in all cases of suspected liver disease.
4. Other liver function studies - Serum protein, A/G ratio, alkaline phosphates, and transaminases should be obtained as part of a chemical screening battery.

B. Endoscopy: When varices are suspected in spite of negative x-rays, esophagoscopy is useful. The procedure can be done on the operating table just prior to laparotomy if necessary. When both varices and peptic ulcer are seen on x-ray, esophagoscopy may help to decide which is bleeding. Fiberoptic esophagogastroscopy and gastroduodenoscopy are highly valuable procedures when done by experienced people and are more effective than x-ray in identifying the actual source of upper gastrointestinal bleeding. Fiberoptic endoscopy can be performed under topical anesthesia and is feasible if the patient is not bleeding massively.

C. X-ray Findings: The cause of upper gastrointestinal bleeding can be demonstrated on x-ray in about 75% of cases. When the diagnosis is in doubt, emergency barium examination of the upper gastrointestinal tract should be done immediately. The examination is only postponed if there is active bleeding or shock.

Treatment.

A. General Measures: The patient should be under the observation of both an internist and a surgeon from the outset. Bed rest, mild sedation if necessary, and regular recording of BP, pulse, respiration, temperature, and urine output are instituted. Vitamin K_1 is given empirically.

A nasogastric tube is placed in the stomach. If massive bleeding has occurred recently, gross blood or "coffee-ground" (guaiac positive) material will be aspirated. The stomach is lavaged with iced saline until the returns are clear. The tube is placed on suction with intermittent lavage with iced saline to remove blood and clots until the patient is able to resume oral intake.

B. Blood Replacement: Treatment of shock by blood transfusion is begun without delay (see p. 22). Hct. or Hgb. determinations are done every few hours until stabilized. The objective of blood replacement is to relieve shock and restore the Hct. to 35% and the Hgb. to 12 Gm./100 ml. The volume of blood required to accomplish this must be estimated empirically. Assume that blood volume is 75 ml./Kg. body weight and calculate the patient's normal blood volume. If moderate shock is present (e.g., BP is 70-90, pulse rate 110-130, and there are clinical signs of hypovolemia), give transfusions equivalent to 25% of the normal blood volume. If shock is severe with BP below 70, the initial volume of blood transfusion will probably need to be 40-50% of normal blood volume. The patient should be resuscitated rapidly and completely. Poor response usually means continued bleeding (see below) or inadequate replacement.

C. Medical Measures: Acid peptic digestion is a causative or aggravating factor in most cases of massive upper gastrointestinal hemorrhage, including varices. Bland feedings and oral medications for ulcer are begun as soon as shock and nausea have subsided. Continued slight bleeding is no contraindication to the following regimen:
   1. Diet - Hourly feedings (on the hour) around the clock of 90 ml. of half milk and half cream (Sippy Stage I). Three to 6 Gm. of sodium chloride may be added to each quart of milk and cream mixture to prevent salt depletion. The diet may be advanced over the next few days as tolerated to purêed bland foods.
   2. Antacids - Aluminum hydroxide gel–magnesium trisilicate mixture (Tricreamalate®, Gelusil®, etc.), 15-30 ml., is given hourly (on the half-hour), alternating with the milk and cream mixture.
   3. Other medications indicated include anticholinergics and mild barbiturate sedation.

D. Management of Bleeding Esophageal Varices: When varices are the cause of bleeding, special measures are indicated (see p. 470).

E. Indications for Emergency Operation: Except when esophageal varices are the cause of bleeding, emergency surgery to stop active bleeding should be considered under any of the following circumstances:
   1. When the patient has received 1000 ml. or more of blood but shock is not controlled or recurs promptly.
   2. When acceptable BP and Hct. cannot be maintained with a maximum of 500 ml. of blood every 8 hours.
   3. When bleeding is slow but persists more than 2-3 days.
   4. When bleeding stops initially but recurs massively while the patient is receiving adequate medical treatment.
   5. When the patient is over 50. It has been shown that the death rate from exsanguination in spite of conservative measures is greater in the older age group and rare in patients under 40. Massive bleeding is less well tolerated and is less likely to stop in older patients, who will therefore require operative intervention more frequently.

Prognosis.

The overall mortality of about 14% indicates the seriousness of massive upper gastrointestinal hemorrhage. Fatality rates vary greatly, depending upon the etiology of the bleeding. Hemorrhage from duodenal ulcer causes death in about 3% of treated cases, whereas in bleeding varices the mortality rate may be as high as 50%. When patients treated conservatively for massive gastrointestinal bleeding are followed for 5-7 years, recurrent bleeding is reported in about one-third. The incidence of recurrent bleeding in duodenal and gastric ulcer is even higher, and the bleeding from gastric ulcer tends to be more severe. Recurrent bleeding after definitive surgical treatment of massive gastrointestinal bleeding does occur, but the incidence is low. These findings plus recent improvements in operative technics and surgical management are responsible for the trend in certain centers toward earlier surgical intervention in massive gastrointestinal bleeding, particularly in patients with ulcer disease.

DISEASES OF THE ESOPHAGUS

Dysphagia is the most frequent complaint in esophageal disease. This symptom, no matter how mild, should always be investigated by esophageal x-rays with contrast medium. If there is a lesion which requires further evaluation or if roentgenography is negative and dysphagia continues, esophagoscopy is advisable. Biopsy specimens can be obtained through the esophagoscope when indicated.

ESOPHAGEAL TRAUMA

Esophageal injury caused by an external crushing force is associated with serious damage to other viscera; penetration of the esophagus by missiles, sharp objects, or instruments may cause little injury to other structures. Rupture of the lower esophagus sometimes occurs as a result of violent vomiting or perforation of an esophageal ulcer. Immediate diagnosis and surgical repair are essential to prevent overwhelming mediastinal and pleural infection, although very small rents produced by instrumentation (e.g., esophagoscopy, bougienage) may sometimes be successfully treated by intensive penicillin and streptomycin therapy. A swallow of soluble contrast medium, e.g., methylglucamine diatrizoate (Gastrografin®) (never barium), under fluoroscopy and esophagoscopy, are useful diagnostic procedures in doubtful cases.

Chemical burns of the esophagus are treated by daily bougienage to prevent dysphagia after the danger of perforation has passed.

DIVERTICULA OF THE ESOPHAGUS

Pulsion diverticula of the esophagus due to herniation of mucosa and submucosa through a weakened portion of the muscle wall may occur either at the pharyngoesophageal junction or just above the diaphragm. Traction diverticula, resulting from the traction of an adjacent inflammatory process (usually tuberculous adenitis), occur occasionally at the midthoracic level but rarely cause symptoms or require treatment.

Pharyngoesophageal (Hypopharyngeal) Diverticula.

These project from the posterior wall of the hypopharynx just above the cricopharyngeus muscle and usually veer to the left of the midline. They rarely occur before middle age. Symptoms and signs consist of dysphagia, regurgitation of food (often that eaten several days previously), and gurgling noises in the neck on swallowing or on pressure over the diverticulum. Cough from tracheal irritation is common; aspiration pneumonia may result from overflow of the diverticulum; and nutritional deficiency may develop if there is serious interference with swallowing. Treatment is by one-stage excision.

Supradiaphragmatic Diverticula.

These are rare. Dysphagia, regurgitation of previously ingested food, and substernal or back pain are the chief complaints. Diagnosis is made readily on barium study. Treatment is by one-stage transthoracic excision.

CARDIOSPASM

In idiopathic dilatation of the esophagus (achalasia, cardiospasm, mega-esophagus, etc.), the entire esophagus down to its distal few cm. may assume huge proportions. The terminal, relatively narrowed portion may show either atrophy or hypertrophy of the muscle layers, but there is no actual obstruction and the defect appears to be a dystonia of the esophagus related to absence or diminution of the ganglion cells of Auerbach's plexus. When the esophagus is not markedly enlarged, fluoroscopic studies with the patient supine will reveal that the defect is a failure of a moving peristaltic wave to develop in the body of the esophagus and of the vestibule to relax normally on swallowing. Spot films of the distal esophagus typically show the point of narrowing as a symmetrically tapered cone. Esophagoscopy will confirm that there is no organic stricture at the vestibule, which usually dilates readily to allow passage of an instrument into the stomach. All ages are affected, but the condition is most common in early adult life.

Clinical Findings.

Dysphagia, regurgitation of previously ingested food, and epigastric or subxiphoid pain are common symptoms. Overflow from the esophagus may produce aspiration pneumonia. Some patients become severely malnourished. Barium study of the esophagus is usually diagnostic, but carcinoma of the cardiac end of the stomach occasionally causes esophageal obstruction with proximal dilatation. When the diagnosis is in doubt, esophagoscopy and biopsy of the cardia are mandatory.

Treatment.

Low-residue diet (see p. 146) and mild sedative drugs may suffice to control mild symptoms. Conservative management should be tried at the outset in early cases who may be able to eat adequately if freed from emotional stress. No drugs are useful for relaxing the sphincter. Amyl nitrite inhalation (or nitroglycerin, 0.4 mg. sublingually) may transiently relax the sphincter, but these agents are of little practical value in management. About 80% of patients can be permanently relieved by one or more dilatations with the hydrostatic dilator, but this method of treatment requires skill and experience. Approximately 20% of cases require operation. The Heller procedure (myotomy of the distal, narrow portion of the esophagus) is the least dangerous and most successful. Other operations which result in regurgitation of gastric contents into the lower esophagus are complicated by a high incidence of peptic esophagitis, which may be more disabling than the original disease.

PEPTIC ESOPHAGITIS

Inflammation of the distal esophagus caused by reflux of gastric juice produces heartburn and substernal pain on swallowing. Ulceration, stricture, hemorrhage, and, rarely, perforation are the major complications. There are 2 predisposing conditions: the peptic ulcer diathesis and hiatus hernia. Diagnosis is made by x-ray and esophagoscopy.

When peptic disease is an aggravating factor, dietary and drug therapy should be given as for peptic ulcer (see p. 429) and the patient should sleep on pillows in the semi-reclining position. Small hiatus hernia with mild esophagitis is treated similarly; larger and more symptomatic hernias require surgical repair. Peptic esophagitis associated with shortening of the esophagus, cicatricial stricture, or traction-type hiatus hernia is best managed by an ulcer regimen and dilatation with mercury bougies. Mild strictures can usually be managed with intermittent dilatations. Intractable strictures require resection. Simple resection of the stricture with esophagogastrostomy results in recurrence because reflux persists and gastric acidity is not reduced. Vagotomy should be performed when the stricture is resected. A number of different methods of restoring continuity of the gastrointestinal tract after resection of stricture have been successfully employed. Interposition of a segment of jejunum or colon between the esophagus and the stomach combined with pyloroplasty has proved satisfactory. Another approach is to perform esophagogastrostomy, antrectomy, and either gastroduodenostomy or gastrojejunostomy. The objectives of surgical treatment are to (1) minimize gastroesophageal reflux, (2) eliminate gastric acidity, and (3) ensure rapid emptying of the stomach.

ESOPHAGEAL NEOPLASMS

Dysphagia is the universal early symptom of neoplastic diseases of the esophagus. X-ray and esophagoscopy with biopsy establish the diagnosis.

Benign Tumors.

Benign esophageal tumors are rare; leiomyomas (most common), fibromas, lipomas, and cysts are treated by local excision.

Malignant Tumors.

Epidermoid carcinoma is the commonest esophageal tumor. Lesions above the lower third spread to regional nodes (beyond the limits of surgical removal) so early that resection is rarely more than palliative. Surgical resection may occasionally be successful but, in general, x-ray therapy is the preferred method of management in tumors above the lower third. Lesions of the lower third of the esophagus should be removed surgically when there is no evidence of metastasis. The five-year survival rate after resection of carcinoma of the lower third of the esophagus is about 30%. Obstruction of the esophagus by incurable carcinoma can often be relieved temporarily by x-ray therapy with or without esophageal dilatations. It may be possible for feeding purposes to pass a small tube through the lesion into the stomach by endoscopy when severe dysphagia prevents adequate oral intake. Placement of a large inlying tube (e.g., Celestin tube) through the obstructing lesion may relieve dysphagia significantly and contribute to palliation (Sanfelippo, P. M., and P. E. Bernatz, S. Clin. North America 53:921-926, 1973). Gastrostomy may be justified when other methods of feeding fail and the general condition of the patient is good.

Adenocarcinomas of the cardiac end of the stomach frequently invade the distal esophagus and may be confused with esophageal carcinoma.

DISEASES OF THE STOMACH AND DUODENUM

PEPTIC ULCER

Ten per cent of people have peptic ulcer during their lifetime. It is most common in young and middle aged adults, and men are affected 4 times as often as women. Diagnoses based on x-ray examination reveal a 9:1 preponderance of duodenal over gastric ulcer, but autopsy diagnoses show an equal incidence of the 2 types.

The etiology is not known, but the action of acid and pepsin on the gastroduodenal mucosa of constitutionally susceptible persons undoubtedly plays a role. Acute ulcers may occur following prolonged administration of corticotropin or corticosteroids, reserpine, phenylbutazone, and salicylates, or following intracranial injury or disease, massive infection, severe burns, and other forms of stress. A severe ulcer diathesis known as the Zollinger-Ellison syndrome may be caused by a non–beta cell, non–insulin-producing islet cell tumor of the pancreas (see p. 485).

Peptic ulcer must be suspected in any case of chronic dyspepsia. The most characteristic complaint is gnawing, "hunger-like" epigastric pain occurring one-half to several hours after eating which is relieved by food or alkalies. Emotional stress is an aggravating factor. Remissions and relapses are common. The physical examination is usually negative, although mild tenderness in the epigastrium may be present. Diagnosis is established by gastrointestinal x-rays. Fiberoptic gastroduodenoscopy is a valuable diagnostic method for visualizing the ulcer.

Medical Management.

The conservative management of peptic ulcer consists of bland diet, antacids, anticholinergics, mild sedatives, rest, and psychotherapy.

A. Diets: These range from the strict Sippy Stage I regimen for acute and complicated ulcers to the more liberal six-meal bland diet.
B. Antacids: Aluminum hydroxide–magnesium salt combinations are most effective (e.g., Maalox®, Tricreamalate®, Gelusil®).

During the first stage of management of severe ulcers, the antacid, 15-30 ml., is given hourly on the half hour and the feeding (90 ml.) of milk and cream is given hourly on the hour throughout the day and when awake at night. When used with an ambulatory regimen and bland diet, the antacid is most conveniently given in tablet form 90 minutes after meals and at any other time that ulcer distress occurs.

C. Anticholinergic Agents: Tincture of belladonna is preferred for oral use; atropine is used when parenteral administration is desirable. Numerous synthetic parasympatholytics are available as belladonna or atropine substitutes (e.g., Pro-Banthine®) which do not have CNS side-effects, but it is difficult to substantiate any other therapeutic advantages for them.

D. Other Measures: Regular eating habits and adequate rest are essential. Bed rest and hospitalization may be advisable in severe cases. Mild barbiturate sedation is often helpful. Coffee and other caffein-containing beverages, alcohol, and tobacco are eliminated. Mental and emotional conflicts should be treated by psychotherapy.

Indications for Surgical Treatment.

Ninety per cent of peptic ulcers respond well to medical management; the remainder require surgical treatment. Indications for surgery are as follows: (1) intractability, (2) perforation, (3) hemorrhage, (4) obstruction, and (5) gastric ulcer with suspicion of malignancy.

A. Intractability: When symptoms persist or recur frequently in spite of appropriate medical therapy, or when the patient is unable for some reason to cooperate in an effective program, surgical treatment should be considered.

B. Perforation: This complication occurs in about 2% of ulcer patients. There is usually (but not always) a past history of ulcer symptoms. Prompt treatment is essential; the over-all mortality for perforated ulcer ranges from 5-10%, but is only 1-2% with early treatment.

1. **Diagnosis** - The onset of severe epigastric or generalized abdominal pain is sudden. The pain may be referred to the top of one or both shoulders (phrenic irritation). Boardlike rigidity of the abdomen with epigastric or generalized tenderness and absent or markedly diminished peristalsis are typical. Occasionally, localization of maximum tenderness in the right lower quadrant suggests appendicitis (see p. 418). The patient tends to lie still with knees flexed to minimize the pain. Temperature and BP may be subnormal immediately following perforation, but fever develops gradually. Leukocytosis is moderate to marked, and serum amylase and urinary diastase may be moderately elevated. Pneumoperitoneum is noted on upright chest or lateral decubitus abdominal films in about two-thirds of patients. X-ray examination of the stomach and duodenum with water-soluble iodine-containing contrast medium such as methylglucamine diatrizoate (Gastrografin®) is a valuable procedure if the diagnosis is in doubt or if it is suspected that the perforation has sealed off, making operation unnecessary. Acute pancreatitis, acute cholecystitis, appendicitis, perforation of another abdominal viscus, diaphragmatic pleurisy,

and coronary thrombosis are the principal disorders which must be considered in the differential diagnosis.

2. Emergency measures - A gastric tube is passed immediately and placed on constant suction; treat as for acute peritonitis (see p. 403). Operation, if indicated, should be carried out as soon as the patient's condition has been stabilized by fluid replacement and other measures.
3. Treatment - There are 3 possible types of therapy: (1) nonoperative treatment, (2) simple closure, and (3) emergency gastric surgery. Most patients are best managed by one of the latter 2 methods.
   a. Nonoperative treatment - Nonoperative treatment consists of constant gastric suction, antibiotics, and other measures for acute peritonitis (see p. 403). Other than those patients who are too ill for any type of surgical procedure or whose ulcers perforate in circumstances where surgical facilities are not available, only a small group are treated electively by the nonoperative method. This type of management may be preferred in 2 types of cases if Gastrografin® x-ray examination shows that the perforation is no longer leaking: (1) in early cases in whom signs of peritonitis have been mild and are subsiding rapidly; (2) in patients seen 24 hours or more after perforation whose abdominal and systemic condition is stabilized or improving (consistent with sealed perforation).
   b. Simple closure of the perforation - This is the safest and most widely applicable mode of treatment and should be employed on all poor risk patients with leaking perforations and when the peritoneum is heavily contaminated or definitive gastric surgery is technically difficult.
   c. Emergency gastric surgery - A definitive operation for cure of the peptic ulcer diathesis may be undertaken on the patient with perforated duodenal or gastric ulcer under the following conditions: (1) the patient is a good surgical risk; (2) the peritoneum is not excessively contaminated; and (3) the operation is not unduly difficult technically. For perforated gastric ulcer, partial gastrectomy is preferred. For perforated duodenal ulcer, pyloroplasty and vagotomy is the simplest and safest procedure although antrectomy-vagotomy or partial gastrectomy is advocated by some.
4. Postoperative and after-care - Postoperatively the patient is treated for acute peritonitis (see p. 403). Diet is advanced as tolerated to a six-meal bland diet. Intensive medical management for ulcer should be carried out for at least 3 months and as long thereafter as the symptoms warrant except in those patients treated by a definitive operative procedure for cure of ulcer disease. This latter group usually requires no special medical regimen after recovery from the operation.
5. Prognosis - About one-third of patients treated by simple closure or nonoperative methods will be asymptomatic or will have only mild symptoms in the future; one-third will have symptoms requiring medical management; and one-third will ultimately require surgery.

C. Massive Hemorrhage From Peptic Ulcer: See p. 422.

D. Pyloric Obstruction:

1. Diagnosis - There is usually a past history of ulcer symptoms culminating in recurrent vomiting, frequently of food eaten at the previous meal. Weight loss, dehydration, metabolic alkalosis, and hypokalemia are late signs of depletion. Tympanitic epigastric fullness may be present, with visible peristalsis in the distended stomach. The diagnosis is confirmed by barium meal: pyloric obstruction is present if there is significant gastric retention of barium in 6 hours or any residual barium after 24 hours. Obstructing neoplasm must be excluded. A fasting gastric content of more than 100 ml. on aspiration is usually indicative of obstruction.

   Pyloric obstruction due to edema and spasm will respond to medical measures. It must be distinguished from obstruction due to scarring, which requires surgical treatment.

2. Treatment -

   a. Medical measures - These should be given a trial in most cases, with the patient at bed rest in a hospital if possible.

      (1) Diet - Begin with Sippy Stage I diet and advance to Sippy II, III, and IV as tolerated.

      (2) Medications - Give sedative and antacid drugs as for uncomplicated ulcer.

      (3) Fluids and feeding - Oral intake will at first usually require intravenous supplementation. Electrolyte balance should be reestablished (see p. 150).

      (4) Gastric aspiration and indications for operation - With the patient on Sippy I diet, aspirate the stomach in the morning and again in the evening and measure intake and output carefully. If the patient is improving, intake will exceed output by a little more each day. When less than 100 ml. are recovered by aspiration, aspirations are made only p.r.n. and the diet gradually advanced. If the volume of aspirated residuum fails to decrease rapidly over a 3-5 day period, cicatricial stenosis is present and surgery is indicated.

   b. Surgical treatment - The stomach should be thoroughly decompressed by constant gastric tube drainage or suction for a few days preoperatively. Gastric resection or other definitive operation for ulcer should be done. Gastroenterostomy is a compromise procedure advisable only in elderly patients with long-standing cicatricial obstruction and low free acid content who will not tolerate more extensive surgery. Such cases are rare.

E. Gastric Ulcer: The symptoms of duodenal and gastric ulcer are similar. However, gastric ulcer tends to occur in older persons and is less related to hyperacidity than duodenal ulcer. Normal or low free acid is common in gastric ulcer. Eight to 20% of benign-appearing gastric ulcers prove to be carcinoma. For this reason the patient with gastric ulcer should be treated intensively and kept under close observation. Medical management is the same for gastric as for duodenal ulcer.

1. Signs of malignancy in gastric ulcer -

   a. Achlorhydria - Absence of free acid after histamine is virtually never found in benign ulcer.

b. Malignant cytology - The finding of malignant cells by Papanicolaou smear of gastric washings indicates the presence of neoplasm.

c. X-ray appearance - A malignant ulcer frequently appears as a filling defect in a crater or a mass. Location on the greater curvature is highly suggestive of cancer. The wall neighboring a malignancy often has diminished pliability. The size of the ulcer is of little diagnostic significance, as benign lesions can be very large.

d. Fiberoptic gastroscopy - Benign ulcers are cleanly punched-out with a smooth base; malignant ulcer may have a heaped-up, irregular margin, and there may be bleeding from the base. Gastroscopic biopsy permits histologic diagnosis of very early malignancies and should be done on all suspicious lesions.

e. Failure of response to treatment - Many malignant gastric ulcers satisfy none of the above criteria. Failure to respond rapidly to 3 weeks of intensive medical therapy for ulcer is strong evidence for carcinoma. On the other hand, good response does not rule out malignancy since ulcer in cancer can heal over temporarily. For this reason, all gastric ulcers should have follow-up x-ray examinations about 3 weeks, 6 weeks, 3 months, and 6 months from the beginning of treatment and thereafter as symptoms indicate. Recurrence of ulcer under medical management suggests carcinoma; about 16% of recurrent gastric ulcers prove to be neoplastic.

2. Indications for operation - Gastric resection is indicated when gastric ulcer exhibits any of the above signs of malignancy or fails either to heal completely or to show marked regression after 3 weeks of intensive medical care. If duodenal ulcer is also present, vagotomy should be done at the time of gastrectomy. In addition, perforation, obstruction, and massive hemorrhage should be treated surgically according to the criteria outlined on p. 430.

Operations for Peptic Ulcer.

The objective of surgical treatment in duodenal ulcer is the marked reduction or elimination of free gastric hydrochloric acid with maximum preservation of gastrointestinal function. The 2 procedures which most successfully meet these specifications are (1) pyloroplasty and vagotomy and (2) antrectomy and vagotomy. Partial (two-thirds) gastric resection is also a highly effective operation but has the disadvantages of reducing the gastric reservoir and of failing to interrupt the cephalic or nervous phase of gastric secretion which is mediated by the vagus nerves. For these reasons, vagotomy with pyloroplasty or antrectomy is now generally preferred as definitive treatment for duodenal ulcer. The morbidity and mortality are also slightly less than with gastric resection. Vagotomy with pyloroplasty offers definite advantages in the emergency treatment of the poor risk patient with a bleeding duodenal ulcer. The ulcer bed is well exposed for direct suture, and minimal dissection and trauma are involved.

Gastric ulcer is treated by partial gastrectomy with either gastroduodenostomy (Billroth I) or gastrojejunostomy (Billroth II) to restore continuity. Vagotomy is added if duodenal ulcer is also present.

The mortality of these operations for peptic ulcer when done electively should not exceed 1-2%.

Postoperative Care.

Nothing is given by mouth for 24-48 hours. Diet is then increased gradually, beginning with 30 ml. of fluid per hour. Gastric suction is maintained for 24-48 hours postoperatively, and ambulation is begun on the first postoperative day. Milk of magnesia and mineral oil by mouth or a low saline enema on the third or fourth postoperative day will aid in establishing bowel regularity if needed.

Early Postoperative Complications.

A. Duodenal Stump Leakage: Sudden, severe upper abdominal pain on the third to seventh postoperative day (occasionally later) is characteristic. The patient is prostrated and acutely ill, with rising fever and WBC. Marked rigidity of the upper or entire abdomen is usual, and may be difficult to evaluate because of the presence of the incision. Radiation of pain to the shoulder (phrenic referral) is suggestive of stump or suture-line leakage.

Treatment is by immediate placement of drains or, preferably, sump suction in the region of the leak. Attempts to resuture the duodenal stump are unsuccessful. If adequate external drainage is provided and the afferent jejunal loop is unobstructed, the duodenal leak tends gradually to close.

B. Gastric Retention: Failure of the gastrojejunostomy or gastroduodenostomy to function promptly occurs to a significant degree in about 5% of cases.

Gastric distention must be avoided during the early postoperative period. The patient's stomach should be aspirated if he feels "full" or nauseous after removal of the tube. Treatment of gastric retention consists of resuming gastric suction for 24-48 hours. The gastric tube is then left on gravity drainage and the first-day gastrectomy diet is resumed. The tube is clamped for the first half hour after feeding and then unclamped for the remaining half hour. Drainage volume is recorded. The feeding volume is increased and the tube is clamped for longer intervals or removed as volume of drainage diminishes.

Hypernatremia, hypokalemia, and hypoproteinemia are precipitating or aggravating conditions which should be relieved. The functioning of the stoma should be checked by barium x-ray study if obstruction persists more than a few days. Reoperation must be seriously considered if total gastric retention persists more than 10 days, although conservative treatment may be successful after periods of several weeks.

Sequelae of Gastric Surgery.

A. Marginal Ulcers: Marginal ulcers develop in about 5% of patients operated on for duodenal ulcer, and may be controlled by a medical ulcer regimen. If this fails, a vagotomy may be done or a more adequate gastrectomy performed. Gastrojejunocolic fistula is the most serious complication of marginal ulcer and should be suspected when persistent pain or ulcer symptoms, vomiting, diarrhea, and nutritional depletion develop following gastrectomy with gastrojejunostomy. Diagnosis is readily made by gastrointestinal x-rays. Fiberoptic gastroscopy is particularly useful in visualizing the gastrojejunostomy and in distinguishing ulceration from postoperative deformity. Treatment is by resection of the fistula after careful preparation of the patient.

B. Dumping Syndrome: The so-called "dumping syndrome" occurs after 5-10% of resections. It is characterized by the development, shortly after eating, of sweating, warmth, flushing, nausea, palpitation, and faintness. Diarrhea may or may not be present. The etiology is obscure, but the syndrome may be caused by acute reduction in plasma volume or by excitation of autonomic reflexes due to rapid filling of the jejunum. Symptoms can usually be controlled by a regimen consisting of frequent low-residue feedings, avoidance of high-carbohydrate foods, restriction of fluids during meals, and lying down after eating. Anticholinergics, mild sedation, and reassurance may have value. Dumping symptoms may occur for a few weeks or months after gastric surgery and then disappear spontaneously. Rarely, such an operative procedure as conversion of a Billroth II (gastrojejunostomy) to a Billroth I (gastroduodenostomy) may be indicated in an attempt to control dumping.

C. Other Sequelae: Failure to gain or actual loss of weight occurs in 15-30% of patients after an adequate gastric resection. Failure normally to assimilate iron, fat, carbohydrate, or protein may occur. The more radical the gastrectomy, the higher the incidence of these disturbances. Management is with frequent feedings and supplementary iron and vitamin therapy. Diarrhea occurs in about 7% of vagotomized patients and is treated by nonspecific measures.

NEOPLASMS OF THE STOMACH

Benign Neoplasms of the Stomach.

These are rare and usually asymptomatic, although leiomyoma, the commonest benign tumor, may cause obstruction or bleeding. Single or multiple adenomatous polyps are probably precancerous lesions. Lipomas, fibromas, hemangiomas, aberrant pancreatic tissue, and a variety of other benign lesions have been reported.

All benign gastric neoplasms should be excised so that differentiation from malignancy can be made by microscopic study.

Malignant Neoplasms of the Stomach.

A. Adenocarcinoma: This common lesion is the third most frequent cause of death from cancer in the United States, being exceeded only by carcinoma of the lung and intestine. Over the past 30-40 years, there has been an unexplained drop in the incidence of gastric cancer in the United States. For some reason gastric cancer is a more common disease in such countries as Japan, Iceland, Finland, and Chile than in the United States. Ninety-five per cent of cases occur in persons past 45 years of age, and two-thirds of the patients are men. Gastric polyps, chronic gastritis, pernicious anemia, and achlorhydria may be precursors. There may be a family history of gastric cancer.

The earliest symptoms are deceptively vague, consisting usually of anorexia or slight dyspepsia. When such complaints (or other forms of indigestion) last more than 3 weeks in a previously well person over 45 years of age, carcinoma of the stomach should be suspected and gastrointestinal x-rays obtained. Fiberoptic gastroscopy with biopsy often provides a histologic diagnosis. The physical examination is negative except in advanced disease, when weight loss, anemia, an abdominal mass, and progressive gastric malfunction commonly develop.

Surgical resection is the only curative treatment. Signs of metastatic disease include a hard, nodular liver, enlarged left supraclavicular (Virchow's) nodes, skin nodules, ascites, rectal shelf, and x-ray evidence of osseous or pulmonary metastasis. Blood alkaline phosphatase determination, radioisotope liver scan, needle biopsy of the liver, and peritoneoscopy are diagnostic methods that may be used to evaluate the liver for possible metastases. If there is no evidence of liver or other distant metastases, exploration is indicated. The presence of an abdominal mass is not a contraindication to laparotomy, since bulky lesions can often be totally excised. The operative mortality in partial gastrectomy for cancer is about 6%, with a 27% five-year survival rate; for total gastrectomy, the mortality is about 9% with a 14% five-year survival rate. Palliative resection or gastroenterostomy is occasionally helpful in pyloric obstruction. X-ray therapy and chemotherapy may occasionally have temporary palliative effects.

B. Leiomyosarcoma: This is a rare tumor with a tendency to hemorrhage. It usually produces little gastric distress, even though large, and anemia may be the chief sign. Leiomyosarcomas grow slowly, are slow to metastasize, and seldom recur after adequate excision; the prognosis is therefore much more favorable than with carcinoma.

C. Lymphosarcoma: The signs and symptoms of lymphosarcoma are similar to those of carcinoma. The differential diagnosis is usually made only after microscopic examination. Resection should be followed by radiation therapy. The resectability and survival rates for lymphosarcoma are higher than for carcinoma.

DUODENAL DIVERTICULUM

True duodenal diverticula are noted frequently as an incidental finding on x-ray examination, usually on the mesenteric border. They rarely cause symptoms, but may do so if retention within the sac results in infection, ulceration, hemorrhage, or perforation. Duodenal diverticulum usually requires no treatment.

DISEASES OF THE JEJUNUM AND ILEUM

EXTERNAL SMALL BOWEL FISTULAS

Clinical Findings.

The commonest causes of external small bowel fistula are accidental or surgical trauma, leaking intestinal suture lines or duodenal stump closure, strangulation or obstruction of the small intestine, peritoneal sepsis, and regional enteritis. The fistula can be demonstrated by the appearance in the wound of methylene blue or indigo carmine administered by mouth; or by x-ray examination after ingestion of barium or after injection of methylglucamine diatrizoate (Gastrografin®) or other radiopaque medium into the fistulous tract.

Treatment.

Conservative measures are employed to support the patient during spontaneous closure or, in large or distally obstructed fistulas, in preparation for laparotomy. If nutrition and fluid balance are well maintained, gradual closure over a period of weeks can be expected in most cases. Hyperalimentation may be very valuable in providing parenteral nourishment and in reducing the volume of gastrointestinal secretions.

A. Maintenance of Fluid and Nutritional Balance: High jejunal fistulas may seriously deplete the patient within a few hours. Strict accounting of fluid intake and output and quantitative replacement are essential.

B. Local Care of the Fistula: Collection of fistulous drainage and prevention of skin excoration by intestinal secretions are major problems. A suction catheter over or in the fistula can often be employed. Occasionally it is possible to glue a plastic ileostomy bag to the skin to pick up drainage. It may be advantageous to place the patient prone on a Bradford frame and allow the fluid to drop down into a basin when skin irritation is otherwise uncontrollable. From the outset the skin around a fistula should be carefully protected. For this purpose, it may be helpful to apply one of the following to the skin surface: karaya powder mixed with zinc oxide ointment, Stomahesive®, silicone ointment (e.g., Silicote®), zinc oxide ointment, 10% powdered aluminum in zinc oxide ointment, or a watery paste of kaolin or Fuller's earth. Exposure of the skin to the drying effect of a desk lamp several times daily is useful.

C. Surgical Treatment: Continuous copious drainage caused by a large fistula or by obstruction of the bowel distally is an indication for surgical repair. Resection of the fistula or enteroenterostomy around it, with later resection of the involved bowel, is usually required. Preoperative placement of a Miller-Abbott or other long intestinal tube through the nose down to the fistula is an aid in identifying the proximal limb of the fistula at operation.

REGIONAL ENTERITIS
(Regional Ileitis, Regional Enterocolitis, Crohn's Disease)

This granulomatous inflammatory disease of unknown etiology

may occur in any portion of the gastrointestinal tract, but is most commonly seen in the terminal ileum. Multiple, segmental involvement is not unusual. The colon is involved in about 40% of cases, usually (but not always) in association with small bowel involvement. The highest incidence is between the ages of 20 and 40. Marked thickening of the bowel wall and adjacent mesentery are characteristic pathologic features. Recurrence, fistula formation (internal or external), local perforation with abscess, and malabsorption are the most frequent complications. Clinically, regional enteritis is usually a chronic disease, but it may also occur in an acute form.

Clinical Findings.

The acute form often presents as an acute surgical abdomen with fever, leukocytosis, and abdominal tenderness (usually in the right lower quadrant). There may be a past history of diarrhea and intestinal colic which is helpful in the differentiation from appendicitis. An indefinite boggy mass may be palpable. If regional enteritis is suspected, an emergency barium enema with reflux into the ileum should be obtained and may establish the diagnosis. When the rectum is involved, biopsy of the mucosa may reveal the granulomatous changes typical of regional enteritis. Perirectal and perianal abscesses and fistulas may develop as a complication of the disease.

Patients with chronic regional enteritis usually give a history of recurrent, generalized abdominal pain, diarrhea, and weight loss. Fever, anemia (hypochromic, occasionally macrocytic), and occult blood in the stools are also common. In many cases an appendectomy will have been done because of abdominal pain. Occasionally there is a palpable mass or gross rectal bleeding. Segmental narrowing of the bowel lumen is often demonstrable on gastrointestinal x-rays, and is characteristic when present. Recurrent or increasing obstruction of the small bowel is the indication for surgery in about 80% of operations for regional enteritis.

Amebiasis, tuberculous enteritis, and neoplasm must be considered in the differential diagnosis.

Treatment.

A. Medical Measures: The objective of conservative management is to maintain nutrition by a high-caloric, low-residue, bland diet with vitamin and iron supplements. Raw fruits and vegetables should be avoided. Diarrhea is controlled with nonspecific medications.

   The poorly absorbed sulfonamides may be helpful, specifically salicylazosulfapyridazine (Azulfidine®), 1-1.5 Gm. 4-8 times daily with meals or food. The drug is usually given in courses of 2 weeks on and one week off. With improvement the dosage may be reduced to 0.5 Gm. t.i.d. Penicillin and the tetracyclines are best avoided except in perforation or abscess formation because of their tendency to produce candidal or enterococcic diarrhea.

   Corticosteroids are valuable for use in preoperative preparation of the severely ill patient and for treatment of exacerbations of the disease not otherwise controllable.

B. Surgical Treatment: A mistaken diagnosis of appendicitis may lead to laparotomy in the acute stage. The appendix is removed unless regional enteritis involves the cecum or neighboring ileum, in which case appendectomy is not done for fear of fistula formation. Resection of the acute process in the bowel is usually not indicated unless there is significant obstruction or impending perforation. Permanent remissions occur more frequently in the acute than in the chronic form of the disease.

Chronic regional enteritis which is intractable to medical treatment or is complicated by obstruction, bleeding, or fistula formation should be treated by resection of the involved bowel. The mortality rate for surgical treatment ranges from 2-14%. In recent years surgical mortality rates have been generally low, chiefly due to improved preoperative and postoperative care. It is now considered safe to resect involved bowel rather than to perform simple short-circuiting procedures such as ileocolostomy. If the colon is the primary site of involvement, ileostomy usually leads to subsidence. The recurrence rate after surgery is 20-60%.

NEOPLASMS OF SMALL BOWEL

Benign Small Bowel Tumors.

These include lipomas, leiomyomas, fibromas, benign carcinoids, polyps, and hemangiomas. Growth is very slow. These tumors produce symptoms by bleeding, obstruction, or by functioning as the leading point of an intussusception. Surgical excision is indicated. Islands of aberrant pancreatic tissue may occur in the bowel wall and be grossly indistinguishable from neoplasms.

Gastrointestinal polyposis associated with melanin spots on the oral mucosa, lips, and digits is a rare but important familial condition (Peutz-Jeghers syndrome). The diagnosis can be readily inferred from the characteristic pigmentation. The polyps in this syndrome rarely become malignant and do not require removal unless they cause a complication such as intussusception or bleeding.

Malignant Small Bowel Neoplasms.

The most important of these are adenocarcinoma, carcinoid (argentaffinoma), and lymphoma (most commonly lymphosarcoma and reticulum cell sarcoma). Malignant tumors in the upper portion of the small bowel are most likely to be adenocarcinoma or carcinoid; those in the lower portion, lymphoma. Small bowel malignancies tend to occur in somewhat younger age groups than gastric and colon carcinomas. Initial symptoms are often vague and misleading, consisting of intermittent abdominal pain or colic suggestive of partial obstruction. Vomiting may occur, and melena is occasionally present. An abdominal mass may be palpable. Acute intussusception may develop. Early diagnosis depends upon a high index of suspicion and insistence on complete and careful x-ray study of the entire small bowel.

Treatment is by resection. Postoperative radiotherapy is of value in lymphoma but in none of the other tumors.

Carcinoid occurs in any part of the gastrointestinal tract, most commonly in the appendix where its behavior is usually benign. The next highest incidence is in the small bowel. Malignant carcinoid with hepatic metastases may produce a syndrome consisting of a peculiar flushing and cyanosis, transient patchy skin lesions, diarrhea, dyspnea, and right-sided cardiac valvular disease. These clinical developments are caused by an excess of serotonin (5-hydroxytryptamine) secreted by the tumor, combined with a failure of the normal detoxification of the hormone by the involved liver. Examination of the urine for 5-hydroxyindoleacetic acid (a serotonin end-product excreted by the kidneys) should be performed in suspicious cases. The test may also be of value as an index of recurrence during the follow-up after resection of malignant carcinoid.

DISEASES OF THE COLON AND RECTUM

Diagnostic Procedures.

In addition to the routine work-up (see p. 402), patients with significant large bowel symptoms should be investigated by means of 1 or more of the following procedures: (1) Examination of the stools for occult blood, ova, and parasites, and culture for enteric pathogens; (2) anoscopy; (3) sigmoidoscopy with smear, culture, or biopsy of suspicious lesions; (4) barium enema with or without air contrast study; (5) visualization of the entire colon by the fiberoptic colonoscope, through which biopsies can be taken.

Preoperative Preparation.

A. General Measures: When a difficult exposure at operation or an unusual degree of postoperative ileus is anticipated, a long intestinal tube should be passed well into the ileum preoperatively. In less complicated cases a gastric tube is inserted on the morning of colon surgery. If the operative field in the pelvis will be obscured by a full bladder, or if urinary retention is to be expected postoperatively (as after a combined abdominoperineal resection), a Foley catheter should be inserted before surgery and placed on constant drainage.

B. Bowel Preparation: The colon should be prepared before any elective operation during which it might have to be opened. The essential features of the preoperative colon preparation are a minimum-residue diet, laxatives, enemas, and (optionally) oral antibacterial agents.

If the colon is not obstructed, the following regimen produces satisfactory conditions within 48 hours:

1. Diet - Liquid diet without milk for 2 days before operation (see p. 144).
2. Laxative - Sodium phosphate solution, 15 ml., or effervescent sodium phosphate, 15 Gm., in water by mouth at 8:00 a.m. and 8:00 p.m. on the second day before the operation and at 8:00 a.m. on the day before the operation; or 30-45 ml. castor oil at 8:00 a.m. on the second day before operation.
3. Enemas - Saline irrigations until the returned fluid is clear on each of the 2 days before the operation in the evening; no enema on the morning of operation.
4. Antibacterial drugs (optional) - For example, neomycin, 4-6 Gm. daily by mouth in divided doses may be given for

1-2 days preoperatively. This drug is not absorbed from the gastrointestinal tract and is very effective in reducing or eliminating normal colonic bacteria. However, a high incidence of staphylococcal enterocolitis (see p. 451) has been observed after its use (Altemeier and others, S. Clin. North America 45:1087, 1965).

It should be emphasized that the most important measures to reduce septic complications after open colonic surgery are based on elementary surgical principles: thorough mechanical cleansing of the bowel preoperatively, meticulous aseptic technic and field protection during operation, preservation of blood supply, avoidance of tension on suture lines, utilization of closed anastomosis when feasible, and protection of questionable suture lines by proximal colostomy. Antibacterial agents within the bowel or systemically administered are adjuncts only and may be omitted entirely in the preparation of the colon with results comparable to those obtained with their use.

DIVERTICULOSIS AND DIVERTICULITIS

Diverticulosis is rare in persons under 40 years of age, but the incidence increases with age and it is probable that more than half of people over 80 have diverticula. The lesions are confined to the sigmoid in 40% of cases. Only a very small proportion of those with diverticulosis develop diverticulitis. The site of diverticulitis is in the sigmoid in about 90% of cases. Genetic or other factors appear to play a role because the incidence of diverticulosis varies in different populations.

Clinical Findings.

The major symptoms of chronic diverticulitis are changes in bowel habits (constipation, diarrhea, or flatulence), recurrent left lower quadrant pain and tenderness, and, occasionally, rectal bleeding. Acute sigmoid diverticulitis is characterized by the rapid onset of severe left lower quadrant pain, tenderness, and signs of peritoneal irritation. Fever and leukocytosis are usually present. An inflammatory mass is frequently palpable in the left lower quadrant. Fistula formation between the sigmoid colon and the bladder may cause urinary tract infection and the passage of flatus per urethra.

Definitive diagnosis can usually be made by barium enema. Differentiation from carcinoma is occasionally difficult or impossible. Coexistent cancer and diverticulosis may produce a confusing clinical picture. Sigmoidoscopy should always be done, even though the inflammatory changes of diverticulitis are usually above the reach of the sigmoidoscope.

Treatment.

A. Medical Measures:
   1. Chronic - About 75% of patients with chronic diverticulitis will improve on low-residue or normal diet, anticholinergic drugs, and control of constipation with colloid laxatives.

2. Acute diverticulitis is treated as for acute peritonitis (see p. 403). It is important to give antibiotics (see Chapter 6). Most attacks can be controlled by conservative measures. Surgery during an acute episode should be avoided if possible.

B. Surgical Treatment: Resection is indicated if any of the following occur: (1) perforation; (2) fistula formation to the bladder, bowel, or elsewhere; (3) obstruction; (4) massive hemorrhage; and (5) chronic or recurrent acute symptoms. If there are no contraindications, resection is advisable for patients who have persistent annoying symptoms or more than 1 acute attack. This policy will lower the incidence of serious complications of the disease, which may require complex and staged procedures.

When possible, operation should be deferred until the local inflammatory reaction has subsided on medical management. This "cooling off" period usually requires 3-6 months after a severe acute attack.

Emergency operation (because of persistent local sepsis) during an acute episode should usually be limited to the establishment of a diverting transverse colostomy and drainage of abscesses if present.

If the disease has reached an advanced stage, with fistula formation or severe local induration and scarring, a transverse colostomy is necessary so that the distal bowel can remain at rest for several months before resection is attempted. The necessity for staged operations has diminished in recent years.

Prognosis.

The over-all mortality for the surgical treatment of diverticulitis is about 6%. When local inflammation has subsided, colon resection with primary anastomosis can be accomplished with a mortality rate of about 1%. Patients usually remain asymptomatic after an adequate resection for diverticulitis. (Colcock, B. P., S. Clin. North America 48:543, 1968.)

ULCERATIVE COLITIS

Clinical Findings.

Ulcerative colitis usually begins between 20 and 30 years of age. The cause is not known. Onset is commonly with diarrhea (often bloody), fever, and weight loss. The initial attack may be mild or severely fulminant; the disease often becomes chronic, with recurrent periods of diarrhea and prostration which lead to semi-invalidism and such complications as colonic perforation, cirrhosis, arthritis, perianal fistulas, malnutrition, or carcinoma. Cancer of the colon develops in 10-30% of cases of over 10 years' duration.

Diagnosis is usually apparent on sigmoidoscopy because the disease involves the upper rectum in about 95% of cases. On sigmoidoscopy in early cases, the mucosa appears edematous and hyperemic, and bleeds easily; irregular superficial ulcerations develop later. In the early stages, barium enema reveals typical ulcerations. Shortening of the colon, loss of haustration, and tubular configurations are signs of advanced disease.

In the differential diagnosis of ulcerative colitis, other causes of diarrhea must often be considered, including amebiasis, dysentery, tuberculous enteritis, sprue, and regional enteritis.

A severe fulminating form of ulcerative colitis is seen occasionally. It is characterized by abdominal pain, distention, severe bloody diarrhea, prostration, fever, leukocytosis, and marked dehydration. Death may occur from peritoneal sepsis, hemorrhage, or overwhelming toxemia. "Toxic" dilatation of the colon is a particularly serious complication in which there is grave danger of colonic perforation. These patients must be observed very carefully and usually require surgery.

Treatment.

A. Medical Measures:

1. Severe, fulminating colitis - Treatment of this acute, necrotizing infection consists of appropriate parenteral fluid therapy, systemic combined antibiotic therapy, blood transfusions, and sedation. When severe systemic symptoms persist, corticotropin or cortisone may give dramatic relief. **Caution:** These drugs may mask symptoms of perforation or sepsis.

   Emergency ileostomy is rarely necessary.

2. Chronic, debilitating colitis - These patients should have a bland diet from which all foods discovered to aggravate the diarrhea have been eliminated. Medications should include anticholinergics, mild sedatives, and nonnarcotic antidiarrheal drugs. Oral nonabsorbable antibacterial agents such as salicylazosulfapyridazine (Azulfidine®) (2-8 Gm./day) may be of benefit. When fever and systemic signs of sepsis are present, parenteral combined antibiotic therapy is indicated (see above).

   Steroid therapy is very effective in inducing remissions and is definitely indicated in severe forms of the disease. Corticotropin may be given to the hospitalized patient as an I.V. drip (20-40 units over a period of 8 hours). Alternatively, give hydrocortisone (100-300 mg./day), prednisone or prednisolone (20-80 mg./day), or equivalent. These drugs may be given parenterally if not tolerated initially by mouth. When response is satisfactory, dosage is gradually reduced over weeks or months. For long-term treatment with a negligible risk of hyperadrenocorticism and other complications of steroid therapy, give hydrocortisone hemisuccinate (100 mg.) or prednisolone phosphate sodium (Hydeltrasol®), 20 mg. in 100 ml. of saline once or twice daily by slow rectal drip or retention enema.

B. Surgical Treatment:

1. Indications - Surgery should be advised only after a thorough trial of medical management, but must not be delayed until the patient is terminal or debilitated. Operation is indicated if the patient is disabled by recurrent attacks, malnutrition, or impairment of general health. Complications such as arthritis, ulcerative dermatitis, hepatitis, nephritis, acute and subacute colonic perforation, colonic obstruction, hemorrhage, and intractable perianal infection are additional indications for surgery. Because chronic ulceration is a precursor of a highly malignant type of cancer, severely diseased bowel should be removed. Until this can be done, barium enema and sigmoidoscopy should be carried out every

6 months. Symptoms suggestive of malignancy (e.g., rectal bleeding, abdominal pain, or change in bowel habits) are often ignored by these patients, who have usually had such complaints for years.

2. Preoperative preparation - Intensive medical treatment as outlined above is employed. Significant blood and protein losses due to diarrhea commonly occur and require repeated transfusions of whole blood. Normal Hgb. and plasma protein levels should be restored before operation if possible. In severe cases corticotropin or cortisone is administered preoperatively for as long as required (usually one to several weeks) to induce a temporary remission. If corticosteroid therapy is instituted, it must be administered after operation and discontinued gradually.
3. Operations for ulcerative colitis - Ileostomy alone may be indicated as a life-saving measure in fulminating disease. Usually the procedure of choice is ileostomy with subtotal colectomy or, if the patient's condition permits, ileostomy with proctocolectomy in one stage. There is no loss of sexual function if the dissection is kept close to the rectum. The entire colon and rectum should be removed eventually except in selected patients with limited localized involvement of the colon; in this small group, segmental resection of the colon may be adequate.

Prognosis.

Medical management in refractory ulcerative colitis has a mortality rate of 10-20%, and the same group of patients can now be operated on with a mortality of less than 5%. Patients with ileostomies can lead normal lives and, if the entire colon and rectum have been removed, are usually cured.

Complications of Ileostomy.

A. Skin Irritation: This is the most common complication. Its prevention depends upon constant protection of the skin by a properly fitting ileostomy appliance. A plastic bag is cemented to the skin around the ileostomy at the operating table and changed as often as necessary during the following week to prevent contact of ileal contents with the skin. A permanent device is then used. If skin excoriation develops, the same measures may be used as in small bowel fistula (see p. 437).

B. Excessive Fluid Loss: Copious fluid stools may occur from the ileostomy immediately postoperatively or intermittently at any time thereafter. Patients should be warned of this possibility and cautioned to seek hospitalization if fluid loss is marked. Prompt correction of electrolyte imbalance is essential. Partial obstruction of the ileostomy or the ileum should be suspected. Insertion of a well lubricated gloved finger or soft rectal tube into the ileostomy may relieve a temporary local obstruction or dysfunction. Antidiarrheal agents and low-residue diet are usually indicated.

C. Prolapse: This is usually a late complication related to inadequate internal fixation of the ileum or to relaxation of the abdominal ring. If prolapse is recurrent and severe, a new ileostomy should be made; excision of the prolapsed ileum will not cure the condition. Wound herniation, when marked, also requires a new ileostomy.

D. Stricture and Fistula at the Skin Level: These may be early or late complications. They are due to errors in surgical technic or to chronic infection, and require local revision of the ileostomy.

E. Mechanical Obstruction: Small bowel obstruction may be an early or late complication. Surgical intervention as for other forms of small bowel obstruction may be necessary (see p. 412).

ADENOMA OF COLON AND RECTUM*

Adenomas are benign neoplasms. Two major types in the colon and rectum are recognized: simple adenoma and villous adenoma. The former are common and the latter rare. These lesions are not to be confused with familial polyposis of the colon (see p. 446).

Simple adenomas are pedunculated polyps (adenomatous polyps) found in the colon in about 9% of autopsies. Two-thirds are in the rectum and sigmoid; the remainder are scattered elsewhere. These lesions were once thought to be precancerous, but they almost certainly are not. Malignant change is seen occasionally in the superficial cells, but invasion of the basement membrane and base of the polyp is rare.

Villous adenomas are sessile lesions which are usually localized to the rectum or sigmoid and tend to occur at an older age than simple adenomas. They may involve an extensive area of the surface of the mucosa, occasionally extending around the bowel or for 6-10 cm. along its length. The incidence of superficial malignant change and of invasive cancer of the base is higher than in simple adenoma.

Clinical Findings.

Painless, slight rectal bleeding is the commonest symptom, but most adenomas are asymptomatic. Villous adenoma may produce a large quantity of mucus, and frequent mucous diarrhea may be a complaint. Sigmoidoscopy and double contrast barium enema are done on all patients suspected of having a polyp. The colon should always be studied by x-ray when an adenoma is found in the rectum. Before laparotomy for adenoma in the colon, the double contrast barium enema should usually be repeated to verify the original findings. The entire colon can be visualized in most cases by fiberoptic coronoscope, through which biopsy and total removal of polyps can be accomplished.

Treatment.

Adenomas of the colon and rectum should be completely removed and examined microscopically; fragments of the lesion may not be representative. If the lesion is benign or if noninvasive malignancy is present, complete local excision is adequate. Invasive carcinoma (as indicated by involvement of the base of the adenoma) must be treated as outlined for carcinoma (see p. 447).

A. Adenomas Within Reach of the Sigmoidoscope or Colonoscope:

---

*Rare benign neoplasms of the colon and rectum (lipoma, angioma, fibroma, leiomyoma, carcinoid) will not be discussed.

1. Very small adenomas or mucosal excrescences are completely excised with the cold biopsy forceps and the base fulgurated with diathermy.
2. Pedunculated simple adenomas are held under tension with grasping forceps while the base is coagulated with the diathermy. The base is then divided with a diathermy snare or with a biopsy forceps and coagulated.
3. Villous adenomas can be removed with an electric snare or a double-loop diathermy resector. Coagulation and piecemeal removal of small lesions of this type is occasionally justifiable if multiple biopsies with the cold forceps show no evidence of malignancy. When villous adenomas can be delivered through the anus for complete submucosal surgical excision and closure with chromic catgut, this is the preferred method of treatment.

B. Adenomas Above the Reach of the Sigmoidoscope or Colonoscope: All of these lesions require laparotomy after bowel preparation (see p. 440). They are usually excised locally through a colotomy. If cancer is suspected, frozen sections are obtained, but the choice of treatment can usually be based on the gross appearance. Because simple adenomas are frequently multiple, careful palpation of the entire colon at operation is essential. The surgeon may wish also to pass a sterile sigmoidoscope through colotomies for examination of the interior of the bowel.

Follow-up.

Simple adenomas rarely recur, but villous lesions not uncommonly do so because of inadequate local removal. All patients with adenoma within reach of the sigmoidoscope should be followed by endoscopy every 3 months for the first 6 months and every 6-12 months thereafter. Examination with double contrast barium enemas or colonoscope every 12-18 months is advisable after removal of an adenoma of the colon.

FAMILIAL INTESTINAL POLYPOSIS

This is a rare hereditary disease characterized by innumerable adenomatous polyps in the colon and rectum. Patients with this disorder usually develop cancer of the large bowel, sometimes at a very early age. The condition is transmitted as a heterozygous dominant mendelian trait. The following are additional important features: (1) Males and females are affected equally, and both may transmit the disease. (2) It is probable that only those who have inherited polyposis can transmit it. (3) In polyposis families, usually only one-half of the children inherit the disease. (4) The severity of the disease and the tendency to develop cancer of the colon or rectum vary considerably in different families. (5) When polyposis develops early in life, cancer frequently occurs within 10-15 years; whereas when polyposis develops later the precancerous incubation period is longer. All patients with polyposis do not give a family history of the disease, but the danger of malignancy is the same in these sporadic cases.

Clinical Findings.

Diarrhea and bleeding from the bowel are the 2 most common

symptoms. The diagnosis can always be made by sigmoidoscopy and the extent of involvement determined by double contrast barium enema. A negative barium enema, however, does not exclude the presence of multiple small sessile polyps in the colon. A careful family history should always be taken and other members of the family, who may be asymptomatic, advised to have an examination. The only disorder likely to be confused with polyposis is the pseudopolyposis of ulcerative colitis, but the differentiation can usually be made by history, sigmoidoscopy, and biopsy.

Treatment.

Colectomy (with preservation of only the distal 15 cm. of the rectum) and end-to-end ileoproctostomy is the treatment of choice. Residual rectal polyps can be removed by excision and electrocoagulation through the sigmoidoscope. Such patients require lifelong follow-up at intervals of 6 months.

Evidence of carcinoma on biopsy of a rectal polyp is an indication for combined abdominoperineal resection. When a patient cannot be adequately followed, total proctocolectomy and ileostomy should be done initially.

Adenomas in the rectal stump disappear or regress after total colectomy and low ileorectal anastomosis.

CARCINOMA OF COLON AND RECTUM

Carcinoma is the only common malignancy of the colon and rectum. Lymphoma, malignant carcinoid, melanoma, fibrosarcoma, and other types of sarcoma do occur but are very rare. The treatment of all is essentially the same.

Carcinoma of the colon and rectum causes more deaths than any other form of cancer. The only known predisposing causes are familial multiple polyposis, chronic ulcerative colitis, chronic lymphogranuloma venereum, chronic granuloma inguinale, and, probably, schistosomiasis. Males are affected more commonly than females in a ratio of 3:2. The highest incidence is in patients about 50 years of age, but occasional cases have been reported in younger persons and even in children. The anatomic distribution of cancer of the large bowel (based on a study of about 5000 cases) is approximately 16% in the cecum and ascending colon, 5% in the transverse colon, 9% in the descending colon, 20% in the sigmoid, and 50% in the rectum.

One-half to two-thirds of all lesions of the colon and rectum lie within reach of the examining finger or sigmoidoscope and therefore can be biopsied on the first visit.

Clinical Findings.

Symptoms vary depending upon whether the lesion is in the right or the left side of the colon. In either case, a persistent change in the customary bowel habit almost always occurs and should invariably alert the physician to investigate the colon. An acute abdominal emergency may be precipitated by perforation or intussusception. The definitive diagnostic procedures in all cases are sigmoidoscopy and barium enema. Fiberoptic colonoscopy will permit visualization and biopsy of lesions in the proximal colon.

A number of immunologic tests for the detection of gastrointestinal cancer are under investigation. High levels of an antigen, designated as carcinoembryonic antigen, have been found in the serum of certain patients with adenocarcinoma of the colon. Cancer detection and treatment by immunologic methods are important new areas of investigation (LoGerto, P., and others, S. Clin. North America 52:829-837, 1972; Griffen, W. O., Jr., and W. R. Meeker, S. Clin. North America 52:839-846, 1972.)

A. Carcinoma of the Right Colon: Because the fecal stream is fluid and the bowel lumen large in the right half of the colon, symptoms of obstruction occur less frequently than in left-sided tumors. Flatulence is often the only initial complaint. This may progress to cramplike pain, occasionally simulating cholecystitis or appendicitis. Secondary anemia with associated weakness and weight loss is found in half of patients with right colon lesions. The stools are usually positive for occult blood, but rarely show gross blood. The patient is likely to have diarrhea. The first indication of cancer may be the discovery of a palpable mass in the right lower quadrant.

B. Carcinoma of the Left Colon: Obstructive symptoms predominate, particularly increasing constipation. There may be short bouts of diarrhea. Occasionally the first sign is acute colonic obstruction. A small amount of bright red bleeding with bowel movements is common, and anemia is found in about 20% of cases. At times a mass is palpable. About half of cases give a history of weight loss.

Treatment.

The most effective curative treatment in cancer of the large bowel is wide surgical resection of the lesion and its regional lymphatics after adequate bowel preparation (see p. 440) and appropriate supportive measures. When a significant degree of mechanical obstruction is present, a preliminary transverse colostomy or cecostomy may be necessary. Even though the lesion is incurable, palliative resection may be of value to relieve obstruction, bleeding, or the symptoms of local invasion. Superficial and localized cancers of the rectum (Dukes' type A lesions) can be cured by electrocoagulation, an old method being revived for treatment of early rectal cancer and for palliative use in patients who are too debilitated to withstand resection.

Management of the Bladder After Combined Abdominoperineal Resection.

Postoperative urinary retention occurs in one-fourth of abdominoperineal resections and persists longer than 3 months in 10% of cases. Formerly this was regarded as neurogenic, but present opinion holds that mechanical factors are largely responsible. Some degree of prostatism is frequently present, and is aggravated by loss of support of the base of the bladder, vesical neck, and prostatic urethra, so that the physiologic balance is disturbed and the bladder decompensates.

Constant bladder drainage with a Foley catheter is maintained for 7 days after a combined abdominoperineal resection. If by this time the patient is fully ambulatory and convalescence is normal, the catheter is removed in the morning and voiding is attempted.

The amount of residual urine is determined that afternoon or evening. If more than 150 ml. are present, either the catheter is replaced for 48 hours or the patient is catheterized several times at 8-10 hour intervals. Even if voiding seems satisfactory, the patient should be catheterized for residual urine once daily for 2-3 days. If voiding is poor, bethanechol chloride (Urecholine®) may be helpful (see p. 92). In patients whose general condition and convalescence are satisfactory, ineffective conservative treatment should not be prolonged more than 3 weeks. Transurethral resection of the prostate is then done with immediate excellent results in about 90% of patients.

Care of the Colostomy.

The commonest permanent colostomy is the sigmoid colostomy made at the time of combined abdominoperineal resection. Abdominal distention must be avoided postoperatively by gastric tube suction until bowel activity returns. This is essential because tension on the colostomy involves the danger of retraction.

Colostomy irrigation is begun about one week after operation. Each day, a well-lubricated catheter (No. 22 F.) is gently inserted about 15 cm. (6 in.) into the colostomy and 500-1000 ml. of water are instilled from an enema can or bag held 30-60 cm. (1-2 feet) above the colostomy. After the bowel has become accustomed to regular enemas, evacuation will occur within about one-half hour after the irrigation and the enema may usually be given every other day. Some individuals have regular movements without irrigation. A small gauze or disposable tissue pad worn over the colostomy, held in place by a wide elastic belt or ordinary girdle, is usually all the protection required during the day. Irritation of the colostomy stoma is lessened by a light coating of petrolatum before the dressing is applied. Dilatation of the colostomy is unnecessary when colonic mucosa is sutured to the skin in accordance with current technics of operation. Commercial colostomy kits make care simple and convenient.

Three important principles of colostomy management are routine time for bowel evacuation; complete emptying after irrigation; and regulation of diet to avoid diarrhea. The patient with a colostomy can live a normal life.

Stricture, prolapse, and wound hernia are late colostomy complications requiring surgical correction. Skin irritation is less likely to occur than with ileostomy.

Prognosis.

Over 90% of patients with carcinoma of the colon and rectum are suitable for either curative or palliative resection, with an operative mortality of 3-6%. The over-all five-year survival rate after resection is about 50%. If the lesion is confined to the bowel and there is no evidence of lymphatic or blood vessel invasion, the five-year survival rate is 60-70%. When the lesion is discovered on careful periodic examination before onset of symptoms, the five-year survival rate in rectal carcinoma is about 90% after resection. Local recurrence of carcinoma in the anastomotic suture line or wound area occurs in 10-15% of cases. The incidence of local recurrence can be decreased if special precautions are taken at operation to avoid implantation of malignant cells. About 5% of patients develop multiple primary colon cancers. Early identification of resectable local recurrence or a new neoplasm depends upon careful follow-up with sigmoidoscopy and barium enema every 6 months for 2 years and yearly thereafter.

RECTAL PROLAPSE

Partial or incomplete rectal prolapse consists of eversion of the rectal mucosa. It can be differentiated from hemorrhoids by the fact that the ridges of mucosa are arranged concentrically instead of radially, as is characteristic of hemorrhoidal prolapse. In complete prolapse, all layers of the rectal wall are involved and a considerable segment of bowel may be everted through the relaxed anal canal. Concealed prolapse consists of an intussusception of the rectum within the rectum and without protrusion through the anus.

Prolapse occurs most commonly in young children or in persons past middle age. Many patients are old and debilitated. The underlying cause is a weakness in the supporting structures. The diagnosis is usually obvious. In suspected concealed prolapse, it is advisable to do a rectal examination with the patient standing because the intussusception may be reduced in the horizontal position.

Conservative treatment is often successful in young children. The patient should lie down to defecate, and the buttocks should be firmly strapped together at other times. Partial prolapse in older patients may respond to multiple submucosal injections of quinine and urea hydrochloride (5% solution); this should be attempted only by one experienced with the method. If this fails, the partial prolapse may be amputated by the Buie technic.

More than 50 operations have been devised for complete rectal prolapse and the recurrence rate is variously reported to be from 5-35%, indicating that successful treatment is difficult. Repair may be carried out by the abdominal or by the perineal approach. The abdominal operation consists of freeing the rectum from the hollow of the sacrum, suturing it high to supporting structures to obliterate the cul-de-sac, and resectioning redundant bowel. The perineal procedure is probably preferable because it can be performed on elderly and debilitated patients with relatively less risk. It consists of amputation of redundant rectosigmoid, obliteration of the sliding hernial sac, and reconstruction of the perineal floor from the perineal approach (Altemeier and others, Arch. Surg. 89:6, 1964).

AMEBIASIS OF THE COLON

Amebiasis of the colon is of surgical significance chiefly because it sometimes mimics other conditions. Fulminating amebic colitis may resemble ulcerative colitis and may result in perforation (usually of the cecum) or hemorrhage. Amebic granuloma or "ameboma" is a complication of chronic amebiasis and involves any part of the colon, but particularly the cecum or rectum. Differentiation from carcinoma may be difficult.

The diagnosis is established by sigmoidoscopic and stool examinations. Acute amebiasis is usually associated with superficial ragged ulcerations in the upper rectum within reach of the sigmoidoscope. Motile amebas are found on fresh smears from these ulcers. In chronic intestinal amebiasis, amebic cysts are present in the stools but may be difficult to find.

Treatment is with antiamebic drugs. Surgical measures may rarely be required in the management of complications.

STAPHYLOCOCCAL ENTEROCOLITIS

Staphylococcus aureus enterocolitis is a complication most commonly encountered in patients receiving broad-spectrum antibiotics. Systemic treatment with a combination of penicillin and one of the tetracyclines and colonic preparation with neomycin appear to be the 2 regimens most frequently associated with the development of enterocolitis.

The clinical picture usually consists of diarrhea, fever, and leukocytosis in a patient receiving broad-spectrum antibiotic therapy. Abdominal pain, nausea, vomiting, and bloody stools occur occasionally. Shock and overwhelming sepsis are rare but dangerous possibilities. Elderly or debilitated patients and those who have had gastrointestinal operations seem to be particularly susceptible.

The diagnosis is made on the basis of the clinical findings and the identification of staphylococci on direct smear and of Staphylococcus aureus on culture of the stools. These examinations should be done as soon as the condition is suspected, and the organism should be tested for antibiotic sensitivity. Sigmoidoscopy should be performed to visualize the friable, sticky pseudomembrane which forms on the bowel wall and to obtain stool for Gram stained smears, which will show a profuse increase of gram-positive cocci. Antibiotic and other therapy should be started without awaiting cultures in fulminating cases.

Treatment consists of symptomatic measures to stop diarrhea, control of electrolyte imbalance, and antishock therapy. The offending antibiotics must be discontinued. Pending completion of of sensitivity studies on cultures, specific antistaphylococcal therapy is given. If the patient is not vomiting and does not have ileus, excellent results can be obtained with oral administration of either vancomycin (0.5 Gm. every 4 hours) or oxacillin (1 Gm. every 6 hours). Vancomycin is not available for oral administration, but the intravenous preparation can be given by mouth. For parenteral administration, the drug of choice is oxacillin or methicillin, 4-6 Gm. daily in divided doses. In patients with penicillin sensitivity, give either vancomycin, 0.5 Gm. every 6 hours I.V., or cephalothin, 4-6 Gm. I.M. daily.

Recovery is usually prompt, but staphylococcal enterocolitis is potentially very serious and deaths may occur when a fulminating infection complicates the course of other serious disease.

DISEASES OF THE ANAL CANAL

HEMORRHOIDS

Internal hemorrhoids are varices of that portion of the venous hemorrhoidal plexus which lies submucosally just proximal to the dentate margin. External hemorrhoids arise from the same plexus but are located subcutaneously immediately distal to the dentate margin. There are 3 primary internal hemorrhoidal masses: right anterior, right posterior, and left lateral. Three to 5 secondary hemorrhoids may be present between the 3 primaries. Portal obstruction and pregnancy are important specific causes of hemorrhoids, but in most cases the etiology is obscure. Straining at stool, constipation, prolonged sitting, and anal infection are contributing factors and may precipitate complications such as thrombosis. Diagnosis is suspected on the history of protrusion, anal pain, or bleeding and confirmed by proctologic examination.

Carcinoma of the colon or rectum not infrequently aggravates hemorrhoids or produces similar complaints. Polyps may present as a cause of bleeding which is wrongly attributed to hemorrhoids (see p. 446). For these reasons the treatment of hemorrhoids is always preceded by sigmoidoscopy and, when there are suspicious bowel symptoms or the patient is over 40, by barium enema. When portal hypertension is suspected as an etiologic factor, investigations for liver disease should be carried out. Hemorrhoids which develop during pregnancy or parturition tend to subside thereafter and should be treated conservatively unless persistent after delivery.

The symptoms of hemorrhoids are usually mild and remittent, but a number of disturbing complications may develop and call for active medical or surgical treatment. These complications include pruritus, leakage of mucus, recurrent protrusion requiring manual replacement by the patient, fissure, infection, or ulceration, prolapse and strangulation, and secondary anemia due to chronic blood loss. Carcinoma has been reported to develop very rarely in hemorrhoids.

Conservative treatment suffices in most instances of mild hemorrhoids, which may improve spontaneously or in response to low-roughage diet and regulation of the bowel habits with mineral oil or other nonirritating laxatives to produce soft stools (see p. 837). Local pain and infection are managed with warm sitz baths and insertion of a soothing anal suppository such as Anusol® 2 or 3 times daily. Ethyl aminobenzoate (benzocaine) and similar types of anal ointments should be avoided so as not to sensitize the patient to these agents.

Prolapsed, strangulated internal hemorrhoids should generally be treated by immediate hemorrhoidectomy. Attempts to reduce the edematous, necrotizing masses of hemorrhoidal tissue are usually unsuccessful. If surgery is not possible for some reason, the condition can be treated by bed rest with the foot of the bed elevated, hot sitz baths, sedatives, and antibiotics if needed for local sepsis. Pain and swelling will gradually subside over 5-6 days, but it may be 2 weeks before the anal area is comfortable. Hemorrhoidectomy is required later in most cases.

For severe symptoms or complications, complete internal and external hemorrhoidectomy is advisable and is a highly satisfactory procedure when properly done. Excision of a single external hemorrhoid, evacuation of a thrombosed pile, and the injection treatment of internal hemorrhoids fall within the scope of office practice.

Evacuation of Thrombosed External Hemorrhoid.

This condition is caused by the rupture of a vein at the anal margin, forming a clot in the subcutaneous tissue. The patient complains of a painful lump, and examination shows a tense, tender, bluish mass covered with skin. If seen after 24-48 hours when the pain is subsiding - or if symptoms are minimal - hot sitz baths are prescribed. If discomfort is marked, removal of the clot is indicated. With the patient in the lateral position, the area is prepared with antiseptic and 1% procaine or lidocaine is injected intracutaneously around and over the lump. A radial ellipse of skin is then excised and the clot evacuated. A dry gauze dressing is held in place for 12-24 hours by taping the buttocks together, and daily sitz baths are then begun.

Injection Treatment of Internal Hemorrhoids.

This method is most suitable for small internal hemorrhoids which bleed or for palliation of large hemorrhoids in patients who are unable to undergo operation. Injection therapy should never be used on external hemorrhoids or in the presence of infection. Quinine and urea hydrochloride (5% solution) or sodium morrhuate (5% solution) may be used as the sclerosing agent.

Technic: With the patient in the left lateral position the internal hemorrhoid is visualized with the anoscope. A few drops of sclerosing solution are injected through a No. 20 gauge needle into the center of each internal hemorrhoid under direct vision. Care is taken to make the injection above the mucocutaneous line, as injection or seepage of the solution beneath the skin causes severe pain. If the injection is made too superficially, the mucosa will blanch and necrosis may follow. Each internal hemorrhoid is treated at each visit; a total dose of 1 ml. is rarely exceeded on any single occasion.

The actual injection is practically painless, although mild pain may begin in about 30 minutes and last for an hour or so; this can be relieved by heat or lying down. Symptoms are often relieved by the first treatment, but maximum benefit will often require 5-6 treatments at intervals of 1-2 weeks. Bleeding can be controlled in 90% of cases, and protrusion is relieved in over half. Complications are minimal if the proper technic is used, and drug reactions are rare. Some induration can often be felt in the hemorrhoid for a few days after treatment; further injections should be delayed until this has subsided, or the injection site may slough.

CRYPTITIS AND PAPILLITIS

Anal pain and burning of brief duration with defecation is suggestive of cryptitis and papillitis. Digital and anoscopic examination reveals hypertrophied papillae and indurated or inflamed crypts. Treatment consists of mineral oil by mouth; hot sitz baths; anorectal ointment or suppository (Anusol®) after each bowel movement; and local application of 5% phenol in oil or carbolfuchsin compound to the crypts. If these measures fail, surgical excision of involved crypts and papillae should be considered.

FISSURE-IN-ANO

Acute fissures represent recent breaks in the anal lining caused

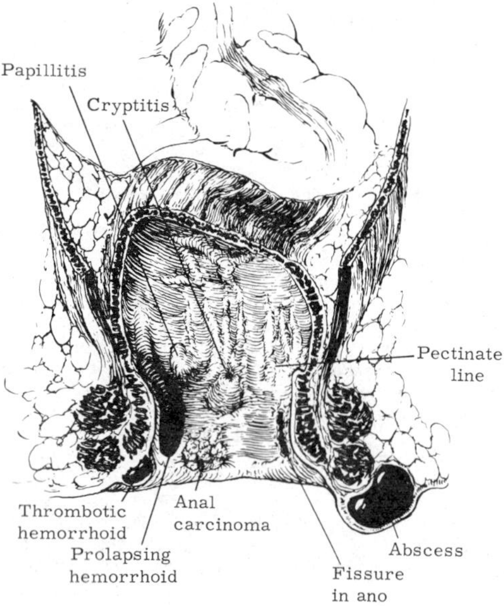

Common Lesions of the Anal Canal

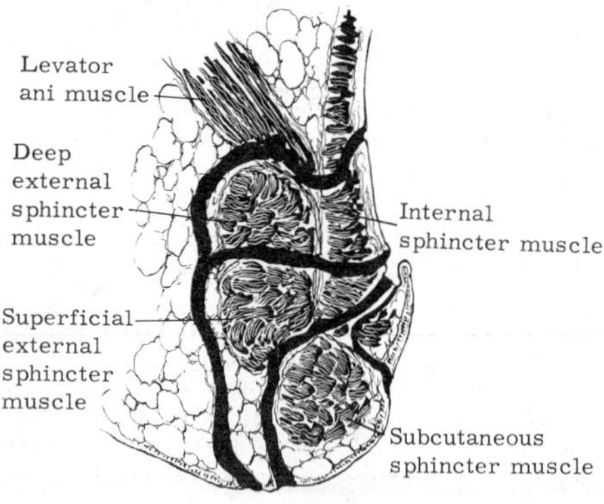

Cross-section of Muscles of Anal Wall Showing Usual Paths of Anal Fistulas

by the trauma of bowel movements. They usually clear if bowel movements are kept regular and soft (e.g., with mineral oil). The local application of 1% gentian violet solution or a mild styptic such as 1-2% silver nitrate may be of value.

Chronic fissure is characterized by (1) acute pain during and after defecation; (2) spotting of bright red blood at stool with occasional more abundant bleeding; (3) tendency to constipation through fear of pain; and (4) the late occurrence of a sentinel pile, hypertrophied papilla, and spasm of the anal canal (usually very painful on digital examination). Regulation of bowel habits with mineral oil or other stool softeners, sitz baths, and anal suppositories (e.g., Anusol®), twice daily, should be tried.

If conservative measures fail, the stretching of the sphincter up to 4 fingers under general anesthesia should be done as an outpatient procedure. Recurrences after this are probably 15-20%, but the morbidity is minimal. If the sphincter-stretching operation fails, or as a primary procedure, the fissure may be excised along with the sentinel pile and hypertrophied papilla and the sphincters stretched and partially incised. Postoperative care is along the lines of preoperative treatment.

ANAL ABSCESS

A perianal abscess should be considered the acute stage of an anal fistula until proved otherwise. The abscess should be adequately drained as soon as it has localized. Hot sitz baths may hasten the process of localization. The patient should be warned that after drainage of the abscess he may have a persistent fistula. It is painful and fruitless to search for the internal opening of a fistula in the presence of acute infection. If the systemic reaction is marked, broad-spectrum antibiotics may be indicated.

FISTULA IN ANO

About 95% of all anal fistulas arise in an anal crypt and they are often preceded by an anal abscess. If an anal fistula enters the rectum above the pectinate line and there is no associated disease in the crypts, ulcerative colitis, rectal tuberculosis, lymphogranuloma venereum, cancer, or foreign body should be considered in the differential diagnosis.

Anal fistula is associated with the chronic purulent discharge from the fistulous opening on the skin near the anus. There is usually local itching, tenderness, or pain aggravated by bowel movements. Recurrent anal abscesses may develop. The involved crypt can occasionally be located anoscopically with a crypt hook. Probing the fistula should be gentle because false passages can be made with ease, and in any case demonstration of the internal opening by probing is not essential to the diagnosis.

Treatment is by surgical incision or excision of the fistula under general anesthesia. If a fistula passes deep to the entire anorectal ring so that all the muscles must be divided in order to extirpate the tract, a 2-stage operation must be done to prevent incontinence.

PRURITUS ANI

Among the common causes of anal itching are intertrigo, discharges from fistulas, folliculitis, fungal infection, including the common tinea cruris and monilial dermatitis (secondary to administration of broad-spectrum antibiotics); drug eruption, contact dermatitis from local applications, primary dermatosis such as psoriasis or seborrheic dermatitis; parasitic infestation such as pediculosis pubis, scabies, and enterobiasis (pinworms); and psychogenic causes.

Treatment should be specific whenever possible, but symptomatic therapy is usually necessary. Sensitizing agents (e.g., anesthetics and antihistamines) should be avoided. When the skin is hot and inflamed, ice-cold normal saline dressings and calamine liniment are applied. If there is only mild skin inflammation, simple calamine lotion with 0.25-0.5% menthol and 0.5-1% phenol may be used; or a bland application such as hydrophilic ointment with 0.25-0.5% menthol and 0.5-1% phenol. Hydrocortisone ointment is often very effective. In severe cases (rare), oral or parenteral cortisone therapy may be indicated. Sedatives and soporifics may be required. Local cleanliness, talc applications to promote dryness, and avoidance of sweating and chafing are helpful. Do not use x-ray therapy or local injections of anesthetic agents. The only indications for surgical treatment are local lesions such as hemorrhoids, fistulas, and fissures which may be contributing to the pruritus.

ANAL CONDYLOMAS

These wart-like papillomas of the perianal skin and anal canal flourish on moist, macerated surfaces, particularly in the presence of purulent discharge. They are not true tumors but are infectious and auto-inoculable, probably due to a virus. They must be distinguished from condyloma lata caused by syphilis. The diagnosis of the latter rests on the positive serologic test for syphilis or the discovery of Treponema pallidum on dark-field examination.

Treatment consists of careful application of 25% podophyllin in tincture of benzoin to the lesion (with bare wooden or cotton-tipped applicator sticks to avoid contact with uninvolved skin). Condylomas in the anal canal are treated through the anoscope and the painted site dusted with powder to localize the application and minimize discomfort. Electrofulguration under local anesthesia is useful if there are numerous lesions. Local cleanliness and the frequent use of a talc dusting powder are essential.

Condylomas tend to recur. The patient should be observed for several months and advised to report promptly if new lesions appear.

BENIGN ANORECTAL STRICTURES

Congenital.

Anal contracture or stenosis in infancy may result from failure of disintegration of the anal plate in fetal life. The narrowing is treated by careful repeated dilatation, inserting progressively larger Hegar dilators until the anus admits first the little and then the index finger.

Traumatic.

Acquired stenosis is usually the result of surgery or trauma which denudes the epithelium of the anal canal. Hemorrhoid operations in which too much skin is removed or which are followed by infection are the commonest cause. Constipation, ribbon stools, and pain on defecation are the most frequent complaints. Stenosis predisposes to fissure, low-grade infection, and occasionally fistula.

Prevention of stenosis after radical anal surgery is best accomplished by local cleanliness, hot sitz baths, and gentle insertion of the well-lubricated finger twice weekly for 2-3 weeks beginning 2 weeks after surgery. When stenosis is chronic but mild, graduated anal dilators of increasing size may be inserted daily by the patient. For marked stenosis a plastic operation on the anal canal is advisable.

Inflammatory.

A. Lymphogranuloma Venereum: This disease is the commonest cause of inflammatory stricture of the anorectal region. Acute proctitis due to lymphatic spread of the organism occurs early, and may be followed by perirectal infections, sinuses, and formation of scar tissue (resulting in stricture). Frei and complement fixation tests are positive.

The tetracycline drugs are curative in the initial phase of the disease. When extensive chronic secondary infection is present or when a stricture has formed, repeated biopsies are essential because epidermoid carcinoma develops in about 4% of strictures. Local operation on a stricture may be feasible, but a colostomy or an abdominoperineal resection is often required.

B. Granuloma Inguinale: This disease may cause anorectal fistulas, infections, and strictures. The Donovan body is best identified in tissue biopsy when there is rectal involvement. Epidermoid carcinoma develops in about 4% of cases with chronic anorectal granuloma.

The early lesions respond to tetracyclines. Destructive or constricting processes may require colostomy or resection.

ANAL INCONTINENCE

Obstetric tears, anorectal operations (particularly fistulotomy), and neurologic disturbances are the most frequent causes of anal incontinence. When incontinence is due to surgery or trauma, surgical repair of the divided or torn sphincter is indicated. Repair of anterior laceration due to childbirth should be delayed for 6 months or more after parturition.

SQUAMOUS CELL CARCINOMA OF THE ANUS

These tumors are relatively rare, comprising only 1-2% of all malignancies of the anus and large intestine. Bleeding, pain, and local tumor are the commonest symptoms. Because the lesion is often confused with hemorrhoids or other common anal disorders, immediate biopsy of any suspicious mass or ulceration in the anal area is an essential diagnostic precaution. These tumors tend to become annular, invade the sphincter, and spread upward into the rectum.

Except for very small lesions (which can be adequately excised locally), treatment is by combined abdominoperineal resection. Radiation therapy is reserved for palliation and for patients who refuse or cannot withstand operation. Metastases to the inguinal nodes are treated by radical groin dissection when clinically evident. The five-year survival rate after resection is about 50%.

DISEASES OF THE BILIARY SYSTEM AND LIVER

CHOLELITHIASIS

The high incidence of gallstones in the general population accounts for the clinical frequency of cholecystitis. Autopsy studies show that 32% of women and 16% of men past the age of 40 have gallstones. The incidence of calculi rises sharply at around 40 years of age. Pregnancy is an important predisposing cause of gallstones, and obesity may also be a contributing factor; hence the description of the typical gallbladder patient as ''female, fat, and forty.''

Gallstones usually consist of cholesterol, calcium bilirubinate, calcium carbonate, or a mixture of these. About 90% of the stones associated with chronic cholecystitis are of the mixed variety, whereas the preceding 3 types of ''pure'' calculi may be seen in a relatively normal gallbladder. Calcium bilirubinate stones tend to occur, sometimes at an early age, in such diseases as congenital hemolytic anemia and sickle cell anemia as a result of increased bilirubin in the bile.

Infection plays an important role in both cholelithiasis and cholecystitis. Chronic, low-grade bacterial involvement of the gallbladder produces cellular debris on which the various salts precipitate in the early stages of mixed stone formation. When mechanical obstruction of the cystic duct occurs, invasive infection of the distended gallbladder is common. Bacteria of intestinal origin (streptococci, coliform bacteria, and staphylococci) can be cultured from about half of calculous gallbladders removed at operation.

Gallstones are asymptomatic in two-thirds of cases, being discovered incidentally at operation or autopsy or on x-ray films. The management of asymptomatic gallstones is controversial, but most surgeons advise prophylactic removal of the gallbladder if the patient is a good surgical risk. This opinion is based on the fact that at least one-third to one-half of these patients subsequently develop severe symptoms or complications such as acute cholecystitis or common duct stone. The chance of developing cancer of the gallbladder in the presence of cholelithiasis is less than 1%.

ACUTE CHOLECYSTITIS

Cholecystitis is associated with gallstones in over 90% of cases.

Acute cholecystitis is usually superimposed on a chronic process and is precipitated by obstruction of the cystic duct by a stone (or, rarely, by edema in the absence of calculi). There is rapid development of a tense, edematous, inflamed gallbladder. Infection often follows as a result of invasion by resident organisms.

Clinical Findings.

A. Symptoms and Signs: A past history suggestive of chronic cholecystitis (see p. 460) can often be obtained. The acute attack is frequently precipitated by a heavy meal and begins with right upper quadrant pain which usually radiates to the right infrascapular region. Pain is agonizingly severe, prostrating, and associated with vomiting.

Right upper quadrant tenderness is invariably present, and in most cases is associated with local muscle spasm and rebound tenderness. The tensely distended gallbladder is frequently palpable. Minimal jaundice is occasionally present in the absence of common duct obstruction. Marked jaundice indicates choledocholithiasis or liver damage.

Low-grade or moderate fever is present.

B. Laboratory Findings: Moderate leukocytosis (10,000-20,000 WBC) is typical. Serum bilirubin levels of 1-4 mg./100 ml. (and occasionally higher) may be seen in the absence of common duct obstruction; clinical jaundice appears when the bilirubin exceeds 2.5 mg./100 ml. Serum alkaline phosphatase may be moderately elevated in acute cholecystitis in the absence of common duct stone. In general, however, elevation of bilirubin and alkaline phosphatase are highly suggestive of common duct stone. Slight elevation of the serum amylase may rarely be noted.

C. X-ray Findings: Gallstones are found on plain abdominal x-rays in about 25% of cases of acute cholecystitis. Intravenous cholecystography may be a useful emergency diagnostic procedure. If the gallbladder fills, acute cholecystitis is ruled out.

Differential Diagnosis.

The disorders most likely to be confused with acute cholecystitis are perforated peptic ulcer (see p. 429), acute pancreatitis (see p. 477), appendicitis in a high-lying appendix (see p. 418), perforated carcinoma or diverticulum of the hepatic flexure, liver abscess, liver congestion, acute viral hepatitis, and pneumonia with pleurisy on the right side. The diagnosis of uncomplicated acute cholecystitis is usually not difficult because of the definite localization of pain and tenderness in the right upper quadrant and the characteristic right infrascapular radiation.

Complications.

The following complications of acute cholecystitis are more likely to occur in diabetics and in patients over 50 with a long history of biliary tract disease. Common duct stones are also more frequent in the latter group.

A. Gangrene of the Gallbladder: Continued marked or progressive right upper quadrant pain, tenderness, muscle spasm, fever, and leukocytosis after 24-48 hours are suggestive of severe inflammation and possible gangrene of the gallbladder. Necrosis may occasionally develop without definite signs, especially in the obese abdomen.

Minor perforations of the gallbladder are frequently walled off by omentum, with or without the development of a localized abscess. Perforation into the free peritoneal cavity results in bile peritonitis which may be associated with shock and rapid deterioration of the patient's condition. Rarely, considerable sterile bile may accumulate intraperitoneally without marked signs. The incidence of perforation of the gallbladder is about 8%.

B. Cholangitis: Intermittent high fever and chills are the major signs. Common duct stone may be a contributing cause.

Treatment.

Acute cholecystitis will subside on a conservative regimen in the majority of cases. Cholecystectomy can then be scheduled 6 weeks to 3 months later when the patient's general condition is optimal and the technical difficulties of operation minimized. If, as occasionally happens, recurrent acute symptoms develop during this waiting period, cholecystectomy is indicated without further delay. When a program of conservative therapy is elected for acute cholecystitis, all patients (particularly the diabetic, the obese, and the elderly) must be watched carefully for signs of gangrene of the gallbladder.

Operation for acute cholecystitis is mandatory when there is evidence suggestive of gangrene or perforation. Operation during the acute stage is also justified as a means of reducing over-all morbidity in good risk patients in whom the diagnosis is unequivocal. It is best to defer operation, if possible, in the presence of acute pancreatitis or common duct stone.

A. Conservative Treatment: During the acute period while the patient is being evaluated, the abdominal examination and WBC should be repeated several times daily. The principles of treatment are the same as in acute peritonitis (see p. 403), with the addition of an anticholinergic drug such as parenteral atropine or oral belladonna. Meperidine (Demerol®) is the analgesic of choice, since morphine produces spasm of the sphincter of Oddi. Antibiotics are administered in all except mild, rapidly subsiding cases.

B. Surgical Treatment: When surgery is elected for acute cholecystitis, cholecystectomy is the operation of choice with an operative mortality of about 1% in experienced hands. The common duct should also be explored if indicated (see p. 464). In the poor risk patient or when technical difficulties with cholecystectomy arise, cholecystostomy is the safest procedure.

CHRONIC CHOLECYSTITIS

Clinical Findings.

A. Symptoms and Signs: When significant complaints occur they fall into 2 general categories: (1) chronic dyspepsia with belching, flatulence, nausea, and other nondescript forms of indigestion, usually aggravated by fatty foods and heavy meals;

and (2) recurrent "biliary colic" characterized by attacks of right upper quadrant pain radiating to the right infrascapular region, lasting a few minutes or hours, occasionally accompanied by vomiting, and often precipitated by dietary indiscretion.

There are no specific physical findings except for transient, mild right upper quadrant tenderness during attacks of biliary colic. If hydrops of the gallbladder is present (rare), the tense, nontender organ can usually be palpated with ease.

B. Laboratory Findings: None are diagnostic. Serum bilirubin and liver function tests should be done, especially if common duct stone or liver disease is suspected.

C. X-ray Findings: Oral cholecystography is the most important diagnostic procedure. The presence of gallstones on plain films or cholecystography is presumptive evidence of cholecystitis. When there is simply nonfilling of the gallbladder, cholecystography is repeated with a double dose of the test medium. Alternatively, an intravenous cholecystogram can be ordered, particularly if common duct stone is suspected. If the gallbladder fails to visualize on the second examination, it is probably diseased. Cholecystography is unreliable when there is significant liver dysfunction (BSP retention greater than 20%), common duct obstruction (serum bilirubin above 5%), malabsorption of the test material, or in the presence of an acute abdomen from any cause.

The noncalculous gallbladder which fills poorly and empties sluggishly is not a surgical problem, but because small stones may be easily overlooked in such cases, cholecystography should be repeated if symptoms are especially suggestive of gallbladder disease. Sensitivity to iodine is the only contraindication to cholecystography.

Differential Diagnosis.

If there are attacks of typical biliary colic and x-ray evidence of cholelithiasis or a nonfunctioning gallbladder, the diagnosis is not difficult. When nonspecific dyspeptic symptoms are the chief complaint of the patient, it is necessary to consider other gastrointestinal conditions. Among these are nervous dyspepsia, peptic ulcer, gastritis, chronic pancreatitis, and carcinoma of the stomach, pancreas, hepatic flexure, liver, or gallbladder. It is a good rule to obtain an upper gastrointestinal barium study on patients with suspected gallbladder disease because of the frequent coexistence of other pathology (especially peptic ulcer).

Complications.

The complications of chronic cholecystitis with cholelithiasis include acute cholecystitis, common duct stone, cholecystenteric fistula, pancreatitis, and carcinoma of the gallbladder.

Treatment.

A. Medical Measures: Symptomatic treatment of chronic cholecystitis is indicated when operation is contraindicated or refused. This consists of a low-fat diet (with avoidance of all foods discovered to cause distress), an anticholinergic agent such as tincture of belladonna, and a bile acid preparation such as dehydrocholic acid (Decholin®), 0.5 Gm. ($7\frac{1}{2}$ gr.) 3 times daily after meals.

B. Surgical Treatment: The most satisfactory treatment for symptomatic, calculous cholecystitis is removal of the gallbladder. Choledochostomy may also be indicated.

Postoperative Complications of Cholecystectomy.

The incidence of postoperative complications is about 8%. Most of the complications are common to other major abdominal operations. The following are peculiar to gallbladder surgery:

A. Bile Drainage: A Penrose (rubber tissue) drain is customarily placed in the subhepatic space near the foramen of Winslow and brought out through a stab wound at operation. This drain is usually shortened on the fourth to sixth days and removed on the seventh day. Persistent drainage of bile along the drain indicates interruption of an accessory bile duct, leakage of the cystic duct stump, or damage to the common duct, and the drain is removed more slowly. If the stools are at the same time acholic, common duct obstruction by ligature or calculus must be suspected and early exploration considered. Signs of peritoneal irritation associated with excessive bile drainage indicate bile peritonitis requiring immediate laparotomy to stop the leak or improve drainage. In the absence of peritonitis or common duct injury or obstruction, a biliary fistula will tend to close and may be treated expectantly.

B. Jaundice: Jaundice which develops in the immediate postoperative period suggests common duct injury, retained common duct stone, or hepatic failure. Injured ducts should usually be repaired at once if the diagnosis can be made and technical skills are adequate for this difficult task. Otherwise, delayed repair is safer. Retained stones, if small, will sometimes pass on the biliary flush routine (see p. 466). In partial obstruction, intravenous cholangiography will delineate the ducts.

C. "Postcholecystectomy Syndrome": This vague but widely used term is used to denote that situation in which the patient continues to have symptoms of chronic biliary tract disease after cholecystectomy. The cause may be common duct stone, a long remnant of cystic duct, chronic pancreatitis, or stenosis of the sphincter of Oddi. Functional or organic gastrointestinal disturbance existing preoperatively - and for which the gallbladder was mistakenly removed - should be suspected. The patient whose gallbladder was removed for noncalculous chronic cholecystitis is a likely candidate for this "syndrome." Treatment depends on etiology. If none is found, a medical program as for chronic cholecystitis can be tried (see p. 460).

Prognosis.

The over-all mortality following cholecystectomy is less than 1%. However, biliary tract surgery is more complicated and hazardous in elderly patients; in patients over 70, cholecystectomy probably has a mortality of 5-10%.

Following a properly performed operation, the patient usually is asymptomatic and requires no special diet or regimen.

CHOLEDOCHOLITHIASIS

About 10% of patients with gallstones have choledocholithiasis.

The percentage rises with age, and the incidence in elderly people may be as high as 50%. Common duct stones usually originate in the gallbladder but may also form in the common duct. The stones are frequently "silent," as no symptoms result unless there is some obstruction.

Clinical Findings.

A. Symptoms and Signs: A history suggestive of chronic cholecystitis can usually be obtained. The additional features which suggest the presence of a common duct stone are (1) frequently recurring attacks of biliary colic, (2) chills and fever associated with the attacks of colic, and (3) a history of jaundice. Jaundice, which may be transient, is usually first noted within 1-2 days after an attack of colic. Occasionally there is no pain associated with the jaundice.

The presence of jaundice is strong evidence for common duct stone in a patient with a history of chronic gallbladder disease. Epigastric tenderness may occur during attacks of colic. Otherwise there are no specific abdominal signs.

B. Laboratory Findings: Liver function tests should be performed in all cases (see p. 468). Bilirubinuria and elevation of serum bilirubin are present if the common duct is obstructed. Elevation of the serum alkaline phosphatase is especially suggestive of obstructive jaundice. Because BSP retention is increased by duct obstruction, this test does not evaluate hepatocellular function under these circumstances. Prolongation of the prothrombin time begins to occur when bile is excluded for more than a few days from the gastrointestinal tract. When marked obstructive jaundice persists for several weeks, liver damage occurs and differentiation of obstructive from hepatocellular jaundice becomes progressively more difficult.

C. X-ray Findings: In the absence of significant jaundice, intravenous cholangiography will usually visualize the common duct. When jaundice is marked, plain abdominal x-rays are studied for biliary calculi.

D. Cholangiography: Percutaneous transhepatic cholangiography is occasionally useful in distinguishing common duct obstruction from hepatocellular disease in the jaundiced patient. The procedure should be performed only when the blood clotting mechanism is normal and - if an obstructed biliary system is found - should be followed by immediate laparotomy because of the risk of bile peritonitis due to leakage from the puncture site. Fiberoptic duodenoscopy with cannulation of the common duct under direct vision is a promising technic for obtaining a cholangiogram in difficult diagnostic problems of jaundice.

Differential Diagnosis.

The commonest cause of obstructive jaundice is common duct stone. Next in frequency is carcinoma of the pancreas, ampulla of Vater, or common duct. Metastatic carcinoma (usually from the gastrointestinal tract) and direct extension of gallbladder cancer are other important causes of obstructive jaundice. Hepatocellular jaundice can usually be differentiated by history, clinical findings, and liver function tests.

Complications.

A. Biliary Cirrhosis: Prolonged common duct obstruction causes severe liver damage; hepatic failure or portal hypertension may be the ultimate result in untreated cases.

B. Cholangitis: The incidence of bacteria in common duct bile is 75% when calculi are present; the organisms most frequently cultured are Escherichia coli, Enterobacter aerogenes, Streptococcus faecalis, and Proteus vulgaris. Ascending infection is frequent in common duct stone, adds to liver damage, and may rarely lead to multiple liver abscesses.

C. Hypoprothrombinemia: Patients with obstructive jaundice or liver disease may bleed excessively at operation as a result of hypoprothrombinemia. If the prothrombin deficiency is due to faulty vitamin K absorption, the following preparations are of value: (Parenteral administration is preferred to ensure complete absorption.)

1. I.V. or subcut. - Give one of the following:
   a. Phytonadione (Mephyton®), 10 mg. (1/6 gr.) daily, is the drug of choice.
   b. Menadione sodium bisulfite (Hykinone®), 10 mg. (1/6 gr.) daily, may be used if phytonadione is not available.
2. Orally - Give one of the following:
   a. Menadiol sodium diphosphate (Synkayvite®), 5 mg. b.i.d., is the preferred oral agent. It is water-soluble and is absorbed from the intestinal tract in the absence of bile.
   b. Menadione, 5 mg. (1/12 gr.) b.i.d., p.c. If there is obstructive jaundice, supplementary bile salts such as ox-bile extract capsules or tablets must be given concomitantly. The dosage of ox-bile extract is 300 mg. per 1 mg. of menadione.

Treatment.

Common duct stone is treated by cholecystectomy and choledochostomy.

A. Preoperative Care: Emergency operation is rarely necessary; a few days devoted to careful evaluation are well spent.

1. Liver function should be evaluated thoroughly (see p. 468).
2. Prothrombin time should be restored to normal by parenteral administration of vitamin K preparations (see above).
3. Diet should be advanced as tolerated. A low-fat diet is best tolerated. High-carbohydrate, high-protein intake is desirable when possible.
4. Vitamin supplements should be given (see p. 132).
5. Cholangitis, if present, should be controlled with antibiotics.

B. Indications for Common Duct Exploration: At every operation for cholelithiasis the advisability of exploring the common duct must be considered. Operative cholangiography via the cystic duct is a very useful procedure for demonstrating common duct stone. Any of the following evidences of common duct stone may be an indication for choledochostomy:

1. Preoperative findings suggestive of choledocholithiasis include history or presence of obstructive jaundice; frequent attacks of biliary colic; cholangitis; history of pancreatitis; and an intravenous cholangiogram showing stone, obstruction, or dilatation of the duct.

2. Operative findings suggestive of choledocholithiasis are palpable stones in the common duct; dilated or thick-walled common duct; gallbladder stones small enough to pass through the cystic duct; and pancreatitis.

C. Postoperative Care:
1. Antibiotics - Postoperative antibiotics are not administered routinely after biliary tract surgery. Cultures of the bile are always taken at operation. If biliary tract infection was present preoperatively or is apparent at operation, an empirically chosen antibiotic is administered postoperatively until sensitivity tests on culture specimens are available.
2. Management of the T-tube - Following choledochostomy a simple catheter or T-tube is placed in the common duct for decompression. It must be attached securely to the skin or dressing because inadvertent removal of the tube may be disastrous. A properly placed tube should drain bile at the operating table and continuously thereafter; otherwise it is blocked or dislocated. The volume of bile drainage varies from 100-1000 ml. daily (avg., 200-400 ml.). Above-average drainage may be due to obstruction at the ampulla (usually edema), increased bile output, low resistance or siphonage effect in the drainage system, or a combination of these.
3. Cholangiography - A cholangiogram through the T-tube should be done on about the seventh or eighth postoperative day. Under fluoroscopic control, a radiopaque medium is aseptically and gently injected until the duct system is outlined and the medium begins to enter the duodenum. The injection of air bubbles must be avoided since on x-ray they resemble stones in the duct system. Spot films are taken. If the cholangiogram shows no stones in the common duct and the opaque medium flows freely into the duodenum, clamp the tube overnight and remove it by simple traction on the following day. A small amount of bile frequently leaks from the tube site for a few days. A rubber tissue drain is usually placed alongside the T-tube at operation. This drain is partially withdrawn on the fourth day and shortened daily until it is removed completely on about the seventh day.

Retained Common Duct Stone After Choledochostomy.

The reported incidence of retained stone varies from 2-25%. The frequency is decreased by good operative technic and by operative cholangiography. The residual stone is usually discovered on postoperative cholangiography. Some authorities do not believe that there is at present any effective method of dissolving retained stones by injections or irrigations into the common duct (Longmire, W. P., Jr., and D. C. Rangel, Advances in Surgery 4:105-161, 1970). Others have reported success. Recognizing that it is usually necessary to advise operative removal of a retained common duct stone, the following procedures may be of value in selected cases and are reported by their proponents to have been successful in about one-third of cases.

A. Management With T-tube in Place: The stone may be fragmented or dislodged by the method of Pibram (Surg., Gynec., & Obst. **60**:55, 1936): After preliminary aspiration of bile, first 0.5-1 ml. of ethyl ether and then 1-2 ml. of liquid paraffin are injected slowly into the T-tube. The tube is clamped. If painful pressure develops, the clamp is released. This procedure may be repeated one or more times daily for a number of weeks.

Five ml. of a mixture of two-thirds ethyl ether and one-third ethyl alcohol may be used instead of ether. (Walters and Wesson, Surg., Gynec., & Obst. **65**:595, 1947.)

B. Management Without T-tube: A stone remaining after removal of the T-tube can often be visualized by I.V. cholangiography. The following three-day biliary flush regimen may induce passage of the stone (Best, Ann. Surg. **128**:348, 1948):
   1. Dehydrocholic acid (Decholin®), 0.75 Gm. (12 gr.) q.i.d. (p.c. and h.s.) for 3 days, then 0.5 Gm. (7½ gr.) b.i.d. thereafter. Patients who tend to form recurrent stones should be kept indefinitely on this or similar medication.
   2. Magnesium sulfate, 1 tsp. in water each morning.
   3. Two tablespoonfuls of pure cream or olive oil before the noon and evening meals and h. s.
   4. Nitroglycerin, 0.6 mg. (1/100 gr.) placed under the tongue before each meal on the first and third days.

The above procedure may also be of value while the T-tube is still in place. Under these circumstances, the tube is kept clamped to permit intraductal pressure to build up. The tube is irrigated each day with warm olive oil after 0.6 mg. (1/100 gr.) of nitroglycerin has been dissolved under the tongue. The flush regimen may be repeated several times if cholangiograms reveal a persistent stone.

DIFFERENTIAL DIAGNOSIS OF JAUNDICE

The evaluation of the jaundiced patient should be thorough and expeditious. A primary objective is to distinguish "surgical" jaundice (i.e., jaundice caused by obstruction of the extrahepatic biliary system) from jaundice due to a medical condition. Liver function tests are performed routinely in the presence of jaundice (see p. 468), but must be interpreted in the light of an accurate history and physical examination. A series of x-rays of the gastrointestinal tract is usually obtained. Intravenous cholangiography will visualize the bile ducts in 90% of cases with serum bilirubin value below 1 mg./100 ml. If the serum bilirubin is above 4 mg./100 ml., opacification of the ducts can be expected in only 9%. With BSP retention below 10% in 45 minutes, opacification can be expected in 96% of injections; whereas if the BSP retention is above 40%, the ducts will visualize in only 26%. Percutaneous transhepatic puncture of a bile duct for cholangiography may be helpful in obscure cases of common duct obstruction when safer diagnostic methods prove inadequate. The procedure should only be used when the patient has been prepared for surgery. All bile and contrast medium are aspirated at the end of the procedure to minimize the danger of bile leakage, which is a potential hazard of this examination. Fiberoptic duodenoscopy and cannulation of the common duct provides an alternative and promising approach to cholangiography when facilities for this procedure are available.

When the diagnosis remains obscure in spite of these studies, several courses of action are open. It may be elected to observe the progress of the patient with repeated stool examinations for bile and weekly liver function tests. A needle biopsy of the liver may be considered unless contraindicated by a bleeding tendency or the possibility that marked biliary obstruction will cause bile leakage from a liver puncture. In spite of all measures, diagnosis is impossible in about 5% of cases and laparotomy is necessary to distinguish surgically correctible jaundice from other types.

Classification of Jaundice.

A. Hepatocellular: Caused by cirrhosis, toxins (viral or chemical), abscess (amebic, pyogenic, fungal), anoxia (congestive heart failure), or tumors.
B. Obstructive: Caused by either extrahepatic obstruction or intrahepatic obstruction.
C. Hemolytic: Caused by excessive blood destruction.
D. Congenital hyperbilirubinemia (constitutional hepatic dysfunction and Dubin-Johnson syndrome).

Hepatocellular vs. Obstructive Jaundice.

It is frequently difficult to distinguish hepatocellular from extrahepatic obstructive jaundice when obstruction has been present for several weeks with resultant hepatic damage. In some cases obstructive jaundice may persist for 4-6 weeks before liver injury occurs, but in other instances a shorter interval is sufficient.

A. Clinical Findings Suggestive of Hepatocellular Jaundice:
   1. Viral hepatitis - Characteristic features of viral jaundice are vague upper abdominal pain, nausea, low-grade fever, diffuse liver tenderness and enlargement, and a history of contact with infectious hepatitis or of receiving an injection of a blood product 45-120 days previously. Pruritus is rare. The hepatitis-associated antigen (HAA or Australia antigen) may be present in long-incubation ("serum") hepatitis.
   2. Portal cirrhosis - Cirrhotics usually have a history of known chronic liver disease, and alcoholism is frequent. Chronic weakness and dyspepsia are common symptoms. Cirrhosis may be associated with palmar erythema, spider hemangiomas, gynecomastia, testicular atrophy, splenomegaly, ascites, dilated abdominal veins, hemorrhoids, and esophageal or gastric varices.
   3. Drug-induced liver damage - Many drugs are hepatotoxic; drug-induced liver disease may therefore mimic infectious hepatitis or obstructive jaundice. Although most patients recover without serious complications, there have been fatalities. There are instances in which jaundice occurs and the differential diagnosis is difficult. The introduction of new drugs into medicine has increased the incidence of such problems. Examples of relatively new hepatotoxic drugs are halothane and chlorpromazine; there are many others.

B. Clinical Findings Suggestive of Extrahepatic Obstructive Jaundice: Upper abdominal pain occurs in the majority of these patients. Since choledocholithiasis is the commonest cause of obstructive jaundice, the pain often takes the form of biliary colic. Jaundice usually follows an attack of pain. A past history of chronic cholecystitis is frequent. Pruritus and clay-

Laboratory Examinations in
Hepatocellular and Obstructive Jaundice

Tests*	Hepatocellular Jaundice	Uncomplicated Obstructive Jaundice
Bilirubin		
Direct	Increased	Increased
Indirect	Increased	Increased
Urine bilirubin	Increased	Increased
Urine urobilinogen	Increased	Markedly decreased in complete obstruction
Stool urobilin	Unchanged or lowered	Decreased
Bromsulphalein retention	Increased	Increased
Serum protein	Albumin decreased	Unchanged
Alkaline phosphatase	Increased (++)	Increased (++++)
Cholesterol		
Total	Decreased if damage severe	Increased
Esters	Decreased if damage severe	Normal
Prothrombin time	Prolonged if damage severe	Prolonged if obstruction marked
SGPT, SGOT	Increased in hepatocellular damage, viral hepatitis	Usually unchanged, may be increased

*For normal values, see back endsheets.

colored stools are characteristic of obstruction. Cholangitis secondary to obstruction may cause chills and fever. Fluctuating jaundice is usually caused by stone, whereas insidious, progressive jaundice is more characteristic of malignancy. A tensely distended, nontender gallbladder in the presence of jaundice signifies extrinsic (usually neoplastic) obstruction of the common duct (Courvoisier's law).

C. Laboratory Findings: See above.

BENIGN COMMON DUCT STRICTURES

These are relatively rare. About 90% are caused by operative injury during cholecystectomy, and in about 30% of these patients the disorder is fatal. Jaundice or excessive bile drainage in the postoperative period after biliary tract surgery suggests the diagnosis; prompt reoperation should be considered in these cases. Delayed onset of jaundice or cholangitis after biliary tract surgery may be due to stricture but is more likely to be the result of retained or recurrent common duct stone. Inflammatory strictures of the bile duct are occasionally caused by chronic pancreatitis, postbulbar peptic ulcer, or common duct stone.

Surgical relief of the stricture should be recommended before liver damage becomes severe. Operations for repair of traumatic stricture require great technical skill. Even in the best hands, satisfactory results can be expected in little more than two-thirds of these patients. The various procedures employed are end-to-end anastomosis of the bile duct, choledochoduodenostomy, and choledochojejunostomy. Multiple operations are often necessary because of recurrent stricture.

Stenosis of the sphincter of Oddi due to fibrosis may occur with or without associated pancreatitis or calculous disease of the biliary tract. When fibrous stenosis is accompanied by thickening and dilatation of the common duct, the results of sphincterotomy are good; otherwise, sphincterotomy is disappointing. Patients who continue to have biliary tract symptoms after cholecystectomy with or without choledochostomy and who show dilatation of the common duct on cholangiography may have stenosis of the sphincter. Pancreatitis is another possible cause, and in other cases the cause may be obscure. The stenosis may be associated with intermittent or persistent jaundice and elevation of alkaline phosphatase. Stenosis of the sphincter of Oddi has been a controversial entity because of the frequent tendency to make the diagnosis on the basis of insufficient evidence for actual obstruction to the flow of bile as indicated by dilatation and other changes in the common duct. (Thomas, C.G., Jr., Nicholson, C.P., and J. Owen, Ann Surg 173: 845-856, 1971.)

PORTAL HYPERTENSION

Portal hypertension is caused by obstruction of the portal vein. In 80% of cases the block is intrahepatic and is a late result of cirrhosis. Extrahepatic obstruction by thrombosis, atresia, or cavernomatous transformation accounts for the remaining cases. Portal hypertension is of surgical significance when complicated by bleeding from esophageal or gastric varices, by intractable ascites, or by severe hypersplenism (see p. 488). The incidence of hemorrhage from esophageal varices in cirrhosis is about 30%, and the mortality in those patients who bleed ranges from 50-70%.

Clinical Findings.

The diagnosis of portal hypertension is rarely difficult. There is often a history of massive upper gastrointestinal hemorrhage. In cirrhosis, one or more of the following signs is present: esophageal varices, hepatomegaly, splenomegaly, thrombocytopenia, leukopenia, jaundice, or ascites. Liver function tests show impairment. The findings in extrahepatic block are similar except that jaundice, ascites, and markedly impaired liver function are rare.

The diagnostic work-up should include, in addition to routine examinations, an upper gastrointestinal series (with careful observation for esophageal or gastric varices or peptic ulcer), endoscopy, liver function tests, and platelet count. Liver biopsy and bone marrow study are occasionally indicated. Portal venography (by splenic puncture) may demonstrate the site of the portal obstruction and is especially valuable when extrahepatic block is suspected. Splenic pulp pressure can be determined during splenoportography and is a satisfactory measure of the portal vein pressure. A bleeding tendency is a contraindication to splenoportography.

Treatment.

Note: Narcotics and sedatives should be administered (if at all) with great care to patients with liver disease. Small doses may produce coma or respiratory failure.

A. Emergency Treatment of Bleeding Esophageal Varices: Varices are established as the source of bleeding by an immediate and thorough investigation, and general measures are instituted as for other forms of massive gastrointestinal hemorrhage (see p. 330). Intravenous vasopressin may be of temporary value by lowering portal venous pressure. The dosage is 20 units in 100 ml. of 5% dextrose in water over a 10-minute period. Dose may be repeated at 3-hour intervals. The effect is transient.

Arteriography may be useful in determining the site of active bleeding. Following x-ray visualization of the varices, a catheter may be left in the superior mesenteric artery for continuous infusion of vasopressin. This may in some cases result in control of bleeding.

Additional specific therapy consists of balloon tamponade of varices and the prevention of ammonia intoxication.

1. Sengstaken-Blakemore tube - Used for arresting hemorrhage from esophageal varices. The Sengstaken-Blakemore tube can cause irreparable damage to the esophagus or stomach if used improperly.
   a. Technic of introducing tube -
      (1) Attach the tubing of a BP manometer to a "Y" glass tube. Connect one limb of the "Y" to the esophageal balloon, the other to a BP bulb.
      (2) Passing tube - Lubricate the tube with jelly and pass it through the nares into the stomach to the "50 cm." mark. Facilitate swallowing with sips of water.
      (3) Securing tube in esophagus -
         (a) Inflate stomach balloon with 200 ml. of air by means of a syringe, and then clamp this tube.
         (b) Withdraw Sengstaken-Blakemore tube until resistance is felt.
         (c) Inflate the esophageal balloon to a pressure of 25-50 mm. Hg (about 40-60 ml. of air). If 150-200 ml. of air are required to achieve a pressure of 25 mm., deflate balloons and readjust position. Esophageal contractions and respiratory and cardiac impulses may intermittently raise pressure to 70 mm. Hg, but a minimal pressure of 25 mm. should be maintained. Clamp tube of esophageal balloon. Check pressure frequently to detect leakage. Maintain tube on traction by taping a piece of sponge rubber about the tube and securing it snugly against the ala nasi.
   b. Maintenance of tube - Irrigate stomach with iced saline until the returns are clear. Connect stomach tube to constant suction for 24 hours. Irrigate tube hourly. If there is no evidence of bleeding after 48 hours, deflate the balloons in situ for 12 hours. If no further bleeding occurs, remove gently. Observe carefully for further bleeding.
2. Prevention of ammonia intoxication -
   a. Catharsis - Blood is removed promptly from the gastrointestinal tract by administration of milk of magnesia, 60

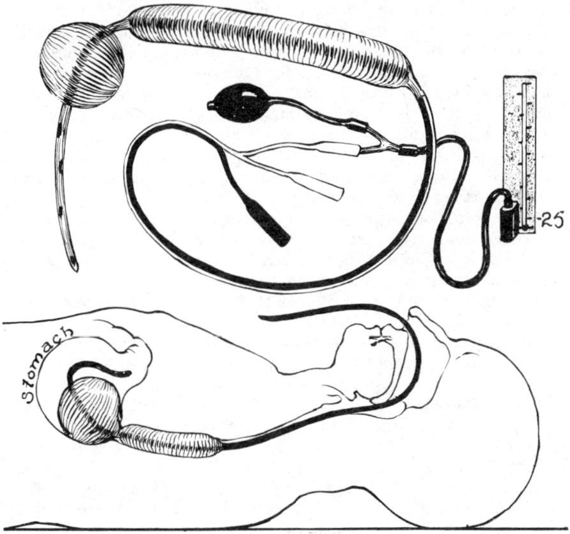

Sengstaken-Blakemore Tube. (Reproduced, with permission, from Krupp, Sweet, Jawetz, Biglieri, and Roe: Physician's Handbook, 17th Ed. Lange, 1973.)

ml. every 2-4 hours, through the Sengstaken-Blakemore tube, until the bowel is clear. Cleansing enemas may also be needed.

b. Intestinal antisepsis - Through the Sengstaken-Blakemore tube, give neomycin, 1 Gm. every hour for 4 hours, then every 4 hours for 2 days. Neomycin, 1 Gm. every 6 hours, is continued thereafter as a maintenance dose as long as necessary to combat ammonia intoxication. Reduction of bacterial flora of the bowel by oral neomycin minimizes the production and absorption of ammonia.

3. Treatment of ammonia intoxication - See p. 474.
4. Indications for operation in bleeding varices - If bleeding cannot be controlled by the Sengstaken-Blakemore tube or other of the above measures and the patient is a reasonable operative risk, an emergency portacaval or splenorenal shunt may be considered. The mortality rate is high in any case and is practically prohibitive in the severe cirrhosis patient with intense jaundice, ascites, and encephalopathy. An alternative approach is the transesophageal ligation of varices followed in a few weeks by an elective portacaval shunt. The mortality rate in emergency operations for bleeding varices is high (25-50%), but this is acceptable in selected good risk patients who continue to bleed in spite of nonoperative treatment.

B. Portacaval Shunt: A history of bleeding from varices is an indication for elective portacaval shunt if liver function tests show acceptable hepatic reserve. The patient is usually a reasonably good operative risk if the serum albumin level is above 3.5 Gm./100 ml.; BSP retention is less than 30% one-half hour after injection; prothrombin time is not in excess of 4 seconds above the normal control; and serum bilirubin is under 1.5 mg./100 ml. In posthepatitis cirrhosis, the BSP retention and bilirubin levels may be somewhat more abnormal without affecting the operative risk adversely.

Chronic ascites may be an indication for portacaval shunt in carefully selected cases which fail to respond to medical measures. A prophylactic portacaval shunt has been recommended by some authorities for prevention of bleeding in patients with varices. There is no evidence that this is justified (Conn, H.O., Medicine 51: 27-40, 1972).

1. Preoperative care - A period of several weeks (or even months) of intensive care will frequently result in sufficient improvement to permit surgical intervention. A low-sodium, 3000 Calorie diet containing 150 Gm. of protein and 75-100 Gm. of fat is prescribed. Commercially available protein or amino acid supplements may be used, but protein intake should be reduced to 0.5 Gm./Kg. body weight if ammonia intoxication is present. Therapeutic doses of vitamin B complex, vitamin C (see p. 132) and vitamin K (see p. 103) are administered. Anemia is corrected by transfusion of whole blood or packed red cells. Ascites, if present, should be eliminated before operation or stabilized as a result of low-sodium diet and diuretic therapy (see Appendix).
2. Shunt operations - The most successful procedures for the relief of portal hypertension are side-to-side or end-to-side anastomosis of the portal vein to the vena cava, or end-to-side anastomosis of the splenic vein to the left renal vein after splenectomy. In extrahepatic block, the splenorenal type of shunt is necessary. Various other types of shunt have been advocated in portal hypertension, but experience with them is limited.
3. Postoperative care - Liver failure is the most serious complication; it occurs postoperatively in 15-20% of patients with cirrhosis, and is fatal in about one-third of those affected. It can be minimized by the following postoperative regimen: (1) Oxygen by nasal catheter at 6-7 L./min. for 24-48 hours; and (2) a minimum of 250 Gm. of glucose daily by vein (as 10 or 25% solution) until oral intake of the preoperative diet (see above) is tolerated. Preoperative vitamin therapy is continued.

   If liver failure develops, oral protein intake is stopped altogether for short periods and then limited to 0.5 Gm./Kg. body weight per day; glucose intake (usually given intravenously) is increased to 300 Gm. or more; and oral neomycin is administered. Transfusions are given as needed to maintain Hgb. above 12 Gm./100 ml.

   Some patients with portacaval shunt tend to develop recurrent ammonia intoxication after heavy protein meals. This may be controlled by a low-protein diet (40 Gm./day) and intermittent administration of neomycin, 0.5 Gm. orally q.i.d. every 3 days for an indefinite period.

Prognosis.

Shunt operations have a mortality of 5-15%. Splenorenal shunt for extrahepatic block is associated with the lowest mortality. About 80% of patients will show reduction in the size of the varices, and liver function may improve after a satisfactory shunt. Recurrent (usually controllable) bleeding occurs in 15-20% of cases; this is more frequent after splenorenal than after portacaval shunts. The incidence of hepatic encephalopathy is greater after portacaval shunt and is a frequent complication in patients with very poor preoperative liver function. (Voorhees, A.B., Jr., Price, J.B., Jr., and R.C. Britton, Am.J. Surg. 119:501-505, 1970; Barnes, B.A., Ann. Surg. 174:76-84, 1971.)

AMMONIA INTOXICATION AND HEPATIC COMA

The syndrome of liver failure occurs most often in patients with chronic hepatic disease who have had gastrointestinal hemorrhage or a portacaval shunt. It may also develop in cirrhotics after major operation or as a terminal stage. Symptoms and signs are largely caused by ammonia intoxication, and the diagnosis is confirmed by the finding of elevated ammonia levels in blood or spinal fluid. The major source of ammonia is the gastrointestinal tract, where the ion is produced by the action of the intestinal bacteria on nitrogenous material (especially blood and protein). Normally, ammonia is detoxified by conversion to urea in the liver and, to a lesser extent, by transamination reactions in the peripheral tissues. A damaged liver cannot cope with an increased ammonia load such as results in bleeding esophageal varices. After portacaval shunt and in patients with portal hypertension who have developed collateral portal-systemic channels, the portal blood bypasses the liver and carries ammonia directly into the general circulation. Such patients may have episodic ammonia intoxication related to heavy meals.

Clinical Findings.

There is usually an obvious precipitating cause such as massive gastrointestinal hemorrhage, severe surgical stress in a cirrhotic, or excessive protein intake in a patient with a portacaval shunt. Administration of ammonium salts (especially ammonium chloride) in cases with depressed liver function may also produce this condition.

The stages of ammonia intoxication range from mental confusion, dysarthria, and irrational behavior to lethargy, somnolence, stupor, and frank coma. One early characteristic sign is a flapping tremor of the hands which also occurs in uremia and respiratory acidosis. In early liver failure the deep tendon reflexes are hyperactive. There are also increased muscle tone, restlessness, and twitching movements. In the late phases, generalized or focal convulsions may accompany the stupor. As coma deepens the respirations become stertorous and the pupils dilated; the muscles become flaccid prior to death. Progressive jaundice and increasing ascites are often noted. Blood and spinal fluid ammonia levels are elevated.

Treatment.

If ammonia intoxication is threatened or precipitated by massive bleeding, the measures outlined for the treatment of tamponade and varices are instituted (see p. 470). Under other circumstances, the general principles of management include:

A. Limitation of Protein Intake: Oral protein is stopped altogether or limited to 0.5 Gm./Kg. body weight daily.

B. High Carbohydrate Intake: Carbohydrate intake is maintained at 300 Gm. daily, usually by administration of supplementary glucose (10-25% solution) I.V.

C. Catharsis: Blood and other protein should be removed as rapidly as possible from the gastrointestinal tract by means of cathartics and enemas. (Cathartics should be administered through the Sengstaken-Blakemore tube if one is in place.) Milk of magnesia, 60 ml. every 2-4 hours, or sorbitol (70% solution), 30 ml. every 6 hours, or magnesium citrate, 120 ml. every 8 hours, is effective. Cleansing tap water enemas may be given concurrently until the gastrointestinal tract is clear.

D. Intestinal Antisepsis: Neomycin, 1 Gm. every 6 hours orally or by tube, until ammonia levels are normal. Neomycin, 1% solution, can be given by retention enema (500-1000 ml.) if oral administration is impossible.

E. Lactulose: Recent studies suggest that lactulose (a disaccharide of galactose and fructose), when administered orally as a flavored syrup containing 50% lactulose, is associated with prevention or reduction of hepatic encephalopathy in postshunt patients. If further experience confirms these preliminary findings, lactulose may be an important addition to the limited armamentarium available for the treatment of recurrent encephalopathy (Brown, H., Trey, C., and W. V. McDermott, Jr., Arch. Surg. 102:25-27, 1971).

Prognosis.

The mortality in hepatic failure is at least 30%. This can be reduced only by early and intensive treatment.

TUMORS OF THE LIVER AND BILIARY TRACT

Benign tumors of the liver and biliary tract are rare and are usually incidental findings at operation or autopsy. The commonest benign liver tumor is cavernous hemangioma, which usually presents beneath the liver capsule as multiple purplish, nodular, compressible masses. No treatment is necessary. Papillomas, adenomas, and lipomas occur throughout the biliary system and are treated by excision. They may be visualized by cholecystography.

Primary Carcinoma of the Liver.

This is rare in the United States but relatively common in Africa and the Orient. It is primarily a disease of adults 40-50 years old, but a peak incidence also occurs in infancy and childhood. It is more frequent in males.

The possible etiologic factors are cirrhosis, malnutrition, parasites, chronic irritation, hemochromatosis, and congenital defects. Three histologic types can be distinguished: malignant hepatoma, malignant cholangioma, and a mixed type (malignant cholangiohepatoma). Hepatoma is usually the most rapidly progressive.

Early in the disease there are no pathognomonic symptoms. Later, abdominal pain and enlargement of the liver are noted. Occasionally there is fever. A needle or open liver biopsy establishes the diagnosis.

The prognosis is grave but not always hopeless, as it is possible in rare cases to resect the lesion. Metastatic liver cancer is very common and must be differentiated from primary tumor.

Adenocarcinoma of the Gallbladder.

About two-thirds of carcinomas of the extrahepatic biliary system arise in the gallbladder. The majority of patients are over 50, and 75% are women. Gallstones are present in 90% of cases and are considered the most important etiologic factor. This is one of the reasons why prophylactic removal of the calculous gallbladder is advisable unless there is some contraindication (see p. 458).

The early symptoms are those of chronic cholecystitis, which is invariably present (see p. 458). Later, pain is often continuous, and a mass in the gallbladder region may be palpable. Jaundice usually occurs eventually.

Cancer of the gallbladder is almost always fatal, although a few five-year survivals have been reported. Radical cholecystectomy with resection of the gallbladder bed or partial hepatectomy should be attempted when the tumor is sufficiently localized.

PYOGENIC LIVER ABSCESS

Pyogenic abscess of the liver is usually secondary to intraperitoneal sepsis. The intestinal flora is commonly involved. Malaise, fever, and right or left upper quadrant pain are usually present. The pain often radiates to the top of the ipsilateral shoulder. Prostration and high spiking fever occur as the infection progresses. Although local signs depend somewhat upon the location of the abscess, an enlarged, tender liver and direct shock tenderness over the lower rib cage are frequently found. Leukocytosis is marked and may aid in differentiation from uncomplicated amebic abscess, in which the WBC usually shows minimal elevation. Jaundice is a late sign. Upright chest and abdominal films should be scrutinized for such suggestive signs as elevation of the diaphragm, fluid in the chest, enlargement or tumefaction of the liver, and abscess cavity with air fluid level. A radioisotope scan of the liver will show a defect in large abscess.

Treatment is by incision and drainage with care to avoid contamination of the pleural and peritoneal cavities. Needle aspiration should be done only under direct vision at exploration. Antimicrobial therapy is based on culture and sensitivity studies. It is important to differentiate pyogenic from amebic abscess of the liver because the treatment is different.

AMEBIC LIVER ABSCESS

Clinical Findings.

Amebic abscess is caused by trophozoites of Entamoeba histolytica which reach the liver from the cecal region by way of the portal system. It occurs in less than 3% of persons with amebiasis, and is most common in young adult males. The most frequent location is in the right lobe near the dome. Abscess formation is preceded by amebic hepatitis. The symptoms and signs of amebic abscess are similar to those of pyogenic abscess. A history of dysentery is obtained and amebas in the stools are demonstrated in only 20-25% of cases. The WBC is slightly elevated and liver function tests are usually normal unless the abscess becomes chronic, in which case increasing leukocytosis and hepatic dysfunction become apparent. The complement fixation test for amebiasis is useful. To avoid overlooking amebas in the stools, 3 stool examinations with at least one following the use of a saline cathartic are advisable; if negative, proctoscopic examination is indicated to determine if amebic ulcerations are present.

The complications of hepatic amebiasis are (1) secondary infection of the abscess, (2) pleuropulmonary complications (empyema, bronchohepatic fistula, pulmonary abscess), and (3) rupture into the peritoneal cavity. Exploratory needle puncture of the liver is employed when the diagnosis is doubtful or when secondary infection of the abscess is suspected. Liver scan after intravenous administration of radioactive isotope may be helpful in localizing an abscess prior to drainage.

Treatment.

A. Medical Measures: The following therapeutic routine is applicable in the majority of cases. If a clinical diagnosis of amebic abscess is made and there is no indication for needle aspiration or surgery, the patient is given both chloroquine and emetine concurrently. Chloroquine is administered orally, 1 Gm. daily for 2 days and then 0.5 Gm. daily for the next 26 days. Emetine, 65 mg. I.M. daily for 10 days, is the average adult dose. When emetine is used in this manner, the patient should be at bed rest in the hospital with frequent electrocardiograms. Therapeutic response to this combination of drugs is usually quite prompt and is of diagnostic value. Repetition of the course after a drug holiday of 2 months may be desirable, but emetine should be given for only 6 or 7 days on the second occasion. If secondary infection in the amebic abscess is suspected, antibiotics should be added to the antiamebic therapy.

If there is no improvement on drug therapy, or if a definite abscess is likely from the clinical picture, an exploratory puncture of the liver under local anesthesia is done with a spinal needle, using strict aseptic technic. Care must be taken to avoid the pleural and peritoneal cavities. If amebic pus (usually reddish-brown) is obtained, the abscess is evacuated completely with a small trocar (14-16 gauge). The pus is cultured and smeared for pyogenic bacteria and amebas. No antiamebic drug is injected into the cavity. Systemic drug therapy is begun or continued. Repeat aspiration may be required.

Intestinal amebiasis should be assumed to be present and treated. A satisfactory program for asymptomatic or subacute amebiasis of the colon consists of diiodohydroxyquin, 650 mg. 3 times daily for 21 days, plus chloroquine, 500 mg. (salt) twice daily for 2 days; then give 250 mg. twice daily for 19 days plus oxytetracycline, 250 mg. 4 times daily for 10 days.

B. Surgical Treatment: Surgical drainage, by an extrapleural, extraperitoneal route, is employed only when one of the complications of amebic abscess occurs or when the abscess cannot be satisfactorily evacuated by trocar.

DISEASES OF THE PANCREAS

ANNULAR PANCREAS

The nature and severity of the symptoms produced by this congenital lesion are related to the degree of duodenal obstruction which it causes. When obstruction is marked, persistent vomiting occurs immediately after birth. Mild duodenal narrowing may not cause symptoms until adulthood. The 4 major complications accompanying the anomaly are duodenal obstruction, peptic ulcer, acute or chronic pancreatitis, and biliary obstruction. Frank peptic ulceration in the duodenum or stomach accompanied by typical ulcer symptoms is present in the majority of adult patients. The diagnosis is confirmed by barium studies.

Treatment is surgical. In infants and in some adults, duodenojejunostomy is performed. Partial gastrectomy is advisable if peptic ulcer is present. It is important to avoid a direct attack on the pancreas itself; most of the surgical fatalities have occurred as a result of attempts to divide the pancreatic ring.

ACUTE PANCREATITIS

The cause of acute pancreatitis is not clearly established and may not be the same in all cases. It is probably precipitated by increased intraductal pressure such as occurs (1) in pancreatic duct obstruction, (2) when pancreatic secretion is copious after a heavy meal, or (3) when bile flows back into the pancreatic ductal system through a common channel at the junction of the common and pancreatic ducts. Pressure sufficient to rupture the tiny ductules in the pancreas releases pancreatic enzymes into the tissues, where they are activated and produce a severe inflammatory reaction. Two varieties occur: acute edematous pancreatitis and the more severe, fulminating, and often fatal acute hemorrhagic pancreatitis.

Clinical Findings.

Although this disorder may occur in any age group, it is most frequently seen in persons between 30 and 50. A past history of chronic cholecystitis or previous attacks of acute pancreatitis can often be obtained. Many patients with acute pancreatitis are alcoholics. Postoperative pancreatitis, particularly after gastroduodenal or biliary tract surgery, is not unusual. Hyperparathyroidism and familial hyperlipemia are 2 conditions which may be associated with an increased incidence of pancreatitis. The pancreas is occasionally involved in mumps.

A. Symptoms and Signs: In acute edematous pancreatitis the onset is relatively rapid, with severe epigastric pain which is usually referred through to the back and lower scapular regions. Nausea and vomiting almost always occur. Abdominal signs include tenderness over the pancreas, mild muscle spasm, and diminished peristalsis. Tachycardia and low-grade fever are usually present. There may be mild, transient jaundice.

In acute hemorrhagic pancreatitis, the symptoms and signs are greatly intensified. Shock occurs and may be rapidly fatal. Edema and discoloration appear in the flanks in some cases. Hypocalcemic tetany and hyperglycemia are not unusual. If the patient survives the acute necrosis, he may form a pancreatic pseudocyst or abscess with sequestration of the pancreas.

B. Laboratory Findings: The following are suggestive of acute pancreatitis: moderate to marked leukocytosis, increased Hgb. and Hct. values indicative of hemoconcentration, increased blood sugar, and decreased serum calcium.

The elevated serum amylase level is a more specific sign of pancreatitis than any other laboratory test, but it must be considered only a useful adjunct to clinical evaluation. It usually reaches its highest value within 24 hours of onset of acute pancreatitis, and may return to normal within 48 hours or remain elevated for several days. The degree of elevation does not correlate well with the severity of the condition. Many acute abdominal conditions and even morphine administration will also cause the serum amylase to rise (occasionally to high levels) in the absence of pancreatic disease. Serum lipase tends to rise in acute pancreatitis, reaches its greatest concentration later than the amylase, and persists longer. Urinary diastase output usually increases when serum amylase rises, and should be determined on a timed two-hour urine specimen in order to estimate the hourly quantitative excretion. Urinary diastase may be increased in the presence of normal serum amylase if renal excretion of the enzyme is efficient. When kidney function is poor, urinary diastase may fail to rise.

Abdominal tap is particularly useful. As little as a fraction of 1 ml. of abdominal fluid may be diluted to show an elevated amylase content. Titration for free acid and examination for bile may be of value in differentiating pancreatitis from perforated ulcer.

C. X-ray Findings: Survey films of the chest and abdomen should be obtained. Basal pneumonitis, pleurisy, or pleural effusion, usually on the left side, may accompany acute pancreatitis. The abdominal x-ray often discloses an isolated, gas-filled "sentinel loop" of small intestine in the middle or upper abdomen; or a more diffuse paralytic type of ileus may be present. Radiopaque gallstones or pancreatic calcifications may be revealed.

Differential Diagnosis.

Acute cholecystitis, choledocholithiasis, and perforated peptic ulcer are most likely to be confused with pancreatitis. In each of these disorders the serum amylase may rise, but usually to a lesser extent than in acute pancreatitis. Mesenteric thrombosis and acute hemorrhagic pancreatitis often produce the same type of profound collapse. The diagnosis of pancreatitis can usually be made without resort to laparotomy.

Complications.

Pancreatic pseudocyst occasionally occurs as a complication of acute pancreatitis. The presence of a pseudocyst is indicated by the appearance of a mass in the region of the pancreas and, in some cases, by persistent elevation of serum amylase, WBC, and temperature. Pancreatic abscess or hemorrhage secondary to necrosis may be serious sequelae of acute hemorrhagic pancreatitis.

Treatment.

A. Medical Measures: The initial treatment of acute pancreatitis is nonoperative, and the same regimen is employed as in acute peritonitis (see p. 403). Nasogastric tube suction is indicated. For relief of pain, use meperidine, 100-150 mg. I.M. every 3-4 hours. Opiates cause spasm of the sphincter of Oddi and should not be used. An anticholinergic drug, such as atropine, is given every 4-6 hours parenterally. Antibiotics (e.g., ampicillin or cephalothin) are advisable in severe cases. Hypocalcemic tetany is treated with calcium gluconate, 1 Gm. in 10% solution I.V., as often as necessary to control the manifestations.

Of great importance in acute hemorrhagic pancreatitis is the intensive treatment of the profound shock which often occurs. Loss of blood, plasma, and fluid into the retroperitoneal space is severe, requiring multiple whole blood and plasma transfusions. Hydrocortisone (e.g., Solu-Cortef®), 100-200 mg. I.V. every 4-6 hours for several doses, may be of some value if BP cannot be maintained by fluid replacement and vasopressor drugs.

Blood and urine sugar levels should be determined and insulin administered on the basis of urine test if diabetes develops (see p. 76).

B. Surgical Treatment: Operative treatment in the acute stage is reserved for a few carefully selected patients with hemorrhagic pancreatitis who are going progressively downhill in spite of completely adequate supportive care and in whom there is the chance that drainage of fluid or necrotic debris from the lesser omental sac or the peripancreatic tissues may change the course of the disease. Such procedures may rarely avert a fatal outcome.

When acute pancreatitis is unexpectedly found on exploration for an acute abdomen, it is usually wisest to close without intervention of any kind. If the pancreatitis appears mild and cholelithiasis is present, cholecystostomy or cholecystectomy may occasionally be justified. In general, patients who receive the least intra-abdominal manipulation have the least morbidity and mortality after laparotomy for unsuspected pancreatitis.

The development of a pancreatic abscess is an indication for prompt drainage, usually through the flank. If a pseudocyst develops, it often requires surgical treatment (see p. 481).

Prognosis.

The mortality in acute hemorrhagic pancreatitis is probably

about 33%, and in edematous pancreatitis about 5%, although reported statistics show a very wide range. Postoperative pancreatitis has a mortality of 40-50%. The efficacy of careful nonoperative management has been proved in a series of 82 patients treated medically with an over-all mortality of only 1.3% during the acute stage of the disease (H.L. Bockus, Gastroenterol. **34**:467, 1958). All patients with pancreatitis should eventually have cholecystography, cholangiography, and upper gastrointestinal x-rays. Surgical disease of the biliary system should be corrected, and stenosis of the sphincter of Oddi, if present, should be relieved by sphincterotomy in order to reduce the likelihood of future attacks.

CHRONIC RELAPSING PANCREATITIS

Some individuals, about a third of whom are alcoholics, have repeated attacks of pancreatitis. Once an attack of pancreatitis has occurred, the chance of recurrence is about 50%. Progressive fibrosis and varying degrees of destruction of functioning glandular tissue occur as a result. Pancreaticolithiasis and obstruction of the duodenal end of the pancreatic duct are often present. Cholecystitis is present in about 50% of patients with chronic pancreatitis. Hyperparathyroidism and familial hyperlipemia should be ruled out. Males are affected 6 times as often as females.

Clinical Findings.

Recurrent attacks of epigastric and left upper quadrant pain with referral to the upper left lumbar region are typical. Anorexia, nausea, vomiting, constipation, and flatulence are common. Abdominal signs during attacks consist chiefly of tenderness over the pancreas, mild muscle guarding, and paralytic ileus. Serum amylase and bilirubin are often elevated during acute attacks. Glycosuria may be present. Plain films often show pancreaticolithiasis and mild ileus. A cholecystogram may reveal biliary tract disease, and upper gastrointestinal series may demonstrate a widened duodenal loop. Attacks may last only a few hours or as long as 2 weeks; pain may eventually be almost continuous.

Steatorrhea as indicated by bulky, foul, fatty stools and other types of intestinal malabsorption may occur in chronic pancreatitis. Fecal fat content should be determined in these cases.

Complications.

Narcotic addiction is common. Other frequent complications include diabetes mellitus, pancreatic pseudocyst or abscess, obstructive jaundice, steatorrhea, malnutrition, and peptic ulcer.

Treatment.

Correctible coexistent biliary tract disease should be treated surgically.

A. Medical Measures: A bland, low-fat diet and anticholinergic drugs should be prescribed. Alcohol is forbidden because it frequently precipitates attacks. Mild sedatives may be helpful. Narcotics are avoided. Malabsorption is treated with pancreatin (e.g., Viokase®), 2 Gm. t.i.d., p.c., orally. Every effort is made to manage the disease medically.

B. Surgical Treatment: When conservative measures fail, surgical intervention must be considered. There is no agreement as to the procedure of choice, and operations must be strictly individualized. The objectives of surgical intervention are to eradicate biliary tract disease, ensure a free flow of bile into the duodenum, and eliminate obstruction of the pancreatic duct. Sphincterotomy of the sphincter of Oddi may be of value if stenosis is present. When obstruction of the duodenal end of the duct can be demonstrated by operative pancreatography, dilatation of the duct or resection of the tail of the pancreas with implantation of the distal end of the duct by pancreaticojejunostomy may be successful. Anastomosis between the longitudinally split duct and a defunctionalized limb of jejunum without pancreatectomy may be in order. In advanced cases it may be necessary, as a last resort, to do subtotal or total pancreatectomy.

Prognosis.

This is a serious disease and often leads to chronic invalidism. The prognosis is best when patients with acute pancreatitis are carefully investigated with their first attack and are found to have some remediable condition such as chronic cholecystitis and cholelithiasis, choledocholithiasis, stenosis of the sphincter of Oddi, or hyperparathyroidism. Surgical relief of these aggravating conditions may prevent recurrent pancreatic disease. (Warren, K.W., and J.C. Mountain, S. Clin. North America 51:693-710, 1971.)

PANCREATIC CYST

The commonest type of pancreatic cyst is the pseudocyst which is secondary to pancreatitis or trauma. It is formed by the accumulation of pancreatic juice in the retroperitoneal space or lesser sac as a result of rupture of the pancreatic ducts.

Other types of pancreatic cyst are quite rare and include (1) true cysts which are lined by cuboidal or low columnar epithelium and contain yellow fluid; and (2) neoplastic cysts which may be benign (cystadenoma) or malignant (cystadenocarcinoma).

Clinical Findings in Pancreatic Pseudocyst.

There is a history of trauma or pancreatitis. Epigastric pain and a palpable, tense, tender mass are usually observed. Anorexia and weight loss are common. Chills and fever may occur. Jaundice is present in 5-10% of patients. Serum amylase will usually not be elevated except during an attack of pancreatitis. Diabetes is occasionally found. Plain abdominal films will show a mass, and calcium in its wall may be visible. Barium study of the stomach and colon may show compression of these organs by the cyst. The duodenal loop may be widened by a cyst of the head of the pancreas. Tumor of the kidney must in some cases be ruled out by excretory or retrograde urography.

Treatment.

Pseudocysts are rarely suitable for total removal. The measures most widely recommended are simple drainage with a Pezzer catheter (especially for poor risk patients and infected cysts); and, preferably, internal drainage by cystogastrostomy or by cystojejunostomy using a Roux-Y limb of jejunum.

TRAUMATIC INJURIES OF THE PANCREAS

Injury to the pancreas is rare. In penetrating wounds, other structures are invariably damaged also. Operative injury to the pancreas may occur, especially during gastrectomy or splenectomy. Hemorrhage and leakage of pancreatic secretions are the commonest complications of pancreatic trauma which require treatment.

When pancreatic leakage is suspected, drainage is mandatory; the fistula which often develops as a consequence of drainage tends to close spontaneously in a few weeks or months. Meanwhile it should be treated like bowel fistula (see p. 437). Meticulous attention to nutrition and fluid balance is necessary to prevent serious depletion in these patients. The pancreatic juice, if copious, should be collected in a suction reservoir and returned by nasogastric tube. Administration of propantheline bromide (Pro-Banthine®) or tincture of belladonna orally will depress the external secretion of the pancreas and reduce the drainage. If a significant amount of secretion is lost, replacement therapy with pancreatin, 2 Gm. 3-4 times daily orally after meals, will improve digestive function. Definitive surgical treatment of a persistent pancreatic fistula consists of implantation of the duct or tract into the duodenum or jejunum.

Blunt trauma may be followed by the delayed appearance of a pseudocyst (see p. 481). Elevation of serum amylase after abdominal trauma is suggestive but not pathognomonic of pancreatic damage.

CARCINOMA OF THE HEAD OF THE PANCREAS AND THE PERIAMPULLARY AREA

Carcinoma is the commonest neoplasm of the pancreas. About 75% are in the head and 25% in the body and tail of the organ. Carcinomas involving the head of the pancreas, the ampulla of Vater, the common bile duct, and the duodenum are considered together because they are usually indistinguishable clinically.

Clinical Findings.

Abdominal pain, jaundice, weight loss, and a palpable gallbladder are the most frequent findings in these tumors. Pain, which is present in over 70%, is often vague and diffuse in the epigastrium and is rarely comparable to biliary colic. Later, more persistent, severe pain develops and often radiates to the back. This usually indicates that the lesion has spread beyond the pancreas and is inoperable. The jaundice is obstructive and must be differentiated from the hepatocellular type (see p. 468). Unfortunately, it is rarely possible to make the diagnosis before jaundice occurs. Diarrhea is seen occasionally, and thrombophlebitis in the legs is a rare sign. It is a useful clinical rule (Courvoisier's law) that jaundice associated with a palpable gallbladder is indicative of obstruction by neoplasm. On rare occasions the gallbladder may not be palpable because of cystic duct obstruction or contraction of the gallbladder secondary to chronic infection. Occult blood in the stools occurs more frequently in tumors of the ampulla. Barium study of the duodenum may show deformity such as widening or indentation of the loop. Fiberoptic duodenoscopy may allow visualization and biopsy of ampullary lesions. Angiography will occasionally provide evidence of a pancreatic tumor.

Treatment.

Abdominal exploration is usually necessary to confirm the diagnosis and determine resectability, which is about 30%. Radical pancreaticoduodenal resection is indicated for lesions which are strictly limited to the head of the pancreas, periampullary zone, and duodenum. When radical resection is not feasible, cholecystojejunostomy is performed to relieve the jaundice. A gastrojejunostomy is also done if duodenal obstruction is expected to develop later.

Prognosis.

Carcinoma of the head of the pancreas has a very poor prognosis; fewer than 10% of resected cases survive 5 years. Lesions of the ampulla, common duct, and duodenum are more favorable with a five-year survival rate from 20-40% after resection. The operative mortality of radical pancreaticoduodenectomy is 10-15%.

CARCINOMA OF THE BODY AND TAIL OF THE PANCREAS

About 25% of pancreatic cancer arises in the body or tail. There are no characteristic findings in the early stages. The initial symptoms are vague epigastric or left upper quadrant distress. Anorexia and weight loss usually occur. Later, pain becomes more severe and frequently radiates through to the left lumbar region. A mass in the mid or left epigastrium may be palpable. The spontaneous development of thrombophlebitis in the legs is suggestive. Angiography may occasionally be of diagnostic value. The diagnosis is usually made only by abdominal exploration. Resection is rarely feasible, and cure is rarer still.

INSULIN-PRODUCING ISLET CELL TUMOR
(Insulinoma, Insulinogenic Betacytoma)

Islet cell tumors of the pancreas may be benign (90%) or malignant, and functioning or nonfunctioning. About 75% occur in the body and tail and 25% in the head of the pancreas. Most of these neoplasms are only 1-2 cm. in diameter; multiple tumors occur in 5-10% of benign cases. Over 90% of the tumors removed at operation are functioning. They are composed of beta islet cells and hence are termed insulinogenic betacytoma. This is to be expected because the diagnosis is usually suggested by hypoglycemia. The majority of patients are under 30; persons past 60 are seldom affected. Rarely, the tumors arise in aberrant pancreatic tissue in the duodenum, stomach, or gastrosplenic omentum, so that a thorough abdominal search must be made if a suspected lesion is not found in the pancreas.

Clinical Findings.

The classical clinical triad consists of (1) a history of attacks of hunger, weakness, sweating, and paresthesia coming on during the fasting state; (2) fasting blood glucose level of 50 mg./100 ml. or less during attacks; and (3) immediate recovery on administration of glucose.

A. Symptoms and Signs: The symptoms produced by functioning islet cell tumors depend entirely upon excessive insulin secretion and the resultant hypoglycemia. Attacks of hypoglycemia are usually precipitated by fasting or overexertion, and often begin with a feeling of intense hunger. Agitation, perspiration, pallor, dizziness, and weakness are early symptoms which may progress to confusion, stupor, excitement, disorientation, drunken behavior, delirium, mania, tonic and clonic spasms, convulsions, and coma. Obesity may result from the excessive carbohydrate ingested to prevent attacks.

B. Laboratory Findings: The only typical change is a fasting blood glucose level below 50 mg./100 ml. during attacks.

C. Special Tests:

1. Prolonged fasting - This is the most reliable diagnostic procedure. The patient receives no food and only water or black coffee with saccharin for up to 72 hours. In almost all patients with insulinoma this regimen will cause the blood glucose to fall below 30 mg./100 ml. and symptoms of hypoglycemia will occur. About one-third of patients with functioning tumor will develop symptoms within 12 hours, and two-thirds by 24 hours. In over 90% of patients, a symptomatic attack will be precipitated within 48 hours by fasting, and exercise will invariably hasten the onset.
2. Tolbutamide test - One Gm. of sodium tolbutamide (Orinase®) is injected **slowly** I. V. in 20 ml. of normal saline solution. In patients with insulinoma, the blood glucose level usually falls to 50-80% of the fasting level in 30 minutes and remains low for several hours; in nonorganic or functional hyperinsulinism the blood glucose level falls to hypoglycemic levels and then rises to normal levels in 1-2 hours. This rapid screening test is not without danger, and at times must be interrupted by the administration of I. V. glucose to prevent severe convulsions and coma. While atypical curves are noted in some patients with insulinoma, an entirely normal response would speak against this diagnosis. (Fajans and others, J. Clin. Endocrinol. 21:371, 1961.)
3. Fasting plasma insulin - In most patients with betacytoma, insulin assays of plasma by either immunochemical or bioassay technic are inappropriately high after an overnight fast. Abnormally high levels of plasma insulin concomitant with prolonged hypoglycemia due to I.V. tolbutamide are highly suggestive of insulinoma.
4. Selective angiography - The location of insulinoma at operation can be quite difficult. Therefore, preoperative arteriography should be considered, for it frequently indicates the site of the tumor (Alfidi, R. J., and others, Surg. Gynec. Obstet. 133:447-452, 1971.).

Differential Diagnosis.

The most important differentiation is that between organic and functional hyperinsulinism. Severe hypoglycemia after an overnight fast may occur in disorders of glycogen storage, Addison's disease, pituitary insufficiency, hypothyroidism, hepatic failure, congestive failure, and severe primary renal glycosuria. Hypoglycemia may also occur in conjunction with large extrapancreatic tumors, most frequently retroperitoneal or thoracic, with the histologic picture of sarcomas or fibromas.

Treatment.

Emergency treatment of hypoglycemic attacks consists of the oral or I. V. administration of glucose solution.

When the insulinoma cannot be found in the pancreas, it is essential to search carefully in all possible sites of ectopic pancreatic tissue such as the gastrocolic, gastrohepatic, and gastrosplenic ligaments and along the entire gastrointestinal tract. If still no tumor is found, it is justifiable to resect the body and tail of the pancreas.

Surgical cxploration should be carried out when the diagnosis is established, as delay may permit mental deterioration as a result of repeated attacks of hypoglycemia. An intravenous drip of 10% glucose is started before operation and continued throughout the procedure to prevent hypoglycemia. Operative mortality is about 4% and complete relief is obtained in 90% of patients with benign tumors.

Surgery has little to offer in the treatment of the rare malignant islet cell carcinoma with metastases. Palliative effects have been reported with streptozotocin, an antibiotic which selectively destroys pancreatic beta cells. The usefulness of this agent, which is still under investigation, is limited by severe renal and hepatic toxicity.

ULCEROGENIC ISLET CELL TUMOR
(Zollinger-Ellison Syndrome)

In 1955 Zollinger and Ellison described a syndrome of fulminating peptic ulcer diathesis, and gastric hypersecretion, accompanied in some patients by severe diarrhea. The cause of the syndrome was found to be a non–beta cell, non–insulin-producing islet cell tumor or hyperplasia of the pancreas which secretes a gastrin-like hormone of very high potency. Subsequent experience has shown that about 60% of the lesions are malignant (two-thirds having metastases at the time of discovery) and 40% are benign. Three-fourths of the benign lesions are adenomas and one-fourth are hyperplasia of the islets alone. It has been observed that the pancreatic adenomas may occasionally be associated with adenomas of other endocrine glands such as the pituitary, thyroid, parathyroid, and adrenal (multiple endocrine adenomatosis). The islet cell carcinoma associated with Zollinger-Ellison syndrome is of low-grade malignancy and may occasionally regress spontaneously or after total gastrectomy.

Clinical Findings.

A. Symptoms and Signs: Severe ulcer diathesis or rapid recurrence of peptic ulcer after adequate gastric surgery is suggestive.

Intractable diarrhea, with or without ulcer symptoms, may be a major complaint. There are no characteristic physical findings.

B. Laboratory Findings: A 12-hour gastric secretion exceeding 1500 ml. and containing in excess of 100 mEq. of free hydrochloric acid supports the diagnosis. The augmented histamine test is very useful. In normal or routine ulcer patients, injection of histamine causes a marked increase in acid production. In patients with ulcerogenic tumors, the baseline acid secretion is already high and may not increase significantly after histamine injection. Serum gastrin level is an important confirmatory immunochemical test; it should be obtained when possible.

C. X-ray Findings: Giant rugae in the stomach, gastric hypersecretion, and atypical location of peptic ulceration are suggestive. Duodenal ileus and hypertrophy of duodenal and jejunal mucosa may be seen.

D. Liver Scan: Preoperative radioisotope liver scan for metastases should be considered.

Treatment.

The pancreas and its environs should be carefully examined at operation in all patients undergoing surgery for peptic ulcer, particularly those with a suspicious history or when active ulcerative disease has recurred after previous operation. The regional lymph nodes and the liver should be scrutinized for metastases.

The surgeon should strongly suspect Zollinger-Ellison syndrome on the basis of preoperative data. If the diagnosis is confirmed by removal of a pancreatic tumor or by the finding of lymph node or liver metastases, it is necessary to decide on the appropriate operative procedure. There have been a few reports of control of the ulcer diathesis by successful resection of a pancreatic adenoma or by removal of the proximal stomach (containing the parietal cells), with preservation of the antrum and pylorus. However, certain control of the disease only follows total gastrectomy, especially if metastases from the pancreatic tumor are not excised.

DISEASES OF THE SPLEEN

The normal functions of the spleen include the following: (1) hematopoiesis in the embryo; (2) lymphocyte formation throughout life; (3) removal of worn-out and damaged blood cells from the circulation, (4) production of antibodies, (5) humoral regulation of the bone marrow, and (6) storage of red cells and iron. In the absence of the spleen, these functions are assumed by the remainder of the reticuloendothelial system; splenectomy has no permanent adverse effect except in those rare cases when the spleen has become an important site of extramedullary hematopoiesis (e.g., in myeloid metaplasia with myelofibrosis).

Following splenectomy there is usually a transient rise in the erythrocyte, leukocyte, and platelet counts. Postoperatively, the platelet count should be determined daily until it is consistently below 1 million/cu. mm. If the thrombocytes exceed 1.5 million, a systemic anticoagulant (heparin or dicoumarol) may be required to prevent spontaneous thromboses.

Indications for Splenectomy.

The medical indications for splenectomy are frequently dependent on response to other forms of treatment. Each case must be carefully studied from the hematologic point of view. Close cooperation of the internist and surgeon is essential to the proper selection and management of these patients.

A. Surgical Indications: Rupture of the spleen (see p. 406), splenic cysts and tumors, wandering spleen, and splenorenal shunt.

B. Medical Indications: Primary hypersplenism (congenital hemolytic anemia, idiopathic thrombocytopenic purpura, primary splenic neutropenia, primary splenic panhematopenia), secondary hypersplenism, or autoimmune hemolytic anemia.

C. Miscellaneous Indications for Splenectomy: Removal of massive spleens associated with medical conditions such as Gaucher's disease, malaria, and schistosomiasis may be indicated for mechanical reasons and because mild hypersplenism is often present.

Contraindications to Splenectomy.

The current tendency is to liberalize the indications for splenectomy; this operation has proved beneficial in carefully selected cases in many disorders which were formerly thought to be contraindications. Before splenectomy is undertaken for any of the medical diseases, it must be demonstrated that the spleen is affecting the hematologic picture adversely or that mechanical symptoms justify the operation. Splenectomy should not be performed in Mediterranean anemia (thalassemia) and sickle cell anemia unless a hemolytic factor is prominent.

In general, removal of the spleen is contraindicated in pernicious anemia, polycythemia, the lymphomas, and agnogenic myeloid metaplasia.

CYSTS AND TUMORS OF THE SPLEEN

Cysts of the spleen are very rare and are of 3 types: (1) primary (true) cysts, (2) secondary cysts (pseudocysts), and (3) parasitic (echinococcus) cysts. They are usually asymptomatic unless they become large enough to cause abdominal discomfort. Calcification in the cyst wall may aid in diagnosis by x-ray. Treatment is by splenectomy.

Primary neoplasms of the spleen are even more rare than cysts. Hemangioma is the most frequent benign tumor. Sarcoma of the lymphoma group is the commonest malignancy. Splenectomy is curative in hemangioma, but five-year survival after removal of the spleen for sarcoma is unusual.

WANDERING SPLEEN

In this disorder the spleen has a long pedicle and floats free in the peritoneal cavity. It may become twisted on its pedicle. Treatment consists of splenectomy.

PRIMARY HYPERSPLENISM

Primary hypersplenism is characterized by depression (or excessive destruction) of one or more of the formed elements of the blood as a result of splenic overactivity. Depending on which blood elements are involved, the following conditions may result: (1) Congenital (primary) hemolytic anemia (erythrocytes), (2) idiopathic thrombocytopenic purpura (platelets), (3) primary splenic neutropenia (neutrophils), and (4) primary splenic panhematopenia (all elements). In all of these conditions except idiopathic thrombocytopenic purpura, splenectomy is the treatment of choice.

Congenital (Primary) Hemolytic Anemia (Congenital Hemolytic Jaundice; Hereditary Spherocytosis).

Onset of symptoms may occur any time between infancy and 40-50 years of age. A familial history is important. The most typical feature is acholuric jaundice. Weakness and malaise are the commonest complaints except during hemolytic crises, when marked hemolysis is associated with nausea, vomiting, abdominal pain, and rapid increase in jaundice. Remissions and exacerbations are characteristic of this disease. Calcium bilirubinate biliary calculi are common as a result of high biliary bilirubin output, and may produce symptoms of cholelithiasis. Chronic leg ulcer over the internal or external malleolus is an uncommon complication, but it may be the chief complaint and will persist for years until splenectomy is performed. The spleen is usually enlarged and may be huge but it may not be palpable in mild cases.

The clinical diagnosis requires laboratory confirmation. Microcytic anemia is present, and erythrocyte counts below 1 million may be seen after hemolytic crises. Spherocytosis, reticulocytosis of 5-20%, and increased red cell fragility are found. Bone marrow studies showing erythroid hyperplasia are essential to rule out other forms of anemia. Indirect serum bilirubin and urine and stool urobilin are increased. Bile is not present in the urine. Red cell survival studies using the patient's own blood labeled with Cr^{51} will show a greatly shortened red cell life span and sequestration in the spleen of Cr^{51} from destroyed cells.

Splenectomy is the only satisfactory treatment. Surgery should be deferred, if possible, until after early childhood because of the probability of increased susceptibility of children to severe bacterial infection after splenectomy. At operation, look carefully for accessory spleens and be prepared to remove the gall bladder if stones are present. Cortisone or corticotropin may be useful to tide a patient over a hemolytic crisis. Preoperative transfusions should be avoided because they tend to precipitate a hemolytic crisis. Once a splenic artery is ligated at operation, it is safe to begin blood replacement.

Idiopathic Thrombocytopenic Purpura.

The cause of idiopathic thrombocytopenic purpura is an autoimmune process in most if not all cases. Platelet agglutinins are commonly found. This disease is seen in 2 forms: (1) an acute, self-limiting illness in infants and children in which remissions usually occur after a few weeks or in some cases as long as a year; and (2) a chronic process in young adults, more commonly women, which may have a remission but often requires splenectomy.

Symptoms and signs vary with the severity of the thrombocytopenia and consist of easy bruising, an otherwise asymptomatic skin rash (petechiae), bleeding from the body orifices or into the subcutaneous tissues, weakness, and loss of weight. Hemorrhage into the brain is the most serious complication, and occurs in 1-5% of cases. The spleen is rarely enlarged; if splenomegaly is present, some other disease such as leukemia should be suspected.

Thrombocytopenia is invariably present, and the blood platelet count may be reduced to 50,000/cu. mm. or lower. The tourniquet test produces multiple petechiae (Rumpel-Leede phenomenon). Bleeding time is prolonged, clotting time is normal, and clot retraction is delayed or absent. Prothrombin consumption is defective. Hyperplasia of the megakaryocytes of the bone marrow is always found, and erythroid hyperplasia is usually observed to a degree consistent with the anemia. The finding of marrow hyperplasia is an essential point in the differentiation of idiopathic from secondary purpura.

Spontaneous recovery is the rule in children; in this age group splenectomy should thus be reserved for uncontrollable bleeding and chronic, recurrent purpura which fails to respond to corticotropin or cortisone. In older patients the danger of intracranial hemorrhage is greater, and splenectomy is indicated if corticosteroids fail to induce a remission.

The platelet count rises promptly after splenectomy and often doubles within the first 24 hours. Splenectomy is considered successful only when the platelet counts have remained normal for at least 2 months. Following splenectomy the response to corticotropin or cortisone may be improved even though thrombocytopenia may be incompletely corrected. Permanent remission follows removal of the spleen in 80-90% of cases.

SECONDARY HYPERSPLENISM

The same cytopenias caused by primary hypersplenism may also be produced by secondary hypersplenism. The splenic dysfunction and enlargement in secondary hypersplenism, however, are caused by chronic diseases such as leukemia and other lymphomas, tuberculosis and other chronic infections, sarcoidosis, Gaucher's disease, and congestive splenomegaly.

Hemolytic anemia is the most common form of secondary hypersplenism. Secondary splenic neutropenia, secondary splenic panhematopenia, and secondary thrombocytopenic purpura also occur.

Although splenectomy does not affect the outcome of the chronic disease which is responsible for the secondary hypersplenism, the hematologic improvement which follows splenectomy justifies surgery in selected cases when other forms of therapy fail. A thorough hematologic work-up preoperatively is essential, and it should be demonstrated that the spleen is contributing to the destruction of the blood elements involved.

ACQUIRED HEMOLYTIC ANEMIA

There are 2 types of acquired hemolytic anemia: (1) idiopathic, in which autoantibodies of the agglutinin or hemolysin type are consistently found and the Coombs (human antiglobulin) test is positive; and (2) symptomatic, which is secondary to poisoning by some toxic agent (e.g., lead, sulfonamides) or malignancy (especially lymphoma). In the idiopathic variety of acquired hemolytic anemia spontaneous remissions may occur, and the manifestations can sometimes be controlled with corticotropin or cortisone. If corticosteroids are not effective, splenectomy should be considered although it is successful in only about 40% of cases. In the symptomatic type of acquired hemolytic anemia, splenectomy may be helpful when there is no response to treatment of the underlying disease or to the administration of corticosteroids.

The response to splenectomy is much less predictable in acquired than in congenital hemolytic anemia. Radioisotope methods have proved valuable in assessing the role of the spleen in hemolysis. Scanning over the spleen, liver, and precordium after injection of autogenous red cells tagged with Cr^{51} shows excessive localization of radioactivity in the spleen when it is the site of excessive red cell destruction, in which case splenectomy will probably be beneficial.

ABDOMINAL HERNIAS

The following types of hernia involve the abdominal organs: (1) External abdominal hernia is any abnormal protrusion through the walls of the peritoneal cavity. This type of hernia presents to the outside, where it is usually visible and palpable. (2) Internal hernia is a protrusion of abdominal viscera into one of the internal abdominal fossae. (3) Diaphragmatic hernia is a protrusion of abdominal contents through a normal or abnormal opening in the diaphragm into the chest.

Hernias may be congenital or acquired. Acquired hernias are the result of trauma, increased intra-abdominal pressure, or abnormal relaxation of normal structures. A hernia may be reducible or irreducible (incarcerated). A strangulated hernia is an irreducible hernia whose blood supply is obstructed, so that the contents will become gangrenous within a few hours unless reduced. The complications of hernia consist of strangulation and the functional disturbances secondary to protrusion or incarceration. Because of the high incidence and possible serious consequences of these complications, surgical repair of most hernias is advisable.

EXTERNAL ABDOMINAL HERNIA

The relative incidence of external hernias is indirect inguinal (60%), direct inguinal (15%), umbilical (9%), incisional (9%), femoral (3%), epigastric (2%), and all others (2%). Those illnesses which cause intermittent or chronic increase of intra-abdominal pressure, such as persistent cough or bladder neck or intestinal obstruction, should be sought for in older patients who develop or suddenly incarcerate a hernia. The treatment of external hernia is surgical. Trusses, binders, and belts are palliative measures reserved for the occasional patient who refuses or is unable to withstand operation.

Indirect Inguinal Hernia.

An indirect hernia consists of the protrusion of abdominal contents through the internal inguinal ring into a congenital diverticulum of peritoneum. This peritoneal sac is the unobliterated processus vaginalis which accompanies the descent of the testis in the male and fixation of the ovary in the female. The sac may be short or may extend into the scrotum to communicate with the tunica vaginalis of the testis. Although indirect hernia may occur at any age, it is more prevalent in the younger age group. There are 2 peaks of incidence of indirect hernia: during the first year of life and during the ages between 10 and 30. It is 9 times more common in males than in females.

A soft, nontender mass in the groin is the usual presenting complaint. Characteristically, this disappears on lying down and reappears on standing, or may be forced out by coughing or straining. Local burning or aching is common. Indirect hernias may extend to the bottom of the scrotum, but direct hernias rarely do so. Occasionally, a hernia is noted for the first time after an episode of sudden strain or severe coughing.

The hernia is best demonstrated by examination of the patient in the standing position. The scrotal skin is invaginated with the index finger until the fingertip is within the external inguinal ring. With the hernia reduced, a sudden cough by the patient will then force the hernia against or past the examining finger and demonstrate its oblique course down the length of the inguinal canal. Digital pressure over the internal inguinal ring will prevent the descent of an indirect hernia, whereas the bulge will still be felt if the hernia is direct. It is often impossible on physical examination to distinguish between direct and indirect hernia, and for practical purposes the distinction is of little importance. Hernias are often bilateral, and (especially in the older age group) direct and indirect hernias ("pantaloon" hernias) may occur together. Indirect hernias are occasionally "sliding," i.e., a viscus (usually the colon) forms part of the wall of the hernial sac. This type of hernia is frequently large and difficult to reduce.

The disorders most likely to be confused with hernia are hydrocele (distinguished by transillumination), varicocele, and inguinal nodes.

Surgical repair is the only satisfactory treatment, and can be done with minimal risk at all ages. Hernias should be repaired unless the patient's general health or advanced age make operation inadvisable. Under these circumstances symptoms can usually be controlled by a properly fitting truss. When a hernia is strangulated, as indicated by incarceration, local pain, and signs of intestinal obstruction, emergency operation is necessary. Following hernia repair the patient is restricted to light activity for 6 weeks to 3 months, but in the average case no restrictions of any kind need be imposed thereafter. The recurrence rate after indirect inguinal hernioplasty is less than 1% in the hands of experienced surgeons. Higher rates are reported in many series.

Direct Inguinal Hernia.

The symptoms, signs, and treatment of direct inguinal hernia are essentially the same as in indirect hernia. Direct hernia often appears as a globular bulge in the region of the external inguinal ring and reduces immediately on recumbency. Direct hernias are rare in females. The tissues involved in direct hernia are usually less suitable for repair than in indirect hernia, and recurrence rates are generally higher (8-50%). However, when careful anatomic repair is carried out, recurrence rates can be reduced to 1-5%.

Femoral Hernia.

A femoral hernia passes through the femoral ring and down the femoral canal to become subcutaneous in the fossa ovalis. It is more common in persons of middle age and is 4 times as frequent in females. These hernias are frequently overlooked, especially in obese individuals, because of their small size. The neck of the femoral sac is invariably small, and incarceration or strangulation of its contents is therefore not unusual.

The diagnosis of femoral hernia should always be considered in unexplained intestinal obstruction. Urinary symptoms, such as dysuria, frequency, or hematuria, will occasionally precede by several months any palpable evidence of a femoral hernia.

Differentiation from inguinal hernia can usually be made with ease by noting the anatomic landmarks. Femoral lymphadenitis may be difficult to distinguish from a strangulated femoral hernia because a tender mass is typical of both. An inflammatory lesion in the lower extremity, genitalia, or perineal region should be sought as a possible cause of lymphadenitis.

Surgical repair is the treatment.

Umbilical Hernia

Adult umbilical hernia is not uncommon, but occurs less frequently than the infantile type (see p. 247). The diagnosis is made with ease by inspection and palpation. The fully developed adult umbilical hernia is prone to incarceration and strangulation and should be repaired surgically.

Epigastric Hernia.

These hernias occur almost entirely in the linea alba between the xiphoid and the umbilicus. The hernia consists of a small mass of fat from the falciform ligament of the liver. Local discomfort is usually present even with very small hernias, and pain secondary to the hernia may be mistaken for that of peptic ulcer or cholelithiasis. Most of these hernias are irreducible and tender. Treatment is by surgical repair.

Incisional Hernia.

Incisional hernias are as various as the abdominal wounds from which they arise, usually as a result of inadequate closure, dehiscence, or infection. Symptoms consist of protrusion and discomfort. Because these hernias tend to increase in size and become more difficult to manage, they should be repaired when the diagnosis is made.

Pelvic Hernia.

Hernias of the pelvic wall and floor are very rare. Obturator hernia leaves the pelvis through the obturator canal; sciatic hernia through the greater sciatic notch; pudendal hernia through the inferior sciatic notch; and perineal hernias through the pelvic diaphragm. These hernias are rarely palpable externally, and are of importance only as unusual causes of intestinal obstruction.

Other External Abdominal Hernias.

Semilunar (Spiegel's) hernia is a protrusion of preperitoneal fat between the aponeurotic fibers of the transversus abdominis, usually at the level of the linea semicircularis. These are very rare and are easily repaired.

A lumbar hernia may occur (1) through the inferior lumbar triangle of Petit, which lies just above the superior margin of the posterior crest of the ilium; or (2) through the superior lumbar triangle of Grynfeltt, which lies just below the distal end of the twelfth rib. These hernias probably begin with the protrusion of retroperitoneal fat into a small neurovascular foramen. They are rare, but must be kept in mind as a possible cause of a mass or pain in the lumbar region. Surgical repair is the treatment.

INTERNAL HERNIA

Internal hernias are very rare. Herniation may occur through the foramen of Winslow or into the paraduodenal or other deep peritoneal recess. A traumatic rent in the omentum or mesentery may provide the hernial ring. Internal hernia must occasionally be considered in the differential diagnosis of intestinal obstruction.

DIAPHRAGMATIC HERNIA

A diaphragmatic hernia consists of the protrusion of one or more abdominal viscera into the thoracic cavity through an aperture in the diaphragm. Large congenital defects of the diaphragm with massive herniation of abdominal viscera usually cause severe symptoms in newborns and require immediate operation (see p. 228). Smaller congenital defects of the parasternal, pleuroperitoneal, or esophageal hiatal region may be the cause of symptomatic hernias in adults or may be incidental findings on x-ray. Clinically, the most frequent and important diaphragmatic hernias are the hiatal and the traumatic.

Esophageal Hiatus Hernia.

The common diaphragmatic hernia seen in adults is associated with an enlarged esophageal hiatus. There are 2 common types: (1) the sliding hernia, in which the cardio-esophageal junction moves upward into the chest, pushing the lower esophagus before it; and (2) the para-esophageal hernia, in which the cardio-esophageal junction tends to remain at its normal level while a portion of the fundus herniates into the thorax alongside the esophagus. A very rare type of hernia is associated with a congenitally short esophagus in which the stomach extends upward through the hiatal opening to join the shortened esophagus in the chest.

Many of these hernias are asymptomatic and are discovered incidentally. The commonest symptoms are probably related to esophagitis and consist of substernal or epigastric distress and heartburn. Discomfort is often made worse by lying down after eating. Nausea and vomiting and dysphagia occur occasionally. Significant bleeding may occur and may be either massive or continuous, and may result in hypochromic anemia.

Physical examination is negative.

Barium study of the upper gastrointestinal tract establishes the diagnosis. Esophagoscopy is often indicated to determine the presence and degree of esophagitis.

Peptic ulcer, chronic cholecystitis, intra-abdominal malignancy, and coronary artery disease must be considered in the differential diagnosis. One must beware of attributing symptoms of a more serious underlying disorder to a hiatus hernia which is found incidentally on upper gastrointestinal x-rays.

Asymptomatic hernias require no treatment. Small hernias with mild symptoms usually respond to an ulcer-type regimen consisting of bland diet, antacids, and anticholinergic drugs. The patient should avoid lying down after meals and should sleep with the head of his bed elevated to minimize the reflux of gastric secretions into the esophagus. When there is a history of significant bleeding or when symptoms persist in spite of conservative measures, repair of the hernia by either the abdominal or the thoracic approach should be recommended.

Traumatic Diaphragmatic Hernia.

Most traumatic hernias involve the tendinous dome of the left diaphragm because the right lobe of the liver tends to protect the right leaf and seal any defects which occur there. Hernias may result from either penetrating or crushing injuries. Traumatic hernias do not have a peritoneal sac. Symptoms usually develop immediately after trauma, but in some instances may not appear for years. Complaints are chiefly respiratory or gastrointestinal, resulting from pulmonary compression or alimentary obstruction.

Diagnosis is established by x-ray.

Treatment is by reduction of the hernia and repair of the defect.

13 . . .

Gynecology

EXAMINATION OF THE GYNECOLOGIC PATIENT

A complete history should be taken on all gynecologic patients. Particular emphasis should be placed on menstrual history, past pregnancies, past gynecologic disorders, and the presence or absence of vaginal discharge, vaginal bleeding, or pelvic pain.

A complete physical examination should also be done, with special attention to the vaginal and combined rectovaginal examination.

Besides the routine blood and urine examination the following tests and examinations are of value:

Gynecologic Laboratory Tests.

A. Vaginal Discharge: Hanging drop or direct saline microscopic examination for Trichomonas vaginalis and (with a few drops of 10% KOH added to clear the debris) for yeast cells.

B. Exfoliative Cytology: (See also p. 506.) Exfoliated material in the posterior vaginal fornix and cervix is collected, smeared on a slide, and fixed immediately. The interpretation of the stained slide for the determination of malignant cells or endocrine status requires special training.

C. Tissue Biopsy: Varies from biopsy of a cervical lesion in the office to endometrial biopsy via dilatation and curettage in the operating room.

D. Tests of Endocrine Function: These are used to test hormonal function and include vaginal cell cornification, the cervical smear fern test, and biologic tests for pregnancy or endocrine gland function.

LEUKORRHEA

Leukorrhea may be defined as a nonbloody discharge from the vagina, usually white but at times yellowish. Normal vaginal "discharge" is clear or white (due to the presence of desquamated epithelium) and is normally present in an amount sufficient to lubricate the vaginal walls; occasionally there may be a small amount of overflow, usually at the time of ovulation.

Trichomonas Vaginalis Vaginitis.

Trichomonas vaginalis causes a vaginal discharge which is heavy, yellow, nonviscous, frothy, has an offensive smell, and is associated with vulval itching. The vaginal mucosa is erythematous and dotted with small areas averaging 5 mm. in diameter which are more red than the surrounding tissue ("strawberry mucosa"). The diagnosis is made by inspecting a small amount of the discharge microscopically.

About 90% of cases will respond to 1 course of trichomonacide treatment. In stubborn cases the organism may be found in the bladder or in the deep cervical mucus glands; conization of the cervix may prove to be beneficial in the latter case.

The most effective means of treatment is with metronidazole (Flagyl®), a systemic agent that reaches the foci of infection in the deeper cervical and paraurethral glands. It is now apparent that the male partner, although asymptomatic, is commonly a carrier of T. vaginalis; both partners should therefore be treated. A dose of 250 mg. twice daily for the male and 250 mg. 3 times daily for the female is usually adequate. A vaginal suppository containing 500 mg. of metronidazole is available; it can be used in conjunction with the oral medication, in which case the oral dose for the female should be decreased to 250 mg. twice daily. If the infection recurs, a second course of metronidazole may be given. Adverse reactions are uncommon and usually mild but, because of an occasional occurrence of leukopenia, 2 courses of treatment should be at least 4 weeks apart, and a precautionary white blood count should be obtained.

Fungal Vaginitis.

Mycotic vaginitis is caused by yeast-like organisms which are often found normally in small numbers in the vagina but which tend to overgrow following antibiotic therapy, in diabetes mellitus, or spontaneously.

The mucosa is intensely inflamed, and the discharge is "cheese-like" in masses of white material. Microscopic examination of a sample of this vaginal discharge shows mycelia and conidia.

The treatment of mycotic vaginitis is usually simpler than that of trichomonal infection. Two to 4 thorough paintings of the vagina and vulva with a 2% aqueous solution of gentian violet or nightly insertion of 1 nystatin (Mycostatin®) vaginal tablet following a vinegar douche for 15 nights will usually effect a cure. Propion-Gel® or Aci-Jel® inserted vaginally, following a water douche, each night for approximately 3 weeks, will cure most cases also.

Noninfectious Leukorrhea.

Leukorrhea at times takes the form of profuse clear mucus which is obviously not infected. This is usually due to a chronically irritated cervix, especially in the endocervical canal.

Treatment is by cauterization of the cervix with silver nitrate or, rarely, with the electrocautery unit. Conization of the cervix may be necessary to decrease the number of mucus-producing glands.

Bacterial Leukorrhea.

Simple bacterial invasion of the intact vagina does not itself cause leukorrhea since the normal nonpathogenic flora will usually overwhelm any pathogens which gain entrance. However, an infected lesion of the vagina or cervix may cause leukorrhea. Specific antibiotics are indicated.

Miscellaneous Rare Causes of Leukorrhea.

Endometritis and fallopian tube inflammation or malignancy may cause leukorrhea. An excess of normal mucus may occur with chronic pelvic congestion or in association with emotional disorders.

Leukorrhea in children, although not commonly seen, is often due to the presence of a foreign body in the vagina. Rectal or x-ray examination should reveal the foreign body.

Gonorrheal Leukorrhea in Children.

Gonorrheal vulvovaginitis occurs only in children, since the mature vaginal epithelium seems to resist infection by this organism. Treatment is by specific antibiotics.

DISORDERS OF THE EXTERNAL FEMALE GENITALIA

IMPERFORATE HYMEN

Imperforate hymen is a rare disorder which may escape detection until the menarche. The onset of menstruation without an avenue of egress for the blood causes distention of the vagina (hematocolpos) and, if not relieved, distention also of the cervix (hematotrachelos), the corpus uteri (hematometra), and the fallopian tubes (hematosalpinx). The symptoms are pain, increasing with each episode of endometrial desquamation; the absence of external bleeding; and, in extreme cases, lower abdominal swelling. Diagnosis is made by finding the bulging, intact hymen. Treatment consists of simple incision of the hymen, with revision to prevent recurrence.

A hymen that is not completely imperforate but that is too small to allow coitus is often found during premarital examination. In most instances the hymen is thin, and the patient can be instructed to dilate the introitus with her fingers for 2-4 weeks. If that much time is not available, an incision can be made at the 6 o'clock position (see p. 498, top), using local anesthesia. Bleeding is not serious, and adhesion of the incised surface can be prevented by means of a lightly placed petrolatum gauze pack. If time is not a factor and finger dilatation is hindered by an inordinate amount of fibrous tissue, a series of 1-2 mm. nicks can be made at the edge of the hymen (see p. 498, bottom). This procedure is relatively painless if the area is benumbed by the "pressure anesthesia" of preliminary stretching, especially if a local anesthetic ointment is used and if the knife edge is quite sharp.

KRAUROSIS VULVAE

Kraurosis vulvae is a degeneration of the subcutaneous fat of the vulvar area; consequent stretching and thinning of the overlying skin produces varying degrees of localized itching and burning. Medical treatment consists of (1) local estrogen therapy in the form of cream or as a vaginal suppository inserted nightly; (2) vitamin A, 50,000 units t.i.d. orally for several months; and (3) cortisone ointment, applied locally one to three times a day as necessary for the control of symptoms. Surgical treatment consists usually of plastic alteration of the introitus to overcome dyspareunia. Vulvectomy may be necessary in extreme cases (see Leukoplakic Vulvitis, below).

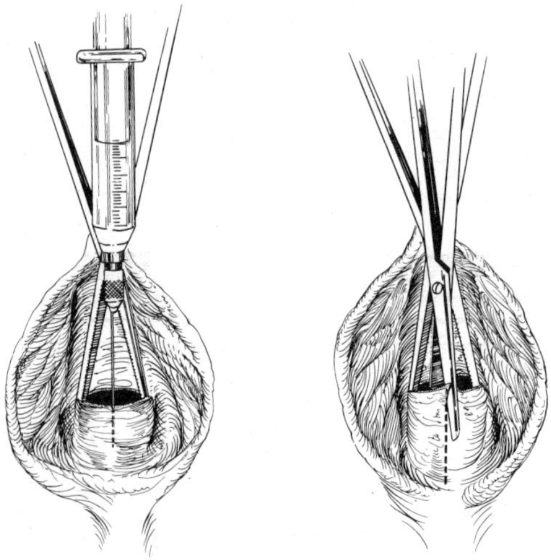

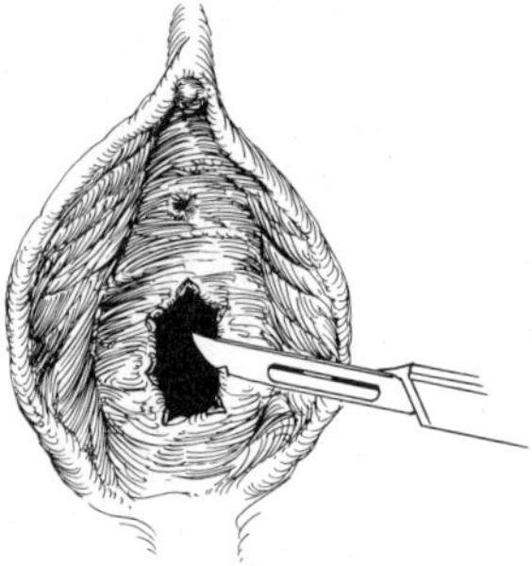

Two Technics of Hymenotomy

LEUKOPLAKIC VULVITIS

Leukoplakic vulvitis is a chronic disorder of unknown cause affecting part or all of the vulva and characterized by white plaques of parchment-like skin. It usually seems (like kraurosis) to be associated with a lack of estrogen and so is most commonly seen in postmenopausal women. The symptoms are pruritus, burning, and dyspareunia.

Leukoplakic vulvitis might well be considered a precancerous lesion, since up to 25% of cases of carcinoma of the vulva have been reported as occurring in an area of leukoplakia. The lesion often responds to local treatment with an estrogen, cortisone, or testosterone ointment; if it does not, biopsy is indicated.

Leukoplakia tends to recur.

BENIGN NEOPLASMS OF THE EXTERNAL GENITALIA AND VAGINA

Cysts.

Sebaceous cysts of the vulvar area are quite common. They may be as large as 4-5 cm. in diameter (usually smaller), are firmly cystic, and are fixed to surrounding tissue. They are not tender unless bruised or secondarily infected. Treatment is by extirpation or by marsupialization and silver nitrate cauterization of the cyst wall.

Wolffian duct cysts are congenital remnants which are usually found in the anterior lateral portion of the vulva (especially near the clitoris). They are typically small, thin-walled, and pedunculated. Treatment is by surgical removal.

Solid Tumors.

Solid benign tumors of the vulva may be composed of any tissue found in the area (leiomyoma, fibroma, lipoma, angioma, hidradenoma, or papilloma). A presumptive diagnosis can be made by inspection of the tumor. Histologic examination of the excised tumor (or biopsy, if malignancy is suspected) will lead to definitive diagnosis.

Condyloma acuminata is a rather common papillomatous growth of epithelium which varies in size from a small "wart" to an extensive distribution of isolated growths or a confluent mass covering the entire vulvar, perineal, anal, and upper thigh areas. It is sometimes seen also in the vagina and on the epithelium of the cervix. Originally termed "venereal wart" because it commonly coexists with gonorrhea, it may occur as a result of chronic local irritation due to persistent vaginal discharge from any cause.

Microscopically, the tumor is a papilloma with great masses of stratified squamous epithelium (often in whorls, with central degeneration), giving an epithelial pearl-like appearance. The firm basement membrane which is always present differentiates this lesion from malignant papilloma.

The lesions may be extirpated surgically or destroyed by electrocoagulation. The local application of podophyllin, 20-25% in an oil or ointment base, usually causes the warts to disappear, but the lesions are apt to recur if the original source of vulvar irritation is not removed.

MALIGNANT NEOPLASMS OF THE EXTERNAL GENITALIA AND VAGINA

Carcinoma of the Vulva.

Carcinoma of the vulva may be secondary to a primary lesion of one of the other genital structures, but this is rare. Primary carcinoma of the vulva, comprising about 3% of all gynecologic cancers, is usually found in women 60-70 years of age. Diagnosis is not difficult since inspection of the vulva reveals the lesion and a biopsy specimen for histologic examination can be quickly obtained. The neoplasm is nearly always epidermoid, and may display any degree of anaplastic activity.

The treatment of vulvar carcinoma is radical surgical removal (including all regional lymph nodes), since the lesion has usually proved to be resistant to irradiation. Operative treatment is often remarkably successful. Five-year survival rates as high as 90% have been reported, but 50% is the more common experience.

DISORDERS OF THE FEMALE URETHRA

INFLAMMATORY URETHRAL DISORDERS

The para-urethral glands (Skene's) may become abscessed (often as a result of gonorrheal infection), and should be drained, if possible, by locating and opening the ducts through the urethral mucosa. This disorder may be simulated by a urethral diverticulum, which may have been formed by a previous abscess. The diverticulum may be diagnosed by endoscopic examination or x-ray films using contrast media. Treatment of diverticulum is by surgical excision and reconstruction.

PROLAPSE OF THE URETHRA

Prolapse of the urethral mucosa resembles and may be difficult to differentiate from neoplastic tissue. Reduction may be attempted, but resection must be resorted to if this is not successful. Since the prolapsed mucosa may bring the ureteral orifices down with it, the exact location of the ureteral orifices should be demonstrated by urography before resection is performed.

NEOPLASMS OF THE URETHRA

Neoplasms are occasionally seen in the urethra. Caruncle, usually seen in women past the menopause, is a benign tumor of the urethral meatus which presents as a red, raspberry-like tumor. It is quite painful and tender. Diagnosis depends upon microscopic examinations of an excised specimen. There are 3 histologic types: papillomatous, angiomatous, and granulomatous. Treatment is by resection, which may be technically difficult because of the great vascularity of the region.

Carcinoma of the urethra is uncommon and sarcoma is rare. They are differentiated from caruncle by biopsy. Treatment is by radical surgical extirpation unless the lesion has progressed to the incurable stage, in which case palliative irradiation may be useful.

DISORDERS OF BARTHOLIN'S GLAND

ABSCESS OF BARTHOLIN'S GLAND

Bartholin's gland may be acutely infected by the gonococcus or other pathogen, resulting in an extremely painful abscess. The abscess frequently ruptures spontaneously by the time it reaches 5 cm. in diameter, or it may be drained by incision at any time when it becomes fluctuant. However, since incision and drainage are frequently followed by recurrence of the abscess or by the formation of a cyst, marsupialization is preferable. Marsupialization is accomplished by making an adequate incision and assuring patency of the gaping wound by suturing the abscess wall to the adjacent skin with interrupted fine absorbable sutures. A small pack may be maintained in the cavity for 1-2 days, but this is usually not necessary. Healing is rather slow, but the cosmetic result is surprisingly good and recurrence is rare.

If the patient should present herself before the abscess "points," it may be aborted in most instances by a simple office procedure. The pus is evacuated as thoroughly as possible by aspiration and the patient is maintained on broad-spectrum antibiotic therapy for 4-10 days. If aspiration is inadequate or if pus accumulates again in 1-2 days, aspiration must be repeated.

CYST OF BARTHOLIN'S GLAND

A cyst of a Bartholin's gland may develop following infection as a result of obstruction of the draining duct by scarring. An uninfected cyst is not harmful, but it may be annoying to the patient. Aspiration is rarely successful; surgical excision or marsupialization is usually necessary.

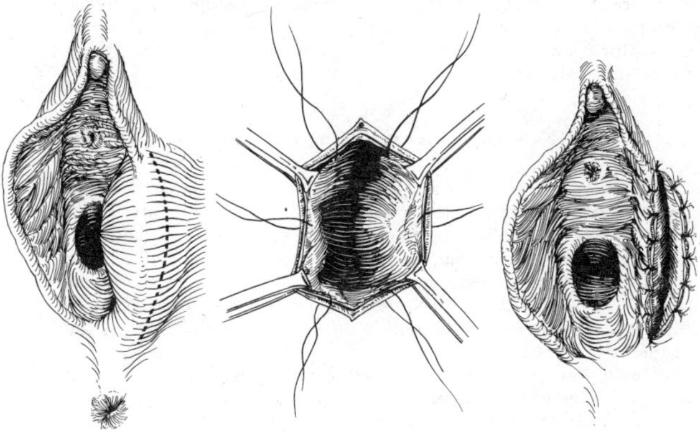

Marsupialization of Bartholin's Cyst

CARCINOMA OF BARTHOLIN'S GLAND

Carcinoma (adenocarcinoma) of Bartholin's glands is occasionally seen. An epidermoid form may occur which most likely originates in the transitional epithelium of the duct. The carcinoma presents as a localized mass which is painless unless secondary infection occurs. Treatment consists of radical bilateral vulvectomy and inguinal node resection.

DISORDERS OF THE VAGINA

CONGENITAL DISORDERS OF THE VAGINA

If congenital vaginal septa or constricting bands interfere with coitus or childbirth, plastic repair is indicated. More serious congenital disorders such as total absence of the vagina are rarely encountered. Proper management includes accurate diagnostic measures to ascertain the patient's genetic sex; psychiatric evaluation of the patient's libido (psychic sex); and often extensive and expert plastic surgical procedures.

INJURIES TO THE VAGINA

Traumatic lesions of the vagina are most commonly caused by the instrumentation involved in attempted criminal abortion. The inept abortionist (often the patient herself) may force an instrument into the vagina as far as possible, thus injuring or perforating the posterior fornix. If perforation has occurred, exploratory laparotomy may be indicated to rule out injury, infection, or chemical irritation. Suturing usually suffices to repair the defect.

In some cases of attempted abortion the vaginal lesion may be a caustic burn caused by the insertion of potassium permanganate tablets or other chemicals. These usually burn a hole in the mucosa which may penetrate up to 2 cm. in depth. Bleeding may be brisk, but can be controlled by suturing.

NEOPLASMS OF THE VAGINA

Gartner's duct cysts arise in unobliterated remnants of the lower portion of the wolffian duct, and thus are seen only in the anterolateral portion of the vagina. These cysts are usually small and asymptomatic, but may become large enough to cause dyspareunia. Treatment is by surgical removal. Microscopic examination of the cyst wall shows the cuboidal ciliated epithelium of the wolffian remnant, which may be flattened by the internal pressure of the cyst.

Inclusion cysts may be formed by infolding of the epithelial surface following obstetric or surgical tissue disruption. The infolded mucosa desquamates, producing a cyst of thick white material. These cysts are rarely large or symptomatic, but they may be excised easily if annoying.

The relatively rare solid benign tumors of the vagina are composed of any of the tissues usually found in the area: myoma, fibroma, papilloma, and myxoma. If there are no symptoms, surgical removal is indicated only to rule out malignancy by histologic examination of the specimen.

Primary carcinoma or sarcoma is rarely seen. Bleeding, especially postcoital, is the presenting sign. Biopsy is required. Lymphatic spread is early and rapid, and local extensions often cause fistulas. The survival rates following radical surgical procedures have not been encouraging; the usual method of treatment is irradiation, but the five-year survival rate is only about 20%.

DISORDERS OF THE CERVIX

CONGENITAL LESIONS OF THE CERVIX

Congenital atresia or even absence of the cervix may occur, but congenital cervical lesions are usually associated with abnormalities of the corpus of the uterus and will be considered in that section.

TRAUMA TO THE CERVIX

Traumatic cervical lesions are nearly always the result of instrumentation or childbirth. In the former case the damage can be seen by inspection and appropriate surgical repair instituted. The bilateral cervical tearing associated with one or more deliveries tends to change the cervical os from a small round opening 5 mm. in diameter to a transverse opening. These tears may be so deep that anterior and posterior "lips" gape open and expose the mucosa of the cervical canal. This tends to cause an excess of mucus production, usually the only symptom. Moderate lesions can be treated in the office by cauterization of the angles of the cervix. More extensive disruptions will require plastic surgical repair.

INCOMPETENT INTERNAL OS OF THE CERVIX

Incompetent internal cervical os is a disorder in which the internal os fails to hold a pregnancy, giving way in the second trimester or early in the third trimester. The condition may be congenital or may be due to the trauma of a previous delivery or a too forceful instrumental cervical dilatation. The incompetence of the os can be demonstrated, after complete postpartum uterine involution, if a sound or dilator more than 7 mm. in diameter can be passed into the canal. The defect may also be demonstrated by radiographic means, but this is rarely necessary.

Treatment is by surgical repair. This may be performed by the excision of a small wedge of tissue at the internal cervical os followed by repair of the defect with firmly-placed chromic sutures; or by strengthening the tissues of the cervix by the implantation of fibrosis-producing irritants or the insertion of a firm band of Mersilene® (see p. 504), a synthetic material made especially for the purpose. Mersilene® can also be put into place while the patient is pregnant if abortion due to this defect is a threat. The fetal salvage rate by any of these methods is at least 50% (higher in the hands of experienced obstetricians).

INFLAMMATORY DISORDERS OF THE CERVIX

Inflammation of the cervix may be acute, as in acute gonorrhea, but this is quite rare. Chronic nonspecific cervicitis, however, is one of the most common lesions seen in the gynecologist's office.

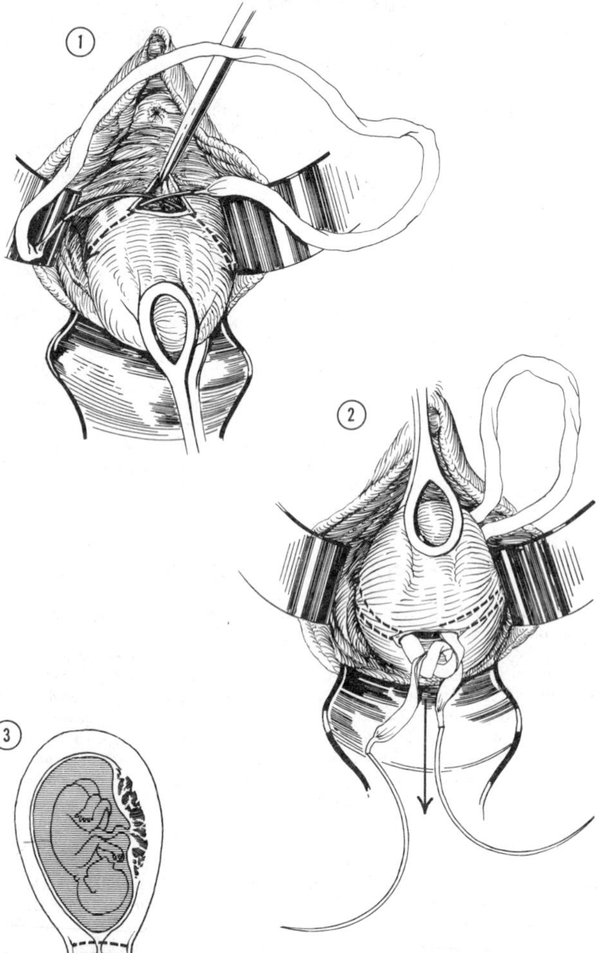

Shirodkar Cerclage of Cervix With Incompetent Os

The chronically irritated tissue of the portio vaginalis area surrounding the external cervical os, normally covered by stratified squamous epithelium, becomes overgrown by the cylindric mucus-producing cells of the cervical canal, producing the 2 characteristics of the lesion: Leukorrhea and a reddened surface which looks like an erosion. If the lumens of the mucus-producing glands of the cervix become occluded, retention cysts (nabothian cysts) are formed. Microscopically, the submucosal connective tissue is infiltrated by round cells, plasma cells, and sometimes by polymorphonuclear cells. The gland epithelium is often replaced in some areas by a stratified squamous epithelium (epidermidalization) which may be difficult to distinguish from carcinoma.

Mild cervicitis may be treated by local caustic (silver nitrate) applications, carefully applied. Severe cervicitis may be treated by destruction of the overgrown cylindric epithelium by electrocautery so that a normal squamous epithelium can develop. Cauterization can be performed in the office without anesthesia since the cervix has few nerve-ends sensitive to heat. The cautery tip is stroked over the surface of the cervix in a radial pattern and may be inserted 1-2 cm. into the cervical canal if necessary. Light pressure on the cautery tip is usually advisable since the lesion is rarely deep in the tissues. Cauterization of the endocervix should be judiciously performed because excessive scar tissue might cause stenosis of the cervix. Stenosis can be prevented by monthly passage of a uterine sound until patency of the cervical canal is assured.

In extreme cases, conization of the cervix should be performed (see p. 508).

Other inflammatory lesions of the cervix such as tuberculosis or the granulomatous venereal diseases occur rarely. Diagnosis depends upon biopsy and specific tests.

Stricture of the cervix may follow inflammation or the treatment of inflammation, but since stricture may also be caused by tissue proliferation malignancy must be ruled out. During the menacme the symptoms are lower abdominal pain and cramping due to hematometra; the postmenopausal patient may have the same symptoms plus fever (due to pyometra) or may have no symptoms. Treatment is by dilatation, which may be sufficiently difficult to warrant hospitalization and anesthesia.

Leukoplakia of the cervix, not often seen, is considered by some to be the same precancerous lesion as leukoplakia of the vulva (see p. 498), but this view is not supported by statistics. Even so, the lesion should be biopsied and, if not malignant, observed repeatedly for evidence of malignant change.

CERVICAL POLYP

The most common benign neoplasm of the cervix is the cervical polyp, a localized area of endocervical epithelium which enlarges until it becomes pedunculated. Polyps may be single or multiple, and vary from 1-2 mm. to 7-8 cm. in diameter. Contact bleeding (coitus, douching) commonly occurs, and there may be an excessive nonbloody discharge.

The polyp should be removed, usually by simply twisting it off and lightly cauterizing its base. If numerous polyps are seen high in the cervical canal, it may be necessary to dilate and curet the canal under anesthesia. The polyps should be examined microscopically for malignancy.

CERVICAL CARCINOMA

Carcinoma of the cervix is the commonest (55%) of all female pelvic malignancies. Two to 3% of all cervices become carcinomatous, usually in patients between the ages of 45 and 55. Recent evidence suggests that cervical carcinoma is more common in women who have had prolonged exposure to the smegma bacillus (especially those who were quite young at the time of first sexual exposure) and who have had several children than in women who have had no contact with smegma (virgins, Jewish women) or have had no children.

The carcinoma may be adenomatous (5%) or epidermoid (95%); the gross appearance, symptoms, and management do not differ in the 2 types.

Clinical Findings.

A. Symptoms: The symptoms, in the usual order of appearance, are abnormal discharge, bleeding (especially contact), and, in the later stages, pain. Most other symptoms are the result of extension of the disease.

B. Signs: Inspection usually discloses an eroding (or, at times, benign-appearing) lesion which bleeds easily, but there may be no visible lesion. On palpation the cervix usually has a hard consistency; it may or may not be nodular. In the later stages of the disease, extension of the mass may be felt as it grows into the parametrial area or the vagina, bladder, or rectum.

C. Laboratory Findings: The diagnosis may be suggested by the vaginal "smear test," but must be proved by biopsy.

1. The Papanicolaou smear test consists of smearing a slide with desquamated cervical epithelial cells found in the vaginal fornix and the cervix and then fixing, staining, and examining the cells for malignant change. Several methods of preparing the slides have been developed, and various systems of reporting the findings are in use; it is important for each physician to prepare his slides in the manner advised by his cytologist and to have a complete understanding of the significance of the cytologist's report.

   The Papanicolaou smear should be part of the routine examination of women in the cancer age group. It is considered accurate in 95-98% of cases of carcinoma of the cervix and in 60-90% of cases of carcinoma of the corpus, but it is unreliable in carcinoma of the tube and of no value in the diagnosis of ovarian malignancy. In any case it is a screening test only, to be verified by biopsy if positive.

   A technic of taking and mailing Papanicolaou smears is described in "Cytology and Cancer of the Cervix," American Cancer Society, 1957, but each physician who treats women patients should work with a competent cytologist and should follow his instructions in the performance of this vitally important procedure.

2. Biopsy of the cervix may be done by the use of a punch biopsy forceps specially designed for the purpose or by knife or scissors excision of the tissue. A specimen should be obtained from each of the 4 quadrants of the cervix. It is often preferable to do a conization of the cervix, particularly if no definite lesion is visible. By whatever method the biopsy is taken, adequate tissue is essential and the area of the squamo-columnar junction must be represented.

Clinical Classification.

Once the diagnosis is made, the carcinoma must then be "staged." Since the method of treatment employed varies with the degree of extension of the malignancy and since the comparison of results obtained by various methods depends upon an agreed terminology, a classification into clinical "stages" has been developed. The following International Classification, an outgrowth of the League of Nations Classification, is now used almost exclusively.

Stage 0: Carcinoma in situ (also termed intraepithelial carcinoma or preinvasive carcinoma). In Stage 0 the carcinoma has not extended past the basement membrane of the epithelium.

Stage I: The carcinoma has extended past the basement membrane but is confined to the cervix.

Stage II: The carcinoma extends past the cervix into the parametrial tissues or the vagina, but has not reached the pelvic wall or the lower third of the vagina.

Stage III: The carcinoma has reached the pelvic wall or the lower third of the vagina.

Stage IV: The carcinoma has extended into the rectum, the bladder, or any other area beyond those previously defined.

The "stage" is properly included in the disease nomenclature, e.g., "carcinoma, epidermoid, of cervix, Stage II."

Repeated attempts have been made to "grade" the tumor according to its microscopic appearance, with the object of basing the selection of methods of treatment on the degree of anaplasticity of the cells. No practical application of this categorization is completely dependable at this time.

Treatment.

A. Stage 0: Stage 0 is usually treated by total hysterectomy, but this degree of malignancy does not necessitate removal of the adnexa. Cervical amputation or conization (see p. 508) may be adequate to remove an intraepithelial lesion, and this might be considered should the patient desire future pregnancy. However, she should be made aware of the possible inadequacy of this treatment and should be advised to return at frequent intervals for visual and cytohistologic examination.

B. Stages I-IV: When adequate facilities and personnel are available, radium and/or external irradiation therapy is usually preferred. The best method of radiation therapy is to deliver a minimum of 6000 R to the cervix and the areas of lymphatic spread at the sides of the cervix. However, some gynecologists prefer radical pelvic surgery: extirpation of the uterus with a

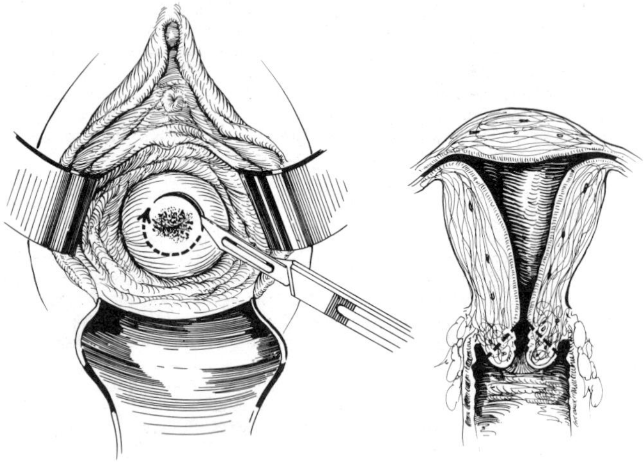

Conization of the Cervix

cuff of vagina, tubes, ovaries, the regional lymph nodes, and all intervening tissue which may contain channels of lymphatic spread or points of direct extension. The surgical approach is generally used in situations where radiotherapy has been tried without complete success or where surgical personnel have demonstrated their ability to carry out this radical procedure without a prohibitive operative mortality rate.

Prognosis.

Using the best methods of treatment available at this time, the following five-year survival rates are to be expected:

Stage 0:	100%
Stage I:	70-90%
Stage II:	35-60%
Stage III:	5-15%
Stage IV:	0%

CERVICAL SARCOMA

Botryoid ("grape-like") sarcoma is a rare dysontogenetic cervical lesion which is usually found in early life (at times even at birth) or after the menopause. It presents as a mass of red or purplish polypoid structures, which may fill the vagina. Histologically the tumor is composed of various embryonic tissues (e.g., striped muscle, cartilage, nerve tissue) in the mass of malignant connective tissue cells. Surgical removal and/or irradiation may be employed in treatment, but cures are rarely reported.

Sarcoma of the cervix composed of round or spindle cells has been reported, but these are so extremely rare that they will not be discussed here.

DISORDERS OF THE CORPUS UTERI

CONGENITAL LESIONS OF THE UTERUS

Congenital lesions of the uterus are not uncommon; some type occurs in 1-2% of all women. The anomaly is due to failure of complete fusion of the two müllerian ducts, which produces various degrees of reduplication of the genital structures. Failure of development of one müllerian duct results in uterus unicornis or uterus bicornis unicollis with one horn rudimentary. Failure of development of both müllerian ducts results in hypoplasia of the uterus, varying in degree from minor (infantile uterus) to marked (absence of the uterus).

The clinical significance of these disorders varies with the type of anomaly: amenorrhea with absence or marked hypoplasia of the uterus, relative or absolute infertility, and interference with the development of a pregnancy or dystocia at the time of delivery. Many patients, however, achieve conception and uncomplicated parturition despite anomalous genitalia.

Plastic surgical procedures on uteri of adequate size are often successful in correcting infertility or dystocia. Hormonal treatment of uterine hypoplasia has been disappointing.

TRAUMATIC DISORDERS OF THE UTERUS

Perforation of the wall of the uterus during dilatation and curettage is the only significant uterine trauma of appreciable incidence. If, during this procedure, the instrument should penetrate the wall and the patient goes into shock, immediate laparotomy is indicated for the purpose of controlling hemorrhage and repairing or removing the damaged uterus or other abdominal viscera. If, as is more often the case, the perforation does not produce untoward symptoms, observation is all that may be required and an uneventful recovery is to be expected.

MYOMAS OF THE UTERUS

Myomas of the uterus ("fibroids"), composed of smooth muscle cells of the uterine corpus, are found in about 20% of all white women over 30 years of age; colored races are more commonly afflicted. The etiology is not known, but since these tumors appear during the menacme and stop growing with the menopause, the ovarian hormones have been incriminated. Myomas are associated with infertility, but no pathogenetic relationship has been established.

Myomas can occur singly but are usually multiple. They vary in size from "seedlings" to massive growths filling the abdominal cavity and weighing up to 100 lb. According to their position in the uterine wall, these tumors may be characterized as submucous, intramural, or subserous (submucous and subserous myomas may be pedunculated). A myoma may also grow to the side of the uterus between the leaves of the broad ligament (intraligamentary myoma).

Clinical Findings.

A. Symptoms: Many patients with uterine myomas have no symptoms even when the tumor is of considerable size; other women present only as infertility problems. Symptoms, when present, depend upon the size and position of the growths. Submucous myomas tend to cause abnormal bleeding by eroding the mucosal surface on the same or opposite side or by interfering with the normal vascular pattern of the overlying endometrium. If submucous myomas are large or pedunculated they may cause pain, especially of the dysmenorrhea type. Subserous myoma in itself causes no bleeding and no pain, but it may disrupt the menstrual pattern by interfering with normal ovarian function and may cause pain if it presses upon an adjacent structure. A pedunculated tumor may become twisted, precipitating an acute abdominal crisis.

B. Signs: The physical examination will disclose a tumor of palpable size, but other firm pelvic tumors may also present similar pelvic masses. A submucous myoma would not be apparent to the examiner's hands; it may be suspected if the uterus is enlarged, if other types of myoma are present, or if an abnormal mass is felt in the uterine cavity with the probing tip of a uterine sound or curet.

Differential Diagnosis.

In the management of myomas of the uterus, it must be borne in mind that bleeding from the uterus, even in the presence of myomas, may be due to other causes (specifically, carcinoma).

Treatment.

In most cases the best treatment is total hysterectomy. If the patient desires future pregnancy and if the uterus is sufficiently intact so that pregnancy may be anticipated, myomectomy may be preferred. However, the pregnancy rate following myomectomy is disappointingly low, and the recurrence rate due to growth of unexcised "seedlings" is high. The growth of the tumor may be halted by irradiation castration, but this method of treatment is not commonly used today. Myomas which are not too large, are not growing rapidly, and are asymptomatic may be kept under frequent observation in the expectation that no complication will occur and that tumor growth will stop after menopause.

Course and Prognosis.

Degenerative changes may occur, usually as a result of alterations in vascularity. The types of degeneration are (1) hyaline, (2) cystic, (3) calcific, (4) suppurative, (5) necrotic ("red"), (6) fatty, and (7) sarcomatous. The degeneration may cause pain due to necrosis, but is otherwise of no clinical significance except for the 0.5-1% which become sarcomatous (see Sarcoma, p. 512).

ADENOMYOSIS OF THE UTERUS

Adenomyosis of the uterus is the extension into the myometrium of benign endometrium. When extensive, the growths cause a diffuse uterine enlargement which is rarely sufficient to be noticeable upon bimanual pelvic examination. Microscopically, endometrial tissue is scattered throughout the myometrium, and the extension of this tissue from the surface of the uterine wall can sometimes be traced. The symptoms are pain with menstruation and, in some cases, increased menstrual flow. Bimanual examination, especially at the time of menses, discloses a tender, boggy uterus.

The usual treatment is hysterectomy, but the suppression of endometrial growth by progestogens sometimes controls the symptoms.

CARCINOMA OF THE CORPUS

Carcinoma of the corpus uteri involves the endometrium. It occurs almost as frequently as carcinoma of the cervix, usually in the age group from 50 to 60. Histologically the tumor is usually an adenocarcinoma, with marked overgrowth of endometrial tissue and typical malignant cell changes. Occasional variations in appearance (e.g., "squamous cell carcinoma") are seen. Growth of the tissue into the uterine cavity eventually produces bleeding. Extension into the wall of the uterus may be minimal or marked. Lymphatic or hematogenous spread to other pelvic organs or distant sites is typically late.

The presenting symptom is nearly always abnormal bleeding; the postmenopausal bleeder is particularly apt to have carcinoma. (**Note**: One in 5 of such patients will have carcinoma.) There may be abnormal discharge, and pain is a late symptom.

Since excessive or prolonged exposure to estrogens is associated with greater than normal incidence of uterine carcinoma, this tumor should be watched for especially in the patient with a history of late menopause, endometrial hyperplasia, or the diabetes-obesity-hypertension triad.

The definitive diagnosis can be made only by the microscopic examination of endometrium obtained by curettage or biopsy. At present the Papanicolaou smear test is not as reliable for corpus carcinoma as it is for cervical carcinoma.

Treatment and Prognosis.

Treatment consists of total hysterectomy and bilateral salpingo-oophorectomy in early cases; lymphadenectomy also may occasionally be indicated.

Some gynecologists prefer to irradiate the uterus prior to surgery in the belief that irradiation prevents spread of the tumor, but recent statistics indicate that this may not be necessary, especially in early cases, since surgery alone in this group has a five-year survival rate of up to 90%. If there is any indication that the malignancy involves the entire uterus (enlarged uterus) or extends to adjacent organs, preoperative irradiation is indicated. If intercurrent disease or poor physical condition contraindicates surgery, intracavitary radium and external irradiation may be used; fairly good results (five-year survival rates up to 50%) have been reported.

The management of the patient should be individualized, depending upon the clinical impression of the extent of the disease.

Large doses of progesterone (e.g., hydroxyprogesterone caproate [Delalutin®]) for the relief of the symptoms of extensive, incurable corpus carcinoma have resulted in temporary remission in about 30% of patients. The usual dose is 1 Gm. I.M. 3 times a week until remission is demonstrated, whereupon the dosage is reduced to about 0.5 Gm. per week depending upon the response. Dosage must be individualized; if no results are apparent in 1 month, this method of therapy should be considered to be of no value.

SARCOMA OF THE UTERUS

Sarcoma may arise from any of the connective tissue elements of the uterus, but it most commonly originates in a myoma (0.5-1% of myomas). Abnormal vaginal discharge and bleeding are the only symptoms until the growth reaches a noticeable size or causes pressure pain in an adjacent structure; unusually rapid growth of a myoma should alert the physician to its presence. A negative Papanicolaou smear is unreliable as a diagnostic aid.

Treatment.

Treatment is by surgical removal of the entire uterus and both tubes and ovaries. Since sarcoma is usually not discovered until operation, it is essential that all myomas be bisected for inspection at this time so that the surgeon can remove all of the internal genital structures if the malignancy is discovered. If a report of sarcoma is not received from the pathologist until several days after supravaginal hysterectomy, the cervical stump should receive a course of irradiation. Supravaginal hysterectomy, however, is rarely indicated today. The total uterus should almost always be removed, and there can certainly be no justification for failing to remove the cervix in a postmenopausal patient with a growing tumor of the uterine corpus.

DISORDERS OF THE FALLOPIAN TUBES

ACUTE PELVIC INFLAMMATORY DISEASE

Infection of the fallopian tubes is extremely common during the menacme but rare in women who have ceased to menstruate. The most common infecting organisms are the gonococcus and streptococcus, but staphylococci, Escherichia coli, and occasionally tubercle bacilli may also be found. Salpingitis may occur (independently of venereal infection) in the immediate postpartum period as puerperal sepsis and accompanying abortion as septic abortion.

In most instances of salpingitis the infection spreads rapidly throughout the pelvis ("pelvic inflammatory disease"). The contralateral tube is involved within 24 hours, and within 72 hours the infection will spread to the entire uterus, all adnexal structures, and the parametrial lymphatic, vascular, and areolar tissues. As the process continues there is infection of the adjacent visceral and parietal peritoneum. Pelvic thrombophlebitis is common, and embolism may occur. As the body defenses come into play, the infection will become walled off by the formation of abscesses. These may involve a tube (pyosalpinx) or a tube and ovary (tubo-ovarian abscess), or may lodge in the cul-de-sac as a "pelvic abscess." Eventually the abscesses become sterile, the purulent elements are absorbed, and the dilated tube - now a thin-walled sac - becomes filled with a clear, sterile fluid (hydrosalpinx). The pelvic abscess, if untreated, usually ruptures spontaneously into the posterior fornix of the vagina, occasionally into the abdominal cavity, or, more commonly, into the rectum or bladder.

Clinical Findings.

Inflammation causes pelvic pain, fever, chills and sweats. Vomiting, bloating, and constipation result as pelvic peritonitis develops. Pelvic examination reveals an excruciatingly tender pelvis, with a mass or masses if the walling off process has begun. If peritonitis has developed there will be a rigid abdomen, rebound tenderness, and decreased peristalsis. The WBC will be high with a marked shift to the left, and the sedimentation rate will be accelerated.

Treatment.

Medical treatment consists of appropriate antibiotics in adequate amounts, usually a broad-spectrum antibiotic or a combination of antibiotic drugs. When this condition is extremely acute it is an indication for massive doses of antibiotics: tetracycline, 0.5 Gm. every 4 hours; or up to 60 million units of penicillin and 2 Gm. of streptomycin per 24 hours, until the infection is under control. Other measures include absolute bed rest and fluid replacement. Should a pelvic abscess "point" in the posterior vaginal fornix, the fluctuant, bulging area should be incised (colpotomy) and rubber drains placed in the cul-de-sac for 4-7 days or longer.

If the infection can be halted by antibiotics before an abscess has formed, a definitive cure may be obtained.

For marked destruction of the reproductive organs ("pelvic cripple"), the usual surgical procedure is removal of both tubes and the uterus. An involved ovary should also be removed, but a normal ovary should be left in place unless there is some other reason for its removal.

Prognosis.

Before the era of antibiotic therapy the mortality rate of pelvic inflammatory disease was as high as 25% in some series. Although the mortality rate is now almost negligible, this is still a serious disease since it causes infertility and may become chronic with recurrent acute exacerbations (see below).

CHRONIC PELVIC INFLAMMATORY DISEASE

Chronic pelvic inflammatory disease is nearly always preceded by the acute disease. In many instances an acute attack which has apparently been cured by antibiotics will recur. The patient may be completely free of symptoms and abnormal physical findings except during repeated acute attacks, or there may be residual pelvic "soreness" between acute attacks which causes dysmenorrhea and dyspareunia and forces the patient to limit her activities ("pelvic cripple"). Although antibiotic therapy may be effective during an acute exacerbation, surgical removal of the involved structures is usually the only method of relief for the pain and disability brought on by recurrent or chronic pelvic inflammatory disease.

TUBERCULOUS SALPINGITIS

Tuberculosis of the pelvis (usually secondary to tuberculosis elsewhere) most commonly involves the fallopian tubes first and most extensively. Although tuberculous infection of the tubes has been reported in 5% of all cases of pelvic inflammatory disease, its incidence is decreasing. It rarely becomes acute, more often presenting the symptoms and signs of chronic pelvic inflammatory disease. Since it involves the tubes primarily, it is sometimes found in the patient whose only complaint is infertility.

The disease is diagnosed at surgery or in the pathology laboratory. The typical tubercles on the peritoneal surface of the tubes will, of course, indicate the true nature of the inflammatory process, but these are not commonly present.

In the past treatment has been surgical removal of all pelvic organs. However, antituberculosis drugs should be tried first in patients who desire future pregnancies.

NEOPLASTIC DISEASE OF THE FALLOPIAN TUBES

Carcinoma (adenocarcinoma) of the fallopian tubes is not common. Because it may not cause bleeding or desquamation of tumor cells to and through the uterus and cervix, the chances of making an early diagnosis on the basis of abnormal bleeding or a positive Papanicolaou smear are remote. The patient may notice gradually intensifying one-sided pelvic pain. A growing adnexal mass, especially in a postmenopausal patient, must be investigated surgically.

The only treatment is surgical removal, but the cure rate is only about 5-10% and most of these few successes are with early tumors discovered during surgery for some other condition.

Parovarian cysts (wolffian remnants) may develop in the mesosalpinx and may reach such a size that removal is indicated. It is not possible by pelvic examination to differentiate between an ovarian and a parovarian cyst. This is immaterial, however, since cysts of a certain size (see p. 515) must be removed.

Parovarian cysts are rarely malignant.

DISORDERS OF THE OVARIES

The ovaries may be small or absent as a result of congenital maldevelopment; and they may become involved in pelvic inflammatory disease (see p. 512). Aside from these abnormalities, ovarian disorders are almost exclusively neoplastic in origin.

OVARIAN TUMORS

Because ovarian tumors are so varied in type and because our knowledge of the origins of some of them is incomplete, it is not possible to develop a completely satisfactory system of classification. The classification used here is chosen primarily for its clinical usefulness.

Cystic Tumors.

A. Nonneoplastic:

1. Follicle cysts - These are caused by failure of the normal follicle to rupture or failure of the incompletely developed follicle to be reabsorbed. They rarely grow to more than 5 cm. in diameter or persist longer than 60 days; a larger or more persistent ovarian cyst should be considered pathologic. Symptoms are produced by follicle cysts only in the uncommon event of torsion or rupture with hemorrhage. The cysts are usually reabsorbed spontaneously.
2. Corpus luteum cysts - Usually caused by an excess amount of bleeding into the corpus luteum cavity. This may be associated with pregnancy, and very large lutein cysts occasionally accompany hydatidiform mole. Corpus luteum cysts may cause a delay in menstruation; otherwise symptomatology and course are as described for follicle cysts.
3. Germinal inclusion cysts - Incidental findings at microscopic examination of ovaries; of no clinical importance.
4. Endometrial cysts - See Endometriosis, p. 521.

B. Neoplastic:

1. Benign -
    a. Pseudomucinous cystadenomas - These may become huge, are usually multilocular, and contain a clear, more or less viscid fluid. They are lined by tall columnar cells, and goblet cells are usually present also. This suggests the most commonly accepted theory of their histogenesis: that these cysts are teratomas composed entirely of entoderm. Another theory is that they originate in Brenner tumors (see p. 516). Except for their size, the cysts are symptomless unless torsion or accidental rupture occurs. Treatment is by surgical removal.
    b. Serous cystadenomas - These usually do not grow to such huge proportions, are often unilocular, and have a tendency toward papillary excrescences on both their outer and inner surfaces. They are lined by cuboid or short columnar cells, many of which are ciliated. Small calcareous deposits (psammoma bodies) are often seen. These tumors arise from invaginations of the germinal epithelium of the surface of the ovary. They should be removed surgically.
    c. Dermoid cysts - These are cystic teratomas consisting primarily of well-differentiated ectodermal elements (hair, teeth, sebaceous material) but often containing some mesodermal structures also. They probably arise as a parthenogenetic process in the ovarian ova, but other theories of their origin have not been disproved. Diagnosis is often made by the radiographic demonstration of teeth in the tumor. Torsion of the pedicle of a

dermoid cyst is common, since these heavy growths often stretch the pedicle to surprising lengths. The cysts should be removed by shelling out if possible; by oophorectomy if necessary. Since bilateral cysts occur in about 25% of cases, the contralateral ovary should be inspected carefully and bisected if necessary.

2. Malignant -
   a. Cystadenocarcinoma - These may be pseudomucinous or serous. There is no way of diagnosing cystadenocarcinoma preoperatively, but since 5-10% of pseudomucinous and 25% of serous cystadenomas are malignant at the time of surgery, all ovarian cysts which are over 5 cm. in diameter or persist for 60 days should be removed. About 10% of all ovarian tumors are cystic carcinomas; about half of these are bilateral. When ovarian malignancy is discovered, total hysterectomy and bilateral salpingo-oophorectomy is indicated. The presence of metastatic implants upon the peritoneum is an unfavorable sign; although irradiation is often of value postoperatively in prolonging the period of regression, cure is not to be expected. The intraperitoneal injection of one of the new chemotherapeutic antineoplastic agents may also be of value.
   b. Dermoid cysts - Malignant degeneration of a dermoid cyst occurs rarely (see Teratoma, p. 517.)

Solid Tumors.

A. Benign:
   1. Fibroma of the ovary - An uncommon tumor which may grow to huge size and produces symptoms only by its size or by torsion of its pedicle, except for the rare occurrence of Meigs' syndrome: ovarian fibroma with ascites and hydrothorax (usually right-sided). (It is now known that the ascites and hydrothorax, or hemoperitoneum and hemothorax, may be found in association with any pelvic tumor, benign or malignant.) Treatment is surgical.
   2. Brenner tumors - These moderately-sized neoplasms are usually indistinguishable grossly from ovarian fibromas; histologically, they are studded with nests of epithelial cells within dense fibrous tissue, probably originating from Walthard's cell rests. Diagnosis and management are as described for fibroma (above). Recently, a few cases of malignant Brenner tumors have been reported.
   3. Other rare tumors - Rarely, such other solid, benign tumors as angioma may be encountered. The symptomatology is not characteristic, and the diagnosis and classification depend upon surgery and pathologic examination.

B. Malignant:
   1. Carcinoma - Primary solid carcinoma may take any of several histologic forms which are indistinguishable from each other on gross examination. It has no characteristic color, size, shape, or consistency; and can best be described merely as a solid ovarian tumor which metastasizes and is more likely than a benign tumor to bear evidence of rapid or irregular growth and invasion of its own capsule.

It accounts for about 5% of all ovarian tumors; about half are bilateral. Diagnosis and treatment are as described for cystadenocarcinoma (see p. 516).

2. Sarcoma - Sarcoma of the ovary is rare. The clinical approach to the problem is as for carcinoma (above).
3. Teratoma - Teratomas of the ovary are not common, but must be considered when an ovarian tumor is found in a young woman. Like dermoid cyst, this tumor is probably an example of "imperfect parthenogenesis," consisting of a variety of embryonic tissues which may grow in any conceivable combination of imperfect structures. Metastasis to nearby structures, especially the peritoneum, tends to occur early. One of the tissues in the tumor may grow rapidly, overwhelming the other tissues and thus presenting a tumor which apparently is composed of a single tissue. Struma ovarii, the thyroid tumor of the ovary, is 1 example; pseudomucinous cystadenoma may be a teratoma in which the entoderm has overgrown all other tissues. The treatment of these tumors is by surgical excision, and the prognosis is poor.
4. Metastatic carcinoma - Metastasis to the ovary occasionally occurs from the uterus or adjacent pelvic structures or from the gastrointestinal tract (especially the pylorus). It may take the form of a Krukenberg tumor: a firm, smooth, nonadherent, usually bilateral growth which tends to retain the original ovarian contour. This is a mucin-producing tumor, and microscopic examination often shows mucinous cells in which the mucin has flattened the nuclei against the cell wall to produce the typical "signet cells."

Embryonic or Dysontogenetic Tumors.

These are sometimes referred to as functioning tumors or special tumors.

A. Feminizing, Granulosa–Theca Cell Tumors: (Either or both cell types may be found.) These tumors account for almost 10% of all ovarian malignancies. They may occur at any age; a few have even been reported in prepuberal girls. Since the cells are nearly always functional, the prepuberal patient may demonstrate sexual precocity and the postmenopausal patient may report vaginal bleeding, whereas the woman in the reproductive age group will usually complain of some form of menstrual irregularity - often alternating amenorrhea and heavy bleeding. These tumors must be considered malignant, although the survival rate from granulosa cell tumors is at least 50% and that from theca cell tumors almost 100%. The tumor may recur many years later, and lifetime follow-up is necessary.

   The recommended treatment is total hysterectomy and bilateral salpingo-oophorectomy, but more conservative measures may be resorted to in a younger woman who desires future pregnancy and who has an apparently well-confined unilateral tumor. This is a calculated risk of which the patient should be aware. Careful observation is essential.

B. Masculinizing, Arrhenoblastomas (Sertoli–Leydig Cell Tumors): These comprise less than 1% of ovarian neoplasms, and usually occur during the reproductive period of a woman's life. There are no unique gross characteristics. Histologic examination may show a well-differentiated Sertoli cell tubular pattern with interspersed Leydig cells, or there may be an undifferentiated, sarcoma-like appearance. The tumors are not often bilateral, but are malignant in about 20% of the cases reported. They usually exert a masculinizing effect: breast atrophy, enlargement of the clitoris, voice changes, hirsutism, and amenorrhea. The tumor should be removed surgically, and the other pelvic organs should be removed at the same time unless the patient desires future pregnancy and there is good clinical evidence of lack of malignancy. The prognosis is good in most instances.

C. Gynandroblastoma (Mixed Tumor): This rare neoplasm is composed of elements of both granulosa–theca cell tumor and arrhenoblastoma, and may cause any combination of feminizing and masculinizing symptoms. As our knowledge of the histogenesis of ovarian neoplasms increases, we may find that this puzzling tumor will be reclassified.

D. Dysgerminomas (Germinomas, Seminomas): Dysgerminomas are tumors of embryonic germ cells which, because they are still sexually undifferentiated, produce no endocrine-induced changes. (This tumor may also be found in the male, in which case it is called a seminoma.) It is usually malignant and accounts for about 4% of malignant ovarian tumors; about one-third are bilateral. The tumor most commonly occurs between the ages of 10 and 30. The patient may present a picture of retarded sexual development. Any treatment short of total hysterectomy and bilateral salpingo-oophorectomy should be undertaken only with the reasoned consent of the patient.

E. Other Rare Types: There are several rare ovarian tumors (e.g., hypernephromas, adrenal-like tumors, and luteomas) which can only be diagnosed at surgery. Because they are so rare, further discussion in the space available is not feasible.

DISTURBANCES OF MENSTRUATION

Normal menstruation usually starts (menarche) at age 9-17 (avg., 13); it continues (menacme) until cessation (menopause) at about age 45-55 (avg., 47-50). About 50 ml. of blood, mixed with desquamated cells and lacking the ability to clot (fibrinolysins), will be passed in a period of 2-7 days at intervals of 22-35 days.

Variations From Normal Menstruation.

A. Amenorrhea: (Absence of menstruation.)

1. Primary amenorrhea - (Without previous menstruation.) Primary amenorrhea may be said to exist if the menarche has not occurred by the age of 18; it must be differentiated from cryptomenorrhea, in which endometrium is desquamated from the uterine wall but is retained within the vagina by some (usually congenital) obstruction, e.g., imperforate hymen. Primary amenorrhea may be caused by congenital absence or marked hypoplasia of the uterus and/or ovaries; adrenogenital syndrome; adiposogenital dystrophy (Fröhlich's syndrome); any constitutional deficiency such as anemia or tuberculosis; or marked emotional disturbances.

2. Secondary amenorrhea - (Following previous menstruation.) With the exception of congenital abnormalities, the causes of secondary amenorrhea are the same as of the primary forms. However, endocrine derangements caused by defeminizing or masculinizing tumors are more apt to occur after the menarche and thus are more apt to be seen in association with secondary than with primary amenorrhea.

B. Hypomenorrhea: (Scanty flow with a normal cycle.) Hypomenorrhea differs from amenorrhea principally in degree. Some women report a scanty flow throughout the menacme. Except for infertility, this condition usually is of no significance, and treatment by extraneous hormone augmentation produces no lasting effect.

C. Menorrhagia: (Excessive flow with a normal cycle.) This disorder is much more common than hypomenorrhea or amenorrhea and is of vastly greater clinical significance. Several common clinical disorders are associated with menorrhagia:
1. Constitutional factors, such as hypothyroidism or thrombocytopenia or other clotting deficiencies of the blood.
2. Polyps of the cervix or of the endometrium.
3. Irregular shedding of the endometrium is a failure of the uterus to desquamate completely within the first 4 days of menstrual flow.
4. Neoplasms in the pelvis.
5. Chronic endometritis (rare).
6. Adenomyosis (see p. 511).

D. Oligomenorrhea: (Infrequent menstruation, i.e., prolonged cycle, but with normal flow.) This may be a precursor of amenorrhea, and any of the pathologic conditions discussed under that heading should be borne in mind. In other instances, oligomenorrhea seems merely to be a normal variation which is of no importance except that it may limit fertility.

E. Polymenorrhea: (Frequent menstruation, i.e., short cycle, but with normal flow.) A cycle of less than 22 days, not commonly seen, is apt to accompany pelvic inflammatory disease or endocrine disturbances. Treatment is by correction of the primary disorder.

F. Metrorrhagia: (Noncyclic bleeding from the uterus.) The term is merely a descriptive one, used to denote the symptom of bleeding from the uterus.

MISCELLANEOUS CAUSES OF ABNORMAL UTERINE BLEEDING

ANOVULATORY CYCLE

The anovulatory cycle is a failure of ovulation during the menacme. The cycle is usually prolonged (may be markedly so), the flow may be heavy (see below), and there is almost never any pain even if the woman usually suffers from severe menstrual cramps. Some women have occasional anovulatory episodes with no significant change in cycle or flow.

ENDOMETRIAL HYPERPLASIA

Hyperplasia of the endometrium is proliferation of endometrium without the "ripening" effect of progesterone. It is the result of excessive or (more usually) prolonged exposure to estrogens, whether caused by an anovulatory cycle, an estrogen-producing ovarian tumor, or medical administration of estrogens. There is usually a history of amenorrhea followed by profuse bleeding (can be almost exsanguinating). Pain is seldom present.

Curettage controls the bleeding and provides tissue for microscopic examination.

If the disorder is caused by an ovarian tumor which can be removed, prompt cure is easily obtained. Commonly, however, endometrial hyperplasia is caused by anovulatory cycles of unknown etiology, and treatment is hormonal. The patient is "cycled" by giving her estrogen from days 5 through 24 and progesterone from day 15 through 24; this regimen usually results in withdrawal bleeding 2-5 days after cessation of therapy. The routine can be repeated for 3-6 months, following which the patient often maintains her regular cycle.

Most dysfunctional bleeding problems can be corrected by the use of progestogens, which are amazingly effective in regulating the menstrual cycle and controlling excessive bleeding. The principle is the same as stated in the paragraph above, but the routine is simpler for the patient to follow. The "sequential" system is a package of 20-21 pills, each containing an estrogen; the pills that are to be taken the last 5-6 days also contain a progestogen. The series is started on day 5 of the menstrual cycle. In the "combined" system, each pill contains both estrogen and progestogen, and this method is usually more effective in decreasing the amount of menstrual flow. The "combined" pill may also be started on day 5 of each cycle. More simply, it may be taken for 21 days of each 28, with a 7-day period during which no medication is taken. Either of these 2 methods is simple and effective in regulating the menstrual cycle and flow, but the patient should understand that ovulation is nearly always inhibited and that pregnancy rarely occurs while she follows this regimen.

STEIN-LEVENTHAL SYNDROME

The Stein-Leventhal syndrome consists of amenorrhea (or oligomenorrhea) accompanied by obesity and hirsutism in the presence of enlarged polycystic ovaries.

The accepted treatment is surgical removal of a wedge-shaped section of each ovary. About 80% of the patients so treated will revert to normal menstrual cycles.

DYSMENORRHEA

Dysmenorrhea (painful menses) may be primary (cause not discernible) or secondary to some other condition (e.g., myoma of the uterus, endometriosis).

Numerous theories of the cause of primary dysmenorrhea have been advanced and many methods of treatment advocated, but the condition has not yet been satisfactorily explained and control is frequently inadequate. It may manifest itself in various ways, and treatment must be adjusted accordingly.

(1) Pelvic congestion causes a chronic, nonspastic, nagging, "heavy" generalized pelvic discomfort which is rarely seen in young nulliparas or in postmenopausal women but is common in parous women between the ages of 30 and 50. The pain is absent or minimal during the first half of the menstrual cycle, developing after ovulation and gradually becoming more pronounced as the time of menstruation is approached. Treatment consists of correcting thyroid deficiency, if present, or of decreasing the fluid retention with a low salt diet and diuretics. Complete control of the pain is not commonly achieved, however.

This syndrome may be caused (or aggravated) by the presence of varicosities in the veins that drain the uterus and course laterally between the leaves of the broad ligaments. In this instance, temporary relief can be obtained by bed rest in Trendelenburg's position; hysterectomy is curative, but the condition is rarely serious enough to warrant such a drastic measure.

(2) Uterine ischemia due to myometrial or vascular spasm is believed to cause the type of dysmenorrhea that presents as a spastic, intermittent, often severe pain that appears with the onset of menstrual flow. Antispasmodic agents are indicated, but the response is frequently disappointing; phenobarbital or tranquilizing drugs used in conjunction will increase their efficacy. This type of dysmenorrhea is rarely seen in parous women.

(3) Endocrine factors may be involved in dysmenorrhea, as evidenced by the numerous reports of control of pain by the use of estrogens or progesterone in the premenstrual period. The basis for this approach is not firm, and results are apt to be disappointing.

However, it has long been noted that the spastic type of dysmenorrhea does not occur with the bleeding that follows an anovulatory cycle; successful treatment is often achieved by reproducing this phenomenon. Diethylstilbesterol, 0.1 mg., or one of the newer progestogens, will prevent ovulation if taken daily from day 5 through day 24 of the cycle, and the subsequent "menstrual period" is usually not accompanied by significant pain.

If the pain of primary dysmenorrhea does not respond to any of the methods of treatment described above, analgesics may be given. If these are not sufficient to control the discomfort, surgery may be resorted to: hysterectomy if the patient is nearing the menopausal age, or presacral neurectomy for a patient who desires future children. The success rate of neurectomy is about 80-90%.

ENDOMETRIOSIS

Endometriosis is the ectopic occurrence of endometrium. When endometrium invades the myometrium the disorder is termed endometriosis interna or adenomyosis (see p. 511). Endometrium found elsewhere in the body is called endometriosis externa. The ectopic tissue in endometriosis externa is usually in the pelvis (pelvic endometriosis), but it may be found in laparotomy scars, the umbilicus, bladder, the intestinal tract, or almost anywhere in the body. In the pelvis, the most common locations are the ovaries, tubes, the uterosacral ligaments, and the pouch of Douglas, although ectopic endometrial tissue may be seen in any of the genital structures. Endometriosis externa is found in about 15% of women who undergo pelvic operations.

Pathologically, the disease is due to the growth of the ectopic endometrium, usually with intermittent desquamation, under the influence of the ovarian hormones. If growth is in an enclosed space, such as the ovary, repeated episodes of desquamation cause the formation of a cyst containing old blood ("chocolate cyst") which gradually increases in size to a usual maximum diameter of about 10 cm. Surface implants on any tissue cause dense scarring, which draws in the surrounding area and gives a "puckered" appearance which may be white (scarring) or blue (desquamation).

The most common symptom is pain, usually beginning about 1 week before menstruation and reaching its peak with the onset of flow. The site, intensity, and character of the pain depend upon the location and extensiveness of the growth. Implants are commonly in the cul-de-sac, and the pain therefore tends to be low in the midline of the pelvis. Symptoms other than pain may also occur: an implant in the bladder may cause frequency of urination; one in the intestinal tract may cause diarrhea and cramps, etc. Pelvic examination will reveal a mass if the disease has progressed to the stage of cyst formation, but in the earlier stages there may be no palpable abnormalities other than tenderness. An almost pathognomonic finding is tenderness, often with nodularity, of the uterosacral ligaments. This is demonstrated by rectovaginal examination, raising the cervix with the index finger in the vagina to stretch the uterosacral ligaments and facilitate their identification by the middle finger. The clinical diagnosis of endometriosis is usually made on the basis of the history and physical findings; definitive diagnosis depends upon finding the lesion at surgery.

Treatment.

Since the lesion depends upon ovarian hormones for its growth, castration by surgery, irradiation, or spontaneous menopause will cause regression. However, this is often undesirable, as when the patient wishes to avoid sterility.

A. Medical Treatment: Medical management will not cure but usually should be tried first as a palliative measure unless a mass is present. For practical purposes, analgesics and treatment of pelvic congestion are the most dependable medical measures.

The most effective nonsurgical "treatment" is pregnancy, which halts the process for almost a year. This process may be mimicked by the induction of a "pseudo-pregnancy" with a progestogen. The progestogen is given daily for 9-12 months, gradually increasing the daily dose as necessary to prevent bleeding. A typical experience would be: norethynodrel and ethinyl estradiol (Enovid®), 5 mg. daily; at 4-8 weeks, the patient begins to bleed slightly, and the dose is increased to 10 mg. daily. In 3-6 weeks, bleeding recurs, and the dose is increased to 15 mg. a day. The gradual increase in dosage is repeated as necessary whenever bleeding occurs. At the end of the pseudopregnancy, the daily dose will be in the range of 30-60 mg. The more recently developed (and lower dose) progestogens will probably work as well as Enovid®. After cessation of therapy, the endometrial implants may remain dormant for a period of several months to a year or more. Experience with this method of management is still scanty, and the results are unpredictable.

B. Surgical Treatment: Hysterectomy and bilateral salpingo-oophorectomy is the surgical procedure of choice if the disease is widespread or if the patient is nearing the menopause and has no desire for future pregnancies. Irradiation castration is not recommended except in the most unusual circumstances. Conservative treatment is indicated for the younger woman who wishes future pregnancies, leaving intact all or part of one ovary, a tube, and the uterus if possible. When operating upon a patient with endometriosis who desires future pregnancies, the surgeon's task is to attempt to preserve and repair tissues, not merely to remove them. This "conservative" type of operation may be inadequate, and further surgery may be necessary at a later date; but if the patient has a complete understanding of the situation it is often worth trying.

In the patient who has had total ablation of the ovaries but who still has endometriosis, exogenous estrogens given for the purpose of controlling the menopausal syndrome will rarely cause recrudescence of the implants.

RETRODISPLACEMENT OF THE UTERUS

The normal position of the uterus is considered to be anteflexion, but in about one-third of women it will be either retroverted (turned backward on its transverse axis) or retroflexed (bent backward).

The retrodisplaced uterus does not commonly cause any symptoms. Occasionally, however, retrodisplacement causes low backache, dysmenorrhea, menorrhagia, and/or dyspareunia.

A pessary will bring relief. The pessary may be worn intermittently - 1-2 months at a time, with a period between for the purpose of sparing the vaginal mucosa - until the menopause, after which time the malformation rarely causes discomfort. In rare instances it may be advisable to suspend the uterus surgically, but the failure rate of this procedure is high.

PELVIC RELAXATION

Relaxation of the tissues of the female pelvis occurs to some degree in most women, although it is often asymptomatic. Weakening of the tissues may be due to congenitally poor tissue tone, neurogenic deficiency (e.g., occult anterior spina bifida), and/or childbirth lacerations. Relaxation of tissues in specific areas causes specific disturbances:

Prolapse of the uterus, caused by a relaxation of the uterine supports (especially the cardinal and uterosacral ligaments), may be first degree (early), second degree (cervix to the introitus), or third degree (cervix past the introitus). The only symptom is a "dragging sensation" in the pelvis.

Urethrocele, a sagging of the urethra caused by relaxation of the lower portion of the pubocervical fascia, produces stress incontinence and urgency of urination.

Cystocele, a bulging or prolapse of the bladder caused by weakening of the entire pubocervical fascia, encourages cystitis, frequency, and urgency of urination.

Rectocele, an anteriorly-directed bulging of the rectum due to weakness of the fascial tissues overlying the rectum produces constipation which may be relieved by the patient by finger pressure in the vagina.

Enterocele, a true hernia of the peritoneum of the pouch of Douglas, extending caudad into the rectovaginal septum, may produce pelvic heaviness but often causes no symptoms.

Perineal relaxation is a lack of firm tissues at the introitus caused by a weakening of all fascial planes and muscles of the area. Although this condition may be due to nonobstetric causes, childbirth lacerations are the most common factor. The tearing of the tissues may have been subcutaneous, in which case scars will not be apparent upon inspection, but the more common finding is a perineal laceration which has left its telltale scar. Symptoms are pelvic heaviness and dragging.

Treatment.

Surgical repair by any of several technics (e.g., the Manchester operation, with or without vaginal hysterectomy) is usually the treatment of choice, but the failure rate is high since relaxation of pelvic tissues is commonly seen in women with an inborn tendency toward poor tissues. Even in the best hands, about 10% of operative results are less than satisfactory no matter what technic is used.

A pessary may be used if the patient is unable to withstand surgery. Special exercises of all the perineal muscles may be beneficial if the patient performs them faithfully.

FISTULAS

The most commonly seen fistulas involving the female genital tract are rectovaginal, vesicovaginal, and urethrovaginal fistulas. They should be watched for in association with malignancy or following pelvic surgery or radiotherapy, and are occasionally seen following trauma (e.g., difficult delivery).

The most common complaint is incontinence of urine, feces, or intestinal gas; other symptoms are not commonly present. The lesion can usually be seen by vaginal inspection, but the aperture may be so small or so well concealed in folds of mucosa that it is not easily discovered. In these instances the suspected origin of the tract can be filled with a methylene blue solution and the vagina inspected for emergence of the dye.

Small, recent fistulas may close spontaneously, especially if healing is encouraged by a freshening of the wound edges, silver nitrate, and diversion of the urinary or fecal stream by catheter or tube. Usually, however, the only effective treatment is surgical repair. This may be very difficult, and the failure rate is high.

OBSTETRIC PROBLEMS

ABORTION

Abortion is defined as termination of pregnancy before the fetus becomes viable (about 28 weeks); it occurs in about 10-15% of all pregnancies, usually in the second or third month. Habitual abortion is said to exist after 3 successive spontaneous abortions.

Classification and Treatment.

A. Spontaneous Abortion:
   1. Threatened abortion - Bleeding and cramps, with the cervix dilated 1 cm. or less. Treatment consists of bed rest, sedation, and analgesics.
   2. Inevitable abortion - The cervix is now dilated to 1 cm. or more, or the membranes rupture. A conservative course may be followed and complete abortion awaited if bleeding is not too severe. Otherwise, dilatation and curettage are indicated.
   3. Incomplete abortion - Part of the products of conception (usually the fetus) has been expelled, but part (usually placental fragments) remains behind. Treatment consists of dilatation and curettage.
   4. Complete abortion - The entire contents of the uterus have been expelled. Since nothing remains behind but decidua basalis and parietalis, which will spontaneously desquamate, no treatment is indicated. If excessive bleeding and/or cramps occur after a diagnosis of complete abortion has been made, then the diagnosis was in error and dilatation and curettage are indicated to remove retained fragments.

B. Induced Abortion:
   1. Therapeutic - Indicated for reasons of maternal health or inevitable fetal malformation. (State laws vary regarding therapeutic abortion; the physician should be aware of the law in his state before initiating treatment.)
   2. Criminal - Dilatation and curettage should be performed if abortion is incomplete, and massive doses of broad-spectrum antibiotics given if there is evidence of sepsis.

C. Septic Abortion: Abortion at any stage or of any type complicated by infection.

D. Missed Abortion: Intrauterine retention of a dead embryo for 2 months or more. Dilatation and curettage are indicated if spontaneous abortion does not occur after estrogen-induced withdrawal bleeding.

E. Habitual Abortion: Three consecutive spontaneous abortions.

Prognosis for Future Pregnancies.

An uncomplicated spontaneous abortion, when due to a blighted ovum (rather than to an abnormality of the maternal structures), does not compromise future pregnancy.

HYDATIDIFORM MOLE

Hydatidiform (vesicular) mole is a benign proliferation of the trophoblast which produces cystic degeneration of the villi and, usually, fetal death. It occurs once in about 2000 pregnancies in the U.S.A. Grossly, the hydropic villi appear as vesicles a few mm. to about 2 cm. in diameter, but the basic pathologic process is seen microscopically as a marked proliferation of the trophoblast, which explains some of the symptoms and diagnostic findings of the disease.

The presence of a mole might be suspected if the uterus enlarges either more rapidly or more slowly than would be expected with a normal pregnancy; if there is bleeding; if lutein ovarian cysts (due to stimulation from the hyperplastic trophoblast) are present; if the fetal skeleton is absent; or if a high titer of chorionic gonadotropin is present (demonstrated by a positive pregnancy test on an unusually small amount of test material).

Hydatidiform mole should be removed immediately by curettage. If the mole is larger than the size of a three-month pregnancy, induction of labor should be attempted; if unsuccessful, abdominal hysterotomy is probably a safer procedure than curettage. After evacuation of the mole, the patient should be observed closely for 2 years with repeated pregnancy tests. A positive test in the absence of another pregnancy indicates malignant degeneration (see Chorio-epithelioma, below).

CHORIO-EPITHELIOMA

Chorio-epithelioma or choriocarcinoma, a rare condition, is a malignancy of fetal trophoblast which may be seen following term delivery or abortion but is usually a complication of hydatidiform mole. Although over 50% of cases of chorio-epithelioma result from moles, only 1-2% of moles lead to chorio-epithelioma. This neoplasm is extremely malignant; early invasion and metastasis to distant sites (especially the lungs) is the rule.

Diagnosis is made during the two-year follow-up care recommended for all cases of hydatidiform mole. The patient is watched for new growths in the vaginal mucosa, abnormal bleeding, or persistently positive pregnancy tests. If chorio-epithelioma is found in the uterus, immediate hysterectomy and bilateral salpingo-oophorectomy is indicated plus the surgical removal of any metastatic lesion which can be completely removed. Postoperative irradiation is usually considered advisable, but statistical proof of its value is lacking.

The prognosis traditionally has been poor, but the advent of chemotherapy has increased the chances for cure to better than 50%. Strenuous efforts to control the disease should be made even in apparently hopeless situations, using a combination of surgical removal and methotrexate and other chemotherapeutic agents.

ECTOPIC PREGNANCY

An ectopic pregnancy is one which follows implantation of an ovum on any surface other than the uterine cavity, usually in the tube but occasionally in the ovary, the cervix, or the peritoneum.

TUBAL PREGNANCY

Tubal gestation occurs about once in 250 pregnancies, often secondary to a congenital or inflammatory tubal abnormality.

Clinical Findings.

A. Symptoms and Signs: Pain is usually unilateral at first. It increases in severity and becomes generalized with any leakage into the peritoneal cavity. Pain becomes acute when the tube ruptures. Vaginal bleeding is irregular in amount and does not occur at the expected time of menstruation. Shock will be present if tubal rupture results in marked hemorrhage.

The mass in the pelvis is usually quite tender (sometimes excruciatingly so), may or may not be fixed, and tends to grow. The uterus itself is usually soft and often somewhat enlarged.

After implantation of the ovum, the course of the condition depends upon the effects produced by the invading trophoblast, as follows:

1. In most instances the growing ovum stretches the tube to the point where it suddenly ruptures, causing extensive internal bleeding. This produces severe pain, shock, and the clinical picture of an acute abdomen due to internal hemorrhage.
2. The ovum may die soon after implantation; the patient's pain, which may have been of any degree of severity, will then gradually subside and there will be no further ill effects.
3. If the ovum was implanted near the end of the tube, it may grow to 1-3 cm. in diameter and then be extruded out of the fimbriated end of the tube into the cul-de-sac ("tubal abortion"). When this happens the character of the pain will change: unilateral discomfort will suddenly become acute, spread to both lower quadrants and the rectum, and then will gradually subside over a period of about 1 month. Internal bleeding is rarely severe, and surgery is seldom indicated.
4. The invading trophoblast may reach the serosa of the tube without having ruptured a vessel of significant size; internal bleeding usually develops so slowly that the abdominal crisis is avoided. In this instance the pain is usually constant and more or less disabling, but operative intervention is often delayed because there is no crisis and no definite diagnosis. The pain usually persists until the disorder is corrected at surgery.
5. The growing trophoblast may invade through the tube wall without causing sufficient pain to bring the patient to surgery, and may then grow along the tube, broad ligament, and often the adjacent structures (uterus, pelvic wall, intestine) as an abdominal pregnancy (see p. 529).

B. Laboratory Findings: A pregnancy test may be either positive (trophoblast functioning) or negative (trophoblast not functioning); endometrial biopsy or curettage may or may not demonstrate decidual endometrium for the same reason.

C. Special Examinations: Free blood in the peritoneal cavity can be demonstrated by needle aspiration through the cul-de-sac. Culdoscopy is useful in the diagnosis of ectopic pregnancy in selected cases; however, since a previous pelvic infection so often is the cause of a tubal pregnancy, the tube is apt to be adherent to the peritoneum of the cul-de-sac, which renders culdoscopy of no value.

Differential Diagnosis.

Tubal pregnancy must be differentiated from pelvic inflammatory disease, ovarian cyst, and threatened or incomplete abortion of an intrauterine pregnancy.

Treatment.

Treatment consists of surgical excision of the mass and reconstruction of the tube if technically feasible, or removal of the entire tube if necessary. If it seems certain that tubal abortion or spontaneous death of the embryo in the tube has occurred, observation may be indicated, but the patient should be in the hospital and the physician should be prepared for surgery at any time. When there has been a tubal rupture, bleeding may be massive; transfusion and antishock measures are important adjuncts to the surgical procedure.

OTHER FORMS OF ECTOPIC PREGNANCY

Interstitial Pregnancy.

Interstitial pregnancy is a pregnancy in that portion of the fallopian tube which lies in the wall of the uterus. The unilateral enlargement may be delineated by bimanual pelvic examination if the patient is not too obese.

Because of the thick myometrium, rupture may not occur until the embryo has grown for several months. Rupture is a serious matter since the uterine and ovarian arteries are often involved. Surgical excision of the cornua of the uterus before rupture can occur is advisable.

Cornual Pregnancy.

A cornual pregnancy is one in which the ovum was implanted in the uterine horn. If severe symptoms or rupture occurs, interstitial pregnancy is the more likely diagnosis. Cornual pregnancy often causes sacculation of that portion of the uterus, with consequent adjustment and term pregnancy.

Cervical Pregnancy.

Implantation of the ovum in the cervical mucosa usually precipitates pain and bleeding early in pregnancy. The bleeding may assume critical proportions if the pregnancy progresses past 3 months. If evacuation through the vagina and packing do not control bleeding, hysterectomy is indicated.

A similar clinical picture may be presented by the imprisonment of a spontaneously aborted ovum in the cervical canal because of a stricture of the external os of the cervix (cervical abortion). Dilatation of the external os will permit the delivery of the abortus.

Ovarian Pregnancy.

Ovarian pregnancy presents a clinical picture identical with that of pregnancy of the fimbriated end of the tube, and treatment is the same, i.e., surgical removal.

Abdominal Pregnancy.

Abdominal pregnancy may occur as a primary nidation or, secondarily, when a tubal pregnancy grows through the wall of the tube and extends over the peritoneal surface to adjacent structures. It may go to term, although the course of the pregnancy usually includes episodes of pain and bleeding. Suspicion should be aroused by prolonged pregnancy, failure of the cervix to efface and begin dilatation, and abdominal palpation of fetal small parts.

Treatment is by laparotomy. If the blood supply to the placenta cannot be completely controlled by ligature, the placenta should be left in situ, attached wherever it is situated. If spontaneous absorption does not occur, the placenta will wall off and liquefy, and can be drained later.

14 . . .

Urology

GENERAL PRINCIPLES OF DIAGNOSIS

The essential steps in the workup of the urologic patient are (1) a history and physical examination, (2) a routine laboratory evaluation, and (3) excretory urograms. The laboratory tests should include a stained smear of the urinary sediment and a PSP test.

In certain instances more definitive investigative procedures may be necessary, e.g., passage of urethral catheters or sounds, cystometry, special radiographic technics, cystoscopy, ureteral catheterization, and retrograde urograms.

UROLOGIC LABORATORY EXAMINATION

Urethral Discharge.

Urethral discharge should be examined immediately in saline for trichomonads. It should then be stained and examined microscopically for bacteria.

Urinalysis.

A. Collection of the Specimen: In the male a "midstream" specimen must be obtained. In the female a similar "midstream" or catheterized specimen can be collected.

B. Immediate Examination: Immediate examination is imperative. A normal urine specimen contains not more than 1-2 red or white cells/low power field. Whether pus cells are present or not, the sediment must be stained with methylene blue since chronic urinary tract infections are apt to be apyuric (and asymptomatic). If pus cells are present but no bacteria can be found in the stained smear, acid-fast stains are indicated.

The presence of bacteria on a stained smear implies that there are at least 10,000 organisms/ml. of urine; this is pathognomonic of clinical infection.

C. Quantitative Cultures: More than 1000 colonies/ml. makes the diagnosis of urinary infection if the urine has been collected properly and plated immediately. Sensitivity tests may be indicated. Cultures for tubercle bacilli should be utilized in patients suspected of having urinary tuberculosis.

D. Sulkowitch's Test: This test affords a rough estimate of the amount of calcium in the urine. To 5 ml. of urine add 2 ml. of Sulkowitch's reagent. A slight cloud implies a small amount of calcium; the rapid formation of a very dense cloud means hypercalcemia until proved otherwise.

Renal Function Tests.

A. Morning Specific Gravity: If this is 1.024 or higher in the absence of massive proteinuria, total renal function is good.

B. The PSP (Phenol Red) Test: This test accurately measures total renal function and makes possible an estimation of the amount of residual urine. Do not force fluids before or during the test. The patient should void just before the injection of exactly 1 ml. of the dye (use tuberculin syringe).

Regardless of the volume of urine, the normal amount of PSP excreted in one-half hour is 50-60%. Recovery of less than this amount means either impaired renal function or vesical or bilateral ureteral obstruction or ureterovesical reflux. In this instance, a second half-hour specimen should be collected. If there is no residual urine, the second specimen should contain 10-15% of the dye. If more than this is recovered, residual urine is present; the amount of residual urine can then be estimated as shown by the following example:

First half-hour = 35 ml. = 30%
Second half-hour = 25 ml. = 25%

The curve is "flat," yet the one-hour total is good; renal function is therefore normal and residual urine is present. Since the first specimen should have contained 50-60% of the dye, the residual urine is 30-35 ml.

C. Tests for nitrogen retention should be performed if the PSP excretion is less than 30% in one-half hour.

Radiography.

A. Noninstrumental:
1. Plain film of the abdomen (KUB) - This may show evidence of a ruptured viscus, gallstones, bowel obstruction, differences in size or position of the kidneys, calcifications, and diseases of bone (e.g., metastatic carcinoma).
2. Excretory urograms - These films will establish the diagnosis of most urologic diseases of the kidneys and ureters.
3. Retroperitoneal pneumograms - Oxygen or CO_2 introduced into the presacral space will usually reveal the kidneys and adrenals in sharp contrast. Tomography is essential to the diagnosis.
4. Gastrointestinal studies - These are useful in differential diagnosis. Retroperitoneal masses (e.g., enlarged kidney) may displace intraperitoneal organs.
5. Renal angiograms - These will demonstrate renal tumors or cysts and stenosis of the renal arteries.

B. Instrumental:
1. Urethrograms - A viscous radiopaque solution instilled into the urethra will reveal the caliber of the urethra, fistulas, and enlargement of the prostate.
2. Cystograms - The instillation of radiopaque material into the bladder will demonstrate rupture of that organ, vesical diverticula, and ureteral reflux. The latter is best demonstrated if a film is exposed during the act of voiding. Posterior urethral valves are best demonstrated by this technic.

3. Retrograde urograms - If excretory urograms are not diagnostic or if maximum detail is essential, catheters may be passed to the renal pelves through the cystoscope. Concentrated radiopaque solution can then be introduced into the renal pelves. In addition, bacteriologic studies can be made of the urine specimens from each kidney and separate renal function tests can be done.

Instrumental Examination of the Urinary Tract.

A. Catheter: The urethral catheter is useful for exploration of the urethra and the measurement of residual urine.

B. Sounds: Metal sounds may be used to diagnose urethral stricture.

C. Cystoscope and Panendoscope: These instruments permit inspection of the urethra and bladder as well as manipulation of ureteral stones, biopsy of vesical tumors, and catheterization of the ureters.

URINARY OBSTRUCTION AND STASIS

Etiology.

Congenital anomalies, more common in the urinary tract than in any other organ system, are the most frequent causes of obstruction or stasis. These include ureteral stenosis, vesicoureteral reflux, posterior urethral valves, and meningomyelocele. In adult life many acquired obstructions occur. The common causes are urethral stricture secondary to infection or injury, prostatic disease, ureteral reflux, vesical tumor or local extension of cancer (e.g., cervix), and stone.

Clinical Findings.

A. Symptoms and Signs:

1. Lower and mid tract (urethra and bladder) - The principal symptoms are hesitancy, lessened size and force of the stream, terminal dribbling, and urinary retention. Rectal examination may show atony of the sphincter (which suggests interruption of the sacral roots) and enlargement or cancer of the prostate. Evidence of distention of the bladder may be found on suprapubic percussion.
2. Upper tract (ureter and kidney) - The principal complaints are pain in the flank, hematuria (from stone), and gastrointestinal symptoms. If infection ensues there may be chills, fever, and vesical irritability. Such a complication presumes the presence of vesicoureteral reflux. If advanced bilateral hydronephrosis is present, the only symptoms may be those of uremia. An enlarged kidney may be found. Cancer of the cervix or prostate may invade the bladder, thus occluding one or both ureteral orifices. A large pelvic mass (e.g., a gravid uterus) can compress the ureters.

B. Laboratory Findings: Anemia secondary to chronic renal infection or uremia may be noted. Pus and bacteria may be found in the urine. If unilateral hydronephrosis exists, the PSP excretion will be normal. Depression of PSP excretion implies bilateral renal damage, vesicoureteral reflux, or vesical or bilateral ureterorenal residual urine. If bilateral renal damage is severe, nitrogen retention will be demonstrated.

C. X-ray Findings: A plain film of the abdomen may show enlargement of the renal shadows (hydronephrosis), calcific bodies suggesting urinary stones, or metastases to bone. Excretory urograms will establish the diagnosis unless renal function is so poor that the radiopaque fluid is not excreted, in which case high-dose infusion urography should be employed. They will demonstrate dilatation of the upper tract and will localize calcific bodies in or outside of the urinary tract. The accompanying cystogram may reveal trabeculation and diverticula if the obstruction is distal to the bladder. Vesical tumors, nonopaque stones, and large intravesical prostatic lobes may cast radiolucent shadows. A film taken immediately after voiding may show residual urine.

Retrograde cystography may show changes in the bladder wall caused by distal obstruction. If the ureterovesical valves are incompetent, excellent ureteropyelograms will be obtained because of ureteral reflux. A film taken during the act of voiding increases the incidence of demonstrable reflux.

Retrograde urograms may be necessary to more clearly delineate the site and type of ureteral obstruction.

D. Instrumental Examination: Passage of a catheter will be arrested by a stricture. Catheterization may reveal residual urine. Cystoscopy (or panendoscopy) will permit visualization of a urethral stricture, enlarged prostate, obstructing vesical tumors, and vesical changes secondary to distal obstruction (e.g., trabeculation). If the ureteral orifices are incompetent, their degree of weakness can be estimated from their morphology. The most incompetent orifices are wide open and gaping. Catheters may be passed to the renal pelves for estimation of function of each kidney, the presence of renal infection, and retrograde pyelograms.

Differential Diagnosis.

A mass in one or both flanks suggests polycystic disease, tumor, or hydronephrosis. Such a finding requires radiologic study.

Complications.

Infection is the principal complication of stasis.

Treatment.

A. Relief of Obstruction:
1. Lower tract obstruction - Urethral strictures must be dilated or corrected surgically. Bladder neck (prostatic) obstruction may require surgical intervention. If vesicoureteral reflux is present or persists after relief of distal obstruction (e.g., posterior urethral valves), ureterovesicoplasty may be necessary.
2. Upper tract obstruction - If tortuous, kinked, dilated or atonic ureters have developed secondary to lower tract obstruction or ureteral reflux (so that they are themselves obstructive), vesical drainage may not protect the kidneys from progressive damage. Temporary nephrostomy (or cutaneous loop ureterostomy) may then be indicated. Re-

gression of severe ureteral changes may then allow removal of the nephrostomy tube or restoration of ureteral continuity.

The relief of obvious ureteral obstruction (e.g., ureteral stone) is mandatory. If tests of renal function and urography show that one kidney is badly damaged, nephrectomy may be necessary.

B. Eradication of Infection: Every effort must be made to combat secondary infection. If infection has been severe and prolonged, antibiotic therapy may be unsuccessful unless vesicoureteral reflux or the cause of obstruction is corrected.

Prognosis.

If renal function is fair to good, if the obstruction can be corrected, and if infection can be eradicated, the prognosis is generally excellent.

INFECTIONS OF THE GENITOURINARY TRACT

The "nonspecific" infections are a group of diseases having similar manifestations and caused by gram-negative rods (e.g., Escherichia coli, Proteus vulgaris) or, less commonly, gram-positive cocci (e.g., Streptococcus faecalis, Staphylococcus aureus). The "specific" infections are caused by specific bacteria (e.g., Mycobacterium tuberculosis, Neisseria gonorrhoeae), each of which causes a clinically unique disease.

The factors contributing to infection are (1) the presence of obstruction and stasis, (2) the presence of a foreign body (e.g., renal stone), (3) ureterovesical reflux, and (4) lowered body resistance.

ACUTE PYELONEPHRITIS

Acute pyelonephritis is manifested by severe aching over the involved kidney and symptoms of cystitis. The temperature reaches 102-104° F. (38.9-40° C.), often with chills. Nausea and vomiting are usually present. Tenderness over the kidney, muscle spasm, abdominal distention, and rebound tenderness may be noted. The WBC is elevated and the percentage of neutrophils increased. Urinalysis reveals white blood cells and bacteria. Quantitative cultures are positive. Sensitivity tests may be helpful in refractory cases. Renal function tests are normal.

Excretory urograms are usually normal. Their value lies in demonstrating the presence of obstruction or the possible presence of vesicoureteral reflux as the cause of the infection. Once the urine becomes sterile, a cystogram should be done, since pyelonephritis implies the presence of reflux.

Urinalysis and urography differentiate pyelonephritis from pancreatitis, appendicitis, and gallbladder disease.

Treatment.

A. Specific Measures: A sulfonamide or a broad-spectrum antibiotic is indicated. If the patient does not respond to treatment in 48 hours, either the wrong drug is being used or obstruction is present. Change to a more promising drug (as judged by sensitivity tests) and take excretory urograms.

B. Follow-up Care: Even after clinical response, the urinary sediment must be examined for pathogens for at least 2 months.

Prognosis.

The prognosis is good if response to antibiotics is complete. If obstruction or vesicoureteral reflux is present but undiagnosed, recurrences are to be expected. Such abnormalities may require surgical correction.

CHRONIC PYELONEPHRITIS

Chronic pyelonephritis is a common disease which often goes undiagnosed. Unsuspected chronic pyelonephritis is found in 3-5% of autopsies. Diabetics and those patients with vesicoureteral reflux are particularly susceptible.

Clinical Findings.

A. Symptoms and Signs: There are apt to be few if any symptoms except at the time of exacerbation, when the patient may complain of fever, back pain, and vesical irritability. If the disease is advanced and bilateral, the presenting symptoms may be those of uremia. There are usually no physical findings.

B. Laboratory Findings: The WBC may be elevated during acute exacerbations. The urinary sediment often contains few if any white cells, but some bacteria can always be found on the stained smear. The finding of bacteriuria, however, is not pathognomonic of pyelonephritis; its most common cause is cystitis. Quantitative cultures and sensitivity tests must be performed.

The PSP or other renal function tests will be normal in unilateral renal infection. If total renal function is depressed, bilateral damage, vesicoureteral reflux, or urinary stasis must be assumed.

C. X-ray Findings: Excretory urograms may be normal in the early stages. As parenchymal scarring progresses, renal size is diminished; the infundibula narrow and obstruct the calyces, which become dilated (clubbed); decreasing function causes delayed appearance and lack of concentration of the radiopaque substance. Voiding cystograms will usually show ureterovesical reflux, which is the most common cause of chronic pyelonephritis.

D. Instrumental Examination: Cystoscopy may show changes in the bladder typical of chronic infection. The introduction of ureteral catheters will identify the site of infection and permit retrograde urography. The function of each kidney can be measured by the PSP test run for a period of 15-30 minutes.

Differential Diagnosis.

Renal urinalysis and urography differentiate chronic pyelonephritis from recurrent acute cystitis, chronic cystitis, and tuberculosis.

Complications.

Hypertension and stone formation are the principal complications. Uremia may supervene if the disease is bilateral.

Treatment.

A. Specific Measures:
   1. Medical - Intensive antimicrobial therapy is needed. The choice of drug depends upon sensitivity tests. The drug should be given for 2-4 weeks or longer and followed by "suppressive" therapy with small daily divided doses of one of the sulfonamides, nitrofurantoin, or acidified methenamine for months. In a significant number of cases chronic renal infection cannot be eradicated; suppressive therapy with small doses of chemotherapeutic drugs is then necessary for months or years.
   2. Surgical - Correction of obstruction (e.g., ureteral stenosis) or reflux is essential. It may be necessary to remove a badly damaged kidney.

B. Treatment of Complications: When renal function is impaired bilaterally, a urine output of at least 1500 ml. is necessary to facilitate the removal of metabolic waste products.

Prognosis.

Prognosis should be guarded, for medical treatment usually fails to cure the infection, particularly if vesicoureteral reflux is not corrected. Fortunately, the usual etiologic bacteria do not rapidly destroy renal tissue; longevity may not therefore be jeopardized.

ACUTE CYSTITIS

In the female, cystitis is commonly caused by ascent of bacteria up the urethra and follows sexual intercourse by 36-48 hours. In men, cystitis is never primary but occurs only as a complication of prostatitis, pyelonephritis, or vesical residual urine (e.g., enlarged prostate). Infections of the bowel may involve the bladder by contiguity, e.g., diverticulitis.

Symptoms and signs include urethral burning on urination, urgency, frequency, and, often, terminal hematuria. Fever is low-grade or absent unless prostatic or renal infection is present. A history of recurring attacks suggests chronic cystitis or pyelonephritis, prostatitis, urinary stasis, or vesicoureteral reflux. Rectal examination may reveal an atonic anal sphincter (neurogenic bladder) or an enlarged or cancerous prostate. The gland should not be massaged during the acute phase of the vesical infection. Urinalysis shows pus and bacteria; red cells are often present. Renal function is normal.

Urinalysis and response to treatment differentiate acute cystitis from chronic prostatitis, chronic cystitis, and tuberculosis. Cystoscopy will reveal vesical neoplasm.

Acute pyelonephritis may develop if there is ureterovesical reflux.

The sulfonamides are the most useful drugs for the treatment of acute cystitis. If they fail to sterilize the urine in 14 days, a thorough urologic investigation is indicated.

In the absence of stasis, acute cystitis resolves promptly with medical therapy. If infection recurs, the underlying cause must be determined.

Prophylaxis in the female consists of complete voiding immediately after intercourse. Should this fail, prescribe 1 Gm. of a sulfonamide or 800,000 units of penicillin G to be taken immediately after the act.

CHRONIC CYSTITIS

Chronic cystitis is often secondary to chronic renal infection or residual urine. Complaints may be those of constant or recurring mild vesical irritability, or there may be none at all.

Few or no pus cells may be found in the urine; nevertheless, the stained smear will show bacteria. Cultures will be positive. Renal function tests are normal. Excretory urograms are normal in uncomplicated cystitis. The post-voiding film may show residual urine. The attempted passage of a large catheter (22 F.) may reveal urethral stricture or vesical residual urine. Cystoscopy may demonstrate evidence of cystocele, vesical stone, or bladder neck obstruction.

Urinalysis, urography, bacteriologic examination of renal urine, and response to therapy differentiate this disease from chronic pyelonephritis and tuberculosis.

The sulfonamides may be tried first, but they often fail to cure long-standing infections. If infection still persists, cultures and sensitivity tests should be obtained. Antibiotic treatment must be intensive and prolonged (3-4 weeks). Simple drug therapy often fails to eradicate the infection unless steps are taken to treat the cause.

ACUTE PROSTATITIS AND PROSTATIC ABSCESS

Acute prostatic infection is often hematogenous in origin. It usually resolves with or without treatment, but in rare cases progresses to abscess formation. Vesical irritability is extreme. High fever is to be expected. Urinary retention may occur. Rectal examination may reveal an enlarged, hot, tender prostate; massage is contraindicated at this time.

Leukocytosis is present. Urinalysis shows white and red blood cells and bacteria.

Rectal examination differentiates from acute pyelonephritis and prostatic enlargement. If an abscess forms, it may rupture into the urethra or perineum. Surgical drainage may be necessary.

The tetracyclines (see Chapter 6) are the drugs of choice. Response is usually prompt. A few weeks later, the residual infection must be treated (see Chronic Prostatitis, p. 538).

The prognosis is good, though some residual chronic prostatitis is to be expected.

CHRONIC PROSTATITIS

Prostatic infection often has a hematogenous source, but bacteria can also ascend the urethra or descend from the bladder or kidney. An acute prostatitis frequently becomes chronic.

There are usually no symptoms. Symptomatic prostatitis may cause urethral discharge or vesical irritability from secondary cystitis. The presenting complaint may be acute epididymitis. The presence of epididymitis implies prostatitis. The prostate may feel normal or may have areas of induration. Prostatic massage will produce a secretion containing pus cells. The urine may be infected. Excretory urograms may show prostatic calculi or vesical residual urine.

Cystitis in men is always secondary to renal or prostatic infection or residual urine. A PSP test (for residual urine), urinalysis, and examination of prostatic secretion will make the differentiation. Complications include urethritis, cystitis, and epididymitis.

Response to chemotherapeutic agents is not spectacular, but they should be employed. Secondary cystitis usually responds rapidly.

Prostatic massage performed at intervals of 10-14 days (2-3 times) promotes drainage. Intercourse should be encouraged for the same reason.

Chronic prostatitis in itself causes little harm, but its complications do. For this reason, prostatic massage should be done in all men undergoing physical examination so that asymptomatic infection can be discovered and treated.

URETHRITIS IN THE MALE

Acute urethritis may be caused by nonspecific bacteria, viruses, trichomonads, or gonococci. The symptoms are urethral discharge and, at times, burning on urination. The infection may be secondary to prostatitis.

The discharge should be examined in saline for trichomonads and stained for nonspecific organisms and gonococci. The prostatic secretion should be examined for pus; if infection is present, 2-3 prostatic massages should be given at intervals of 10-14 days.

Nonspecific urethritis usually responds to antibiotics (e.g., tetracycline) given for 1 week. Gonorrhea seldom fails to clear when an injection of 2.4 million units of repository penicillin is given.

If the discharge reveals pus without organisms on a stained smear, Mycoplasma pneumoniae infection may be assumed. This is apt to respond best to tetracycline or erythromycin. If trichomonads are found, metronidazole (Flagyl®), 250 mg. orally twice daily, should be administered for 10 days. The sexual partner should also be treated; a condom should be used.

ACUTE EPIDIDYMITIS

Acute nonspecific epididymitis is usually secondary to prostatitis. The fibrosis which occurs with healing may obstruct the ducts. If bilateral, sterility may ensue.

The symptoms include marked pain and swelling of the epididymis. The swelling equally involves the testicle. Fever may be as high as 102-104° F. (38.9-40° C.). Symptoms due to secondary cystitis may be present.

Only in the early stages can the enlarged, tender epididymis be felt separate from the testis. The scrotal skin is often reddened and adherent to the inflammatory mass. Prostatic massage is contraindicated in the acute stage, since it may make the epididymitis worse. Urinalysis may show infection.

Acute epididymitis must be differentiated from tuberculosis, testicular tumor, torsion of the spermatic cord, and mumps orchitis.

Treatment consists of cold compresses, antimicrobial drugs, and bed rest with support to the scrotum. Analgesics are required for pain. If the patient is seen within a few hours of onset, procaine block of the spermatic cord may significantly hasten resolution.

ACUTE ORCHITIS

Acute orchitis (and associated epididymitis) most commonly occurs as a complication of mumps. It is most often unilateral.

The symptoms and signs include painful swelling of the testicle, fever, and parotitis. Except for leukocytosis, the laboratory evaluation is normal.

Acute orchitis must be differentiated from acute epididymitis (see above) and torsion of the spermatic cord.

The main complication is atrophy and, if bilateral, infertility. Androgenic function, however, is maintained.

Infiltration of the spermatic cord with 1% procaine may abort the disease and thus protect spermatogenesis. Bed rest, analgesics, cold compresses, and scrotal support are also helpful.

GENITOURINARY TUBERCULOSIS

Genitourinary tuberculosis is a disease of young adults. The infecting organism is Mycobacterium tuberculosis, which reaches the genitourinary organs by the hematogenous route. The kidney is most often affected. Secondary descending involvement of the ureter, bladder, prostate, and epididymitis is common.

The renal lesion is typified by caseation and ulceration of the mucosa of the calyces. Calcification is often present.

In the early stages, the bladder merely shows the nonspecific change of hyperemia. Later, tubercles appear in the mucosa; they may coalesce and ulcerate. In the healing process, fibrosis may be marked; ureteral occlusion or vesicoureteral reflux may result.

The infection often descends to the prostate, which becomes nodular secondary to the fibrosis caused by healing; the seminal vesicles likewise may be indurated. Similar changes may develop in the vas and epididymis. Rarely, the epididymal infection may involve the testis by direct extension.

Clinical Findings.

A. Symptoms and Signs: The renal lesion is usually silent. Symptoms of cystitis are the common complaint. Only occasionally is tuberculous epididymitis painful.

Evidence of extra-urologic tuberculosis may be noted. A thickened, nontender epididymis may be found, and is often associated with a nodular vas deferens. A draining scrotal sinus may be present. Rectal examination may reveal induration and nodularity of the prostate and ipsilateral seminal vesicle.

B. Laboratory Findings: Pus without organisms on culture or on a methylene blue stain of the urinary sediment means that tuberculosis is present until proved otherwise. Acid-fast stains will reveal tubercle bacilli in 60% of cases. Cultures for tubercle bacilli and guinea pig inoculation are positive in almost every case of urinary tuberculosis.

Renal function is normal unless the infection is bilateral and severe. A negative tuberculin test in an adult speaks against the diagnosis.

C. X-ray Findings: A chest film may show active or healed tuberculous lesions. A KUB may reveal punctate calcification in the renal parenchyma. Excretory or retrograde urograms may show "moth-eaten" (ulcerated) calyces, obliteration of calyces, or a straight ureter due to contracture from scarring. A voiding cystogram may reveal ureteral reflux secondary to contracture of the bladder.

D. Instrumental Examination: Cystoscopy may reveal the typical tubercles; biopsy may establish the diagnosis. Ureteral catheterization will afford separate urine specimens for bacteriologic study.

Differential Diagnosis.

Acid-fast stains and excretory urography differentiate tuberculosis from chronic nonspecific cystitis or pyelonephritis.

Nonspecific epididymitis is very painful at onset; tuberculous epididymitis is usually not. The finding of pyuria with tubercle bacilli is diagnostic. Excretory urograms may show the typical renal lesion.

Complications.

If vesical involvement is severe, secondary fibrosis may cause ureteral occlusion or ureteral reflux with hydronephrosis. Bilateral epididymitis will cause infertility. The testis may be destroyed by direct extension.

Treatment.

Tuberculosis of the genitourinary organs must be treated as a generalized disease. It must be assumed that an active primary focus also exists.

Triple drug therapy is indicated for a minimum of 2 years: (1) Cycloserine, 250 mg. twice a day by mouth; (2) sodium aminosalicylate (PAS), 15 Gm. orally per day in divided doses; (3) isoniazid (INH), 100 mg. 3 times a day by mouth. Pyridoxine, 100 mg./day in divided doses, will counteract the vitamin B_6 depletion effect of isoniazid.

If no gross pyelographic change is present, nephrectomy is not indicated. Bilateral infection can only be treated by medical measures. However, if only one kidney is involved and shows definite ulceration of one or more calyces, nephrectomy should be done after

2-4 months of medical treatment. The urine must be examined carefully by stain of sediment, culture, and guinea pig inoculation for Mycobacterium tuberculosis for years, since relapse is not uncommon.

Vesical infection usually responds well to antimicrobial therapy. If severe vesical contracture occurs, diversion of the urine (e.g., ureteroileal-cutaneous conduit) or ileocystoplasty (to increase bladder capacity) may be necessary.

Prognosis.

If the disease is limited to one kidney and if the bladder and seminal tract are not involved, the outlook is excellent.

CHEMOTHERAPEUTIC AND ANTIBIOTIC TREATMENT OF UROLOGIC INFECTIONS

Choice and Dosage of Drugs.

In order to cure infections of the urinary tract, particularly those in the chronic stage, standard therapeutic dosages of anti-infective drugs should be administered for at least 2 weeks and preferably longer. In order to suppress an incurable infection, one-half to one-fourth of this dose should be administered for many months or years.

The most useful drugs in the treatment of nonspecific infections are the sulfonamides and the tetracyclines. Most acute infections respond to them; if they do not, a chronic infection or urinary stasis may be present and further examination is required, including sensitivity tests. These may indicate the usefulness of another drug.

Despite prolonged use of the most appropriate antibiotic, long-standing chronic infection is often refractory. Suppressive therapy for months or years should then be instituted. Small doses of a sulfonamide or one of the urinary antiseptics (e.g., nitrofurantoin, methenamine mandelate) are effective.

URINARY STONES

Urinary lithiasis may occur in association with metabolic diseases (e.g., cystinuria, gout, hyperparathyroidism) or can be secondary to infection. Many cases are idiopathic. Calculi are most common in men.

RENAL AND URETERAL CALCULI

Clinical Findings.

A. Symptoms and Signs: Nonobstructive stones usually cause no symptoms. A small stone in the ureter or kidney is apt to cause agonizing renal pain and colic radiating along the course of the ureter. Gross hematuria is not uncommon.

Tenderness over the kidney may be noted. Marked abdominal distention due to paralytic ileus is a common secondary finding in patients with ureteral stone.

B. Laboratory Findings:
   1. Urinalysis - Red cells are commonly found; white cells and bacteria may be present. Oxalate, phosphate, uric acid, or cystine crystals may be seen.
      A Sulkowitch test may reveal hypercalciuria, which suggests hyperparathyroidism. If the stone is only mildly radiopaque, if there have been many recurrences, or if there is a family history of lithiasis, a qualitative test for cystine in the urine should be done.
      On a low-calcium diet (no dairy products), the total urinary calcium should not exceed 175 mg./24 hours. Higher values suggest hyperparathyroidism or idiopathic hypercalciuria.
   2. Renal function tests - The PSP will be normal unless there is bilateral obstruction or infection.
   3. Special blood chemistry studies - Fasting serum calcium, phosphorus, and proteins should be determined, particularly if the Sulkowitch test is strongly positive. Determination of the tubular reabsorption of phosphate may be indicated; it is low (40-80%) in hyperparathyroidism.
      Serum uric acid tests may reveal hyperuricemia; evidence of gout may suggest uric acid stone.
   4. Stone analysis - Stones passed previously should be analyzed. This is important when outlining prophylactic treatment.

C. X-ray Findings: A KUB will afford presumptive evidence of stone since 90% are radiopaque. Excretory urograms accurately localize the radiopaque body in the urinary tract and depict the degree of obstruction or renal damage caused by the stone.

D. Instrumental Examination: Cystoscopy for diagnostic purposes is seldom necessary if excretory urograms are satisfactory.

Differential Diagnosis.

Urography differentiates lithiasis from acute pyelonephritis and renal or ureteral tumor. Bacteriologic examination differentiates from renal tuberculosis.

Complications.

Infection occasionally develops secondary to a renal or ureteral stone. Obstruction at the ureteropelvic junction or in the ureter, caused by a stone, leads to progressive hydronephrosis.

Treatment.

A. Conservative Treatment:
   1. Renal stone - No treatment is indicated for pelvic or calyceal stones that cause few or no symptoms and produce no obstruction. Most staghorn calculi are best left alone since they are usually nonobstructive and seldom cause pain.
   2. Ureteral stone - The majority of stones that reach the ureter will pass by themselves.

B. Cystoscopic or Surgical Measures:
   1. Renal stone - If a renal stone is obstructive or is associated with disabling pain or recurrent infection, it should be removed surgically. Nephrectomy may be necessary if obstruction and infection have markedly impaired renal function.

2. Ureteral stone - Cystoscopic manipulation or ureterolithotomy is necessary if progressive hydronephrosis develops, if persistent infection supervenes, or if the stone is judged to be too large to pass spontaneously.

Prophylaxis.

A. Specific Measures:
1. Calcium stones - Primary hyperparathyroidism requires parathyroidectomy. Eliminate milk and cheese from the diet if the Sulkowitch test remains strongly positive. If the urine is uninfected, the incidence of recurrence is reduced if potassium acid phosphate, 3-6 Gm. daily, is given. This decreases the excretion of calcium in the urine. In the presence of chronic pyelonephritis, however, give hydrochlorothiazide (Hydro-Diuril®), 50 mg. twice daily.
2. Phosphate stones - Acidification of the urine markedly increases the solubility of calcium or magnesium ammonium phosphate.
3. Oxalate stones - A low-oxalate diet may decrease the amount of oxalate in the urine. Give phosphate (see above).
4. Metabolic stones - These include cystine and uric acid stones, both of which are insoluble in acid urine; the urinary pH should be raised to 7.5 or higher in order to increase their solubility. In addition to an alkaline-ash diet, alkaline drugs (e.g., sodium and potassium citrate) are usually necessary. It is advantageous to limit the purines in the diet of uric acid stone formers. Severe cystinurics will require a low-methionine diet (restriction of sulfur-containing amino acids), since methionine is the precursor of cystine. Penicillamine, 4 Gm./day, may abolish cystine from the urine. Allopurinol (Zyloprim®) may be required to prevent uric acid stones. The dose is 300 mg. every 12 hours.

B. General Measures: A large fluid intake will keep the solutes dilute. Infection should be combatted; obstruction and stasis should be corrected. Avoid prolonged recumbency.

Prognosis.

Renal stone recurs in a significant number of cases, and the prognosis is therefore guarded. The patient must be followed carefully for years. The real danger from stone is renal damage caused by obstruction and infection.

VESICAL CALCULI

Vesical calculi almost always occur as a complication of other urologic disease. Ninety-five percent occur in men. The most common cause is vesical residual urine which is infected by urea-splitting organisms. In the Far East and India, primary vesical stones are commonly seen in children. The cause is thought to be vitamin B_6 deficiency. After their removal, recurrence is rare.

Clinical Findings.

A. Symptoms and Signs: The patient may complain of sudden interruption of the stream of urine and pain radiating down the urethra as the stone rolls onto the bladder neck. Hematuria is not uncommon.

B. Laboratory Findings: The urine is usually infected. Red cells are often noted. Excretion of PSP may be depressed because of residual urine.

C. X-ray Findings: Vesical stones are usually visible on a plain film.

D. Instrumental Examination: A catheter may be arrested by a urethral stricture. If it passes to the bladder, it will usually recover infected residual urine. A urethral sound passed to the bladder may cause a "click" when it hits a stone. Cystoscopy will clearly visualize the calculi and help in the diagnosis of the primary cause.

Differential Diagnosis.

Cystoscopy differentiates vesical stone from vesical tumor and extravesical calcifications seen on x-ray.

Complications.

A small stone may become lodged in the urethra.

Treatment.

A. Small stones can be removed by cystoscopic means. Larger ones can be crushed with the lithotrite transurethrally. If the stone is very large, cystotomy may be necessary. Most such stones, however, are removed in conjunction with prostatectomy.

B. Treatment of Complications: Infection cannot be eradicated until the stone and its cause are removed.

Prophylaxis.

Stasis (e.g., prostatic obstruction) and infection, whether primary or secondary, must be eradicated. Early mobilization of injured patients will do much to prevent vesical calculi.

Prognosis.

The rate of recurrence of vesical stone is low if the primary cause is successfully treated.

INJURIES TO THE GENITOURINARY TRACT

INJURIES TO THE KIDNEY

Renal injuries are not common but are potentially serious and may be complicated by trauma to other organs or structures. The renal injury may range from a mild ecchymosis, bruise, or contusion to laceration or rupture.

Clinical Findings.

A. Symptoms and Signs: Pain in the renal area may be obscured by the severity of other injuries. Hematuria is usually present.

Shock or signs of hemorrhage may be noted. Ecchymoses and tenderness over the renal area may be found. A mass felt or percussed in the flank may represent hematoma, urinary extravasation, or both. A progressively falling blood pressure implies persistent bleeding.

B. Laboratory Findings: The Hct., when followed serially, is of the greatest importance; progressive anemia means progressive hemorrhage. Red cells are usually found on urinalysis.

C. X-ray Findings: A KUB may show grayness of the renal area and loss of the renal and psoas shadows if perirenal fluid (urine, blood) is present.

As soon as shock has been treated, excretory urograms should be taken. If the urogram shows evidence of injury to one kidney (e.g., no visualization, extravasation), it is important to note that the contralateral kidney is normal since emergency nephrectomy might have to be considered.

Renal angiography may prove helpful in choosing definitive surgical treatment.

D. Instrumental Examination: Cystoscopy, ureteral catheterization, and retrograde urography are seldom necessary.

Differential Diagnosis.

Trauma to the lumbar area and fractures of the ribs, spine, or transverse processes may cause local symptoms suggesting renal injury. In these injuries, hematuria is absent and urograms normal.

Complications.

Excretory urograms should be obtained 3-6 months after any renal injury for the purpose of diagnosing ureteral stenosis with secondary hydronephrosis, or atrophy of the kidney due to injury or thrombosis of the renal artery. Serial BP readings should be obtained. Post-trauma hypertension may develop secondarily to stenosis of the renal artery.

Treatment.

A. Emergency Measures: Treat shock and hemorrhage.

B. Surgical Treatment: 10-20% of injured kidneys may require surgical intervention because of persistent bleeding. The laceration may be sutured, but nephrectomy may be necessary if injury is severe and the other kidney is normal.

C. Treatment of Complications: Perinephric infection requires surgical drainage. Late complications may indicate the need for nephrectomy or repair of ureteral stenosis.

Prognosis.

In contusions, the prognosis is excellent. When rupture occurs, serious complications may supervene.

INJURIES TO THE URETER

Ureteral injuries most often occur accidentally during difficult and extensive pelvic surgery.

Clinical Findings.

A. Symptoms and Signs: Persistence of abdominal distention and lack of peristalsis past the second or third postoperative day suggest the possibility of ureteral injury. Signs of peritonitis may be elicited. Urine may be seen draining from the wound or the vagina.

B. Laboratory Findings: Blood counts and urinalysis are of little value. The PSP may be depressed if one ureter is occluded.

C. X-ray Findings: A plain film of the abdomen may reveal grayness in the pelvis if extravasation has occurred. Excretory urograms may reveal extravasation. If the ureter has been completely occluded, the renal pelvis and calyces may receive no radiopaque fluid but progressive increase in density of the renal parenchyma may be noted. Retrograde ureterograms will reveal the site of obstruction.

D. Instrumental Examination: Ureteral catheterization will demonstrate patency or obstruction.

Differential Diagnosis.

Urinary specific gravity, PSP test, cystoscopy, renal isotope scanning, and urograms differentiate bilateral ureteral injuries from acute renal failure as a cause of oliguria or anuria.

Complications.

These include urinary fistula, ureteral stenosis with hydronephrosis, renal infection, and peritonitis.

Treatment.

Reanastomosis over a splinting catheter or "T" tube is highly successful. Reimplantation into the bladder - or a tube formed of adjacent bladder wall - usually affords a good result.

If the injury is discovered late and hydronephrosis is advanced, nephrectomy may be the operation of choice.

Prophylaxis.

The surgeon operating in the pelvis must identify the ureters in order to prevent ureteral injury. When difficult or extensive abdominal procedures are anticipated, indwelling ureteral catheters should be placed just prior to the operation for ease of identification.

Prognosis.

Prognosis is best when the ureter is repaired at the time of injury. Delayed repair is less successful because of the fibrous tissue reaction and renal damage from obstruction.

INJURIES TO THE BLADDER

The bladder may be injured by external forces or during surgery.

Clinical Findings.

A. Symptoms and Signs: Gross hematuria and suprapubic pain are to be expected. Shock and evidence of local trauma may be noted. Suprapubic and rebound tenderness are usually found.

A large suprapubic mass may be felt. Rectal examination may reveal a large boggy mass above the prostate.

B. Laboratory Findings: Urinalysis reveals blood.

C. X-ray Findings: A KUB may reveal pelvic fracture. Increased grayness of the vesical area suggests extravasation. Excretory urograms will survey the kidneys for injury.

A retrograde cystogram is the most dependable test for vesical injury. Frank extravasation may be demonstrated.

Differential Diagnosis.

Injury to other urologic organs is differentiated from vesical injury by appropriate x-ray technics.

Complications.

Rarely, the degree of hemorrhage may endanger life. Delay in diagnosis may lead to severe sepsis. Evidence of injury to other organs must be sought.

Treatment.

A. Emergency Measures: Treat shock and hemorrhage.

B. Specific Measures:

1. Extraperitoneal rupture - Drain the site of injury surgically. Open the peritoneum and explore the intraperitoneal organs for injury. An indwelling urethral catheter should be placed.
2. Intraperitoneal rupture - Close the tear transperitoneally if possible. Both an indwelling urethral catheter and a cystostomy tube should be utilized.

Prognosis.

If the diagnosis is made and proper treatment instituted within 6-12 hours, morbidity and mortality will be minimal.

INJURIES TO THE MEMBRANOUS URETHRA

This portion of the urethra is enclosed in the ligamentous urogenital diaphragm attached to the pubic bone. Fracture of this bone often results in tears of this portion of the urethra.

Clinical Findings.

A. Symptoms and Signs: Urethral bleeding is common. The patient may be unable to void. Pain may be present in the lower abdomen or perineum. A tender suprapubic mass (blood, urine, or both) may be felt. Rectal examination may reveal a large boggy mass; the prostate may be avulsed and dislocated upward.

B. Laboratory Findings: The urine is usually grossly bloody.

C. X-ray Findings: A plain x-ray may show fracture of the pelvic bones. A urethrogram may reveal the site of injury. If a catheter can be passed to the bladder, a cystogram should be done to rule out vesical damage.

D. Instrumental Examination: A catheter may be arrested at the site of injury.

Differential Diagnosis.

Other urologic injuries are differentiated by appropriate x-ray technics.

Complications.

Hemorrhage and urinary extravasation are the serious early complications. The common late complication is urethral stricture. Impotence is not uncommon.

Treatment.

A. Emergency Measures: Treat shock and hemorrhage.
B. Specific Measures: If a catheter can be passed to the bladder it should be left in place for 14-21 days. If a catheter is arrested at the site of injury, suprapubic repair over a Foley catheter should be done. One lb. of traction should be placed on the end of the catheter to approximate the ends of the urethra if it cannot be reconstituted by suture. The area should be drained.
C. Treatment of Complications: Periodic urethral sounds (to 24 F.) are indicated for at least one year to prevent stricture formation.

Prognosis.

The immediate mortality is low. Stricture may develop.

INJURIES TO THE BULBOUS URETHRA

Straddle injuries to the bulbous urethra cause bleeding and urinary extravasation which may spread to the scrotum and penis. There is local pain. Urination may cause extravasation. Urethral bleeding is common. A mass is present in the perineum. Ecchymosis of the penile and scrotal skin appear later.

Hematuria is present. The WBC may be elevated if infection ensues. A urethrogram will demonstrate the site and degree of injury. With minor injuries, a catheter may pass to the bladder. Arrest of the catheter suggests the presence of more serious damage.

The early complications are perineal hematoma and urinary extravasation. The late complication is urethral stricture.

If the patient can void and there is no urinary extravasation, no treatment is necessary. In more severe injuries, the passage of a catheter should be attempted. If this is successful, the catheter should be left indwelling for 3 weeks. If not successful, surgical repair over a splinting catheter is necessary.

If perineal urinary extravasation and hematoma formation are extensive, drainage may be necessary.

All patients suffering from urethral injury require periodic sounding to prevent stricture formation.

INJURIES TO THE PENDULOUS URETHRA

The pendulous urethra is most commonly injured by instruments used for the treatment of severe urethral stricture. Some urethral bleeding is to be expected. If the injury has been severe, the catheter may be arrested.

If urination is unaffected, no treatment is necessary. Severe bleeding may require the placement of a large catheter. In more severe injuries, an indwelling catheter should be left in place for 14 days. Surgical repair (over a catheter) may rarely be necessary.

Postoperatively, sounds should be passed periodically. The only sequel is urethral stricture.

TUMORS OF THE GENITOURINARY TRACT*

Neoplasms of the prostate gland, bladder, and kidneys are among the most common abnormal growths. Tumors of the testis are highly malignant and afflict young men. Neoplasms of other genitourinary organs are rare.

ADENOCARCINOMA OF THE KIDNEY (Grawitz's Tumor; Hypernephroma)

About 80% of renal neoplasms are adenocarcinomas, and two-thirds of these occur in men. They apparently arise from adenomas or renal tubule cells. Benign tumors are relatively rare.

Most metastases occur by way of the blood stream to the liver, lungs, and the long bones. Regional lymph nodes and at times the supraclavicular nodes may also be involved.

Clinical Findings.

A. Symptoms and Signs: Painless total gross hematuria is the most common symptom. An abdominal mass noted by the patient may be the presenting complaint.

   A mass in the flank may be found. It is usually firm and is often nodular.

B. Laboratory Findings: The cardinal sign is microscopic or gross hematuria. Erythrocytosis and elevation of LDH in the urine may be found.

C. X-ray Findings: A KUB may show an enlarged kidney. Excretory urograms show calyceal distortion from a space-occupying mass. If these films are not diagnostic, retrograde urograms may be necessary. Renal angiography will help differentiate cyst from tumor.

D. Instrumental Examination: If the patient has gross hematuria when seen, immediate cystoscopy is mandatory. Bloody efflux from one ureteral orifice is an invaluable sign.

Differential Diagnosis.

Urography differentiates this tumor from hydronephrosis, polycystic disease, and extrarenal tumors. Differentiation from simple cyst is often difficult but may be made by renal angiography or angionephrotomography.

Complications.

These include metastases and hydronephrosis from ureteral compression.

---

*Embryoma of the kidney (Wilms's tumor) is discussed in Chapter 7.

Treatment.

Nephrectomy is indicated in the absence of metastases. Although these tumors are radioresistant, irradiation may be utilized for local recurrence or osseous metastases.

About 35% of patients are alive 5 years after nephrectomy.

TUMORS OF THE RENAL PELVIS AND URETER

Histologically, tumors of the renal pelvis and ureter resemble tumors of the bladder. They may be benign but are usually malignant. The pelvic tumors comprise 10% of renal neoplasms. Ureteral tumors are relatively rare. Secondary similar tumors are apt to be found distal to the primary growth (including the bladder).

Metastases involve principally the regional lymph nodes.

Hematuria is the commonest complaint. There may be pain if the tumor is obstructive or if clots pass down the ureter. Red cells are commonly found in the urine. An obstructive tumor may lead to infection. Excretory urograms will disclose a space-occupying lesion in the pelvis or ureter. Retrograde urograms may be indicated if excretory urograms are equivocal. Cystoscopy may reveal blood emanating from a ureteral orifice. Search should be made for "satellite" vesical tumors. A Papanicolaou smear usually reveals tumor cells in the urine.

Adenocarcinoma of the kidney may also cause hematuria. Urograms should establish the diagnosis.

Nonopaque stone can mimic pelvic or ureteral tumor on urograms. The differentiation may only be made at surgery.

Unless metastases are present, complete ureteronephrectomy with removal of a cuff of periureteral bladder wall is indicated.

With benign tumors the prognosis is excellent. The outlook for patients with well differentiated tumors is fair; those with anaplastic neoplasms usually die of metastases within 2 years.

TUMORS OF THE BLADDER

Vesical tumors are relatively common. At least 75% occur in men after the age of 50. The cause is not known, but there is increasing evidence that carcinogens in the urine are etiologic factors.

Clinical Findings.

A. Symptoms and Signs: Hematuria is the most common symptom. Secondary infection may develop. Perivesical spread causes constant suprapubic pain.

There is usually little to be found on abdominal examination unless a large tumor is present. On rectal or vaginal examination, fixation and induration may be noted at the base of the bladder.

B. Laboratory Findings: Secondary infection of the urine is common. Bleeding is apt to be intermittent, and for this reason red cells may not always be found on urinalysis. Renal function tests are normal unless bilateral ureteral obstruction has developed.

C. X-ray Findings: Excretory urograms may show ureteral obstruction. On the cystogram, a space-occupying lesion may be noted. Careful search for a primary renal pelvic or ureteral tumor should be made.

D. Instrumental Examination: Cystoscopy makes the diagnosis.

E. Cytology: A Papanicolaou smear will usually reveal malignant cells.

Differential Diagnosis.

Hematuria due to other causes is differentiated by appropriate diagnostic technics (e.g., cystoscopy, urography).

Complications.

Secondary infection of the bladder is common. Hydronephrosis may occur as a result of ureteral occlusion. Urinary retention may supervene if the tumor occludes the bladder neck.

Treatment.

A. Specific Measures: Transurethral resection will cure the less invasive lesions and control some of the less well differentiated growths. Cystectomy is indicated for the more invasive low to medium grade tumors without demonstrable metastases. This requires urinary diversion (e.g., ureterosigmoidostomy).

B. Radiation Therapy: The high-grade anaplastic tumors respond best to this mode of treatment. About 25% will be controlled at 5 years. Should this fail, cystectomy should then be done.

C. Local Chemotherapy: The instillation of thiotepa, 60 mg. in 60 ml. of water, into the bladder once a week for 4-6 weeks, may control or eradicate the more differentiated and superficial tumors. A series of such treatments may be required.

D. Treatment of Complications: Control of secondary infection should be attempted. Nephrectomy may be indicated for an infected hydronephrotic kidney.

Prognosis.

The well-differentiated papilloma may recur or new tumors may form; periodic cystoscopy is therefore imperative for 3-5 years. Later recurrences may be less well differentiated and more malignant.

The prognosis for sessile infiltrating carcinomas is poor even though radical treatment (radiotherapy or surgery) is employed.

BENIGN PROSTATIC HYPERPLASIA

The term "benign prostatic hyperplasia or hypertrophy" is a misnomer since it is not the prostate itself but the prostatic periurethral glands which undergo hyperplasia and in so doing compress the true prostate laterally to form the "surgical" capsule.

Clinical Findings.

A. Symptoms and Signs: The syndrome of "prostatism" includes hesitancy and straining in initiating urination, loss of force and caliber of the stream, terminal dribbling, and (usually) frequency and nocturia. The degree of the latter 2 symptoms depends upon the volume of residual urine and the presence or absence of complicating infection. Rupture of dilated veins at the bladder neck may cause hematuria. Acute urinary retention may develop.

A suprapubic mass may be found if a great deal of residual urine is present. The prostate may or may not be enlarged and may be of any consistency from soft to firm. (Stony hardness means cancer until proved otherwise.)

B. Laboratory Findings: Urinalysis may reveal infection. If the first half-hour PSP specimen contains 50-60% of the dye, there is no residual urine. If less than this is excreted, there is either residual urine or impaired renal function.

C. X-ray Findings: Excretory urograms may reveal complicating hydronephrosis or vesical calculi. Cystography may show vesicoureteral reflux (rare).

D. Instrumental Examination: Catheterization immediately after voiding will measure residual urine. Cystoscopy will reveal the degree of prostatic enlargement, the secondary changes in the bladder wall (e.g., trabeculation), and calculi.

Differential Diagnosis.

Benign prostatic hypertrophy must be differentiated from neurogenic bladder and cancer of the prostate.

Complications.

Obstruction leads to infection of the bladder, kidneys, or prostate. Vesical calculi may form.

The obstruction may cause vesical diverticula. Hydronephrosis may occur from trigonal hypertrophy or when a ureterovesical valve becomes incompetent.

Treatment.

A. Conservative Treatment: Mild to moderate prostatism may be considerably relieved by 3-4 prostatic massages given every 2 weeks. Massages are of value also in reducing edema due to prostatitis, if present. Intercourse should be encouraged to promote drainage. Secondary infection should be treated with antimicrobial drugs.

The patient should be cautioned to void as soon as the desire is noted and not to drink a large volume of fluid in a short time.

Catheterization is mandatory for acute urinary retention. If spontaneous voiding does not then occur, a catheter may be left indwelling for 3 days; a permanent indwelling catheter may be the treatment of choice for the poor-risk patient.

B. Surgery: Four procedures are available: (1) transurethral prostatectomy for the smaller glands; (2) suprapubic; (3) retropubic; and (4) perineal prostatectomy, for the larger glands.

Prognosis.

Surgical removal of the obstructing tissue has a low mortality and should relieve most symptoms.

CARCINOMA OF THE PROSTATE

Cancer of the prostate is rare before the age of 60. The cause is not known, but growth of the neoplasm is influenced by sex hormones.

Most cancers arise in the "surgical" capsule (the true prostatic tissue). The tumor finally grows into the seminal vesicles and surrounding tissues.

These malignancies spread via the perineural lymphatics to the regional lymph nodes. Metastases also occur through the veins, particularly the vertebrals, and most commonly involve the bones of the pelvis. Visceral spread is also seen.

Clinical Findings.

A. Symptoms and Signs:
   1. Early - The presenting symptoms are usually from obstruction, and are similar to those described in the discussion of benign enlargement. Rectal examination discloses a firm, usually flat plaque in the prostatic capsule on its lateral edge. It is usually not raised above the surface of the gland.
   2. Late - There may be complaints referable to local spread or metastases: pain in the low back radiating down one or both legs, edema of one or both legs, enlarged supraclavicular nodes, and loss of weight. The entire gland is usually stony hard and often nodular and fixed. The seminal vesicles may be involved.

B. Laboratory Findings: Anemia may be extreme if bone marrow is replaced by tumor. Urinalysis may show infection. In the early stages of obstruction, renal function is unimpaired. With bilateral ureteral obstruction, renal function will be depressed.

   Serum acid phosphatase is often increased when local extension or metastases have occurred. Serum alkaline phosphatase and urinary LDH may also be elevated when osseous metastases develop.

C. X-ray Findings: X-rays or radioisotope scan of the pelvic bones may reveal metastases. On radiographs, they are usually osteoblastic.

D. Instrumental Examination: Catheterization will measure the residual urine. Cystoscopy will reveal the degree of obstruction and the secondary changes in the bladder wall.

E. Biopsy: If the lesion is extensive and incurable, perineal needle biopsy is indicated before palliative treatment is instituted. The tissue removed on transurethral resection also affords tissue for pathologic diagnosis.

Differential Diagnosis.

Benign prostatic hyperplasia can usually be differentiated by palpation of the prostate. Osteoblastic metastases or elevation of serum acid phosphatase establishes the diagnosis of cancer.

Benign prostatic nodules may be caused by tuberculosis, chronic prostatitis, or prostatic calculi. Biopsy may be necessary to differentiate these lesions from cancer.

Complications.

In addition to the changes secondary to the obstruction, spontaneous fractures may occur at the sites of metastases, e.g., spine with paraplegia.

Treatment.

A. Specific Measures: Any prostatic nodule which may represent an early carcinoma should be biopsied; if pathologic examination is positive, radical prostatectomy should be considered.

B. Palliative Measures:

1. Antiandrogen therapy (for men whose tumors are too advanced for radical surgery) -
   a. Estrogen medication - Diethylstilbestrol, 1 mg. daily.
   b. Orchiectomy.
   c. Medical adrenalectomy (with corticosteroids) when the tumor becomes androgen-independent. This may afford comfort for a few months.
2. Radiotherapy to the prostate gives promise of reasonable control.
3. For symptomatic osseous metastases, local radiotherapy, or androgens followed by P^{32} by mouth, may afford relief.
4. Transurethral resection may be necessary if vesical neck obstruction is severe.

Prognosis.

Radical prostatectomy will cure half of cases when the lesion is localized, but the "early" lesion is relatively rare. Palliative treatment affords considerable temporary relief for most patients. The majority die within 3 years; a few may be controlled for 10 years or more.

TUMORS OF THE TESTIS

With rare exceptions, all testicular tumors are malignant. Most occur in men between the ages of 20 and 35 years. The most common type is the seminoma. Second in incidence is embryonal carcinoma. Many of these tumors elaborate chorionic gonadotropins; this finding is usually associated with hyperplasia of the Leydig cells. The true teratoma is composed of both epithelial and mesenchymal components.

Interstitial cell tumors are rare and benign. They secrete both androgen and estrogen, which causes precocious sexual maturation in boys and gynecomastia in men. The rare Sertoli cell tumor is benign and feminizing; gynecomastia is the rule.

The common sites of metastases are the preaortic lymph nodes, lungs, and liver.

Clinical Findings.

A. Symptoms and Signs: The most common symptom is painless enlargement of a testicle. Gynecomastia may be noted with those tumors which elaborate gonadotropins. Symptoms due to metastases include an abdominal mass, pain from bowel or ureteral obstruction, and loss of weight.

The testis is usually enlarged, firm, smooth, and heavy. Squeezing such a lesion fails to elicit typical testicular pain. Ten percent are associated with secondary hydrocele.

B. Laboratory Findings: The presence of urinary chorionic gonadotropins means that a chorio-epithelioma is present. Urinary 17-ketosteroids are elevated with Leydig cell tumor.

Urinary estrogens may be increased with both Leydig and Sertoli cell tumors.

C. X-ray Findings: Excretory urograms may show displacement or obstruction of the ipsilateral ureter caused by involved lymph nodes. Lymphangiography may demonstrate lymphatic involvement. A chest film to seek out metastases should be routine.

Differential Diagnosis.

Hydrocele is cystic and transilluminates. However, hydrocele in a young man should be aspirated so that definitive palpation of the testis can be done. Spermatocele is a cyst which lies free above the testis. It contains sperm. Gumma of the testis is rare. A positive serologic test for syphilis should suggest the diagnosis.

Complications.

The complications arise from metastases. A ureter may become occluded by pressure from involved lymph nodes.

Treatment.

If testicular tumor cannot be ruled out, orchiectomy should be done through an inguinal incision. The cord should be divided at the level of the internal ring.

X-ray therapy to the regional lymph nodes (iliac and preaortic) is indicated in all cases; seminomas are quite radiosensitive. Metastatic chorionic tumors may be palliated by chemotherapeutic agents.

Radical retroperitoneal lymph node resection should be considered for all but seminoma and chorio-epithelioma. It is contraindicated in any type when gross metastases are demonstrated.

Prognosis.

The prognosis is poor if there are obvious metastases, chorionic gonadotropins in the urine (choriocarcinoma), or hyperplasia of the interstitial cells. Seminoma offers the best prognosis; chorio-epithelioma the poorest.

TUMORS OF THE PENIS

Tumors of the penis are epidermoid in type. The majority arise on the glans under a redundant foreskin. Metastases involve the subinguinal, inguinal, and later the iliac nodes.

Biopsy is mandatory for all suspicious penile lesions. Darkfield examination will differentiate tumor from chancre.

Tumors of the penis require amputation at least 1.5 cm. proximal to the growth, though the smaller lesions (up to 1 cm. in diameter) are curable by irradiation. In the absence of lymphadenopathy, radical groin (lymph node) dissection is not necessary.

The prognosis is good in small epitheliomas. It is poor when lymph nodes are extensively involved.

DISORDERS OF THE PERIRENAL AREA

Disorders of the perirenal area include enlargements and tumors of the adrenal glands (see pp. 564-574) and connective tissue neoplasms. The majority involve the adrenal glands (e.g., tumors and hyperplasia), and most of these cause endocrinologic symptoms and signs (e.g., paroxysmal hypertension, virilism).

Diagnosis is corroborated and the tumor localized by the usual technics of urologic diagnosis. A KUB may reveal the mass. Urograms may more clearly delineate displacement of the kidney.

Retroperitoneal gas insufflation usually outlines the extrarenal mass. Angiography is also useful in diagnosis. Gastrointestinal series and barium enema may demonstrate displacement of a portion of the enteric tract.

NEUROGENIC BLADDER

Normal vesical function depends upon the presence of an intact nerve supply, both motor and sensory. The most common cause of neurogenic bladder is trauma to the spinal cord. Other causes include degenerative neurologic disease and congenital anomalies.

The detrusor vesical muscle is innervated by parasympathetic (pelvic) nerves S2-4. The external voluntary sphincter is supplied by the pudendal (somatic) nerves S2-4. Sensory fibers travel with the pudendal nerve, the pelvic nerve and the sympathetics (T9-L2). The micturition center in the sacral cord lies at the level of the T12-L1 vertebral bodies. Fractures above that level will produce an upper motor neuron lesion (spastic bladder and legs); at or below that level, a lower motor neuron reaction will be observed (flaccid bladder and legs).

Cystometry affords information about the type and degree of the neurologic deficit. A catheter is passed to the bladder and attached to a manometer. Water is then allowed to fill the bladder slowly. Intravesical pressures are recorded related to the volume of fluid in the bladder. Normally, as the bladder fills, intravesical pressure remains fairly constant until a volume of 350-400 ml. is reached, at which time an involuntary detrusor contraction occurs, causing a sharp increase in intravesical pressure which forces the catheter out. The stream is forceful and there is no residual urine.

Trauma to the spinal cord or cauda equina initially causes "spinal shock," wherein both flaccid paralysis, vesical atony, and anesthesia are present below the level of the injury. This state may last for a month or even a year. The result is overflow incontinence. An indwelling catheter is therefore necessary. If the injury involves the sacral cord or cauda equina, flaccidity will persist. Should the injury be above the sacral segments, increasing spasticity of both the extremities and bladder will develop as shock subsides.

A. Spastic Neurogenic Bladder: The lesion lies above S2-4. Vesical capacity is diminished, intravesical pressure is high, and spasm of the striated external sphincter (and the pelvic floor) causes increased resistance to flow. In addition, involuntary contractions of the detrusor lead to precipitate, cerebrally uncontrollable voiding. Neurologic examination will establish the site of the lesion. Stimulation of the skin of the abdomen, genitalia, or thighs may trigger involuntary voiding. If the injury involves the upper thoracic or cervical cord, an overdistended bladder (plugged catheter) may excite hyperactive autonomic reflexes: severe hypertension, bradycardia, and pilomotor and sudomotor responses above the level of injury.

Periodic excretory urograms and cystograms should be done to observe for hydroureteronephrosis secondary to hypertrophy of the trigone or vesicoureteral reflux. In the presence of infection, vesical or renal calculi may develop. Cystometry will reveal a hyperactive detrusor and high intravesical pressure. Vesical capacity tends to be diminished, and there is some residual urine.

If vesical capacity is large, the patient need do no more than trigger voiding by stimulating the skin of the lower abdominal or genital area. If capacity is small, an indwelling catheter may be needed. If the external sphincter is hyperspastic, leading to a large amount of residual urine, pudendal neurectomy should be considered. If involuntary spasm of the legs accompanies urination, it may be necessary to convert the neurologic lesion from an upper to a lower motor neuron lesion. This will increase bladder capacity and permit manual expression of urine, and will also stop the spastic reaction of the legs. Urinary diversion may be considered if progressive renal damage is noted.

B. Flaccid Neurogenic Bladder: The lesion involves the conus (S2-4) or the cauda equina. The micturition reflex arc is destroyed. Thus, vesical capacity is increased and detrusor activity is impaired, leading to significant residual urine. Urethral resistance is decreased; overflow incontinence is therefore to be expected. The sense of fullness is absent. Suprapubic pressure will cause the urine to flow. Neurologic examination will delineate the neurologic lesion. Flaccidity of muscles and anesthesia will be found if the lesion is complete.

Periodically, excretory urograms and cystograms should be obtained seeking such complications as calculi, hydroureteronephrosis, and vesicoureteral reflux, though their incidence is less than that seen with the spastic bladder. Cystometry will show a bladder of increased capacity, absence of detrusor contractions, and a large volume of residual urine.

If the lesion is complete, urine is passed by manual suprapubic pressure; residual urine, however, is the rule. Attempts at vesical emptying should be carried out every 2 hours to protect detrusor tone. In the presence of vesicoureteral reflux, manual expression of urine is contraindicated; the placement of an indwelling catheter should be considered. If the amount of residual urine is large, it may be necessary to do transurethral resection of the vesical neck. If this does not suffice, destruction of the external sphincter may be indicated. A collecting device will then be needed.

Prognosis.

The major threat to these patients is renal damage from hydronephrosis, vesicoureteral reflux, calculosis, and pyelonephritis.

Periodic urograms and tests of renal function are essential. Progressive damage may ultimately require urinary diversion.

DISORDERS OF THE KIDNEYS*

POLYCYSTIC KIDNEY DISEASE

Polycystic kidneys are usually larger than normal. Cysts of various sizes are scattered throughout and cause progressive impairment of function. In severe cases, death occurs during infancy. The remainder present themselves for diagnosis and treatment after the age of 40 years.

Clinical Findings.

A. Symptoms and Signs: The very weight of the kidneys may cause pain. Hematuria is common. In the stage of renal insufficiency, complaints may include headache, nausea and vomiting, weakness, and loss of weight (uremia).
   One or both kidneys may be palpable. Hypertension is often found. Fever may accompany pyelonephritis or infection of a cyst.

B. Laboratory Findings: Anemia secondary to uremia may be found. Proteinuria and hematuria are the rule. Pus cells and bacteria are common. The PSP or tests of nitrogen retention will reveal some functional impairment.

C. X-ray Findings: Both kidneys are usually significantly enlarged on the KUB. Urograms reveal marked bilateral calyceal distortion. In case of doubt, renal angiography is indicated.

D. Instrumental Examination: If renal function is poor, retrograde urograms may be required for diagnosis.

Differential Diagnosis.

Bilateral simple cysts may deform a few calyces, but calyceal distortion is more bizarre in polycystic disease and total renal function is depressed; hypertension is a common finding.

Complications.

Pyelonephritis and hypertension are common complications.

Treatment.

A. General Measures: Give a low-protein diet, and force fluids so that urinary output is 1500 ml./day if there is impairment of renal function.

B. Treatment of Complications: Pyelonephritis must be rigorously treated. An infected cyst may require drainage. If a cyst compresses the ureter it should be unroofed or aspirated in order to relieve obstruction.

Prognosis.

If the disease presents in childhood, the prognosis is poor. Patients in middle age are apt to die of uremia within 5-10 years after the diagnosis is made.

---

*See Index for Renal Infection, Tumors, etc.

SIMPLE (SOLITARY) CYST

Simple cysts are the most common space-occupying lesions of the kidneys. They are usually unilateral and single. As such a cyst grows, it may destroy renal parenchyma. Calcification of the cyst wall is occasionally seen. About 10% contain hemorrhagic fluid; half of these have papillary tumors on their walls.

Flank pain may be present. The cyst may be palpable. Urinalysis and renal function are usually normal. Urograms will show distortion of the adjacent calyces.

Renal carcinoma is differentiated from cyst by urinalysis (hematuria) and, at times, aortography; polycystic disease is differentiated by widespread bilateral calyceal distortion and depressed renal function.

Spontaneous infection of a simple cyst is rare. Sudden hemorrhage into a cyst causes severe pain. The bleeding may come from a complicating tumor on the cyst wall.

Surgical exploration is indicated because the differentiation between cyst and cancer of the kidney is difficult even with angiography and because 5% of cysts have tumors on their walls. Treatment consists of excision of the extrarenal portion of the cyst.

Without complications, the prognosis is excellent if the cyst is excised. In untreated cases progressive damage to the kidney may occur.

RENAL FUSION

About one out of 1000 people have some type of renal fusion, the most common being the horseshoe kidney. Less frequently, the total renal tissue develops as one mass ("cake kidney") situated in the midline or in one flank. In either case, 2 separate ureters drain the kidney.

Most of these patients have no symptoms. A few may have ureteral obstruction secondary to aberrant vessels, which are always present. Hydronephrosis and secondary infection then develop.

Urograms will usually be diagnostic. The pelves of a horseshoe kidney are situated on the anterior surfaces of the renal masses. The lower calyces extend onto the psoas muscles (in the isthmus). Two pelvicalyceal systems may be noted in the "cake" kidney with both ureters entering the organ.

No treatment is necessary unless obstruction or other complication is demonstrated.

RENAL HYPERTENSION

Most cases of hypertension are of unknown etiology. Coarctation of the aorta, polycystic kidneys, glomerulonephritis, and periarteritis nodosa are often accompanied by high BP.

Renal ischemia may cause hypertension. The etiologic factors include chronic pyelonephritis and stenosis of the renal artery or its branches. The onset of hypertension developing before the age of 30 or after 50 suggests the presence of renal ischemia. The patient with malignant hypertension is also suspect.

Urinalysis may reveal infection. Total renal function is usually normal. Excretory urograms may show changes compatible with chronic pyelonephritis or some delay in excretion with poor concentration of the radiopaque material on the 2-3 minute film. Hyperconcentration of the radiopaque material in the ischemic kidney on the 5-10 minute films implies renal ischemia. A difference of as little as 1 cm. in the length of one kidney shadow on x-ray should suggest renal artery stenosis.

Ureteral catheterization permits evaluation of the function of each kidney. Significant tests include urine volumes, PSP, and the concentrations of sodium, potassium, and creatinine. An ischemic kidney excretes at least 50% less water, has at least a 15% lower sodium concentration, and excretes less PSP than its mate. However, the concentrations of creatinine, potassium, and PSP are increased due to the marked reabsorption of water by the ischemic organ. For the same reason, if a radiopaque fluid is given intravenously, the specific gravity of the urine from the ischemic kidney will rise significantly higher than that from the normal kidney.

The Stamey test is similar in that the infusion of a combination of urea, ADH and PAH will reveal an increased concentration of PAH from the hypotensive kidney.

The radioisotope renogram is also a useful screening test for unilateral renal ischemia (or chronic pyelonephritis). A scintillation scan may show evidence of impaired transport of the isotope (I^{131}) from the cortex to the pelvis in the ischemic kidney.

Aortography is indicated if renal ischemia is suspected. It will reveal the caliber of the renal arteries.

Treatment consists of nephrectomy if the affected kidney is atrophic. Endarterectomy or another acceptable vascular surgical procedure is indicated if the involved kidney is near normal size and significant stenosis of the renal artery is demonstrated.

A large number of hypertensive patients may be cured of hypertension (or significantly improved) when renal ischemia is corrected or the atrophic kidney removed.

DISORDERS OF THE BLADDER

EXSTROPHY OF THE BLADDER

Exstrophy of the bladder is a complete ventral defect of the urogenital sinus and the overlying skeletal system. The posterior bladder wall is continuous with the abdominal skin. The rami of the symphysis pubis are widely separated. Hydronephrosis with infection is common. Treatment usually consists of diversion of the urinary stream (e.g., ureterosigmoidostomy) and excision of the bladder. The associated epispadias must also be repaired. Reconstruction of the bladder and its sphincters has met with little success.

VESICAL FISTULAS

The bladder may communicate with the bowel or vagina. Vesicointestinal fistulas are secondary to intestinal malignancy, tuberculosis, or diverticulitis. Vesicovaginal fistula usually occurs following a gynecologic procedure (e.g., Wertheim operation) or in the advanced stage of cervical carcinoma.

Vesicointestinal fistulas are distinguished by the fact that the patient may pass gas and feces with the urine. In vesicovaginal fistulas there is constant drainage of urine through the vagina.

Treatment of vesicointestinal fistula usually requires proximal colostomy followed by resection of the primary lesion and closure of the bladder. Repair of vesicovaginal fistulas may be performed either vaginally or suprapubically, depending upon the site of the opening.

DISORDERS OF THE PENIS AND MALE URETHRA

POSTERIOR OR PROSTATIC URETHRAL VALVES

Posterior or prostatic obstructing valves consist of folds of mucosa on the floor of the prostatic urethra.

Symptoms are usually those of sepsis. The observed urinary stream is of poor caliber. A distended bladder may be felt. Anemia from infection or uremia is common. The PSP excretion is low, and nitrogen retention in the blood is usually found.

Excretory urograms will reveal marked changes in the bladder (i.e., trabeculation), and dilatation of the ureters and kidneys if there is sufficient function to excrete the iodide. A cystogram often reveals bilateral ureteral reflux. A voiding urethrogram may delineate the urethral valves in a dilated elongated prostatic urethra.

Cystoscopy will show trabeculation of the bladder wall and diverticula. The valves may be visualized with the panendoscope.

Treatment consists of destruction of the valves. Ureteral reflux may require prolonged urethral or suprapubic catheter drainage and, later, repair of the ureteral valves. For advanced upper tract dilatation, nephrostomy drainage may be necessary.

Some of these children die ultimately in uremia.

HYPOSPADIAS

The hypospadiac penis presents ventral curvature distal to the urethral meatus, which is proximal to its usual position. The meatus may open as far back as the perineum. In the latter instances, the scrotum is bifid, and there may be a cyst of the prostatic utricle. Associated cryptorchism is not uncommon.

No surgical treatment is necessary unless the degree of curvature with erection precludes sexual intercourse or if the orifice is so far back that semen cannot be deposited deep in the vagina.

EPISPADIAS

Epispadias is less common than hypospadias but is more disabling because urinary incontinence is usually present. The urethra opens proximal to the glans but on the dorsum of the penis, usually at the abdominopenile angle. Dorsal curvature is the rule. It should be noted that epispadias is a mild degree of exstrophy.

Treatment consists of correction of the urinary incontinence, straightening of the penis, and urethroplasty. If urinary continence cannot be gained, diversion of the urine may be necessary.

PHIMOSIS

Phimosis is the inability to retract the foreskin over the glans. Treatment consists of circumcision, but if acute inflammation is present preliminary incision in the dorsum of the foreskin may be necessary.

PARAPHIMOSIS

In paraphimosis the foreskin, once retracted behind the glans, is prevented from being drawn forward again by a tight preputial ring. This leads to compression of blood vessels and therefore edema of the glans. A dorsal slit in the constricting ring should be made. Circumcision should be done later.

URETHRAL STRICTURE IN THE MALE

Acquired urethral stricture is usually secondary to a "straddle" injury or a late complication of gonorrhea. Its development may follow urethral trauma secondary to the use of the resectoscope (transurethral prostatectomy).

Clinical Findings.

A. Symptoms and Signs: There is loss of force and caliber of the stream. Urinary retention may occur. Cystitis or pyelonephritis may be present. Periurethral induration may be felt at the site of stricture. An abscess may be noted.

B. Laboratory Findings: Pus and bacteria are often found in the urine. The PSP excretion may be diminished if renal damage is present.

C. X-ray Findings: A urethrogram will reveal the degree and site of the stricture. Fistulas may be demonstrated. Excretory urograms may reveal urinary calculi or chronic pyelonephritis.

D. Instrumental Examination: A catheter or sound of average size (22 F.) will be arrested by the stricture. Cystoscopy, after dilatation of the stricture, will show hypertrophy of the vesical muscle and signs of infection.

Differential Diagnosis.

Prostatic obstruction may cause similar symptoms, but in this instance a catheter passes to the bladder with ease.

Carcinoma of the urethra will be diagnosed by biopsy.

Complications.

Prostatitis, cystitis, pyelonephritis, and urinary stones are common complications. Periurethral abscess may develop at the stricture site and may rupture through the skin, causing a fistula.

Treatment and Prognosis.

If a 20 F. sound is arrested, attempts to pass a filiform should be made. If this is successful, moderate dilatation can be accomplished with followers of increasing sizes. Further dilatations with larger followers can then be done every 3-4 days. As an alternative, an indwelling catheter can be passed to the bladder after the initial dilatation and replaced every 2-3 days with a catheter of the next largest size.

The stricture must be dilated at appropriate intervals or gradual contracture will occur. In a few cases the urethra will be too fibrous to permit dilatation; in these instances surgical repair will be necessary.

Most strictures can be kept open by periodic dilatations. The prognosis depends upon the secondary effects upon the kidneys.

DISORDERS OF THE TESTES, SCROTUM, AND SPERMATIC CORD

CRYPTORCHISM

Strictly speaking, the cryptorchid testis is one which has been arrested along the path of normal descent (e.g., in the inguinal canal or prepubic area), whereas an ectopic testis is one which has wandered off the path (e.g., to perineum or the root of the penis). Ten percent of newborns have cryptorchism, but most descend spontaneously during the next few weeks. Three per cent are cryptorchid at puberty.

The spermatogenic (but not the Leydig) cells are quite sensitive to body temperature, and progressive damage can be demonstrated from the age of 6 years on. About 10% of cryptorchid testes have intrinsic defects which will, of course, not respond to therapy.

One or both testes are absent from the scrotum. The scrotum on the affected side is underdeveloped. The testis may be palpable above the scrotum, but it cannot be manipulated into the sac. Inguinal hernia is commonly associated. Differentiation from retractile testes (physiologic cryptorchism) is made on the basis of normal development of the scrotum on both sides and the fact that the testis may be pushed into the scrotum (proving that the length of the spermatic cord is normal).

Complications include inguinal hernia (75%) and, occasionally, torsion of the spermatic cord (see p. 564). Malignant growth seems to be more common in the undescended testis.

Treatment must be instituted by the age of 5 or 6 years. Chorionic gonadotropin, 5000 I.U., I.M., should be given daily for 5 days. If this fails, orchiopexy must be done.

Success of treatment is measured by fertility. The man with one untreated cryptorchid testis produces fewer sperm than normally. Untreated bilateral maldescent causes sterility.

SPERMATOCELE

Spermatocele is a small painless cystic mass usually situated just above the testicle. It arises from tubules that connect the rete testis to the epididymis. Surgical excision is not necessary unless the mass is so large that the patient requests treatment.

HYDROCELE

A hydrocele is a collection of fluid within the tunica vaginalis which may develop secondary to injury, epididymitis, orchitis, or testicular tumor. It is common in newborn infants, but spontaneous cure is the rule in these patients.

Hydrocele is painless; it is cystic and transilluminates. If it develops without apparent cause in a young man it should be aspirated to make certain that it is not secondary to a testicular neoplasm.

No treatment is usually required. If the patient complains of a dragging sensation, periodic aspiration may be sufficient. If the hydrocele refills rapidly after aspiration, surgical excision of the parietal layer of the tunica vaginalis is indicated.

TORSION OF THE SPERMATIC CORD

Torsion of the spermatic cord usually occurs in boys just after puberty. Atrophy of the testis will usually occur unless detorsion is accomplished within 3-4 hours. Symptoms include local pain and swelling and often nausea and vomiting. Scrotal edema is common. Torsion of the spermatic cord must be differentiated from acute epididymitis. Treatment consists of surgical detorsion. At surgery the parietal tunica vaginalis of the other testis should be excised as well to prevent its torsion later.

SURGERY OF THE ADRENAL GLANDS*

PHEOCHROMOCYTOMA (Chromaffinoma)

Pheochromocytomas are functionally active chromaffin tumors which are usually benign. They are rare, usually occurring in no more than 7 per 1000 patients who are screened for this potentially

---

*By John H. Karam, MD.

curable form of hypertension. The sex incidence is equal, and the tumor may appear at any age (most commonly between ages 30 and 50). In over 90% of cases, the tumors are located beneath the diaphragm, most often in or near adrenal glands but occasionally along the aorta, in the sympathetic chain, in the organ of Zuckerkandl, or the urinary bladder. Rare occurrences in the posterior mediastinum or the skull have been reported. The tumors occur bilaterally in 10% of adult patients and slightly more frequently in children, especially when a familial incidence is present.

Malignancy has been reported to occur in 10% of cases, but a diagnosis of malignant pheochromocytoma requires demonstration of metastatic tumor growing within nonchromaffin tissue since the histologic appearance alone is not a reliable criterion of malignancy.

Clinical Findings.

A. Symptoms and Signs: Clinical findings are due to the excessive secretion of catecholamines which produce characteristic pharmacologic effects. Norepinephrine is considered to be predominantly an alpha-adrenergic stimulator, although in large doses it possesses some beta-adrenergic effects as well. Alpha-adrenergic effects result in constriction of arterioles and venules, which increases peripheral vascular resistance and thereby elevates the systolic and diastolic blood pressure. Epinephrine has both alpha-adrenergic and beta-adrenergic effects, the latter resulting in increased inotropic and chronotropic effects on the heart as well as in glycogenolysis and fatty acid mobilization, which contribute to an increased basal metabolic rate.

Typical paroxysmal manifestations are severe headache, blurring of vision, palpitations, nausea and vomiting, epigastric or substernal pain, profuse sweating, dyspnea, pallor, tremulousness, and apprehension. The skin of the extremities may become cold, clammy, and mottled. Attacks may be precipitated by emotion, trauma, or other stress, and can vary in frequency from several times daily to only once or twice a year. Hypertension may be paroxysmal or sustained, or sustained with paroxysms of higher pressures. Pheochromocytoma is often overlooked as a cause of high blood pressure and should be suspected if any of the following characteristics are present: (1) Hypertension that is paroxysmal, extreme, widely fluctuating, recent in onset, or occurring in the young. (2) Hypertension occurring unexpectedly during induction of anesthesia or during an operative procedure. (3) Hypertension associated with symptoms of hypermetabolism, weight loss, or hyperglycemia, with neurofibromatosis, or with medullary carcinoma of the thyroid.

B. Laboratory Findings: The discovery of the major metabolic pathways of the catecholamines has led to considerable progress in the diagnosis of pheochromocytoma. In addition to technics that measure urinary catecholamines, it is now possible to measure their major metabolites such as metanephrine, normetanephrine, and vanillylmandelic acid (VMA). VMA determination is particularly useful for screening large numbers of hypertensive patients, since it is normally excreted in large enough quantities to be measured with simple colorimetric methods rather than the less widely available fluorometric technics required to detect the catecholamines. Furthermore, VMA is not affected by the metabolic products of methyldopa (Aldomet®), a widely used antihypertensive agent that produces falsely high values for either urinary catecholamines or the metanephrine-normetanephrine metabolites. Since occasional cases have been reported in which tumors failed to produce high levels of VMA, urinary catecholamines or metanephrine-normetanephrine metabolites should also be measured in hypertensive patients with any of the clinical features of pheochromocytoma.

Measuring metanephrine-normetanephrine or urinary catecholamines reveals whether the tumor is secreting predominantly epinephrine or norepinephrine. This information is useful in localizing the tumor and planning proper preoperative care. Tumors secreting large amounts of epinephrine are located in or adjacent to one of the adrenal glands in 95% of cases, whereas those producing only norepinephrine are extra-adrenal in as many as one-third of cases. Because of the myocardial stimulation action of epinephrine and its predominantly unopposed peripheral vasodilating effects, the epinephrine-secreting tumors can be especially hazardous during surgery as regards cardiac arrhythmias and vascular collapse, and they require special preoperative management.

False-positive values can be obtained using fluorometric methods in patients who have been taking fluorescent compounds such as quinidine, vitamin preparations, and tetracyclines. Vanillin (in the form of food flavoring) or coffee may interfere with VMA measurements. The catecholamine content of bananas and sympathomimetic nasal sprays can elevate the results of all methods, and the same is true of acute stress such as increased intracranial pressure, electric shock therapy, and myocardial infarction.

Blood and urine glucose are often elevated in patients with pheochromocytoma, and a diabetic glucose tolerance test is present, associated with decreased serum insulin levels. After excision of the tumor, this carbohydrate intolerance usually disappears.

C. Special Diagnostic Procedures:

1. Drug tests - Before the development of reliable methods to measure catecholamines and their metabolites, a great deal of reliance was placed on pharmacologic tests such as the use of an alpha blocker, phentolamine, to reduce an elevated blood pressure, or of histamine or (preferably) glucagon to provoke an attack in a normotensive patient. At present, there is less need for these tests, whose diagnostic accuracy is less than 75% and which can be hazardous to the patient if there is an acute fall or rise in blood pressure. The biochemical methods outlined above offer a convenient diagnostic approach which is almost 100% accurate and is without risk.
2. X-ray examinations - Localization of the tumor with intravenous urograms combined with nephrotomography has been possible in 50% of cases. If aortography is indicated, it should be done only **after** the diagnosis is established and the patient is well controlled with alpha-adrenergic and

possibly beta-adrenergic drugs. This is essential to reduce the hazard from excessive catecholamine release during the testing procedure.

Treatment.

Once the diagnosis of pheochromocytoma has been established, the patient should be carefully prepared for surgery. Potentially fatal complications at surgery include the following: (1) excessive rises in blood pressure, which may induce cerebral hemorrhage or pulmonary edema; (2) cardiac arrhythmias, especially if epinephrine secretion is high; and (3) a precipitous fall in blood pressure once the tumor is removed. Great progress has been made in reducing surgical mortality from as high as 45% before 1950 to 13% from 1950 to 1960, and down to 1-5% presently. This reduction can be attributed to improvement in diagnostic methods, permitting earlier surgical intervention; more effective drugs for control of hypertension and arrhythmias; and a heightened awareness of the problem of hypovolemia resulting from chronic vasoconstriction in many of these patients. By preoperative administration of alpha-adrenergic blocking agents such as phentolamine (Regitine®), a short-acting agent, or phenoxybenzamine (Dibenzyline®), a longer-acting agent, it is possible to reduce the BP and permit gradual reestablishment of the blood volume. Because of its longer duration of action, smoother control, and fewer side-effects, phenoxybenzamine has proved to be the superior agent for preoperative management as well as for chronic treatment of patients with inoperable metastatic pheochromocytoma. The drug requirement must be titrated in each patient; the usual dosage range is 100 mg. of phenoxybenzamine in 2-3 divided doses.

In addition to the chronic preoperative medication with alpha-adrenergic blocking agents, it is important to avoid anesthetic agents such as cyclopropane, ether, or curare, which increase sympathetic activity. Halogenated hydrocarbons are the anesthetics of choice - particularly methoxyflurane (Penthrane®). Just before and during the operation, hypertension is controlled by frequent repeated intravenous injections of 1-5 mg. of phentolamine (10 mg. in 100 ml. of saline). Because of their relatively short duration of action, beta-adrenergic blocking agents have not been advocated in preoperative management except in cases of severe sinus tachycardia or recurrent arrhythmias. However, 2-3 mg. of propranolol (Inderal®) administered intravenously during surgery has been most effective in curtailing ventricular arrhythmias or extreme tachycardia. Combined alpha and beta blockade reduces the chances of hypertensive crises and death from ventricular arrhythmias but complicates the anesthetist's task by removing some of the classic signs of blood loss and overtransfusion. An anterior abdominal approach is advocated by most surgeons, and the abdomen and pelvis should be explored for multiple tumors, particularly in children and familial cases. Timely repletion of blood volume by administering whole blood or human albumin, beginning with the skin incision, has been most useful in preventing the vascular collapse which often follows successful removal of the tumor. Difficulty in maintaining normal levels of BP without vasopressors during or after operation usually indicates that blood volume has not been effectively restored. Using central venous pressure as a guide, blood should be administered promptly and in adequate quantity to combat hypovolemic hypotension.

If the tumor has been successfully treated, urinary catecholamines or metabolites should return to normal by one week postoperatively. However, reevaluation at regular intervals is recommended, since additional pheochromocytomas may occur.

CUSHING'S SYNDROME
(Adrenocortical Hyperfunction)

The metabolic and clinical changes of Cushing's syndrome are caused by excessive secretion of adrenocortical hormones due to (1) bilateral adrenocortical hyperplasia (60-65%), (2) adrenocortical tumor (30%), or (3) no demonstrable anatomic lesion of the adrenals (5-10%). Bilateral hyperplasia usually occurs without other recognizable endocrine lesions, but it can occur less commonly either in association with a basophilic or chromophobic pituitary tumor or with carcinoma of nonadrenal, nonpituitary origin - so-called ectopic ACTH-producing carcinomas. These latter are most often either undifferentiated "oat cell" carcinoma of the lung, or are thymomas, but have originated in many other entodermal sites, including the esophagus, colon, pancreas, biliary tree, or thyroid. Adrenal tumors, which are usually unilateral, may either be benign adenomas or, in less than half of cases, carcinomas. Rarely, bilateral nodular lesions occur which behave with the autonomy found in tumors yet retain certain histologic features of hyperplasia.

Cushing's syndrome is most common in women between 20 and 40 years of age. The cause of adrenal hyperplasia is unknown in most instances. A malfunctioning hypothalamic control center where corticotropin-releasing factor is produced in excess and not suppressed by the usual physiologic levels of cortisol has been suggested.

Clinical Findings.

A. Symptoms and Signs: Weakness, menstrual irregularity or amenorrhea, moon facies, "buffalo hump," truncal obesity, hirsutism, plethora, hypertension, back pain, acne, psychiatric disturbances, easy bruisability, purple striae, and diabetes are the most characteristic manifestations. Virilization is usually marked in carcinoma of the adrenal.

B. Laboratory Findings: Typical hematologic features are mild polycythemia and slight leukocytosis with neutrophilia and relative lymphopenia (less than 15% of total WBC). When carcinoma is the cause, anemia and hypokalemic alkalosis are more common.

While increased levels of metabolic products of cortisol generally appear in the urine of patients with Cushing's syndrome, this is not a specific finding and can occur in hypermetabolic states as well as obesity. Unfortunately, a plasma measurement of 17-hydroxycorticosteroids is also not definitive, since it is not always raised significantly above normal in patients with Cushing's syndrome and can be greatly elevated by oral contraceptives or pregnancy, which increase corticosteroid-binding globulin.

For screening patients, particularly in differentiating those with exogenous obesity from Cushing's disease, suppression tests have proved most useful. A synthetic steroid with marked glucocorticoid activity, dexamethasone, will inhibit pituitary production of ACTH in normal individuals when given at 11 p.m. in a dosage of only 1 mg. Accordingly, if the level of plasma cortisol is below 5 μg./100 ml. at 8 a.m. the following morning, the diagnosis of Cushing's disease can be ruled out. If it is above this level, in the absence of obvious physical or emotional stress, the most definitive diagnostic test to establish Cushing's syndrome is the demonstration of more than 200 μg. of free cortisol in a 24-hour collection of urine.

Once Cushing's syndrome is diagnosed, it is necessary to determine whether it is dependent on pituitary ACTH or if it is autonomous. Accordingly, a suppression test with a high dose of dexamethasone (2 mg. every 6 hours) for 8 doses has been shown to suppress the pituitary-dependent cases, such as bilateral hyperplasia, but will not affect the urinary cortisol metabolites of patients with autonomous neoplasms, whether adrenal or extra-adrenal. Nonsuppressible patients with Cushing's syndrome who respond to ACTH usually have benign adenomas, and their prognosis for successful therapy is the best of all the types of Cushing's syndrome.

A recently developed radioimmunoassay of plasma ACTH offers great promise as a most convenient way of differentiating the various types of Cushing's syndrome. Slightly high values with absence of diurnal variation occur in those patients with bilateral hyperplasia, while patients with adrenal tumors have undetectable levels, and those with extra-adrenal tumors show extreme elevations.

However, until ACTH assays are more prevalent, the use of a metyrapone test is recommended which blocks cortisol production acutely in all forms of Cushing's syndrome. Five hundred mg. of metyrapone (Metopirone®) are given hourly from 7 a.m. through 12 noon for 6 doses and a 24-hour urine is collected. A plasma ACTH increase can either be assayed directly, which indicates pituitary-dependent bilateral hyperplasia, or indirectly by demonstrating a rise in urinary metabolites of a cortisol precursor, tetrahydrodeoxycortisol, which is readily detected by all standard urinary corticosteroid determinations. This test provides the same information as the large-dose dexamethasone suppression test while eliminating the need to administer excessive glucocorticoids to patients with Cushing's syndrome who are already on the borderline of impending psychosis, peptic ulceration, and excessive protein catabolism.

C. X-ray Findings: Generalized osteoporosis of the skull and ribs with compression fractures of the spine can occur in any patient, especially if the diagnosis is delayed. This is most severe in prepubertal or postmenopausal cases. The sella turcica is almost never enlarged preoperatively. Nephrotomography after intravenous urography may suffice for preoperative localization of the adrenal lesion; however, a combination of arteriography and retroperitoneal gas insufflation has been advocated as the most definitive localizing technic for difficult cases.

Treatment.

The treatment of choice for Cushing's syndrome appears to be adrenalectomy - unilateral for adrenal neoplasms and bilateral and total for adrenal hyperplasia. When a tumor has been diagnosed and localized to one side, a lumbar approach is preferable, whereas with bilateral hyperplasia most surgeons advocate a transabdominal approach and total adrenalectomy. Following total adrenalectomy, lifelong substitution therapy with corticosteroids is required; pituitary adenoma may be present and later become clinically apparent in about 10% of adrenalectomized patients who develop severe pigmentation secondary to increased elaboration of melanophore-stimulating hormone (MSH) by a pituitary adenoma. Despite these disadvantages of total adrenalectomy, it has proved far superior to attempts at subtotal adrenalectomy, which were characterized by frequent recurrences of Cushing's syndrome, necessitating further surgery without significantly reducing the incidence of postoperative enlargement of a pituitary adenoma.

Attempted irradiation or surgical ablation of the pituitary in cases of pituitary-dependent hyperplasia has not proved successful and is not generally recommended except in the rare patient who manifests an enlarged pituitary fossa. Optimal preoperative preparation for adrenalectomy consists of diabetes control and correction of hypokalemia by administering potassium chloride, 3-6 Gm. daily, in divided doses for 1 week. Antacid therapy should be instituted to minimize the effects of surgical stress on any existing tendency toward peptic ulceration. An intravenous drip containing 100 mg. of hydrocortisone hemisuccinate (Solu-Cortef®) or hydrocortisone phosphate is begun before the induction of anesthesia in patients with autonomous adrenal tumors whose endogenous ACTH production is defective, and at the time of the skin incision in patients with bilateral adrenal hyperplasia. Postoperatively, 50-75 mg. of the above rapidly acting hydrocortisone preparations are administered intravenously by slow drip or intramuscularly every 6 hours to provide a total of 300 mg. of hydrocortisone on the day of operation - 200 mg. on the first postoperative day and 100 mg. over each of the subsequent 2 postoperative days. Hydrocortisone is then given orally with gradual reduction of dosage over the next 7-10 days. Patients with total adrenalectomy require permanent replacement therapy with 30-40 mg. of hydrocortisone in daily divided doses and often require supplementary mineralocorticoids in the form of 0.1 mg. of fludrocortisone (Florinef®) to maintain normal blood volume and electrolyte balance. After excision of a unilateral tumor, the maintenance dose of hydrocortisone is gradually reduced over 3-4 weeks to reach a final regimen of 5-10 mg. of hydrocortisone just prior to stopping treatment completely. Forsham recommends that this be given in a single morning dose during the last week of withdrawal to minimize inhibition of the endogenous ACTH, which is gradually resuming control of the reviving normal adrenal gland.

Special postoperative attention is required in patients with Cushing's syndrome since the presence of high levels of glucocorticoids preceding and during the immediate postoperative period adds to the hazard of infection, wound dehiscence, stress-induced peptic ulcer, and psychosis. Respiratory complications are increased postoperatively by the pendulous obese abdomen with weak, flabby musculature and elevated diaphragms. In addition, a slight increase in coagulability of the blood, with danger of infarction and thromboembolism, seems to occur coincident with the fall in the very high levels of glucocorticoids after successful therapy. Any of the signs of acute adrenal insufficiency (hypotension, tachycardia, or hyperthermia) are indications for increasing the intravenous hydrocortisone replacement while carefully examining for other causes.

The prognosis after excision of adrenal adenoma is good. However, to verify that the tumor was truly benign, urinary steroid measurements should be made every 6 months for several years after removing a functioning tumor. After total adrenalectomy for hyperplasia, pituitary chromophobe adenoma may become clinically apparent. Therefore, it is advisable to obtain x-rays for enlargement of the sella turcica and to check the visual fields periodically, especially if hyperpigmentation develops. Patients with evidence of a pituitary tumor require pituitary irradiation and, if this is unsuccessful, hypophysectomy.

The prognosis for adrenal carcinoma is poor. Its presence should be suspected in any patient with Cushing's syndrome who has a history of recent onset of symptoms that have progressed rapidly and who has physical features of virilization, hypokalemic alkalosis, relatively high levels of blood and urinary corticosteroids containing measurable levels of tetrahydrodeoxycortisol, and high levels of 17-ketosteroids in base-line urines, and who fails to increase corticosteroid production after ACTH administration.

Rarely, malignant tumors of the adrenal cortex are feminizing, with increased urinary excretion of estrogenic substances.

Cancer chemotherapy with specific adrenal cytolytic agents such as mitotane (Lysodren®; o,p'DDD) has generally proved unrewarding. Aminoglutethimide, an agent that block steroidogenesis, reduces the corticosteroid production but does not restrict the growth of carcinomatous tissue. Likewise, total adrenalectomy in cases of inoperable ectopic ACTH-producing carcinoma may alleviate the weakness and severe electrolyte imbalance but has little effect on prolonging survival.

ADRENOGENITAL SYNDROME

The adrenogenital syndrome is characterized by virilization that is clinically apparent only in females or in prepubertal males. The 2 major sources of endogenous androgens are the adrenal gland and ovary, and disorders of either can produce virilization. **Adrenal virilism** is produced by adrenocortical hypersecretion of androgens which include both the weak androgenic 17-ketosteroid hormones and the highly potent androgen, testosterone. This hypersecretion can result from either Cushing's syndrome, as discussed in the previous section, or may be caused by a congenital or, occasionally, an acquired deficiency of certain key hydroxylating enzymes required for cortisol biosynthesis. In the latter case, with inadequate levels of cortisol, feedback inhibition of pituitary ACTH production is subnormal, and the greater trophic stimulation of the adrenal cortex results in the development of hyperplastic tissue which overproduces androgens, including testosterone.

Congenital adrenal hyperplasia is an autosomal recessive defect which is usually manifested in childhood as precocious puberty, producing macrogenitosomia praecox in boys and pseudohermaphroditism in girls. Height is increased at first, but these children will eventually be shorter than normal. The acquired form of this syndrome is clinically evident in the adult female, who has an enlarged clitoris, small breasts, hirsutism, amenorrhea, acne, deepening of the voice, and increased muscular development with a male habitus.

In the most commonly recognized form of congenital hyperplasia, there is a deficiency of the 21-hydroxylating enzyme. When this defect is partial, compensatory hyperplasia usually results in the production of enough cortisol and mineralocorticoids to meet basal requirements, and the clinical manifestation is only that of **simple virilism.**

If the defect is more complete, so that compensation is inadequate, the associated mineralocorticoid deficiency results in **virilization with a salt-losing tendency.** Infants with this defect may present a clinical picture of severe addisonian crisis in the neonatal period. The diagnosis of 21-hydroxylase deficiency can be confirmed by finding a low or normal level of 17-hydroxycorticosteroids in the urine, associated with elevated excretion of both 17-ketosteroids and pregnanetriol.

In the less common 11-hydroxylase deficiency, the androgen excess is associated with an accumulation of deoxycorticosterone, which often presents as virilization with hypertension. Patients with this defect have steroid hypertension, which is usually reversible when the adrenal is suppressed. The confirmatory laboratory findings consist of a high 17-ketosteroid excretion associated with an elevation of 17-hydroxycorticosteroids as well, due to excessive accumulation and excretion of the immediate precursor to cortisol, 11-deoxycortisol (compound S). Urinary excretion of pregnanetriol is normal or only slightly increased. Patients with 11-hydroxylase deficiency can be distinguished from those with Cushing's syndrome by demonstrating that excessive 17-hydroxycorticosteroid excreted in the urine is largely made of tetrahydro S, and that total 17-hydroxycorticosteroid excretion is readily suppressed by the second day of dexamethasone (0.5 mg. every 6 hours for 8 doses), a dosage too small to suppress patients with Cushing's syndrome.

The treatment of adrenal virilism due to defective cortisol biosynthesis is mainly medical. It consists of restoring physiologic levels of circulating corticosteroids, thereby suppressing the excess ACTH with its consequent androgen overproduction. The use of prednisone or prednisolone has been recommended. The adult dose should not exceed 12.5 mg. daily administered in 3 unequally divided doses as follows: 5 mg. in the morning, 2.5 mg. at noon, and 5 mg. at bedtime. This schedule provides effective suppression of ACTH during the crucial hours after midnight. Adequate treatment is manifested by a return of urinary pregnanetriol and 17-ketosteroid excretion to normal or subnormal levels, as well as clinical regression of many of the virilizing features. It is important to make the diagnosis early, while virilization is still reversible. Clitoridectomy and plastic vaginal repair may be needed for reconstruction of the external genitalia in cases of pseudohermaphroditism.

Surgical treatment is indicated in patients with adrenal virilization due to adrenocortical malignancies and in most cases of ovarian virilism such as arrhenoblastoma, hilar cell tumor, or in certain patients with Stein-Leventhal syndrome.

PRIMARY HYPERALDOSTERONISM

Aldosterone is a potent mineralocorticoid produced by the zona glomerulosa of the adrenal cortex. Primary hyperaldosteronism, or autonomous hypersecretion of the hormone, is distinguished from secondary hyperaldosteronism, wherein the adrenal cortex is responding appropriately to an external stimulus such as the renin-angiotensin system. In most cases of primary hyperaldosteronism, a single well-capsulated adrenocortical adenoma is responsible. These are quite small, being less than 16 mm. in diameter in two-thirds of cases, and seem to occur in the left adrenal gland at least twice as often. Females predominate in a ratio of 2.6:1, with most patients being between 30 and 50 years of age. Bilateral nodular hyperplasia of the adrenals has recently been noted to occur with relatively high frequency in cases of primary hyperaldosteronism (at least 20%, to as high as 45% in one large series), and has been termed "idiopathic" or "pseudoprimary" hyperaldosteronism.

Clinical and Laboratory Features.

Hypertension without edema is characteristic of primary hyperaldosteronism, and Conn has emphasized the 4 most common symptoms of this syndrome as muscle weakness, polydipsia, headache, and nocturnal polyuria. Other features of the disease are orthostatic hypotension, tetany, and a relatively mild retinopathy. Laboratory abnormalities include hypervolemia and hypokalemic alkalosis in the presence of a normal or elevated serum sodium. Occasionally hypokalemia may not be apparent in cases of long-term sodium restriction, and can be unmasked by a few days of salt loading to restore the capacity of the distal renal tubule to excrete potassium excessively. On the other hand, diuretic therapy should be discontinued before any special emphasis is given to the finding of hypokalemia associated with hypertension. Since hormonal assays for screening of all hypertensive patients are not practical at present, they should be reserved for those hypertensive patients with some of the clinical features of the syndrome. Additional diagnostic aids suggesting hyperaldosteronism include (1) an inappropriately high urinary excretion of potassium in excess of 30 or 40 mEq./L., despite hypokalemia, and (2) correction of hypokalemia after 100 mg. of spironolactone (Aldactone®) 4 times a day for 3 days, a dose that does not raise serum K^+ in control subjects.

Final confirmation of hyperaldosteronism requires the direct demonstration that aldosterone is being produced excessively. The value for aldosterone excretion is most meaningful when the patient has been restored to normokalemia, after which potassium supplementation is discontinued for 3 days while 100 mEq. or more of sodium is being administered. Under these conditions, urinary excretion exceeding 20 μg. of aldosterone per day is indicative of hyperaldosteronism.

The next diagnostic step requires differentiation between primary hyperaldosteronism and secondary aldosteronism due to renovascular hypertension. While the latter often causes a more severe retinopathy and possibly an abdominal bruit, further diagnostic maneuvers are often required to establish the proper diagnosis. One investigator has advocated a suppression test wherein the autonomous aldosteronoma does not reduce its secretion during plasma volume expansion after 3 days of deoxycortisone acetate (10 mg. I.M. twice daily) on a high-sodium diet, whereas patients with secondary hyperaldosteronism decrease their daily aldosterone excretion well into the normal range.

It has been noted that while spironolactone corrected the hypokalemia of both the primary and secondary varieties, its use for 3-5 weeks normalized the BP only in those patients with the primary disease due to an aldosteronoma.

However, the most definitive way to characterize hyperaldosteronism is to determine the plasma renin activity, which is high in secondary hyperaldosteronism and low in the primary form. Improved assays of renin utilize the production of angiotensin I, which is measured by immunoassay after incubation of the patient's plasma with a stock plasma containing renin substrate. The pathognomonic laboratory finding for primary aldosteronism is a low plasma renin activity despite at least 4 hours' ambulation while on a low sodium intake in a patient who also has abnormally high aldosterone production while on a high sodium intake. At present, it is virtually impossible to distinguish patients with primary hyperaldosteronism caused by an aldosterone-producing adenoma from those with "idiopathic," bilaterally involved adrenals.

Treatment.

Primary hyperaldosteronism is treated surgically. Due to the small size of aldosteronomas, their localization is extremely difficult by standard x-ray methods, and requires special technics such as adrenal phlebograms or measurement of aldosterone concentration in adrenal venous effluents obtained during venous catheterization. With localization of the tumor to one gland, the surgeon has the option of using a posterolateral approach for unilateral adrenalectomy, eliminating the need to enter the peritoneal cavity, as well as avoiding the manipulation, mobilization, and occasional removal of normal adrenal tissue in the search for very small tumors. Preoperative electrolyte imbalance should be corrected by administering 8 Gm. of potassium chloride daily in divided doses over a period of 3-10 days, while restricting dietary sodium to reduce urinary potassium loss. Spironolactone is of help in the preoperative repletion of body potassium as well as in correcting the hypertension in some patients. Postoperatively, sodium supplements or, in rare cases, 50-100 μg. of fludrocortisone (Florinef®) daily for several weeks may be required to counteract the hypoaldosteronism that commonly occurs while the remaining suppressed adrenal gland gradually recovers normal mineralocorticoid function. Hypertension returns to normal in at least 70% of patients and improves in most of the others, with only about 5% being unimproved. Likewise, glucose tolerance, which is often slightly impaired in primary hyperaldosteronism, also returns to normal after successful therapy. In patients with "idiopathic" hyperaldosteronism, even total adrenalectomy seldom reduces their hypertension, although normalization of their electrolytes is the rule.

15...

Vascular Surgery

CONGENITAL VASCULAR DEFECTS

CONGENITAL ARTERIOVENOUS FISTULA

The multiple embryonic communications between the arterial and venous trunks occasionally persist as one or more direct or indirect connections between the artery and vein. These fistulas may not be clinically apparent for years.

The lower extremity is most frequently involved, but the vessels of the arm, neck, head, and brain are sometimes affected. Lesions in the extremities are most frequently around the joints. Multiple communicating channels, often involving long segments of vessels, make the condition difficult and often impossible to treat.

Lesions may exist as (1) lateral communications between the artery and vein, without altering the continuity of the main vessels; or (2) 1 or more arteries terminating in a plexus of veins. Capillary and cavernous hemangiomas are closely related disorders.

Clinical Findings.

Many of the local and systemic alterations noted in acquired arteriovenous fistulas are frequently present in the congenital form also (see Chapter 7, Pediatric Surgery).

A. Symptoms and Signs: The involved artery and vein become enlarged, tortuous, and thin-walled to a degree depending upon the number and size of the communications. The skin temperature is higher over the fistula. Very occasionally a thrill may be felt and a bruit heard. There may be increased hair and sweating in the region of the fistula, and the bones of the involved extremity may be abnormally long or eroded. Birthmarks in the area are common.

   Chronic venous obstruction secondary to the fistula may manifest itself by varicose veins and stasis pigmentation, and distal ulceration may occur. Cardiac dilatation may eventually appear, although it is less frequent and pronounced than in the acquired form where the parasitic circulation through the fistula is usually larger.

B. Laboratory Findings: The oxygen saturation of the venous blood in the extremity with the fistula is higher than that of samples taken from the normal side.

C. X-ray Findings: Angiograms before or during surgery will sometimes give useful information, although the results are often confusing.

Treatment.

A. Conservative Treatment: When the communications are present in the lower extremities, pressure on the superficial veins by elastic bandages or stockings make it more difficult for the blood to flow from the artery into the superficial veins. The secondary varicose veins may be at least partially controlled.

B. Surgical Treatment: Direct surgical correction is seldom possible, and even when attempted it may have to be done in stages. Proximal ligation of the largest artery involved is not successful; the communications themselves (they are usually multiple) must be dissected out and ligated. In the rare case of single fistula or where the abnormalities are confined to a limited and readily accessible area, surgical correction by dividing the communications is of value.

VASCULAR INJURIES

ACUTE ARTERIAL INJURIES

The diagnosis of vascular injury may be difficult, but an arterial injury is usually present if the following findings are present: The injured extremity is pale, waxy, mottled, cold, or cyanotic. No pulsations can be felt distal to the injured area. (Distal pulsations do not rule out a vascular injury, however.) Varying degrees of sensory loss may be present, from hypesthesia to anesthesia. External hemorrhage may or may not be present; if it is not, the injured limb is often swollen in the wounded segment whereas the uninjured extremity is not. Ischemia of the muscles distal to the injury will usually cause severe pain and partial or complete loss of muscle function.

A cold, pulseless limb may also be the result of shock, crushing or contusing blows, or exposure. Accurate diagnosis may not be possible until debridement is undertaken, although a wound in the region of a large vessel should always arouse suspicion of an arterial injury.

Treatment.

Regardless of the type of injury, the control of hemorrhage, adequate blood replacement, and restoration of arterial blood flow as soon as possible are the major objectives in management.

The best results are obtained when blood flow is reestablished by arterial repair within 10 hours from the time of injury, but successful repairs have been achieved even after 24 or more hours.

A. Emergency Measures:

1. Control of hemorrhage - If a tourniquet has been necessary, an attempt should be made during the period of resuscitation to replace it with an adequate pressure dressing. A pneumatic tourniquet should be avoided if possible during repair, although it may be necessary during part of the procedure.

   If the wound is large, the ends of the bleeding artery may be directly secured by surgical clamps, taking care to occlude the vessel close to the lacerated ends.

2. Preoperative care of an ischemic extremity - Shock should be energetically treated with adequate blood replacement. A prolonged surgical procedure should usually be deferred until shock is controlled. **Note:** Do not use vasoconstrictor drugs or local heat, and do not elevate the extremity.

Adequate immobilization in a well-padded splint is important. It is probably best to keep the limb at room temperature.

An x-ray of the injured area may be of value to determine the presence of fractures or foreign bodies. An emergency arteriograph may be of value in certain cases in determining the presence or extent of a distal arterial injury.

B. Surgical Treatment:

1. Debridement of the wound should be done as described in Chapter 1, Trauma and Emergencies. Infection is one of the most serious complications that can occur in relation to vascular surgery; the artery wall may become soft and suture lines may leak or disrupt.
2. Arterial suture - Care should be taken to make sure that an artery has not been injured in more than one place and that the posterior wall has not been injured also.

   Suture repair of a lacerated artery is suitable only for small, cleanly lacerated injuries; contused, irregular arterial wounds should be treated by excising the damaged area and a 5-10 mm. segment of apparently normal vessel wall on both sides. An end-to-end anastomosis should be done if technically feasible; if not, a graft should be used and should be of autogenous vein if possible. The manufactured arterial prostheses are unsatisfactory in contaminated wounds; if infection occurs, the presence of the foreign body will prevent the eradication of the infection. Secondary hemorrhage may occur at the anastomotic site and the graft will ultimately have to be removed to eliminate the infection.

   The concomitant vein should be preserved when possible; if it has been damaged, it may have to be ligated.

   Care should be taken to cover the repaired artery, using muscle tissue if possible. If the injury is in a joint area, that area should be splinted for 2-3 weeks.

   Bounding pulses may be noted in the distal arteries at the close of the procedure; occasionally pulses will not be noted for a few hours after the repair even though there is clinical evidence of capillary circulation. If, on the other hand, there is no evidence of return of circulation an hour or so after completion of a grafting procedure, arteriography should seriously be considered to determine if thrombosis has occurred, and the wound may have to be re-explored and the artery examined.
3. Arterial ligation - Ligation of a major artery in an extremity should be reserved for the rare case with arterial injury which will not tolerate the more prolonged surgery required for primary repair or where there has been such extensive soft tissue or bony injury that the repaired or grafted artery cannot be covered by soft tissue.
   a. A single artery in the lower arm or lower leg can be ligated; if two are injured, an attempt should be made to repair one of them even though the success rate in these small vessels is low.

b. Back bleeding from the distal end of a divided artery does not always give an accurate indication of adequacy of collateral circulation.
c. In borderline cases, intermittent sympathetic blocks at six-hour intervals may be of importance in the early postoperative period. If block is effective, an emergency sympathectomy may be of value.

4. Associated fractures - Casts should be cut to allow ready access to the repaired vessel in case secondary hemorrhage should result. Traction should be applied with extreme care so as not to disrupt the anastomosis.
5. A pulsating hematoma which does not increase progressively in size and is associated with a small or distant skin wound will go on to form a false or traumatic aneurysm; in this case, surgical correction of the defect may be deferred for weeks or months. Under ideal conditions, it may be elected to do an immediate exploration and arterial repair.

Prognosis.

Prognosis for survival of a limb which has sustained a severe arterial injury depends upon the following:

A. Duration of Impaired Oxygenation: In general, injuries which are repaired within 10 hours have the most favorable prognosis.
B. Management: Simple ligation of a major artery has a high subsequent amputation rate (50-75%), whereas the amputation rate in cases where arterial continuity has been restored is only about 10%.
C. Associated Injuries: If there is a fracture at or below the level of the arterial injury, the prognosis for survival of the limb is considerably worse.

TRAUMATIC ARTERIOVENOUS FISTULA

An arteriovenous fistula may result from a clean-cut knife wound or a through-and-through bullet wound which produces injury to both artery and vein but usually little associated damage to other structures. In most cases bleeding can be controlled by only slight pressure, and pulsating hematomas may be mild and temporary because the artery bleeds more easily into the vein than into the tissues. Since the artery is often only partially divided, gangrene may not be imminent; and if the circumstances do not demand immediate surgery there are several advantages to delaying surgery until the initial wound has healed and the tissue reaction has subsided: (1) The hazards of operating through contaminated tissue are avoided. (2) Surgery may be difficult because the anatomy is altered by the associated hemorrhage. (3) More adequate collateral circulation develops in a number of weeks. (4) Spontaneous closure of a fistula occasionally occurs.

However, if the injury is associated with a progressively expanding hematoma, or if there is marked and progressive vascular insufficiency of the extremity, emergency surgery may be needed in order to save the limb or the patient's life.

Clinical Findings.

In an unrepaired traumatic arteriovenous fistula a progressive dilatation of the vessels closely associated with the fistula occurs. Collateral circulation gradually develops around the lesion. The larger the fistula, the greater the amount of collateral circulation which develops, and the artery distal to the defect will often enlarge as a result of blood flowing into it from the enlarged collateral channels. If the fistula is large, the direction of blood flow in the artery just distal to the fistula will be toward the fistula and the low-pressure venous circulation beyond. Arteriosclerotic changes gradually occur in the proximal artery, in the fistula, and occasionally in the vein. A palpable thrill and an audible bruit are usually present.

Complications.

A. Varicose veins and sometimes ulcers may develop in the extremity distal to the fistula, and considerable edema and fibrosis may be present secondary to the impaired venous return.

B. Cardiac Manifestations: Centrally located fistulas are more dangerous than a fistula of the same size in a more peripheral part of the vascular tree; this is because the volume of flow through a fistula is greater in the centrally located lesions.

   1. Tachycardia is present, which slows if the fistula is temporarily occluded (Branham's sign). The diastolic pressure is lowered by the persistent reduction of the peripheral resistance caused by the fistula, and an increased pulse pressure results. "Water-hammer" pulse may be noted.
   2. The total blood volume of the body gradually increases to compensate for the blood flow through the fistula.
   3. Cardiac dilatation and, to a lesser extent, hypertrophy result from the increased venous return and cardiac output.
   4. High output cardiac failure may result which can lead to death.

Treatment.

Repair of the defect should be carried out soon after the initial wound has healed and the tissue reaction has subsided in order to prevent local or cardiac complications.

The fistula should be excised and, if possible, a primary anastomosis carried out between the ends of the artery. A vein graft or artery prosthesis should be used if any degree of tension is required to bring the vessel ends together. The vein is usually ligated above and below the fistula, although it should be repaired and preserved if possible.

DEGENERATIVE AND INFLAMMATORY ARTERIAL DISEASES

ANEURYSMS OF THE THORACIC AND UPPER ABDOMINAL AORTA

Progress in antibiotic therapy has reduced the incidence of syphilitic aneurysms; most thoracic aneurysms are now arteriosclerotic in nature. Very rapid deceleration, as in an automobile or airplane accident, can result in a tear of the thoracic aorta just beyond the origin of the left subclavian artery. Cystic medial necrosis, a poorly understood and relatively rare degenerative condition, may lead to a thoracic aneurysm in relatively young people.

Clinical Findings.

Manifestations depend largely on the position of the aneurysm and its rate of growth.

A. Symptoms and Signs: There may be no symptoms. Substernal, back, or neck pain may occur, as well as symptoms and signs due to pressure on (1) the trachea (dyspnea, stridor, a brassy cough), (2) the esophagus (dysphagia), (3) the left recurrent laryngeal nerve (hoarseness), or (4) the superior vena cava (edema in the neck and arms; distended neck veins). The findings of regurgitation at the aortic valve may be present.
B. Laboratory Findings: Serologic tests for syphilis may be positive.
C. X-ray Findings: X-ray examination (several views) and perhaps fluoroscopy, tomography, esophagography, and angiocardiography are the chief means of arriving at a diagnosis.

Differential Diagnosis.

The differential diagnosis between an aneurysm and a mediastinal tumor can sometimes be made only at thoracotomy, and even then the diagnosis may be difficult since some aneurysms are so filled with old gelatinous thrombotic material that pulsations may not be a prominent feature.

Treatment.

Aneurysms of the thoracic aorta often progress, with increasing symptoms, and finally rupture. Resection of the aneurysm is now considered the treatment of choice if technically feasible and if the patient's general condition is such that the major surgical procedure can be done with an acceptable risk. This is especially true if the aneurysm is large and is associated with symptoms. Small, asymptomatic aneurysms, particularly in poor-risk patients, are perhaps better followed by periodic examinations and treated surgically only if there is progressive enlargement or the development of symptoms.

A. Saccular Aneurysms With Narrow Necks: These can usually be removed at the neck without cross-clamping the aorta; the aorta can then be closed with a series of sutures at the junction of the neck of the sac with the aorta.
B. Larger Saccular and Fusiform Aneurysms: These require resection of the aneurysm with an aortic graft to the defect. Temporary occlusion of the aorta is necessary, and this interrupts the blood flow to the spinal cord, kidneys, and sometimes the brain. Among the technics which have been used to maintain circulation to vital areas during the period of occlusion are (1) extracorporeal circulation by means of a pump oxygenator (for aneurysms of the ascending aorta and sometimes the arch); (2) a temporary shunt from the aorta above to the aorta below the aneurysm; and (3) pumping of blood from the left atrium to the femoral artery (for aneurysms located distal to the arch in the descending thoracic aorta).

DISSECTING ANEURYSMS OF THE AORTA

The dissection may begin as a primary tear of the intima of an atherosclerotic ascending aorta or, less commonly, of the aorta distal to the arch. Hypertension is often an etiologic factor. Dissection may arise as a result of degenerative changes in the media of the aorta (cystic medial necrosis), which may result in intramural bleeding; the resulting hematoma may lead to a tear of the intima. Blood may then flow out of the lumen into the wall of the aorta. In either case, the blood dissects in the media of the artery, and external rupture usually occurs in hours, days, or weeks. Intraluminal rupture may occur with the establishment of a reentry opening, and the patient may survive with blood flowing through both the lumen of the aorta and the new channel in the aortic wall.

Clinical Findings.

A. Symptoms and Signs: Severe, persistent pain of sudden onset is usually present, most often in the chest and occasionally radiating to the back, abdomen, and hips. Shock may be present. Partial or complete occlusion of the arteries to the brain or spinal cord may lead to CNS findings. Peripheral pulses and blood pressures may be diminished and unequal and murmurs may appear over the aortic valve area or over the arteries.

B. X-ray Findings: X-rays may show widening of the thoracic aorta with progressive changes. Angiocardiography, by means of a catheter passed into the right side of the heart, may show the double lumen. Hemorrhage into the pericardial sac may result in an enlarged cardiac silhouette. Pleural effusion may occur, usually on the left side.

C. Electrocardiography: Ecg. may help differentiate this condition from an acute myocardial infarction.

Treatment.

The aim of surgery is to prevent further intramural dissection and eventual rupture by creating a reentry from the dissecting intramural channel to the true lumen of the aorta. If dissection starts in the descending thoracic aorta, this segment of vessel can be replaced by a prosthesis. A temporary shunting maneuver is usually necessary to protect the spinal cord while the thoracic aorta is clamped.

The emergency surgical approach to this serious problem has been associated with a high mortality rate, and, when hypertension is present (as it usually is), an active medical approach with hypotensive drugs may in many cases prove to be more satisfactory. The objective of medical treatment is to lower the blood pressure and diminish the pulsatile flow from the heart. This may convert the acute condition to a chronic or stable one, possibly with rechannelization. The drug presently recommended is trimethaphan (Arfonad®) intravenously to reduce the systolic blood pressure to about 100 mm. Hg. This infusion is maintained for about 48 hours, by which time oral antihypertensive agents such as guanethidine (Ismelin®) and reserpine will have taken effect to maintain a relative hypotension.

Chest x-rays, peripheral pulses and murmurs, heart sounds, and the CNS must be checked frequently; if the condition fails to stabilize, surgery may still be employed provided a team and equipment for cardiac bypass is available.

Prognosis.

Without treatment the mortality is very high; death usually occurs in days or weeks unless treatment is prompt and adequate. Some patients can be saved by surgical means or by hypotensive therapy.

ANEURYSMS OF THE ABDOMINAL AORTA

The vast majority of aneurysms of the abdominal aorta are below the origin of the renal arteries and often involve the common iliac arteries. Aneurysms of the upper abdominal aorta are rare. Most aneurysms of the distal aorta are arteriosclerotic in origin and fusiform in shape.

Clinical Findings.

A. Symptoms and Signs: Three phases can be recognized:

1. Asymptomatic - A pulsating mid and upper abdominal mass may be discovered on a routine physical examination, most frequently in men over 50 years of age. As a general rule, surgical resection should be advised even for asymptomatic aneurysms, particularly if the aneurysm is large. Although small aneurysms (less than 7 cm.) also rupture, surgery may occasionally be withheld if the patient is a poor operative risk and especially if he has a significant cardiac, renal, or distal peripheral obliterative vascular disease. If the aneurysm increases in size or becomes symptomatic, operative intervention should seriously be considered.
2. Symptomatic - Pain varies from mild mid-abdominal discomfort to severe constant or intermittent abdominal and back pain requiring narcotics for relief. Intermittent pain may be associated with a phase of enlargement or intramural dissection. Pain is an unfavorable prognostic sign which usually justifies early surgery. Peripheral emboli and thrombosis, which commonly complicate the more distal aneurysms, are infrequent in abdominal lesions.
3. Ruptured - Rupture of an aneurysm almost always causes death in a few hours or days and is therefore an indication for immediate surgical intervention. Pain is usually severe. Because the dissection is most often into the retroperitoneal tissues, which offer some resistance, shock and other manifestations of blood loss may at first be mild or absent; but free uncontrolled bleeding inevitably follows, resulting in death. There is an expanding, pulsating abdominal and flank mass, and subcutaneous ecchymosis is occasionally present in the flank or groin. Massive gastrointestinal hemorrhage from the aneurysm through a fistula into the distal duodenum can occur. About half of the patients with ruptured aortic aneurysm can be saved by immediate surgery.

B. Laboratory Findings: Cardiac and renal function should be evaluated by means of Ecg., urinalysis, and BUN determination.

C. X-ray Findings: Calcification in the wall of the aneurysm will usually outline the lesion on anteroposterior and lateral plain films of the abdomen. In some cases the position of the aneurysm in relation to the renal arteries can be identified by intravenous urograms, but more often the examination is inconclusive. Bony erosion of the vertebrae seldom occurs with abdominal aneurysms. Translumbar aortograms are seldom employed; the aneurysm may be ruptured by the procedure, and the information gained regarding the upper limits of the lesion may be inaccurate since a thrombus often occupies most of the aneurysm. If distal arterial occlusive disease is suspected, an aortogram may be indicated to obtain more accurate knowledge of the extent of the distal disease.

Treatment.

Surgical excision and grafting of the defect is indicated on all aneurysms of the distal aorta except when the lesion is very small and asymptomatic or when the general condition of the patient is so poor that the surgical risk is greater than the risk of rupture.

Prognosis.

Complications and mortalities following surgery are most often associated with myocardial infarction, acute renal failure, hemorrhage from one of the anastomoses, and distal arterial thrombosis. The mortality following elective surgical treatment is 5-10%; after the aneurysm has ruptured, surgical mortality is about 50%.

ANEURYSMS OF THE VISCERAL BRANCHES OF THE ABDOMINAL AORTA

The hepatic, splenic, and more rarely the renal and superior mesenteric arteries occasionally are subject to aneurysmal changes. Treatment is by resection with or without reestablishment of circulation depending upon the nature of the aneurysm and the importance of the vessel.

FEMORAL AND POPLITEAL ANEURYSMS

Aneurysms of the femoral or popliteal arteries are not uncommon. They are usually arteriosclerotic in origin, in which case they may be multiple and are often bilateral. They may also be due to trauma. Syphilitic or mycotic aneurysms occur occasionally, the latter after an episode of bacteremia or, more often, from a septic embolus.

Clinical Findings.

The diagnosis is usually not difficult, although a lesion in the popliteal area may go unnoticed until attention is focussed on the area by a complication of the aneurysm.

A. Symptoms and Signs: The cardinal finding is a firm, pulsating mass in the femoral or popliteal area, often associated with a bruit. Pulsation may not be present if thrombosis has already taken place. The distal circulation may be impaired, especially if the gelatinous thrombus which so frequently fills most of the aneurysm has partially or completely occluded the central lumen or if emboli from this thrombus have blocked 1 or more of the distal vessels.

B. X-ray Findings: X-rays with arteriography may be helpful in outlining the extent of the aneurysm and the status of the peripheral vessels, although the central gelatinous thrombus which is so often present may make interpretation difficult.

Complications.

Rupture can occur, and often results in loss of the limb and, occasionally, death. Complete thrombosis causes distal gangrene in about one-third of popliteal aneurysms. Emboli to the distal vessels from the thrombus lining the wall of the aneurysm often cause ischemic changes or gangrene. Thrombophlebitis can occur as a result of pressure obstruction of a neighboring vein. Pressure on the tibial or peroneal nerves may produce pain in the lower leg.

Treatment and Prognosis.

Surgical excision of the aneurysm with grafting of the defect is the treatment of choice in all except very small femoral or popliteal aneurysms or in patients who are poor surgical risks. The incidence of loss of limb following resection and grafting is low. Thrombophlebitis is a not infrequent postoperative complication even though care is taken to avoid injuring or dividing the neighboring veins. In the popliteal area, venous ligation may be necessary.

CAROTID ARTERY ANEURYSMS

Aneurysms of the carotid artery are relatively rare. The bifurcation of the common carotid is often involved. Pressure symptoms and pain are sometimes present, and a pulsating mass is readily seen and felt. The complications include rupture, thrombosis, or emboli from the aneurysm to the cerebral vessels.

Treatment.

Small fusiform aneurysms may be wrapped with strips of fascia lata. Larger aneurysms must be resected, and a graft is often required to bridge the defect. Since surgery may be complicated by CNS damage, an internal shunt should be employed during the period of occlusion.

OCCLUSIVE DISEASE OF THE AORTA AND ILIAC ARTERIES

Occlusion of the aorta and the iliac arteries begins most frequently just proximal to the bifurcation of the common iliac arteries as atherosclerotic changes in the intima and media, often with associated perivascular inflammation and calcified plaques in the media. Progression is usually in a proximal direction, involving first the aortic bifurcation and then the abdominal aorta up to the region of the renal vessels. Narrowing progresses to complete thrombotic occlusion, which often extends from just below the renal arteries to the distal common iliac arteries. Although atherosclerosis is a generalized disease, occlusion tends to be segmental in distribution, and when the involvement is in the aorto-iliac vessels there is often minimal atherosclerosis in the more distal external iliac and femoral arteries. The best candidates for direct arterial surgery are those with localized occlusions with relatively normal vessels above and below.

Men between the ages of 30 and 60 are most commonly affected. Cardiac and renal diseases and hypertension are often associated with this defect.

Clinical Findings.

A. Symptoms and Signs: Intermittent claudication is almost always present in the calf muscles and is usually present in the thighs and hips as well. It is most often bilateral and progressive, so that by the time the patient seeks help the pain may be produced by walking a block or less. Difficulty in having or sustaining an erection is a common complaint in men. Coldness of the feet may be present; rest pain is infrequent.

Femoral pulses are absent or weak. Pulses distal to the femoral area are usually absent. Pulsation of the abdominal aorta may be palpable. A palpable thrill or bruit over an artery is usually indicative of narrowing of the lumen at that site or proximally. Atrophic changes of the skin, subcutaneous tissues, and muscles are usually minimal or absent. Dependent rubor and coolness of the skin of the foot are minimal.

B. Laboratory Findings: Cardiac and renal function should be evaluated preoperatively to determine the degree of coronary and degenerative renal disease.

C. X-ray Findings: A translumbar aortogram gives much valuable information regarding the level and extent of the occlusion and the condition of the vessels distal to the block. Significant plaques in the posterior wall of the vessel may not be clearly defined by the arterial study; this circumstance should be kept in mind in the overall evaluation of a case. The possibility of a complication from this procedure must be weighed against the importance of the information to be gained, but it is usually indicated. Anteroposterior and lateral films of the abdomen and sometimes of the thighs will give some information regarding the degree of calcification in the vessels. An intravenous urogram is desirable.

Treatment.

Surgical treatment is indicated if claudication interferes appreciably with the patient's activities or work. The objective of treatment is reestablishment of blood flow through the narrowed or occluded aorto-iliac segment. This can be achieved by arterial prosthesis or thrombo-endarterectomy.

A. Arterial Graft (Prosthesis): Arterial prosthesis, bypassing the occluded segment, is probably the treatment of choice in the more extensive aorto-iliac occlusions.

B. Thrombo-endarterectomy: This is perhaps of most value when the occlusion involves only a short segment of artery.

C. Sympathectomy: A bilateral lumbar sympathectomy should usually be added to the direct arterial procedure.

Complications of Treatment.

The complications most frequently encountered are (1) hemorrhage from the suture line, (2) thrombosis of the prosthesis or the endarterectomized artery or of vessels in the legs, (3) postoperative oliguria or uremia, (4) myocardial infarction from preexisting coronary artery disease, (5) infection around the prosthesis, often with the development of a false aneurysm associated with one of the anastomoses, and (6) alterations in sexual function.

Prognosis.

The operative mortality is relatively low and the immediate and long-term benefits are usually marked. There is generally relief of all or most of the claudication and in many cases return of all of the pulses in the legs. Sexual function in the male may or may not be improved.

OCCLUSIVE DISEASE OF THE FEMORAL AND POPLITEAL ARTERIES

In the region of the thigh and knee the vessels most frequently blocked by occlusive disease are the superficial femoral artery and the popliteal artery. Atherosclerotic changes usually appear first at the most distal point of the superficial femoral artery where it passes through the adductor magnus tendon into the popliteal space. In time the whole superficial femoral artery and the proximal popliteal artery may become occluded, but often the common femoral and profunda femoral arteries are patent and relatively free from disease. The postoperative status of the popliteal artery and its 3 main branches (the anterior and posterior tibial arteries and the common peroneal artery) is important since early or late postoperative thrombosis will occur if moderate or marked atherosclerosis in this area prevents an adequate and rapid blood flow through the area, into the leg and foot.

Clinical Findings.

As a rule the changes are initially more advanced in one extremity than the other, although similar changes often appear later in the other extremity.

A. Symptoms and Signs: Intermittent claudication, which often appears upon as little exertion as walking one-half to 1 block, is confined to the calf and foot. If rest pain is also present, arterial disease is extensive and the prognosis is poor. Atrophic changes in the lower leg and foot may be quite definite, with loss of hair, thinning of the skin and subcutaneous tissues, and diminution in the size of the muscles.

   Dependent rubor and blanching on elevation of the foot is usually present. When the leg is lowered after elevation, venous filling on the dorsal aspect of the foot may be slowed to 15-20 seconds or more. The foot is usually cool or cold.

   The common femoral pulsations are usually of fair or good quality, but no popliteal or pedal pulses can be felt.

B. X-ray Findings: X-rays of thigh and leg may show calcification of superficial femoral and popliteal vessels. A femoral arteriogram will show the location and extent of the block and the status of the distal vessels, but often it is important to know the condition of the aorto-iliac vessels also since a relatively normal flow of blood into the extremity as well as adequate open vessels to carry the blood into the lower leg and foot are important in determining the success of an arterial procedure. A translumbar aortogram will give information on the condition of the iliac, femoral, and popliteal vessels; the same information can sometimes be gained by the transfemoral study if the patient performs the Valsalva maneuver while 30 ml. of contrast material are rapidly injected into the iliac artery up to the bifurcation of the aorta.

Treatment.

Surgery is indicated (1) if intermittent claudication interferes significantly with the patient's work or essential activities or (2) if pregangrenous or gangrenous lesions appear on the foot and it is hoped that a major amputation can be avoided.

A. Arterial Graft: An autogenous vein graft using a reversed segment of the great saphenous vein - or, if an adequate vein is not available, an arterial prosthesis - can be placed, bypassing the occluded segment, using end-to-side anastomoses both proximally and distally.

B. Thrombo-endarterectomy: Thrombo-endarterectomy with removal of the central occluding core can be carried out by means of specially designed instruments which dissect in the cleavage plane in the wall of the diseased artery. Part of the media and the adventitia is left. The arteriotomies may be closed by means of a patch of vein so as not to narrow the lumen at that point. This may sometimes be used when the occluded segment is very short.

C. Arteriography done at the time of surgery (at the completion of the grafting or endarterectomy procedure) may reveal technical defects which can then be corrected, thus forestalling thrombosis during the postoperative period.

D. Although heparin is usually used locally and in the distal vessels during surgery, most prefer not to use it in the postoperative period because of hematomas and associated complications. Low molecular weight dextran may be used in situations where there is a likelihood of postoperative thrombosis.

E. When iliac or common femoral occlusive disease exists as well as distal femoral and popliteal occlusions, it is probably better to relieve the obstructions in the larger, proximal arteries and thus to deliver more blood to the profunda femoris than to operate on the smaller distal vessels where the chances of success are less favorable. This is especially true if the inflow of blood is diminished by the more proximal occlusive disease.

F. Sympathectomy: Lumbar sympathectomy may be used as an adjunct to grafting or endarterectomy or as the sole measure if a direct operation is thought inadvisable. It can be done a few days before or at the same time as a direct procedure; the vasodilator effect of sympathectomy may improve the circulation to the foot and lower leg, especially if there is considerable arterial disease in the vessels of the lower leg or foot.

Prognosis.

Thrombosis of the "bypass" graft or of the endarterectomized vessel either in the immediate postoperative period or months or years later is relatively frequent in the superficial femoral-popliteal area. This is particularly true if one or more of the 3 terminal branches of the distal popliteal artery are occluded or badly diseased. For this reason it is usually not performed for mild or moderate claudication, and many of these patients will go for years without much progression of their symptoms or the development of ischemia or gangrene. The chances of success are even less in patients with ischemia, but the procedure is often justified for at least some limbs can be saved from amputation. Failure of the graft or the endarterectomy does not usually make the condition of the limb worse than it was before the procedure.

OCCLUSIVE DISEASE OF THE ARTERIES IN THE LOWER LEG AND FOOT

Occlusive processes in the lower leg and foot may involve, in order of incidence, the tibial and common peroneal arteries and their branches to the muscles, the pedal vessels, and occasionally the small digital vessels. Symptoms depend upon the vessels that are narrowed or thrombosed, the suddenness and extent of the occlusion, and the status of the proximal and collateral vessels. The clinical picture may thus vary from slowly developing vascular insufficiency coming on over months or years and sometimes resulting ultimately in atrophy, ischemic pain, and finally gangrene, to a rapidly progressive and extensive thrombosis resulting in acute ischemia and often gangrene.

Clinical Findings.

Although all of the possible manifestations of vascular disease in the lower leg and foot cannot be described here, there are certain significant clinical aspects which enter into the evaluation of these patients.

A. Symptoms:

1. Claudication - Intermittent claudication is the commonest presenting symptom. Aching fatigue during exertion usually appears first in the calf muscles; in more severe cases a constant or cramping pain may be brought on by walking only a short distance. Less commonly the feet are the site of most of the pain. Pain that lasts longer than 10 minutes after rest suggests some other disease, such as arthritis. The distance that the patient can walk before pain becomes severe enough to necessitate a few minutes' rest gives a rough estimate of circulatory inadequacy: 2 blocks (400-500 yards) or more is mild, 1 block is moderate, and half a block or less is severe.
2. Rest pain - Rest pain may be due to sepsis or simple ischemia. The former is usually throbbing, whereas ischemia usually produces a persistent, gnawing ache with occasional spasms of sharp pain. Rest pain first comes on in bed when the foot is warm, and some relief is obtained by uncovering the foot and placing it in a dependent position. In more advanced stages the pain may be constant and so severe that even narcotics may not relieve it. Ischemic neuropathy is an important factor in this condition. The patient may request amputation.

3. Muscle cramps - Sudden painful contractions that last only a few minutes but leave a soreness for minutes or days in a pulseless leg are usually caused by the arterial disease.

B. Signs:

1. Absence of pulsations - Careful palpation over the femoral, popliteal, dorsalis pedis, and posterior tibial arteries should be done to determine if pulsations are present. Although the popliteal pulse may be present, both pedal pulses are usually absent. The dorsalis pedis pulse is congenitally absent in 8% of people, but the posterior tibial pulse is always present unless the artery is diseased even though obesity or edema may make it difficult to find. The examiner may have trouble telling which pulsations are his own and which are the patient's. Exercise or nitroglycerin may speed the patient's pulse and make the difference more apparent. Exercise in certain patients with arterial disease may make pedal pulses disappear.

   Claudication and atrophic changes can occur in patients with palpable pedal pulses. If the popliteal pulse is present, a direct surgical approach on the vessels of the lower extremity is not likely to be of any value.

2. Color changes in the feet - Normally the skin of the feet is warm and pale as a result of the rapid flow of blood through the arterioles, and few of the capillaries are filled. Skin irritation leads to capillary filling and the skin becomes red. Defective blood supply causes anoxic paralysis of the capillaries and a bluish-red skin.

   The rate of return of color following blanching induced by local pressure is an inaccurate index to circulatory adequacy because the blood which returns on release of the pressure does not necessarily represent oxygenated blood that is flowing through the area.

   a. Pallor upon elevation - If pallor appears rapidly upon elevation of the foot from the horizontal - or if it appears when the leg is only slightly raised, the circulatory status is poor.

   b. Flushing time - Color normally returns in a few seconds to a foot placed in a dependent position after 1-2 minutes of elevation to 70-90° with the patient lying on his back. The poorer the collateral circulation, the longer the interval before flushing begins to appear in the toes. In general, if dependent flushing (or reactive hyperemia) begins in the toes within 20 seconds, the arterial disease is mild and the collateral circulation probably adequate, and the extremity may be salvaged by lumbar sympathectomy. If flushing time is over 20 seconds - and especially if it appears only after 45-60 seconds - the arterial disease is extensive and sympathectomy will be of little or no value.

   c. Dependent rubor - Beefy redness of the toes or foot on dependency is frequently present in occlusive disease of this area, but it may not reach its full extent until a minute or more after the leg has been placed in the dependent position. Dependent rubor represents ischemic paralysis of the capillaries in the skin, and implies moderate or severe arterial occlusive disease.

d. Rubor of stasis - When almost complete stasis in the distal vessels occurs, with venous as well as arterial thrombosis and extravasation of red blood cells, redness of the toes and forefoot may develop which may not completely disappear on elevation of the leg. Usually, however, there is pallor of the skin surrounding the red area in the elevated leg. This disorder is often associated with severe pain and is more commonly noted in thromboangiitis obliterans than in atherosclerosis.

e. Patchy cyanosis and pallor indicates a severe degree of ischemia; it is seen frequently following acute thrombosis or recent embolus.

3. Venous filling time - If the valves in the saphenous system are competent, venous filling is a valuable gauge of collateral circulation of the foot. If the veins on the dorsum of the foot begin to fill in 30 seconds or less after the leg is placed in a dependent position after having been elevated for about 1 minute, the borderline pregangrenous extremity with arterial occlusions distal to the popliteal artery can probably be saved by sympathectomy. After complete obstruction of a major artery, the venous filling time may be as long as 90 seconds.

4. Local tissue changes - Diminished arterial flow causes wasting of the subcutaneous tissues of the digits, foot, and lower leg. Hair is lost over these areas, the skin becomes smooth and shiny, and the nails become thickened and deformed. Infections are common following minor injuries or even without injury at the edge of a nail or under a thick callus. Once established, infection may become indolent and chronic with the formation of an ischemic ulcer which is often located over a pressure point of the foot; or the infection may lead to localized or progressive gangrene. Local heat should not be used in the treatment of such an infection.

5. Skin temperature studies - Skin temperature and plethysmographic studies may be of value in calibrating the degree of vasoconstrictor activity, and in certain borderline cases may help determine whether lumbar sympathectomy will be of value. A rough clinical test may be carried out by exposing the leg to room temperature for a few minutes. If arterial circulation is inadequate the leg will feel quite cool.

6. Sweating - Sweating is under the control of the sympathetic nervous system and is therefore an index to the degree of autonomic activity in the extremity. If a patient with occlusive disease still notes sweating of his feet, some degree of sympathetic activity is present and lumbar sympathectomy is likely to be of benefit.

C. X-ray Findings: Films of the lower leg and foot may show calcification of the vessels and thinning of the bones. If there is a draining sinus or an ulcer close to a bone or joint, osteomyelitis may be apparent on the film. If fairly strong popliteal pulses can be felt, arteriography is not likely to be of much value as a guide to surgical treatment; sometimes, however, the status of the femoral or popliteal arteries must be evaluated in this way.

Arterial Disease in Diabetic Patients.

Atherosclerosis develops oftener and earlier in patients with diabetes mellitus, especially if the disease has been poorly controlled over a period of years. Either the large or small vessels may be involved, but occlusion of the smaller vessels is relatively more frequent than in the nondiabetic forms. These are the vessels that do not qualify for direct arterial surgery. The care of the diabetic patient who develops occlusive arterial disease of the foot and lower leg is more difficult. The resistance to infection seems to be less, and the control of diabetes may be more difficult in the presence of infection. Anemia and hypoproteinemia are not infrequently present in moderate or severe diabetes and tend to be resistant to therapy; tissue ischemia may be made more severe by this anemia, and blood transfusions may be necessary. Anesthesia of the toes and distal foot (due to diabetic neuropathy) predisposes to injury and secondary infection. Visual defects due to diabetic retinopathy make care of the feet more difficult and injuries more likely.

Treatment.

A. Intermittent Claudication:

1. The patient should be instructed to walk slowly, take short steps, avoid stairs and hills, and to stop for brief rests to avoid pain.
2. Lumbar sympathectomy is the surgical treatment of choice. It is most likely to be of benefit if the popliteal pulse is palpable, but it may still be of value when only the femoral pulse can be felt in the leg. A flushing time or venous filling time of 20 seconds or less when the leg, blanched by a period of elevation, is placed in the dependent position is a favorable sign; if flushing or venous filling is delayed more than 30 seconds, there is much less chance that sympathectomy will be of any benefit. If sweating of the feet occurs, the operative result is likely to be favorable. More refined objective evidence for or against the operation may be obtained in constant temperature rooms and by means of the plethysmograph.
   a. Walking capacity following sympathectomy may never improve or may not improve for weeks or months since the increased collateral flow to the muscles develops gradually. The improvement in skin circulation, with a dry, warm foot, is often apparent within a few hours.
   b. Because bilateral sympathectomy may result in considerable paralytic ileus in older patients, 2 procedures with 5-7 days between is probably more satisfactory and can be done with a low mortality.
   c. A frequent and annoying sequel to sympathectomy is an unexplained neuralgia down the lateral aspect of the thigh which develops usually by about the tenth postoperative day. The pain may be mild or severe, and may last for days or weeks. The treatment is symptomatic, and the neuralgia always ultimately disappears.

B. Circulatory Insufficiency in the Foot and Toes: Sympathectomy may be indicated even when the femoral pulse is absent (in conjunction with direct arterial surgery in the ileofemoral arteries) or when pregangrenous changes are present in the toes. Moderate or marked rest pain usually implies such advanced changes that the procedure will often be of little or no benefit. The operation usually results in a dry, warmer foot, and the additional collateral flow offers some protection to the leg should further vascular occlusions occur.

C. Infections, Ulcers, and Gangrene of the Toes or Foot:

1. Early treatment of acute infections - Place the patient at complete bed rest with the leg in a horizontal or slightly depressed position. An open or discharging lesion should be covered with a light gauze dressing, but tape should not be used on the skin. Culture and sensitivity studies should be obtained if there is any purulent discharge, but if advancing infection is present an appropriate antibiotic should be started immediately. Purulent pockets should be gently drained.

   Ulcerations covered with necrotic tissue can often be gently debrided and prepared for spontaneous healing or grafting with wet dressings of sterile saline changed 2-3 times a day.

   Treat diabetes and anemia, if present.

2. Early management of established gangrene - In most instances an area of gangrene will progress to a point where the circulation is sufficient to prevent progressive tissue death. The process will at least temporarily demarcate at that level. This can be encouraged by measures similar to those outlined in the preceding section on the treatment of acute infection. If the skin is intact and the gangrene is dry and due only to arterial occlusion, antibiotics should be withheld. If infection is present or if the gangrene is moist, antibiotics should be used in an effort to limit the process and prevent septicemia.

   If the gangrene involves only a segment of skin and the underlying superficial tissue, sympathectomy and, if possible, an artery graft may reverse the process. The necrotic tissue can be removed and the ulcer grafted or allowed to heal as outlined above in the section on ulcers. If the hoped for healing does not occur and amputation is resorted to, it can sometimes be carried out at a more distal level because of these procedures.

3. Amputations for gangrene -
   a. A toe which is gangrenous to its base can sometimes be amputated through the necrotic tissue and left open; this procedure may be employed to establish adequate drainage when there is active infection with undrained pus in addition to the gangrene.
   b. When the distal part of the toe is gangrenous and there is sufficient circulation in the proximal toe, a closed amputation can be carried out after the area has become well demarcated and inflammation has subsided.
   c. Transmetatarsal amputation can be considered if the gangrene involves 1 or more toes down to but not into the foot and if the circulation in the distal foot seems adequate to support healing.
   d. Amputation below the knee may be employed in patients with a palpable popliteal pulse or even without femoral and popliteal pulses if there is good collateral circulation around the knee (as indicated by a warm and well-nour-

ished lower leg) when gangrene or ischemia in the foot is so severe or so distributed that local amputation (as outlined above) is not feasible. The preservation of the knee and proximal part of the lower leg is most important in that a more useful prosthesis can then be applied and the patient can turn in bed with greater ease, and amputation at that level should always be attempted provided there is a reasonable chance of success: Immediate postoperative fitting of a prosthesis and early ambulation appears to aid in the rehabilitation, but careful and precise technics must be employed.

e. Amputation above the knee (through the distal thigh in the supracondylar area) is indicated in patients with advanced peripheral vascular disease requiring amputation because of gangrene or severe ischemic pain. Even if the femoral artery is obliterated, there will be sufficient collateral circulation to allow healing provided gentle technic with good hemostasis is used.

f. Guillotine amputation - Infection with bacteremia or septicemia occasionally develops secondary to gangrene of the lower extremity. This can usually be controlled only by emergency amputation above or below the knee. In such a situation, it is often wise to leave the stump open so that it can heal by secondary intention or be revised or reamputated when the infection has been controlled.

Prophylaxis of the Complications of Impaired Circulation.

A. General Measures:

1. Care and control of cardiac disease, diabetes mellitus, anemia, hypoproteinemia, and obesity. A diet low in calories, saturated fatty acids, and cholesterol and high in unsaturated fatty acids is probably of value.
2. Tobacco should be prohibited for nicotine is a vasoconstrictor.
3. Undue exertion and fatigue are not desirable. Walking should be allowed only to the point of pain and not beyond.
4. Alcoholic beverages in moderation may be of value.
5. Warm clothes should be worn.
6. Elevation of the head of the bed on 4-inch blocks increases the circulation in the feet.
7. Properly prescribed Buerger's exercises may be of value.

B. Local Measures:

1. The patient should be instructed about the dangers of foot infections and injuries; if sensation is altered, the significance and dangers of this should be discussed. Warn the patient that he should consult a physician promptly even in the event of minor injuries or infections. Direct heat should not be applied to ischemic areas.
2. Lanolin should be rubbed on the skin each night to keep it pliable and free of fissures and thick calluses; the nails should be trimmed straight across and not too short in order to prevent ingrown nails; thick calluses and corns should be trimmed by a chiropodist or physician; and extremes of temperature should be avoided.
3. Socks (preferably soft wool) should be changed once a day. Shoes should be well fitted; great care should be taken in breaking in new shoes. The patient should never go barefoot.

OCCLUSIVE DISEASE OF THE EXTRACRANIAL ARTERIES

The symptoms of cerebrovascular insufficiency may vary from transient dizzy spells to sudden complete hemiplegia and death. In the majority of patients the stenosis or occlusion is in the intracranial arteries and thus is not amenable to surgical correction, but in approximately one-third of cases disease of one or more of the extracranial vessels is responsible for either the major stroke or, more frequently, the transient ischemic attacks.

Arteriosclerosis is the usual cause of extracranial arterial occlusive disease and the process is frequently segmental in nature, involving typically the proximal portions of the internal carotid and vertebral arteries; less commonly, the intrathoracic segments of the major aortic branches may be involved. The significant occlusive process may be limited to a short segment of one vessel, or 2, 3, or 4 vessels may be involved. Consequently, the integrity of all the vessels supplying the brain should be assessed in evaluating symptoms thought to be due to cerebral or brain stem ischemia on the basis of a reduction to below a critical point of the total blood flow to the brain.

Occlusions of the great vessels at the aortic arch can also occur as a result of syphilitic aortitis or of a nonspecific arteritis which occurs in young women.

Clinical Findings.

A. Symptoms and Signs: There is no completely consistent correlation between the clinical findings and the degree and location of the occlusive arterial processes. Arteriography is therefore of major importance, and generally it is desirable to demonstrate the 4 vessels to the brain since multiple lesions are common. It is also valuable to define the intracranial vessels before concluding that an extracranial arterial lesion is the cause of the neurologic abnormalities.

1. In insufficiency related primarily to the carotid vessels, the symptoms are usually those of supratentorial involvement: weakness of the extremities or face, anesthesia, motor aphasia, mental confusion, memory deterioration, personality changes, hemiplegia, and coma. Pulsation in the internal carotid artery cannot be accurately palpated clinically, but a bruit over the carotid bifurcation is an indication of stenosis of the internal carotid in that area. If no bruit is present, the vessel may be normal, extremely narrow, or occluded.
2. Insufficiency related primarily to the vertebral and basilar vessels results in subtentorial symptoms such as vertigo (especially on standing up) and unsteady gait.
3. Eye manifestations - Transient episodes of altered vision or blindness (especially when walking) may occur. Bilateral visual disturbances suggest the vertebral system, whereas monocular alterations suggest ipsilateral carotid stenosis with ulceration and microemboli from the ulceration to the retinal vessel. There may be decreased intraoptic arterial pressure on the side of the major carotid occlusive disease as measured by ophthalmodynamometry.
4. Occlusive lesions of the great vessels arising from the aortic arch may produce intermittent claudication in the arm, di-

minished or absent pulsations in the common carotid or axillary vessels, BP differences in the 2 arms, or a bruit over the supraclavicular areas.

Subclavian steal syndrome occurs when the proximal left subclavian or the innominate artery is completely occluded and some of the collateral blood flow to the arm comes through the vertebral artery on the involved side as a retrograde flow with a resultant reduction of the total blood supply to the brain. Exercise of the arm may thus be associated not only with claudication but with dizzy spells or other CNS symptoms.

B. X-ray Findings: Arteriography is the most accurate diagnostic procedure and should usually consist of a series of studies which include all 4 arteries to the brain. Most favor an aortic arch study first, usually by means of a catheter inserted into the arch through the right axillary or brachial artery or one of the femoral arteries, usually using the percutaneous method of catheterization (Seldinger technic).

Treatment.

A. Indications: Surgery may restore a more normal blood flow to the brain, and improvement may result if the total blood flow or the circulation in the circle of Willis has not been adequate. Surgery may provide some future protection to the brain from damage due to a progression of the arterial disease with further reduction of total blood flow, or from emboli to the brain originating in the areas of stenosis. Stenoses that narrow the lumen less than 50% are not significant and should be left alone unless there is good evidence that an ulcer in that area is the source of recurrent emboli. "Prophylactic" surgery on stenotic vessels in patients with no CNS symptoms is seldom indicated.

1. Emergency surgery - Emergency surgery for acute stroke has been disappointing, and fatal postoperative bleeding into an area of infarcted brain is not infrequent. In most cases, particularly if the patient is in coma or semicoma, arterial studies and surgery should probably be deferred until the condition has stabilized and the collateral circulation has become better established.
2. Elective surgery - Patients with transient ischemic attacks or constant mild neurologic defects - or those who have recovered well from a major vascular insult - should be evaluated for surgery.
3. Withhold surgery - Patients with complete hemiplegia who show no signs of recovery will probably not be benefited by an operation to improve the blood supply to the damaged brain. If the occlusion of the internal carotid artery is complete and is more than a few hours old, the vessel will probably be thrombosed beyond the cervical segment of the internal carotid artery. Surgery to reestablish flow through this vessel is usually unsuccessful.

B. Surgical Treatment:

1. Stenosis at the level of the carotid bifurcation, the most common lesion, is treated by endarterectomy. If there is danger of narrowing the origin of the internal carotid artery

when closing the arteriotomy, patch angioplasty may be employed.

2. Innominate, common carotid, or proximal subclavian stenosis or occlusion may often be treated by a relatively simple shunting procedure in the neck by means of a graft from one major artery in the neck to another. The intrathoracic procedure which must sometimes be employed to bypass the occluded segment with a graft from the aorta to the neck vessel is a procedure of much greater magnitude with a considerably higher mortality.
3. Stenosis of the proximal 1-2 cm. of the vertebral artery is a difficult surgical problem which may be approached by opening the subclavian artery opposite the origin of the stenotic vertebral vessel or by using a vein patch to enlarge the lumen of the endarterectomized proximal vertebral artery. The results have been disappointing.
4. Consideration must be given to the protection of the brain during the operative vascular occlusion. When the vessels are exposed under local anesthesia, a preliminary test period of occlusion may indicate that collateral flow to the brain is insufficient, in which case a shunt to ensure a continued flow of blood to the brain may be used. General anesthesia, with or without hypercarbia or an internal shunt, is being used more frequently now, and reliable criteria are still being sought to determine which patients require an internal shunt during endarterectomy.

Prognosis.

Although the surgical procedures can be carried out in the properly selected patients with an acceptable mortality and complication rate, it has not been proved conclusively that surgery results in a prolongation of life. Transient ischemic attacks can usually be eliminated, even though the individual may not be permanently protected from a major stroke in the future.

RENAL ARTERY STENOSIS

Stenosis of a renal artery can cause progressive hypertension which may be relieved if an unobstructed blood flow is restored to the kidney. The renal pressor mechanism functions whenever a portion of the kidney is perfused by an inadequate blood flow. Atherosclerosis is the most common cause, but congenital stenosis of the renal artery does occur and may account for hypertension on this basis in children or young adults. Stenosis of 1 or both renal arteries can result from a thickening of the media of the artery referred to as fibromuscular hyperplasia, and this condition can account for hypertension in the young or middle-aged individual (especially in women).

Clinical Findings.

A. Symptoms and Signs: Renal artery stenosis should be considered in any patient with rapidly developing, severe hypertension, especially if the diastolic pressure is high or if a bruit can be heard over the area of a renal artery, and in the following types of cases:

1. Hypertension which has its onset either in old people or in those under 30 years of age.
2. Hypertension which develops or progresses after an episode of flank or abdominal pain.
3. Hypertension in patients in whom intravenous urograms reveal a definite difference in the size of the kidneys (more than 1 cm.) or in the time taken for the nephrogram to appear or the first sign of the contrast media to appear in each renal pelvis (frequent films in the first 10 minutes and a larger dose of contrast media may be necessary to determine the degree of difference).

B. X-ray Findings: Although a difference between the 2 kidneys may be noted on an intravenous urogram and, if present, may be a significant finding, a difference may not be detected and a normal study does not rule out renal artery disease. Retrograde transfemoral aortography, with the tip of the catheter placed at or just below the orifices of the renal arteries, may reveal stenosis of one or both of the renal arteries. This is probably the most valuable single study and certainly should be carried out in any patient considered operable in whom the diagnosis of renal artery stenosis is seriously entertained.

C. Laboratory Findings: Isotope renography, using one, 2, or 3 different isotopes to define separate aspects of renal blood flow and function by means of the scintillation camera, is a relatively simple screening procedure. Differential renal excretion studies are now generally considered too difficult to perform with sufficient accuracy to yield reliable results. Measurement of circulating renin or angiotensin may become of value as a screening test.

Treatment.

The treatment of choice in the carefully selected patient is the reestablishment of normal blood flow to the kidney; if this cannot be done, nephrectomy should be performed provided the other kidney is free from disease. The direct procedure on the artery may involve (1) an artery graft from the aorta to the renal artery distal to the stenosis; (2) endarterectomy of an atherosclerotic area; or (3) anastomosis of the splenic artery to the renal artery beyond the stenotic area (if the defect is in the left side).

If the diagnosis is accurate and surgical correction of the defect is successful, a normotensive state is achieved in many of these cases. In the very arteriosclerotic patient over 50 or 60, the surgical mortality is high enough so that medical management or nephrectomy should be seriously considered rather than direct arterial surgery.

CELIAC AND SUPERIOR MESENTERIC ARTERY DISEASE

Although slight narrowing of the orifices of these vessels is rather common, sufficient occlusion to produce symptoms is relatively rare.

Clinical Findings.*

A. Symptoms and Signs: Pain, usually postprandial (abdominal angina), and malabsorption of food without demonstrable gastrointestinal lesions are the principal manifestations. The abdominal pain may be quite variable, and diarrhea may occur. Vascular insufficiency in other areas reinforces the diagnosis. A systolic murmur above the umbilicus may result from superior mesenteric artery stenosis.

B. X-ray Findings: Arteriography of the individual visceral arteries may demonstrate the lesion. Occlusive disease of more than one of the 3 major arteries to the gastrointestinal tract is usually present before arterial insufficiency advances enough for symptoms to develop.

C. Exploratory laparotomy for obscure abdominal complaints in elderly patients should involve a careful examination of the visceral vessels to the gut.

Treatment.

A bypass graft from the aorta to the artery distal to the stenosis or endarterectomy of the occluding atherosclerotic lesions at the origin and proximal part of the superior mesenteric artery or the celiac artery is the usual approach to this problem at the present time. In some cases, however, reimplantation of the superior mesenteric artery lower in the aorta may be employed.

THROMBOANGIITIS OBLITERANS
(Buerger's Disease)

Buerger's disease is an episodic and segmental inflammatory and thrombotic process of the arteries and veins, principally in the limbs. It is seen most commonly in men between 25 and 40 years of age. The effects of the disease are almost solely due to occlusion of the arteries. The symptoms are primarily due to ischemia, complicated in the later stages by infection and tissue necrosis. The inflammatory process is intermittent, with quiescent periods lasting weeks, months, or years.

The differential diagnosis between Buerger's disease and atherosclerotic peripheral vascular disease may be difficult or impossible. The differentiation is sometimes based on the age at which symptoms first appeared. It is now known, however, that atherosclerosis can appear in young adults, and the diagnosis of thromboangiitis obliterans is thus made less frequently now than formerly. Other conditions which must be considered in the differential diagnosis are scleroderma, Raynaud's disease, acrocyanosis, frostbite, and neuromuscular conditions resulting in pain in the hands or feet.

The arteries of the legs are most commonly affected. The plantar and digital vessels and those in the lower leg (especially the posterior tibial artery) are most frequently involved. Occlusion of the femoral-popliteal arteries does not often occur. In the upper extremity, the distal arteries are most commonly affected. Different arterial segments may become occluded in successive episodes; a certain amount of recanalization occurs during quiescent periods.

---

*The manifestations of acute thrombosis of the superior mesenteric artery are discussed on p. 416.

Superficial migratory thrombophlebitis is a common early indication of the disease.

The etiology is not known, but a history of smoking is almost always obtained and little or no progress can be made in treatment if the patient continues to smoke.

Clinical Findings.

The signs and symptoms are primarily those of arterial insufficiency, and the differentiation from arteriosclerotic peripheral vascular disease may thus be difficult. Although the 2 diseases are similar in many ways, the following findings suggest Buerger's disease:

A. The patient is a man between 20 and 40 years of age who smokes.
B. There is a history of migratory superficial segmental thrombophlebitis, usually in the saphenous tributaries rather than the main vessel. If there is an active thrombotic process as manifested by a superficial, red, tender cord, a biopsy of such a vein will often give microscopic proof of Buerger's disease.
C. Intermittent claudication is common and is frequently noted in the palm of the hand or arch of the foot. Rest pain is common and, when present, is persistent and gnawing or aching, often interfering with sleeping and eating. This pain tends to be more pronounced than in the patient with atherosclerosis. Numbness, diminished sensation, and pricking and burning pains may be present as a result of ischemic neuropathy.
D. The color of the digits and the distal foot may remain relatively unchanged by posture; the skin may not blanch on elevation, and on dependency the intensity of the rubor is often more pronounced than that seen in the atherosclerotic group. The distal vascular changes are often asymmetric, so that not all of the toes are affected to the same degree.
E. Trophic changes may be present, often with painful indolent ulcerations along the nail margins.
F. There is usually evidence of disease in both legs and possibly also in the hands and lower arms. There may be a history or findings of Raynaud's phenomenon in the fingers or distal foot.
G. The course is usually intermittent, with acute episodes followed by remissions. When the collateral vessels as well as the main channels have become occluded, an exacerbation is more likely to lead to gangrene and amputation. The course in the patient with atherosclerosis tends to be less dramatic and more persistent.

Treatment.

The principles of therapy are the same as outlined for atherosclerotic peripheral vascular disease; but the long-range outlook is better in patients with Buerger's disease, so that when possible the approach should be more conservative and tissue loss kept to a minimum.

A. General Measures: Smoking must be given up; the physician should be emphatic and insistent on this point. The disease is almost sure to progress if this advice is not heeded.
B. Surgical Treatment:
   1. Sympathectomy is useful in eliminating the vasospastic manifestations of the disease and aiding in the establishment of

collateral circulation during the acute phase. It is also helpful in relieving the milder or moderate forms of intermittent claudication and rest pain and may aid in healing following amputation of a toe.

2. Arterial grafts - If the femoral pulse is present and the popliteal pulse is absent, a femoral arteriogram should be taken to assess the feasibility of using a graft. However, arterial grafting procedures are not often indicated in patients with Buerger's disease because there is usually not a complete block in the iliofemoral region.
3. Amputation - The indications for amputation are similar in many respects to those outlined for the atherosclerotic group (see p. 592), although the approach tends to be somewhat more conservative from the point of view of the preservation of tissue. Most patients with Buerger's disease who are managed carefully do not require amputation. The results of amputation of the middle 3 toes are better than those achieved by amputation of the great and little toes. It is almost never necessary to amputate the entire hand, although fingers must occasionally be removed.

   If there is evidence of both large and small vessel disease, the results of conservative management are poor and amputation is frequently necessary. Pain may become so severe that the conservative approach must be discarded.

Prognosis.

Except in the case of the rapidly progressive form of the disease - and provided the patient stops smoking and takes good care of his feet - the prognosis for survival of the extremities is good. Thromboangiitis obliterans rarely results in death.

ACUTE ARTERIAL OCCLUSION

Arterial occlusion can result from an embolism or from a thrombosis, usually in a previously diseased artery but occasionally in an acutely traumatized artery. In an older individual with both arteriosclerotic vascular disease and cardiac disease, the differentiation may be difficult. The signs and symptoms depend on the artery occluded, the organ or region supplied by the artery, and the adequacy of the collateral circulation to the area. Acute occlusion in an extremity usually results in the findings of acute ischemia distal to the site of occlusion. Occlusions in other areas result in such conditions as cerebrovascular accidents, intestinal gangrene, and renal or splenic infarcts.

1. ARTERIAL EMBOLISM

Arterial embolism usually occurs as a complication of rheumatic heart disease, myocardial infarction, bacterial endocarditis, or congestive heart failure; about two-thirds of cases are associated with atrial fibrillation. In about 10% of patients no source of the embolus is clinically evident, and in this group the differential diagnosis between embolism and thrombosis may be difficult.

Emboli tend to lodge at the bifurcation of an artery and usually occur in the arteries of the lower extremities, although the arteries of the upper extremities, brain, or viscera are occasionally involved.

Clinical Findings.

In the extremity the initial symptoms are usually pain (sudden or gradual in onset), numbness, coldness, and tingling. Signs include absence of pulsations in the arteries distal to the block, coldness, pallor or mottling, hypesthesia or anesthesia, and weakness or paresis of the limb.

Treatment.

Immediate embolectomy is the treatment of choice in most cases. It should be done within 12 hours if possible; if more than 10-12 hours have passed - and particularly if it appears that the limb will survive without embolectomy - anticoagulant therapy without surgery is often the safer approach. This is also the case if tissue necrosis has already developed (ultimately requiring amputation).

A. Emergency Preoperative Care:
   1. Heparin sodium, 5000 units I.V., should be given as soon as the diagnosis is made or suspected in an effort to prevent distal thrombosis. The effect of this dose will usually be dissipated by the time the patient has been transported to the hospital and to surgery. If a delay of 4-5 hours is anticipated, 3000-4000 units should also be given I.M.
   2. A sympathetic block should not be attempted once heparin has been given, and it is better to emphasize heparin and surgery at the earliest moment rather than to risk the delay involved in a blocking procedure. If surgery must be delayed or if the patient is considered inoperable, a sympathetic block may be tried before heparin is given.
   3. Keep the extremity at or below the horizontal plane. Do not apply heat or cold to the involved extremity (but heat to an uninvolved arm may help produce a reflex vasodilatation). Protect from hard surfaces and overlying bedclothes.
   4. Arteriography may be of value either before or during surgery. There may be more than 1 embolus in an extremity; x-ray studies may help locate a distal embolus or determine the extent of a secondary thrombosis.

B. Surgical Treatment:
   1. Use local anesthesia for embolectomy of a vessel of an arm or leg; general anesthesia if the abdomen must be opened.
   2. Extraction of the embolus - Control of the artery above and below the embolus must be achieved before extraction of the clot. Care must be taken not to dislodge the embolus to a more distal segment during the exposure of the artery.

      Local arterial spasm, if present, is best treated by the application of a solution of papaverine hydrochloride, 2%.

      A distal thrombosis or a second embolus, lodged in one of the more peripheral arteries, may be removed by means of an arterial catheter with a small, inflatable balloon at the tip which can be inserted through the arteriotomy into the distal arteries. After the balloon has been inflated, the catheter is withdrawn, removing the embolus or thrombus. This can be repeated several times until adequate back bleeding has been obtained and the arterial tree seems clear of occlusive material. Fogarty or balloon tip catheters can also be used to extract emboli lodged at a site proximal to the arteriotomy; an embolus in the iliac artery may thus be removed through a common femoral arteriotomy or one at the aortic bifurcation through bilateral common femoral arteriotomies. By this technic a general anesthetic can often be avoided.

C. Postoperative Care: Anticoagulants should usually be withheld for a few days postoperatively because their early use often results in a hematoma in the wound.

Disappearance of a distal pulse in the early postoperative period usually requires reexploration in an attempt to remove a thrombus or a new embolus.

Prognosis.

Arterial embolism is a threat not only to the limb but also to the life of the patient. The emergency surgery is poorly tolerated by patients with major cardiac disease and the mortality rate is high.

Mortality increases with the size of the embolus; aortic and iliac emboli are the most dangerous. Cerebral or visceral vessels may be occluded by emboli which complicates the management of the peripheral embolus. Emboli associated with hypertensive or arteriosclerotic heart disease have a poorer prognosis than those arising from rheumatic valvular disease in younger patients. Emboli recur in almost half of the entire group of patients, and in over half of those with atrial fibrillation.

In patients with atrial fibrillation an attempt should be made to restore normal rhythm with quinidine or cardioversion, although this is usually possible only in patients with recent or transitory fibrillation. Long-term anticoagulant therapy may diminish the danger of further emboli. Heart surgery is justified in selected cases with removal of thrombus from the left atrium and correction of the mitral stenosis.

2. ACUTE ARTERIAL THROMBOSIS

Acute arterial thrombosis generally occurs in an artery in which the lumen has become almost obliterated by the gradual deposition of atherosclerotic material in the wall of the artery, often resulting in a channel which is 90% or more obliterated. Blood flowing through such a narrow, irregular, or ulcerated lumen may clot, leading to a sudden complete occlusion of the narrow segment. The thrombosis may then propagate either up or down the artery to a point where the blood is flowing more rapidly in a less diseased segment with open collateral branches. Occasionally the thrombosis is precipitated by the displacement of an arteriosclerotic plaque by the blood stream which then blocks the lumen. Inflammatory involvement of the arterial wall with narrowing of the channel (as in thromboangiitis obliterans) and chronic mechanical irritation of the artery (as with a cervical rib) may also lead to acute thrombosis. Thrombosis in a diseased artery may be associated with an episode of hypotension, acute trauma, or cardiac failure; polycythemia will also increase the chance of thrombosis.

The chronic, incomplete arterial obstruction usually results in the establishment of some collateral flow. Further flow develops relatively rapidly through the collaterals once complete occlusion has developed. The extremity may go through an extremely critical period of hours or several days, however, while the collateral circulation develops around the block. The survival of the tissue distal to the block will depend on the development of adequate collateral, and this in turn depends on the location and length of the arterial thrombosis and whether such undesirable abnormalities as shock, heart failure, anemia, or hemoconcentration can be corrected promptly.

Clinical Findings.

The local findings in the extremity are usually very similar to those described in the section on arterial embolus. Differential points to check include the following: (1) Are there other manifestations of advanced occlusive arterial disease in other areas, especially the opposite extremity (bruit, absent pulses, secondary changes)? (2) Is there a history or are there findings or a recent episode of atrial fibrillation, or a myocardial infarction? If so, an embolus is more likely than a thrombosis. (3) Laboratory findings: Ecg. and serum enzyme studies may give added information regarding the cardiac state and its likelihood as a source of an embolus. (4) X-ray findings: An emergency arteriogram may be of value in making a more accurate differential diagnosis and in planning the therapy.

Treatment.

Whereas emergency embolectomy is the usual approach in the case of an early occlusion from an embolus, a nonoperative approach is frequently used in the case of thrombosis for 2 reasons: (1) The segment of a thrombosed artery may be quite long so that rather extensive and difficult surgery may be required to deal with the obstruction by thrombo-endarterectomy or artery graft. (The removal of a single embolus in a normal or near normal artery is in comparison usually relatively quick and definitive.) (2) The extremity is more likely to survive without the development of gangrene because some collateral circulation has usually formed during the stenotic phase before the acute thrombosis. (In the case of embolus, this is usually not the case and the block is most often at a major arterial bifurcation occluding both branches, and associated arterial spasm is usually more acute.)

The treatment is therefore as outlined under emergency preoperative care for the arterial embolus (see p. 600), followed by observation for hours or days. Usually, gradual improvement in the circulation of the distal areas of the extremity will be noted. If this does not occur and if tissue necrosis seems likely, emergency surgery may be considered, particularly if x-ray studies reveal that there is a reasonable chance of success. (See p. 601.) If they do not, sympathectomy may save the extremity (though anticoagulation must be discontinued temporarily if surgery is employed).

Prognosis.

Limb survival usually occurs with acute thrombosis of the iliac or superficial femoral arteries; gangrene is more likely if the popliteal is suddenly occluded, especially if the period between occlusion and treatment is long or if there is considerable arterial spasm. If the limb does survive the acute occlusion, a period of observation and evaluation is usually possible, with the late treatment and prognosis as defined on pp. 587-588.

VASOSPASTIC DISORDERS

RAYNAUD'S PHENOMENON AND DISEASE

Raynaud's phenomenon (secondary) or disease (primary) is characterized by intermittent attacks of pallor or cyanosis - or pallor followed by cyanosis - in the fingers (and rarely the toes) precipitated by cold or occasionally by emotion. Early in the course of the disease, only 1 or 2 fingertips may be affected; as the disease progresses, all of the fingers down to the distal palm may be involved. The thumbs are rarely affected. General as well as local body cooling is usually necessary. Recovery usually begins near the base of the fingers as a bright-red return of color to the cyanotic or pale digit. Sensory changes which often accompany the vasomotor manifestations include numbness, stiffness, diminished sensation, and aching pain. If there is organic narrowing or obstruction of the digital vessels, the condition may progress to atrophy of the terminal fat pads and the digital skin, and gangrenous ulcers may appear near the fingertips which may heal during warm weather.

Raynaud's phenomenon may be primary, with no organic occlusion of the arteries, or may occur as a manifestation of severe or chronic cold injuries, vibration injuries, scleroderma and certain other collagen diseases, neurologic disorders affecting the arms, obliterative vascular disease of the atherosclerotic or thromboangiitis obliterans type, thoracic outlet problems, and ergot poisoning.

Raynaud's disease is much rarer than Raynaud's phenomenon. It appears first between the ages of 25 and 45, almost always in women. Its earlier manifestations are similar to those described for Raynaud's phenomenon, but the disorder is progressive, with early trophic changes (skin atrophy or sclerodermatous changes, irregularity of nail growth, wasting of the finger pads, and small, painful, recurrent necrotic ulcers at the tips of the fingers which may in time lead to shortening of the fingers). Symmetric involvement of the fingers of both hands is the rule but the thumbs are rarely affected. The spasm gradually becomes more frequent and prolonged. Gangrene of the whole finger is rare, and the peripheral pulses are normal.

Treatment.

A. General Measures: The body should be kept warm, and the hands especially should be protected from exposure to cold; much use should be made of gloves. Injuries to the fingers should be avoided, since wounds heal slowly and infections are hard to control. Softening and lubricating lotions should be used to control the fissured dry skin. Smoking should be stopped.

B. Medical Treatment: There may be some benefit from (1) methyldopa (Aldomet®), 1 Gm. orally daily; (2) nitroglycerin, 0.3 mg. sublingually 10 minutes before exposure to cold; or (3) papaverine (Pavabid Plateau Capsules®), 150 mg orally every 12 hours.

C. Surgical Treatment: Although the duration of benefit of dorsal sympathectomy to dilate the cutaneous vessels of the fingers may be limited, this is still the most effective method of treatment for Raynaud's phenomenon or disease. Symptoms in the fingers tend to recur in 2-5 years with the gradual return of sympathetic activity. Sympathectomy is of no value in advanced severe cases.

VASOMOTOR DISORDERS ASSOCIATED WITH TRAUMA
(Sudeck's Atrophy, Causalgia)

Sudeck's atrophy is an acute atrophy of the bones of an extremity which usually comes on after minor injury, especially to the ankle or wrist. Symptoms and signs of vasomotor hyperactivity include pain of a burning type made worse by movement, edema, local heat, and swelling. The limb may ultimately become cold, cyanotic, and wasted, with stiffness of the joints. Secondary fractures occasionally occur in the atrophic bones.

Prophylaxis consists of adequate early treatment of sprains. The early manifestations are usually treated by physical therapy: mild heat, light massage, and gentle movement of the joints. A walking type of plaster cast for the foot and ankle region may be of value.

In severe and chronic forms, sympathectomy may give relief.

Causalgia, which is characterized by intense burning pain and vasodilatation in an extremity, is a rare disorder caused by partial division or bruising of a peripheral nerve (usually the median nerve) or involvement of the nerve in scar tissue. The injury may be trivial. The pain is distal to the point of injury but not confined to the course of the nerve, and may not appear for a few days or weeks. Pain is initiated by light touch, temperature changes, or movement of the limb. The skin becomes red, smooth, devoid of wrinkles and hair, scaly, and cold, with disuse atrophy of the bones. If severe nervous and mental manifestations are prominent, local or operative procedures will probably be of no value.

Treatment.

A. Conservative Treatment: Keeping the affected area cool and protected from stimuli is the treatment of choice even though the patient often demands more aggressive therapy, since the disorder usually subsides after a year or so.

B. Surgical Treatment: Sympathectomy may be of value if a sympathetic block gives relief, and this is usually the treatment of choice if operative measures are required. Division of the nerve proximal to the site of irritation gives relief but denervates the area supplied by the nerve. Reamputation of a painful stump is often followed by recurrence of symptoms in the new stump. Spinothalamic tractotomy is a desperate measure which is not always successful.

DEGENERATIVE AND INFLAMMATORY VENOUS DISEASE

VARICOSE VEINS

Varicose veins develop predominantly in the lower extremities, and consist of abnormally dilated, elongated, and tortuous alterations in the saphenous veins and their tributaries. These vessels lie immediately beneath the skin and superficial to the deep fascia and so do not have as adequate support as the veins deep in the leg, which are surrounded by muscles. In many cases there is an inherited defect in the walls or valves of the veins which leads ultimately to the formation of varicosities. Other contributory factors are prolonged standing over a number of years, pregnancy, obesity, and perhaps aging.

Secondary varicosities can develop as a result of obstructive changes in the deep venous system following thrombophlebitis, or occasionally as a result of proximal venous occlusion due to neoplasm. Congenital or acquired arteriovenous fistulas are also associated with varicosities.

The great saphenous vein and its tributaries are most commonly involved, but the small saphenous vein is occasionally affected. There may be 1 or many incompetent perforating veins in the thigh and lower leg, so that blood can reflux into the varicosities not only from above, by way of the saphenofemoral junction, but also from the deep system of veins through the incompetent perforators. Largely because of these valvular defects, venous pressure in the superficial veins does not fall appreciably on walking; over the years the veins progressively enlarge and the surrounding tissue and skin develop secondary changes such as fibrosis, chronic edema, and pigmentation. Atrophic changes take place in the skin.

Clinical Findings.

A. Symptoms: Extensive varicose veins may produce no subjective symptoms, whereas minimal varicosities may produce many symptoms. Aching or burning discomfort, fatigue, or pain in the lower leg brought on by periods of standing are the most common complaints. Cramps may occur, but intermittent claudication and coldness of the feet are not associated with varicose veins. One must be careful to distinguish between the symptoms of arteriosclerotic peripheral vascular disease and those of venous disease, since occlusive arterial disease usually contraindicates or modifies the operative treatment of varicosities. Itching from an associated eczematoid dermatitis may occur in the region of the veins.

B. Signs: Dilated, tortuous veins beneath the skin in the thigh and leg are generally readily visible in the standing individual, although in very obese patients palpation and percussion may be necessary to detect their presence. Secondary tissue changes may be absent even in extensive varicosities; but if the varicosities are of long duration, brownish pigmentation and thinning of the skin above the ankle are often present. Swelling may occur, but extensive swelling and fibrosis in the subcutaneous tissues of the lower leg usually denote the postphlebitic state.

C. Special Examinations:

1. Percussion test with the patient standing - Percussion over the varicosities with 1 hand while palpating along the course of the vein with the other will show the course of the varicosities.
2. Trendelenburg's test - Of use in determining the competence of the valves at the saphenofemoral junction and in the communications between the superficial and deep vessels.
   a. With the patient supine, elevate the leg. If there is no organic venous obstruction, varicosities will empty immediately.
   b. Place a rubber tourniquet around the upper thigh and ask the patient to stand.
      (1) If the long saphenous vein remains empty for 30 seconds or more and then fills very slowly from below over a period of 1-2 minutes, the saphenofemoral valve is incompetent, the valves in the communicating veins are competent, and the blood is flowing through them in the right direction (superficial to deep). On release of the tourniquet, if the veins fill rapidly from above, the incompetence of the proximal valves is confirmed.
      (2) If the varicosities fill rapidly, the communicating veins between the deep and the superficial vessels are incompetent and blood is refluxing into the varicosed vessels. If, on release of the tourniquet, no additional filling of the varicosities occurs, the valves in the saphenous vein close to the saphenofemoral junction are competent; if further distention of the varicosities occurs when the tourniquet is released, the valves at the upper end of the long saphenous vein are also incompetent.
3. Perthes' test may be used to determine if the saphenous valves are competent, if the communicating valves are competent, or if deep venous obstruction is present. With the patient standing, a tourniquet is applied to the thigh so as to occlude the superficial but not the deep veins of the leg; the patient is then required to walk for 5 minutes.
   a. If the veins collapse, the communicating veins are competent. If, on releasing the tourniquet, the veins fill relatively slowly (35-60 seconds), the saphenofemoral valve is also competent.
   b. If the veins remain unchanged, the valves of the communicating and saphenous veins are incompetent and the pressure in the 2 systems is the same.
   c. If the veins become more prominent and pain develops, the deep veins are obstructed and the valves of the communicating veins may be incompetent. This conclusion should be checked by a venogram, and surgery on the superficial veins should not be performed if the deep system is blocked.

Complications.

A. Ulceration will often result from a blow to the thin, atrophic, pigmented skin of the lower leg or ankle region, and such a lesion often becomes chronic, scarred, and painful. Treatment consists of rest and elevation of the leg and saline compresses until healing has occurred. A skin graft may be necessary. If the patient must remain ambulatory, firm compression of the lower leg and foot as afforded by Unna's boot or a compression boot dressing may be used. Recurrences are common.

B. Thrombophlebitis, starting in the varicosities and occasionally extending into the deep system, may occur.
C. Bleeding, which may be profuse, may occur if a venous-cutaneous fistula develops; hemorrhage generally stops if the limb is elevated and pressure is applied to the area.

Differential Diagnosis.

Primary varicosities should be differentiated from those secondary to obstruction or incompetence in the deep system of veins; surgery in the case of the latter conditions is often of little or no benefit and the patient must still use elastic stockings to control the chronic edema even though the varicosities may be eliminated. Venography may occasionally be of value in determining the condition of the deep venous system.

Treatment.

Varicosities tend to progress, and some form of therapy must be instituted if progressive changes and complications are to be avoided. Only surgery can provide prolonged relief from varicose veins when the saphenofemoral valve is incompetent.

A. Conservative Treatment:
   1. Elastic stockings and intermittent elevation of the legs is the best therapeutic approach in very old or poor-risk patients, in patients who refuse surgery or have to put it off, and sometimes in women with mild or moderate varicosities who are going to have more children (since better long-term results can be obtained in women who are not going to become pregnant again). Elastic stockings may also be of value in those patients who already show a tendency toward varicosities or whose families have a high incidence of varicosities, especially if they must spend many hours standing.
   2. Injection treatment of varicosities with sclerosing solutions to produce thrombosis of the segment of vein should be reserved for treatment of short segments which remain after adequate surgery. The recurrence rate after injection therapy is high, and complications can occur (e.g., local reactions and infections around the vein, deep thrombophlebitis).

      Technic: A very fine (No. 25) needle is inserted into the varix with the leg dependent; after the needle is inserted the leg can be placed in the horizontal position. After drawing blood back into the syringe to make sure the needle is in the vein, and after the vein is relatively free of blood, 1-2 ml. of a sclerosing solution is injected. The needle is withdrawn, and digital pressure is applied for 2-3 minutes above and below the area of injection to hold most of the solution where its effect is most desired. Only 2-3 areas should be injected at each office visit.

B. Surgical Treatment: High ligation at the saphenofemoral junction, with stripping of the vein, is the treatment of choice. Multiple low ligations of the secondary branches, taking care to interrupt all incompetent perforating veins, should be added to the stripping procedure. In elderly individuals, in those with relatively few varicosities, and in those with chronic ulcerations, the saphenous vein and its branches and associated perforators may be ligated but not stripped; this can be done entirely under local anesthesia, and the postoperative discomfort is usually less.

Postoperatively, ambulation with elastic bandages is encouraged on the day of surgery if local anesthesia is used, or the next day if general anesthesia is used. Standing or sitting is not desirable for 10-14 days, and when the patient is in bed the leg should be elevated.

Prognosis.

All patients should be informed that even thorough and extensive surgery may not remove all varicosities and that additional (more limited) procedures may be necessary either in the early postoperative period or months or years later. If extensive varicosities reappear after surgery, the completeness of the high ligation should be questioned and reexploration of the saphenofemoral area may be necessary.

DEEP THROMBOPHLEBITIS

Thrombophlebitis is a partial or complete occlusion of a vein by a thrombus with a secondary inflammatory reaction in the wall of the vein. It is encountered most frequently in the deep veins in the legs and pelvis in postoperative or postpartum patients between the fourth and the fourteenth days, and in patients with fractures and cardiac disease, especially if confined to bed.

The deep veins of the calf are most frequently involved, but the thrombotic process may start in or progress to the femoral and iliac veins. The site of origin is at times in the pelvic veins or in the great saphenous vein.

Predisposing factors are aging, malignancy, anemia, oral contraceptive drugs, and chronic infection. Perhaps the most prominent etiologic factors in thrombophlebitis are venous stasis and the pressure changes produced in the endothelium of the vein wall as the legs lie for hours supported by the mattress of the bed or operating table. Exposed subendothelial tissue or a variety of intravascular stimuli affecting the blood result in the release of platelet constituents; platelet aggregates form, followed by the deposition of fibrin and (later) red cells, resulting in a propagating thrombus.

Clinical Findings.

There may be no symptoms or signs in the extremity. The patient not infrequently suffers a pulmonary embolus, presumably from the leg veins, without symptoms or demonstrable abnormalities in the extremities.

A. Symptoms: The patient may complain of a dull ache, a tight feeling, or frank pain in the calf or, in more extensive cases, the whole leg.

B. Signs: Typical findings, though variable, are as follows: tenderness and induration or spasm in the calf muscles; slight swelling in the involved calf, as noted by careful measurements; pain in the calf produced by dorsiflexion of the foot

(Homans' sign); and slight fever and tachycardia. When the femoral and iliac veins are also involved, the swelling in the leg may be quite marked. The skin may be slightly cyanotic if venous stasis is severe, or pale and cool if a reflex arterial spasm is superimposed.

Complications.

The major complication of deep thrombophlebitis is pulmonary embolism. A small or moderately large pulmonary embolism may be present without any associated pulmonary symptoms, signs, or x-ray findings. Clinical manifestations, when present, take the form of pleuritic pain, often with a transient friction rub; a dry cough, sometimes associated with hemoptysis; local rales in the area of involvement; a small amount of pleural fluid; and, occasionally, x-ray evidence of pulmonary consolidation. Fever and increased pulse and respiration rates are frequently present. The serum LDH may be elevated.

Massive pulmonary embolism is associated with shock, dyspnea, and cyanosis, and often with transient Ecg. changes characteristic of cor pulmonale. The pulmonary artery pressure is elevated, and pulmonary angiography will demonstrate the embolus in the pulmonary vascular tree. Death may occur in minutes or hours.

Chronic venous insufficiency may ultimately develop in some of these patients.

Treatment.

A. Local Measures and Follow-up Care:
   1. Elevation of the legs by means of absolute bed rest with the foot of the bed on 6-inch blocks and the head of the bed in the horizontal position is maintained during the initial period. After 5-7 days, when the inflammatory aspects have had time to produce a more adherent thrombus - and provided the swelling and local symptoms have largely subsided - walking but not standing or sitting is permitted.
   2. Elastic bandages or stockings are applied from the toes to just below the knees as soon as the diagnosis is made and continued for at least 6-12 months. Bandages and anticoagulants initially, and intermittent elevation of the legs subsequently, will do much to reduce the danger of permanent changes and disability. These measures are even more important if surgical ligation of the femoral vein or the vena cava have been necessary.

B. Medical Treatment (Anticoagulants): (See Appendix.) Anticoagulant therapy is considered to be definitive in most cases of deep thrombophlebitis with or without pulmonary embolism. There is good evidence that the relatively high incidence of fatal pulmonary embolism secondary to venous thrombosis is significantly reduced by adequate anticoagulant therapy. Progressive thrombosis with its associated morbidity is also reduced considerably, and the chronic secondary changes in the involved leg are probably also less severe. The specific drug used depends to some extent on the physician's preferance and experience, but the relative urgency of the situation usually requires the use of heparin initially and in most cases throughout the course of the anticoagulant therapy. If a prolonged course of anticoagulant therapy is considered desirable, a shift may later be made to one of the longer-acting drugs such as warfarin (Coumadin®) or dicumarol.

Anticoagulants should be continued for at least 3 days after subsidence of local pain and tenderness in the involved extremity and until ambulation has been fully established. The rate of subsidence of symptoms is variable, and occasional cases are quite refractory to therapy. Therapy should be continued for at least 10 days for venous thrombosis and 21 days for pulmonary embolism, but therapy may have to be continued for a longer period if signs and symptoms persist.

C. Surgical Treatment:
1. Surgical division or plication with a clip or sutures of the inferior vena cava or occasionally of both common femoral veins must be seriously considered if a patient on adequate anticoagulant therapy has a pulmonary embolism. The chance of additional pulmonary embolism is considerably reduced (though not eliminated) by this procedure, though the operation in a seriously ill patient is not without risk. Although some degree of chronic edema of the legs may develop as a result of this procedure, it can usually be minimized if anticoagulant therapy is resumed 1-2 days following surgery and if follow-up care, consisting of elastic supports to the lower legs and elevation of the legs at intervals during the day and at night, is continued for at least 1 year.
2. In certain cases of massive venous occlusion (phlegmasia cerulea dolens) which have not responded to a trial of a sympathetic block, elevation of the leg, heparin, and fluid and electrolyte replacement, femoral vein thrombectomy to remove the iliofemoral thrombosis may be indicated. This has also been advocated for cases where massive edema without vasospasm exists (phlegmasia alba dolens). If the thrombus has not become adherent (less than 48 hours from the time of onset), normal function of the venous system may be restored and maintained by postoperative heparin. Massive edema and vasospasm have been relieved by this procedure; rethrombosis or pulmonary embolus can occur postoperatively, and the procedure is indicated on only rare occasions.

Prophylaxis.

A. Undue pressure on the calf or thigh during a long operation should be avoided.

B. Patients with a history of phlebitis or with varicose veins should have elastic supports on the legs during and after operation.

C. Preoperative correction of anemia, dehydration, congestive failure, or metabolic disturbances will diminish the incidence of thrombophlebitis.

D. Postoperative exercises of the legs should be started at the close of the operative procedure while the patient is still on the operating table and continued for several days after operation. Early ambulation (but not standing or sitting) is likewise of value. If complete bed rest is necessary, passive or active exercises such as flexion of the toes, ankles, knees, and hips should be instituted and the patient should be encouraged to move frequently in bed. Deep breathing should be encouraged.

E. Elevation of the foot of the bed with the head of the bed in a horizontal position may be of value in patients predisposed to thrombophlebitis.
F. Prophylactic use of anticoagulants, particularly in patients with major fractures, may be indicated, but if this is done the drug should be started during the early phase of hospital care.

SUPERFICIAL THROMBOPHLEBITIS

Superficial thrombophlebitis may occur spontaneously, as in pregnant or postpartum women or in individuals with varicose veins or thromboangiitis obliterans; or it may be associated with trauma, as in the case of a blow to the leg or following intravenous therapy with irritating solutions. It may also be a manifestation of abdominal malignancy such as carcinoma of the pancreas. The great saphenous vein is most often involved. Superficial thrombophlebitis is usually not associated with thrombosis in the deep leg veins. Pulmonary emboli are infrequent but do occur.

Clinical Findings.

The patient usually experiences a dull pain in the region of the involved vein. Local findings consist of induration, redness, and tenderness over the vein. The process may be localized, or it may involve most of the great saphenous vein and its tributaries. If the process is migratory, involving one segment after another, thromboangiitis obliterans should be suspected. The acute inflammatory reaction generally subsides in 1-2 weeks; a firm cord may remain for a much longer period. Edema of the extremity is absent.

Treatment.

If the process is well localized and away from the saphenofemoral junction, treatment consists of moist heat to the area and bed rest in the "legs elevated" position. Anticoagulants are usually not indicated except when the process seems to be very active and there is fear of involvement of the deep system. Phenylbutazone (Butazolidin®), 100 mg. 3 times daily for 5 days, may aid in resolving the acute inflammation.

If the process is very extensive or shows a tendency to proceed upward toward the saphenofemoral junction, or if it is in the proximity of the saphenofemoral junction initially, ligation and division of the saphenous vein at the saphenofemoral junction is indicated. The manifestations usually regress following this procedure, although removal of the involved segment of vein may result in a more rapid recovery.

CHRONIC VENOUS INSUFFICIENCY

Chronic venous insufficiency commonly results from changes secondary to deep thrombophlebitis (the postphlebitis syndrome), but it can also occur as a result of neoplastic obstruction of the pelvic veins or congenital or acquired arteriovenous fistulas.

When insufficiency is secondary to deep thrombophlebitis, the valves in the deep venous channels and sometimes in the perforating veins as well have been destroyed by the thrombotic process and the vessels are often irregular and tortuous. The venous pressure therefore fails to drop when the patient walks; and because the standing venous pressures are not reduced, secondary changes eventually take place in the venules, capillaries, subcutaneous tissues, skin, and superficial veins.

Clinical Findings.

Chronic venous insufficiency is characterized by progressive edema of the leg (particularly the lower leg) and secondary changes in the skin and subcutaneous tissues. The usual symptoms are itching, a dull discomfort made worse by periods of standing, and pain if an ulceration is present. The skin is usually thin, shiny, atrophic, and often brownish. Eczema is often present, and there may be superficial weeping dermatitis of large areas. The subcutaneous tissues are thick and fibrous. Recurrent ulcerations are common, usually just above the ankle; healing results in a thin scar on a fibrotic base. Varicosities often appear and are usually associated with incompetent perforating veins in the mid and upper part of the lower leg.

Treatment.

A. Bed rest with the legs elevated to diminish chronic edema is fundamental in the treatment of chronic venous insufficiency. Subsequent measures to control the tendency toward edema include (1) intermittent elevation of the legs during the day and elevation of the foot of the bed at night; (2) avoidance of long periods of sitting or standing; and (3) the use (for life) of well-fitting elastic supports worn from the toes to just below the knee during the day and evening.

B. Stasis Dermatitis: Eczematous eruption may be acute or chronic and the treatment varies accordingly.
   1. Acute weeping dermatitis -
      a. Wet compresses for 1 hour 4 times daily of either boric acid solution (1 Tbsp./L. of water), potassium permanganate solution (100 mg./L. of water), or Burow's solution (2 tablets/L. of water).
      b. Compresses are followed with a 0.5% hydrocortisone cream in a water-soluble base. (Neomycin may be incorporated into this cream.)
      c. Systemic antibiotics may be indicated if active infection is present.
   2. Subsiding or chronic dermatitis -
      a. Can continue the hydrocortisone cream for 1-2 weeks or until no further improvement is noted.
      b. Zinc oxide ointment with ichthammol (Ichthyol®), 3%, once or twice a day, cleaned off as desired with mineral oil.
   3. Energetic treatment of chronic edema as outlined in sections A and C, with almost complete bed rest during the acute phase.

C. Ulcerations are preferably treated with compresses of isotonic saline solution, which aid in the healing of the ulcer or may help prepare the base for a skin graft; or the lesion can be treated on an ambulatory basis by means of a boot of Unna's paste, Viscopaste®, or Gauztex® on the lower leg after much of the swelling has been reduced by a period of elevation.

D. Varicosities secondary to the obstructive elements and the valvular defects in the deep system of veins may in turn contribute to the undesirable changes in the tissues of the lower leg. Varicosities should occasionally be removed and the incompetent perforators ligated, but the tendency toward edema will persist and the measures outlined above will be required for life. The varicosities can often be treated along with the edema by elastic stockings and other nonoperative measures. If the obstructive element in the deep system is severe, it may be most undesirable to remove superficial channels which may be carrying most of the blood out of the leg. (See Perthes' test, p. 607.) Phlebography may be of value in the more complicated forms of the postphlebitic conditions (and even in certain instances in acute phlebitis) in mapping out by means of x-rays the areas of obstruction or incompetence of the deep veins of the leg. The injection of contrast media is made in a foot vein with a tourniquet at the ankle area occluding the superficial flow and with the patient in a semierect position.

Prophylaxis.

Irreversible tissue changes and associated complications in the lower legs can be prevented through adequate treatment of acute thrombophlebitis with anticoagulants and energetic measures to avoid edema in the subsequent years by means of elastic supports to the lower legs, intermittent periods of elevation of the legs, and elevation of the foot of the bed.

LYMPHEDEMA

The underlying mechanism in lymphedema is impairment of the flow of lymph from an extremity, either as a result of an inflammatory or noninflammatory obstruction of the channels or because of malformations in the vessels themselves. Secondary dilatation leads to incompetence of the valve system, disrupting the orderly flow along the lymph vessels, and results in progressive stasis of a protein-rich fluid with secondary fibrosis. Episodes of acute and chronic inflammation may be superimposed, with further stasis and fibrosis. Hypertrophy of the limb results, with markedly thickened and fibrotic skin and subcutaneous tissue and diminution in the fatty tissue.

Treatment.

There is no very satisfactory treatment for lymphedema, but the following measures can be instituted: (1) The flow of lymph out of the extremity, with a consequent decrease in the degree of stasis, can be aided through intermittent elevation of the extremity, especially during the sleeping hours; and with elastic bandages or supports and massage toward the trunk. (2) Secondary cellulitis in the extremity should be avoided by means of good hygiene and treatment of any trichophytosis of the toes. Once an infection starts, it should be treated thoroughly. (3) Intermittent courses of diuretic therapy, especially in patients with premenstrual or seasonal exacerbations. (4) Surgery is indicated in severe cases when conservative management fails to control the size of the limb or when recurrent attacks of infection cannot be prevented by other means. It is not indicated for cosmetic reasons since the results from that point of view are poor. There is no completely satisfactory operation. A procedure which unites permanently the superficial to the deep lymphatics over a wide expanse by means of buried dermal flaps appears to be the most favorable method thus far devised.

16 . . .

Plastic Surgery

The objective of plastic and reconstructive surgery is the repair of congenital or acquired defects to improve function and appearance. The plastic surgeon is called upon to treat a wide variety of deformities, limited for the most part to the surface tissues but including also the deeper structures of the head, neck, and hands.

Planning a Reconstructive Operation.

A. Make an accurate diagnosis of the deformity. From the standpoint of plastic surgery, this includes a determination of the amount of tissue loss and the degree of distortion, separation, and atrophy or hypertrophy.

B. Consider all possible methods of repair and select one which will achieve the best possible result in the simplest and most direct manner, utilizing neighboring tissues whenever possible.

C. In multiple stage procedures, plan in detail the entire sequence in advance. Pedicle grafts which are to be transferred should be designed to avoid torsion or unnecessary discomfort during all stages of healing.

Principles of Technic.

Gentleness in handling tissues is a very important factor in successful reconstructive surgery; the selection of instruments, suture materials, and procedures is based on this principle.

A. Incisions are made at right angles to the surface, not on the bevel. They should not cross normal flexion or expression creases, but should conform to skin lines of minimal tension whenever possible (see p. 618).

B. Hemostasis must be meticulous. Do not grasp more tissue than necessary with fine mosquito forceps. Use fine ties of 000 or 0000 catgut or the electrocautery.

C. Do not manipulate the skin with forceps; grasp the subcutaneous tissue with fine-tooth forceps or skin hooks.

D. Subcutaneous tissues are closed with fine plain catgut and knots are tied on the deep surface. Avoid tension in closing. Undermine in the subcutaneous plane only as necessary to permit relaxed closure (see p. 619).

E. Skin sutures are placed for accurate approximation after the wound edges have been brought together with catgut. The simplest suture is preferred: interrupted, vertical or horizontal mattress, or subcuticular, according to the situation and the surgeon's preference. Use 00000 or 000000 silk or nylon with an atraumatic needle. The needle should enter and emerge at right angles, close to the wound margins. Sutures should not be tied tightly, to avoid cross hatching.

Sources of Grafts.

A. Autografts are taken from an individual and used upon the same individual, e.g., skin, bone, cartilage, fat, or fascia.

B. Homografts are taken from one individual and used upon another individual, e.g., skin, bone, cartilage, cornea. Homografts of skin are used as a temporary cover in extensive burns. These are rejected after a few weeks except in the case of identical twins.
C. Heterografts are transferred to an individual from a biologically unrelated species, e.g., pigskin epidermal dressings for burn wounds.

SYNTHETIC IMPLANTS

Certain synthetic materials developed in recent years are being used in selected cases as a substitute for bone or cartilage in reconstruction of contour defects. These include dimethyl siloxanes (Silicone®), solid block, sponge, or semifluid; halogenated carbons (Teflon®), solid block or felt; and polyvinyl alcohol sponge. They have the advantage of being nonabsorptive and available in any desired size and shape, and they eliminate the necessity for a second surgical procedure in obtaining autogenous graft materials. However, the implant may be extruded in certain cases if it is not absolutely inert, if infection should occur, if it has sharp edges or is subjected to trauma, or if it is not well covered with normal surface tissues. Cystic formation may also occur, and sponge implants have a tendency to harden and shrink in time. Some of these disadvantages will no doubt be eliminated as research continues.

At present research is being conducted with Dow Corning 360 Medical Fluid Silicone® for soft tissue augmentation. The use of this fluid is at present restricted to certain centers for the purpose of controlled experimentation; recommendations will eventually be made pending the experience and conclusions of these research groups. (**Note:** The use of Silicone® fluid in breast augmentation which has been widely reported both in this country and in Japan is not to be recommended for a variety of reasons. This is not the carefully prepared medical grade Silicone® which is presently being evaluated by Dow Corning. Some of the industrial grades have been tested and found to be toxic; the vast majority have not been tested and should therefore not be used medically.)

SKIN AND PEDICLE GRAFTS

Types of Free and Pedicle Skin Grafts.

A. Free Skin Grafts: These are grafts which are completely removed from one part of the body and applied to another part. They are used to replace skin losses only, and their survival requires a recipient site with a healthy vascular bed. They must therefore not be applied to areas devoid of adequate circulation, on exposed bone or tendon, or on grossly infected wounds. Free grafts are occasionally used to replace large mucous membrane losses, e.g., as a lining for a reconstructed nose. Free skin grafts are of 2 kinds:
   1. Split-thickness (Thiersch) - Split-thickness grafts may be taken from the extremities, abdomen, or back for covering granulating defects, facial defects (temporary or permanent

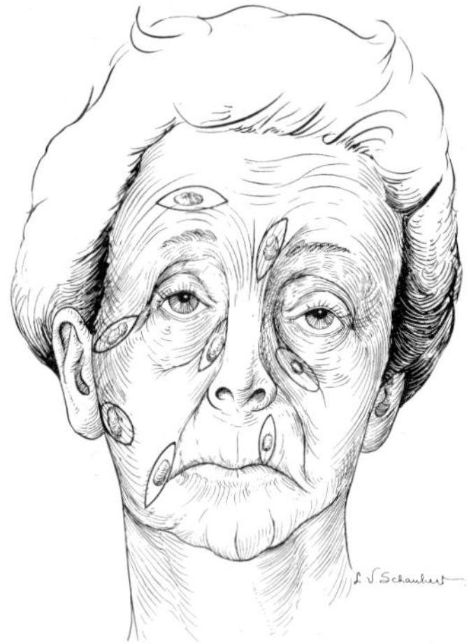

Sites of Elliptical Incisions Corresponding to Wrinkle Lines in the Face. (Reproduced, with permission, from Dunphy and Way [editors], Current Surgical Diagnosis and Treatment. Lange, 1973.)

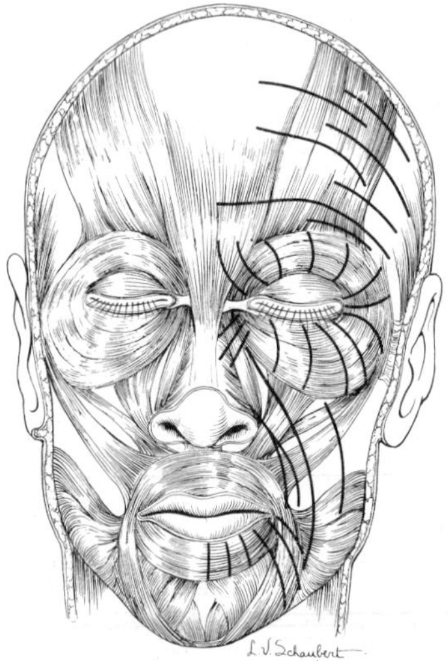

Course of Wrinkle Lines, Transverse to Direction of Facial Musculature. (After Netter.)

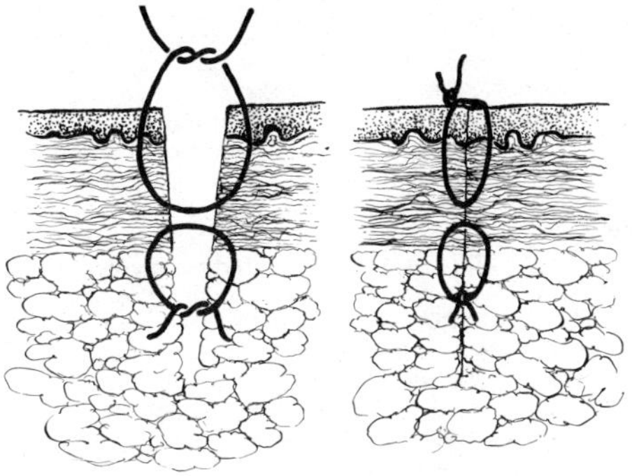

Wound Closure in Layers

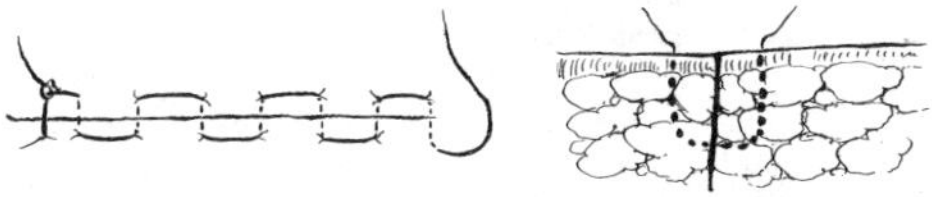

Continuous Horizontal Mattress Sutures

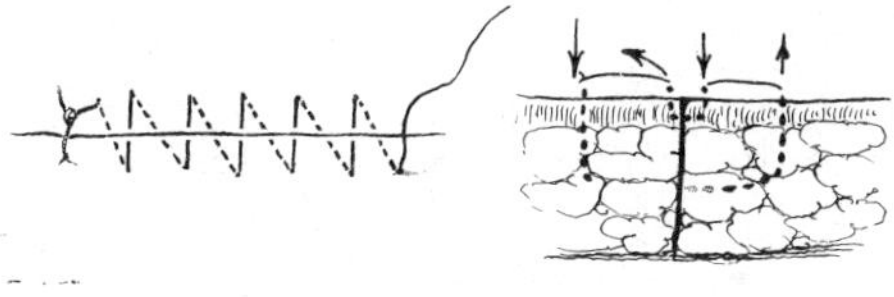

Continuous Vertical Mattress Sutures

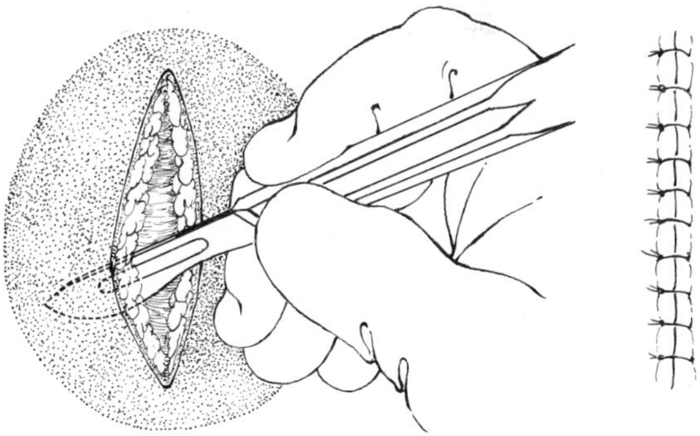

Undermining and Wound Closure. Stippling shows area to be undermined. At right, closure of incisions by interrupted sutures.

covering), for resurfacing the hands, or for inlays. If split-thickness grafts are cut too thin they will contract and wrinkle, but thicker grafts make a good surface covering. Color match is poor. The donor site heals spontaneously.

2. Full-thickness (Wolfe) - Full-thickness grafts may be taken from the postauricular area, the neck, or the supraclavicular region for repair of facial defects or replacement of eyelid tissues. They may be taken from the extremities, the iliac crest, or the abdomen for replacement of the volar surface of the hand. Secondary contraction does not occur, and color match is usually good. The donor site requires closure, either by direct approximation or, if this is not possible, by a split thickness graft.

B. Pedicle Grafts or Flaps: These contain skin and subcutaneous tissue, and must retain a circulatory connection through an attachment at one or both ends. They are used when free grafts are inadequate; to cover exposed bone or tendon; and in instances demanding not only skin but subcutaneous tissue replacement as well. The pedicle attachment must be maintained until a new circulation has developed from the recipient site; this usually requires about 3 weeks.

A pedicle graft may be raised and transferred at one operation, or, if there is any doubt concerning the arterial or venous circulation, a "delaying" procedure may be done. To "delay" a flap means to incise and partially raise the tissue, then replace and suture it in its original site. The objective is not only to test the circulation but to encourage increased blood supply from the pedicle, which will eventually be its only connection.

The circulation of a flap depends upon its arterial supply and its venous return. Should the former be deficient, the flap will become white; if the latter is inadequate, the flap will become blue and edematous, eventually strangulating its circulation entirely. With this in mind flaps should be designed so that the best possible circulation is afforded. The base should be broad, and the length should ordinarily not exceed two and one-half times the width.

Pedicle grafts or flaps are of 2 kinds:

1. Direct pedicle flaps - These are designed, raised, and shifted as a unit. The flap may utilize local neighboring tissues and be shifted or rotated into its new location; or it may be transferred from a distance, as in the case of an abdominal flap transported to the neck by way of an intermediate attachment to the wrist.
2. Tubed pedicle grafts - These form a closed unit which is migrated by shifting first one end of the pedicle and then the other until the graft has reached its destination. An interval of at least 3 weeks is usually necessary between stages. This type of graft requires an additional stage for the construction of the tube. However, because it is a closed unit with no raw surface, the chances of infection and subsequent shrinkage of the graft are minimized and dressings and hospitalization are reduced. The tubed pedicle graft is most often used when multiple transfers are required.

Preparation of a Granulating Wound for Skin Grafting.

A. Debridement: Much time may be saved by mechanical debridement under general anesthesia rather than waiting for gradual separation of the eschar. This seems more satisfactory and is more rapid than enzymatic debridement, which depends upon gradual digestion of necrotic tissue.

B. Interim Management:
   1. Wet dressings of saline or other suitable solution will aid in the preparation of the wound. These should be changed at least every 6 hours for best results. Acetic acid, 0.5-1%, may be added to help control the growth of Pseudomonas organisms.
   2. Antibiotics locally or systemically may be indicated after determination of sensitivity. These drugs should not be continued over prolonged periods.

Procedure at Time of Grafting.

A. General anesthesia is most often used. Local anesthesia may be used if the area to be grafted is small. In this case the donor area is infiltrated with 0.5-1% lidocaine (Xylocaine®) containing epinephrine, 1:100,000 (if not contraindicated). The recipient area should not be infiltrated, since the wound is not sterile and infiltration may contaminate the surrounding tissues.

B. A previously selected donor site is then exposed. This site should be chosen with the following in mind:
   1. If the Thiersch knife is to be used a flat surface is required, preferably the hips or thighs or the medial aspect of the arm. A flat surface is also required for the Brown electrodermatome, but in this case the graft may also be taken from the back. If the Padgett or Reese dermatome is used, the abdomen is also a suitable donor site. Saline may be injected into the tissues of the donor site if bony prominences present a problem.
   2. Hair is not a problem since in taking split skin grafts the follicles remain in the donor area.
   3. In young females, avoid using the thighs or other areas which would normally be exposed in play clothes (unless no other area is available). Some scarring, discoloration, or depigmentation is likely to remain after healing.

C. Prepare the donor area by the technic of skin preparation of the surgeon's preference. Drape and cover the donor area. Prepare well around the recipient site in a similar way, using only saline irrigations for the wound itself. Drape and cover the recipient area.

D. Estimate as accurately as possible the total amount of skin required, and cut the grafts to avoid the hazard of returning to the donor area after working at the recipient site. The depth of the grafts will vary from 0.008 to 0.014 inches in children and from 0.014 to 0.024 inches in adults. Spread the grafts on gauze moistened with saline and cover with gauze. Place the grafts on a table where they will not be disturbed.

E. Dress the donor area and do not return to it.

F. If the granulations are healthy, firm, and flat, they need not be removed. If they are spongy or pale, or if there is considerable deep scarring, the granulations and underlying scar should be removed by scraping with a No. 10 Bard-Parker blade or by actual dissection. If the wound is large and involves an extremity, debridement may be done while bleeding is controlled with a tourniquet; bleeding is thereafter controlled by firm pressure for 5 minutes after the tourniquet is released. If a tourniquet is not used, the bleeding can be controlled by pressure, but blood replacement should be available.

G. Apply the grafts to the dry surface of the wound and spread out under normal skin tension. Suture the grafts to the skin edges with 0000 silk. It is not necessary to puncture the grafts for drainage. After suturing, make certain that no blood has accumulated under the graft. Apply vaseline or xeroform gauze, cover with several layers of flat smooth gauze and a layer of fluffed gauze, and wrap firmly with elastic bandage. Immobilize adjacent joints with a splint or cast. Elevate the part if it is an extremity, and do not disturb the grafts for 8-10 days unless there is drainage or prolonged pain.

   An alternative method of management in selected cases (and particularly in chronic contaminated wounds) is to eliminate dressings entirely, protecting the area with a wire mesh and permitting direct visualization at all times. Any secretions around or under the grafts may then be gently expressed with applicators at once. In many instances grafts which would otherwise be lost may be saved in this way.

H. Any extra skin from the donor area may be rolled in petrolatum gauze and placed in a test tube or glass jar in the refrigerator until the first dressing of the graft.

Dressing the Graft.

On the eighth to the tenth day, remove the splints and dressings and expose the grafts, taking care not to pull them away from the recipient area. Remove sutures. Viable skin will be pink; nonviable skin will be gray. Remove nonviable skin and gently cleanse the area with saline. If a portion of the graft is not viable and the wound is clean, apply the refrigerated skin at the time of the first dressing or a few days thereafter. Reapply dressings and splint again for another week, changing dressings as required. After 2 weeks the grafts should be well enough established so that immobilization is no longer necessary.

Transplantation of Free Skin Grafts.

The free skin graft (as opposed to the pedicle graft, which carries its own blood supply) depends upon the recipient bed for its nourishment until a new blood supply has been established. This nourishment is provided by the tissue fluids, which serve to keep the graft viable until the upward growth of capillaries establishes circulation. The thinner the graft, the more rapidly is new circulation established. It is thus essential that the entire graft be in contact with the recipient bed. A hematoma or purulent drainage under any portion of the graft will interfere with the upward growth of capillaries, and that portion will therefore fail to survive. Meticulous hemostasis, avoidance of infection, and immobilization are prerequisites for successful grafting.

Healing and Innervation.

Healing of the graft is similar to wound healing elsewhere. After 2 weeks, the graft is firmly attached to the bed by connective tissue. A pliable layer of fat will usually be deposited in 3-4 weeks. In 4-6 weeks, sensory nerves will begin to grow in from the periphery; the sense of touch and the perception of pain and temperature appear in that order.

Treatment of Donor Site.

Avoid infection, which will delay healing and may even destroy remaining epithelium and necessitate grafting of the donor site. Two methods are available, either of which will achieve the desired result if contamination of the donor area is avoided.

A. Open Method: Apply a cradle over the wound to prevent contact with bed clothes and allow a natural crust to form. Crusting usually seals off the area in 24-48 hours and separates in 10-14 days.

B. Closed Method: Apply very fine mesh over the wound, such as silk or vaseline gauze. Apply a pressure dressing and allow it to remain in place for 10 days. If healing is delayed, apply 5% scarlet red ointment to stimulate the growth of epithelial cells. In case of contamination with drainage, apply wet saline dressings. Healing usually occurs in 14 days.

CONGENITAL ANOMALIES

CLEFT LIP AND PALATE

Approximately one out of every 750 infants is born with a cleft of the lip or palate (or both). Heredity is a definite etiologic factor. If either parent or a sibling is so affected, the unborn child has a 5% chance of also being affected; when both a parent and a sibling are affected, the risk rises to 15%. Maternal malnutrition, particularly vitamin and mineral deficiencies, and hormonal lack appear also to play a definite role in etiology.

Pathogenesis.

Mesodermal deficiency has been shown to be the important factor in the pathogenesis of cleft lip. (Stark, R.B., Plast. & Reconstr. Surg. **22**:435, 1958.) Normally, there are 3 mesodermal masses in the developing lip and premaxilla which unite to form the upper lip. If one or more of these masses is absent or deficient, a cleft will result, its location depending on the absence of one lateral mass (unilateral cleft), both lateral masses (bilateral cleft), or medial mass (median cleft).

Classification.

The primary palate includes the lip and the premaxilla to the incisive foramen. The secondary palate includes the hard and soft palate posterior to this foramen. Thus, a cleft may involve either the primary or secondary palates or both and may also be either total or subtotal and unilateral or bilateral.

Treatment.

A. Timing of Operation: Closure of the cleft lip is usually done before the infant leaves the hospital; the age of 3 weeks is acceptable if the child is gaining normally.

Operation on the cleft palate is ordinarily done when the child is 12-18 months of age. Most surgeons believe the cleft should be closed before the child learns to speak; others prefer to delay the operation because of possible ill effects on maxillary growth centers.

B. Feeding: Prior to closure of the lip, it may be necessary to assist feedings if the infant has difficulty in sucking; this is

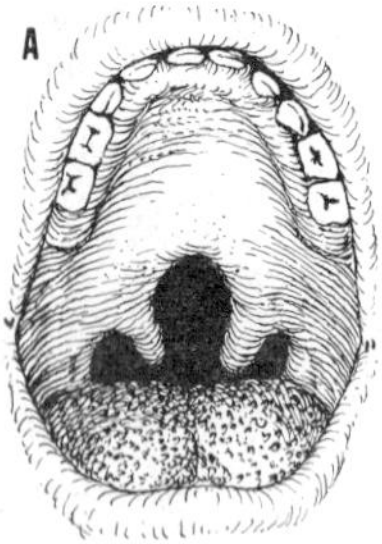

Subtotal Cleft of Secondary Palate

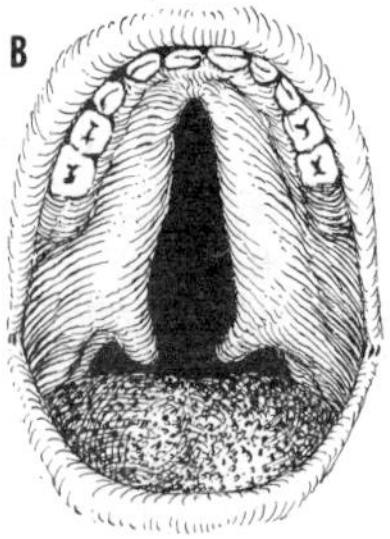

Total Cleft of Secondary Palate

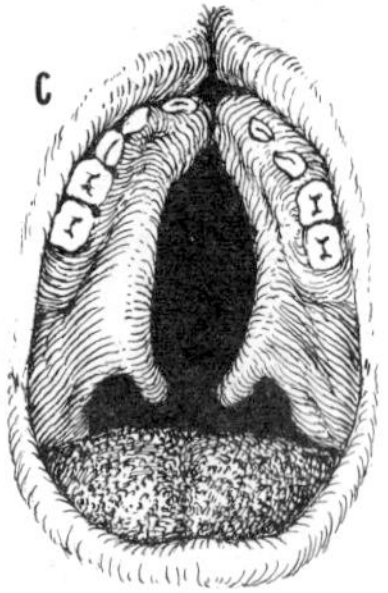

Subtotal Unilateral Cleft of Primary Palate and Total Cleft of Secondary Palate

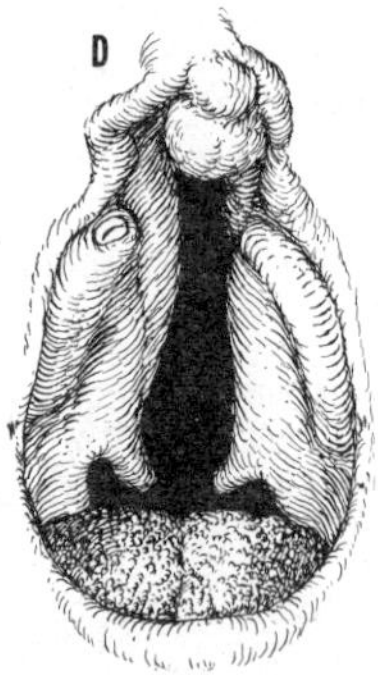

Total Bilateral Cleft of Primary and Secondary Palate

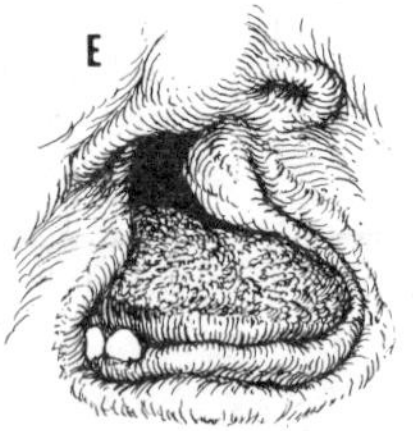

Total Unilateral Cleft of Primary and Secondary Palate

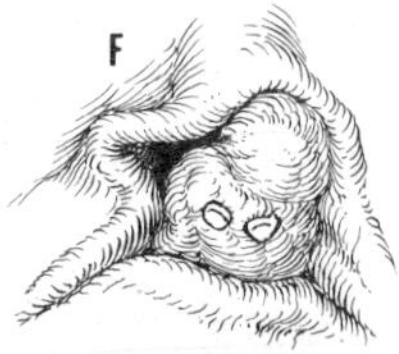

Similar to D

most often noted in complete bilateral clefts. A Breck feeder may be used or, in extreme cases, gavage.

After the lip repair, gavage is usually employed for the first week; thereafter, regular bottle feedings are started.

C. General Principles of Repair:
   1. Cleft lip - There is no actual tissue loss in cleft lip; the problem is to re-form the available lip tissue, which is present but separated. Numerous procedures have given excellent results in experienced hands, notably the procedures of Le Mesurier, Blair and Brown, Tennison, and Millard. Incisions are planned to give a full, normal appearing lip, correcting much of the nostril deformity at the same time.
   2. Cleft palate - In the repair of palatal clefts it is not necessary to obtain bony union but merely to shift the palatal mucoperiosteum to the midline and suture it in place. The objective is not only to obtain closure of the cleft but to ensure adequate length of the soft palate for proper velopharyngeal closure. The procedures of Langenbeck, Wardill, and Veaux, or modifications of them, are most frequently used.

Prognosis.

With refinements in the technic of lip repair, it is possible to obtain excellent results in unilateral cases in one stage. Bilateral repairs are complicated by the protruding premaxilla and prolabium. A satisfactory result may be obtained in these cases, but it is usually necessary to resort to secondary procedures.

The results of cleft palate repair are evaluated on the basis of function. A normal appearing palate may not produce the best speech, and vice versa. Speech training should be begun at the age of 3 years, or as soon as the child will cooperate.

Patients with cleft lip or palate should be brought before a Cleft Palate Panel so that long-term care and follow-up can be planned. Such a panel should consist of the following: (1) dental consultants (dentists, orthodontists, prosthodontists, and pedodontists), (2) plastic surgeons, (3) pediatricians, (4) otologists and otolaryngologists, (5) audiologists, (6) speech therapists, and (7) psychologists, social workers, and vocational advisors.

Secondary and Supplementary Procedures.

A. Nose and Lips: Revision of the nostril deformity may be required. The usual defect is a flattening of the nostril on the cleft side. Minor revision of the vermilion border or cupid's bow may be desirable. In the case of bilateral clefts of the lip, a revision of the nose will probably be necessary since the columella nasi is shortened and the nasal tip is thus pulled downward. Occasionally, in addition to the nasal deformity, the upper lip will be tight and the maxilla underdeveloped. In such cases the rotation of the central portion of the full lower lip into the central portion of the upper lip will produce marked improvement (Abbé-Estlander operation).

B. Palate and Pharynx: Secondary procedures on the palate are indicated when the speech impediment is not correctible by speech therapy. Shortening of the palate with inadequate velopharyngeal closure is the primary cause of the typical cleft palate speech.

Dorrance's method of lengthening the palate consists of raising the entire palate and ligating the posterior palatine arteries at the first stage, and raising and pushing back the palate at the second stage. The VY method has also been used for many years, although the palate cannot be greatly lengthened in this way. In general, these operations do not produce sufficient improvement, since healing and scar contraction counteract some of the added length.

The operation of pharyngeal flap is more satisfactory in this regard. This consists of raising a flap on the posterior pharyngeal wall, usually based superiorly. The flap is then attached to a prepared donor site in the posterior border of the soft palate. On healing, the scar contraction draws the palate posteriorly, which is desirable.

If possible, secondary procedures should be concluded by school age to avoid psychic trauma.

PROTRUDING EARS

This defect is usually bilateral. The auricle may simply protrude from the side of the head to an extreme degree, may be cup-shaped in addition, or the superior border of the helix may overhang ("lopear"). The antihelix is usually not developed, and the auricular cartilage may be misshaped.

Taping the ears in infancy is of no value. Surgery is the only treatment, and should be performed at about 5 years of age (preschool) to avoid psychologic trauma.

Treatment is directed at correction of the abnormality of the cartilage through a postauricular incision. The antihelix is formed by folding the cartilage upon itself, with or without incising the cartilage, depending upon the technic selected.

Occasionally, a separate incision is required along the anterior superior helix to remove or reshape the cartilage in this area (lopear).

MICROGNATHIA

Receding lower jaw may be combined with other congenital defects, especially cleft palate. Serious respiratory and feeding difficulties will occur in extreme cases as a result of posterior displacement of the tongue.

There should be no delay in treatment once the diagnosis has been made. Tracheostomy is sometimes indicated. The operation described by Douglas (Plast. & Reconstruct. Surg. **1**:300, 1946) has been successful in many cases. This consists of suturing the tongue to the buccal surface of the lower lip. With subsequent mandibular growth, the tongue may usually be released in 3-4 months.

NEOPLASMS OF THE SKIN

CAPILLARY HEMANGIOMAS

Port Wine Stain (Nevus Flammeus).

These are usually flat, and vary in color from faint pink to bright red. Nodular outgrowths may occur. Port wine stains may involve any area of the body surface, but they are usually not a problem unless they occur on exposed areas.

These nevi do not regress. Small lesions may be surgically excised and the wound closed by direct approximation or local flaps. Larger lesions would necessitate full-thickness skin grafting, and it is usually preferable to leave them alone (relying on cosmetics to cover them). Tattooing has been used, but a good color match is difficult to obtain.

Port wine stain is not radiosensitive. Local applications of CO_2 snow may only lead to scarring.

Strawberry Birthmark (Hemangioma Simplex).

Strawberry marks are circumscribed, finely lobulated, and elevated, with dilated capillaries, veins, and arterioles (resembling a strawberry). The greater portion may be below the surface. They are most commonly seen on the face, neck, and scalp, but may occur anywhere on the body or face. They may ulcerate as a result of rapid growth or trauma.

Spontaneous regression occurs in a high percentage of cases during the first 7 years (not afterward). However, all do not regress, and even among those which do there may first be a period of rapid growth and ulceration with considerable deformity. A conservative attitude is usually to be recommended; however, in certain cases which show signs of active growth, many surgeons are of the opinion that surgical excision is indicated before the case is complicated by extensive increase in size and ulceration.

Strawberry birthmarks are radiosensitive, but the side effects of radiation must be carefully considered; excessive radiation may produce atrophy of the skin and underlying soft tissues, telangiectasis, or arrested development of bony structures.

Injection of sclerosing solutions will sometimes initiate regression.

Application of CO_2 snow has been used in the treatment of these lesions; however, the effect is inadequate since CO_2 snow blanches out the surface tissues only.

Cavernous Hemangiomas.

These are soft compressible tumors, predominantly venous in character, which contain thin-walled sinus spaces. They may be entirely subcutaneous, in which case the overlying skin usually shows a bluish discoloration, or they may involve skin as well. On the face they cause extensive deformity as well as disturbance of function. Complications (ulceration, infection, and hemorrhage) may be extremely serious.

The endothelium of the sinuses is sensitive to radiation, which initiates interstitial fibrosis and obliteration of the spaces. External radiation, however, may have undesirable side effects such as skin changes or disturbance of bone growth. Radon seeds have proved to be of great value in regulating the dosage to a given area. The usual dosage per seed is 0.1 millicurie. The seeds are inserted through small stab incisions at the periphery of the tumor, and should lie about 1-1.5 cm. apart in all planes.

Sclerosing solutions may be injected into the tumor. This results in obliteration of the area by irritation and fibrosis. The solution need not be injected into a space or the lumen of a vessel since the obliterative reaction may be initiated anywhere in the tumor. Dosage varies from a few minims to 0.5 ml., depending upon the size of the growth and the type of solution used. A marked tissue reaction will result from larger doses, and since more than 1 treatment will usually be required it is well to start with the smaller dose and evaluate the result. An interval of several weeks should elapse before repeating the injection.

Smaller lesions may be simply and effectively treated by surgical excision. Surgery is also frequently indicated following obliteration of these tumors by other methods to improve the cosmetic result.

Cirsoid Angiomas.

These are of the cavernous type, but they also have an arterial circulation by way of arteriovenous fistulas. They pulsate and present a bruit, and may bleed profusely.

Ligation of efferent vessels should precede any other treatment. This is done around the periphery, since ligation of main trunks will not be effective because of abundant collateral circulation. Following ligation, treatment is directed according to the methods described for cavernous hemangiomas.

PIGMENTED NEVI AND MALIGNANT MELANOMA

These cutaneous lesions are composed of nevus cells which have the capacity to form melanin.

Pigmented nevi may be classified histologically as intradermal, compound, junctional, or blue nevi; malignant melanoma may be classified as superficial, invasive, or amelanotic.

Diagnosis.

A. Pigmented Nevi:
   1. Intradermal (resting) - These are circumscribed, smooth or slightly elevated verrucous lesions. They vary in color from light to dark brown and frequently contain hairs. The nevus cells are located in the dermis.
   2. Junctional (active) - These are flat or slightly elevated, smooth, and devoid of hairs. They are usually quite darkly pigmented. There is an active formation of nevus cells in the basal layer of the epidermis (dermo-epidermal junction) but not in the dermis. In a compound nevus, there is also junctional activity, and nevus cells are present in the dermis as well as at the dermo-epidermal junction. These nevi have a malignant potential.
   3. Blue nevus - These are deeply pigmented, slate blue or blue-black, and sharply circumscribed. The melanin pigment is

located in the middle or lower third of the dermis, and the epidermis is normal. Malignancy does not seem to occur in this type of nevus.

B. Malignant Melanoma: It is generally recognized that there are 2 types of malignant melanoma, superficial and invasive, with the former having much the better prognosis. The majority of these tumors arise from a preexisting junctional or compound nevus. Changes in the appearance of such a nevus include growth, increase in pigmentation, bleeding, and inflammatory reaction or ulceration. There is relatively little pigmentation in the amelanotic type, which is occasionally seen. Satellite lesions may appear in the adjacent skin. Metastasis usually occurs first through lymph channels and later through the blood stream.

These tumors are rare before puberty, and when they do occur are often clinically benign. However, malignant types with metastasis are occasionally seen in this age group.

Treatment and Prognosis.

A. Pigmented Nevi: Pigmented nevi which are subject to chronic irritation should be excised prophylactically - particularly the junctional or compound type.

B. Malignant Melanoma: Malignant melanoma requires wide local excision, usually necessitating a skin graft for repair. If regional nodes are clinically positive, a node dissection is also indicated. If the nodes are clinically negative, opinion differs on whether a node dissection is indicated or not.

A 20-year series of 825 patients with melanoma treated at Memorial Center for Cancer and Allied Diseases grouped the survival figures as follows: (1) Melanoma confined to the primary site with negative nodes: 71% 5-year survival, 62% 10-year survival. (2) Melanoma involving the regional lymph nodes: 19% 5-year survival, 12% 10-year survival. (3) Distant metastases: no 5-year survivals.

CARCINOMA OF THE SKIN

Carcinoma of the skin is the most common form of cancer. It is most frequently seen in patients over 40 years of age, but may occur much earlier. Chronic exposure to sun and wind with development of keratotic lesions is a predisposing factor. Skin cancer is therefore most often noted on the face and dorsum of the hands in persons of fair or ruddy complexion.

Classification and Diagnosis.

A. Basal Cell Carcinomas: These may develop on keratotic lesions or on normal skin. They are frequently multicentric, sometimes pigmented, and are most often seen on the scalp, nose, nasolabial fold, eyelids, lips, chin, and forehead. Growth is by extension and infiltration, or may be exophytic, producing large, protruding tumors. Metastasis is rare.

Basal cell carcinomas are usually elevated, circumscribed, "pearly" lesions which later develop into an ulceration with rolled edges. The so-called "rodent ulcer" infiltrates and destroys widely and deeply, whereas the exophytic type develops large outgrowths with relatively little infiltration.

B. Epidermoid (or Squamous Cell) Carcinomas: These usually arise from keratotic lesions and are most frequently seen on the ears, the preauricular, temporal, and malar regions of the face, and on the dorsum of the hands. They may arise on unexposed areas of poor vascularity, such as in unhealed chronic burn scars and ulcerations, areas of radiodermatitis, and on chronic inflammatory lesions. These tumors may be multicentric and may metastasize to neighboring lymph nodes, although this does not often occur on the face. The percentage of metastasizing epidermoid carcinomas is about 5% on the face, 20% on the upper extremities, and 30% on the lower extremities.

Epidermoid carcinomas frequently begin as warty growths on preexisting keratoses which crust over, ulcerate, crust over again, and gradually spread with rolled indurated borders. Extension may be peripheral or deep, or both. Secondary infection is present after ulceration.

Treatment.

Many methods of therapy are in use, including electrocoagulation, escharotics (Mohs), roentgen or Curie therapy, and surgery. The objective of treatment is complete removal or destruction of the tumor, bearing in mind that the first opportunity is the best.

A. Surgical Excision: Complete excision, with microscopic study of the borders of the specimen, is recommended unless surgery is contraindicated. Recurrences are due either to inadequate surgery or to multicentric lesions. In most instances, an immediate repair may be accomplished by direct approximation of the wound or by the use of local flaps. If the resultant wound is very extensive, or if a definitive repair is contraindicated because of the type or location of the tumor, temporary healing may be obtained by means of a split-skin graft.

Regional node dissection is undertaken at the same time when indicated.

B. Roentgen and Curie Therapy: Roentgen therapy is more commonly used than radium in the treatment of carcinoma of the skin because more efficient methods of application and control are available. A balance must be made between insufficient dosage, with recurrence, and overdosage, with resultant radiodermatitis. As in other forms of treatment, results vary according to the experience of the operator.

Radiated tissue is not suitable for use in any subsequent plastic procedure, and this must be borne in mind if later reconstruction is to be considered.

C. Chemosurgery: The Mohs technic of using escharotics under histopathologic control has a place in the treatment of extensive lesions with indefinite boundaries. This method should be reserved for those cases in which other forms of therapy cannot accomplish the same purpose. Reconstruction is undertaken after the tumor has been eradicated.

D. Electrocoagulation is not recommended, inasmuch as superior methods are available. The extent of tumor destruction cannot be accurately controlled with this technic, and recurrence is therefore not infrequent.

FACIAL WOUNDS

Immediate Treatment.

Proper primary care of facial wounds is of great importance, since this tends to minimize the need for later revision of scars. Whenever the general condition of the patient permits, a meticulous repair should be done. Suitable sedation, with either local or general anesthesia, as indicated, will be required. Primary repair may usually done as late as 12-20 hours after injury except in the case of extremely contaminated wounds.

Tetanus prophylaxis is administered as indicated (see p. 208).

A. Cleansing and Debridement: Hexachlorophene or other cleansing agent is used primarily, followed by thorough irrigation with saline. Skin flaps are lifted up to expose pockets, and foreign bodies are searched for and removed. Dirt or grease is removed from the tissues, at times with the aid of dermabrasion.

   Ragged edges and obviously devitalized tissue should be excised. However, one should be conservative in debriding tissues of the face because the excellent blood supply to this area reduces the threat of infection. Bone should be conserved even if it is detached. Portions of facial skin which have lost their blood supply may sometimes be converted to full-thickness grafts and used in the repair. Portions of the ears, nose, or eyelids, if not too badly traumatized, should be trimmed, gently washed in saline, and used in the repair; many times these will survive as composite grafts, and nothing is lost in the attempt. Suturing conforms to the principles described on p. 616. Drainage is usually not required. If there are abraded surfaces, a layer of petrolatum gauze may be applied to the wound. A pressure dressing is then advantageous, with the pressure evenly distributed. Elastoplast® or a head wrap of Kerlix® gauze (or both) is often used for this type of pressure dressing.

B. Repair:
   1. If no tissue is lost - Excise beveled edges to make right angles with the surface of the skin. It is not necessary to undermine the skin. If the suture line crosses a flexion crease which will produce webbing after healing, a small Z-plasty (see p. 636) may be done to avoid the necessity of later revision.
   2. If tissue is lost - Avoid any distortion of features. Avoid tension on suture lines. Several procedures are available for repair of tissue-loss injuries.
      a. Undermining local areas will often provide sufficient tissue for the closure of wounds of moderate size.
      b. Trimming avulsed skin and using it as a free full-thickness graft.
      c. Use of local rotated or interpolated flaps.
      d. Full-thickness skin grafts taken from suitable areas.
      e. Split-thickness grafts may be used in large defects. These may be revised or replaced later if necessary.
      f. For losses involving cavities which cannot be immediately repaired (such as loss of a portion of the nose), suture the skin to the mucous membrane around the margin, wait for healing, and reconstruct later. Similarly, in

loss of a portion of the ear, suture skin to skin. Always replace any avulsed parts of the facial features if the avulsed tissues are available and not too badly traumatized.

C. Postoperative Care of the Wound: Examine the wound after 48 hours and reapply a similar pressure dressing. Look for hematomas and any evidence of infection. If a hematoma is present, sufficient sutures should be removed so that the trapped blood can be expressed. If there is any evidence of infection, obtain culture and sensitivity studies and remove sufficient sutures so that drainage can take place. The appropriate antibiotic should be given in large doses and discontinued as soon as the infection is under control.

Remove sutures early. Half of the sutures may be removed on the third or fourth day and the remainder on the sixth day. The incision line should then be supported with Steri-Strips® for another 10 days.

Prognosis.

Prognosis depends on many factors, including the extent of the original injury, the method used in repair, and the inherent healing powers of the individual tissues. Time will tend to fade and soften scars, smooth contours, and blend grafts with surrounding tissues. An interval of 2 years should elapse before evaluating the final results.

FRACTURES OF FACIAL BONES

The most common types of fractures of the facial bones, in order of frequency, are fractures of the nose, mandible, malar, maxilla, and multiple fractures. All are caused by external force.

Edema may disguise or accentuate the deformity. Inspection and palpation are important guides to diagnosis. These should be supplemented by x-ray examination.

Displacement of bone fragments is determined by the direction of the fracturing force and by muscle pull, as seen in mandibular fractures, where the posterior fragment is displaced upward and the anterior fragment downward.

FRACTURES OF THE NOSE

If nasal fractures are seen early, before massive edema accumulates, they may be reduced at once. If treatment has been delayed it is better to wait until the swelling subsides so that more accurate diagnosis and reduction can be done.

Nasal fractures are usually reduced under local anesthesia, using 1% lidocaine (Xylocaine®) with 1:100,000 epinephrine solution, supplemented with 10% cocaine and epinephrine topically. General anesthesia (administered intratracheally) is preferable in some cases and is essential in children.

After anesthesia has been administered, clear the nose to establish an airway and aid in visualization of interior structures.

Examine the septum for signs of hematoma, and incise and evacuate any clots present.

Types of Nasal Fractures and Treatment.

A. Simple Fractures: Gently disimpact the bones by internal manipulation with Walsham's forceps or a broad elevator. Align bones by a combination of internal pressure and external manipulation with the thumb and index finger.

Packing usually is not required unless persistent bleeding is a problem. In such a case the packing should not be disturbed for at least 3-4 days, since early removal will very likely cause renewed hemorrhage. Wait until the gauze is well saturated with secretions so that it may be removed easily. If a posterior pack is indicated, a No. 14 F. catheter may be inserted through the nostril and the 5 cc. bag inflated. The catheter is then fixed anteriorly with a bolster, and sufficient pressure applied (in combination with the anterior packing) to control bleeding. Although this method is simple and easy to apply, it is probably not as effective in some cases as posterior packing with gauze.

Once the bones have been disimpacted and replaced in normal position, there is no muscle pull which will displace them. Therefore, an external splint is required only for protection. This is left on for 4-5 days.

B. Compound Fractures: Associated lacerations of the nose should be treated at the same time as the fracture. If treatment cannot be given within the first 12-20 hours, however, it is wiser to wait for healing of the skin lacerations before reducing the fracture.

C. Comminuted Fractures: Additional fixation may be required in cases of severe comminution and flattening of the nasal bones. After reduction, a No. 24 stainless steel wire mattress suture may be passed through the fracture sites from one side of the nose to the other. This suture is twisted over large buttons or lead plates, which holds the nasal bones in their advanced position. Care must be taken to avoid pressure points on the skin.

MALAR AND ZYGOMATIC ARCH FRACTURES

The dense body of the malar bone is not readily fractured. Fractures and dislocations most often occur at articulations: the malar frontal suture, the malar maxillary suture along the floor of the orbit, and the zygomatic suture. The anterior wall of the antrum and the zygomatic arch are also frequently involved.

Fracture of the malar and zygomatic arch may cause depression or flatness of the cheek, limitation of motion of the mandible due to mechanical obstruction, diplopia due to displacement of the floor of the orbit, and emphysema due to laceration of the lining of the antrum. X-rays are of great value in diagnosis.

Treatment.

Reduction should be done early if possible, but at least within 2 weeks so that the bones may be readily mobilized. The following alternatives are available:

A. Temporal approach (Gillies), by incision through the temporal fascia and introduction of an elevator under the zygomatic arch.
B. Direct traction on the body of the malar bone by means of a forceps or towel clip.
C. Elevation by the antral approach through a buccal incision.
D. Direct wiring of fracture sites is frequently required when there is considerable displacement.

"BLOWOUT" FRACTURE OF THE FLOOR OF THE ORBIT

This fracture is caused by a sudden increase in intraorbital pressure due to trauma. There is usually associated diplopia due to herniation of the inferior rectus and inferior oblique muscles. The diplopia is most apparent to the patient when he attempts to look upward.

A diagnosis of blowout fracture should not be made on x-ray evidence alone. There must be persistent clinical findings as well before a decision is made to explore the orbit surgically.

Treatment consists of replacement of the herniated structures and closure of the bony defect in the orbital floor. This closure may be obtained by reduction of the bony fragments, by autogenous bone graft, or by foreign implants such as Silicone®.

FRACTURE OF MANDIBLE

Fractures of the mandible most often involve the region of the mental foramen, the angle, and condyle. A fracture in the mental region is often associated with fracture of the angle or condyle on the opposite side.

Displacement is manifested by malocclusion, and depends upon the direction of the fracturing force and upon muscle pull, which tends to elevate the posterior fragment and depress the anterior fragment. Diagnosis depends upon the presence of some or all of the following signs and symptoms: pain and swelling, hemorrhage at the fracture site along the alveolus, crepitus, and displacement. For accurate determination of the degree of displacement and for detection of fractures without displacement, x-ray examination is essential.

Treatment.

Interdental wiring may be used alone or in combination with other methods, depending upon the circumstances. For simple fractures without displacement or those which may be realigned and maintained without difficulty, wiring will be all that is required. Immobilization of the mandible to the maxilla should be maintained for about 6 weeks.

If teeth are absent on one side, an acrylic bite plate may be provided which is attached by a bar to a cap splint on the teeth of the opposite side. The plate contains hooks for interdental fixation.

If the patient is edentulous, his dentures may be utilized after they have been trimmed to fit without pressure points at the fracture site. The lower denture is then immobilized by 4 circumferential wires inserted from below. The upper denture is maintained in place by a wire encircling the zygomatic arch on each side (inserted from above and entering the mouth in the posterior alveolar region) and by an additional wire through the nasal spine (inserted orally). These wires are then twisted around loops provided in the denture. The upper and lower dentures are then wired together.

Fracture of the condyle is usually treated by simple interdental wiring. Even though the displacement is marked, the functional result is usually quite satisfactory.

Isolated fracture of the coronoid is rare and does not affect occlusion, although there may be considerable displacement of the fragment by temporal muscle pull. Simple interdental wiring is indicated.

Pin fixation is usually used for fractures of the body or angle of the mandible when the displacement may be corrected by manipulation but cannot be maintained by interdental wiring alone.

Open reduction is indicated in fractures with marked displacement which cannot be reduced and maintained satisfactorily by other methods. The intraoral approach may be used in fractures of the body of the mandible. The extraoral approach is used for fractures involving the ramus or angle. Two stainless steel wires are inserted through drill holes in each fragment, the bones aligned accurately, and the wires twisted firmly. Interdental wiring is then used for immobilization.

FRACTURES OF THE MAXILLA

Fractures of the maxilla vary from simple unilateral fracture without displacement to complete separation of the entire maxilla. They are frequently associated with severe intracranial injuries and fractures of other facial bones. The care of such fractures may present a serious and complicated problem.

The direction of displacement depends upon the degree and direction of force. The entire maxilla may be displaced downward (by complete detachment), upward into the nasal fossa, or directly backward.

Classification.

A. Le Fort I: Fractures above the level of the apices of the teeth, including the alveolar process, the vault of the palate, and the pterygoid processes.

B. Le Fort II: Pyramidal fracture, through the frontal process, lacrimal bones, floor of orbit.

C. Le Fort III: Craniofacial disjunction, when the fracture extends through the zygomatico-frontal suture and across the floor of the orbits. The entire mid third of the bony structure of the face may be detached from the base of the skull.

Treatment.

A. First Aid: Provide an adequate airway, since massive edema and associated nasal fractures are often present. Tracheostomy may be necessary. Support the maxilla temporarily by external bandaging with muslin or elastic material slung beneath the chin and tied over the head, thus utilizing the lower jaw for partial immobilization.

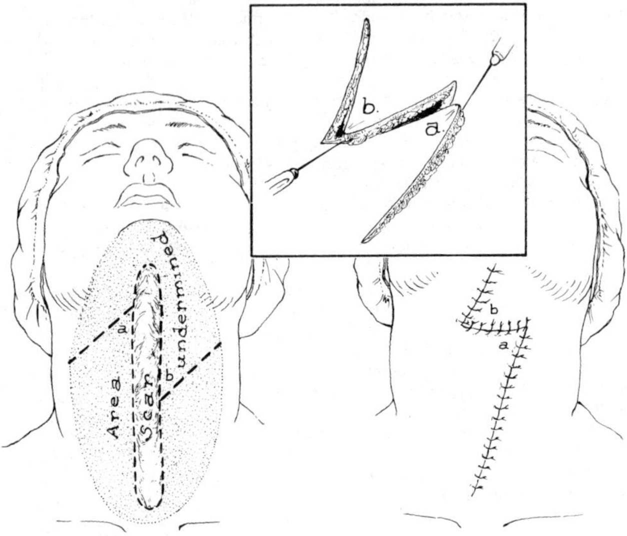

Repair of Anterior Neck Contracture by Z-Plasty. Left: Anterior neck contracture with incisions outlined for Z-plasty. Right: Transposition of flaps. Inset: Detail of flap transposition.

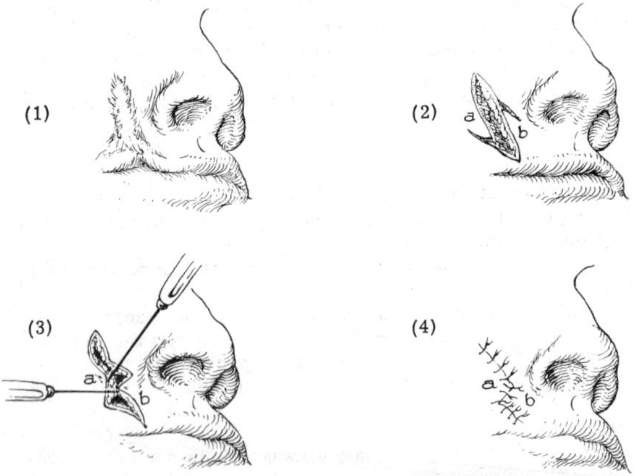

Repair of Scar Contracture of Lip and Cheek by Z-Plasty. (1) The defect. (2) Excision of scar and outline of Z-plasty. (3) Transposition of flaps. (4) Completed closure of wound.

B. Fixation: In simple fractures involving one side only, the maxilla is realigned to correct occlusion and an arch bar is then fitted and wired to the teeth.

In severe fractures with complete mobility of the maxilla, a combination of methods will be required. These will include wiring of the teeth, suspension to higher intact bones, and interdental wiring to the mandible. Associated fractures of the mandible or other facial bones are cared for at the same time. The use of cumbersome head caps and traction is reserved for the few cases in which simpler methods are not sufficient.

C. Feeding in Jaw Fractures: It is not necessary to extract teeth in order to give fluids; a nasogastric tube may be used for the first few days if necessary. A high-protein supplementary formula is used. Foods may also be prepared in a blender for administration in the same way.

SCARS AND CONTRACTURES

HYPERTROPHIED SCARS AND KELOIDS

The hypertrophic scar is raised, red, and indurated. It is confined to the area of the wound. In time, usually after 6 months to 2 years, these scars tend to soften, flatten, and fade.

Overgrowth of connective tissue is frequently seen in third degree burns, especially if allowed to heal by granulation. It also may result from infection, tension, or inaccurate approximation of wound edges. It is more often seen when the scars run across normal tension lines. The anterior chest is particularly prone to overgrowth - so much so that benign lesions should not be removed from this area without due consideration.

It has been noted that the tendency to this scar formation may diminish after puberty.

True keloids, which are most often seen in blacks, tend to invade surrounding tissue. They do not usually improve with time, and may attain tremendous proportions.

Treatment.

The best treatment is prophylactic, by paying close attention to the general principles of repair and by avoiding elective operations in dark-skinned patients in anatomic areas where this type of scar reaction is likely to develop. Prophylactic roentgen therapy may be given as soon as sutures are removed, although its value is debatable. Do not attempt to excise or revise a hypertrophied scar until all reaction has subsided, or it will very likely recur.

Treatment of the true keloid is often unsatisfactory, and recurrence is common. Excision and repair frequently result in a larger keloid. Any attempt at removal is a calculated risk.

Intralcsional injection of triamcinolone into the scar or keloid has often proved to be beneficial. In responsive cases the scar becomes softer, smoother, and smaller.

CONTRACTURES OF THE NECK

These usually result from third degree burns or surgical incisions crossing flexion lines. Contracture is minimized by early grafting of burns, but some degree may develop from contraction of split grafts. The extent of contracture depends on the amount of skin loss; in extreme cases the chin is pulled down to the chest, with ectropion of the mouth and lower eyelids.

Scar tissue must be removed and replaced with normal skin. Minor degrees of contracture may be corrected by Z-plasty (see p. 540).

After excision of all scar tissue, the resultant defect is usually much greater than anticipated, and in severe cases skin grafting will be required. For this purpose, split grafts of uniform thickness give the best result. However, a molded collar must be worn day and night for several months during the contractile period of the grafts. The ultimate result by this method is worth the inconvenience and eliminates the necessity for multiple stage pedicle grafting.

CONTRACTURES OF THE AXILLA

Contractures of the axilla are most often seen following third degree burns, but may result from any type of wound involving skin loss in the axilla or from surgical incisions which cross the normal creases and create webbing.

Moderate contracture may be repaired by 2 plastic flaps if the surrounding tissue is not heavily scarred.

Severe contracture will require complete dissection of scar tissue, and if this is necessary the remaining defect will be quite large. Rotating a flap into this defect and grafting the donor site, when feasible, is superior to the use of a split-skin graft. If insufficient tissue is available for a rotated flap, a free graft will be necessary. Maximal mobilization of the shoulder joint should be attempted at surgery; however, a full range of motion is not always obtainable at the time due to muscle or tendon contracture, which may later yield to active use of the joint.

FACIAL PARALYSIS

Paralysis of the facial nerve involves the muscles of expression and the buccinator. The affected side is without expression, and the deformity is increased by the action of the muscles of the normal side. The mouth droops, the eye cannot close, and mastication is impaired. Speech is also affected.

Treatment.

A. Nerve Repair: Some evidence of spontaneous regeneration should appear within 6 months or not at all. Reinnervation may be attempted by decompression, end-to-end anastomosis, nerve grafts, or anastomosis with hypoglossal or spinal accessory nerves. However, the results are usually disappointing.

B. Mechanical Support:
1. Muscle transplants include slips of the temporalis to the eyelids and of the masseter to the lips. These transplants may become fibrotic in time, losing some of their dynamic action and serving as static support only. The use of the masseter usually affords a fairly good result.
2. Fascial slings - These may be used as static support alone or in combination with the masseter to provide some degree of muscle action. Fascial strips encircle the orbicularis, extending to the unparalyzed side to obtain contralateral pull. These strips are then attached to the masseter muscle or the temporalis fascia to slightly overcorrect the asymmetry. A sling may be inserted in some cases where return of function is ultimately expected to prevent stretching of muscles.
3. Rhytidectomy (face lift) removes sagging excess skin. Lateral tarsorrhaphy protects the cornea.
4. Sectioning of certain muscles of expression on the normal side is sometimes recommended to prevent gross distortion when the facial expression is animated.

COSMETIC PROCEDURES

RHINOPLASTY
(Plastic Surgery of the Nose)

The most common cosmetic defects of the nose are the long hump nose, the twisted nose, the deflected nose, and the saddle nose. Quite minor defects may for certain patients assume an exaggerated importance. An evaluation of the patient's motivation and personality is therefore an important part of the preoperative examination.

Preoperative photographs should always be taken.

The nose should be fully developed (16-18 years of age) before rhinoplasty is performed.

Surgical procedures consist of freeing the skin from the underlying bone and cartilage and altering the nasal framework as indicated, either by bone and cartilage removal or by grafting.

Incisions are closed with plain catgut, leaving adequate openings for drainage to avoid hematoma formation. Packing is lightly inserted to eliminate dead spaces. Adhesive strapping is carefully applied to mold the nose in its new contour; a molded splint of metal or modeling compound is then applied and fixed with adhesive.

Cold compresses over the eyes will help to reduce the edema which is sure to develop. This swelling and discoloration will gradually disappear during the first week.

The packing is removed in 48 hours. Thereafter the nose is cleaned daily of crusts. The splint is maintained for 6-7 days.

The usual length of time before the patient resumes normal activities is 14 days.

RHYTIDECTOMY
(Meloplasty, "Face Lift")

Cosmetic surgery of the aging face is designed to remove redundant skin, thereby smoothing the face and neck and lifting sagging jowls. The "face lift" operation is a major surgical procedure which is not to be undertaken without complete physical and psychologic evaluation. The patient must be warned also that the aging processes cannot be halted by surgery, and that the tissues will continue to sag at a rate which cannot be predicted.

Incisions are placed so that the resultant scars are minimized. Extensive undermining and freeing of facial and neck skin is necessary to obtain a worthwhile result. Care must be taken to avoid injury to the branches of the facial nerve or to the posterior auricular nerve, and bleeding must be meticulously controlled.

After dissection has been completed and hemostasis is satisfactory, the excess skin is pulled upward and excised. The skin incisions are then closed with 00000 black silk and a pressure head dressing is applied. Sutures are usually removed from the preauricular and postauricular incisions on the fifth day; the sutures within the hairline are allowed to remain for 8-10 days.

Edema and discoloration of the face and neck tissues is usually moderate and will disappear in 7-10 days. Patients may ordinarily return to their regular activities at the end of 2 weeks.

BLEPHAROPLASTY
(Correction of Baggy Eyelids)

Blepharoplasty is frequently done in combination with rhytidectomy, but sometimes is done as a separate procedure. Excess skin is excised, as well as any periorbital fat which has herniated through the muscle and come to lie subcutaneously. Removal of skin is conservative, especially in the lower lids, to avoid ectropion.

DERMABRASION

This procedure is used for the removal of superficial foreign bodies resulting from road or industrial accidents, for improvement of facial pitting following acne or chickenpox, and for removal of superficial tattoos. The degree of improvement which can be achieved with this technic will depend upon the depth of the pigmentation. In any pitted skin no more than 50% improvement should be anticipated. This procedure is not advisable in dark-skinned races because of the danger of keloid formation or hyperpigmentation.

17 . . .

Hand Surgery

Any severe hand disorder should be referred to a general, plastic, or orthopedic surgeon who specializes in the hand, if one is available. Only a specialist can adequately manage all of the tissues and structures (skin, muscles and tendons, nerves, vessels, bones and joints) and give the expert care necessary to preserve or restore the function of all systems of this complex mechanism. Most hand problems are caused by trauma, but tumors, neurologic disorders, congenital anomalies, and rheumatic joint and tendon afflictions also contribute to the daily toll of conditions that need treatment. The functional outcome depends on the quality of early and late surgical treatment.

TRAUMA TO THE HAND

Successful management of the injured hand requires constant attention to the essential components of hand function (sensibility, mobility, placement, and power) and a thorough knowledge of how such function may be compromised or threatened by trauma or its treatment. A thorough understanding of the functional anatomy of the upper extremity is often crucial to a successful outcome.

EVALUATION OF THE INJURED HAND

Careful records of history and examination - including, in many instances, a complementary diagram detailing the problem - are invaluable aids in the initial and subsequent treatment as well as in preparing administrative reports on temporary and permanent disability. It is essential to record in precise language everything that one knows about, plans, and actually does for the injured hand. Accurate reports can be prepared only if these details are recorded immediately at the time of evaluation and treatment.

History.

It is necessary to repeat the history taking procedure once or twice to make certain that the data from the patient, his family, his employer, etc. are accurate and complete. Correct diagnosis and plan of treatment of an old or new injury require the following information:

(1) Age, occupation, hand dominance, and pre-existing hand problems, if any.

(2) Chief complaint, its duration, its previous occurrence, and

whether or not it is getting worse, getting better, or remaining static.

(3) The how, where, when, and why of the injury. A detailed history must be taken of the mechanism of injury, the interval between injury and treatment, factors of contamination, and treatment rendered to date.

(4) The status of tetanus prophylaxis and medical allergies.

(5) A review of the patient's past and current state of health and any treatment given.

Physical Examination.

The examination of the total patient may be cursory or complete depending on whether the history raises any relevant questions or whether the patient is to be admitted to the hospital for care.

The examination of the extremity should then determine the following:

A. Pain or Anesthesia: Note the presence, type, and severity of pain. Throbbing pain implies venous congestion and must be relieved by mechanical means rather than by drugs. The patient must be made as comfortable as possible during the examination, often by recumbency. Anesthetic areas should be mapped and confirmed later by retesting.

B. Viability of Tissues: Comparison of capillary filling, color, and temperature with normal skin and the opposite hand should be noted, as well as the quality of the pulse.

C. Deformity: Note any distortion of form by soft tissue swelling (edema, hemorrhage, infection), tumor, or bone displacement.

D. Mobility: Note the status of active and passive mobility. Division of motor nerves or tendons creates characteristic deficits in active motion. Selective testing of muscle units should be done.

E. Wounding: Is the wound tidy or untidy, new or old, bleeding, blood-logged or dry, clean or infected, punctured or incised, deep or superficial, with or without foreign body? Probing should not be done by inexperienced surgeons or in circumstances where help is inadequate, lighting is poor, or proper instruments and facilities are not available. In such cases, probing of a wound should be deferred to the definitive surgeon who is properly equipped. Bleeding can usually be controlled by direct pressure on the bleeding point and the release of tight garments and jewelry. If not, the bleeding point may be isolated under tourniquet (blood pressure cuff) control and carefully ligated without injury to an adjacent nerve. Loupe magnification is often indispensable for this purpose.

F. X-Rays: X-rays (postero-anterior, lateral, and special views) should be selectively taken to determine any abnormality of bone or the presence of a radiopaque foreign body.

Referral and Deferral of Treatment.

The freshly injured hand should be made as comfortable as possible, usually by splinting and elevation. Constrictive dressings must be avoided. A well-padded, light cast around the forearm and hand (like a boxing glove) with the wrist slightly extended and a large soft roll of gauze in the palm between the thumb and fingers often gives the greatest comfort. Pain should also be controlled by analgesics if necessary. Surgical toilet (irrigation and skin preparation) may be rendered and wounds closed loosely and covered with sterile dressings. If there will be more than 2 or 3 hours of delay before definitive care of an open injury can be given, tetanus prophylaxis together with prophylactic intramuscular broad-spectrum antibiotics should be administered by the physician rendering emergency care. A detailed record of the initial diagnosis and treatment should accompany the patient, who should be given nothing by mouth. An amputated part may be wrapped with ice and transferred with the patient.

MANAGEMENT OF THE INJURED HAND

Surgical Facilities.

An operating table, arm board, good light, a magnifying loupe, specialized fine instruments, a pneumatic gauged cuff, and surgical assistance are essential for proper hand surgery. Inexperience, haste, and fatigue are serious and often costly handicaps.

Preparation for Surgery.

The patient should be supine and comfortable, with a well-padded pneumatic tourniquet on the arm. Many surgeons sit, but it is better to elevate the table and stand so that the surgeon can readily shift his position as circumstances require. However, microsurgery of nerves and vessels is done sitting. If pain is not unduly severe, anesthetic paralysis of the arm should be withheld until the skin preparation and draping are completed since the patient's cooperation greatly facilitates these procedures. Skin preparation consists of one paint brush coating of 1-2% iodine, which is then neutralized with alcohol. These solutions should be kept out of the wound and off of the tourniquet and its padding. Sterile waterproof draping is then applied. General or regional anesthesia can then be administered. The freshly injured or infected extremity may then be passively elevated and the tourniquet inflated (to 300 mm. Hg for adults or to 150-250 mm. Hg for infants and persons with very thin arms). Uncontrolled bleeding may necessitate tourniquet control before the anesthesia and skin preparation are administered. Elective surgical cases which are not infected are usually exsanguinated with an elastic roll (e.g., Esmarch bandage) before inflation of the tourniquet. The patient will generally tolerate tourniquet ischemia on the unanesthetized upper arm for 20-30 minutes. When the arm is anesthetized, the tissue tolerance for ischemia is usually $2\text{-}2^1/2$ hours. The tourniquet manometer should be tested for accuracy before use since paralyses have occurred as a result of excessive tourniquet pressure. The tourniquet may be released and reinflated after the reactive hyperemia subsides in procedures demanding prolonged tourniquet time.

Anesthesia.

General anesthesia is preferred for most procedures which last for over 20-30 minutes. Premedication with morphine sulfate and scopolamine (when not contraindicated by allergy or glaucoma) is ideal for its tranquilizing and analgesic effect.

Lidocaine (1-2%) **without** epinephrine injected slowly with a fine needle (e.g., No. 26-30 gauge for the digit) is preferred for local blocks (into the wound) or nerve blocks (axillary, radial, ulnar, median, or digital nerve (see p. 122). Caution is necessary to avoid excessive amounts which will congest the nerve, the hand, or the digit. The skin and fat should still be soft and pliable after the injection. The most one should inject at the base of an adult digit is 2.5 ml.

General Surgical Technics for Fresh Injuries.

Anything that touches the wound must be aseptic and both chemically and mechanically atraumatic. Starch powder should be wiped off of sterile gloves. Sponging should be by dabbing, not wiping. Instruments must be in the best condition and should consist of a selection of fine plastic hooks, retractors, forceps, clamps, scissors, needle holders, atraumatic sutures, and Kirschner wires and drill. Nonreactive material should be stipulated for sutures and ligatures. Monofilament nylon is preferred. The tissues must be kept moist, preferably with lactated Ringer's solution. Hemostasis must be complete.

The 6 fundamental technical precepts of successful dissection in the hand are as follows: (1) Dissect with at least 2 × magnification, tourniquet ischemia, and a needle-point electrocautery available. (2) Dissect from normal tissue into abnormal. (3) Keep the tissues dissected under tension. (4) Keep the margins of the wound suspended by hooks or stay sutures. (5) Once through the dermis with a scalpel, use short-bladed, sharp, fine scissors for dissection and identify and coagulate or ligate all vessels. (6) Spread the tissue gently before cutting, and then cut with precision only the tensed white fascial or fibrous tissue. This will prevent the inadvertent severing of nerves or vessels, which are identifiable by their soft and lax consistency.

A. Irrigation: Gross dirt on the skin should be washed off with soap and water. Skin stains do not necessarily have to be washed off. If the skin is coated with oil, grime, or tar, ether or benzine may be necessary to remove it, but such solutions must be kept out of the wound. Dried blood is most easily removed with hydrogen peroxide. An open wound may be irrigated with water, lactated Ringer's solution, or antibiotic solution.

B. Debridement: The purpose of debridement is the removal of blood clots, nonviable tissue, and foreign bodies which will constitute "dead space." Thus, living tissue can be coapted and grafted tissue can be nourished by capillary invasion. It is occasionally necessary to do this without tourniquet ischemia so that the level of viability can be determined by the scalpel. The hand specialist will know when and how to save debrided tissue for primary or secondary use in reconstructive surgery. The objective of debridement in the primary care of injuries is to preserve function by preserving circulation and curtailing edema and infection. Closing a wound with irregular but viable margins or with primary or delayed split thickness grafting is far preferable to trimming the edges and forcing the closure with tight sutures. Stained but viable tissue and minute fragments of foreign material should not be removed unless the foreign material is known to be caustic.

C. Exposure: (See illustration on p. 645.) Proper evaluation and repair demand anatomic identifiability. Therefore, wound extension beyond scar or blood-discolored tissue is often manda-

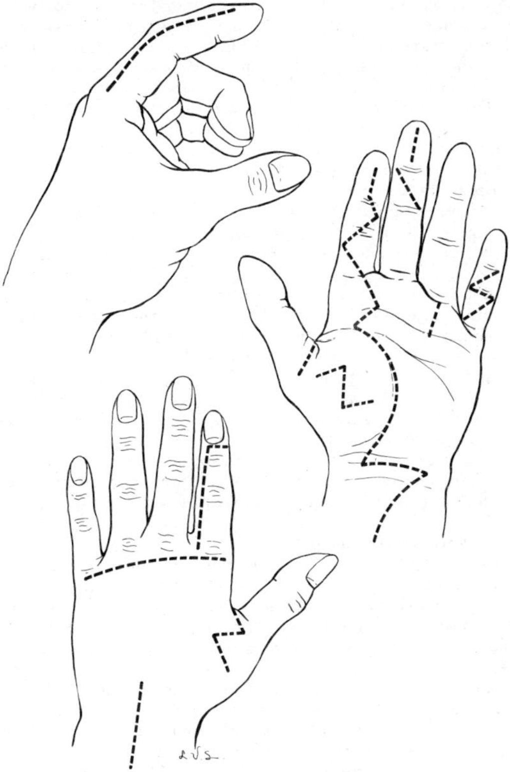

Proper Placement of Skin Incisions. (Reproduced, with permission, from Dunphy and Way [editors], Current Surgical Diagnosis and Treatment. Lange, 1973.)

tory. This should be done without injury to the blood supply, nerves, and tendons and should not predispose to secondary disabling contractures (e.g., scars crossing at right angles to flexion skin creases).

D. What to Repair: After effective debridement and exposure, experience and facilities will determine how much to repair deep to the skin. Skilled primary reparative or reconstructive hand surgery will go far to spare function, time, and expense. Unskilled efforts may do just the opposite. Generally speaking, skeletal distortion should be gently corrected, and if the tissues are not congested and the circulation is good, structures that are easily identifiable and clearly matched should be approximated. Unstable bone alignment often requires Kirschner wires. Sutures of nylon vary in caliber from 8-0 to 10-0 for digital nerves and from 4-0 to 6-0 for tendons and skin. All ligatures are preferably of 4-0 to 6-0 nylon. (Catgut is reactive and therefore should not be used except to close the skin of infants.)

Given satisfactory skeletal stability, the circulation has first priority, skin and fat second, tendons (e.g., long flexor tendons) third, and nerves the last priority in primary repair. One must avoid overloading the already injured tissues with the trauma of surgery itself.

1. Primary repair is that which is done within the first 24-72 hours. If circumstances of wounding suggest heavy contamination (e.g., a tooth, a farmyard, or a sewer inflicted wound), it is probably best to drain the wound and repair nothing primarily. When contamination is minimal but the circulation is impaired (e.g., much swelling)- or if over 8 hours have passed without any surgical toilet or splinting - then it is best to prepare, dress, splint, and elevate the part and administer prophylactic broad-spectrum antibiotics. If within the first 2 weeks there is no evidence of inflammation and the tissues are soft and pliable, delayed primary repair may be considered.
2. Secondary repair is that which follows the first 2 weeks after injury and is usually undertaken after maximal resolution of the swelling and induration that followed the injury.

Wound Closure and Drainage.

A rubber drain prevents the accumulation of serum and blood and forestalls the development of "dead space" and infection. Therefore, drainage should be selectively used in contaminated wounds and severe compound crushing wounds. Drains should be inserted in such a way as to favor gravity drainage from the elevated extremity.

Wounds should never be closed with tension. If tension is unavoidable, it is best to leave the wound open or to graft it. When tension has already built up and uncontrollable throbbing pain has developed, it should be treated by adequate slitting of the skin and fascia.

Most wounds of the hand can be closed with one layer of interrupted or running everting skin sutures. Interrupted sutures are preferred if motion is to start early.

Prophylaxis Against Infection.

This involves prophylaxis against tetanus (see p. 208) and against streptococcal and staphylococcal infections. If the wound is contaminated (not necessarily clinically infected), it should be irrigated with bacitracin solution at surgery and systemic antibiotics should be given for 48-72 hours afterward. The systemic drugs of choice for gram-positive organisms are methicillin, lincomycin, erythromycin, or oxacillin; for gram-negative organisms, kanamycin. Antibiotics must not be regarded as a substitute for the more important fundamental principles of surgical technic and protection of circulation.

Dressings and Splints.

The dressing should serve to keep the soft tissues at rest and

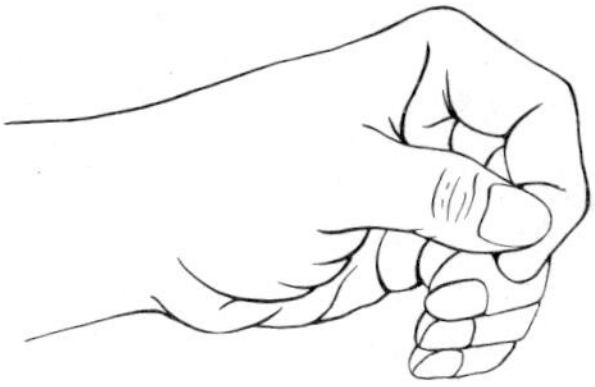

Position of Function of the Hand. (Reproduced, with permission, from Dunphy and Way [editors], Current Surgical Diagnosis and Treatment. Lange, 1973.)

prevent the development of "dead space" by gentle compression that does not obstruct venous return. Soppy wet dressings facilitate drainage of blood and serum. A single layer of fine mesh gauze smoothed out flush with the wound prevents granulation tissue from invading the dressing and facilitates the search for sutures when the dressing is removed. On top of this should be placed wet, loose-meshed gauze which should be tailored to lie flat without folds and ridges. Over this should then be placed a carefully tailored sheet of sponge rubber or plastic (e.g., Reston®) to prevent congestion by the dressing. This in turn is held in place with circumferentially wrapped, loose-meshed gauze (e.g., Kling®, Kerlex®). Care should be taken not to wrap the part too snugly.

Immobilization is mandatory initially in most cases of hand trauma, bearing in mind that prolonged immobilization involves a risk of stiffness. The position in immobilization must never be at the extreme of joint extension or flexion but must generally serve its need, e.g., to relieve tension on a tendon or nerve suture line. Whenever possible, immobilization should be in the **position of function** (see above). This favors circulation and promotes comfort as well as early reestablishment of unimpaired function. It is the posture assumed when the hand holds a small drinking glass and is most readily achieved by putting a soppy-wet roll of gauze (e.g., Kerlex®) in the palm between the thumb and fingers and molding it to them. Loosely wrapped dry cast padding covered with a volar plaster splint (12-16 thicknesses, 1-2 inches wide and 6-8 inches long) from the midpalm across the wrist to the midforearm and held in place with one 3-4 inch wide roll of circumferentially wrapped plaster makes a light and effective splint (see p. 648).

After extensive hand trauma, infection, or surgery, a boxing glove forearm cast is preferred. One may put only part of the hand in such a cast - e.g., the thumb alone, or a combination of any 2 or 3 adjacent fingers. Generally speaking, such splinting is preferred for even severe fingertip injuries (e.g., amputation or crush). If the wrist is immobilized, so is the digit. Flat splints (e.g., tongue blade) and single digit splinting for an extensive injury impose a risk of distortion and stiffness and often fail to relieve pain.

The duration of splinting will vary with the problem and the age of the patient. Repair of nerves and tendons and fractures of phalanges and metacarpals usually require immobilization for 3-4

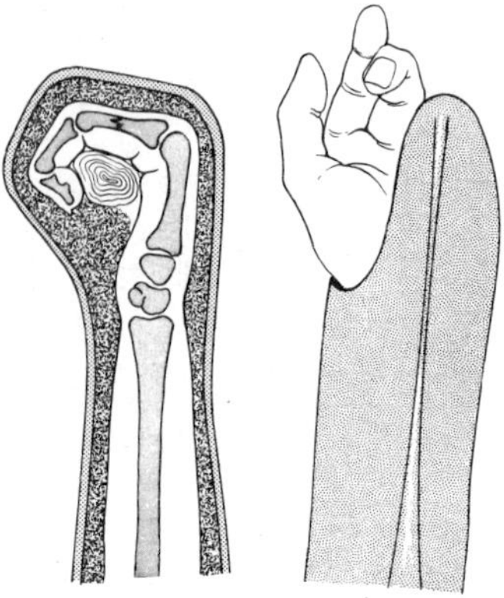

Keeled Cast. (Reproduced, with permission, from Dunphy and Way [editors], Current Surgical Diagnosis and Treatment. Lange, 1973.)

weeks, whereas ganglionectomy and fingertip grafting require only 6-8 days of casting.

Postinjury and Postoperative Care.

A. Control of Circulation: In serious cases where microcirculation is significantly threatened by tissue trauma and congestion, sludging and microthrombosis may be curtailed by administering 1 unit of low molecular weight dextran (dextran 40) daily. It is essential that the hand be constantly elevated in comfort above the heart. There must be no compression or constriction by clothing, jewelry, dressings, casts, or even skin or fascia. Throbbing and brawny induration must be mechanically (not medically) relieved - if necessary, by slitting skin and fascia.

B. Movement: The patient must understand that motion inside a splint is undesirable even though possible and that vigorous movement of the upper extremity may disrupt the tissues being splinted. On the other hand, gentle movement of all unsplinted joints helps the circulation of the whole upper extremity. When immobilization is discontinued, active exercise should be started on an organized routine (e.g., 4 times daily for 15 minutes). The frequency and duration of rehabilitative exercises of the injured part should steadily increase. The more the patient can do on his own and the less he needs the crutch of physical therapy, the better.

C. Chronic Stiffness: Pain is often the chief deterrent to overcoming stiffness caused by tight scars and contracted ligaments. This can sometimes be relieved by the intra-articular and periarticular injection of a small amount of lidocaine mixed with triamcinolone. Passive stretching is also possible by the use of dynamic splints carefully adjusted and tailored to the needs of the specific stiff joints, but these must be worn intermittently rather than continuously and should not be permitted to cause pressure sores, nerve injury, or edema. In selected intractable cases, arthrolysis, tenolysis, or modification of skin scars may be required.

D. Care of the Paralyzed Hand: During the recovery stage following nerve injury, the patient must take care not to injure anesthetic skin and joints by burns, cuts, sprains, and subluxations of joints. Appropriate splints should be used to keep paralyzed muscles from being overstretched and uninvolved muscles from overcontracting without antagonism. An example is the cock-up splint for the wrist and metacarpophalangeal joints in radial nerve palsy.

CONTUSION AND COMPRESSION INJURIES

A blow or a crushing or compressive force to the forearm, hand, or digit can result in severe stiffness and even impairment of nerve function. Impaired circulation in such cases results from bleeding and serous effusion, then swelling, and finally venous obstruction and microvascular thrombosis caused by tissue tension. This can lead to irreversible ischemic fibrosis, as in Volkmann's ischemic paralysis and contracture. It can usually be prevented by attending promptly to throbbing pain and relieving it mechanically. Brawny (rocky hard) congestion must be prevented even if it means slitting the skin and fascia extensively. It is both useless and harmful to try to squeeze infiltrated blood out of tissues, though clearly defined clots can occasionally be extracted.

HAND INFECTIONS

The most common hand infections are caused by gram-positive cocci and develop out of ignorance or neglect of the pathogenic factors. Those tissues and structures whose blood supply is limited or easily impaired (e.g., nail folds, digital fat pads, joints, and tendon sheaths) have the least resistance to infection. Constricting fascia, garments, and jewelry, wounds closed under tension, and dependent position of the hand all favor congestion and the formation of dead space (i.e., seroma and hematoma) which greatly enhance the likelihood of infection of any wound. Most hand infections can be avoided if proper early treatment is given.

The most important preventive measures in the case of hand injuries are (1) preservation of circulation by elevation and immobilization and the avoidance of tension by sutures, dressings, garments, or swelling; (2) facilitation of drainage of potential dead space or contaminated wounds by drains, wet dressings, or zinc oxide; (3) the liberal prophylactic use of local and systemic antibiotics, along with tetanus prophylaxis; and (4) debridement of clots, foreign bodies, and dead tissue.

Adequate immobilization often requires splinting the wrist and even the whole hand. Rapid onset of an infection, marked swelling, or unrelenting, throbbing pain often requires continuous bed rest with the trunk flat so the extremity can be continually at rest and propped up on pillows above heart level.

Erythromycin, methicillin, oxacillin, and lincomycin are currently effective systemic antibiotics for staphylococcal and streptococcal infections. Bacitracin is useful in the wound. Kanamycin is effective for gram-negative organisms.

Incision for drainage should be done adequately over the point of maximum tenderness or fluctuancy and parallel to structures of vital functional importance so they will not be damaged. This requires sufficient anesthesia so that the procedure will be painless, and a blood pressure cuff inflated rapidly to 300 mm. Hg on the upper arm for a bloodless field.

FURUNCLE AND CARBUNCLE

These are common about hair follicles and often require only a bulky zinc oxide compress with or without incision and drainage.

GRANULATING WOUNDS
(Third Degree Burns, Abrasions, Avulsions)

These should be debrided and grafted as quickly as possible. Silver-sulfadiazine and 0.5% silver nitrate compresses are useful antibacterial topical agents.

CELLULITIS

Cellulitis is characterized by throbbing pain, local heat, redness, swelling, and tenderness. Elevation, immobilization, empirical antibiotic treatment, and frequent observation are the crucial elements of care. Surgical release of tension on skin and fascia must be done before brawny induration occurs.

Lymphangitis and lymphadenitis are treated in the same way as cellulitis (see above).

PYOGENIC GRANULOMA

Granulation tissue that forms on wounds should be scraped off flush with the skin and compressed to control bleeding for 12-24 hours. It is then left exposed to the air to dry up if it is less than 1/4 inch in diameter, or grafted with a thin shaving of skin if it is larger.

PYODERMA

Pyoderma is a pus-filled blister which often has a central sinus to a **collar-button abscess.** Treatment consists of unroofing the abscess and applying a bulky zinc oxide compress.

EPONYCHIA, PARONYCHIA, AND SUBEPONYCHIAL ABSCESS

Incipient cases may respond to rest, elevation, and antibiotics.

When drainage is spontaneous, resolution may be expedited by zinc oxide compresses. Surgical drainage of the nail fold can usually be done with a No. 11 pointed scalpel placed flat against the surface of the nail and advanced slowly in a "scratching" fashion into the point of maximum fluctuancy and tenderness. If this is done properly, it is not painful and no blood is drawn - only pus. When the base of the nail floats in pus, it is best to resect it. (See below, left.)

SPACE INFECTIONS

These include infections of the pulp (e.g., felon) and web and of the thenar, hypothenar, midpalmar, dorsal subcutaneous, dorsal subaponeurotic, and quadrilateral (Perona) spaces. It also includes the flexor (digital, radial, and ulnar bursae) and extensor sheath infections. If pain, tissue tension, and tenderness are minimal or slight, incision and drainage may not be necessary and there may be a rapid response to rest, elevation, and antibiotics. The chief function of incision is the release of tension. If pus is drained and if there is involvement over a significantly broad or long space (e.g., tendon sheath), catheter-drip administration of local antibiotics (e.g., bacitracin, 50,000 units in 500 ml. saline) should be considered.

Felon. (See below, right.)

The best drainage of a felon is through a midline longitudinal incision, often only 1-2 cm. long. The vertical septa do not have to be divided. This technic spares the important blood and nerve supply to the digital tip, which may be iatrogenically damaged by the traditional "fishmouth" and "lateral" incisions.

Flexor Tenosynovitis. (See p. 652.)

The diagnosis is established if pain can be elicited by making the tendon move actively or passively within its sheath. The examiner may passively do this by handling (picking up) **only** the patient's finger nail as he extends the distal digital joint. If this can be done painlessly, then the site of infection rests in the skin or subcutaneous fat and spares the sheath.

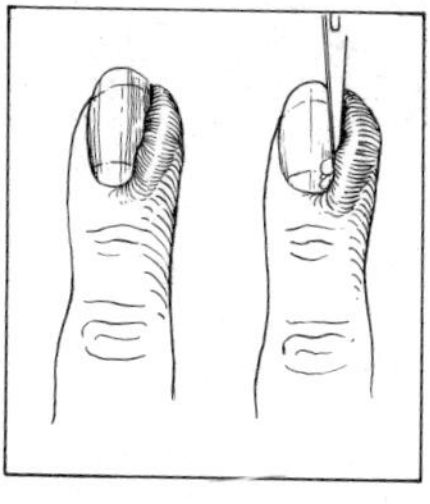

Incision and Drainage of Paronychia

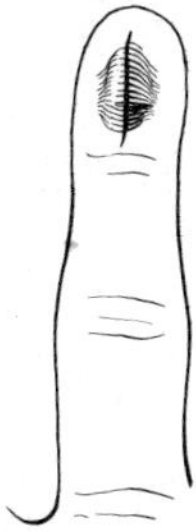

Incision of Felon

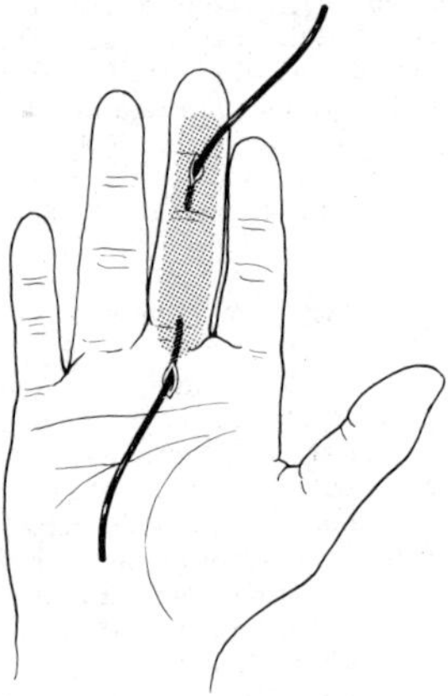

Drainage and Irrigation for Septic Tenosynovitis

Most cases of tenosynovitis that require incision and drainage need only a volar longitudinal incision in the midline of the middle phalanx of the finger (proximal phalanx of the thumb) that does not cross the skin flexion creases with a similarly directed counter-incision in the palm. A fine catheter for antibiotic drip (10 ml./hour) is placed into the distal wound and another catheter (for drainage) into the proximal wound. These are usually removed in 24-72 hours.

Phlegmonous tenosynovitis often destroys digital function unless the flexor sheath is widely opened. This is done through a lateral midaxial incision.

BONE AND JOINT INFECTIONS

These structures have particularly low resistance to infection because circulation is limited and easily compromised. All open wounds of bone and joint must be treated as if infection were present, i.e., with local and systemic antibiotics, immobilization, and elevation. Established osteomyelitis may require hyperbaric oxygen treatments for 1-2 hours daily at 2 atmospheres.

HUMAN BITE INJURIES

Most of these are into the knuckles as a result of fist-fights and should be considered emergencies for prophylactic treatment. When infections become established, they are apt to be very disabling. Wounds of the soft parts should be drained and never fully closed.

MISCELLANEOUS INFECTIONS

Streptococcal Gangrene.

Requires prompt fasciotomy, debridement, and antibiotic treatment.

Tuberculosis.

This is an indolent process which most often involves the synovial tissues of joints and tendons. Cultures may take months to be diagnostic. Good response follows synovectomy and antituberculosis drug therapy.

Fungal Infections.

These involve primarily the nail area. The response to antifungal agents may be good, e.g., griseofulvin systemically and diamthazole (Asterol®), 0.5% ointment locally.

Herpes Simplex.

This usually presents as multiple tiny vesicles about the distal phalanx which may become purulent and even coalesce into a pyoderma. It may need no treatment since it is self-limiting in about 3 weeks. Idoxuridine, a specific antiviral agent, may be useful.

Other Infections.

Gas gangrene, syphilis, deep fungal infections (coccidioidomycosis, blastomycosis, actinomycosis, sporotrichosis), tularemia, yaws, and glanders are rare infections diagnosed by history, chronicity, and identification of stigmas and pathogens.

Leprosy is not so much an infection of the hand as it is a motor and sensory paralyzer requiring extensive prophylactic education against trophic ulceration and sometimes reconstructive surgery.

LACERATIONS AND SKIN AVULSIONS

All wounds should be inspected and closed under tourniquet control. A magnifying loupe should be available. Blood clots should be removed, and easily accessible foreign bodies should be searched for by inspection or probing. It is often impractical and unnecessary to remove all foreign bodies. Secondary removal is often preferable after the surrounding blood has been absorbed. Vessels that need ligation must be identified and isolated, and ligatures must be placed accurately to avoid damage to an adjacent nerve. If continued oozing is expected after the wound is closed, a drain should be inserted. If a full thickness of skin has been lost, the wound may be primarily closed with a skin graft. If oozing is too great, grafting should be delayed for 1 or 2 days. Split-thickness grafts are the most certain to take, but a full-thickness graft may be prepared by defatting an avulsed piece of skin or by taking some from the hairless portion of the groin. Very long reverse flaps and flaps that have been significantly traumatized are preferably defatted and applied as free full-thickness grafts or replaced by a split-thickness graft. Adequate immobilization (see above) is crucial to the successful healing of lacerations and grafts.

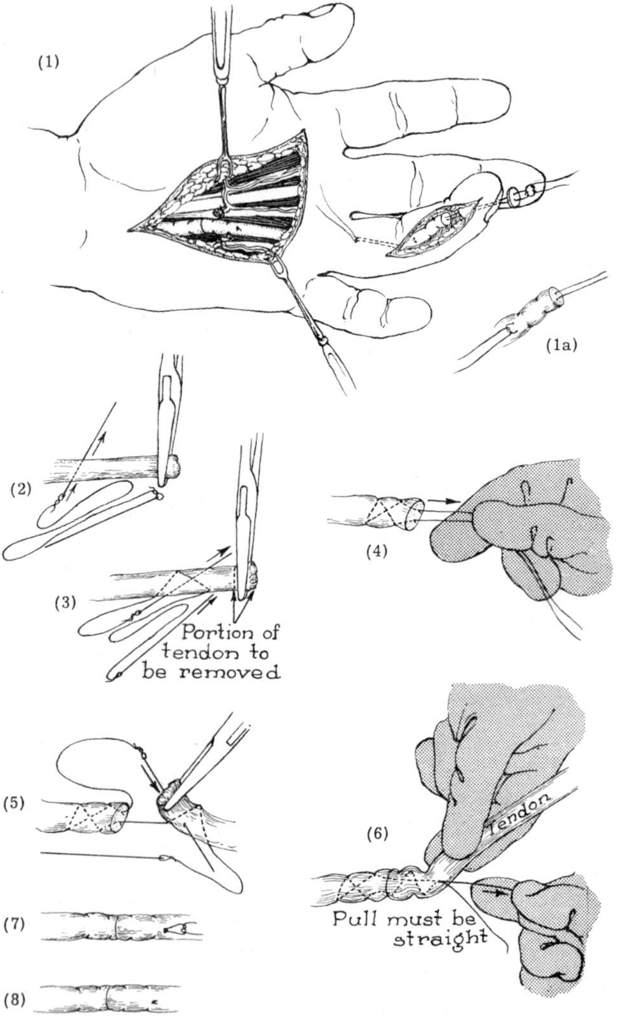

Methods of Flexor Tendon Repair. (1) Exposure and suture of flexor tendons. Within the finger, the pull-out method is used. In the palm, the buried suture technic is used. (1a) Enlarged view of suture placement in finger. (2, 3, 4) Details of suture placement in the proximal tendons. (5, 6, 7, 8) Details of suture placement in the distal end of tendon for buried suture.

TENDON INJURIES

Any laceration must be assumed to have divided a tendon until proved otherwise by inspection of the wound under tourniquet ischemia with prior or simultaneous systematic testing of all tendons as they are actively tensed. An abnormal digital stance created by a tendon injury can often be demonstrated by extreme passive flexion or extension of the wrist. Penetrating glass and metal wounds can damage tendons far in excess of what is apparent and at sites far removed from the skin wound. Tendon constriction is a common cause of pain at the site of the offending tendon sheath (pulley). The pain may coincide with a jog in the excursion of the tendon (usually a flexor tendon, e.g., "trigger finger"); or it may be merely associated with stretch and tension of the synovial sheath when the tendon is tensed (e.g., DeQuervain's stenosing tenosynovitis of the abductor pollicis longus). Tendon rupture is uncommon, but tendon adherence due to adhesions (tenodesis) is common.

Treatment.

Tendon stenosis is usually treated first by injecting a small amount of lidocaine mixed with triamcinolone into the tendon sheath at the trigger point. If that fails, the tendon must be liberated surgically. Ruptures that materially affect digital function often present complex reconstruction problems. Tenolysis can be effective in restoring tendon glide, but early active postoperative movement is always required.

The restoration of function after division of tendons requires the best surgical judgment and skill and the subsequent perseverance of the patient in the rehabilitation effort. Tendon repair must not be at the expense of mobility of uninjured tendons and joints. The surgeon may appropriately elect no treatment, tenorrhaphy, tendon transfer, tenodesis, or arthrodesis. Tenorrhaphy may be done primarily or secondarily by direct suture, by tendon advancement with or without lengthening, or by tendon graft, followed by adequate immobilization for 3-4 weeks. Cases seen late should receive primary wound toilet, closure, splinting, and prophylactic antibiotics. Joints must be freely mobile and skin and fat cover healthy and pliable before tenorrhaphy or tendon transfer is undertaken.

The handling of tendons and their fibro-osseous sheaths should be with the strictest atraumatic technic. Sponges, forceps, clamps, and needles all invite adhesions where they contact these structures. The long flexor tendons require pulleys for mechanical efficiency and to prevent bowstringing; however, in order to make certain that this pulley system does not choke and prevent excursion of a tenorrhaphy callus, enough fibro-osseous sheath must be removed to correspond with the expected amplitude of glide of the callus.

The technic of suturing a tendon must be meticulous. The amount of suturing required depends on the amount of separation of the proximal stump from its distal attachment and the force necessary to hold the suture line. Retraction of the proximal stump may be prevented while placing the tendon suture by skewering the stump with a straight needle. Atraumatic nonreactive 4-0 to 5-0 sutures (e.g., monofilament nylon) should be used and can be threaded (see illustration on p. 656) in a horizontal mattress or once or twice crisscrossing fashion through the tendon stumps. The rim of a ten-

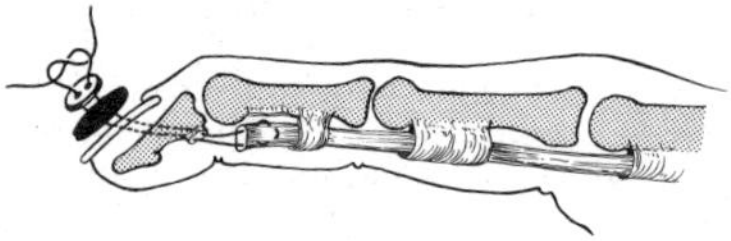

Flexor Tenorrhaphy by Advancement or Graft

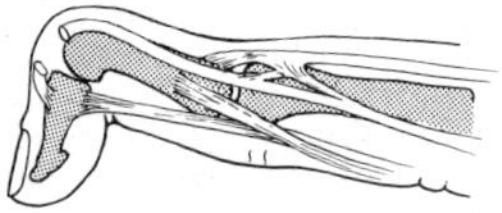

Mallet Finger With
Swan-Neck Deformity

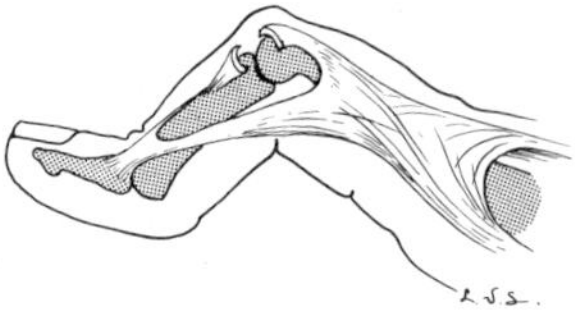

Buttonhole Deformity

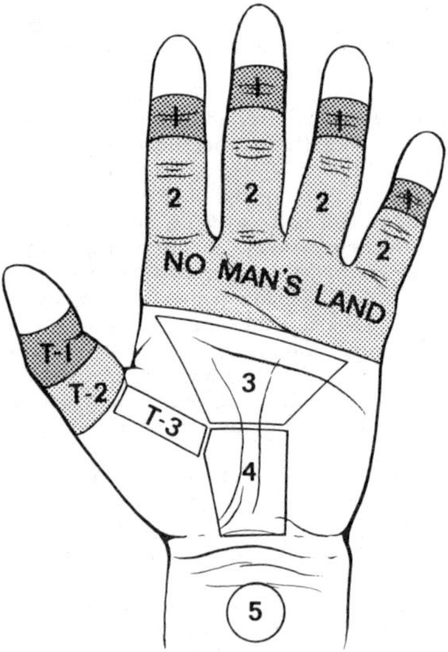

Flexor Tendon Zones

Illustrations at the top of the page are reproduced, with permission, from Dunphy and Way (editors), Current Surgical Diagnosis and Treatment. Lange, 1973.

don juncture may be reinforced and evened up by a 6-0 or 7-0 running over-and-over suture. Nylon sutures are usually buried except when anchoring a tendon into bone, in which case the suture ends may pass through the bone and overlying epithelial layer (e.g., fingernail) to be tied over a padded button and then withdrawn in 3-4 weeks (p. 656, top). When the size of 2 tendons to be joined is disproportionate, the smaller one may be woven once or twice through the larger one.

Immobilization should be in a position that takes tension off the tendon wound without putting any joints in extreme flexion or extension. The wrist is most often the principal joint to be positioned.

A. Extensor Tendon Injury: If injury to an extensor tendon is recognized immediately and proper treatment given, the prognosis for recovered function is usually more favorable than is the case with flexor tendons. This is because there is less sheath to contend with and the overall anatomy of the long extensors is less complex than that of the flexor tendons.

Exposure (often by proximal and distal extension of the wound) is important for the proper assay and repair of the injury. Because retraction of the proximal stump may be physically negligible but functionally significant, reapproximation of ends and immobilization are usually essential.

Positioning alone may satisfactorily restore the continuity. If not, buried 4-0 to 6-0 monofilament nylon sutures are placed as figure-of-eight, horizontal mattress, or (on the dorsum of the hand and forearm) crisscross weaving sutures. Immobilization should be maintained for 3-6 weeks.

Mallet (baseball) finger (p. 656, center left) is a flexion stance of the distal joint resulting from separation of the attachment of the extensor to the distal phalanx. Bone or tendon may be separated, and active extension may be partially or completely lost. A volar padded splint across the distal joint for 6 weeks may be all that is needed in fresh cases. Intractable cases may cause a secondary change in the middle finger joint, which goes into hyperextension (recurvatum), resulting in **"swan neck" deformity.**

Buttonhole (boutonniere) deformity (p. 656, center right) is the converse of the swan neck habitus. It results from blunt or sharp injury to the dorsum of the middle finger joint (or metacarpophalangeal joint of the thumb). By attenuation of the extensor hood, the injured joint fails to extend while the distal joint overextends. Anticipation of the deformity and immobilization of the injured joint in full extension by a padded volar splint or by Kirschner wires for 4-6 weeks is the recommended treatment.

B. Flexor Tendon Injury: Anatomic zones of injury that have important implications for prognosis and management are shown on p. 656, bottom. The principal difference between the zones is not only the existence or nonexistence of a fibrous flexor sheath and its nature but also the number of tendons within it. Thus, in zone 2 of the finger ("no-man's-land"), there is a tight sheath around 2 tendons, one of which (the superficialis) forms a tunnel around the other (the profundus). Because of the unselective involvement of all structures in reparative scar, tendon injuries in this zone often defy subsequent excursion by virtue of intractable tenodesis. Consequently, considerable experience and judgment are required for successful management of such tendon injuries.

Tendon advancement (p. 656, top) with sacrifice of the distal stump is often favored for division of the flexor within 1-1.5 cm of the distal phalanx (i.e., zone 1). It may be combined with tendon lengthening in the case of the flexor pollicis longus. The alternatives to tendon advancement are tenodesis of the distal stump, arthrodesis of the distal joint, or no treatment.

Primary tendon repair (within 72 hours) or delayed primary repair (within 2 weeks) is favored for midpalm (zone 3), wrist (zone 4), and forearm (zone 5) injuries. It is also favored selectively in tidy injuries in the proximal portion of the finger (zone 2). When the wound in this area is untidy or when several weeks or months have elapsed since the injury, a tendon graft is generally preferred in zone 2. Secondary tendon repair (more than 2 weeks after surgery) is frequently possible in zones 3, 4, and 5.

When multiple tendons are divided in one zone, it may be preferable to repair only the more important ones. This is especially true in injuries in zone 2, where the profundus is usually the only one that should be repaired.

Lateral digital incisions may be made to connect the ends of the flexion creases, or volar incisions may cross the fat pads obliquely in a zigzag fashion. Zigzagging is also preferred for opening the palm or wrist. Damage to neurovascular bundles must be avoided. (See illustration on p. 645.)

Priority should be given to repairing flexor tendons before repairing nerves. When dealing with a very bloody palm or digit with both nerve and flexor tendon injury, neurorrhaphy often demands such excessive surgical dissection to even identify a nerve that it is contraindicated as a primary procedure.

Movement of digits within 3 weeks after flexor tenorrhaphy, if permitted at all, must be done very guardedly and under the guidance of trained hand surgeons. After 3 weeks, active motion may progress in a graded fashion. It often takes many months - even up to a year - to regain maximal tendon excursion and joint motion and for the collagen of scar tissue to attenuate and adapt. The patient must be encouraged to persevere and must be made aware of the difficulty and sometimes impossibility of recovering completely normal excursion.

Prognosis.

Excursion after tenorrhaphy or tenolysis depends on the mobility of joints, the remodeling of scar tissue so that it yields to the glide of tendons, adequate strength of muscles, and the perseverance by the patient over a period of many weeks or months of rehabilitative work. Progress may be gauged by serial records of the distance by which digital tips fail to reach points in space (e.g., a straight line in extension or the midpalm in flexion). If there is no sign of improvement during a period of 4 weeks of close supervision beginning 2-3 months after surgery, spontaneous change is most unlikely.

NERVE INJURY

The interruption of nerve conduction following injury may be merely physiologic (i.e., neurapraxia) or it may be anatomic. The

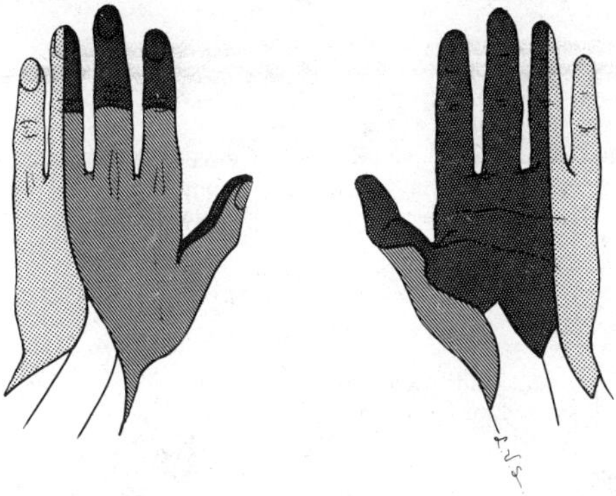

Sensory Distribution in the Hand. Dotted area, ulnar nerve; diagonal area, radial nerve; darker area, median nerve. (Reproduced, with permission, from Dunphy and Way [editors], Current Diagnosis and Treatment. Lange, 1973.)

distinction can often be made early by repeated examination in the first few hours after injury and before any anesthetic is administered.

The median, ulnar, and radial nerves are vital to the function of the hand. They are all mixed (sensory and motor) at the elbow, and the median and ulnar nerves are mixed up to the heel of the hand. A knowledge of innervation is essential to determine the level of an injury. Pain and failure to cooperate may lead to a false diagnosis of motor paralysis, whereas absence of sweating over the distribution of an injured nerve objectively identifies sensory paralysis. Two-point discrimination 3-4 mm. apart, like good sweat, signifies good sensory function.

Bleeding should be initially controlled by compressing and not by clamping. When an arterial tourniquet (e.g., blood pressure cuff to 100 mm. Hg above systolic pressure) can be applied with the patient supine and when ideal facilities are available for the precise visualization of the bleeder and an adjacent nerve, the bleeder can be ligated without iatrogenic injury to a nerve by "blind" clamping.

When blood or scar tissue prevents meticulous exploration, the dissection should extend to normal tissue and then reverse into the zone of injury.

Motor and sensory nerve conduction studies occasionally help to clarify difficult diagnostic problems.

Treatment.

Neurapraxia is treated expectantly. How long to defer the exploration of a nerve depends on the mechanism of injury and the surgeon's estimate of its physical impact on the nerve. If there is no sign of regeneration (i.e., return of muscle function and advancement of Tinel's sign) in 4-6 months, surgical measures (if ap-

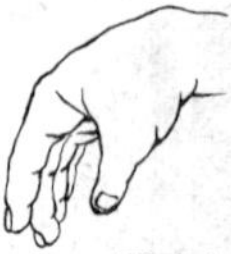

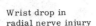

Wrist drop in radial nerve injury

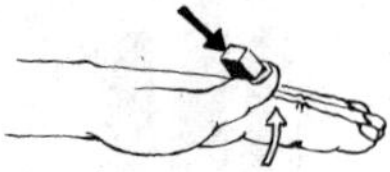

Forceful extension of thumb tip is lost in radial nerve injury

Radial Nerve

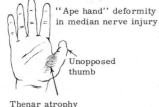

"Ape hand" deformity in median nerve injury

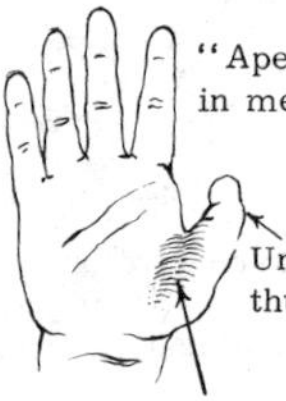

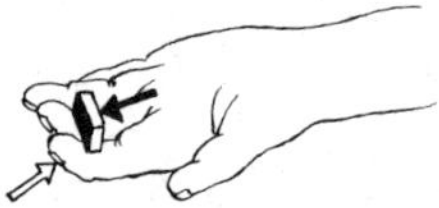

Forceful flexion of tip of index is lost in high median nerve injury

Median Nerve

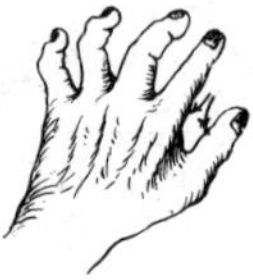

Thumb web atrophy and clawing of ring and little fingers

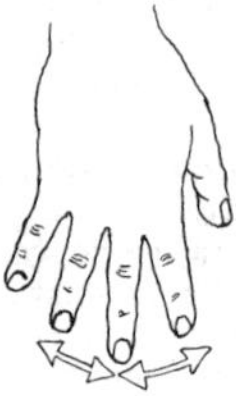

Loss of abduction and adduction in ulnar nerve injury

Ulnar Nerve

plicable) should no longer be deferred. Surgical measures (singly or in combination) may consist of neurolysis, resection of scarred nerve and neurorrhaphy, nerve graft, tendon transfer, tenodesis, arthrodesis, and neurovascular island pedicle flaps.

The sooner a divided nerve is repaired, the better. Regeneration takes months, and after 2 months the motor end plates of the small intrinsic muscles become increasingly resistant to recovery. Neurorrhaphy within a year of injury results in good return of sensory function.

Peripheral neurorrhaphy is highly specialized surgery which

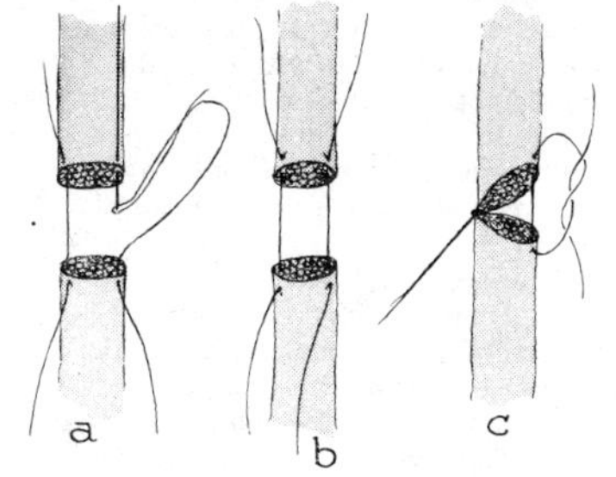

Placement of Initial Sutures in Nerve Sheath and Approximation of Nerve Ends

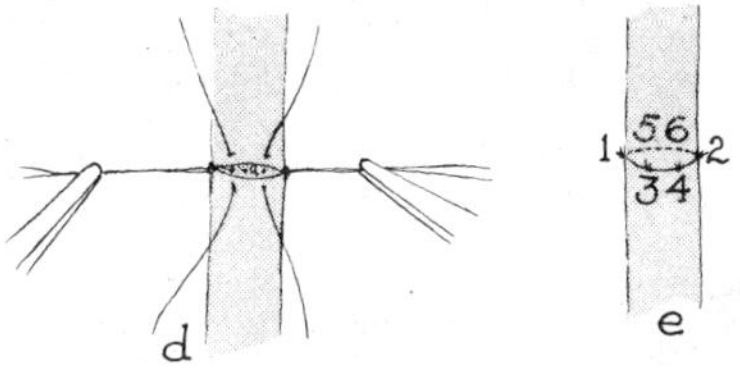

Placement of Additional Sutures in Nerve Sheath. Numbers indicate sequence of suture placement.

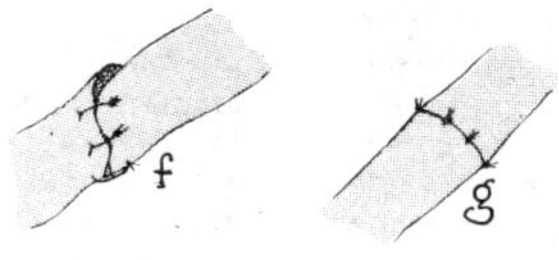

Incorrect (Left) and Correct (Right) Placement of Sutures

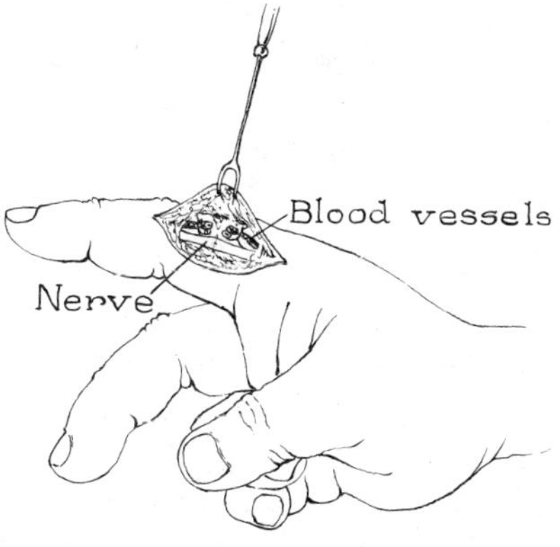

Exposure Showing Sutured Digital Nerve

can only be done properly by the experienced hand surgeon. Fresh cases being referred should have a surgical skin preparation and the extremity should be immobilized and elevated with or without temporary wound closure and prophylactic antibiotics.

Technic of nerve suture. (See illustrations on p. 661.) All peripheral nerve surgery requires loupe and microscopic magnification as well as microsurgical instruments and suture material (i.e., 8-0 to 10-0 atraumatic nylon).

Freshly incised nerves should be approximated without further surgical section of the stumps. Macerated and scarred nerves require razor blade section across normal nerve tissue before approximation. The minimal amount of nerve should be resected.

Anatomic matching of fascicles and epineural vessels in proximal and distal nerve stumps is essential. Sutures should be atraumatic, fine caliber, as few as possible, and placed into the epineurium or perineurium in such a way as to accurately approximate fascicular stumps without overlap, telescoping, furling, and protrusion from the connective tissue sleeve. Tension must be avoided; if it can not be overcome by the positioning of joints, a nerve graft should be considered.

The use of local corticosteroids and the coating of nerve junctures with a thin silicone cuff has helped to reduce neuromal scar formation.

Tension on the suture line must be avoided for 3-4 weeks postoperatively. This usually requires plaster immobilization. Thereafter, joints may be gradually mobilized at a rate inverse to the tension on the nerve juncture.

Prognosis.

A nerve that has been reunited can never regain normal innervation completely. Compensatory factors may subsititue adequately for the deficit so that function may be nearly normal. The principal factors that restrict complete reinnervation are as follows: (1) Inability to reunite and match all divided axons. (2) Distortion due to bleeding, edema, and scar formation. (3) Impairment of circulation and the lack of soft tissue about the injured nerve. (4) Delay in neurorrhaphy. (5) Inexperience in hand surgery.

BURNS OF THE HANDS

Hand burns occur in the following order of decreasing incidence: thermal, friction, electric, chemical, and radiation. The impact on function may be catastrophic. The overall economic loss due to deep second and third degree thermal burns of the hand is a staggering national burden. Preventive safety measures and proper primary therapy can significantly reduce this toll.

While instituting lifesaving measures in the severely burned patient, the upper extremity must simultaneously receive urgent primary attention. Swelling and the loss of the functional arches of the hand must be avoided as much as possible by adequate elevation, by dermatomy and fasciotomy if brawny edema develops, and by immobilization and positioning (wrist in extension, metacarpophalangeal joints flexed, and, in certain instances, proximal interphalangeal joints in extension). The hand must not be allowed to become fixed in the "claw" position. It must be remembered that, "A swollen hand is a claw hand in disguise." The elbow must not be allowed to become fixed in extension and the shoulder in adduction. Whenever possible (and as soon as possible), all joints must be moved actively - often before the burn wound is reepithelialized.

Treatment.

Burns that do not need debridement and grafting (e.g., first and second degree burns) may be treated initially with an ice water bath to relieve pain followed by a soothing cream (e.g., zinc oxide or a proprietary burn remedy such as Kip First Aid Cream®). If the burn is deep second degree, is infected, or is already granulating but not healthy and "clean" enough to graft, it should be coated twice a day with mafenide (Sulfamylon®) or silver-sulfadiazine cream. If neither of these is available, an ointment consisting of 1 part silver nitrate, 5 parts balsam of Peru, 30 parts hydrous lanolin, and 30 parts amber petrolatum - or a coating of zinc oxide - may be applied. Chemical burns are treated initially by copious irrigation with tap water or weak acid (alkali burns) or alkaline (acid burns) solutions.

The chief objective of therapy of deep or extensive burns is to restore effective skin cover and the integrity of deep tissue as rapidly as possible without infection, so that muscle and joint use may be started early and maximal function spared. There is no one rule or one method of accomplishing this, but delay and neglect in the implementation of these principles may lead to permanent disability.

As long as swelling does not prevent adequate active motion and there is no sign of infection, debridement and grafting are not urgent. However, the converse is equally true, and in urgent cases it makes little difference if, during debridement, a small amount of equivocally viable skin is removed in continuity with unequivocally insensitive and lifeless eschar.

Debridement should be followed by a biologic dressing (autograft, homograft, or heterograft) as soon as hemostasis is adequate to prevent dead space under the graft - usually in 24-48 hours. Immobilization for 24-48 hours is essential so that there will be no shift of the graft on its bed.

Careful immobilization and protection of the hand with or without a dressing may preclude the need for sutures to hold the graft in place. Continuous wet dressings inside a waterproof seal (e.g., plastic bag) often avoid the need for "rolling out" grafts in the first 24-48 hours.

The thinner (i.e., 10/1000 inch) and smaller (i.e., 1/8-1/4 inch) the grafts are, the surer they are to take. "Mesh" grafts are suitable substitutes for postage stamp grafts, but they must be sutured in place. Sheets of skin are favored for "clean" wounds with good hemostasis. If the margins lie along lines of stretch, they should be zigzagged with skin darts.

Functional Disabilities Due to Hand Burns.

Scar falls in the wake of burns and leads to a host of characteristic digital deformities (e.g., clawing, buttonhole, swan neck, mallet), adduction contracture of the thumb, and a multitude of other extension and flexion joint contractures. Proper splinting may prevent and reconstructive procedures may correct many deformities.

FRACTURES, DISLOCATIONS, AND LIGAMENT INJURIES

The history of the degree of force and the mechanism of injury to the hand is essential to the recognition and evaluation of these injuries. X-rays in the anteroposterior and lateral planes as well as comparative views of the opposite hand are often indispensable for accurate diagnosis, planning treatment, and estimating the chances of recovery. Pain, distortion, or abnormality of motion (hypermobility or reduced mobility) is usually but not always present. Swelling may mask distortion, and distortion may be mistaken for swelling.

Treatment should be directed at restoration of proper alignment, painless movement, and stability with forceful use of the involved parts. Ultimate function of the hand, not radiologic perfection, is what is most important, and functional considerations must dictate the timing and choice of treatment. For example, irreversible and disabling stiffness may be the price of a "perfect" reduction and union of a fracture that has been manipulated too much and immobilized too long. For this reason, in selected cases, it is best to start guarded movement early, particularly in "heavy-handed" and older individuals. If closed reduction requires force, it is often best to do an open reduction or settle for imperfect alignment.

Initial immobilization should assume the position of maximal function in order to minimize the impact of stiffness. The test of adequate immobilization is freedom from pain. With few exceptions, if one finger needs immobilization, one or more adjacent fingers should also be splinted as well as the wrist. Soft gauze, cast padding, and plaster are generally far better for making a custom-fitting splint than boards, sticks, or metal or plastic material. The surgeon must beware of splinting all joints of a digit in extension for fear of stiffness and rotational deformities and must guard against the hazards of traction technics, i.e., stiffness and pressure necrosis.

Internal fixation with Kirschner wires should be considered when there is marked instability and when one wishes to allow motion of neighboring tendons and joints. Joints are usually secured with one oblique wire, whereas bones often need one longitudinal wire with another one placed obliquely to prevent rotation.

Open bone and joint injuries should be treated with prophylactic local or systemic antibiotics (or both). When skin and fat cover is lost, it should be replaced by suitable free grafts or pedicle transfer of local or distant skin.

Fracture treatment generally takes precedence over tendon repair, but this does not mean that easily accessible tendon ends should not be reapproximated as a primary procedure.

FRACTURES OF THE HAND AND WRIST

Wrist Fractures.

Every apparent sprain of the wrist should be considered a fracture until shown to be otherwise by total subsidence of pain or negative follow-up x-rays in 8-10 days. The 3 most common fractures of the wrist are the result of sudden forceful hyperextension or radial deviation.

A. Colles' Fracture: The deformity consists of dorsal displacement of the joint surface of the radius, recession of the radial styloid, and fracture of the ulnar styloid. One must watch for compression of the median nerve with numbness over its distribution in the hand. Reduction requires anesthesia and should be gentle. It need not be radiologically perfect. Immobilization in a long arm cast for 4 weeks and a forearm cast for 2 weeks is usually adequate. Digital motion should be started immediately. Temporary disability commonly persists for 4-6 months or more. Residual traumatic arthritis may be unavoidable and require surgery (e. g., ulnar styloidectomy or wrist fusion).

B. Navicular (Scaphoid) Fracture: Pain is maximal in the anatomic snuff box and on radial deviation of the wrist. Reduction is seldom necessary. Immobilization is usually maintained by means of a long arm cast that includes the metacarpophalangeal joint of the thumb for 4 weeks and a short arm cast for an additional 2 weeks. Many patients are then ready to return to work. When there is no x-ray evidence of union, months of immobilization may be necessary. If union does not occur or if aseptic necrosis develops, surgery must be considered and may consist of bone grafting, radial styloidectomy, silicone implant substitution, wrist fusion, or other procedures. Such cases may have traumatic arthritis and 6-12 months of disability. Special x-ray views are essential to rule out these fractures.

C. Triquetral Fracture: Fracture of the triquetrum is usually a small chip dorsal fracture seen only on the lateral x-ray view. Pain and tenderness are localized to the dorsal-ulnar aspect of the carpus and are often of short duration, requiring only a forearm cast for 1-3 weeks.

Metacarpal Fractures.

Metacarpal fractures are often undisplaced. When displacement does occur, the distal segment is usually pulled volarward so that the fracture is bowed to the dorsum (see below). Manipulation and reduction are often difficult and are not necessary for minor distortions (e.g., 20-40 degrees of bowing). Rotation at the fracture site must be prevented by keeping adjacent fingers furled side by side in functional flexion for 3-4 weeks. Open reduction and longitudinal Kirschner wire fixation are advocated for unstable fractures. A forearm cast may be necessary to the metacarpophalangeal joint level or may involve the entire length of the digits. Metacarpophalangeal joints must be splinted in flexion to avoid disabling stiffness.

Bennett's fracture is one at the base of the thumb metacarpal.

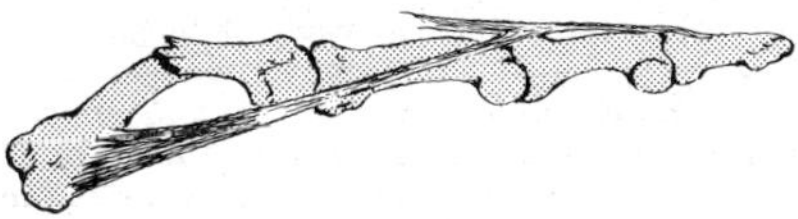

Dorsal Bowing of Metacarpal Fracture

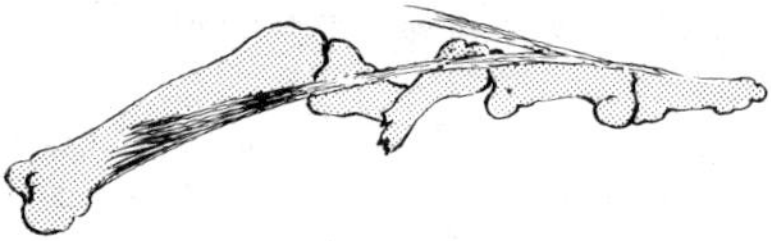

Volar Bowing of Phalangeal Fracture

Proximal and Middle Phalangeal Fractures.

The most common distortion of these fractures is opposite to that of metacarpal fractures. Here the distal segments are pulled dorsally, causing a volar bowing of the fracture site (see illustration). Extension of the wrist and flexion of the metacarpophalangeal joint give the relaxation needed for reduction. This, together with side-to-side splinting to the adjacent finger and forearm boxing glove casting for 3 weeks, usually gives sufficient immobilization. Internal fixation with Kirschner wires - and even open reduction - may be necessary for accuracy of reduction and for very unstable fractures and intra-articular fractures. If joint integrity cannot be reestablished in articular fractures, positioning for a "spontaneous" functional fusion is required or, occasionally, silicone joint-spacer arthroplasty is undertaken. Very small chip fractures are only treated for the pain they cause. Intra-articular fracture fragments involving less than a third of the articular surface are often resected.

Distal Phalangeal Fractures.

These present the least hazard to function once pain has subsided (usually in 3-4 weeks). They are often comminuted and open. Intramedullary fixation with a No. 18 or 19 hypodermic needle on a 10 ml. syringe barrel is sometimes necessary for displaced shaft and intra-articular fractures, but most cases require only external splinting. This may be achieved by forearm-to-fingertip casting for several days, followed by a digital guard. Open "bursting" type injuries are often too tense to tolerate sutures and should be simply "molded" with fine mesh wet gauze before casting.

DISLOCATIONS OF THE HAND AND WRIST

Most dislocations occur as a result of hyperextension injuries and can be reduced by a combination of traction and hyperextension and by manipulating the displaced parts back into position. If reduction is impossible without force, open reduction is required.

Dislocations of the Wrist.

Severe injuries of the wrist may cause dislocations about the navicular and lunate bones. The inexperienced eye may easily fail to notice the abnormality in the x-ray unless it is compared with exactly the same view of the opposite wrist. The navicular is often fractured as well as dislocated, whereas the lunate is simply dislocated volarward, where it tends to compress the median nerve and cause dysesthesia. Primary closed reduction under anesthesia is usually successful, but surgery must be resorted to if this fails. Immobilization is generally for 4-6 weeks.

Finger Dislocations.

Finger dislocations may occur at any joint and usually involve the dorsal displacement of the distal bone on the proximal one. The proximal interphalangeal joint is most commonly dislocated. The patient often reduces it immediately himself. When closed reduction is not possible in a fresh case, it means that the head of the more proximal bone has become trapped in a noose formed by displaced tendons, ligaments, and even bands of fascia. The volar plate occasionally fails to clear the joint during reduction and blocks flexion. In other instances, the volar plate has been avulsed so that the phalanx of its origin tends to redislocate. All such difficulties can only be managed surgically. Simple dislocations which are easily reduced and do not tend to redislocate (as verified by x-ray) need very little or no splinting beyond the patient's own tendency to favor the part.

LIGAMENTOUS INJURIES
(Sprains and Ruptures)

Any ligament may be sprained or torn. However, before making a diagnosis of a sprain of the wrist, one must rule out fracture by repeated x-rays. Desmitis (inflammation of a ligament) is a common cause of wrist pain and responds well to rest and trigger point lidocaine and triamcinolone injections.

Abduction force to the metacarpophalangeal joints and abduction or adduction force to the proximal interphalangeal joints are the most common sources of such injuries. Local pain and evidence of relaxation by clinical and x-ray examination under stress are diagnostic. A small piece of bone is sometimes avulsed. If large, it may require removal.

Most of these injuries are treated by splinting. An injured finger may be strapped to the adjacent normal one. Prolonged immobilization invites stiffness, which itself is a cause of pain.

Total avulsions of the collateral ligaments of the metacarpophalangeal joint of the thumb should be repaired if fresh and reconstructed if old.

AMPUTATIONS

Loss of all or part of a digit is always a shocking experience for the patient, who often brings in the amputated part in the hope that it can be reimplanted. This is rarely feasible or indicated. Any amputation composed of more than just skin requires anastomosis of an artery and vein if it is to survive. Except in tidy injuries at or proximal to the wrist, such reimplantations are rarely successful. The part should be kept sterile and ice cold if a patient is referred to a hand surgeon for possible reimplantation.

The functional impact of an amputation depends on the digits involved and the plane and extent of the loss. Thus, volar-radial fingertip loss and volar-ulnar thumb tip loss (the surfaces that oppose for pinch) are often disabling amputations. The concepts of hand breadth for stability of grasp and digital length (especially of the thumb and the finger closest to it) for effectiveness of pinch must always be considered in planning salvage and reconstruction. Above all, the amputation stump must be rendered pain-free and with durable skin cover. Fingers that are intractably stiff, anesthetic, painful, or too short are often amputated by the surgeon if that will enhance overall function of the hand. Custom molded prosthetic devices that provide a hook or enhance pinch may be used

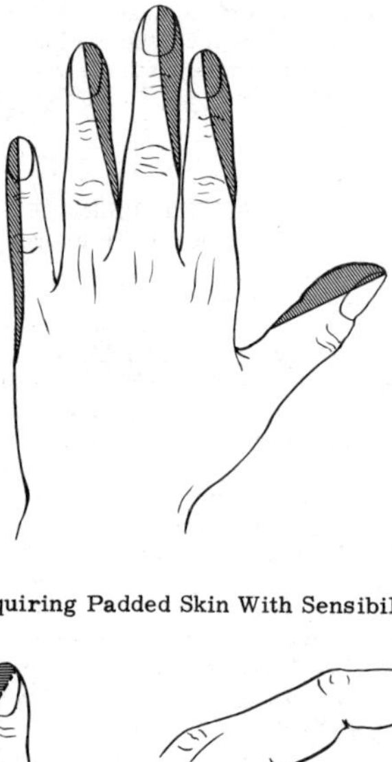

Areas Requiring Padded Skin With Sensibility

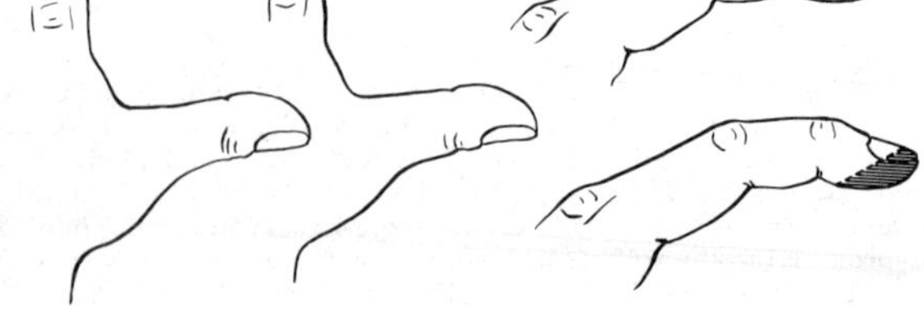

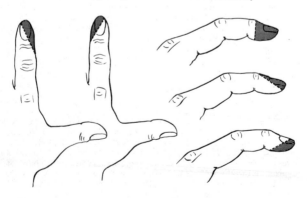

Planes of Distal Digit Amputation

in selected cases. Other prostheses worn for their cosmetic value have no functional usefulness and are generally discarded by the patient after a time.

STUMP CLOSURE

Clots and nonviable or usable tissue should be debrided, but any part or tissue of reconstructive value should be saved. Closure should never be under tension. Bleeders should be meticulously distinguished and separated from nerves by the use of loupe magnification and tourniquet control. Ligatures should be of nonreactive material such as fine nylon. Protruding bone should either be covered with a pedicle flap or rongeured back. Cartilage does not have to be removed. Nerve stumps must be recessed or transferred (preferably into a bed of fat or muscle) well away from bone stumps or pressure points. Tendons should not be sutured over amputation stumps. Local and systemic antibiotics should be used freely.

The loss of a fingertip is the most common amputation. The surest closure of such wounds is by means of a split thickness onlay graft. Grafting should be done primarily unless active bleeding prevents it, in which case grafting must be deferred for 24-48 hours. The donor site is most often the volar-ulnar aspect of the proximal forearm, which is regionally anesthetized before the graft is taken with a razor blade. Anesthesia is required for the digit only if it must be debrided of clots and other debris. The procedure is done under tourniquet control (blood pressure cuff at 300 mm. Hg). The graft may be held in place with fine narrow strips of mesh gauze and carefully tailored and applied with gauze and plastic (e.g., Reston®) or rubber secured with adhesive strips (e.g., Steri-Strips®). The digit is then immobilized - alone if it is the thumb, or with an adjacent finger if it is a finger - by a well-padded forearm circumferential cast which is worn for a week. Constrictive dressings and garments are avoided, and the extremity is kept elevated. Such grafts survive more often than full thickness skin grafts and invariably take on a satisfactory recipient bed. In time they shrink 50% or more so as to draw normal skin over the defect for satisfactory function.

The experienced hand surgeon may selectively employ other grafting technics consisting of local or distant pedicle flaps. When amputation stumps remain sensitive, the pain may subside with fingertip percussion. If not, surgical revision may be necessary.

MISCELLANEOUS HAND DISORDERS

DESMITIS, TENDINITIS, AND MYOSITIS

Inflammation of ligaments, tendons, or muscles may cause pain and tenderness in many areas of the elbow, forearm, wrist, and hand. Examples of this are **lateral** and **medial epicondylitis** and **myositis crepitans**. Repetitive or excessively vigorous effort often initiates the process, but in some cases no cause can be identified. Treatment includes local slow injection of a mixture of lidocaine and triamcinolone, systemic anti-inflammatory agents, rest, and, in acute severe cases, temporary immobilization.

Constrictive conditions commonly impair nerve and tendon function. **Carpal tunnel syndrome** is characterized by pain and numbness radiating along the median nerve due to its compression in the carpal tunnel. The cause is most commonly nonspecific and consists of an anatomic predilection combined with factors of aging or a shift in the water content of tendons and ligaments. However, it may also result from swelling and space consumption by repetitive effort, trauma, rheumatoid disease, tumor, etc. A similar state may affect the ulnar nerve in its tunnel at the elbow or the carpal level.

Constriction of tendons occurs for similar reasons where they are most snugly tethered by the sheath-pulley systems. The most common stenosing tenosynovitis occurs at the level of the proximal pulleys of the digital flexors in the distal palm as a **"trigger finger or thumb,"** and about the radial styloid as **DeQuervain's tenosynovitis.**

Initial treatment for most of these conditions is local injection of a mixture of lidocaine and triamcinolone (3:1) into the affected space but not into a nerve. Failure to respond after 2 or 3 injections combined with appropriate rest of the part (e.g., splinting) justifies surgical release of the constriction.

GOUT AND OSTEOARTHRITIS

Pain, limitation of motion, and deformity are the complaints that lead to treatment of these conditions. Gout is most often controlled by colchicine or allopurinol (Zyloprim®). Tophi are sometimes resectable. The pain of osteoarthritis can be helped by local triamcinolone and systemic anti-inflammatory agents. Disabling stiffness can often be corrected by appropriate arthroplasties.

RHEUMATOID HAND DISORDERS

This disease of unknown cause affects the hand in many ways. The hand surgeon is able to improve its appearance and function, and, in many instances, can forestall disabilities by appropriate excisional, incisional, and reconstructive technics. These include the resection of nodules, synovectomy, tenovaginotomy, and a host of tenoplasty and arthroplasty procedures to correct such deformities as ulnar drift, swan neck, buttonhole, intrinsic plus, etc.

DUPUYTREN'S CONTRACTURE

This is a thickening of the palmar fascia of unknown cause. It is commonly mistaken for a callus or tendon problem. It may involve any portion of the fascia and may develop insidiously over years or rapidly in weeks. It may be tender, but the most common complaint is of a lump in the palm or inability to extend the involved digits (usually the ring and little fingers). Treatment is surgical and for the most part consists of excision of the involved fascia. Skill is important to avoid neurovascular injury and postoperative stiffness (e.g., a frozen hand). Occasionally, one may prefer a subcutaneous fasciotomy of a discreet longitudinal band if the skin around it is soft and pliable. Recurrences are not uncommon.

TUMORS

Malignancies in the hand are rare. The most common one is squamous carcinoma of the dorsal skin in Caucasians with chronic exposure to sunlight which can generally be cured with local excision.

Warts (verrucca vulgaris), ganglions, inclusion cysts, and soft tissue giant cell tumors (xanthomas) are the most common tumors. All may recur if inadequately treated. Warts may be electrodesiccated or treated with a 40% salicylic acid pad. The others should be meticulously operated on under tourniquet and magnification conditions.

18 . . .

Neurosurgery

GENERAL PRINCIPLES

A detailed history and thorough neurologic examination are the most important steps in arriving at a diagnosis and selecting the proper therapy in neurologic diseases. Special attention by direct and/or leading questions should be given to headache, visual difficulties, episodes of loss of consciousness, impairment of higher intellectual functions, weakness, incoordination, sensory disturbances, etc. The chronology of the history may reveal a steady progression or fluctuation of symptoms.

Ophthalmoscopic examination is an important part of the neurologic survey. It is usually unwise to use mydriatics, as the size of the pupils and their reaction to light are valuable signs of changes in intracranial pressure. If a mydriatic must be given for better visualization of the retina, a note to this effect should be made in the patient's chart so that subsequent examiners will know the cause of the pupillary changes. **Never artificially dilate the pupils in head injuries.**

History taking and neurologic examination are designed to answer 2 questions: (1) Where is the lesion? and (2) What type of lesion is it? Additional diagnostic studies are usually required for definitive diagnosis.

Skull X-rays.

In 50% of cases the presence of a brain tumor can be inferred by examination of plain films of the skull. The plain film is therefore a most important preliminary study. At least 5 views should be taken: anteroposterior, posteroanterior, right and left lateral, and a half-axial view to visualize the area about the foramen magnum. Stereoscopic views are helpful also. When lesions about the base of the skull are suspected, tomograms may demonstrate them even though the routine skull films are normal. Skull x-rays should be taken in all cases of significant head injury to visualize fractures, depressed bone, foreign bodies, pineal shift, etc., and for medicolegal purposes.

Spine X-rays.

Anteroposterior, lateral, and right and left oblique films should be taken of the appropriate spinal region when there is clinical indication of injury or disease involving the vertebrae and/or spinal cord. Tumors and other space-occupying lesions may be shown by foraminal enlargement, increase of interpedicular distance, erosion or osteoblastic changes, calcification, or adjacent (paravertebral) soft tissue changes.

Electroencephalography.

EEG's are indicated in the following circumstances: (1) When there are episodes of alteration in consciousness, to aid in the differentiation of convulsive seizures from syncope, and in carotid sinus syndrome. (2) Following serious head injuries, serial examination has considerable prognostic value. (3) When the presence of a focal cerebral lesion is suspected, serial examination may be helpful.

Lumbar Puncture.

Lumbar puncture is used to obtain information concerning 1 or all of the following: (1) Intracranial pressure; (2) CSF protein, cells, and glucose; (3) serology; (4) evidence of subarachnoid hemorrhage; and (5) bacteriologic and viral studies and agglutination reactions. In general, the following information should be obtained in every lumbar puncture: (1) Initial pressure. (2) Gross appearance: 1 ml. of CSF is placed in each of 3 test tubes and the color and clarity of the first tube is compared with that in the last tube. A cell count should be done on the last tube. (3) Final pressure. **Note:** The Queckenstedt test should be carried out **only** in cases with suspected space-consuming lesions in the spinal canal and **never** in patients with suspected intracranial lesions.

A. Contraindications:
   1. Increase in CSF pressure (as determined by the presence of papilledema) - The danger in this situation is that the reduction of pressure occasioned by the escape of CSF at the time of puncture or after the needle is withdrawn may produce (1) herniation of the medial-inferior temporal lobes into the incisura tentorii or (2) herniation of the cerebellar tonsils into the foramen magnum. Either may cause serious complications or death due to sudden compression of vital brain stem structures.
   2. In cases where spinal cord tumor is suspected, lumbar puncture should be done only when all arrangements have been made to perform a myelogram if a total manometric block is found. If this is not done, all available fluid below the spinal fluid block may be inadvertently drained off, in which case the crucial myelogram required later may be impossible to obtain.

B. Technic: Lumbar puncture may be done with the patient in the sitting position but is usually carried out as follows:
   1. The patient is placed on his side with his legs, thighs, and neck flexed so that the spinal column is well "bowed out" toward the operator.
   2. The skin is suitably prepared with an antiseptic solution and infiltrated with a local anesthetic.
   3. A No. 20 lumbar puncture needle is introduced between the spinous processes of the selected interspace (L3-L4). The needle must be perpendicular to the skin. As the needle is advanced through the interspinous ligament, one can usually feel a "pop" when the needle point penetrates the ligamentum flavum; at this point the stilet should be partially withdrawn to see if CSF appears. If not, the stilet is reintroduced, the needle gently advanced a few mm., and the stilet again partially withdrawn until CSF is obtained. The stilet is then immediately replaced to prevent loss of CSF.

4. The stilet should never be completely withdrawn, since loss of CSF may be extremely dangerous in the presence of increased intracranial pressure or spinal cord tumor. A three-way stopcock adjusted to prevent flow is carried in the left hand and the stilet slowly removed with the right hand so that the stopcock can be immediately inserted in the needle hub to prevent loss of fluid. (An alternative method is to remove the stilet when the ligamentum flavum has been penetrated and to attach the stopcock and water manometer to the needle. As the needle is advanced and the arachnoid penetrated, the fluid pressure can immediately be determined and fluid loss and sudden changes in pressure prevented.)
5. The patient should slowly straighten his legs and neck so that intracranial pressure can be measured accurately. Flexion of the legs will compress the abdomen, which in turn may raise the intraspinal pressure; and flexion of the neck may compromise the venous return in the jugular system and also produce rises in pressure. If a spinal block is suspected, the Queckenstedt test should be done at this point by recording the pressure again after an assistant has compressed both jugular veins for 10 seconds. After release of jugular compression the pressure should be recorded at ten-second intervals for 30 seconds. With normal dynamics the pressure should promptly rise and fall. With a complete block there will be no change. Partial block causes an incomplete and slow rise and fall.
6. After measurement of CSF pressure as above, 1 ml. samples should be collected in each of 3 test tubes drop by drop under manometric control. If there is more blood in the first tube than the third, the blood is due to traumatic spinal tap, whereas in subarachnoid hemorrhage the fluid in all 3 tubes will be the same color. The only certain way to differentiate between a "bloody tap" and true hemorrhage into the CSF is to centrifuge the specimen immediately after it is obtained. If the supernatant is clear and not xanthochromic, the bloody CSF is only the result of a traumatic puncture.
7. The final pressure is recorded, the needle withdrawn, and a small dressing applied. The patient should remain flat in bed for 12-24 hours.
8. The cell count should be done immediately on tube No. 3 and the remaining specimens sent to the laboratory for pertinent chemical analyses.

Other Tests.
The information obtained from the history, neurologic examination, and the above-mentioned diagnostic tests is then used to determine what additional diagnostic tests may be required, e.g., pneumoencephalography, cerebral angiography, ventriculography, and brain scintiscan.

SPECIAL FEATURES IN MANAGEMENT

Neurosurgical patients frequently present the most difficult and involved management problems, both preoperatively and postoperatively. In many cases adequate management requires the attending surgeon's personal observation and evaluation of the patient **as often as every 2 hours or even continuously.** Sudden changes in intracranial pressure may produce an emergency situation in a matter of minutes or hours. Seizures or even status epilepticus may occur suddenly. Dilatation of a pupil, increasing obtundation, or progressive hemiparesis may develop in a matter of minutes.

Increased Intracranial Pressure.

This is a common and critical problem in neurosurgery. It will always be a complication in expanding intracranial lesions if sufficient time elapses before the patient seeks medical attention. The brain can compensate for a surprising amount of distortion which comes on slowly, but decompensation can occur swiftly if rapid changes in intracranial pressure occur. The patient may become unresponsive and moribund in a matter of minutes.

Increased intracranial pressure may be caused by (1) cellular and/or vascular injury or disease, producing cerebral swelling (so-called ''cerebral edema''); (2) space-occupying lesions (e.g., neoplasms, hematomas, abscesses); (3) obstructions of ventricular and CSF pathways; or (4) interference with venous drainage from the intracranial cavity (e.g., tumor encroachment, thrombosis of dural sinuses), and (5) miscellaneous infrequent causes.

A. Symptoms and Signs: Headache, alteration in consciousness (from slight decrease in higher intellectual functions to deep coma), nausea and vomiting, papilledema (which may lead to blindness), extraocular muscle palsies (abducens: medial deviation of the eye; oculomotor: dilatation of a pupil may be a sign of transtentorial herniation of the temporal lobe).

B. Treatment:
   1. Preoperative and postoperative - Restrict fluid intake. The intravenous administration of osmotic diuretics (30% urea or mannitol) over a period of 30-60 minutes may be valuable.
   2. During surgery the most effective means of combatting increased intracranial pressure is by surgical removal of the causative lesion as completely and rapidly as possible. If total removal is not possible, as complete as possible subtotal removal (internal decompression) is indicated. The rapid infusion of 30% mannitol is also extremely valuable in correcting this dangerous situation. If the intracranial pressure continues to be obviously increased after surgical treatment of the causative lesion, external decompression can be done by leaving the dura mater partially or completely open and by removing part or all of the bone flap.
   3. Constant ventricular drainage by means of an inlying ventricular catheter is sometimes useful as a temporary measure to reduce increased intracranial pressure due to CSF block.
   4. The most effective means of reducing increased intracranial pressure caused by brain edema or edema in a space-occupying lesion is the use of dexamethasone.

Seizures.

Aura, onset, type of seizure, and postictal state may provide significant diagnostic clues to the localization of causative factors. A major seizure may be the precipitating factor causing sudden deterioration in a patient with increased intracranial pressure (see above). Postoperative seizures indicate either localized cerebral edema from surgical trauma, or a hematoma. If an extradural, subdural, or intracerebral hematoma is suspected, cerebral angiography or reoperation is mandatory.

Medical treatment consists of anticonvulsant drugs in a dosage sufficient to control seizures. The usual regimen is diphenylhydantoin (Dilantin®), 0.1 Gm. (1½ gr.) every 4-6 hours orally, or 0.15 Gm. (2½ gr.) I.V. Anticonvulsants may be given alone or in combination with intravenous barbiturates.

Other Supportive and Symptomatic Measures.

Because of impaired consciousness, paresis, etc., neurosurgical patients may be unable to take care of their own bodily needs.

A. Airway Obstruction: If the level of consciousness is severely depressed, frequent tracheopharyngeal aspiration is required to maintain an adequate airway. Tracheostomy should be done as soon as obstruction of the airway is imminent (see p. 251).

B. Urinary Retention: Continuous indwelling catheter drainage is usually required. The catheter should be changed every 7 days and urinary output maintained at a minimum of 1500 ml./day if renal function is normal. Prolonged use of an inlying catheter almost invariably causes a lower urinary tract infection, but antibiotic therapy should be withheld until systemic symptoms appear.

C. Decubitus Ulcers: The comatose, paraplegic, or quadriplegic patient is extremely susceptible to the formation of decubitus ulcers (sacral, over the greater trochanters, heels, elbows, etc.). These can be prevented by proper nursing care (see p. 105).

D. Restlessness: Restlessness is a frequent problem, particularly in patients with severe head injuries, and a search should be made for an obvious cause such as a distended bladder, blood in the CSF, hypoxia, etc. The most effective medications are small doses of chloral hydrate, paraldehyde, and the ataraxic drugs. NEVER USE NARCOTICS, PARTICULARLY IN PATIENTS WITH HEAD INJURIES.

E. Fluid Balance: Fluid intake should be sufficient to ensure adequate urinary output. Fluid balance and requirements in the neurosurgical patient are no different than in other areas of surgery, but certain dangers are peculiar to the neurosurgical patient:

1. Production or accentuation of cerebral edema by overhydration, with resultant hyponatremia, may cause increasing stupor and mimic postoperative bleeding. The appropriate treatment is to give 300 ml. of 3% saline I.V.
2. Diabetes insipidus may follow severe head injuries or intracranial surgery.
3. Fluid balance in the comatose or postoperative patient should be closely followed by daily weighing of the patient, careful recording of intake and output, and frequent determinations of blood electrolyte levels. Fortunately, in neurosurgical patients, nasogastric tube feeding is well tolerated and should be instituted as soon as possible to prevent the

difficulties encountered with intravenous feedings. In the immediate preoperative or postoperative state, in acute head injuries, etc., cerebral edema or "brain swelling" may be effectively treated with corticosteroids such as dexamethasone, 10 mg. I.V., followed by 4 mg. every 6 hours. The dosage is gradually reduced when the acute phase has passed. This therapy is dangerous, of course, in a patient with a history of peptic ulcer or active peptic ulcer, or other disorders which contraindicate the use of corticosteroid drugs.

CONGENITAL LESIONS OF SURGICAL IMPORTANCE

A clear understanding of the embryology of the CNS is essential in evaluating congenital lesions involving the nervous system. The formation of the neural groove begins at the mid-embryo, and closure progresses both rostrally and caudally. As the tube is formed it separates from the ectoderm and comes to lie within the mesoderm. Since the nerve tissue is formed from the ectoderm and early comes to lie within the mesoderm, malformations of the nervous system are frequently accompanied by malformations of mesodermal tissue as well as the skin (ectodermal) and its appendages.

CRANIUM BIFIDUM

Failure of the bones of the skull to unite at the midline is usually discovered at birth since the bones of the skull in the midline are easily palpable. The diagnosis should be substantiated by skull x-rays. Cranium bifidum must be differentiated from separation of normal sutures due to raised intracranial pressure. The defect is rarely of significant size unless there is associated protrusion of the dura, arachnoid, or brain (cranial meningocele or meningoencephalocele).

Treatment is not usually required. If the defect is extensive, cranioplasty is indicated to protect the underlying brain, utilizing bone, plastic, or tantalum mesh. This procedure should be deferred for about 4 years until the period of rapid growth of the skull bones has passed.

CRANIOSTENOSIS
(Craniosynostosis)

The cause of premature bony fusion of the cranial sutures is not known. Normally, the bones of the skull are separated at birth and become joined in a fibrous union at the suture lines after 3-6 months of age; bony union does not normally occur before the fifth or sixth decade.

Early recognition of premature fusion of the sutures is important because brain weight more than doubles in the first year of life.

The growth of the skull is caused by the growth of the brain, and if the sutures fuse prematurely normal brain growth will be hampered. Surgical intervention is essential to permit normal mental development.

Clinical Findings.

The principal clinical feature of craniostenosis is deformity of the cranial contour; the type of deformity is dependent upon the suture or sutures involved, as follows (in order of frequency of occurrence): (1) sagittal suture - dolichocephaly or scaphocephaly; (2) coronal suture - brachycephaly; (3) all sutures - oxycephaly.

Treatment and Prognosis.

The only treatment is surgical. The operation consists of removing a linear strip of bone, 1-2 cm. wide, following the line of (and including) the involved suture. Polyethylene film or tubing is then sutured over the edge of the bone in an attempt to delay regrowth; the periosteum should be widely resected to further delay regrowth.

The outlook for normal mental development is good if the diagnosis is made during the first few months of life and surgery is done before the rapid increase in brain growth is impaired. The operation may have to be repeated, since regrowth sometimes occurs in spite of vigorous efforts to prevent it.

ENCEPHALOCELE

Grouped under this term are all lesions which cause protrusion of meninges (with or without neural tissue) and neural tissue from their normal intracranial location. About 75% of all encephaloceles are in the occipital area. Most protrude extracranially in the midline, but protrusion not uncommonly occurs in the nasopharynx, nasal cavity, or orbit.

The sac may be large, with a narrow stalk, but is more commonly sessile in shape. On examination it is difficult to determine if the mass contains neural structures or only fluid; transillumination with a bright light in a darkened room will show neural masses as shadows against the homogeneous red glow of the fluid.

The objective of surgery is to expose the neck of the mass and the cranial defect; to open the sac and replace neural contents within the cranial cavity (or amputate the neural tissue if it is excessive or abnormal); and to obtain a water-tight dural closure. Large bony defects can then be repaired with wire mesh, plastic, or bone, but this is rarely required.

DERMAL SINUS TRACTS

Dermal sinus tracts are due to incomplete embryonal separation of the neural tube from the overlying ectoderm; this creates a persistent connection between the skin and the CNS or its investing membranes or bone. Since closure and separation of the neural tube proceeds caudally and rostrally from about the midpoint of the embryo, persistent dermal sinus tracts occur most commonly at either extremity of the neural tube, i.e., the anterior or posterior neuropore. Midline cutaneous defects most commonly occur in the sacral area. Most sacral midline cutaneous defects are of no neurosurgical significance, as they extend no deeper than the sacral fascia (pilonidal cysts). If they extend into the subarachnoid space through a bony defect (spina bifida), the tract may serve as a pathway of infection; meningitis is a frequent complication.

The diagnosis is usually suggested by the accompanying cutaneous defect (dimple, port wine stain, hair tuft, etc.). There may be a history of recurrent bouts of meningitis.

Surgical excision should be done to prevent meningitis.

HYDROCEPHALUS

Hydrocephalus is enlargement of the CSF pathways as a result of an increase in the amount of fluid under elevated pressure. In infants this causes progressive enlargement of the head.

Hydrocephalus may be due to (1) a decrease in the normal rate of CSF absorption; (2) over-production of CSF (rare); (3) obstruction to the normal flow of fluid by a congenital lesion such as occlusion of the aqueduct of Sylvius, occlusion of the foramens of Luschka and Magendie, or obstruction of the basilar cisterns, as may occur in the Arnold-Chiari malformation. The absorptive bed over the surface of the hemisphere may function improperly, leading to a decrease in the normal rate of CSF absorption. Other causes include neoplasm and inflammation due to hemorrhage or infection.

Clinical Findings.

The diagnosis of hydrocephalus is made on the basis of abnormal and progressive enlargement of the head. If the diagnosis is in doubt, repeated measurements of the occipital bregmatic circumference should be compared with standard charts. The fontanel is usually wide, tense, and nonpulsating. The frontal bosses are prominent, and sclera may be visible above the iris in the natural position of gaze as the eyeballs are displaced downward by pressure on the thin orbital roofs. Symptoms of increased intracranial pressure are often present: irritability, vomiting, somnolence, etc. If the cortex is very thin, transillumination of the head with a bright light in a darkened room will permit passage of light through the head. Complete transillumination occurs in far-advanced hydrocephalus with only a shell of cortex remaining and in hydranencephaly (hydrocephalus with partial absence of brain). If complete transillumination occurs, attempts at surgical correction of hydrocephalus are not warranted. Where a reasonably thick cortical mantle remains, no transillumination occurs.

Before a decision can be made regarding the proper therapy, the type of hydrocephalus must be established. In obstructive hydrocephalus there is no communication between the ventricular system and the absorptive bed. In communicating hydrocephalus there is free communication between the ventricles and the subarachnoid space in the spinal canal. To determine the type and, if possible, the cause of hydrocephalus, the following steps should be carried out with the patient in the lateral decubitus position: (1) Subdural taps should be done to make certain that enlargement of the head is not caused by subdural hematoma. A No. 20 short-beveled pediatric spinal needle is inserted into the subdural space through the lateral angle of the anterior fontanel or the coronal suture well away from the midline. (2) If no blood is recovered on subdural tap, the needle should be cautiously advanced until the ventricle is entered. The depth at which the ventricle is entered should be recorded, as this is a measurement of the thickness of the remaining cerebral mantle. A manometer is then fixed to the needle and the pressure recorded. One ml. of neutral PSP or indigo carmine is then injected into the ventricle. A lumbar puncture is immediately performed and the time required for the dye to appear in the lumbar space recorded. If no dye appears within 20 minutes, the hydrocephalus is said to be an obstructive type. Air ventriculography is then carried out by replacing sufficient ventricular fluid with air in 10 ml. increments. This exchange is carried out until 30-50 ml. of fluid have been withdrawn. Skull x-rays are then taken with the head in various positions to demonstrate the entire ventricular system. The ventriculogram is done (1) to demonstrate the width of the cortex and (2) to rule out a neoplasm and, if possible, to establish more definitely the cause of the hydrocephalus. As a general rule, if the cortex is less than 1 cm. thick, the prognosis for normal development is poor and operative correction is probably not justified.

Treatment.

Occasional cases will arrest spontaneously. Repeated lumbar punctures (in communicating hydrocephalus) or ventricular taps (in obstructive hydrocephalus) can be used to tide the patient over until definitive management can be carried out. Numerous operative procedures have been devised, but none are uniformly successful. Removal of the choroid plexus is occasionally effective. Several shunting procedures are available to direct the CSF to an area where it may be excreted or absorbed. The choice of shunting procedure depends to some extent on the type of hydrocephalus: in obstructive hydrocephalus the fluid must be taken from the ventricular system, whereas in communicating hydrocephalus the fluid can be taken from the lumbar subarachnoid space. The fluid can then be shunted into either the peritoneal or the pleural cavity. A subarachnoid ureteral shunt to direct the fluid from the lumbar subarachnoid space into the ureter is effective in communicating hydrocephalus but entails the loss of a normal kidney and the difficulties that can arise because of the fluid and electrolyte loss since the CSF is thus excreted from the body.

At the present time the most promising procedure is to create a shunt directly from the ventricular system into the right atrium of the heart. A valve inserted in the tubing prevents reflux of blood into the ventricle. No fluid is lost from the body, and the absorption of the fluid is not dependent upon an absorptive bed, as is the case with pleural and peritoneal shunts. The disadvantages of this procedure are (1) chronic low-grade infection of the distal end, resulting in subacute bacterial septicemia with all its attendant complications; and (2) blockage of the system by clotting on the distal end, which occasionally occurs and which requires surgical revision.

Prognosis.

In hydrocephalus secondary to neoplasm or inflammation, the

lesion causing the hydrocephalus determines the prognosis. The prognosis of congenital hydrocephalus has become more favorable with the development of the newer shunting procedures, but long-term follow-up will be required before positive statements can be made. Nevertheless, it can be stated categorically that a properly functioning ventriculo-atrial shunt, if inserted early enough, will allow subsequent normal development.

PORENCEPHALY

This is a circumscribed cavity in cerebral tissue which communicates with the ventricle. The most common clinical findings are seizures and, at times, enlargement of the head, which may be asymmetric, particularly as viewed by x-ray. Surgical treatment is indicated only when seizures cannot be controlled by anticonvulsant drug therapy.

ARNOLD-CHIARI MALFORMATION

This consists of (1) elongation and caudad projection of the cerebellar tonsils through the foramen magnum; (2) elongation (and kinking) of the medulla into the cervical canal, so that the fourth ventricle frequently opens into the cervical spinal subarachnoid space; and (3) downward displacement of the cervical spinal cord, so that the cervical nerve roots run upward to their foramens of exit instead of along their normal horizontal course. The etiology is not known, but in cases with spina bifida, meningocele, and meningomylocele, fixation of the spinal cord at the level of the malformation probably prevents the normal cephalad migration of the cord and thus causes downward displacement of the structures in the posterior fossa.

Hydrocephalus is often present, as well as congenital anomalies of the cervical vertebrae, e.g., fusion of 1 or more of the cervical vertebrae, resulting in a short neck (brevis colli); lower cranial nerve palsies, cerebellar disturbances, and/or pyramidal and posterior column disturbances.

The hydrocephalus and other symptoms may be relieved by posterior fossa decompression with high cervical laminectomy. At that time the cerebellar tonsils can be lifted out of the cervical spinal cord to allow the normal flow of CSF around the basilar cisterns; occasionally it may be necessary to amputate the cerebellar tonsils. The adhesions between the cerebellum and the spinal cord can be lysed as an aid to reestablishment of normal CSF flow. If these measures are ineffective in relieving the hydrocephalus, a shunting procedure may be required.

PLATYBASIA
(Basilar Impression)

This is a developmental defect in which there is upward displacement of the cervical vertebral column into the base of the skull so that the odontoid process projects into the cranial cavity. Other bone anomalies are frequently associated, e.g., occipitalization of the atlas, misshapen foramen magnum, and fusion of the cervical vertebrae.

Symptoms rarely develop prior to adult life. Neurologic signs are those of compression of the cervical spinal cord, with weakness, ataxia, sensory loss, sphincter disturbances, etc. The diagnosis is established by x-rays of the skull and cervical vertebrae. Platybasia is said to be present when, on a good lateral view of the skull, the odontoid process is seen to project more than 5 mm. above a line drawn from the posterior rim of the foramen magnum to the posterior edge of the hard palate (Chamberlain's line).

Treatment is directed toward decompression of the area of the foramen magnum by suboccipital craniectomy and cervical laminectomy. Recovery of function is occasionally excellent, but in most cases arrest is all that can be accomplished. An occasional case may be more successfully treated by the anterior approach with removal of the odontoid process.

SYRINGOMYELIA (AND SYRINGOBULBIA)

A syrinx is a central cavitation of the spinal cord and/or the brain stem. This is usually found in the cervical and upper thoracic cord, but it may occur also at various levels in the brain stem. Syringomyelia or syringobulbia is believed to be due either to congenital maldevelopment or neoplastic proliferation of the glial cells around the central canal of the spinal cord.

The classical clinical finding is the dissociated loss of pain and temperature sensation in a "jacket" distribution involving the upper extremities, shoulder girdles, and upper thorax, with relative preservation of touch perception. This is produced when the cavitation disrupts the decussating pain fibers in the commissures around the central canal. Associated findings are weakness of the muscles of the upper extremities, particularly the intrinsic muscles of the hands, with visible atrophy and fasciculations. Some degree of long tract involvement in the lower extremities is often present. X-rays of the cervical or thoracic spine may reveal erosion of the pedicles or increase in the interpedicular distances. Contrast myelography may demonstrate widening of the spinal canal at the involved segments, or the spinal cord may be so widened so as to produce a total block to the flow of the contrast medium.

Treatment is by laminectomy and decompression (with or without drainage of the cystic area by needle aspiration), myelotomy (incision into the cord through the posterior median fissure), or an attempt to establish permanent drainage of the cavity to slow the progression of the symptoms. X-ray therapy is advocated by some. The prognosis is guarded, although decompression and/or x-ray therapy may slow the progression of symptoms. The process seems at times to run its course with periods of relative quiescence.

SPINA BIFIDA OCCULTA

This is a defect in the laminar arch, usually asymptomatic, which most often occurs in the lumbosacral area. Associated anomalies in the skin overlying the bifid spine and malformations of the lower extremities (varus, valgus, or cavus deformities of the feet) are often present. Urinary incontinence, weakness, atrophy, sensory loss in the lower lumbar area and along the distribution of the sacral nerve roots, and other neurologic defects may be noted.

Contrast myelography may demonstrate an intraspinal mass, usually a lipoma.

Treatment is indicated only when there are associated neurologic findings, and consists of complete laminectomy with removal of any intraspinal mass (lipoma, dermoid, etc.). Care must be taken to preserve nerve tissue. Electric stimulation is helpful in differentiating nerve filaments from fibrous strands. If a thickened filum terminale is discovered, this should be sectioned. The aim of surgery is to prevent further neurologic damage. Restoration of lost function is not likely to occur.

MENINGOCELE AND MYELOMENINGOCELE

A meningocele is a protrusion of meninges containing CSF through the defective neural arch. If neural elements are present, the lesion is then termed a myelomeningocele. All sizes and shapes of protrusions may occur, from a simple flat meningocele covered with a parchment membrane level with the skin to huge sessile masses with significant portions of neural tissue exposed on the surface (spinal rachischisis). They most commonly occur in the lumbosacral area, but may occur at any level and occasionally protrude anteriorly into the pelvic, abdominal, or thoracic cavities. It is often difficult or impossible to differentiate between simple meningocele and meningomyelocele, but transillumination of the mass with a bright light in a darkened room may reveal the shadows caused by neural elements. Neurologic deficits (sensory, motor, and sphincter disturbances) establish the lesion as a myelomeningocele.

The objective of surgery is cosmetic removal of the mass and prevention of further neurologic deficits. The lesion should be removed in all cases if it is technically feasible and if the neurologic deficit does not preclude relatively normal development. Infants with spinal rachischisis and complete paraplegia should not be operated on until they are at least 6 months old; those who do not survive have overwhelming defects and associated anomalies which would have made them unacceptable candidates for surgery. A meningocele or meningomyelocele which has ruptured and is leaking CSF should be repaired on an emergency basis if the neurologic loss is not overwhelming. Otherwise in most instances operation can and should be delayed until there is sufficient skin covering the lesion to ensure a satisfactory skin closure. Progressive hydrocephalus should be surgically corrected before the repair of the meningocele, since increased CSF pressure threatens to break down the repair.

The prognosis depends upon the extent of the associated neurologic deficit and the severity of associated anomalies.

HEAD INJURIES

Injury to the head frequently results in brain injury, and the extent of brain damage determines the treatment and prognosis.

The management of injuries to the scalp and skull is dictated by the type and degree of underlying brain damage and associated injuries in other parts of the body.

Emergency management is as follows:

1. Establish and maintain adequate respiratory exchange.
2. Control hemorrhage.
3. Treat shock.
4. Examine the patient quickly but thoroughly to ascertain the type and degree of all injuries.
5. Splint long bone fractures. **Note:** Do not reduce or apply casts; only splinting is warranted.
6. Evaluate the type and severity of the nervous system injury.
7. Do not move the patient for any reason (e.g., to obtain x-rays, for transportation to another hospital or to a private room) until the extent of all injuries is known and until the immediate threats to life (respiratory embarrassment, hemorrhage, etc.) have been controlled and the patient's condition stabilized.

Injury to the brain results from rapid deceleration, acceleration, and/or the shearing-rotational effects of a blow to the head. These mechanisms may produce (1) concussion, a temporary loss of consciousness with no permanent organic brain damage; (2) contusion, bruising of the brain; or (3) laceration, a frank disruption of brain substance. These 3 types of brain injury can occur singly, but are more commonly seen in varying combinations. Contusion may be local, causing focal signs and symptoms such as hemiparesis or aphasia; or generalized, with widespread damage to the brain. Increased vascular permeability in contusion produces cerebral "edema" or swelling. In severe head injuries decreased respiratory exchange leads to further anoxia and hypercapnia, resulting in cerebral vasodilatation, all of which contribute to further cerebral swelling.

Initial Evaluation of the Extent of Nervous System Injury.

Every case of head injury should be treated as potentially serious. As soon as practicable after the patient has been admitted to the hospital and his condition stabilized, a thorough neurologic examination should be performed. The following should always be noted and recorded.

A. Level of Responsiveness: Note response to spoken voice, shouted voice, and painful stimuli.
B. Size of pupils and response to light.
C. Ability to move the extremities voluntarily or in response to painful stimuli.
D. Degree and equality of the deep tendon reflexes.
E. Presence of superficial reflexes.
F. Presence of abnormal reflexes (e.g., Babinski response).
G. Direct inspection of the entire head for abrasions, swelling, laceration, etc.
H. Presence of bloody or CSF drainage from nose or ears.
I. Ophthalmoscopic examination, if possible. **Note:** Never artificially dilate the pupils in head injury.

The findings of this initial examination must be accurately recorded, as the indications for surgery depend to a great extent upon the observed variations from this initial baseline examination. The most important factor in management of severe head injuries is frequent observation, and the most sensitive sign of improvement or deterioration is change in the level of responsiveness. X-rays of the skull should be taken in every case of significant injury to the head, but removal to the x-ray department should be deferred until the patient's condition is stabilized. X-rays of the cervical spine should be taken if there is evidence of injury to that area or if the patient is still unconscious on admission. Lumbar puncture should not be done unless specifically indicated. Where an intracerebral or extracerebral (subdural, extradural) hemorrhage is suspected, immediate cerebral angiography is a most useful diagnostic study.

GENERAL POSTOPERATIVE MANAGEMENT OF HEAD INJURIES

After definitive care of the more specific aspects of head injuries, one is frequently left with a comatose patient who has received a massive brain injury (contusions and/or lacerations). Hypoxia and hypercapnia must be prevented, since they cause intracranial vascular dilatation and add to cerebral swelling. Continuous intranasal oxygen is usually indicated, but frequent pharyngeal aspiration to keep the airway clear at all times and, if secretions accumulate rapidly, tracheostomy are the most effective measures to prevent hypoxia. Some neurosurgeons are now advocating prolonged hypothermia to a body temperature of approximately 31° C. as a means of preventing anoxic damage to the brain by reducing its oxygen requirement.

Intravenous mannitol or urea, 150-300 ml. of 30% solution, can be used to reduce brain swelling, but should never be used until one is absolutely certain that there is no expanding intracranial clot; administration of urea will immediately expand a hematoma and produce disastrous results. Urea should therefore not be used until multiple bur hole exploration has ruled out hematoma.

For further details on the management of the comatose patient, see p. 31. Early application of rehabilitation technics by the physical therapy department may greatly shorten the period of rehabilitation.

SCALP INJURIES

The scalp is an extremely vascular structure, and injury may cause serious hemorrhage. Bleeding is usually best controlled with a simple pressure dressing of several 4 × 4 gauze sponges placed over the wound and held firmly in place by a circumferential dressing. Arterial bleeding can be controlled by firm finger pressure along the edges of the wound, or a hemostat can be attached to the galea and allowed to hang down over the skin edge in such a way as to pull the galea firmly against the skin and compress the bleeding vessels. All wounds of the scalp should be closed as soon as possible unless they overly a depressed fracture or penetrating wound of the skull. If either of these is present, the patient should be taken to the operating room and the skin wound treated in conjunction with the definitive treatment of the fracture.

Scalp Lacerations.

Always shave at least 1 inch beyond all edges of the wound. Wash the area around the wound thoroughly with surgical soap, taking care to wash away from the wound. (If the laceration is large it is best to place a 4 × 4 gauze sponge in the wound to prevent debris from entering.) Cleanse the wound thoroughly with repeated irrigations of warm normal saline or Ringer's solution. Infiltrate the circumference of the wound with local anesthetic about 1 inch away from the wound edges. Remove foreign bodies which may lead to infection or leave unsightly tattoos. Minimal debridement should include all devitalized tissue, taking care not to cut away so much tissue that closure will be difficult or impossible.

The wound can be closed with multiple interrupted vertical mattress sutures of stainless steel wire or with a double layer of interrupted sutures of the galea and skin. Technic should be meticulous.

Avulsions of the Scalp.

Avulsions of the scalp usually include all layers down to the periosteum. These injuries should be treated only by experienced personnel with complete operating room facilities. The surrounding area should be shaved and thoroughly irrigated. If the avulsion is small, the ragged edges can be sparingly trimmed; closure can often be accomplished by tripod extension or modified Z-plasties. If the denuded area is large the surrounding area should be shaved; the wound is then repeatedly and thoroughly irrigated and covered with a single layer of fine mesh (burn) gauze. A large dressing of "fluffies" or mechanic's waste is placed over this and a firm circumferential dressing applied to exert even pressure over the area. Delayed closure via a plastic procedure will then be required 8-10 days later. If the bone is completely denuded of all soft tissue, a small split-thickness graft can be applied as a temporary measure and covered with lightly impregnated fine mesh gauze to protect the bone until delayed closure can be safely carried out.

SKULL FRACTURES

Skull fracture per se is not a more serious injury than fracture of any other bone; it is the injury to the brain that determines the prognosis in head injuries. Death due to severe brain injury may follow head injury in which there is no evidence of skull fracture; and patients with extensive "egg-shell" fractures of the skull may have no neurologic deficit or other permanent ill effects.

Fractures may be classified according to (1) whether the skin overlying the fracture is intact (simple) or broken (compound); (2) whether there is a single fracture line (linear), several fractures radiating from a central point (stellate), or fragmentation of bone (comminuted); and (3) whether the edges of the fracture line have been driven below the level of the surrounding bone (depressed) or not (nondepressed).

Simple Skull Fractures (Linear, Stellate, or Comminuted Nondepressed).

These fractures are of clinical importance if they have crossed major vascular channels in the skull such as the groove of the middle meningeal artery or the major dural venous sinuses. If these vessels are torn, epidural or subdural hematomas may form; and all patients with these types of fractures should be kept under close observation until it can be ascertained that no such bleeding is occurring. A fracture which extends into the accessory nasal sinuses or the mastoid air cells is considered to be compound, since it is in communication with the external surface of the body.

Depressed Skull Fractures.

Depressed stellate or comminuted fractures require surgical elevation, but if there are no untoward neurologic signs and the fracture is closed, surgery can be delayed until a convenient time.

Compound Skull Fractures.

As soon as his general condition warrants, the patient with a depressed compound skull fracture should go to surgery where complete neurosurgical facilities and a trained neurosurgeon are available. Emergency treatment consists merely of applying a sterile compression dressing. The wound should not be closed, and no attempt should be made to remove any foreign body protruding from the wound until the patient is in the operating room and all preparations have been made for craniotomy, as catastrophic hemorrhage may occur when the tamponading effect of the foreign body is no longer present.

Linear or stellate, nondepressed compound fractures can be treated by simple closure of the skin wound after thorough cleansing. Compound fractures with severe comminution of underlying bone should be treated in the operating room, where proper debridement can be carried out. Mature judgment is required in deciding whether small pieces of bone completely denuded of blood supply should be removed before the wound is closed. If possible, the dura should be inspected to make certain that no laceration has been overlooked. Basal skull fractures may cause rhinorrhea or otorrhea if the dura and arachnoid are torn, and may also cause bleeding from the nose or ears if mucous membranes or skin are torn. When such bleeding occurs it is often difficult to tell if blood is admixed with CSF. A presumptive diagnosis of CSF leakage can be made by placing a drop of the bloody discharge on a cleansing tissue; if CSF is present there will be a spreading yellowish-orange ring around the central red stain of blood. A patient with otorrhea or rhinorrhea should be kept in bed for at least 10 days with his head elevated about 35° and strongly cautioned not to blow his nose for fear of forcing contaminated material from the nose or ear into the cranial cavity. Prophylactic antibiotics may be used. In about 80% of cases, these CSF leaks will close spontaneously within 8-10 days. If CSF drainage persists, the point of leakage should be ascertained and repaired via craniotomy.

TRAUMA TO THE MENINGES

Head injury with or without skull fracture may cause tears in the major or minor vascular channels coursing through the meninges and lead to serious intracranial hemorrhage. Tears in the dura should always be repaired to afford water-tight closure (to lessen the chance of infection or epileptogenic scar formation).

EPIDURAL HEMATOMA

Hemorrhage between the inner table of the skull and the dura mater most commonly arises from a tear in the middle meningeal artery produced by a linear fracture in the temporal region when the fracture line crosses the arterial groove. Since the bleeding is under arterial pressure, it gradually strips the dura from the undersurface of the bone; this produces more bleeding as the small bridging veins from dura to bone are torn. The hematoma thus increases in size rapidly and severely compresses the cerebral cortex, producing contralateral hemiparesis or hemiplegia. As the hemisphere is further compressed, the medial portion of the temporal lobe (uncus and hippocampal gyrus) is forced through the incisura tentorii (compressing the third cranial nerve and thus producing dilatation of the pupil on the same side) and the brain stem is shifted toward the opposite side of the tentorial notch. If the brain stem compression reaches significant degree, venous hemorrhages into the stem will lead to irreparable neurologic deficits or death.

In rare cases epidural hematoma may arise from venous channels in the bone at the point of fracture or from lacerated major dural venous sinuses. Since venous pressure is too low to dissect the dura from the bone, venous hematomas usually form only when a depressed skull fracture has stripped the dura from the bone and left a space in which the hematoma can form.

The classic case presents a history of a blow to the head (which may or may not be of sufficient force to bruise the overlying skin), leading to unconsciousness for a brief interval. As the patient regains consciousness he may have no untoward neurologic symptoms and be perfectly clear mentally; this is the so-called lucid interval. In a matter of minutes or hours, as the rapidly forming hematoma enlarges sufficiently to severely compress the cerebral hemisphere, there is a gradual deterioration of conscious level progressing to coma and death if the hematoma is not immediately evacuated. As the conscious level deteriorates the pupil on the side of the lesion dilates and a contralateral hemiplegia occurs.

The mortality rate in epidural hematoma is high despite the fact that this is potentially a completely curable lesion. The problem is that these patients are either not seen by a physician (since head injury is felt to be too mild) or, more commonly, because they are seen during the lucid interval and discharged to bed rest at home. The patient is then assumed to be asleep when actually the hematoma has increased in size, producing coma instead of sleep; not uncommonly this type of patient is found dead in bed the next morning. Any patient with a history of a blow on the head leading to unconsciousness, even for a brief interval, should therefore have a thorough neurologic examination and skull x-rays. If x-rays show a fracture, he should be hospitalized and his conscious level checked at least every hour. Any impairment of the sensorium is an indication for immediate bur hole exploration in the operating room. **This is a true emergency,** for if surgery is delayed until brain stem hemorrhages occur the patient is likely to remain decerebrate even though the clot is surgically evacuated.

In those cases with a history of a blow to the head followed by unconsciousness, even though no fracture is demonstrated, a reliable relative should be instructed to awaken the patient at least hourly to make certain he is arousable and not comatose.

SUBDURAL HEMATOMA

Subdural hematomas occur most commonly (1) when the veins running from the cortex through the subdural space to the superior sagittal sinus near the midline are torn or (2) when an intracerebral hematoma communicates with the subdural space. The bleeding then occurs between the arachnoid and the dura into the subdural space. Since the arachnoid is only loosely attached to the dura, these hematomas can attain tremendous size even though the bleeding is of venous (low-pressure) origin.

Acute Subdural Hematomas.

Acute subdural hematomas occur only in severe head injuries, probably as a result of frank lacerations of the pia and arachnoid of the cortex and subsequent bleeding into the subdural space. They are usually thin, as the overwhelming injury to the brain often produces cerebral swelling, frequently with great increase in pressure. This makes it impossible for a hematoma of venous origin to attain significant size. These lesions are usually discovered during bur hole exploratory surgery on severely injured patients. Evacuation rarely produces significant change in the patient's condition, as the major neurologic deficit is produced by the widespread cerebral contusion and/or laceration.

Subacute Subdural Hematomas.

These are also due to brain contusion and laceration. Because the brain injury is not overwhelming and brain swelling not great, the hematoma may become large enough to produce symptoms. Progressive hemiparesis, obtundation, aphasia, etc. often appear 3-10 days after the injury. Evacuation of the clots may improve the patient's condition, and the degree of ultimate recovery depends upon the extent of brain damage produced at the moment of injury.

Chronic Subdural Hematomas.

Chronic subdural hematomas are most common in infants and in adults past middle age. They are commonly produced by tearing of the veins that bridge the subdural space as they pass from the convexity of the cortex into the superior sagittal sinus. The hematoma becomes encased in a fibrous membrane, usually liquifies, and gradually enlarges. A history of head injury may be lacking, as the blow is often quite minimal. The history is usually one of progressive mental or personality changes with or without focal symptoms (progressive hemiplegia, aphasia, etc.). Papilledema may be present. These findings often suggest a diagnosis of brain tumor, and the hematoma may be discovered by angiography or bur hole placement preparatory to ventriculography. Subdural hematomas can mimic almost any disease affecting the brain and its coverings.

Treatment consists of drainage of the clot or fluid contained in the subdural space. Many feel that evacuation through multiple bur holes is sufficient; others advocate evacuation through a craniotomy so that the subdural membranes (fibrous capsule) can be widely resected to offer a better prognosis for return of normal mental function and to discourage re-formation of the hematoma.

Echo-encephalography is an extremely valuable diagnostic tool for rapidly surveying patients with acute head injuries and as an aid to the diagnosis of an expanding intracranial hematoma. This device uses pulsed ultra-sound energy to identify the position of the midline cerebral structures. A shift of the midline suggests the presence of a hematoma in the third ventricle.

Subdural Hygromas.

These are collections of clear or yellow-stained fluid in the subdural space. Their mechanism of production has not been completely explained, but most neurosurgeons agree that they form through a tear in the arachnoid which allows CSF to escape into the subdural space and to be held there by a postulated ball valve action of the tear.

Hygromas produce symptoms of subdural hematoma.

Treatment consists of draining the subdural space through multiple bur holes.

Traumatic Subarachnoid Hemorrhage.

Traumatic laceration of vessels in the subarachnoid space is the most common cause of subarachnoid hemorrhage. The diagnosis can be made by collection of uniformly bloody CSF on lumbar puncture, or on the basis of nuchal rigidity, positive straight leg raising tests, and a positive Brudzinski response. No surgical treatment is indicated.

BRAIN INJURY

Direct injuries to the brain, as contusions or lacerations, are not amenable to surgical treatment. Some neurosurgeons feel that in profound injuries, where experience has shown that the temporal and frontal lobe tips are the most seriously injured portions, resection of these severely contused portions of cerebrum may be indicated. Intracerebral hematoma may occur as a result of trauma, usually in association with lacerations; if they are of significant size, surgical evacuation is indicated.

INJURIES TO THE SPINE*

Fractures and fracture-dislocations of the vertebrae are usually the result of acute hyperextension and hyperflexion of the spine. Penetrating injuries may occur as a result of gunshot or stab wounds, etc. Concussion of the spinal cord produces temporary physiological interruption of function without anatomically demonstrable changes. Contusion of the cord usually occurs at the site of a fracture-dislocation or penetrating wound. Laceration, disruption, or dissolution of part or all of the spinal cord is usually the result of severe fracture-dislocations or penetrating wounds.

---

*Only those spine injuries which are accompanied by neurologic manifestations will be discussed here. See also Chapter 19, Orthopedic Surgery.

Clinical Findings.

The neurologic loss in trauma to the spinal column may be partial or complete and transient or permanent. The usual clinical findings are as follows: (1) Immediate flaccid paralysis of the extremities and complete areflexia below the level of the injury due to "spinal shock." Spinal shock may persist for hours, days, or months, depending upon the severity of the injury and the presence of anemia, hypoproteinemia, urinary tract infection, etc. (2) Complete or partial loss of any or all modalities of sensation below the level of the lesion. (3) Urinary retention. (4) Paralytic ileus with abdominal distention. (5) In cervical lesions below C4, there is frequently respiratory difficulty since in this situation the intercostal musculature is paralyzed and breathing is purely diaphragmatic. (6) Loss of sweating below the level of the lesion. (7) Point tenderness over the fracture site, with or without gibbus or crepitus. (8) X-rays may be negative or may demonstrate simple fracture or complete fracture dislocation with marked comminution.

Diagnosis is usually not difficult, but in severe brain injuries with loss of consciousness areflexia is frequently present initially and spinal cord injury may be overlooked. It is imperative in all severe head injuries that x-rays be taken of the cervical spine to be certain that cervical fracture-dislocation is not present.

Treatment.

A thorough neurologic examination must be performed as soon as possible after injury to establish the level and degree of functional loss. Spinal cord injury must be assumed until there is definite proof that none has occurred. Do not move the patient until the full extent of the injury is known, since the spinal cord may be irrevocably damaged by careless handling.

Obtain a detailed description of the accident, as management may depend upon whether the injury was caused by hyperflexion, hyperextension, or a direct blow. Examine for associated injuries.

If cervical fracture is suspected, place sandbags at both sides of the head to prevent motion and apply halter traction with 6-10 lb. of weight as emergency splinting measures. At least 4 and preferably 6 persons are required to lift the patient onto a Stryker or Foster turning frame, taking care to allow no distortion of the spine.

Ask the patient to void; if he is unable to do so, catheterize with a No. 14 or No. 16 Foley catheter and leave it in place.

As soon as the patient's general condition warrants, obtain adequate x-rays of the spine. The physician should always accompany the patient to the x-ray department and remain with him until satisfactory anteroposterior and lateral views have been obtained. The patient should not be turned for the purpose of x-ray, as adequate projections can be obtained with the cross-table technic.

If a cervical fracture or fracture-dislocation is found on x-ray, skeletal tong traction should be immediately instituted. This can be carried out in the x-ray room or, preferably, in an operating room which has an x-ray unit.

Some neurosurgeons feel that laminectomy is almost never indicated; others feel it is always indicated. However, the weight of authoritative opinion is that laminectomy should be done in any of the following circumstances: (1) if there is progressive neurologic loss, (2) if total block of the vertebral canal is shown by a positive Queckenstedt test, (3) if x-rays show bone fragments or foreign bodies depressed into the spinal canal, or (4) if there is a direct penetrating missile wound of the spinal column. If laminectomy is decided upon, it should be carried out as soon as the patient's condition is stable and immediately life-threatening associated injuries have been dealt with. If the injury is cervical, skeletal tong traction should be instituted immediately and maintained during surgery.

PROTRUDED (HERNIATED) INTERVERTEBRAL DISKS

The protrusion may consist of a posterior or lateral bulge of the weakened but intact annulus fibrosus produced by a partially dislocated nucleus pulposus, or part of the entire nucleus may extrude into the spinal canal through a rupture in the annulus.

PROTRUSION OF LUMBAR INTERVERTEBRAL DISKS

Clinical Findings.

A. Symptoms and Signs: All but 5-10% of protrusions occur at the last 2 lumbar interspaces. There is usually a history of progressively more prolonged episodes of back pain with or without leg pain. The pain characteristically spreads to the gluteal region and then down the posterior or posterolateral aspect of the thigh and calf; is aggravated by coughing, sneezing, or straining; and may be relieved by rest. The patient will limp to favor the painful leg, and will tend to carry himself with a "list" either away from or toward the side of the protrusion. Other significant symptoms and signs include spasm of the paravertebral muscles; flattening of the lumbar spine with loss of the normal lordosis; limitation of back motions by pain, particularly on forward flexion; and tenderness to deep pressure over the interspace involved.

B. Neurologic Examination:
   1. Straight leg raising produces leg pain and frequently back pain which can be accentuated by dorsiflexion of the foot (further stretching of the sciatic nerve and roots).
   2. Reflexes - The ankle reflex is diminished or absent (more common with protrusion at the L5-S1 interspace impinging on the first sacral nerve root). The knee reflex may be diminished with herniations at the L3-L4 interspace.
   3. Motor evaluation - Weakness of dorsiflexion, plantar flexion, and inversion or eversion of the foot may be found with herniations at the lower 2 lumbar interspaces. Weakness of the quadriceps may be present with L3-L4 lesions.
   4. Sensory evaluation - Sensory status varies from no loss to complete analgesia in the distribution of the root involved.

C. X-ray Findings: Plain films may be normal or may show narrowing of the involved interspace, arthritic "lipping" of the adjacent vertebral bodies, and/or arthritic changes around the zygoapophysial joints.

D. Special Examinations:
1. Myelography is the most commonly used and most valuable test. Iophendylate (Pantopaque®) is the contrast medium most often used. Three to 21 ml. of medium are instilled into the lumbar thecal sac and the dye observed fluoroscopically as it flows over the suspected interspaces. Permanent films record the extent and level of the lesion.
2. Electromyography can be used to identify the involved nerve root by demonstrating denervation fibrillation potentials in the muscles supplied by the root.
3. Diskograms are rarely employed. Diatrizoate (Hypaque®) is injected directly into the disk. A normal disk will accept 0.5 ml. or less; pathologic disks may accept 2 or 3 ml., and injection frequently reproduces the patient's clinical pain. X-rays confirm disruption of the disk by demonstrating diffusion of opaque material.

Differential Diagnosis.

Protrusion of lumbar intervertebral disks must be differentiated from tumor, subluxation of facets, and rheumatoid spondylitis.

Treatment.

A. Conservative Measures: Many cases can be tided over an acute episode by conservative measures. Supportive treatment includes analgesics for pain and strict bed rest with boards between springs and mattress to prevent sagging. Bilateral leg traction or pelvic traction may help to reduce muscle spasm. The patient is often more comfortable in the modified Fowler's or contour position. After the acute pain subsides, a progressive resistance physical therapy program should be instituted to strengthen the back, abdominal, and leg muscles and to instruct the patient in the proper way of using his back muscles to prevent straining injuries. Back support with a corset brace or flexion body cast may be useful when back pain is severe and chronic.

B. Surgical Measures: Surgery is indicated when complaints are too severe for conservative treatment or when there are progressive signs of neurologic involvement. If the patient does not respond favorably to a trial of conservative treatment, laminectomy and simple excision of protruding nucleus pulposus is sufficient in most cases.

PROTRUSION OF CERVICAL INTERVERTEBRAL DISKS

Clinical Findings.

A. Lateral Protrusions: Patients with lateral cervical protrusions give a history of frequent bouts of pain involving the neck, shoulder, and scapular region (ultimately accompanied by lancinating root pain into the arm or hand) which is accentuated by straining. Paresthesias into the fingers are common: into the first and second digits if the root of C6 is involved; the third digit if the root of C7 is involved; and the fourth and fifth digits if C8 is involved. Examination reveals restricted neck motions, absence of cervical lordosis, spasm of the neck muscles, hypesthesia in root distribution to the arm and hand,

and weakness in the muscle supplied by the involved root. Arm reflexes are often decreased: diminished biceps reflex if C6 is involved; diminished biceps and triceps reflexes if C7 is involved; and diminished triceps reflex if C8 is involved.

X-rays may be normal if the protrusion is recent, or may show a narrowed interspace and/or hypertrophic lipping and narrowing of the root foramens. Iophendylate (Pantopaque®) myelography (see p. 693) reveals a defect of the root sleeve.

B. Midline Protrusions: With midline protrusions there may be no history of root pain; a common presenting complaint is spastic paraparesis with or without urinary hesitancy or incontinence. Signs of pyramidal tract involvement are apparent in the lower extremities; if the cervical roots are involved there will be signs of muscle weakness or atrophy and reflex and/or sensory changes in the upper extremities. Less commonly, there is impairment of ability to perceive pinprick up to the high thoracic level due to spinal cord compression. X-rays reveal marked interspace narrowing, often at several levels, with extensive bony proliferation at the posterior edges of the vertebrae. Myelography shows midline bar deformities.

Treatment.

A. Conservative Measures: Bed rest with continuous halter traction initially; as symptoms subside, a felt or metal neck brace may be helpful.

B. Surgical Measures: In lateral protrusions simple removal of the fragment through the posterior hemilaminectomy approach gives good results. In midline protrusions the operation of choice in recent years has been laminectomy over the involved area with sectioning of the dentate ligaments on both sides to allow the spinal cord to be displaced posteriorly and thereby relieve the anterior compression on the cord. Anterior diskectomy and intervertebral fusion (through the paratracheal approach) has produced excellent results in both lateral and midline disk protrusions. In midline bar protrusions surgery usually prevents progression of neurologic loss and may partially restore lost function.

PERIPHERAL NERVE INJURIES

Injuries to the peripheral nerves may be caused by lacerating injuries, fractures of the long bones, crushing injuries of the extremities, or penetrating or perforating wounds. These injuries may cause partial or complete anatomic separation of the nerve, destruction of the nerve with the nerve sheath remaining in continuity (as in crush injuries), or temporary impairment of function without actual destruction of nerve tissue (as in concussion injuries).

Clinical Findings.

Trauma to the peripheral nerves causes complete or partial loss of sensory and/or motor function in the structures innervated by the nerve involved. The diagnosis is made by individual testing of the muscles in the involved extremity to determine which are paretic and to what extent. The area of sensory loss should be outlined on the skin and a photograph or drawing entered in the record. There may be extremely painful dysesthesias referred to hypalgesic areas. After the acute phase of the injury has passed, percussion over the stump or suture site evokes a tingling sensation which is projected into the anesthetic area in the distribution appropriate to the nerve involved (Tinel's sign). In old nerve injuries the nails and skin may show severe trophic changes, and painless ulcers may be present as a result of injuries or burns to anesthetic skin. After 21 days (the time required for complete degeneration of nerve distal to the point of injury), electromyography shows denervation fibrillation potentials, increased chronaxie, failure to react to faradic stimulation, and absence of voluntary contraction.

Treatment.

A. Initial Treatment of Acute Injuries: If the patient is seen within 6-8 hours after injury and there is little surrounding soft tissue injury and minimal contamination, primary end-to-end anastomosis can be carried out in the operating room (never in the emergency room). If the injury is of the crushing type or has resulted in a jagged laceration with a great deal of soft tissue injury, no attempt should be made to carry out primary anastomosis. In these cases the nerve ends (distal and proximal) should be tagged with wire sutures for later identification and the wound treated appropriately; delayed anastomosis should be carried out 18-21 days later, at which time degeneration of nerve distal to the wound will be complete and the Schwann cell tubules will be ready to accept outgrowing neurofibrils. At this time it will be possible to determine how much of the nerve ends are nonviable, resect back to healthy nerve, and, if necessary, mobilize the nerve above and below so that end-to-end anastomosis can be carried out.

B. Old Nerve Injuries: If the initial injury resulted in complete loss of function and primary nerve repair was not attempted, anastomosis will usually give good results as long as 1-2 years after the injury. In incomplete nerve injuries seen weeks or months after injury, mature judgment is required to decide which of the following surgical approaches is indicated: (1) extrinsic neurolysis (lysis of scar external to the nerve) and/or intrinsic neurolysis (lysis of scar within the nerve sheath); or (2) resection of the neuroma followed by neurorrhaphy. Where primary anastomosis is impossible, improved results have been obtained recently in severe nerve injuries by the use of homografts and a millipore sheath around the graft. This technic offers much promise for the future.

CENTRAL NERVOUS SYSTEM NEOPLASMS

INTRACRANIAL NEOPLASMS

Brain tumors occur in all age groups with approximately equal distribution up to the age of 70 years. Two-thirds of all brain tumors in children occur in the subtentorial space (posterior fossa), whereas 80% of brain tumors in adults occur in the supratentorial space. Certain brain tumors are found almost exclusively in childhood (medulloblastoma); others are found almost exclusively in adults (glioblastoma multiforme). Brain tumors almost never metastasize outside the CNS. Brain tumors are found in 1% of hospital admissions and perhaps as many as 2% of autopsies.

Classification and Approximate Frequency.

Gliomas, 45%; meningiomas, 15%; pituitary tumors, 12%; tumors of nerve sheaths, 8%; blood vessel tumors, 5%; congenital tumors, 5%; and metastatic tumors, 2-5%. Miscellaneous tumors account for the remainder.

Clinical Manifestations of Brain Tumors.

The diagnosis of brain tumor is made on the basis of the history, neurologic examination, and appropriate laboratory tests, and is confirmed by special diagnostic tests. In any suspected case of brain tumor a careful ophthalmoscopic examination should be made. If papilledema is present, spinal puncture should not be done. If papilledema is not present and a brain tumor is suspected, a carefully performed spinal puncture can be quite helpful, since by carefully measuring the pressure one can determine if increased pressure is present which has as yet not produced papilledema. One or a combination of the special diagnostic tests discussed below are usually carried out to confirm a strong suspicion of brain tumor, to localize the lesion as accurately as possible, and to gain as much information as possible preoperatively concerning the character of the tumor.

A. Symptoms and Signs: These depend upon the location and rapidity of growth of the tumor and the age of the patient. Symptoms and signs are produced by the local mass effect of the tumor or by secondary effects such as edema and obstruction of the flow of CSF.

1. General or secondary effect - The increased intracranial pressure produced by any space-occupying intracranial mass leads to the classic triad of (1) headache, commonly located in the vertex, worse in the morning after prolonged recumbency, and frequently relieved by standing up; (2) nausea and vomiting; and (3) papilledema. Increased intracranial pressure may also cause personality changes, convulsions, cranial nerve palsies, and even homonymous hemianopsia as the posterior cerebral artery passing over the edge of the tentorium is compressed by the tense brain. These signs and symptoms, then, are not necessarily of localizing or even lateralizing value since they can be produced by pressure alone. The focal signs of the brain tumor depend upon its location (e.g., temporal lobe, cerebellum, third ventricle) and on whether it is situated on the surface or in the deeper tissues.

   The most common presenting complaint is also dependent upon the location of the tumor, its cell type, rapidity of growth, etc. Whether the presenting complaint is headache, convulsions, hemiparesis, or visual or gait disturbances, it is imperative to determine if there is a history of progression - no matter how rapid or slow - as it is progression of symptomatology which justifies the strong suspicion of brain tumor and the confirmatory studies outlined below.

2. Focal effects - In diagnosing brain tumors, one asks first where the lesion is and second what type of lesion it is. The clinical manifestations of tumors in various locations in the brain are discussed below as a guide to determining where the lesion is; the remainder of this section will be devoted to brief discussions of individual types of tumors as a guide to determining what type of lesion it may be.
   a. Frontal lobe - Involvement of the frontal lobes usually produces personality changes (inappropriate behavior, loss of social inhibitions) and mental changes. These findings are easily confused with those produced by increased pressure, but if increased pressure is present there will also be headache, nausea and vomiting, and papilledema. If the posterior portions of the frontal lobe are involved, the patient may show forced grasping and, if the motor areas of the cortex or subcortical areas are involved, varying degrees of hemiparesis on the contralateral side, increased deep tendon reflexes, and a positive Babinski reflex; if the tumor is in the dominant frontal lobe, expressive aphasia may be manifest. If convulsions occur they are frequently of the adversive type (head and eyes turned toward the side opposite the lesion). Tumors arising anteriorly beneath the frontal lobes may cause anosmia.
   b. Parietal lobe - Involvement of the parietal lobe tends to produce contralateral paralysis accompanied by defects in the appreciation of the weight, texture, size, and shape of objects. Ability to perceive and localize pinprick on the side of the body opposite the lesion may be impaired (astereognosis). Parasagittal tumors (involving the paracentral area) may cause spastic paralysis of the contralateral leg or, as the tumor enlarges, paraplegia and urinary incontinence. Tumors low in the parietal area may produce visual field defects. If the dominant hemisphere is involved, global aphasia will be present.
   c. Occipital lobe - Occipital lobe tumors are relatively uncommon. Visual field defects are the major symptom, and tend to be more congruous than visual field defects produced by lesions in the temporal lobe. (Complete homonymous hemianopsia has no localizing value since it can be produced by a lesion anywhere from the chiasm to the occipital lobe.) Isolated visual hallucinations may occur, or they may appear as part of a generalized seizure.
   d. Temporal lobe - "Temporal lobe seizures" are a common manifestation of temporal lobe tumors. There may be classical uncinate fits accompanied by unpleasant olfactory sensations, often with lip smacking and loss of contact with surroundings. A generalized seizure may follow. The seizure may take the form of momentary episodes of staring of which the patient is not aware, a feeling of unreality, and extreme familiarity (déjà vu) or unfamiliarity with surroundings at the time of the attack. Distorted perceptions of sounds, objects, sizes, or

shapes may be noted. Visual field defects are common and tend to be incongruous. If the dominant temporal lobe is involved, receptive aphasia or auditory agnosia may occur.

e. Posterior fossa - Tumors in the posterior fossa produce early symptoms by involvement of the cerebellum, brain stem, and cranial nerves, and, as a rule, by obstruction of the flow of CSF.
   (1) Cerebellum - A tumor arising in a hemisphere of the cerebellum causes ataxia of gait and incoordination of the ipsilateral arm and leg. Nystagmus is common. The principal manifestation of a tumor involving primarily the midline of the cerebellum is often ataxia of the trunk, with unsteadiness and falling even while sitting; incoordination of the arms is less frequent. Cranial nerve palsies, particularly of those nerves innervating the extraocular muscles, are prone to occur.
   (2) Brain stem (intramedullary) tumors produce increased intracranial pressure late; the most common symptoms and signs are multiple cranial nerve palsies, nystagmus, and incoordination and paresis of extremities.
   (3) Cerebellopontine angle tumors (presenting in the angle formed by the petrous ridge, tentorium, cerebellum, and brain stem) - The vast majority arise from the vestibular portion of the eighth cranial nerve (e.g., "perineural fibroblastoma," neurinomas, neurilemmomas). The classical symptomatology is tinnitus on the involved side followed by nerve deafness. Involvement of the seventh cranial nerve produces facial palsy; involvement of the fifth cranial nerve may give rise to numbness or paresthesias in the face and loss of the corneal reflex. Involvement of the cerebellum causes ataxia, dysmetria, and nystagmus.
   (4) The midbrain is usually involved secondarily by tumors arising from nearby structures (e.g., the pineal gland), but may be involved directly. Tumors in the pineal region frequently produce direct pressure on the roof structures of the midbrain, difficulty in upward gaze (Parinaud's syndrome), and impairment of the pupillary light reflex; involvement of the red nucleus area produces ataxia, incoordination, and intention tremor.

f. Sellar region - Tumors arising in the pituitary gland may produce hyperfunction of portions of the gland (acromegaly) or, more commonly, hypofunction, leading to loss of libido, pubic and axillary hair, etc. Appropriate laboratory tests confirm the hypopituitarism. As sellar tumors enlarge they encroach on the optic chiasm and produce a characteristic bitemporal hemianopsia.

B. Special Examinations:

1. Pneumoencephalography - With the patient in the sitting position and usually under local anesthesia, a spinal puncture is carried out and a measured amount of air is introduced (and a comparable amount of fluid withdrawn) to adequately fill the ventricular system and subarachnoid pathways to give good visualization of the intracranial structures. Mul-

tiple x-rays are taken of the skull in varying positions. This test is never used if intracranial pressure is known to be increased.

2. Ventriculography - Utilizing local anesthesia, bur holes are placed in symmetric positions, 4 cm. to each side of the midline in the posterior parietal region, and special needles introduced into the atrial region of the lateral ventricles. Air is then exchanged for the fluid and multiple x-rays are taken with the skull in various positions. This test is used when there is increased intracranial pressure.
3. Carotid and/or vertebral angiography - The appropriate artery is injected with a contrast medium (50% Hypaque®) while serial x-rays are rapidly taken. This test is used to localize the tumor, either by indicating a tumor "blush," or by inference, indicating which arteries or veins are shifted out of their normal position. More recently, with the availability of image intensification and catheter technics, selective opacification of the individual cerebral vessels (i.e., internal or external carotid) is possible, and it results in less morbidity and greater accuracy in diagnosis.
4. Radioactive brain scan - A radioactive isotope of Hg, As, technetium, or iodinated serum albumin, for example, is injected intravenously and the head is subsequently scanned by a scintillation counter, positron camera, or other technic. A positive localizing diagnosis can be made in about 85% of cases depending upon the type and location of the tumor.
5. Electroencephalography - This is helpful in the recognition of certain brain tumors involving the cerebrum since it may indicate a focal pathologic process. The localization thus arrived at is never accurate enough for purposes of surgical treatment.

Treatment of Brain Tumors.

In general, the treatment of all brain tumors is surgical exploration and excision through a craniotomy or craniectomy centered as accurately as possible over the tumor. The tumor should be completely removed if this can be done without producing a serious neurologic deficit. If total removal is not possible, subtotal removal should be as radical as is feasible for the purpose of decompression. If the location of the tumor precludes direct surgical attack (e.g., third ventricle or pontine) and it blocks the flow of CSF, shunting of the CSF from the lateral ventricles to the cisterna magna (Torkildsen procedure) should be carried out. Postoperative x-ray radiation may be of considerable value in some tumors and of no value in others. Chemotherapy of primary and metastatic brain tumors, although still in the experimental stage, shows promise.

INTRACRANIAL GLIOMAS

All tumors which arise from the interstitial cells of the CNS are included in this category.

Glioblastoma Multiforme.

Glioblastoma multiforme (about 25% of gliomas), the most malignant of all primary tumors of the brain, arises in the white matter, grows rapidly, and has a strong tendency to cross to the opposite hemisphere. These tumors are highly cellular and pleomorphic, with many mitoses. The most common sites of occurrence are the frontal, parietal, and temporal lobes, and the highest incidence is in the age group from 40 to 60.

Glioblastoma multiforme can rarely (if ever) be completely removed, and is resistant to x-ray therapy. Life expectancy is usually less than 1 year after diagnosis.

Astrocytoma.

Astrocytomas make up approximately 35% of all gliomas. They are composed of adult astrocytes, are relatively slow-growing, and frequently blend diffusely with the surrounding brain. In children they occur predominantly in the cerebellar hemisphere and are often cystic. In adults, astrocytoma occurs most often in the frontal, parietal, and temporal lobes.

In adults these tumors are often impossible to remove completely, as they extend into vital deep structures. Most astrocytomas are not radiosensitive, and survival is usually only 3-6 years. Survival may be extended by reoperation. Cystic or solid cerebellar astrocytomas can often be completely excised, and recurrence is uncommon.

Medulloblastoma.

Medulloblastomas comprise about 10% of all gliomas. They occur almost exclusively in children 4-8 years of age, usually boys (3:1). They are composed of small, round, deeply staining cells, arise from the lateral wall or roof of the fourth ventricle, and frequently seed to other parts of the nervous system.

Complete surgical removal is not possible. These tumors are initially radiosensitive and literally "melt" with the first full course of treatment. However, they become radioresistant, and survival beyond 5 years is not common.

Ependymomas.

Ependymomas (about 10% of gliomas) arise most commonly in the wall and floor of the fourth ventricle, but can arise in the lateral ventricles.

Complete removal, particularly of those in the fourth ventricle, is rarely possible, and operative mortality is high. With subtotal removal, however, a survival span of 5 years is not uncommon. Ependymomas arising from the choroid plexus in the lateral ventricles may be totally removable.

Ependymomas are amenable to x-ray therapy.

Oligodendrogliomas.

Oligodendrogliomas (about 5% of gliomas) usually occur in adults. They are composed of uniform cells which have a "halo" around the nucleus and usually arise in the cerebral hemispheres.

Total removal is frequently not possible, and the cells are relatively radioresistant. Average survival is 3-7 years.

Pinealomas.

Pinealomas (2-3% of gliomas) usually occur in young adults and block the flow of CSF early. Surgical removal has an extremely high mortality rate. The treatment of choice is to shunt the CSF around the block (Torkildsen procedure) and administer x-ray therapy. The prognosis for survival is 3-10 years.

MENINGIOMAS

Meningiomas arise from arachnoidal "cap cells" or from stromal cells of the pia arachnoid and dura. The course is usually prolonged and slowly progressive. Meningiomas occur predominantly in the 40-60 age group and frequently produce changes in the overlying bone. Since meningiomas involve the cerebral cortex early in their growth, convulsive seizures are often the first manifestation of their presence. Characteristic locations (in descending order of frequency) are as follows:

A. Parasagittal: Anterior parasagittal meningiomas produce predominantly headache and personality change. Mid-parasagittal meningiomas produce a classic picture of paresis of the contralateral foot with or without cortical sensory change, incontinence of urine, and seizures beginning in the contralateral foot. Posterior parasagittal meningiomas produce headache and visual field defects.

B. Over the Convexity of the Cerebral Hemisphere: Symptoms depend upon the location, but in general these tumors are anteriorly situated and produce mental changes and motor power loss. Tumors in the mid area produce motor and sensory loss, and posteriorly situated tumors produce sensory and visual field losses.

C. Sphenoid Ridge: Meningiomas along the inner third of the sphenoid ridge cause extraocular muscle palsies and visual loss, with optic atrophy. Meningiomas along the middle third of the ridge usually attain a large size before significant symptoms are produced. Ultimate encroachment on the temporal lobe causes temporal lobe fits; encroachment into the frontal lobe produces mental changes. A meningioma occurring along the outer third of the ridge often grows as a flat plate of tumor (en plaque) and produces progressive exophthalmos and a palpable mass in the temporal region.

D. Olfactory Groove: These usually become quite large before clinical manifestations appear (anosmia and personality changes).

E. Less common locations are suprasellar, in the posterior fossa, and in the region of the gasserian ganglion.

Treatment.

Surgical removal is indicated in all cases. Meningiomas are benign tumors, and complete removal is often possible. Even with subtotal removal the prognosis is good.

TUMORS OF THE CRANIAL NERVES

Cranial nerve tumors arise from the sheath of the nerve (schwannomas, neurinomas, and perineural fibroblastomas). The great majority arise from the eighth cranial nerve at the internal auditory meatus (so-called acoustic tumors or cerebellopontine angle tumors).

Total surgical removal is indicated if possible. Where total removal is not possible (because the capsule is intimately adherent to the brain stem), the prognosis with subtotal removal may still be good since some of these tumors grow very slowly. Reoperation can be done when symptoms recur, but the operative mortality is much higher with the second operation.

TUMORS OF THE INTRACRANIAL BLOOD VESSELS

Hemangiomas.

Hemangiomas are actually only malformations with no neoplastic elements, e.g., capillary telangiectasia, which may be multiple and associated with telangiectasis of the skin (Sturge-Weber syndrome). They usually occur in the pons and are usually clinically silent, although occasionally they may produce symptoms if the malformation ruptures or obstructs the flow of CSF. Surgery is indicated only if CSF obstruction occurs with later signs, and consists of bypassing the obstruction with a shunting procedure (ventriculocisternostomy; Torkildsen procedure).

Hemangioblastomas.

These are true neoplasms formed by proliferation of angioblasts. They are usually found in the cerebellum in adults. If there is associated hemangioblastoma of the retina, the disorder is called Lindau-von Hippel disease. Hemangioblastomas in the cerebellum frequently produce a large cyst filled with thick yellow fluid with the tumor represented in the wall of the cyst as a small mural nodule. Symptoms are those of a cerebellar lesion (see p. 698).

Surgical removal of the mural nodule is curative. Solid tumors are difficult to excise completely, and the prognosis is less favorable.

CONGENITAL INTRACRANIAL TUMORS

Craniopharyngioma (Rathke Pouch Cyst).

Craniopharyngiomas are the most common congenital brain tumors (3-4% of all brain tumors). They arise from epithelial cell rests in the region of the infundibular stalk, and consist of squamous epithelium or epithelium of the type seen in developing tooth buds (also called adamantinomas). The cyst may become quite large. Deposits of calcium above the sella turcica can often be seen by x-ray. Symptoms are produced by compression of neighboring structures, and consist of endocrine disorders, visual field defects, and optic atrophy. If the cyst encroaches on the third ventricle, increased intracranial pressure produces headache, nausea and vomiting, and papilledema.

Treatment is by surgical removal, although in the majority of instances total removal is not possible as the capsule is adherent to the hypothalamus or the carotid artery. Aspiration of the cyst and subtotal removal of the capsule carries a low operative mortality, but symptoms soon recur. The long-term prognosis is poor.

Epidermoid Cysts (Pearly Tumors, Cholesteatomas).

Epidermoid cysts arise from embryonic epidermal cells, and are composed of a glistening white fibrous capsule (looks like mother-of-pearl) and squamous epithelium; the center of the cyst is filled with grumous material and cholesterol crystals. Symptoms are usually delayed until adulthood. The cysts tend to occur near the midline.

Treatment is by complete surgical removal, when possible. If the wall is adherent to some vital structure, complete surgical removal is not possible, but long-term survivals have been reported even with incomplete removals.

Dermoids.

These resemble epidermoids but contain dermal structures, e.g., sebaceous glands and hair follicles. Treatment is as for epidermoid cyst.

Teratomas.

Teratomas are derived from 3 germinal layers and may contain caricatures of the structures usually derived from these layers. Symptoms usually occur in childhood, and the lesion may attain huge size.

Where complete removal is possible the prognosis is good; the prognosis is poor if, as is more often the case, the tumor cannot be completely removed.

Chordomas.

These rare, slow-growing neoplasms are persistent remnants of primitive notochord which occur in characteristic location along the base of the sphenoid beneath the pons and extending into the middle fossa and cerebellopontine angle. They produce multiple cranial nerve palsies combined with long tract signs from the pressure on the pons. Marked erosion of the base of the skull is usually visible on basilar x-rays.

Total removal is rarely possible, and the prognosis is poor.

Paraphysial Cysts of the Third Ventricle.

These tumors, located in the anterior portion of the third ventricle and attached to the roof of the ventricle by a stalk, are thought to be derived from the paraphysis. They are cystic, smooth-walled, and lined by cuboidal epithelium. Symptoms are produced by intermittent blockage of flow of CSF through the foramen of Monro. Since the cyst hangs from a stalk, changes in body position may produce (or relieve) sudden violent headache.

Surgical removal is carried out by a transcortical approach to the lateral ventricle and then through the foramen of Monro to reach the third ventricle. The prognosis is good.

Pituitary Tumors.

Pituitary tumors arise from the anterior lobe and may be composed of any of 3 cell types: chromophobic, chromophilic or eosinophilic, and basophilic.

A. Chromophobe adenomas comprise the great majority of pituitary tumors. They are composed of chromophobe cells which have no known secretory function and therefore produce symptoms by compressing the secretory cells of the anterior pituitary; this causes signs of hypopituitarism: loss of libido, decreased cold tolerance, pale skin, and loss of axillary and pubic hair. As the tumor enlarges it balloons the sella turcica to give a characteristic x-ray enlargement and compresses the optic chiasm to produce bitemporal hemianopsia, usually the presenting symptom. The diagnosis can usually be made easily on the basis of the appearance of the patient and visual field and x-ray changes. Laboratory tests can be used to confirm the presence and degree of hypopituitarism.

The primary objective of therapy is to preserve vision. These tumors respond well to x-ray therapy, and in those cases where no visual field involvement is present radiation therapy is the treatment of choice. However, the visual fields should be checked daily during the course of radiation treatment; if the tumor swells and produces visual field defects, surgical removal of the tumor is indicated. Radiation therapy can be utilized postoperatively. In those cases with slight visual field changes it may be difficult to decide whether therapy should be by radiation or surgery. If radiation is chosen, the visual field should be checked daily.

Total removal of these tumors is not often possible, but subtotal removal and radiation therapy offer a very good prognosis.

B. Eosinophilic adenomas which develop before closure of the epiphyses cause gigantism; those which develop in adult life cause acromegaly. They rarely attain sufficient size to produce significant visual field defects. Radiation therapy was formerly the treatment of choice, but it rarely provided longstanding improvement. Surgical treatment by transsphenoidal cryogenic hypophysectomy or hypophysectomy by transfrontal craniotomy is replacing radiation therapy.

C. Basophilic adenomas rarely reach sufficient size to produce local pressure symptoms, and are usually part of a polyglandular involvement producing Cushing's syndrome. They may be removed by hypophysectomy.

Von Recklinghausen's Neurofibromatosis.

This is a heredofamilial disorder characterized by (1) café-au-lait spots, (2) multiple neurofibromas on the peripheral, sympathetic, spinal, and cranial nerves, and (3) multiple brain tumors of all types: meningiomas, neurinomas, gliomas, etc. There is no effective therapy for the disease as a whole, but individual tumors causing disabling symptoms may have to be surgically removed. The long-term prognosis is poor.

INTRASPINAL NEOPLASMS

Intraspinal neoplasms may occur at any level of the cord from the foramen magnum to the sacral canal. The greatest number occur in the thoracic area, as this is the longest subdivision of the cord. They may arise from the spinal cord or its investing sheaths, the nerves or their sheaths, bone, cartilage, fat, blood vessels, fibrous tissue, or as metastatic lesions. Intraspinal neoplasms may occur at any age, but are rare in persons under 10.

These tumors may be grouped for descriptive anatomic purposes as follows: (1) Those arising within the spinal canal and extending extraspinally (or vice versa) through a vertebral foramen (dumbbell tumors); (2) those arising within the spinal canal but not invading the dura or cord (intraspinal extradural tumors); (3) those arising within the dura but not invading the spinal cord (intradural extramedullary tumors); and (4) those arising entirely within the substance of the cord (intramedullary tumors).

In general, the same types of tumors are found in the spinal canal as in the cranial vault, but the frequency of occurrence of individual tumor types is quite different: neurofibromas, 31%; meningiomas, 28%; intramedullary gliomas, 23%; and all others, 18%.

Since 60-70% of intraspinal tumors are benign, early diagnosis and treatment are essential before irreparable spinal cord damage has occurred.

Clinical Findings.

A history of pain in the back with radiation into dermatomal patterns, accompanied by sensory and/or motor loss of a root or long tract type, leads to a clinical diagnosis of spinal cord tumor. When these symptoms are rapidly progressive, surgical treatment is urgent. **This constitutes one of the most important emergencies in neurologic surgery.**

A. History: One of the most important diagnostic findings is a history of more or less relentless progression. It is imperative to establish (1) whether symptoms began abruptly and have not changed significantly since onset, in which case an intraspinal tumor can be ruled out; (2) whether symptoms began abruptly and since that time have been marked by considerable exacerbation and intervals of remission, as one would expect in multiple sclerosis; or (3) whether the onset was vague but progression since onset has been more or less steady, as one would expect in spinal cord tumor.

B. Symptoms and Signs: One of the earliest symptoms of spinal cord tumor is radicular pain, i.e., pain produced by direct or indirect pressure or traction on the posterior (sensory) nerve roots. The pain is often experienced in a peripheral area of the dermatome supplied by the root or roots involved, e.g., tumors of the cervical region may cause pain in the shoulder, arm, or hand. In order to avoid an incorrect diagnosis of disease underlying the point of pain, the physician must secure a careful description of the type of pain. Radicular pain has the following rather distinct characteristics: (1) It is often restricted to the involved dermatomes; (2) it is severe, sharp, and stabbing, superimposed on a background of continuous dull, aching pain; and (3) it is made worse by coughing, sneezing, or straining, worse at night after prolonged recumbency, and temporarily relieved by activity. Paresthesias and/or dysesthesias are variously described as numbness, coldness, tingling, and hot or crawling sensations, also in a radicular pattern.

The sensory loss may follow a root pattern at the level at which the roots are involved by the tumor; and the sensory loss below this level, if present, is of a spinal cord type, i.e., it produces a distinct level of sensory loss with often greater involvement of 1 modality of sensation than another. Motor involvement may be of the upper motor neuron type, i.e., spasticity, hyperreflexia, and extensor plantar response; or of the lower motor neuron type if the tumor involves the cauda equina.

Hesitancy in urination is a frequent early sign of pressure on the spinal cord.

C. X-ray Findings: X-rays of the spine frequently give additional evidence of the presence of a tumor, i.e., erosion, calcium deposition in the tumor, increase in the interpedicular distances, enlargement of the intervertebral foramens, collapse of vertebrae, etc. The diagnosis can be confirmed by positive contrast myelography (see p. 693).

Caution: If in carrying out the preliminary spinal tap a total manometric block is discovered and a block is found to the flow of the contrast material, no attempt should be made to remove the medium since removal of spinal fluid from below the block may lead to "jamming" or descent of the tumor and immediately increase the neurologic deficit.

Treatment and Prognosis.

Surgical exploration and excision is indicated in every case. Most benign tumors can be removed completely. The prognosis for return of function depends upon the location of the tumor, whether it can be removed completely, and the severity and duration of neurologic deficit prior to diagnosis. The prognosis in intramedullary tumors is more guarded, as the hazard of increasing the neurologic deficit rarely permits complete removal. Postoperative x-ray therapy may be beneficial in diminishing the mass of these tumors and preventing further neurologic losses.

METASTATIC INTRASPINAL TUMORS

The spinal cord is not infrequently involved secondarily by metastases to the bones of the spinal column or to the epidural space. These lesions produce secondary compression of the spinal cord and paraplegia. When obvious compression of the spinal cord occurs, laminectomy and decompression should be seriously considered. The patient's general condition and life expectancy, taking into account other metastases and the type and location of the primary tumor, may contraindicate laminectomy. In general, if the patient's life expectancy is felt to be more than several weeks and his general condition is good, decompressive laminectomy is indicated.

PERIPHERAL NERVE TUMORS

Perineural Fibroblastomas.

The most common tumors of the peripheral nerves are those arising in supporting tissue (perineural fibroblastomas). They are usually solitary, well encapsulated, and benign, and may be of any size. Diagnosis is usually suggested by a mass in the periphery. Symptoms include paresthesia or hypesthesia; with tumors of mixed or pure sensory nerves, percussion over the tumor frequently elicits tingling (Tinel's sign). Malignant change (sarcoma) occurs only rarely.

Treatment is by surgical removal. In many cases it is relatively easy to remove the tumor completely from its capsule; in other instances removal may be quite difficult and may cause permanent impairment of function.

Neurofibromas.

Neurofibromas are composed of all the elements of peripheral nerves (axis cylinders, myelin sheaths, and connective tissue).

These may appear as solitary lesions but most commonly are multiple, occurring as part of von Recklinghausen's neurofibromatosis. Multiple excision is rarely indicated, as these tumors cannot be shelled out and surgical removal requires interruption of the continuity of the nerve trunk.

Sarcomatous change (neurogenic sarcoma) is more common in neurofibromas than in sheath tumors. Although neurogenic sarcoma may not be distinguishable clinically from the benign tumors except for the rapidity of its growth, at surgery its sarcomatous characteristics are demonstrated by infiltration of surrounding structures. Distant metastases also occur.

CEREBROVASCULAR DISEASE

Surgical disorders of the cerebral blood vessels produce their clinical effects by 1 of 2 pathologic processes: (1) Occlusion, leading to ischemia, and (2) hemorrhage.

CEREBRAL ISCHEMIA

Any area of the brain may be involved by an ischemic process produced by (1) partial occlusion of an extracranial or intracranial vessel as a result of narrowing of the vessel by atheromatous plaques and/or progressive thrombus formation on these plaques; (2) complete occlusion, usually at the site of atheromatous plaques; or (3) by embolization. These processes occur most commonly at the point of bifurcation of the common carotid artery into the internal and external carotid arteries; at the bifurcation of the internal carotid artery into the middle and anterior cerebral arteries; at the point of origin of the common carotid artery from the aortic arch or innominate artery; and at the point of origin of the vertebral artery. Symptoms are often produced by each new deposition of thrombus as the lumen closes or by episodes of relative hypotension. In the early stages, these attacks are frequently transient and have been termed "little strokes." Symptoms may develop slowly but progressively via hours or days where there is a gradual thrombosis formation, or there may be a sudden and catastrophic onset of symptoms produced by embolization or sudden complete occlusion of the vessel.

Recent studies have indicated that about 15-20% of all cerebrovascular accidents are due to occlusive processes, either incomplete or complete, in the major extracranial vessels in the neck. Because these stenotic lesions are amenable to surgical treatment, diagnosis should be made as early as possible before permanent residuals have occurred.

Clinical Findings.

The diagnosis is suggested by (1) a history of any number of transient "little strokes"; (2) decreased pulsation of either carotid artery in the neck; (3) the presence of a bruit over either carotid bifurcation or over the take-off of the carotid and vertebral arteries low in the neck; and (4) symptoms referable to the area of the brain supplied by the vessels (see below). Ophthalmodynamometry (measurement of intraocular arterial pressure) may be diagnostic if the pressure in the retinal artery on the involved side is significantly lower than that on the other side. Cerebral arteriography is essential to establish the diagnosis. All 4 vessels (both carotid and both vertebral arteries) as well as their origins at the arch of the aorta should be visualized.

A. Internal Carotid Artery: Occlusion usually produces contralateral weakness, subjective numbness, ipsilateral blindness (from involvement of the ipsilateral ophthalmic artery in the temporary ischemic process), and, if the predominant hemisphere is involved, aphasia.
B. Middle Cerebral Artery: Usually the same symptomatology as total internal carotid insufficiency, but no blindness.
C. Anterior Cerebral Artery: Weakness and/or subjective numbness of the contralateral leg and occasionally the arm, and, not infrequently, reflex incontinence.
D. Posterior Cerebral Artery: Hemianopsia, scintillating scotomas, and, if bilateral, temporary cortical blindness.
E. Basilar Artery: Usually bilateral symptoms such as quadriparesis, bilateral paresthesias, ataxia, dysarthria, diplopia, dysphagia, blindness, and frequently unconsciousness.

Treatment.

There is no effective treatment for complete occlusions and no effective surgical treatment for intracranial involvement at the branches of the carotid or vertebral systems.

A. Medical Treatment: Long-term anticoagulant therapy in the hope of preventing further thrombus formation.
B. Surgical Treatment: In partial occlusions of the extracranial portions of the carotid or vertebral arterial systems, surgical therapy is aimed at restoring the blood flow to normal by thromboendarterectomy or bypass procedures. Visualization of the aortic arch and all 4 major vessels in the arch (4-vessel angiography) by catheter technics is a prerequisite for surgical endarterectomy.

CEREBRAL HEMORRHAGE

Spontaneous intracranial hemorrhage may be caused by hypertension, rupture of an intracranial aneurysm, rupture of an arteriovenous malformation, or hemorrhagic disorders. Of these, only hemorrhages due to aneurysms and arteriovenous malformations are of surgical importance. The hemorrhage may be subarachnoid (most common), intracerebral, or subdural (rare).

INTRACRANIAL ANEURYSMS

Most intracranial aneurysms are congenital and most occur on the anterior portion of the circle of Willis, usually at the point of bifurcation of the major arteries (e.g., carotid–posterior communicating). About 10-15% occur in branches of the basilar artery, including the posterior cerebral arteries. In approximately 20% of cases multiple aneurysms are present.

Clinical Findings.

Intracranial aneurysms produce symptomatology by 1 or all of the following processes: (1) Subarachnoid hemorrhage and, less frequently, intracerebral and subdural hemorrhage; (2) pressure on nearby structures, which most commonly produces cranial nerve palsies (third, fifth, second, fourth, and sixth) but may produce symptoms due to ischemia if the aneurysm partially occludes neighboring or parent arteries; and (3) distention of or pressure upon pain-sensitive structures, producing headache, usually orbital or supraorbital.

In subarachnoid hemorrhage due to rupture of an intracranial aneurysm, the mortality with the first episode of bleeding is 30-40%. These most commonly occur as a catastrophic illness in previously healthy individuals 20-40 years of age. The danger of a second hemorrhage is greatest within the first 3 weeks after the initial episode of bleeding. The mortality rate increases with successive hemorrhages. A sudden onset of severe headache with or without loss of consciousness is followed by signs of severe meningeal irritation (stiff neck, photophobia, diffuse headache, irritability, etc.). The diagnosis is established by lumbar puncture, which reveals homogeneously bloody fluid (see p. 673), usually under markedly increased pressure. The aneurysm may also rupture into the brain substance (intracerebral) and thereby produce profound neurologic loss (e.g., hemiplegia, aphasia), coma, or death.

Arteriograms should be taken immediately or as soon as the patient's condition permits.

Treatment.

A. General Measures: Absolute bed rest, maintenance of fluid intake, and mild analgesics to control headache and restlessness.

B. Surgical Measures: If surgical treatment is indicated it should be done as soon as the patient's condition permits.

1. Direct intracranial approach - Treatment is aimed at isolating the aneurysm from the circulation (without producing a neurologic deficit) by (1) clipping the neck of the aneurysm or (2) trapping the aneurysm without compromising the distal circulation of the parent vessel. For example, aneurysm of the anterior cerebral artery proximal to the communicating artery can be trapped by clipping the anterior cerebral artery proximal and distal to the aneurysm, thus leaving the distal anterior cerebral arterial supply intact by virtue of the blood crossing over through the anterior communicating artery. Direct intracranial surgical attack on these lesions has been greatly facilitated by the use of hypothermia.
2. Indirect surgical approach - The purpose of ligation of the carotid artery in the neck is to reduce the intraluminal pressure in the aneurysm and thus reduce the danger of subsequent hemorrhage. In general, this method of treatment is only applicable to aneurysms arising from the internal carotid artery below the circle of Willis, since the collateral circulation from the contralateral carotid artery will maintain high intraluminal pressure in aneurysms above the circle.

CEREBRAL ANGIOMAS

Cerebral angiomas are congenital lesions which may cause (1) subarachnoid or intracerebral hemorrhage (hemorrhage is far less common in angioma than in aneurysm); (2) recurrent convulsive seizures; (3) loss of function of adjacent brain, producing neurologic deficits such as hemiparesis and aphasia; or (4) progressive mental deterioration. Neurologic deficit may be due to hemorrhage, with subsequent gliosis and cyst formation; or shunting of the blood supply away from the brain tissue directly into the venous system, with resultant hypoxia, gliosis, etc.

The diagnosis is suggested by the history, the presence of an audible bruit over the lesion, and intracranial calcification on x-ray. Cerebral angiography is diagnostic.

The only effective method of treatment is surgical removal. The prognosis depends upon the size and site of the lesion (superficial or deep, in the dominant or nondominant hemisphere) and the presence and severity of the preoperative neurologic deficit.

INFECTIONS OF SCALP, BONE, AND BRAIN

PYOGENIC SCALP INFECTIONS

All pyogenic infections of the scalp should be treated vigorously, as there are abundant communications via the venous channels from the scalp to the diploic spaces of the calvaria and from these diploic spaces to the underlying dura, etc. Early and vigorous treatment of scalp infections by warm soaks and antibiotics should be employed to prevent the spread of infection to these deeper structures.

OSTEOMYELITIS OF THE SKULL

Osteomyelitis of the skull occurs most commonly (1) by direct implantation of bacteria into bone by trauma, or (2) by direct extension from infection in contiguous structures, e.g., scalp or sinuses.

A recent or remote history of head trauma or of infection in a nearby structure can usually be obtained, although onset of signs and symptoms may be delayed for a considerable period after the initial insult. Typical manifestations are headache, local evidence of inflammation around the involved area (with or without a draining sinus), and pain upon palpation of the involved area. Generalized systemic effects such as fever, leukocytosis, cervical or suboccipital lymphadenopathy, etc., may not be present. X-rays may be negative early, but later reveal the characteristic mottling or moth-eaten appearance.

Most cases of osteomyelitis can be prevented by proper debridement, sterile technic, and adequate initial therapy in trauma and by prompt treatment of infection of adjacent structures. Vigorous antibiotic therapy is indicated, and should be based on cultures and sensitivity tests. The original infection should also receive appropriate therapy. If the process continues to advance despite antibiotic therapy, all infected bone and a generous margin of normal bone should be excised. Direct instillation of the appropriate antibiotic may be helpful. Cranioplasty should be deferred until at least 6-12 months after all evidence of infection has disappeared.

EPIDURAL ABSCESS

Epidural abscess usually results from direct extension of an overlying infection, although hematogenous spread does occur. The classical findings in cranial epidural abscess are those of a rapidly enlarging space-occupying lesion in association with the symptoms and signs of systemic infection. Spinal abscesses cause sudden, excruciating pain accompanied by rapidly advancing motor paralysis of all functions below the level of the lesion.

This is a critical surgical emergency. In intracranial epidural abscess multiple bur holes are placed to effect complete drainage of all loculated areas. (Adherence of the dura to the suture lines may localize the abscess to a specific area.)

Appropriate antibiotics are given systemically and directly into the epidural space. In the spinal canal the abscess should be completely evacuated and the wound packed open and allowed to granulate in.

The prognosis for life and for the return of lost neurologic function depend upon the virulence of the infective organism and the promptness and vigor of surgical treatment.

SUBDURAL ABSCESS

Subdural abscess is usually the result of direct extension of infection from an overlying area, but may occur following rupture of an intracranial abscess into the subdural space. Since there are no limiting structures in the subdural space these abscesses extend over the entire hemisphere, under the brain, and into the interhemispheral fissure.

The clinical findings are those of a rapidly enlarging space-consuming lesion: lethargy, obtundation, paresis, coma, papilledema, etc. The diagnosis is based upon a history of primary infection and the finding of subdural pus on bur hole exploration.

Treatment is by placement of multiple bur holes so that every portion of subdural space over the hemisphere and in the interhemispheral fissure can be adequately drained. Massive systemic antibiotic therapy is indicated as well as direct instillation of antibiotic into multiple small polyethylene catheters left in the subdural space. The mortality is high.

INTRACEREBRAL ABSCESS

A variety of bacterial organisms as well as animal parasites, yeasts, fungi, and molds may cause intracerebral abscess. Eight out of 10 cases are due to direct extension of infection from the mastoid bone, paranasal sinuses, or middle ear. These cavities are expanded diploic spaces and so have thinned out inner and outer walls that offer slight resistance to the spread of infection. Abscesses caused by direct extension are usually single, whereas the 20% arising from distant sources by hematogenous spread are usually multiple. Half of those which are metastatic from distant foci originate in the lung (bronchiectasis or lung abscess).

Most abscesses begin in the area of least vascularity, about 10-20 mm. below the cortex. In those that originate by direct extension the infectious process incites an osteomyelitis which extends by suppurative retrograde thrombophlebitis along the diploic veins to involve the dura. The underlying arachnoid becomes involved in the inflammatory process and becomes sealed off to prevent lateral spread; the infectious process thus proceeds into brain tissue and the intracerebral abscess forms. During the initial acute stage, the infection is not well sealed off by the brain and cerebritis results. As the process becomes localized, a pseudocapsule develops and gradually is transformed into a true capsule composed of astrocytes and fibroblasts. The surrounding cerebritis and edema subside, and the abscess becomes a chronic one, acting as a space-consuming lesion.

Clinical Findings.

A history of infection of the ears or sinuses, or of a systemic infection, is most important. In a typical case the signs of the original infection in those areas may begin to subside only to be followed by convulsions, increasing headache, and paresis, with progressive lethargy. In the acute phase the patient is toxic with fever, leukocytosis, and an elevated CSF cell count. In the chronic phase, as the process is walled off by the capsule, the toxic symptoms are replaced by signs of a space-consuming lesion. Lumbar puncture may reveal elevation of cell count and protein, but should not be done in the presence of papilledema.

The diagnosis is confirmed by air studies or arteriography. Because the present widespread indiscriminate use of antibiotics frequently masks the characteristic progression of signs and symptoms from the acute through the chronic phases, the possibility of intracerebral abscess must always be kept in mind.

Treatment.

In the acute phase massive treatment with appropriate antibiotics must be given promptly. In the subacute stage, if suppuration is occurring and the infection is well localized, the abscess cavity can be tapped through a bur hole, the pus aspirated, and 1-2 ml. of contrast material such as iophendylate (Pantopaque®) instilled into the cavity. As the macrophages in the wall of the abscess begin to take up the medium, the exact size and location of the abscess can be seen by x-ray; if subsequent tapping or direct instillation of antibiotics is required, the area can thus be accurately cannulated. The abscess may have to be tapped several times during convalescence.

After recovery the abscess wall should be resected if this will not produce a neurologic deficit. In chronic, well-encapsulated abscess, total excision is the treatment of choice.

PAIN

The neurosurgeon is frequently called upon to carry out a pain-relieving surgical procedure for the purpose of relieving chronic pain of known or unknown origin. Every effort must be made to determine the cause of the pain, and every patient who complains of chronic pain which does not have an apparent cause or does not fall into a well-established clinical category must be thoroughly evaluated from the psychiatric point of view before surgery is considered.

The most common painful syndromes requiring surgical pain-relieving procedures are trigeminal neuralgia, glossopharyngeal neuralgia, post-herpetic neuralgia, and pain produced by advanced malignancies.

TRIGEMINAL NEURALGIA
(Tic Douloureux, Trifacial Neuralgia)

The etiology of trigeminal neuralgia is not known. It occurs most commonly in the age group from 40-60.

The type of pain in trigeminal neuralgia is characteristic. It occurs without warning in the distribution of any of the major branches of the trigeminal nerve, and is severe, lancinating, "bright" pain. Each pain is a brief short jab, but attacks frequently come in flurries.

The third division of the fifth cranial nerve is most commonly involved. The paroxysms of pain are most frequent in the spring and fall, and there may be periods of remission lasting for many months. Most patients soon discover that there is an apparent "trigger" area somewhere about the face, mouth, or tongue. When this area is stimulated by touch, chewing, or a cold breeze, the paroxysm results. These patients understandably go to great lengths to avoid stimulating this "trigger" area and may refuse to eat, shave, talk, etc. It is imperative to remember that in true trigeminal neuralgia the pain is not steady or aching, there is no pain between attacks, and there is no loss of sensation in any division of the trigeminal nerve. If there is a demonstrable loss of sensation over the trigeminal distribution, the pain is more likely caused by a tumor in or near the gasserian ganglion.

Treatment.

In the vast majority of cases of true tic douloureux, the pain can be permanently relieved by section of the sensory root of the fifth nerve. However, this leaves the face on the side of the operation permanently anesthetized, and since the cornea on that side is also anesthetized the risk of keratitis must be considered. Surgery should therefore be done only as a last resort and more conservative measures tried first.

A. Conservative Measures:

1. Medical treatment - Diphenylhydantoin sodium (Dilantin Sodium®), 100 mg. ($1\frac{1}{2}$ gr.) t. i. d.-q. i. d. for at least 2 weeks, should be given a trial in all cases, since a significant number of patients report at least temporary relief on this regimen. Carbamazepine (Tegretol®), a relatively new

pharmacologic agent, appears to be effective in controlling the paroxysms of pain in well over 80% of cases.

2. Alcohol block - If the above measures are ineffective, alcohol blocks of the involved division or divisions of the trigeminal nerve should be carried out. The mandibular division is blocked at the foramen ovale, the maxillary division at the foramen rotundum; the only part of the first or ophthalmic division which can be blocked is the supraorbital nerve where it exits in the supraorbital ridge. Alcohol block renders the nerve functionless for varying periods. Relief following the first block frequently lasts 12-24 months, but with each succeeding block the scarring produced about the nerve makes it more difficult to obtain a good block, and relief may last several months or there may be no relief. After 2 alcohol blocks the patient should be advised to undergo surgery.

B. Surgical Measures: The surgical treatment of choice is intracranial section of the sensory root of the trigeminal nerve through the subtemporal approach. Some surgeons advocate compression of the ganglion, exposing and vigorously rubbing but not cutting the ganglion and posterior root; it has been found that this relieves the pain in a significant number of patients and prevents facial and corneal anesthesia. If pain recurs, sectioning of the root is indicated. If the pain is limited to the second and third divisions, subtotal section of the sensory root can be carried out in an attempt to preserve the fibers carrying sensation to the cornea. The prognosis is excellent; in true tic douloureux, complete relief can be obtained in over 95% of cases.

GLOSSOPHARYNGEAL NEURALGIA

The pain of glossopharyngeal neuralgia is of the same type as described for trigeminal neuralgia, but is located in the distribution of the ninth cranial nerve, in the tonsillar fossa, and deep in the neck at the angle of the jaw on the affected side. The diagnosis can be easily confirmed by cocainizing the tonsillar fossa on the affected side; in true tic douloureux this immediately relieves the pain, and pain recurs after the local anesthetic has worn off. Intracranial section of the ninth and the upper 2 filaments of the tenth cranial nerves through a posterior fossa approach gives permanent relief. The prognosis is excellent.

POST-HERPETIC NEURALGIA

In a few cases of herpes zoster there is a persistent severe burning pain in the involved area after the infection has run its course. Chronic inflammatory changes have been shown to be present not only in the posterior root ganglion but also in the ascending pathways in the spinal cord and brain stem carrying the pain impulses. Because these changes are so widespread, surgical procedures designed to interrupt the pain-conducting pathways at a particular level are seldom successful. Relief has been obtained by undermining the skin in a wide margin around the involved area. (If the ophthalmic division of the fifth cranial nerve is involved, a large skin flap is elevated; if an intercostal or other area of the body is involved, the entire area is undercut.) In other cases relief has been obtained by various peripheral neurectomies. Because of the widespread inflammatory changes in the pain-conducting pathways, the simplest procedures should be tried first before resorting to cordotomy or tractotomy in the brain stem; and it may be necessary, as a last resort, to perform a restricted frontal leukotomy.

PAIN PRODUCED BY ADVANCED MALIGNANCIES

Severe pain becomes a problem as inoperable malignancies invade pain-sensitive structures. The pain produced is usually deep, boring, and steady, with sharp, stabbing pains at times superimposed. Relief can be given without loss of vital neurologic function by cutting the fibers responsible for pain transmission at an appropriate level in the peripheral or central nervous system.

Operations for relief of pain in cancer should not be thought of only as a last resort. As soon as chronic pain becomes a problem in operable malignancy, the patient should be evaluated as a candidate for pain-relieving surgery and a decision reached regarding which procedure offers the best chance for success. Large doses of narcotics over prolonged periods create the problem of addiction and induce an undesirable mental dullness and disinterest in life. As a general rule, if, in the clinician's opinion, the patient's life expectancy is longer than 3-6 months, a pain-relieving surgical procedure should be carried out as soon as the pain becomes significant.

The most frequently utilized operation is a cordotomy (spinothalamic tractotomy); the spinothalamic tract in the anterior quadrant of the spinal cord on the side opposite the pain is sectioned at the high thoracic or high cervical level. The patient thus loses the ability to perceive pain and thermal sensation on the contralateral side of the body below the level of the section. For purely unilateral pain involving the midline area, or for bilateral pain, bilateral cordotomy on the contralateral side is all that is required. For pelvic pain involving the midline area, or for bilateral pain, bilateral cordotomy is indicated. For relief of any pain below the level of the xyphoid, a thoracic cordotomy at the T1-T3 level may suffice. To relieve pain in the upper thorax or arm, the cordotomy should be carried out at the C1-C2 level; this "high cervical cordotomy" is favored by many neurosurgeons as the procedure of choice regardless of the level of pain.

It is now possible to accomplish localized destruction of the spinothalamic tract by means of percutaneous cordotomy. This entails inserting a small radio-frequency electrode directly into the anterolateral quadrant of the cord between the lamina of C1 and C2. A controlled lesion is then made by elevating the temperature of the cord by passage of the radio-frequency current through the electrode. This relatively simple and painless procedure has greatly extended the indications for spinothalamic tractotomy.

In pain involving the face, jaw, neck, or brachial plexus the pain fibers can be sectioned in the medulla at the level of the obex.

An alternative procedure is to section the trigeminal, glossopharyngeal, and upper filaments of the vagus nerves intracranially and the upper 3 or 4 posterior cervical roots on the side of the pain.

STEREOTAXIC SURGERY

Within the past several years it has become possible to destroy various nuclear masses and fiber tracts deep within the brain with a high degree of accuracy by utilizing a human stereotaxic apparatus. This consists of a rigid metal frame which can be temporarily firmly affixed to the patient's head by metal pins. Mounted on this frame is an electrode carrier. The electrode can then be inserted into the brain through a properly placed bur hole to any desired depth at any angle. Lesions can then be produced by electrocoagulation, cold and heat, or mechanically, and can be graduated to any size. The nuclear mass or fiber tract selected as the target is localized by use of a coordinate system derived from cadaver material, x-rays, and pneumoencephalography.

The field of stereotaxic surgery is relatively new, but an increasing number of conditions are now being attacked in this manner. The results to date are much better than those obtainable in the past with older technics.

At present, the major application of this technic is in the following conditions:

A. Hyperkinetic movement disorders, e.g., as in parkinsonism, dystonia musculorum deformans, and choreo-athetosis. Lesions are placed in the ventrolateral nucleus of the thalamus, and in the subthalamic region (H field of Forel) on the side of the brain opposite the side of the involved extremities. This operation can be carried out bilaterally if there are severe bilateral symptoms. The introduction of levodopa therapy has reduced the use of thalamotomy in Parkinson's disease, but thalamotomy is still the most effective treatment of the tremor. Surprisingly effective relief can be obtained from the tremor and rigidity in parkinsonism and from the hyperkinesias in dystonia musculorum deformans and choreo-athetosis in properly selected cases.

B. Pain Problems: In cases of advanced inoperable malignancy where the pain is too high to be relieved by standard pain-relieving technics or if more caudad interruptions of pain pathways have failed to give sufficient relief, selective destruction of the nuclear masses within the thalamus concerned with pain transmission has been attempted. When the affective component of the pain response is predominant, stereotaxic destruction of the cingulum or selected frontothalamic pathways has been effective.

C. Stereotaxic surgery of the pituitary gland is increasing in scope. The gland can be safely destroyed (completely or partially, as desired) by a simple stereotaxic approach to the sella turcica via the nose and sphenoid sinus. Such procedures are applicable to treatment of diabetic retinopathy, carcinoma of the breast, tumors of the pituitary gland itself, and other disorders.

19 . . .
Orthopedic Surgery

FRACTURES AND DISLOCATIONS OF THE SPINE

Traumatic injuries to the spine most commonly result from indirect violence such as hyperextension or hyperflexion mechanisms. Direct trauma without an open wound is more likely to cause fracture of the spinous process, and rarely of the lamina. Open fractures are usually due to penetrating injuries, especially those caused by firearms or military missiles.

Fractures of the spine may be classified according to their anatomic location (i.e., body, pedicle, lamina, or muscular process), but classification according to regional location is more useful since neurologic deficit resulting from cord injury depends upon the level at which injury occurs. Spinal injuries are thus classified here as cervical, thoracic, lumbar, sacral, or coccygeal.

In most cases of injury to the spine neither the spinal cord nor the nerve root is injured, but the possibility of such injury, especially in the cervical spine, is always present. Injury to the cord or nerve roots may result from displacement of bone fragments or spinal segments. Neurologic injury may occur at the time of injury or may be the result of subsequent manipulation. Since initial x-rays do not necessarily reflect the degree of displacement which may have occurred, severe neurologic deficit may be present even though only a minor fracture can be demonstrated. The greatest permanent disability caused by injury to the spine is due to associated injury to the spinal cord or the spinal nerves.

FRACTURES AND DISLOCATIONS OF THE CERVICAL SPINE

Concomitant injury to the cord or nerve roots can be expected in about 25% of cases of severe injury to the cervical spine. Fracture of the vertebral body, posterior displacement of fragments of the intervertebral disk, and dislocation account for most cord or nerve root injuries.

The diagnosis is suggested by a history of injury to the cervical spinal region and confirmed by careful physical examination and x-rays. Care must be taken to avoid manipulation of the neck during the initial examination or while making preliminary x-ray studies. If routine films do not confirm the suspected injury, special studies such as laminagraphy may be required. An accurate diagnosis is essential to plan rational treatment.

Compression Fracture of the Cervical Vertebral Body Without Dislocation.

In lateral x-rays compression fracture of the superior plate of the vertebral body without apparent forward dislocation of the segment above is apt to be demonstrated by a wedge-shaped deformity with the apex directed anteriorly. Although films may demonstrate no evidence of dislocation, the possibility of a prior dislocation with disruption of supporting ligaments and followed by spontaneous reduction should be considered.

Compression Fracture of the Cervical Vertebral Body With Dislocation.

Complete anterior dislocation of the cervical spine is observed most commonly with fracture, but may occur without fracture (see below). Compression of the superior plate of the body, with disruption of the intervertebral disk, dislocation of the facet joints, and tearing of the posterior ligaments, accounts for the major lesions. If the facet joints do not dislocate, fracture of the pedicles can permit dislocation.

The lesion can be corrected by unsustained axial traction on the head, but the deformity tends to recur when the force is discontinued. Continuous traction for 3-6 weeks is usually necessary before application of plaster or a brace to permit stabilization by the initial healing process. Because of the complications and discomfort associated with the use of head halter traction for prolonged periods of time, skeletal traction is the method of choice until the deformity has been reduced and stability attained.

Anterior Dislocation of the Cervical Spine.

Partial or complete anterior dislocation of the cervical spine may follow acute flexion injury to the neck. Although bone injury may not be present, disruption of the intervertebral disk and tearing of the interspinous ligaments and ligamentum flavum may occur and allow complete dislocation.

Complete dislocation occurs when the inferior articular processes of the dislocated segment above are displaced anterior to the superior articular process of the segment below. It is likely to be associated with cord injury. If the dislocated articular processes are locked, reduction is difficult even with skeletal traction.

If the inferior articular processes of the segment above are displaced forward but the articular surfaces of the facets remain in partial contact, the dislocation is termed incomplete, or a subluxation. It must be emphasized that x-rays may demonstrate only subluxation in cases where more extensive displacement has occurred but has partially reduced spontaneously since the injury. Any evidence of neurologic deficit should suggest that possibility.

Complete Unilateral Dislocation of the Cervical Spine.

Complete unilateral dislocation is characterized by torsional displacement in which the anatomic relationship of 1 facet joint remains undisturbed while the other is displaced. Closed methods of reduction may not be effective when dislocation is complete. Closed manipulation is hazardous and should be attempted only by a specialist. If treatment by skeletal traction is not successful, open reduction is indicated and should be done before healing makes repositioning impossible. Complete unilateral dislocation is commonly the result of severe injury, and cord damage should always be suspected.

Unilateral Subluxation of the Cervical Spine.

In adolescents unilateral cervical subluxation may occur spontaneously during sleep without appreciable trauma. Rotation of the head and lateral flexion of the neck toward the affected side are restricted, so that the patient holds his head tilted toward the opposite side. The lesion is best demonstrated by lateral stereoroentgenography. Reduction can usually be accomplished by gentle manual traction or by head halter traction using 5 lb. of weight for 24-48 hours. For a few days after reduction the neck should be immobilized and protected by a felt collar.

Atlanto-axial Dislocation in Children.

Spontaneous dislocation of the atlas and axis may occur as a complication of upper respiratory tract infection in children. Spontaneous restriction of active neck motions, irritability, and crying when the neck is examined even by gentle manipulation may alert the examiner to the need for further diagnostic studies, especially x-rays. Initial treatment should be by head halter traction; after the patient becomes ambulatory, bracing may be required. Immobilization should be continued, sometimes for a few weeks, until flexion and extension x-ray films made in the lateral projection demonstrate that stability has been recovered.

Posterior Dislocation of the Cervical Spine.

Posterior dislocation is a rare lesion which may be due to a blow on the forehead causing sudden, acute hyperextension of the neck such as may result from a severe rear-end automobile collision. It is usually associated with severe spinal cord injury.

Comminuted Fracture of the Cervical Vertebral Body.

Comminuted fracture of a cervical vertebral body may occur as a result of a heavy blow on the top of the head which drives the intervertebral disks above and below into the body, causing it to burst. Automobile and diving accidents are recognized causes of this injury. A posterior fragment of the centrum may impinge upon the spinal cord and cause severe injury. Immediate quadriplegia or paraplegia after the accident without prompt evidence of neurologic recovery are indications for emergency laminectomy (see p. 691). If laminectomy is performed, primary spine fusion may be desirable to provide added mechanical stability for the skeletal structures.

Closed treatment is by skull traction until stabilization takes place, usually in 4-8 weeks. The neck is then immobilized in a plaster Minerva jacket until healing is sound. This often takes more than 16 weeks.

Fractures and Fracture-Dislocations of the Atlas and Axis (Epistropheus).

The most common injury involving the first and second cervical vertebrae is fracture of the odontoid process, with anterior dislocation of the atlas with relation to the axis. When displacement occurs, the odontoid process is carried forward with the atlas, and

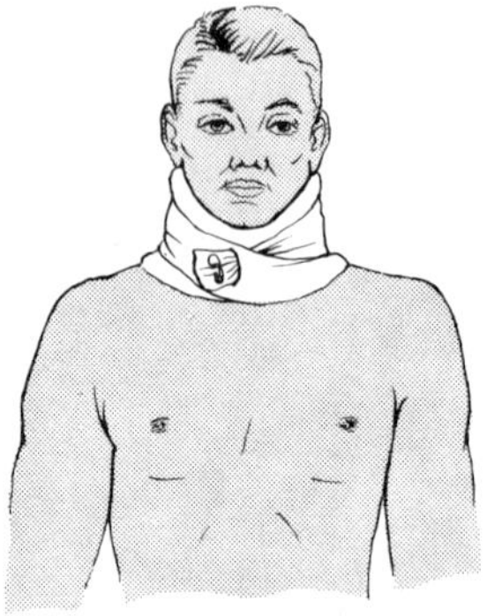

Cervical Collar

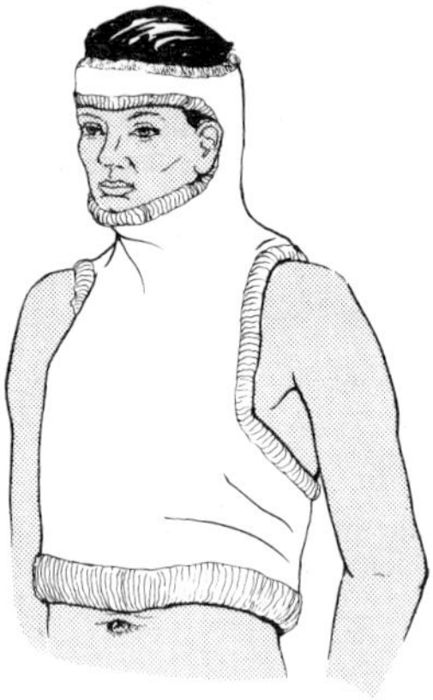

Minerva Jacket

this at least partially protects the cord from being crushed. Reduction can generally be accomplished by skull traction, but plaster immobilization must be maintained for at least 16 weeks since bony healing of the odontoid process is slow. Bony healing may not take place in spite of prolonged immobilization. Operative fusion of the atlas to the axis may be necessary to prevent displacement, with injury to the spinal cord.

Bursting fracture of the atlas (Jefferson's fracture) may also result from a blow on the top of the head. Displacement of the lateral mass takes place when the condyles of the occiput are driven into the atlas. If the spinal cord has not been injured and the fragments are not widely displaced, plaster immobilization for 12-16 weeks may be all that is required. Otherwise, skull traction for 4-8 weeks is required before immobilization in plaster.

Sprains of the Cervical Spine.

When the normal range of motion is exceeded suddenly, a sprain of the cervical spine may result. Cervical sprain occurs commonly in persons in a stationary or slow-moving vehicle that is struck suddenly from behind. The prominent clinical feature of this poorly understood lesion is dull, aching pain in the back of the neck. Pain may not be felt until a few hours after the injury has occurred, and is associated with muscle guarding and restriction of movement. The pain may radiate into the occipital or the interscapular region or down the arm. Posterior cervical tenderness is usually diffuse, and the site of pain poorly defined. If tenderness remains localized and persistent, the possibility of the presence of an occult fracture must be considered. If routine anteroposterior and lateral x-rays have been found to be negative, lateral flexion and extension films should be taken to determine the presence or absence of instability. Occasionally, laminograms will demonstrate an infraction of the lateral mass which cannot be demonstrated by routine x-ray technics. Patients with degenerative arthritis which preexisted the injury may demonstrate restriction of motion in the lower cervical segments. Where litigation or emotional lability is not a factor, symptoms generally respond promptly with conservative measures including immobilization with a cervical collar, radiant heat, massage, and analgesics. Prolonged treatment with diathermy or ultrasound may cause persistence and even accentuation of painful symptoms.

Reduction of Injuries to the Cervical Spine.

A. Skeletal Traction: The head halter is useful for the application of heavy traction for short periods, as may be required during manipulative reduction. In general, the head halter is not suitable for continuous traction because more than 7-8 lb. causes pain in the region of the chin or occiput. When halter traction is used for prolonged periods, the submental region should be carefully padded to prevent pressure necrosis of skin and ulceration. Skeletal traction applied to the skull or zygomatic arches will support 40 lb. of force over prolonged periods without discomfort. Various types of tongs (e.g., those of Barton, Crutchfield, or Roger Anderson) and wires (Hoen) have been designed for this purpose.

   After the skeletal apparatus has been applied, reduction is accomplished by increasing the force of traction under periodic physical examination and x-ray control. Once reduction has been achieved, the force is gradually reduced to 8-12 lb., which is usually sufficient to maintain reduction.

   If closed reduction is not successful, open reduction must be resorted to.

B. Open Reduction and Arthrodesis: When reduction cannot be accomplished by closed methods, open reduction may be successful. If open reduction is required it should be done early, especially if symptoms of cord injury are present (see p. 691).

FRACTURES OF THE THORACIC SPINE

The thoracic spine is comparatively stable. Fracture results either from direct violence, which may involve only a spinous process; or indirect violence, which may result in compression of the body of the vertebra. Occasionally an avulsion fracture of the spinous process of the seventh cervical or first thoracic vertebra is caused by muscle activity ("clay shovelers' fracture").

Compression fractures of the thoracic vertebrae are rare in young children and are caused only by severe trauma in older children. In this age group, therefore, unless there is a positive history of severe trauma, a wedge-shaped deformity in the thoracic spine should suggest pathologic fracture. This must not be confused with Calvé's or Scheuermann's disease or deformity due to traumatic fracture.

Minimal (frequently unrecognized) trauma may cause compression fracture of the body of the thoracic vertebrae in adults with osteoporosis. Disability is not great, and reduction is not indicated. If rest in bed for 3-4 days does not relieve the pain, a surgical corset with shoulder restraints or brace (Taylor or Arnold type) may provide comfort and permit early ambulation.

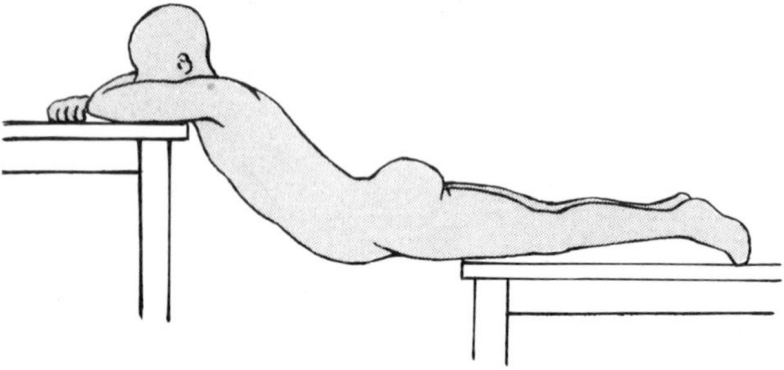

Watson-Jones Technic of Reduction of Compression
Fracture of the Lumbar Spine

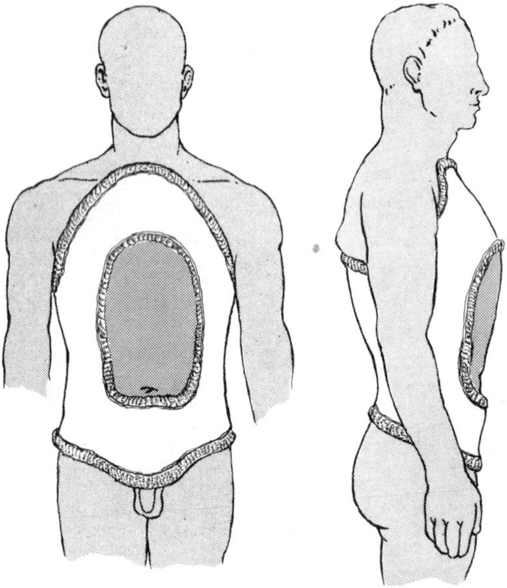

Hyperextension Plaster for Compression
Fracture of the Lumbar Spine

Compression fractures of the thoracic spine caused by severe trauma are characterized by wedge-shaped deformity of the vertebral body. No adequate method has been devised for the reduction of these injuries. However, because of the inherent stability of the thoracic spine, prolonged immobilization is not necessary. In fracture of the upper thoracic region, if immobilization is required for relief of pain, a plaster Minerva jacket may be the only adequate method of external support that will provide relief from pain.

FRACTURES AND FRACTURE-DISLOCATIONS OF THE LUMBAR SPINE

Fractures of the Lumbar Spine.

A. Uncomplicated Compression Fractures: Compression fractures of the vertebral bodies caused by hyperflexion injury are the most common fractures of the lumbar spine and occur most often near the thoracolumbar junction. The widespread use of seat belts in automobiles has been accompanied by an increasing incidence of fractures that occur near the lumbosacral level as the result of accidents. More than one vertebral body is often involved, but deformity may be greatest in one segment. Acute angulation of the spine caused by a compression deformity of the body of a vertebra may be associated with varying degrees of disruption of the facet joints, from sprain to complete dislocation.

Anteroposterior, lateral, and oblique x-rays are required to demonstrate the characteristic lesions such as wedge-shaped deformity of the body and the presence of dislocation of the facets, comminuted fracture of the body, and fracture of the pedicle. Laminagraphy is a useful adjunctive technic for disclosure of lesions that might not be demonstrated by routine x-ray studies.

Treatment depends upon the age of the patient, the presence of preexisting disease, and the severity of injury. In older patients with preexisting degenerative arthritis where there is mild deformity involving no more than one-fourth of the anterior height of the body of the vertebra, the surgeon may elect not to reduce the deformity but merely to place the patient at bed rest for a few days. As soon as acute pain is relieved, the back should be braced and increasing physical activity encouraged within the tolerance of pain. In the more active age group, when the compression deformity involves more than one-fourth of the anterior height of the body of the vertebra, reduction by hyperextension and immobilization in a plaster jacket (see p. 722) is the treatment of choice for these limited and uncomplicated fractures.

B. Comminuted Fractures: Comminuted fracture of the vertebral body is characterized by disruption of the adjacent intervertebral disks and varying degrees of displacement of the fragments. The end plates of the body are forced into the centrum together with the disk. The extent of fragmentation (comminution) of the body depends upon the severity of the causative injury. A large fragment of the body may be displaced anteriorly. Posteriorly displaced fragments are apt to cause compression of the cord or cauda equina; and the facet joints may be fractured or dislocated. Therefore, careful physical and x-ray examinations are mandatory before treatment is instituted.

The method of treatment may be dictated by the extent of bone injury and the presence of neurologic complications. When neurologic involvement is absent and comminution is not manifest by extensive fragmentation, reduction may not be necessary. Under these circumstances, immobilization in a plaster jacket can be adequate treatment. Caution must be taken to determine whether dislocation has occurred or is likely because of posterior element injury (see below). Mobilization of the patient from recumbency should be judiciously controlled by periodic physical and x-ray examinations to determine incipient displacement of fragments which may herald or accompany the onset of neurologic deficit. When the posterior elements are intact and compression of the body has been greater than one-fourth to one-third its former height, reduction by extension of the spine and immobilization in a plaster jacket should be considered for the treatment of young adults. When cord or cauda equina injury has occurred, laminectomy may be indicated (see p. 691), in which case spine fusion may also be performed. Bone healing is likely to be slow, and immobilization should be prolonged until stabilization has occurred. Cautiously executed biplane bending x-ray studies give helpful guidance in determining the soundness of healing and the extent to which mechanical stability is restored.

C. Fracture of the Transverse Processes: Fracture of the transverse processes may result from direct violence, such as a crushing injury, or may be incidental to a more serious fracture of the lumbar spine. It may result also from violent muscle contraction alone. One or more segments may be involved. If displacement is minimal, soft tissue injury is likely to be minor. Extensive displacement of the fragments indicates severe soft tissue tearing and hematoma formation.

Treatment depends upon the presence or absence of associated injuries. If fracture of the transverse process is the sole injury, and if pain is not severe upon guarded motions of the back, strapping and prompt ambulation may be sufficient. If displacement and soft tissue injury are extensive, bed rest for a few days followed by prolonged support in a corset or brace may be necessary and slow symptomatic recovery may be anticipated.

Fracture-Dislocation of the Lumbar Spine.

Severe compression trauma may cause fracture-dislocation with rupture of 1 disk or, if comminution occurs, rupture of 2 disks. Varying degrees of injury to the posterior elements occur, including unilateral or bilateral dislocation of the facets and/or fracture of the pedicles or facets. Accompanying fractures of spinous and transverse processes, and tearing of the posterior ligaments and adjacent muscles can add to the complexity of this severe lesion. The dislocation of the upper segment may be solely in the anteroposterior plane, or it may be complex, with additional displacement in the coronal plane with torsion around the longitudinal axis of the spine.

Careful physical and radiologic examinations are necessary to determine the nature of the injury before reduction is attempted, since associated injury to the cord or cauda equina may be present.

The method of treatment depends upon the type of injury. If there is no neurologic involvement and dislocation was associated with fracture of the pedicles or facets, reduction may be attempted by cautious extension with traction on the lower extremities under x-ray control without anesthesia. When dislocation has been corrected, immobilization in a plaster body cast with a spica extension to incorporate at least one thigh may be necessary for adequate support. Early mobilization of the patient from the recumbent position should be accomplished slowly because displacement of fragments can occur and neurologic complications may result. When reasonable doubt exists, it is preferred to continue recumbency for 8-12 weeks until initial healing has provided mechanical stability. If closed reduction is not successful, or if extension causes neurologic symptoms, the attempt should be abandoned at once in favor of open reduction.

In complete dislocation of one or both facets, reduction can be accomplished by open operation.

FRACTURE OF THE SACRUM

Fracture of the sacrum may accompany fracture of the pelvis. It may also appear as an isolated lesion as a result of direct violence. Linear fracture of the sacrum without displacement should be treated symptomatically. Strapping of the buttocks of males and the wearing of a snug girdle by females can provide some comfort during the acutely painful stage. If the fracture extends through a sacral foramen and is associated with displacement, there may be injury to one of the sacral nerves and consequent neurologic deficit. If the sacral fragment is displaced anteriorly, reduction should be attempted by means of bimanual manipulation. Great care should be exercised to prevent injury to the rectal wall by pressure of the palpating finger against a sharp spicule of underlying bone.

FRACTURE OF THE COCCYX

Fracture of the coccyx is usually the result of a blow on the buttock. No specific treatment is required other than protection. Strapping the buttocks together for a few days may minimize pain. Pressure on the coccygeal region can be avoided by selecting a firm chair in which to sit or placing a support beneath the thighs to relieve pressure. The patient should be warned that pain may persist for many weeks. Fracture-dislocation can be reduced by bimanual manipulation, but recurrence of the deformity is likely. Every effort toward conservative management should be made before coccygectomy is considered for treatment of the painful unhealed or malunited fracture.

FRACTURES OF THE PELVIS

AVULSION FRACTURES OF THE PELVIS

Avulsion fractures of the pelvis include those involving the anterior-superior and anterior-inferior iliac spines and the apophysis of the ischium. The ischial apophysis may be avulsed indirectly by violent contraction of the hamstring muscles in the older child or adolescent. If displacement is minimal, prompt healing without disability is to be expected. If displacement is marked (i.e., more than 1 cm.), reattachment by open operation is justifiable.

FRACTURE OF THE WING OF THE ILIUM

Isolated fracture of the wing of the ilium without involvement of the hip or sacroiliac joints most often occurs as a result of direct violence, such as a crushing injury. With minor displacement of the free fragment, soft tissue injury is usually minimal and treatment is symptomatic. Wide displacement of the free fragment may be associated with extensive soft tissue injury and hematoma formation. Healing may be accompanied by ossification of the hematoma with exuberant new bone formation.

ISOLATED FRACTURE OF THE OBTURATOR RING

Isolated fracture of the obturator ring, involving either the pubis or ischium with minimal displacement, is associated with little or no injury to the sacroiliac joints. This is also true of minor subluxation of the symphysis pubis. Initial treatment consists of bed rest for a few days followed by ambulation on crutches. A sacroiliac belt or pelvic binder may give additional comfort. As soon as discomfort disappears, unsupported weight-bearing may be permitted.

COMPLEX FRACTURES OF THE PELVIC RING

Complex fractures of the pelvic ring are due either to direct violence or to force transmitted indirectly through the lower extremities. They are characterized by disruption of the pelvic ring at 2 points: (1) anteriorly, near the symphysis pubis, manifested either by dislocation of that joint or by fracture through the body of the pubis, by unilateral or bilateral fracture through the obturator ring, or by fracture through the acetabulum; and (2) disruption of the pelvic ring through or in the vicinity of the sacroiliac joint. The disruption can extend partially through the sacroiliac joint as a dislocation and extend into the sacrum or into the adjacent ilium as a fracture. The magnitude of displacement of the fragments may indicate the severity of soft tissue injury. These complex injuries are often associated with extensive hemorrhage into the soft tissues or injury to the bladder, urethra, or intra-abdominal organs. When anterior and posterior disruption are ipsilateral, the entire involved hemipelvis and extremity may be displaced proximally. Anterior disruption may occur on one side, and posterior disruption on the opposite side with wide opening of the pelvic ring.

When severe and complex fractures of the pelvic ring are suspected, the extent of associated injuries must be determined at once by physical and x-ray examination. Shock due to blood loss may be present. Treatment of the fracture by reduction should not be instituted until the extent of associated injuries has been determined. Treatment of some of those injuries may be more urgent than that of the fracture lesion. A careful search for possible injury to bowel, bladder, ureters, and major vessels should be made at the earliest opportunity.

Treatment is based upon the type and severity of the injury. If displacement and soft tissue injury are minimal, a pelvic sling to facilitate nursing care may be all that is required. When the hemipelvis has been displaced proximally, skeletal traction on the distal end of the femur on the affected side with suspension of the extremity may permit reduction.

If the sacroiliac joint has been dislocated and the ilium is rotated posterior to the sacrum, with opening of the anterior fracture, closed reduction can be attempted. Post-manipulation maintenance of reduction is accomplished by a pelvic sling or a short bilateral thigh spica.

INJURIES OF THE SHOULDER GIRDLE

FRACTURE OF THE CLAVICLE

Fracture of the clavicle may occur as a result of direct violence or indirect violence transmitted through the shoulder. Most fractures of the clavicle are seen in the distal half, commonly at the junction of the middle and distal thirds. About two-thirds of clavicular fractures occur in children. Birth fractures of the clavicle vary from greenstick to complete displacement.

Because of the relative fixation of the medial fragment and the weight of the arm, the distal fragment is displaced downward and toward the midline. Anteroposterior x-rays should always be taken, but oblique projections are occasionally of more value. Although injury to the brachial plexus or subclavian vessels is not common, such complications can usually be demonstrated on physical examination.

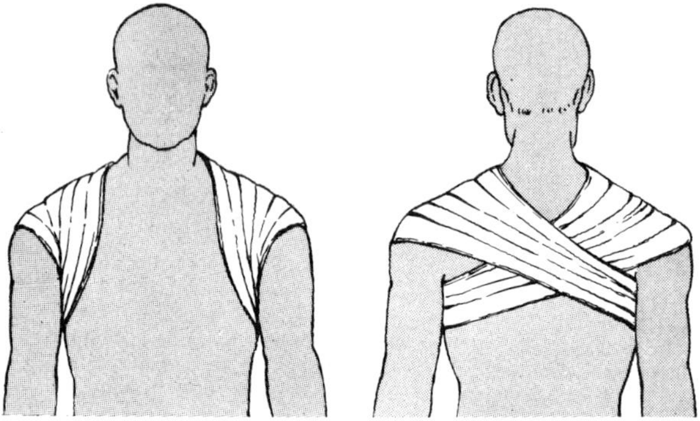

Figure-of-Eight Dressing

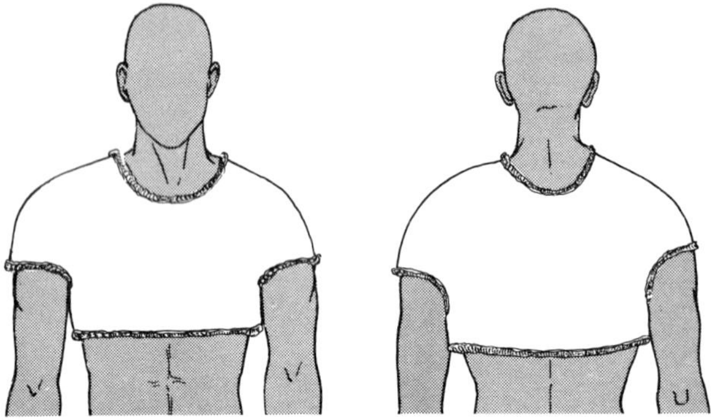

Plaster Shoulder Spica for Fracture of Clavicle

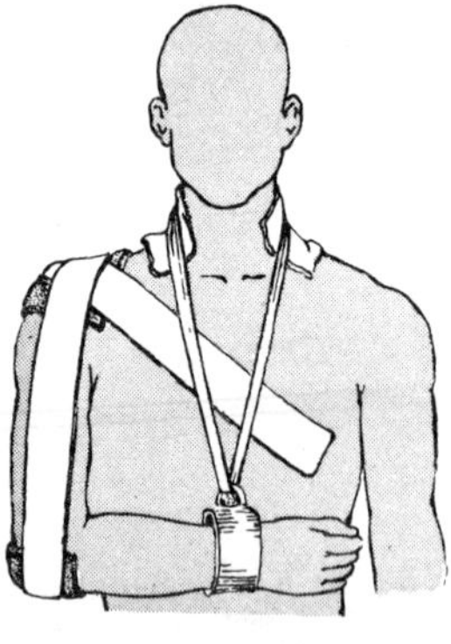

Stimson's Dressing

Treatment.*

A. Without Displacement: Immobilization of greenstick fractures is not required in children, and healing is rapid. Complete fractures should be immobilized for 10-21 days. A figure-of-eight dressing made of sheet cotton and an elastic bandage is adequate. In adolescents and adults, treatment is by immobilization in a sling and swathe for 4-6 weeks.

B. With Displacement: In infants and small children, apply a figure-of-eight dressing of sheet cotton and elastic bandage reinforced with adhesive tape. Healing usually takes 2-4 weeks. Older children and adolescents require reduction by closed manipulation and immobilization with a figure-of-eight dressing reinforced with plaster (see p. 728). Reduction need not be exact, since exuberant callus formation will be partially or completely obliterated by remodeling of bone architecture incidental to the late stage of the fracture reparative process.

C. With Displacement or Comminution (in Adults):

1. Closed reduction - Comminuted fractures of the clavicle with displacement can usually be managed successfully by closed reduction, although in women greater effort must be made to secure accurate realignment without deformity. A plaster shoulder spica (see p. 728) gives more secure immobilization than the figure-of-eight dressing. Immobilization must be maintained for 6-12 weeks. The patient should remain ambulatory if possible, but in some cases the position of the fragments requires bed rest initially, with skin traction applied to the abducted upper arm and a sandbag between the shoulders to permit the distal fragment to fall into position and to aid in maintaining reduction. Recumbency in this position may be necessary for 5-6 weeks or even longer until stabilization has occurred.
2. Open reduction may be justifiable occasionally to prevent delay of healing where there is interposition of soft tissue.

ACROMIOCLAVICULAR DISLOCATION

Dislocation of the acromioclavicular joint may be incomplete or complete. A history of a blow or fall on the tip of the shoulder can often be obtained. The acromial end of the clavicle is displaced upward and backward; the shoulder falls downward and inward. Careful physical examination generally demonstrates this deformity. Anteroposterior x-rays should be taken of both shoulders with the patient erect. Displacement is more likely to be demonstrated when the patient holds a 10-15 lb. weight in each hand. An axillary projection will demonstrate backward displacement of the acromial end of the clavicle.

---

*Fracture of the outer third of the clavicle distal to the coracoclavicular ligaments is comparable to dislocation of the acromioclavicular joint. If the coracoclavicular ligaments are intact and the fragments are not widely displaced, immobilization in a sling and swathe is adequate. If the coracoclavicular ligaments have been lacerated and extensive displacement of the main medial fragment is present, treatment is similar to that advocated for acromioclavicular dislocation.

Incomplete dislocation (subluxation) is associated with only minor tearing of the acromioclavicular ligaments, since complete dislocation requires rupture of the conoid and trapezoid components of the coracoclavicular ligament. These ligaments may be torn within their substance, or may be avulsed with adjacent periosteum from the acromial end of the clavicle.

Treatment.

Unreduced acromioclavicular dislocations usually cause no disability; however, painful post-traumatic arthritis may require excision of the distal 4 cm. of the clavicle. In general, reduction is indicated for both complete and incomplete dislocations.

A. Incomplete Dislocation: When displacement is minimal, initial treatment may be by sling until acute pain from movement and the weight of the upper extremity has been relieved. Stimson's dressing (see p. 728) can be used for injuries of intermediate severity, where displacement is greater than minimal but not complete. It is applied as follows: A strip of 3 inch adhesive tape is applied to the chest anteriorly and carried obliquely upward over the acromial end of the clavicle, which has been padded with felt. An assistant then presses downward on the acromial end of the clavicle and lifts the patient's arm upward and backward. The strip of adhesive is then continued posteriorly along the upper arm and over the elbow, where another felt pad is placed over the olecranon and proximal ulna. The strip is then continued along the anterior aspect of the upper arm, across the acromial end of the clavicle, and posteriorly over the scapula. The hand and forearm are supported by a sling. This dressing must be maintained for at least 4 weeks; frequent adjustment is necessary to maintain immobilization in the correct position. The patient is encouraged to sleep in a semi-reclining position.

B. Complete Dislocation: It is difficult to maintain reduction and adequate immobilization of complete acromioclavicular dislocations by closed methods. Stimson's dressing or its modifications may be used successfully only if the patient can be kept under constant observation and frequent x-ray examinations made. Open reduction with temporary internal fixation offers the best possibility to restore anatomic perfection. Open reduction is most successful if it can be carried out within a few days after the injury. If it is deferred for 3 weeks or longer, the ligaments will have partially healed with elongation, so that the deformity may be expected to recur when immobilization is discontinued.

STERNOCLAVICULAR DISLOCATION

Displacement of the sternal end of the clavicle may occur superiorly, anteriorly, or, less commonly, inferiorly. Retrosternal displacement is rare. Complete dislocation can be diagnosed by physical examination. Anteroposterior and oblique x-rays confirm the diagnosis.

For incomplete dislocation a plaster shoulder spica is adequate. Complete dislocations are not difficult to reduce, but external dressings are not adequate to maintain reduction. Open reduction with repair of torn sternoclavicular and costoclavicular ligaments with or without internal fixation are normally required to maintain adequate reduction of complete dislocations. Additional protection by external immobilization should be continued at least while the internal fixation apparatus is in situ.

Painful symptoms caused by post-traumatic degenerative arthritis from anatomically reduced or unreduced sternoclavicular dislocation may be persistent. Extraperiosteal resection of the medial two-thirds of the clavicle may be necessary to relieve annoying painful symptoms.

FRACTURE OF THE SCAPULA

Unless fracture of the scapula is complicated by dislocation of the shoulder joint, no treatment is usually required except as noted below.

Fracture of the neck of the scapula is most often caused by a blow on the shoulder or by a fall on the outstretched arm. The degree of fragmentation varies from a crack to extensive comminution. The main glenoid fragment may be impacted into the body fragment. The treatment of impacted or undisplaced fractures in patients 40 years of age or older should be directed toward the preservation of shoulder joint function, since stiffness may cause prolonged disability. In young adults especially, unstable fractures require arm traction with the arm at right angles to the trunk for about 4 weeks (see p. 732) and protection in a sling and swathe for an additional 2-4 weeks. Open reduction is rarely required even for major displaced fragments except for those involving the articular surface when associated with dislocation of the humeral head. These fractures are likely to involve only a segment of the articular surface and may be impacted.

Fracture of the acromion or spine of the scapula requires reduction only when the displaced fragment is apt to cause interference with abduction of the shoulder. Persistence of an acromial epiphysis should not be confused with fracture.

Fracture of the coracoid process may result from violent muscular contraction or, rarely, may be associated with anterior dislocation of the shoulder joint.

When fracture of the body of the scapula is caused by direct violence, fractures of underlying ribs may be associated. Treatment of uncomplicated fracture should be directed toward the comfort of the patient and the preservation of shoulder joint function.

FRACTURE OF THE PROXIMAL HUMERUS

Fracture of the Surgical Neck of the Humerus.

Fracture of the surgical neck is the most frequent fracture of the proximal humerus and occurs most often in patients in the older age group. It is commonly the result of indirect violence, a fall in which the hand of the outstretched arm strikes the ground. Swelling of the shoulder region and restriction of motion due to pain are the prominent clinical features. The diagnosis is established by transthoracic and anteroposterior x-rays.

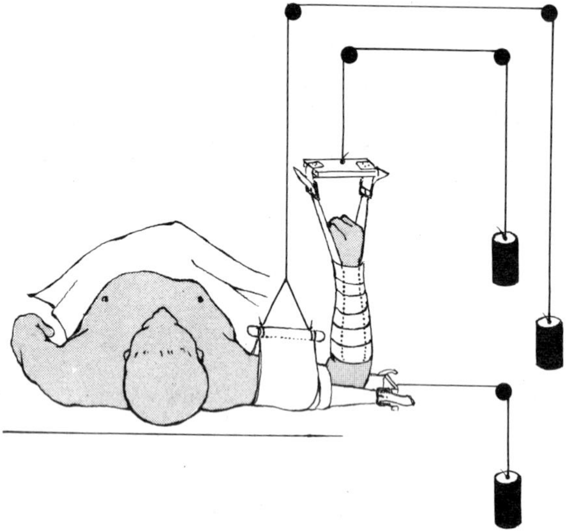

Skin Traction Applied to Upper Extremity

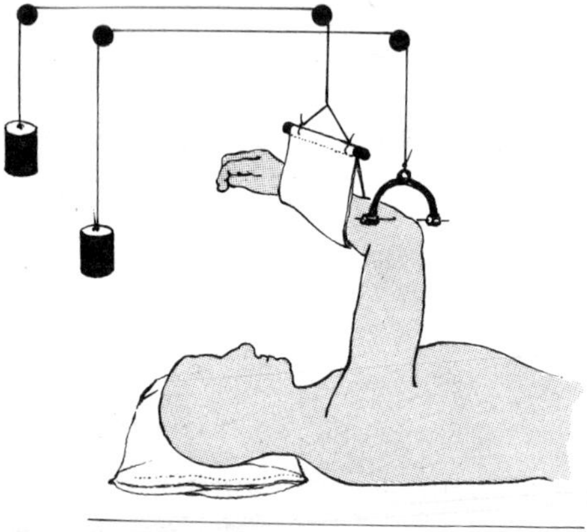

Method of Suspension of Upper Extremity
With Skeletal Traction on Olecranon

Undisplaced fractures require little treatment beyond the use of a sling and guarding of the shoulder until discomfort has disappeared. Restoration of bone continuity normally occurs in 8-12 weeks.

The head fragment may be impacted on the shaft in relative varus or valgus. An impacted fracture in marked varus may cause restriction of abduction, but the deformity is rarely sufficient in the elderly adult to warrant disruption of the impaction and reduction. Impacted fractures of the surgical neck can be treated by means of a sling and swathe with early institution of active motion to preserve shoulder joint function.

Under anesthesia, attempted manipulation of unstable and displaced fractures of the surgical neck without complicating injury is justifiable, but in such instances the lesion must be stabilized by impacting or locking the fragments. When the shaft fragment has been displaced anteriorly and medially (in relation to the head fragment), prompt recurrence of the displacement may follow reduction if the fracture is not stable. Redisplacement is even more likely to occur with an unstable fracture which has been immobilized with the arm in abduction. Continuous traction, either by Buck's extension or by means of a Kirschner wire through the proximal ulna with the arm in abduction, and flexion of the elbow, is advisable when the fracture cannot be stabilized (see p. 732). Traction must be continued for about 4 weeks before partial healing causes stability.

An unstable fracture in varus position may be reduced by traction and abduction of the arm in external rotation, so that the shaft is brought into alignment with the head fragment. In this position the fracture may become stable and can then be immobilized in a spica. To avoid stiffness of the shoulder in abduction, the fracture can be stabilized with 1 or 2 stiff Kirschner wires. This will permit immobilization of the extremity at the side. The wires can be introduced percutaneously and obliquely in the deltoid region through the distal fragment into the head of the humerus with the fracture reduced. With the fragments stabilized, the arm is then brought to the side and immobilized either by a sling and swathe or by a plaster Velpeau dressing (see p. 734). The necessity for open reduction of fracture of the surgical neck to ensure an adequate functional result is uncommon.

Fracture of the Greater Tuberosity of the Humerus.

Fracture of the greater tuberosity of the humerus with no associated injury is apt to be undisplaced, and may require little treatment other than relief of pain and preservation of shoulder joint function. Fracture of the greater tuberosity with displacement is likely to be associated with anterior dislocation of the head of the humerus.

Comminuted Fracture of the Proximal Humerus.

Comminuted fracture of the proximal humerus is not common, but its prognosis is unfavorable. The configuration of the fracture may vary, but 4 main fragments usually can be identified: 2 tuberosities, the head, and the shaft. Since little or no soft tissue attachment to the head fragment remains, avascular necrosis is apt to occur. The head fragment may be completely displaced anterior or posterior to the glenoid, or it may be impacted on the shaft. In eld-

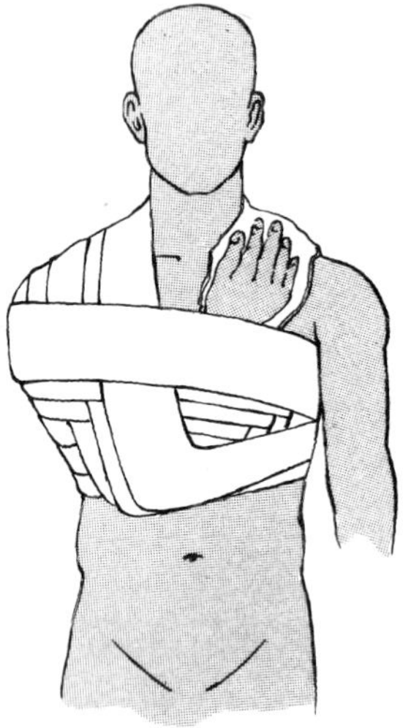

Velpeau Dressing

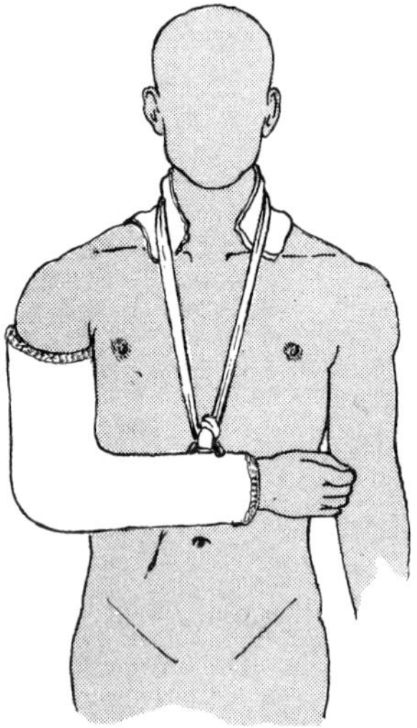

Caldwell's Hanging Cast

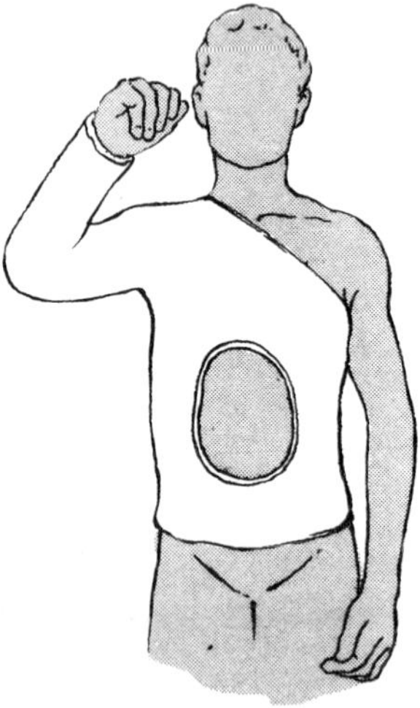

Plaster Shoulder Spica
for Fracture of Humerus

erly patients, if the fracture is impacted and the head fragment is not dislocated, reduction should not be attempted. Early mobilization is indicated to preserve as much shoulder joint function as possible. If the head fragment is dislocated from the glenoid fossa, open reduction offers the best chance of salvaging shoulder joint function. If the blood supply to the head fragment has been destroyed, the fragment may be removed and the upper end of the humerus placed in the glenoid or a prosthesis inserted. The prognosis for optimal functional recovery is poor in these cases.

Separation of the Epiphysis of the Head of the Humerus.

When this injury occurs as a result of birth trauma it is difficult to recognize because of the absence of a bony nucleus in the capital epiphysis. Even though x-ray examination is negative, the injury should be suspected when there is swelling of the shoulder region and limitation of active movements of the arm. Fracture through the epiphysial plate may be encountered in older children. The principles of treatment are the same as for fracture of the surgical neck of the humerus. Open reduction is rarely desirable, and every effort should be made to obtain reduction by manipulation or traction.

DISLOCATION OF THE SHOULDER JOINT

Over 95% of all cases of shoulder joint dislocation are anterior or subcoracoid. Subglenoid and posterior dislocations comprise the remainder.

Anterior Dislocation of the Shoulder Joint.

Anterior dislocation presents the clinical appearance of flattening of the deltoid region, anterior fullness, and restriction of motion due to pain. Both anteroposterior and axillary x-rays are necessary to determine the site of the head and the presence or absence of complicating fracture which may involve either the head of the humerus or the glenoid. Anterior dislocation may be complicated by (1) injury to major nerves arising from the brachial plexus; (2) fracture of the upper extremity of the humerus, especially the head or greater tuberosity; (3) compression or avulsion of the anterior glenoid; and (4) tears of the capsulotendinous rotator cuff. The most common sequel is recurrent dislocation. Before manipulation, careful examination is necessary to determine the presence or absence of complicating nerve or vascular injury. Under general anesthesia, reduction can usually be accomplished by simple traction on the arm for a few minutes or until the head has been disengaged from the coracoid. If reduction cannot be achieved in this way, the surgeon should apply lateral traction manually to the upper arm, close to the axilla, while the assistant continues to exert axial traction on the extremity. This is a modification of Hippocrates' manipulation in which the surgeon exerts traction on the arm while the heel of his unshod foot in the axilla provides countertraction and simultaneously forces the head of the humerus laterally from beneath the acromion.

If neither of the foregoing technics proves successful, Kocher's method may be useful. This maneuver, however, must be carried out gently or spiral fracture of the humerus may result. The elbow is flexed to a right angle and the surgeon applies traction and gentle external rotation to the forearm in the axis of the humerus. The surgeon continues traction to the arm while gentle external rotation about the longitudinal axis of the humerus is applied, using the forearm flexed to a right angle at the elbow as a lever. The maneuver can be completed by displacing the elbow region of the extremity across the anterior chest while traction is continuously exerted and, finally, slow internal rotation of the arm until the palm of the affected side rests on the opposite shoulder.

After closed reduction of an initial dislocation the extremity is immobilized in a sling and swathe for 3 weeks before active motion is begun. If the second episode is the result of minor trauma, the lesion is considered permanent and treated accordingly.

Subcoracoid Dislocation of the Shoulder Joint.

Uncomplicated subcoracoid dislocation can almost always be reduced by closed manipulation. With associated fracture, or when the dislocation is old, open reduction may be necessary. Even when the dislocation is old, however, closed reduction by skeletal traction should be tried before open reduction is elected.

Posterior Dislocation of the Shoulder Joint.

Posterior dislocation is characterized by fullness beneath the spine of the scapula and by restriction of motion in external rotation. An axillary x-ray view demonstrates the position of the head of the humerus in relationship to the glenoid. This uncommon lesion may be reduced by the same combination of coaxial and transverse traction as described for anterior dislocation. Immobilization following an initial episode should be accomplished by plaster spica, with the arm in approximately 30° external rotation and the elbow flexed to a right angle.

Recurrent Dislocation of the Shoulder Joint.

Recurrent dislocation of the shoulder is almost always anterior. Various factors can influence recurrent dislocation. Avulsion of the anterior and inferior glenoid labrum or tears in the anterior capsule remove the natural buttress that gives stability to the arm with abduction and external rotation. Other lesions which impair the stability of the shoulder joint are fractures of the posterior and superior surface of the head of the humerus (or of the greater tuberosity) and longitudinal tears of the rotator cuff between the supraspinatus and subscapularis. Reduction of the acute episodic dislocation is by closed manipulation. Immobilization does not prevent subsequent dislocation, and it should be discontinued as soon as acute symptoms subside, usually within a few days.

Adequate curative treatment of recurrent dislocation of the shoulder, so that unrestricted normal use of the joint is possible, almost always requires plastic repair of the anterior capsulotendinous cuff by operations such as those recommended by Bankhart, Putti and Platt, or Magnuson and Stack.

FRACTURES OF THE SHAFT OF THE HUMERUS

Fracture of the shaft of the humerus is more common in adults than in children. Direct violence is accountable for the major portion of such fractures, although spiral fracture of the middle third of the shaft may result from violent muscular activity such as throwing a ball. The diagnosis is based upon the history and physical examination. Localized tenderness, swelling, and deformity are apparent. Palpation may elicit crepitus. Anteroposterior and transthoracic x-rays show the location and configuration of the fracture. Before initiating definitive treatment, a careful neurologic examination should be done (and recorded) to determine the status of the radial nerve. Injury to the brachial vessels is not common.

Fracture through the metaphysis proximal to the insertion of the pectoralis major is classified as fracture of the surgical neck of the humerus (see p. 731).

Fracture of the Upper Third of the Shaft of the Humerus.

Fractures between the insertions of the pectoralis major and the deltoid commonly demonstrate adduction of the distal end of the proximal fragment, with lateral and proximal displacement of the distal fragment. Medial displacement occurs with fracture distal to the insertion of the deltoid.

Treatment depends upon the presence or absence of complicating neurovascular injury, the site and configuration of the fracture, and the magnitude of displacement.

In infants, skin traction for 1-2 weeks will permit sufficient callus to form so that immobilization can be maintained by a sling and swathe or a Velpeau dressing. Open reduction for the sole purpose of accurate positioning of the fragments is rarely justified in children and adolescents, since slight shortening and minor degrees of angulation will be compensated during growth. Torsional displacement, however, will not be compensated, and must be corrected initially.

In the adult, an effort should be made to reduce completely displaced transverse or slightly oblique fractures by manipulation. An injection of 10-15 ml. of 2% procaine directly into the hematoma at the fracture site will provide adequate anesthesia for manipulation. If the ends of the fragments cannot be approximated by manipulative methods, traction on the skin or skeletal traction with a wire through the olecranon is indicated (see p. 732). In young patients the olecranon wire should be placed opposite the coronoid process to avoid injury to the epiphysis. Traction should be continued for 3-4 weeks until stabilization occurs, after which time the patient can be ambulatory with an external immobilization device.

Fracture of the Middle and Lower Thirds of the Shaft of the Humerus.

Spiral, oblique, and comminuted fractures of the shaft below the insertion of the pectoralis major may be treated by Caldwell's hanging cast, which consists of a plaster dressing from the axilla to the wrist with the elbow in 90° of flexion and the forearm in midposition (see p. 734). The cast is suspended from a bandage around the neck by means of a ring at the wrist. Alignment should be verified on anteroposterior and transthoracic x-rays with the patient standing. Angulation may be corrected by lengthening or shortening the suspension bandage. When lateral convex angulation cannot be corrected by adjustment of the bandage, moving the suspension ring closer to the elbow may be effective. Traction is afforded by the weight of the plaster. The patient is instructed to sleep in the semi-reclining position. As soon as clinical examination demonstrates stabilization (in about 6-8 weeks), the plaster may be discarded and a sling and swathe substituted.

If the configuration of the fracture approaches the transverse and is located between the insertions of the pectoralis major and the deltoid, the distal end of the proximal fragment may be in relative adduction. To prevent recurrence of medial convex angulation and maintain proper alignment, it may be necessary to bring the distal fragment into alignment with the proximal by bringing the arm across the chest and immobilizing it with a plaster Velpeau dressing (see p. 734).

When fracture of the shaft of the humerus is associated with other injuries which require confinement to bed, initial treatment may be by skin or skeletal traction (see p. 732). Continuous supervision is necessary.

Fractures of the shaft of the humerus - especially transverse fractures - may heal slowly. If stabilization has not taken place after 6-8 weeks of traction, more secure immobilization, such as with a plaster shoulder spica (see p. 734), must be considered. It may be necessary to continue immobilization for 6 months or more.

When complete loss of radial nerve function is apparent immediately after injury, open operation is indicated to determine the type of nerve lesion or to remove impinging bone fragments. If partial function of the radial nerve is retained, exploration can be deferred since spontaneous recovery sometimes occurs and may be complete by the time the fracture has healed. Open reduction of closed fractures is indicated also if arterial circulation has been interrupted or (in the adult) if adequate apposition of major fragments cannot be obtained by closed methods, as is likely to be the case with transverse fractures near the middle third of the shaft. When 4-5 months of treatment by closed methods have not resulted in clinical or x-ray evidence of healing, operative treatment may be considered.

INJURIES OF THE ELBOW REGION

FRACTURE OF THE DISTAL HUMERUS

Fracture of the distal humerus is most often caused by indirect violence. Therefore, the configuration of the fracture cleft and the direction of displacement of the fragments are likely to be typical. Injuries of major vessels and nerves and elbow joint dislocation are apt to be present.

Clinical findings consist of pain, swelling, and restriction of motion. Minor deformity may not be apparent because swelling usually obliterates landmarks. The type of fracture is determined by x-ray examination. Especially in children, it is advisable to obtain films of the opposite elbow for comparison.

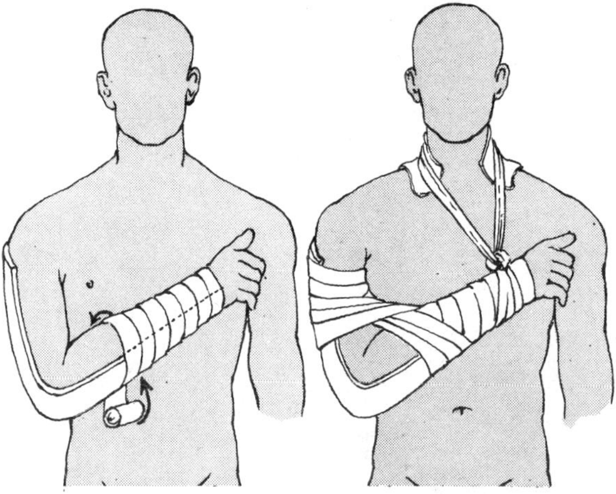

Posterior Plaster Splint for Supracondylar Fracture

Examination for peripheral nerve and vascular injury must be made and all findings carefully recorded before treatment is instituted.

Supracondylar Fracture of the Humerus.

Supracondylar fracture of the humerus occurs proximal to the olecranon fossa; transcondylar (diacondylar) fracture occurs more distally and extends into the olecranon fossa. Neither fracture extends to the articular surface of the humerus. Treatment is the same for both types.

Supracondylar fractures are observed more commonly in children and adolescents, and they may extend into the epiphysial plates of the capitellum and trochlea. Transcondylar fracture is very rare in children.

The direction of displacement of the distal fragment from the midcoronal plane of the arm serves to differentiate the "extension" from the less common "flexion" type. This differentiation has important implications for treatment.

A. Extension Type Fractures: The significant direction of displacement of the distal fragment in the "extension" type of fracture is posterior and proximal. The distal fragment may also be displaced laterally and, less frequently, medially. The direction of these displacements is identified easily on biplane x-ray films. Internal torsional displacement, however, is more difficult to recognize; and unless torsional displacement is reduced, relative cubitus varus with loss of carrying angle will persist.

Displaced supracondylar fractures are surgical emergencies. Immediate treatment is required to combat circulatory embar-

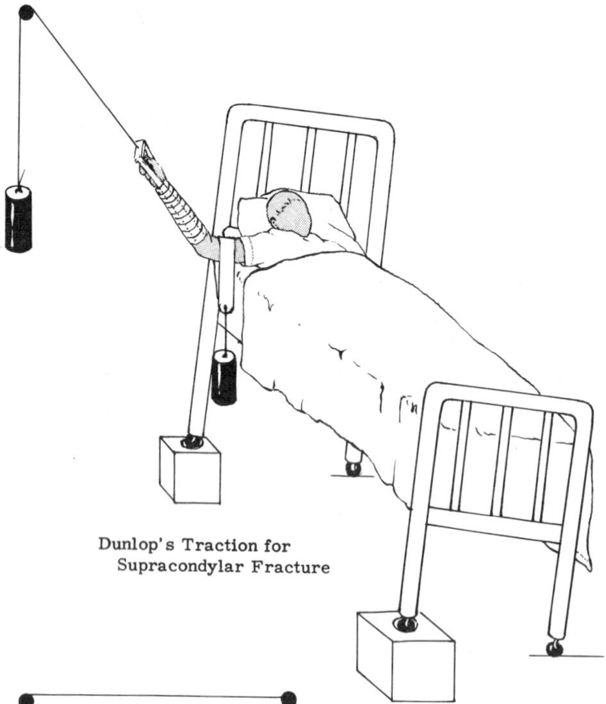

Dunlop's Traction for
Supracondylar Fracture

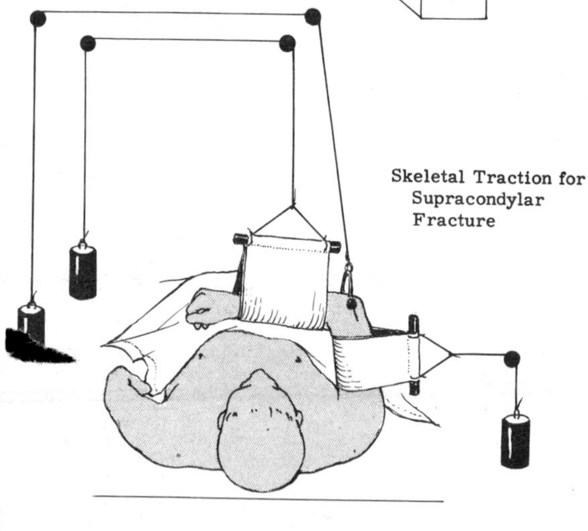

Skeletal Traction for
Supracondylar
Fracture

rassment and to prevent or to avoid further peripheral nerve injury. If hemorrhage and edema prevent complete reduction of the fracture at the first attempt, a second manipulation will be required after swelling has regressed.

1. Manipulative reduction - Minor angular displacements (tilting) may be reduced by gentle forced flexion of the elbow under local or general anesthesia, followed by immobilization in a posterior plaster splint in 45° of flexion (see above). If displacement is marked but normal radial pulsation indicates that circulation is not impaired, closed manipulation under general anesthesia should be done as soon as possible. If radial pulses are absent or weak on initial examination and do not improve with manipulation, traction is indicated (see below). Capillary flush in the nail beds cannot be relied on as the sole indication of competency of deep circulation. After reduction and casting the patient should be placed at bed rest, preferably in a hospital, with his elbow elevated on a pillow and the dressing arranged so that the radial pulse is accessible for frequent observation. Swelling can be expected to increase for 24-72 hours. During this critical period continued observation is necessary so that any circulatory embarrassment which may lead to Volkmann's ischemic contracture can be identified at once. The circular bandage must be adjusted frequently to compensate for initial increase and subsequent decrease of swelling. If during manipulation it was necessary to extend the elbow beyond 45° to restore radial pulses, the joint should be flexed to the optimal angle as swelling subsides to prevent loss of the reduction.

   In children stabilization will take place in 4-5 weeks, after which time the plaster splint may be discarded and a sling worn for another 2 weeks before active motion is permitted. In adults healing is less rapid and immobilization must be continued for 8-12 weeks or even longer before active exercise is permitted.

2. Traction and immobilization - In certain instances supracondylar fractures of the humerus with posterior displacement of the distal fragment should be treated by traction (see p. 732): (1) If comminution is marked and stability cannot be obtained by flexion of the elbow, traction is indicated until the fragments have stabilized. (2) If 2 or 3 attempts at manipulative reduction have been unsuccessful, continuous traction under x-ray control for 1-2 days is justifiable before further manipulation. (3) If the radial pulse is absent or weak when the patient is examined initially and does not improve with manipulation, traction may be necessary to prevent displacement of the fracture and further embarrassment of circulation. During the early phase of treatment by continuous traction, flexion of the elbow beyond 90° should be avoided since this may jeopardize circulation.

B. Flexion Type Fracture: Flexion type fracture of the humerus is characterized by anterior and sometimes also torsional and lateral displacement of the main distal fragment. Treatment is by closed manipulation. A posterior plaster splint is then applied from the axillary fold to the level of the wrist, with the forearm in supination and the elbow in full extension. Elevation is advisable for at least 24 hours or until soft tissue swelling has reached the maximum, after which time the patient may be ambulatory. Immobilization is then continued for 4-6 weeks. When satisfactory reduction cannot be accomplished by closed manipulation, treatment should be by traction with the elbow in full extension until the fragments become stabilized.

Separation of the Distal Humeral Epiphyses.

An uncommon variation of supracondylar fracture is separation of the distal humeral epiphyses with or without appreciable displacement. Sprains of the elbow do not commonly occur in children; injury more often involves the distal humeral epiphyses. X-ray comparison of the injured elbow with the uninjured elbow may show no deviation, but careful physical examination may demonstrate posterior tenderness over the lower epiphyses and also swelling. This combination of swelling and tenderness should suggest epiphysial separation, and warrants protection from further injury by means of a sling worn for about 3 weeks.

The direction of displacement is determined by careful clinical and radiographic examinations. Depending upon the direction of angulation of the osseous nuclei of the capitellum and trochlea (as demonstrated in the lateral x-ray), immobilization is as described for supracondylar fractures.

Intercondylar Fracture of the Humerus.

Intercondylar fracture of the humerus is classically described as being of the "T" and/or "Y" type, according to the configuration of the fracture cleft observed on an anteroposterior x-ray. This fracture is usually seen in adults, commonly as the result of a blow over the posterior aspect of the flexed elbow. Open fracture and other injuries to the soft tissues are frequently present. The fracture often extends into the trochlear surface of the elbow joint, and unless the articular surfaces of the distal humerus can be accurately repositioned, restriction of joint motion, pain, instability, and deformity can be expected.

A. Closed Reduction: If the fragments are not widely displaced, closed reduction may be successful. Since comminution is always present, stabilization is difficult to achieve and maintain by manipulation and external immobilization.
   1. Anterior displacement may be treated first by a combination of continuous skin traction with the elbow in full extension and closed manipulation of the main fragments. If adequate positioning can be achieved in this manner, traction is continued until stabilization occurs. The extremity may then be immobilized in a tubular plaster cast.
   2. Significant posterior displacement requires overhead skeletal traction by means of a Kirschner wire inserted through the olecranon (see p. 732). It may be necessary to apply a swathe around the arm and body for simultaneous transverse traction.

B. Open reduction may be indicated if adequate positioning cannot be obtained by closed methods. A requirement for acceptable results of open reduction and internal fixation is that the fragments be sufficiently large so that they can be fixed to one another. Comminution may be so extensive that satisfactory stabilization cannot be accomplished by current technics of internal fixation. Under such circumstances, it is better to abandon open operation and to accept the imperfect results of closed treatment.

Fracture of the Lateral Condyle of the Humerus.

The 3 major varieties of fracture of the lateral condyle of the humerus are (1) fracture of a portion of the capitellum in the coronal plane of the humerus, with or without extension into the trochlea (seen only in adults); (2) isolated fracture of the lateral condyle without extension into the trochlea; and (3) separation of the capitellar epiphysis (in children).

A. Fracture of the Capitellum: This is characterized by proximal displacement of the anterior detached fragment, and probably occurs as 1 component of a spontaneously reduced incomplete dislocation of the elbow joint. The essential lesion is most clearly demonstrated on lateral x-rays. Closed reduction should be attempted by forcing the elbow into acute flexion. After reduction the extremity is immobilized in a posterior plaster splint with the elbow in full flexion to prevent displacement of the small distal fragment.

When accurate reduction cannot be accomplished by closed technics, open operation may be desirable to avoid subsequent restriction of elbow movement. If the small distal fragment retains sufficient soft tissue attachment to assure adequate blood supply, it may be temporarily fixed to the main fragment in anatomic position by a Kirschner wire. If the articular fragment lacks significant soft tissue bonds, removal is recommended since avascular necrosis is likely to follow.

B. Isolated complete fracture of the lateral condyle without extension into the trochlea* is uncommon, and is not usually associated with major displacement of the detached fragment. The extremity should be supported by a sling. If tense hemarthrosis is present, aspiration may minimize pain. Guarded active motions of the elbow should be initiated as soon as pain subsides.

C. Fracture of the lateral condyle of the humerus in children is essentially separation of the capitellar epiphysis, even though the fracture may extend into the metaphysis and the trochlear epiphysis. If the center of ossification of the capitellum is small, minor displacement may be missed on initial examination; further displacement will then result from unguarded use. The fact that a part of the extensor muscles originates on the fragment is an important factor in displacement.

1. Closed reduction - Minor displacement may be treated by manipulative reduction and external immobilization in a posterior plaster splint which extends from the posterior axillary fold to the level of the heads of the metacarpals. X-rays are taken at least twice a week for the first 3 weeks to determine whether displacement has recurred.
2. Open reduction - When anatomic reduction cannot be

---

*Fracture which involves the entire capitellum and extends into the trochlea is associated with proximal and lateral displacement of the detached fragment and lateral subluxation of the elbow. This lesion is discussed on p. 747.

achieved by 1 or 2 manipulations, open reduction is indicated.

Avulsion of the Medial Epicondylar Apophysis.

Avulsion of the medial epicondylar apophysis in children may occur without dislocation of the elbow. Minor displacement causing localized tenderness and swelling over the medial aspect of the elbow can be treated by immobilization in a sling and swathe for a few days. More extensive injury should be suspected if tenderness and swelling are diffuse. When separation is greater than 1-2 mm., treatment is similar to that for dislocation of the elbow associated with separation of the apophysis (see p. 747).

FRACTURE OF THE PROXIMAL ULNA

Common fractures of the proximal ulna include fracture of the olecranon and fracture of the coronoid process. Fracture of the coronoid process is a complication of posterior dislocation of the elbow joint, and is discussed on p. 746.

Fracture of the olecranon which occurs as the result of indirect violence (e.g., forced flexion of the forearm against the actively contracted triceps muscle) is typically transverse or slightly oblique. Fracture due to direct violence is usually comminuted and associated with other fracture or anterior dislocation of the joint. Since the major fracture cleft extends into the elbow joint, treatment should be directed toward restoration of anatomic position to afford maximal recovery of range of motion and functional competency of the triceps.

Treatment.

The method of treatment depends upon the degree of displacement and the extent of comminution.

A. Closed Reduction: Minimal displacement (1-2 mm.) can be treated by closed manipulation with the elbow in full extension, assisted by digital pressure over the proximal fragment, and immobilization in a volar plaster splint which extends from the anterior axillary fold to the wrist. X-rays should be taken twice weekly for 2 weeks after reduction to determine whether reduction has been maintained. Immobilization must be continued for at least 6 weeks before active flexion exercises are begun.

B. Open reduction and internal fixation are indicated if closed methods are not successful in approximating displaced fragments and restoring congruity to articular surfaces. The extremity is then immobilized in 90° of flexion for at least 6-8 weeks before active flexion exercises are instituted.

FRACTURE OF THE PROXIMAL RADIUS

Fracture of the Head and Neck of the Radius.

Fracture of the head and neck of the radius may occur in adults as an isolated injury uncomplicated by dislocation of the elbow or the superior radioulnar joint. This fracture is caused by indirect violence, such as a fall on the outstretched hand, when the radial head is driven against the capitellum. Care must be taken to obtain true anteroposterior and lateral x-rays of the proximal radius as well as of the elbow joint, since minor lesions may be obscured by a change in position from midposition to full supination during exposure of the films.

A. Conservative Measures: Fissure fractures and those with minimal displacement can be treated symptomatically, with evacuation of tense hemarthrosis by aspiration to minimize pain. The extremity may be supported by a sling or immobilized in a posterior plaster splint with the elbow in 90° of flexion. Active exercises of the elbow are to be encouraged within a few days. Recovery of function is slow, and slight restriction of motion (especially extension) may persist.

B. Surgical Treatment: When the fracture involves the articular surface and is comminuted, or when displacement is greater than 1-2 mm., excision of the entire head of the radius is generally recommended. However, simple removal of a minor fragment of the head which comprises less than a quarter of the articular surface is compatible with recovery of satisfactory elbow function.

Fracture of the Upper Epiphysis of the Radius.

Fracture of the upper radial epiphysis in a child is not a true epiphysial separation since the fracture cleft commonly extends into the neck of the bone. Because the articular surface of the proximal fragment remains intact, the prominent features of displacement are angulation and impaction. Wide displacement of the minor proximal fragment may mean that the elbow joint was dislocated but has reduced spontaneously since the injury.

A. Closed Reduction: Every effort should be made to reduce these fractures by closed manipulation. Several x-rays taken with the forearm in various degrees of rotation should be examined so that the position can be selected which is best suited for digital pressure on the proximal fragment. Anteroposterior and lateral x-rays with the elbow in flexion are then taken; if angulation has been reduced to less than 45°, the end result is likely to be satisfactory.

B. Open Reduction: If closed reduction is not successful, open reduction and repositioning under direct vision is indicated even in the child.

SUBLUXATION AND DISLOCATION OF THE ELBOW JOINT

Subluxation of the Head of the Radius.

This injury occurs most frequently in infants between the ages of 18 months and 3 years, usually when the child is suddenly lifted by his hands with the forearm in pronation. Because of comparative laxity of the interosseous membrane and other supporting ligamentous structures, the direction of displacement of the radial head is distal in the direction of the longitudinal axis of the shaft. It has been suggested that this permits the proximal part of the annular ligament to become infolded between the radial head and the capitellum. In unreduced subluxations, in addition to tenderness about the radial head and restriction of supination, swelling and tenderness may be present in the region of the ulnar head at the level of the inferior radioulnar joint. The infant holds the forearm semiflexed and pronated. If spontaneous reduction has occurred, diagnosis is dependent upon finding slightly restricted supination associated with discomfort. X-rays are not helpful at this stage.

Reduction by forced supination of the forearm can be accomplished easily without anesthesia. The arm should be protected in a sling for 1 week to prevent recurrence.

Dislocation of the Elbow Joint Without Fracture.

Dislocation of the elbow joint without major fracture is almost always posterior. It may be encountered at any age, but is most common in children. Complete backward dislocation of the ulna and radius implies extensive tearing of the capsuloligamentous structures and injury to the region of insertion of the brachialis muscle. The coronoid process of the ulna is usually displaced posteriorly and proximally into the olecranon fossa, but it may be displaced laterally or medially. Biplane x-rays of the highest quality are necessary to determine that no fracture is associated.

Peripheral nerve function must be carefully assessed before definitive treatment is instituted. The ulnar nerve is most likely to be injured.

In recent dislocations, closed reduction can be achieved (under general anesthesia) by axial traction on the forearm with the elbow in the position of deformity. Hyperextension is not necessary. Lateral or medial dislocation can be corrected during traction. As soon as proximal displacement is corrected, the elbow should be brought into 90° of flexion and a posterior plaster splint applied which reaches from the posterior axillary fold to the wrist. Active motion is permitted after 3 weeks.

Closed reduction should be attempted even if unreduced dislocation has persisted for 2 months following the injury.

FRACTURE-DISLOCATION OF THE ELBOW JOINT

Dislocation of the elbow is frequently associated with fracture. Some fractures are insignificant and require no specific treatment; others demand specialized care.

Fracture of the Coronoid Process of the Ulna.

Fracture of the coronoid process of the ulna is the most frequent complication of posterior dislocation of the elbow joint. Treatment is the same as for uncomplicated posterior dislocation of the elbow joint (see above).

Fracture of the Head of the Radius With Posterior Dislocation of the Elbow Joint.

This injury is treated as 2 separate lesions. The severity of comminution and the magnitude of displacement of the radial head fragments are first determined by x-ray. If comminution has occurred or the fragments are widely displaced, the dislocation is reduced by closed manipulation; the head of the radius is then excised.

If fracture of the head of the radius is not comminuted and the fragments are not widely displaced, treatment is as for uncomplicated posterior dislocation of the elbow joint.

Fracture of the Olecranon With Anterior Dislocation of the Elbow Joint.

This very unstable injury usually occurs from a blow on the dorsum of the flexed forearm. Fracture through the olecranon permits the distal fragment of the ulna and the proximal radius to be displaced anterior to the humerus, and may cause extensive tearing of the capsuloligamentous structures around the elbow joint. The dislocation can be reduced by bringing the elbow into full extension, but anatomic reduction of the olecranon fracture by closed manipulation is not likely to be successful and immediate open reduction is usually indicated. Recovery of function is likely to be delayed and incomplete.

Fracture of the Medial Epicondylar Apophysis With Dislocation of the Elbow Joint.

Dislocation of the elbow joint in children may be complicated by avulsion of the medial epicondylar apophysis. The direction of dislocation may have been lateral, posterior, or posterolateral. Physical and x-ray examination may not demonstrate the extent of displacement at the time of injury since partial reduction may have occurred spontaneously. X-rays of the uninjured elbow in similar projections are desirable to compare the exact locations of the 2 apophyses. The free fragment is normally displaced downward by the action of the flexor muscles. If partial spontaneous reduction has occurred, the detached apophysis may be found incarcerated within the elbow joint between the articular surfaces of the trochlea and the olecranon. This may happen also during manual reduction. Ulnar nerve function must be evaluated before definitive treatment is given.

Dislocation of the elbow joint may be reduced by closed manipulation, but accurate repositioning of a widely separated apophysis cannot be achieved by closed methods. Opinion differs concerning the necessity for anatomic reduction of the apophysis if it is not incarcerated within the elbow joint. Some authorities maintain that fibrous healing of the apophysis causes no disability; others anticipate weakness of grasp or subsequent pain as the result of development of a pseudarthrosis between the apophysis and the medial condyle. Exuberant bone formation around the apophysis may cause tardy ulnar paralysis. If it is elected not to reduce displacement of an apophysis outside the elbow joint, the extremity should be immobilized at a right angle for 3 weeks in a tubular plaster cast before active motion is permitted.

If the ulnar nerve has been injured, or if the apophysis cannot be displaced from the elbow joint by closed manipulation, open reduction is advisable.

Fracture of the Lateral Condyle With Lateral Dislocation of the Elbow Joint.

Fracture of the lateral condyle of the humerus with lateral dislocation of the elbow joint must be differentiated from fracture of the lateral condyle with or without posterior dislocation of the joint (see below). Neither lesion is common. A complicating feature of fracture of the lateral condyle with lateral dislocation is inclusion not only of the entire capitellum but also extension of the fracture cleft into the trochlea. This creates an unstable mechanism which cannot be reliably immobilized in either flexion or extension even though closed reduction has been successful. If closed methods of treatment are not adequate, open reduction is recommended.

Fracture of the Lateral Condyle With Posterior Dislocation of the Elbow Joint.

Treatment should be divided into 2 phases. The dislocation should be reduced first by closed manipulation. This maneuver may also simultaneously accomplish adequate reduction of the condylar fracture. If the condylar fragment cannot be adequately repositioned by closed manipulation, open reduction and internal fixation are justifiable to assure anatomic restoration of the articular surfaces.

INJURIES OF THE SHAFTS OF THE RADIUS AND ULNA

FRACTURES OF THE SHAFTS OF THE RADIUS AND ULNA

General Considerations.

A. Causative Injury: Spiral and oblique fractures are likely to be caused by indirect injury. Greenstick, transverse, and comminuted fractures are commonly the result of direct injury.

B. Radiography:
   1. In addition to anteroposterior and lateral films of the entire forearm, including the elbow and wrist joints, oblique views are often desirable.
   2. The lateral projection is usually taken with the forearm in midposition (between complete pronation and supination).
   3. For the anteroposterior projection care must be taken to prevent any change in relative supination of the radius; if this happens, the distal radius will be the same in both views.
   4. Especially in children, films of the uninjured forearm are desirable for comparison of epiphyses and for future reference if growth is impaired.

C. Anatomic Peculiarities: Both the radius and the ulna have biplane curves which permit 180° of rotation in the forearm. If the curves are not preserved by reduction, full rotatory motion of the forearm may not be recovered or derangement of the radioulnar joints may follow.

   Torsional displacement by muscle activity has important implications for manipulative treatment of certain fractures of the radial shaft. The direction of torsional displacement of the distal fragment following fracture of the shaft is influenced by the location of the lesion in reference to muscle insertion. If the fracture is in the upper third (above the insertion of the pronator teres), the proximal fragment will be drawn into relative supination by the biceps and supinator and the distal fragment into pronation by the pronator teres and pronator quadratus. The relative position in torsion of the proximal fragment may be determined by comparing the position of the bicipital tubercle on an anteroposterior film with similar projections of the uninjured arm taken in varying degrees of forearm rotation. In fractures below the middle of the radius (below the insertion of the pronator teres), the proximal fragment characteristically remains in midposition and the distal fragment is pronated; this is due to the antagonistic action of the pronator teres on the biceps and supinator.

D. Closed Reduction and Splinting: With fracture and displacement of the shaft of either the radius or the ulna, injury of the proximal or distal radioulnar joints should always be suspected. The presence of swelling and tenderness around the joint may aid in localization of an occult injury when x-rays are not helpful.

In both adults and children, closed reduction of uncomplicated fractures of the radius and ulna should be attempted. The type of manipulative maneuver depends upon the configuration and location of the fracture and the age of the patient. The position of immobilization of the elbow, forearm, and wrist depends upon the location of the fracture and its inherent stability.

Fracture of the Shaft of the Ulna.

Isolated fracture of the shaft of the proximal third of the ulna (above the insertion of the pronator teres) with displacement is often associated with dislocation of the head of the radius. Reduction of an undislocated transverse fracture may be achieved by axial traction followed by digital pressure to correct displacement in the transverse plane. With the patient supine, the hand is suspended overhead and counter-traction is provided by a sling around the arm above the flexed elbow. After the fragments are distracted, transverse displacement is corrected by digital pressure. With the elbow at a right angle and the forearm in midposition, the extremity is then immobilized in a tubular plaster cast extending from the axilla to the metacarpophalangeal joints. During the first month, weekly examination by x-ray is necessary to determine whether displacement has occurred. Immobilization must be maintained until bone continuity is restored (usually in 8-12 weeks).

Fracture of the shaft of the ulna distal to the insertion of the pronator teres is apt to be complicated by angulation. The proximal end of the distal fragment is displaced toward the radius by the pronator quadratus muscle. Reduction can be achieved by the maneuver described above. To prevent recurrent displacement of the distal fragment, the plaster cast must be carefully molded so as to force the mass of the forearm musculature between the radius and ulna in the anteroposterior plane. Care should be taken to avoid pressure over the subcutaneous surfaces of the radius and ulna around the wrist. Healing is slow, and frequent radiologic examination is necessary to make certain that displacement has not occurred. Stabilization by bone healing may require more than 4 months of immobilization.

An oblique fracture cleft creates an unstable mechanism with a tendency toward displacement, and immobilization in a tubular plaster is not reliable. Open reduction and rigid internal fixation with bone plates or an intramedullary rod are indicated.

Open reduction of uncomplicated fracture of the ulna in children is rarely justifiable because accurate reduction is not imperative; in children under 12 years of age an angular deformity as great as 15° may be corrected by growth. Torsional displacement of uncomplicated fractures of the shaft is not likely to occur. Deformity caused by transverse displacement will be corrected by growth and remodeling.

Fracture of the Shaft of the Radius.

Isolated closed fracture of the shaft of the radius can be caused by direct or indirect violence; open fracture usually results from penetrating injury. Closed fracture with displacement is usually associated with other injury (e.g., fracture of the ulna or dislocation of the distal radioulnar joint). X-rays may not reveal dislocation, but localized tenderness and swelling suggest injury to the distal radioulnar joint.

If the fracture is proximal to the insertion of the pronator teres, closed reduction is indicated. The extremity should then be immobilized in a tubular plaster cast which extends from the axilla to the metacarpophalangeal joints, with the elbow at a right angle and the forearm in full supination (see below).

If the fracture is distal to the insertion of the pronator teres, manipulation and immobilization are as described above except that the forearm should be in midrotation rather than full supination. Since injury to the distal radioulnar joint is apt to be associated with fracture of the radial shaft below the insertion of the pronator teres, weekly anteroposterior and lateral x-ray projections should be taken during the first month to determine the exact status of reduction.

If the configuration of the fracture cleft is transverse rather than oblique, displacement is less apt to take place following anatomic reduction. In the adult, if stability cannot be achieved or if reduction does not approach the anatomic, open reduction and internal fixation are recommended since deformity as a result of displacement of fragments is likely to cause limitation of forearm and hand movements. Children under 12 years of age are likely to recover function provided that torsional displacement has been corrected and angulation does not exceed 15°. Especially if it is

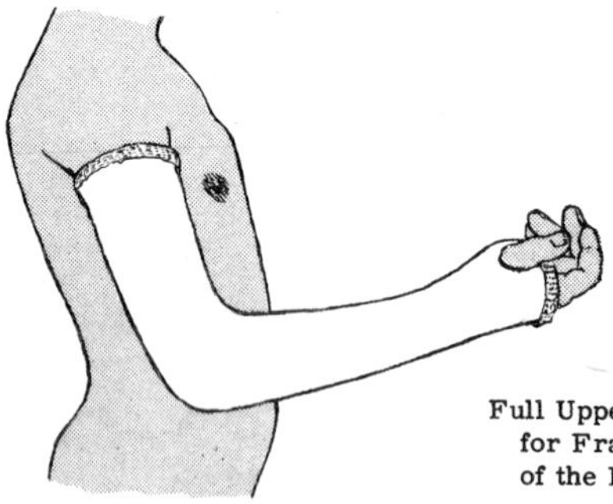

Full Upper Extremity Plaster for Fracture of Both Bones of the Forearm

convex anteriorly, angulation greater than 15° should be corrected in children even though open reduction is required.

In adults, a snug plaster should be maintained for 8-12 weeks or even longer, since healing may be slow. Healing is rapid in children even though reduction is not anatomic; open reduction to promote bone healing in children is not necessary.

Fracture of the Shafts of Both Bones.

The management of fractures of the shafts of both bones of the forearm is essentially a combination of those technics which have been described for the individual bones. If both bones are fractured at the same time, dislocation of either radioulnar joint is not likely to occur. If the configuration of the fracture cleft is approximately transverse, stability can be attained by closed methods provided reduction is anatomic or nearly so. Oblique or comminuted fractures are unstable.

Treatment depends in part upon the degree of displacement, the severity of comminution, and the age of the patient.

A. Without Displacement: In adults, fracture of the shaft of the radius and ulna without displacement can be treated by immobilization in a tubular plaster cast extending from the axilla to the metacarpophalangeal joints with the elbow at a right angle and the forearm in supination (fractures of the upper third) or midposition (fractures of the mid and lower thirds). Immobilization for 8-12 weeks is generally sufficient for restoration of bone continuity in children; immobilization for a longer time is necessary for adults. To avoid late angulation or refracture, the elbow should be included in the plaster until the callus is well mineralized.

B. Greenstick Fractures: Greenstick fractures of both bones of the forearm are common in children.

1. With fractures of the lower third in children under 12 years of age, if angulation is no more than 15° and convex posteriorly, satisfactory correction of the deformity can be expected to occur spontaneously with growth. If angulation is greater than 15° or if the apex is directed anteriorly, deformity should be corrected and the extremity immobilized in a tubular plaster cast extending from the axilla to the bases of the fingers, the elbow at a right angle, the forearm in pronation, and the wrist in the neutral position. Reduction is maintained by snug anteroposterior molding of the plaster over the distal third of the forearm rather than by placing the wrist in volar flexion.
2. Greenstick fracture of both bones proximal to the distal third of the shaft has a tendency toward increased angular deformity if angulation alone is corrected without completion of the fracture. It is recommended that the fracture be completed by sharply reversing the direction of angulation until a palpable "snap" indicates that intact fibers of bone and periosteum on the convex surface have ruptured. The extremity is then immobilized in a plaster cast similar to that used for lower third fractures, with the forearm in semisupination.

C. With Displacement: Although it is not always possible to correct displaced fractures of both bones of the forearm by closed methods, an attempt should be made to do so both in adults and

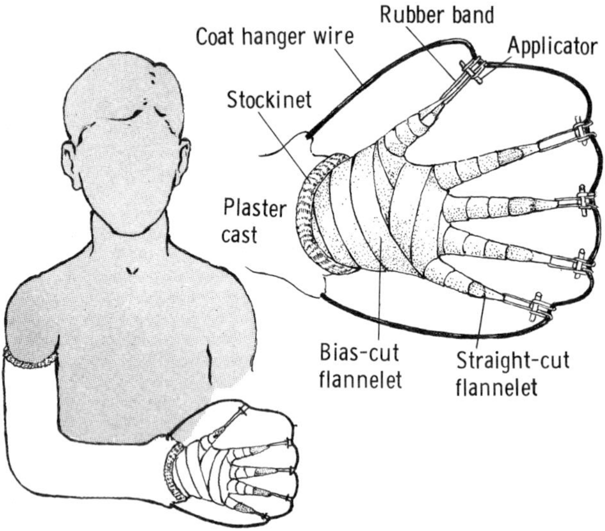

Banjo Splint and Skin Traction for Fracture of the Forearm in Children (Blount)

in children if x-ray studies show a configuration whereby stabilization can be accomplished without operation. Manipulative reduction is recommended if the patient is treated soon after injury and overriding is less than 1 cm. It is essential that good apposition of the fragments of each bone be obtained. Once adequate reduction has been achieved, and while traction is maintained, a padded tubular plaster cast is applied from the bases of the fingers to the axilla.

If treatment is delayed until hemorrhage and swelling have caused induration by infiltration of the soft tissues, or if overriding is more than 1 cm., sustained traction for 2-3 hours will probably be necessary to overcome shortening. Traction on the skin with countertraction on soft tissues are hazardous in these circumstances because of the possibility of decubiti or vascular injury. Skeletal traction is indicated. When correction of the overriding is demonstrated by x-ray, the fragments are manipulated into position under local or general anesthesia. A plaster cast with wires incorporated is then applied and the tension bows maintained to keep the wires taut.

Persistent overriding without angulation in children is not a problem since 0.5 cm. of shortening may be corrected by growth. If overriding of more than 0.5 cm. is demonstrated, continuous skin traction upon the fingers with elastic bands attached to a banjo loop incorporated into the tubular plaster is indicated (see Blount's technic, above).

In adults, if accurate apposition of fragments or stability cannot be achieved in fractures of both bones, open reduction and internal fixation are recommended provided that experienced personnel and adequate equipment are available. Persistent displacement of the fragments of 1 or both bones may be associated with delay of healing, restriction of forearm movements, derangement of the radioulnar joints, and deformity. In those fractures in which open reduction is justifiable in the adult, rigid internal fixation is indicated; a technical pitfall to be avoided is the use of a single wire loop or transfixation screw, a short bone plate attached with unicortical screws, or small intramedullary wires. Even though excellent stability is achieved at operation with internal devices, the extremity should be protected by external fixation until bone healing is well under way.

FRACTURE-DISLOCATIONS OF THE RADIUS AND ULNA

Fracture of the Ulna With Dislocation of the Radial Head.

Fracture of the shaft of the ulna near the junction of the middle and upper thirds may be associated with anterior or posterior dislocation of the head of the radius (Monteggia's fracture). Lateral dislocation of the head of the radius with convex angulation of the shaft of the ulna in the same direction is not common.

A. Closed Reduction:

1. Anterior dislocation of the head of the radius - Although this lesion is usually caused by direct violence upon the dorsum of the forearm, it may also be caused by forced pronation. The annular ligament may be torn, or the head may be displaced distally from beneath the annular ligament without causing a significant tear. The injured ligament may be interposed between the articular surface of the head of the radius and the capitellum of the humerus or the adjacent ulna.

   Closed reduction can be achieved under general anesthesia. Lateral and posteroanterior x-rays are then taken, and a posterior plaster splint is applied from the axillary fold to the head of the metacarpals with the elbow in 45° of flexion (see p. 739) while the films are prepared. If reduction is anatomic, the arm is elevated and observed frequently for signs of circulatory embarrassment for at least 72 hours. Bandages must be adjusted at appropriate intervals to prevent displacement of the splint. As soon as the dressings have been applied, the x-ray examination should be repeated. Examination should be done again on the third day after reduction. Thereafter, for at least 1 month, biplane x-rays are taken once a week. Immobilization is maintained until bone continuity of the ulna is restored; this usually requires 10-12 weeks or even longer, since healing is likely to be slow. Acute flexion of the elbow in plaster should not be decreased before the eighth week.
2. Posterior dislocation of head of the radius - This lesion is caused by direct violence to the volar surface of the forearm. Treatment is by closed reduction. Anteroposterior and

lateral x-rays are then taken, and a tubular plaster cast or stout posterior plaster splint is applied from the metacarpal heads to the axilla with the elbow in full extension and the forearm in midposition. Careful postreduction observation as for anterior dislocation (see above) is essential.

B. Open Reduction: If accurate reduction of the fracture and the dislocation cannot be achieved by closed methods, open reduction by the technic of Boyd is indicated. Plaster immobilization is indicated until bone healing is well under way.

Fracture of the Shaft of the Radius With Dislocation of the Ulnar Head.

In fracture of the shaft of the radius near the junction of the middle and lower thirds with dislocation of the head of the ulna (Dupuytren's fracture, Galeazzi's fracture), the apex of major angulation is usually directed anteriorly while the ulnar head lies volar to the distal end of the radius. (Convex dorsal angulation with the ulnar head posterior to the lower end of the radius is rare.)

A. Closed Reduction: Anatomic alignment is difficult to obtain by closed manipulation and difficult to maintain in plaster, but these technics should be tried before open reduction is used. After reduction, anteroposterior and lateral x-rays are taken and developed before application of the cast. If reduction is adequate, a tubular plaster cast is applied from the axilla to the knuckles with the elbow at a right angle, the forearm in pronation, and the wrist in neutral position. Weekly x-ray examination is indicated during the first month. Immobilization in a snug tubular plaster cast is continued until healing of the radius is complete.

Immobilization of the rare posterior type is with the forearm in supination.

B. Open Reduction: If anatomic reduction cannot be achieved by closed methods, open reduction of recent fracture of the radius is recommended.

INJURIES OF THE WRIST REGION

SPRAINS OF THE WRIST

Isolated severe sprain of the ligaments of the wrist joint is not common, and the diagnosis of wrist sprain should not be made until other lesions, e.g., injury to the lower radial epiphysis (in children) and carpal fractures and dislocations (in adults), have been ruled out. If symptoms persist for more than 2 weeks, and especially if pain and swelling are present, x-ray examination should be repeated.

Treatment may be by immobilization with a volar splint extending from the palmar flexion crease to the elbow. The splint should be attached with elastic bandages so that it can be removed at least 3 times daily for gentle active exercise and warm soaks.

COLLES' FRACTURE

Abraham Colles described the fracture that bears his name as an impacted fracture of the radius 1.5 inches above the wrist joint. Modern usage has extended the term "Colles' fracture" to include a variety of complete fractures of the distal radius characterized by convex volar angulation and by varying degrees of dorsal displacement of the distal fragment.

The fracture is commonly caused by a fall with the hand outstretched, the wrist in dorsiflexion, and the forearm in pronation, so that the force is applied to the palmar surface of the hand. Colles' fracture is most common in middle life and old age.

The fracture cleft may be transverse or oblique, and extends across the distal radius. It may be comminuted, extending into the radiocarpal joint. Displacement is often minimal, with dorsal impaction caused by tilting of the distal fragment and volar convex angulation. As displacement becomes more marked, dorsal and radial tilt of the distal fragment causes increased angulation and torsional displacement in supination of the distal fragment. The normal volar and ulnar inclination of the carpal articular surface of the radius is reduced or reversed.

Avulsion of the styloid process is the usual injury to the distal ulna. Extension of the fracture cleft into the ulnar notch may injure the distal radioulnar articulation. The carpus is displaced with the distal fragment of the radius. Marked displacement at the fracture site causes dislocation of the distal radioulnar and ulnocarpal articulations, and tearing of the triangular fibrocartilage, both radioulnar ligaments, and the volar ulnocarpal ligament. If the ulnar styloid is not fractured, then the collateral ulnar ligament is torn. The head of the ulna lies anterior to the distal fragment of the radius.

Clinical Findings.

Clinical findings vary according to the magnitude of injury, the degree of displacement of fragments, and the interval since injury. If the fragments are not displaced, examination soon after injury will demonstrate only slight tenderness and insignificant swelling; pain may be absent. Marked displacement produces the classical "silver fork" or "bayonet" deformity, in which a dorsal prominence caused by displacement of the distal fragment replaces the normal convex curve of the lower radius and the ulnar head is prominent on the anteromedial aspect of the wrist. Later, swelling may extend from the fingertips to the elbow.

Complications.

Derangement of the distal radioulnar joint is the most common complicating injury. Direct injury to the median nerve by bone spicules is not common. Compression of the nerve by hemorrhage and edema or by displaced bone fragments is frequent and may cause all gradations of sensory and motor paralysis. Initial treatment of the fracture by immobilization of the wrist in acute flexion can be a significant factor in aggravation of compression. Persistent compression of the nerve creates classical symptoms of the carpal tunnel syndrome, which may require operative division of the volar carpal ligament for relief (see p. 657). Other complicating injuries

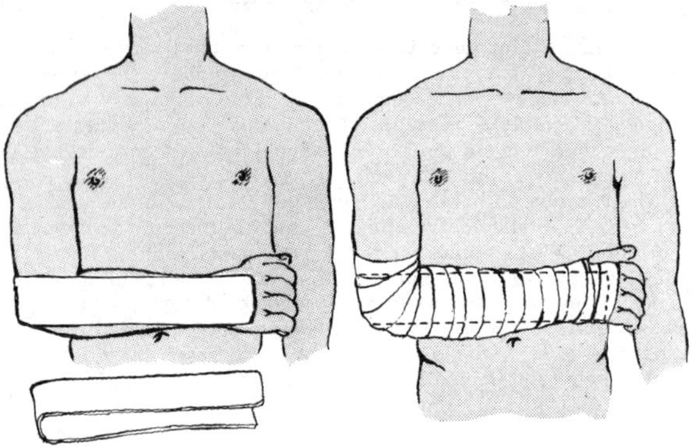

"Sugar Tong" Plaster Splint

Skeletal Distraction for Closed Manipulation of Fracture of the Forearm or Wrist

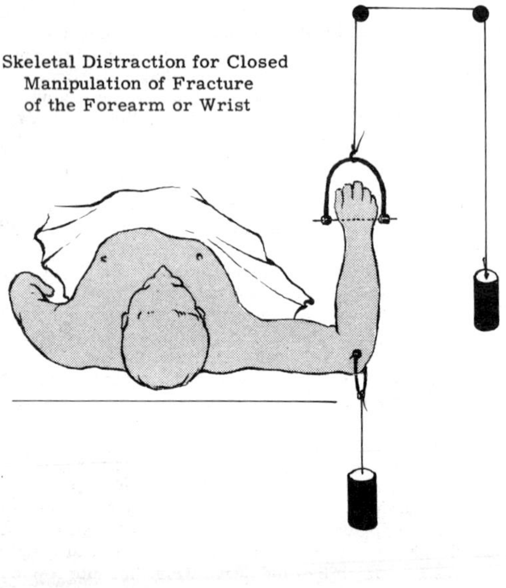

are fractures involving the carpal navicular, the head of the radius, or the capitellum. Dislocation of the elbow and shoulder and tears of the capsulotendinous cuff of the shoulder may be associated.

Treatment.

Complete recovery of function and a pleasing cosmetic result are goals of treatment which cannot always be achieved. The patient's age, sex, and occupation, the presence of complicating injury or disease, the severity of comminution, and the configuration of the fracture cleft govern the selection of treatment.

Open reduction of recent closed Colles' fracture is rarely the treatment of choice. Many technics of closed reduction and external immobilization have been advocated; the experience and preference of the surgeon determine the selection.

A. Minor Displacement: Colles' fracture with minimal displacement is characterized by absence of comminution and slight dorsal impaction. Deformity is barely perceptible, or may not be visible even to a trained observer. In the elderly patient, treatment is directed toward early recovery of function. In young patients, prevention of further displacement is the first consideration.

   Reduction is not necessary. The wrist is immobilized for 3-5 days in a volar plaster splint extending from the distal palmar flexion crease to the elbow. Thereafter the splint may be removed periodically (4-5 times daily) to permit active exercise of the wrist. Soaking the hand and forearm for 15-20 minutes in warm water 2-3 times a day tends to relieve pain and stiffness. The splint can usually be discarded within 2 weeks.

B. Marked Displacement: Early reduction and immobilization are indicated. When reduction has been delayed until preliminary healing is advanced, open reduction may be elected or correction of the deformity can be deferred until healing is sound. The malunion can then be corrected by osteotomy and bone grafting.

   In an old person with complicating arthritis, when impaction causes stability, the mild deformity may be accepted in favor of early restoration of function.

   1. Stable fractures - Colles' fracture is characterized by comminution of the dorsal cortex. Correction of the deformity creates a wedge-shaped area of fragmented and impacted cancellous bone. The base of the wedge is directed dorsally, and there is no buttress to prevent recurrence of displacement. In part, stability is attained by bringing the volar cortices of the fragments into anatomic apposition.

      Muscular relaxation of the extremity can usually be attained more readily under general anesthesia, but local anesthesia is commonly the better choice for the elderly patient.

      Reduction is by manipulation. Success of manipulation is determined by clinical examination. Swelling is dissipated by massaging the volar and lateral aspects of the radius until the subcutaneous border can be palpated. Restoration of the normal convex curve of the distal radius implies that transverse displacement and angulation are absent. Proximal displacement has been reduced if the radial styloid process can be palpated 1 cm. distal to the ulnar styloid.

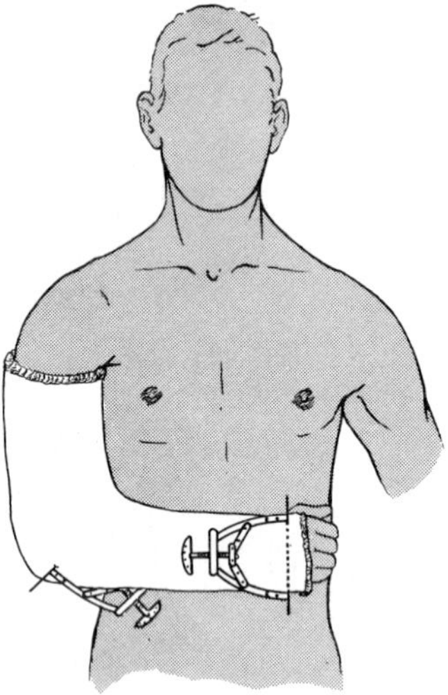

Full Upper Extremity Plaster With Kirschner Wires Incorporated

A lightly padded tubular cast extending above the elbow or a ''sugar tong'' splint (see p. 756), is preferred. The plaster should extend distally only to the palmar flexion crease, with the forearm in midposition and the wrist in slight volar flexion and ulnar deviation. In obese patients, immobilization is more reliable if the elbow is included in the plaster. After the plaster has been applied, it is molded carefully around the wrist until it has set. X-rays are taken while anesthesia is continued. If x-rays show that reduction is not adequate, remanipulation is carried out immediately.

X-ray examination is repeated on the third day and thereafter at weekly intervals during the first 3 weeks. The plaster must remain snug; if loosening occurs after absorption of hemorrhagic exudate, a new cast should be applied.

2. Unstable fractures - If x-rays show extensive comminution with intra-articular extension and involvement of the volar cortex, the fracture is likely to be unstable and skeletal distraction is probably indicated by means of traction on Kirschner wires (see above). Traction is continued while the plaster is applied. To ensure maximal external support, the extremity is immobilized in a tubular plaster cast extending from the axilla to the palmar flexion crease, with the elbow at a right angle, the forearm in midposition, and the wrist in slight ulnar deviation and volar flexion. The Kirschner wires are incorporated in the plaster, and the bows are maintained to hold the wires taut (see above). The wires are left in place for 6 weeks. The fracture is protected for an additional 2 weeks following removal of the wires by a gauntlet or a ''sugar tong'' splint.

Postreduction Treatment.

Frequent observation and careful management can prevent or minimize some of the disabling sequelae of Colles' fracture. The patient's full cooperation in the exercise program is essential. If comminution is marked, if swelling is severe, or if there is evidence of median nerve deficit, the patient should remain under close observation (preferably in a hospital) for at least 72 hours. The extremity should be elevated to minimize swelling, and the adequacy of circulation determined at frequent intervals. Active exercise of the fingers and shoulder is encouraged. In order that the extremity should be used as much as possible, the plaster should be trimmed in the palm to permit full finger flexion.

As soon as the plaster is removed, the patient is advised to use the extremity for customary daily care but to avoid strenuous activity that might cause refracture.

Complications and Sequelae.

Joint stiffness is the most disabling sequel of Colles' fracture. Derangement of the distal radioulnar joint may be caused by the original injury and perpetuated by incomplete reduction; it is characterized by restriction of forearm movements and pain (see p. 761). Late rupture of the extensor pollicis longus tendon is relatively uncommon. Symptoms of median nerve injury due to compression caused by acute swelling alone usually do not persist more than 6 months. Prolonged symptoms can cause the "carpal tunnel syndrome" (see p. 657). Failure to perform shoulder joint exercises several times daily can result in disabling stiffness.

SMITH'S FRACTURE ("REVERSED COLLES")

The distal fragment of the radius is displaced forward and the apex of angulation is directed dorsally so that the normal volar convexity of the lower radius is increased. The ulnar head may be displaced dorsally and there may be derangement of the inferior radioulnar joint.

The fracture can be reduced by closed manipulation, and immobilized with the wrist in dorsiflexion and ulnar deviation.

FRACTURE OF THE RADIAL STYLOID

Forced radial deviation of the hand at the wrist joint can fracture the radial styloid. A large fragment of the styloid is usually displaced by impingement against the carpal navicular. Avulsion of the tip of the styloid by the radial collateral ligament occurs less frequently, and may be associated with dislocation of the radiocarpal joint. If the fragment is large, it can be displaced farther by the brachioradialis muscle, which inserts into it.

Because the fracture is intra-articular, reduction of large fragments should be anatomic. If the styloid fragment is not displaced, immobilization in a plaster gauntlet for 3 weeks is sufficient. If the fragment is displaced, manipulative reduction should be tried. If the distal, smaller fragment tends to displace but can be apposed by digital pressure, percutaneous fixation can be achieved by a medium Kirschner wire inserted through the proximal anatomic snuff-box so as to transfix both fragments. The wrist is then immobilized in a snugly molded plaster gauntlet for 6 weeks. X-ray examination is repeated every week for at least 3 weeks.

If closed methods fail, open reduction is indicated since persistent displacement is likely to cause post-traumatic degenerative arthritis relatively early.

FRACTURE OF THE DISTAL RADIAL EPIPHYSIS

Fracture through the distal radial epiphysial plate in children is the counterpart of Colles' fracture in the adult. Wrist sprain is rare in childhood and should be differentiated as early as possible from fracture of the distal epiphysis. Such an injury is usually caused by indirect violence due to a fall on the outstretched hand. The magnitude of displacement of the epiphysial fragment varies.

In some cases separation and displacement of the epiphysis cannot be demonstrated by radiologic examination and may be quite difficult to identify on clinical examination. The patient may complain of pain in the region of the wrist joint, and slight swelling may be present. Pressure with a blunt object, e.g., the eraser of a lead pencil, may demonstrate maximal tenderness at the epiphysial plate instead of at the wrist joint. Buckling of the adjacent metaphysial cortex manifests greater displacement.

Displacement is posterior and to the radial side. Marked displacement may be accompanied by crushing of the epiphysial plate, tear of the triangular fibrocartilage of the distal radioulnar articulation, displacement of the distal ulnar epiphysis, or avulsion of the ulnar styloid.

Both wrists should be examined by x-ray if injury to the distal radial epiphysis is suspected. Severe injury, crushing the epiphysial cartilage and fracturing the epiphysis, is likely to impede growth and may even lead to early epiphysial fusion; continued growth of the distal ulnar epiphysis produces derangement of the distal radioulnar joint.

If radial deviation of the hand becomes marked, symptomatic Madelung's deformity may result.

Open reduction is rarely necessary. The trauma of the operation superimposed on the injury is likely to cause early arrest of epiphysial growth. Closed reduction by manipulation is usually successful if it can be done within the week following injury. Immobilization is with a plaster gauntlet or "sugar tong" splint. The plaster should be worn for 4-6 weeks. Permanent stiffness due to immobilization of the wrist is not to be feared.

The child should be examined yearly to determine whether there is any growth disturbance.

FRACTURE-DISLOCATIONS OF THE RADIOCARPAL JOINT

Dislocation of the radiocarpal joint without fracture is rare. Dislocation without injury to 1 of the carpal bones is usually associated with fracture of the anterior surface of the radius or the ulna. Comminuted fracture of the distal radius may involve either the anterior or posterior cortex and extends into the wrist joint. Subluxation of the carpus may occur at the same time. The most common fracture-dislocation of the wrist joint involves the posterior or anterior margin of the articular surface of the radius.

Anterior Fracture-Dislocation of the Radiocarpal Joint (Barton's Fracture).

Anterior fracture-dislocation of the wrist joint is characterized by fracture of the volar margin of the carpal articular surface of the radius. The fracture cleft extends proximally in the coronal plane in an oblique direction, so that the free fragment has a wedge-shaped configuration. The carpus is displaced volar and proximally with the articular fragment. This uncommon injury should be differentiated from Smith's fracture by x-ray examination.

Treatment by closed reduction may be successful, especially in cases in which the free fragment of the radius does not involve a large portion of the articular surface. Immobilization is with a tubular plaster cast extending from the palmar flexion crease to above the elbow with the wrist in volar flexion and the elbow at a right angle. Immediate x-rays are taken in 2 projections. If reduction is not anatomic and the fracture is unstable, skeletal distraction may be necessary. Weekly x-ray examination should be repeated during the first month. Skeletal distraction should be continued for 6 weeks or until preliminary bone healing has stabilized the fracture.

Posterior Fracture-Dislocation of the Radiocarpal Joint.

Posterior fracture-dislocation of the wrist joint should be differentiated from Colles' fracture by x-ray. In most cases the marginal fragment is smaller than in anterior injury, and often involves the medial aspect where the extensor pollicis longus crosses the distal radius. If reduction is not anatomic, fraying of the tendon at this level may lead to late rupture.

Treatment is by manipulative reduction as for Colles' fracture and immobilization in a snug plaster gauntlet with the wrist in dorsiflexion.

DISLOCATION OF THE DISTAL RADIOULNAR JOINT

The triangular fibrocartilage is the most important structure in preventing dislocation of the distal radioulnar joint. The accessory ligaments and the pronator quadratus muscle play a secondary role. Complete anterior or posterior dislocation implies a tear of the triangular fibrocartilage and disruption of accessory joint ligaments. Tearing of the triangular fibrocartilage in the absence of major injury to the supporting capsular ligaments causes subluxation or abnormal laxity of the joint. Since the ulnar attachment of the triangular fibrocartilage is at the base of the styloid process, x-rays may demonstrate associated fracture. Widening of the cleft in comparison with the opposite radioulnar joint, which is apparent by x-ray examination, demonstrates diastasis of the radius and ulna if frank anterior or posterior displacement is not present.

Complete anterior or posterior dislocation of the distal radioulnar joint is rare. Medial dislocation is associated with fracture of the radius. The direction of dislocation is indicated by the location of the ulnar head in relation to the distal end of the radius.

FRACTURES AND DISLOCATIONS OF THE CARPUS

Injury to the carpal bones occurs predominantly in men during the most active period of life. Because it is difficult to differentiate these injuries by clinical examination, it is imperative to obtain x-ray films of the best possible quality. The oblique film should be taken in midpronation, the anteroposterior film with the wrist in maximal ulnar deviation. Special views, such as midsupination to demonstrate the pisiform, and carpal tunnel views for the hamate, may be necessary.

Fracture of the Carpal Navicular.

The most common injury to the carpus is fracture of the navicular. Fracture of the carpal navicular should be suspected in any injury to the wrist in an adult male unless a specific diagnosis of another type of injury is obvious. If tenderness on the radial aspect of the wrist is present and fracture cannot be demonstrated, initial treatment should be the same as if fracture were present (see below) and should be continued for at least 3 weeks. Further x-ray examination after 3 weeks may demonstrate an occult fracture.

Three types of fracture are distinguished:

A. Fracture of the Tubercle: This fracture usually is not widely displaced, and healing is generally prompt if immobilization in a plaster gauntlet is maintained for 2-3 weeks.

B. Fracture Through the Waist: Fracture through the narrowest portion of the bone is the most common type. The blood supply to the proximal fragment is usually not disturbed, and healing will take place if reduction is adequate and treatment is instituted early. If the nutrient artery to the proximal third is injured, avascular necrosis of that portion of the bone may occur.

X-ray examination in multiple projections is necessary to determine the direction of the fracture cleft and displacement of the proximal fragment. If the proximal fragment is displaced, it can be reduced under local anesthesia by forced dorsiflexion and radial deviation of the wrist. Immobilization in a plaster gauntlet with the wrist in slight dorsiflexion is necessary. The plaster should extend distally to the palmar flexion crease in the hand and to the base of the thumbnail. If reduction has been anatomic and the blood supply to the proximal fragment has not been jeopardized, adequate bone healing can be expected within 10 weeks. However, such healing must be demonstrated by the disappearance of the fracture cleft and restoration of the trabecular pattern between the 2 main fragments. X-ray examination to verify healing should be repeated 3 weeks after removal of the cast.

C. Fracture Through the Proximal Third: Fracture through the proximal third of the navicular is likely to be associated with injury to the arterial supply of the minor fragment. This can be manifested by avascular necrosis of that fragment. If the lesion is observed soon after injury, reduction and immobilization in a plaster gauntlet will promote healing. The plaster gauntlet should be applied snugly, and must be changed if it becomes loose; it is usually necessary to renew the gauntlet every 4 weeks. X-rays should be taken once a month to determine the progress of bone healing; it may be necessary to prolong immobilization for 4-6 months. The same criteria of radiographic examination as are used for healing of fractures through the waist are used in fractures of the proximal third. It is advisable to make an additional x-ray examination 3-4 weeks after removal of the cast.

If evidence of healing is not apparent after immobilization for 6 months or more, further immobilization will probably not be effective. This is especially true if x-rays show that the fracture cleft has widened and if sclerosis is noted adjacent to the cleft. If the interval between the time of injury and the establishment of a diagnosis is 3 months or more, a trial of immobilization for 2-3 months may be elected. If obliteration of the fracture cleft and evidence of restoration of bone continuity are not visible in x-rays taken after this trial period, some form of operative treatment will be necessary to initiate bone healing. Bone grafting is probably more successful. Prolonged immobilization in a plaster gauntlet is necessary before bony continuity is restored.

If avascular necrosis has occurred in the proximal fragment, bone grafting is less likely to be successful. Although excision of the avascular fragment may relieve painful symptoms for a time, the patient usually notes weakness of grasp and discomfort after prolonged use. Post-traumatic arthritis is apt to develop late.

Prolonged failure of bone healing predisposes to post-traumatic arthritis. Bone grafting operations or other procedures directed toward restoration of bone continuity may be successful, but arthritis causes continued disability. Arthrodesis of the wrist gives the best assurance of relief of pain and a functionally competent extremity.

Fracture of the Lunate.

Fracture of the lunate may be manifested by minor avulsion fractures of the posterior or anterior horn. Careful multiplane x-ray examination is necessary to establish the diagnosis. Either of these lesions may be treated by the use of a volar splint for 3 weeks.

Fracture of the body may be manifested by a crack, by comminution, or by impaction. A fissure fracture can be treated by immobilization in plaster for 3 weeks.

One complication of this fracture is persistent pain in the wrist, slight restriction of motion, and tenderness over the lunate. X-ray examination can demonstrate areas of sclerosis and rarefaction. Impaction or collapse can be accompanied by arthritic changes surrounding the lunate. This x-ray appearance is referred to as Kienböck's disease, osteochondrosis of the lunate, or avascular necrosis.

Fracture of the Hamate.

Fracture of the hamate may occur through the body, and is shown on x-ray as a fissure or compression. Fracture of the base of the hamulus is less common and more difficult to diagnose; special projections are necessary to demonstrate the cleft. If the hamulus is displaced, closed manipulation will not be effective. Prolonged painful symptoms or evidence of irritation of the ulnar nerve may require excision of the loose fragment.

Fracture of the Triquetrum.

Fracture of the triquetrum is caused commonly by direct violence and is often associated with fracture of other carpal bones. Treatment is by immobilization in a plaster gauntlet for 4 weeks.

Dislocation of the Lunate.

Dislocation of the lunate is the second most common injury of the carpus. Dislocation is caused by forced dorsiflexion of the wrist, and the direction of dislocation is almost always anterior. The diagnosis is usually made by x-ray examination. Dislocation may be manifest by dorsal displacement of the capitate while the lunate retains contact with the radius. A further degree of injury is manifested by complete displacement of the lunate from the radius, so that it comes to lie anterior to the capitate and loses its relationship to the articular surface of the radius. If x-ray examination is adequate, the diagnosis can be established easily.

Reduction may be achieved by closed manipulation. X-rays are then taken to determine the success of treatment. If reduction is adequate, the extremity is immobilized in a plaster gauntlet with the wrist in full volar flexion for about 2 weeks. The plaster is then removed and another applied with the wrist in neutral position for an additional 2 weeks. If x-rays show that this manipulative maneuver has not caused reduction, skeletal distraction by means of Kirschner wires may separate the radiocarpal joint sufficiently to permit manipulative reduction (see p. 756). If closed methods are not successful, open reduction should be done promptly.

Dislocation of the Capitate.

Dislocation of the capitate is most often associated with other lesions of the carpus, and is commonly called transcarpal or midcarpal dislocation. The most frequent accompanying injury is fracture of the carpal navicular, in which case the lunate and the proximal fragment of the navicular retain their relationship to the articular surface of the radius whereas the distal fragment of the navicular, the capitate, and the remainder of the carpus are displaced dorsally. Thus the dislocation is retrolunar.

Subluxation of the navicular is less often associated with dislocation of the lunate. The direction of this dislocation is also retrolunar. Fracture of the radioulnar styloid processes is likely to be present also.

X-rays of poor technical quality may not demonstrate the lesion satisfactorily; anteroposterior and true lateral projections are necessary.

The comparatively uncommon midcarpal dislocation can be reduced by closed manipulation if the lesion is uncomplicated and recognized within 10-14 days after injury. Immobilization in a plaster gauntlet with the wrist in slight dorsiflexion for 4 weeks is sufficient for stabilization by early ligamentous healing. If fracture complicates the dislocation, treatment is divided into 2 phases. Reduction of the fracture-dislocation is accomplished by closed manipulation. The navicular fracture is then treated as outlined on p. 762.

INJURIES OF THE HIP REGION

BIRTH FRACTURE OF THE UPPER FEMORAL EPIPHYSES

Birth injury to the upper femoral epiphyses is rare, and the diagnosis by physical examination alone is difficult because the skeletal structures involved are deeply situated. Swelling of the upper thigh and pseudoparalysis of the extremity following a difficult delivery suggest the injury. X-ray examination may demonstrate outward and proximal displacement of the shaft of the femur. Formation of new bone in the region of the metaphysis may be demonstrated in 7-10 days. If displacement has occurred, treatment for 2-3 weeks by Bryant's traction (see p. 776) is recommended. Otherwise, protection by a perineal pillow splint for the same length of time is adequate.

DISPLACEMENT AND SEPARATION OF THE CAPITAL FEMORAL EPIPHYSIS

Displacement of the capital femoral epiphysis due to trauma in the normal child should be differentiated from idiopathic slipped epiphysis (epiphysiolysis, adolescent coxa vara) due possibly to endocrine or metabolic dysfunction. However, between the ages of 10 and 16 years, differentiation may be impossible. Mild injury may cause sudden separation and displacement because of weakening of the plate by antecedent idiopathic disturbance of cartilage growth.

Traumatic separation of the capital femoral epiphysis is rare in normal children, but it may occur as a result of a single episode of severe trauma which otherwise might cause fracture of the femoral neck. The direction of displacement is likely to be the same as in adolescent coxa vara. Although anatomic reduction can be obtained by closed manipulation, immobilization in a plaster spica should not be trusted since redisplacement is possible; internal fixation is more reliable. Traumatic separation of the capital epiphysis associated with dislocation of the hip joint (epiphysis and proximal femur) is a rare lesion with an unfavorable prognosis. Avascular necrosis of the epiphysis is almost certain.

FRACTURE OF THE FEMORAL NECK

Fracture of the femoral neck occurs most commonly in patients over the age of 50. If displacement has occurred, the extremity is in external rotation and adduction. Leg shortening is usually obvious. Motion of the hip joint causes pain. If the fracture is impacted in the valgus position, the injured extremity may be slightly longer than the opposite side and active external rotation may not be possible. If the fragments are not displaced and the fracture is stable, pain at the extremes of passive hip motion may be the only significant finding. The fact that the patient can actively move the extremity often interferes with prompt diagnosis.

Before treatment is instituted, anteroposterior and lateral films of excellent quality must be obtained; if adequate detail is not demonstrated in the initial films, repeated exposure should be made. Gen-

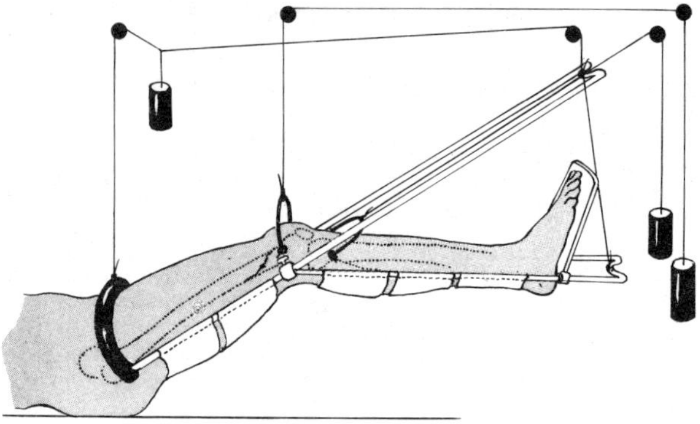

Above: Method of Suspension of Lower Extremity With Skeletal Traction on Tibial Tubercle

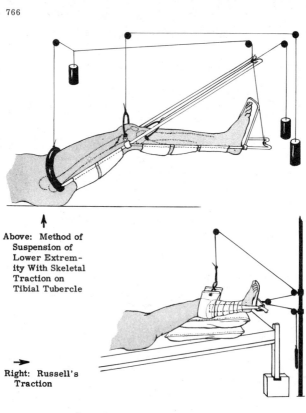

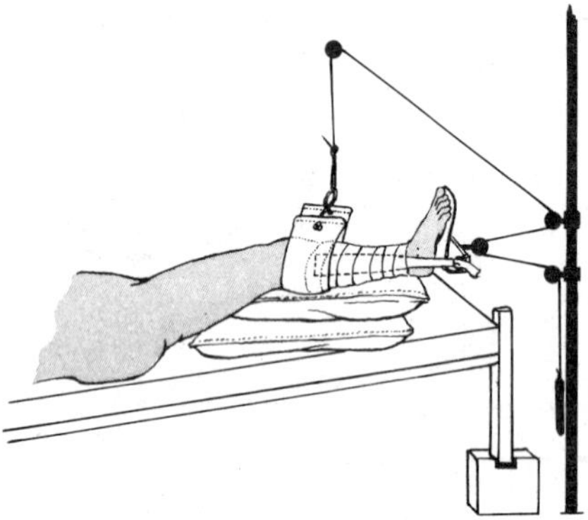

Right: Russell's Traction

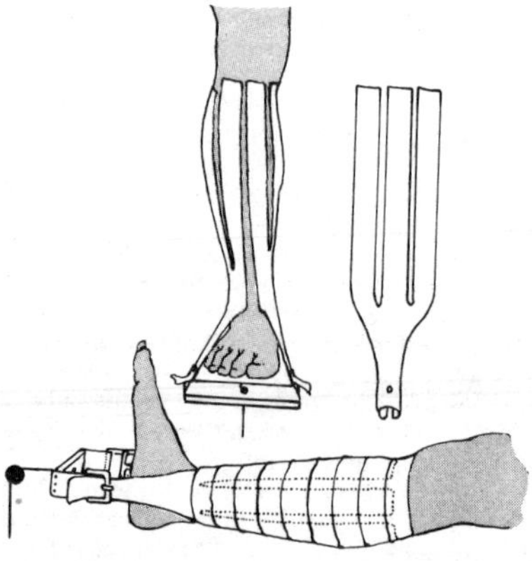

Left: Method of Application of Skin Traction

tle traction and internal rotation of the extremity while the anteroposterior film is exposed may provide a more favorable relation of fragments to demonstrate the fracture cleft.

Fractures of the femoral neck may be classified as abduction or adduction fractures.

Abduction Fracture of the Femoral Neck.

Abduction describes the relationship between the neck and shaft fragment and the head, which creates a coxa valga deformity. Abduction fractures occur most often in the proximal femoral neck adjacent to the head. Displacement is apt to be minimal, and impaction is often present. The direction of the fracture cleft approaches the transverse plane of the body, and the angle is 30° or less (see p. 768). The anteroposterior x-ray may show a wedge-shaped area of increased density whose base is directed superiorly. A good lateral film will demonstrate both the anterior and posterior cortices of the femoral neck. In this plane the neck and shaft fragment may be angulated slightly, so that only the posterior cortex appears to be impacted and the anterior cortices of the fragments appear to be separated.

Impaction is precarious and undependable as a fixation mechanism; if internal fixation is not used, separation may occur before healing is sound. If firm impaction can be demonstrated in both the anterior and posterior x-rays, some surgeons recommend conservative treatment, i.e., bed rest with the extremity in balanced suspension for 4-8 weeks. The patient is then permitted to be ambulatory with crutches, but full weight-bearing is not permitted until complete healing can be demonstrated by x-rays (usually 4-12 months after injury). Other surgeons prefer internal fixation because it permits the patient to be out of bed soon after the operation, even though unsupported weight-bearing is not permitted any sooner than after nonoperative treatment.

If examination in the lateral projection does not show firm impaction of both cortices at the fracture site, closed manipulation and internal fixation are indicated.

Adduction Fracture of the Femoral Neck.

Adduction fracture is characterized by coxa vara deformity. The fracture may be at any level of the neck, and the direction of the fracture cleft approaches that of the sagittal plane of the body. Displacement is usually present. The relatively vertical configuration of the fracture cleft favors proximal displacement of the distal fragment by the force of any axial thrust transmitted through the extremity. The fracture should be considered unstable if the angle between the fracture cleft and the transverse plane of the body is greater than 30° (Pauwels) (see p. 768). Internal fixation is necessary to prevent displacement after reduction since immobilization in a spica or treatment by traction is not reliable.

Adduction fracture of the femoral neck is a life-endangering injury; treatment is directed toward the preservation of life and restoration of function of the hip joint. Some surgeons believe that immediate operative treatment is required; others reply that 1-2 days of evaluation of the general health status of the patient while in traction is associated with a lowered mortality rate.

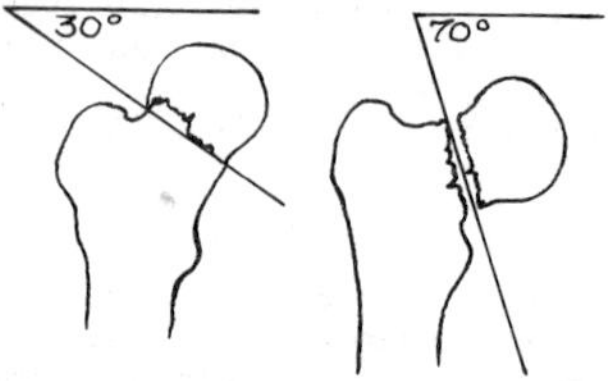

Pauwels' Angles

Preliminary treatment may be by skin or preferably by skeletal traction. X-rays are repeated in 12-24 hours to determine the adequacy of reduction. Comminution which was not evident on the initial examination will often be demonstrated on films taken with the fracture fragments in a more anatomic position.

Open operation is the treatment of choice. If internal fixation is adequate, postoperative immobilization is not necessary. The patient can be free in bed and can be mobilized at an early date; complications are minimized. If fixation is precarious, traction in balanced suspension for 1-4 months may be necessary until preliminary healing gives additional stability.

Weight-bearing should not be permitted until bone continuity is restored and avascular necrosis is not an immediate threat. The agile and cooperative patient may be ambulatory on crutches (but without weight-bearing) within a few days after operative treatment. Crutch walking is hazardous in elderly patients since inadvertent loading is likely to disrupt the fracture relationship.

The most common sequelae of cervical fracture of the femur are redisplacement after reduction, failure of bone healing, and osteonecrosis (avascular or aseptic necrosis) of the head fragment. Post-traumatic arthritis appears relatively late.

Femoral Neck Fracture in Childhood.

Traumatic cervical fracture of the femur in childhood (rare) must be differentiated from congenital coxa vara. Traumatic fracture is usually caused by severe injury. Anatomic reduction by closed manipulation and immobilization in a plaster spica are necessary to prevent deformity. Internal fixation with wires or screws may be necessary. Removal of the fixation apparatus after healing may prevent early fusion of the epiphysis.

Osteonecrosis of the capital epiphysis is a frequent sequel.

TROCHANTERIC FRACTURES

Fracture of the Lesser Trochanter.

Isolated fracture of the lesser trochanter is quite rare but may develop as a result of the avulsion force of the iliopsoas muscle. It occurs commonly as a component of intertrochanteric fracture.

Fracture of the Greater Trochanter.

Isolated fracture of the greater trochanter may be caused by direct injury, or may occur indirectly as a result of the activity of the gluteus medius and gluteus minimus muscles. It occurs most commonly as a component of intertrochanteric fracture.

If displacement is less than 1 cm. and there is no tendency to further displacement (determined by repeated x-ray examinations), treatment may be by bed rest with the affected extremity in balanced suspension until acute pain subsides. As rapidly as symptoms permit, activity can increase gradually to protected weight-bearing with crutches. Full weight-bearing is permitted as soon as healing is apparent, usually in 6-8 weeks. If displacement is greater than 1 cm. and increases on adduction of the thigh, extensive tearing of surrounding soft tissues may be assumed and open reduction is indicated, followed by internal fixation with 2-3 loops of stainless steel wire.

Intertrochanteric (Including Pertrochanteric) Fractures.

These fractures occur most commonly among elderly persons. The cleft of an intertrochanteric fracture extends upward and outward from the medial region of the junction of the neck and lesser trochanter toward the summit of the greater trochanter. Pertrochanteric fracture includes both trochanters, and is likely to be comminuted.

It is important to determine whether comminution has occurred and the magnitude of displacement. These fractures may vary from fissure fracture without significant separation to severe comminution into 4 major fragments: head-neck, greater trochanter, lesser trochanter, and shaft. Displacement may be so marked that the head-neck fragment forms a right angle with the shaft fragment and the distal fragment is rotated externally through an arc of 90°.

Failure of restoration of bone continuity by healing of intertrochanteric fractures is unlikely and the causes are usually apparent. Of the many factors that influence the rate of healing, those of particular significance are inadequate treatment as manifested by incomplete reduction with unsatisfactory apposition of fragments and unsustained immobilization; comminution; and osteopenia (osteoporosis and disuse atrophy). Healing in malposition (varus and external rotation) is abetted by the major stresses that cause displacement (gravity and muscle activity).

Initial treatment of the fracture in the hospital can be by balanced suspension and, when indicated, by the addition of traction. The selection of definitive treatment - closed or operative technics - depends in part upon the general condition of the patient. Because of the elderly age group in which intertrochanteric fracture is likely to occur, multiple system disease is a determinant of the mortality rate and for that reason the incidence of complications is diminished by the avoidance of prolonged recumbency in bed. Some surgeons are of the opinion that delay in open treatment is hazardous to the life of the patient, and they prefer to operate promptly. Others believe that an evaluation of the general health status of the patient should be made and that preliminary treatment of the fracture - reduction by closed technics - can proceed simultaneously.

Undisplaced fractures can be treated by balanced suspension of the lower extremity until the fragments are stabilized by preliminary bone healing. These fractures can also be treated initially by immobilization in a plaster spica. Sufficient healing generally occurs within 2-3 months to permit the patient to follow a bed—wheel chair existence until partial weight-bearing with crutches can be initiated. Unsupported weight-bearing should not be resumed until the fracture cleft has been obliterated by healing.

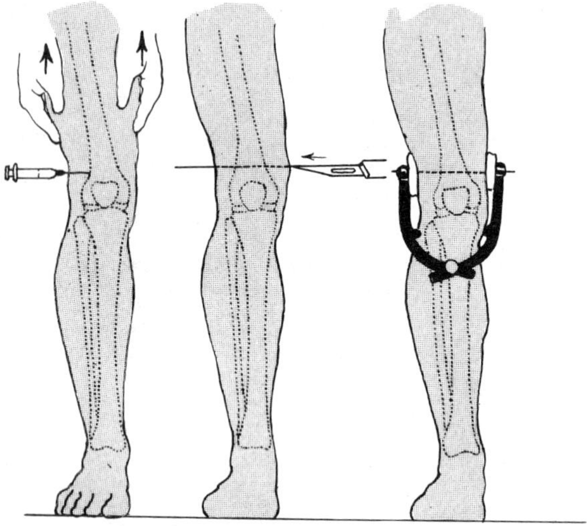

Technic of Insertion of Kirschner Wire in the
Supracondylar Region of the Femur

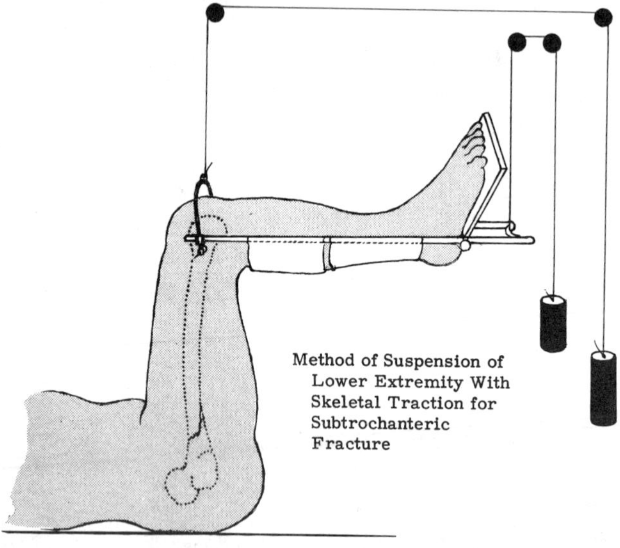

Method of Suspension of
Lower Extremity With
Skeletal Traction for
Subtrochanteric
Fracture

If comminution is present and displacement is significant, skin or (preferably) skeletal traction by a Kirschner wire through the tibial tubercle must be added to provide immobilization and to accomplish reduction. Definitive treatment of the fracture can be given in this way or it can be used as a preliminary to open operation.

Open operation may be done electively or may be mandatory for optimal treatment. Reduction of the fracture can be accomplished by closed technics, or it can be an integral part of the open operation. Some surgeons do not prefer to anatomically reduce unstable fractures caused by comminution of the medial femoral cortex. It is maintained that medial displacement of the upper end of the main distal fragment enhances mechanical stability (although it may cause concomitant varus deformity), and this advantageously permits earlier weight-bearing and more prompt healing. The chief intent of open operation is to provide sufficient fixation of the fragments by a metallic surgical implant so that the patient need not be confined to bed during the healing process.

Intertrochanteric fracture during childhood can be treated by skeletal traction with a Kirschner wire inserted through the lower femur above the epiphysial line (see p. 770) or by closed reduction and internal fixation. Varus deformity should be avoided if possible. The incidence of avascular necrosis of the capital femoral epiphysis following this fracture is high.

SUBTROCHANTERIC FRACTURE

Subtrochanteric fracture due to severe trauma occurs below the level of the lesser trochanter at the junction of cancellous and cortical bone. It is most common in men during the active years of life. Soft tissue damage is extensive. The direction of the fracture cleft may be transverse or oblique. Comminution occurs and the fracture may extend proximally into the intertrochanteric region or distally into the shaft. Muscle is often interposed between the major fragments.

Closed reduction should be attempted by continuous traction to bring the distal fragment into alignment with the proximal fragment. If comminution is not extensive and the lesser trochanter is not detached, the proximal fragment is often drawn into relative flexion, external rotation, and abduction by the predominant activity of the iliopsoas, gluteus medius, and gluteus minimus muscles.

Prolonged skeletal traction by means of a Kirschner wire inserted through the supracondylar region of the femur (with the hip and knee flexed to a right angle) is necessary (see below). X-ray is repeated every 4-8 hours until reduction has been accomplished. If soft tissue interposition is not a factor, reduction can be achieved within 48 hours. Thereafter the extremity is left in this position with an appropriate amount of traction until stabilization occurs, usually in 8-12 weeks. The angle of flexion is then reduced by gradually bringing the hip and knee into extension. After 2-3 months of continuous traction, the extremity can be immobilized in a plaster spica provided stabilization of the fracture has occurred. Weight-bearing must not be resumed for 6 months or even longer, until bone healing obliterates the fracture cleft.

Interposition of soft tissue between the major fragments may prevent closed reduction. Open reduction of this fracture is difficult and should be undertaken early; if treatment is delayed until the third week following injury, extensive bleeding at the fracture site is likely to be encountered.

After open reduction has been performed, internal fixation is required to prevent redisplacement. If comminution is present, or if it is important to avoid prolonged immobilization, biplane fixation is recommended.

The activity status after operation depends upon the adequacy of internal fixation. If fixation is precarious, skeletal traction in balanced suspension should be continued until healing is well under way. Otherwise, if the patient is agile and cooperative, he may be ambulatory on crutches (but without weight-bearing) a few days after the operation.

DISLOCATION OF THE HIP JOINT

Dislocation of the hip joint may occur with or without fracture of the pelvis. It occurs most commonly during the most active years of life as a result of severe trauma. The femoral head can be completely dislocated from the acetabulum only if the ligamentum teres is ruptured.

Posterior Hip Dislocation.

The head of the femur is usually dislocated posterior to the acetabulum while the thigh is flexed, e.g., as may occur in a head-on automobile collision when the passenger's knee is driven violently against the dashboard.

The significant clinical findings are shortening, adduction, and internal rotation of the extremity. Anteroposterior, transpelvic, and, if fracture of the acetabulum is demonstrated, oblique projections are required. Common complications are fracture of the acetabulum, injury to the sciatic nerve, and fracture of the head or shaft of the femur. The head of the femur may be displaced through a rent in the posterior hip joint capsule, or the glenoid lip may be avulsed from the acetabulum. The short external rotator muscles of the hip joint are commonly lacerated. Fracture of the posterior margin of the acetabulum can create an unstable mechanism.

If the acetabulum is not fractured or if the fragment is small, reduction by closed manipulation either by Bigelow's or Stimson's method is indicated.

The success of reduction is determined immediately by anteroposterior and lateral x-rays. Interposition of capsule substance will be manifest by widening of the joint cleft. If reduction is adequate the hip will be stable with the extremity in extension and slight external rotation.

Postreduction treatment may be by immobilization in a plaster spica or by balanced suspension. Since this is primarily a soft tissue injury, sound healing should take place in 4 weeks. Active hip joint movements may be instituted then, but even partial weight-bearing should be deferred for at least 3 months and full weight-bearing for 6 months.

If the posterior or superior acetabulum is fractured, dislocation of the hip must be assumed to have occurred even though displacement is not present at the time of examination. Undisplaced fissure fractures may be treated by bed rest for 3 weeks and avoidance of weight-bearing for 2 months. Frequent examination is necessary to make certain that the head of the femur has not become displaced from the acetabulum.

Minor fragments of the posterior margin of the acetabulum may be disregarded unless they are in the hip joint cavity. Larger displaced fragments often cannot be reduced adequately by closed methods. If the fragment is large and the hip is unstable following closed manipulation, open operation is indicated. If the sciatic nerve has been injured it should be exposed and treated by appropriate neurosurgical technics when the posterior hip joint is exposed. The fragment is then placed in anatomic position and fixed with 1-2 bone screws.

After the operation the patient is placed in bed with the extremity in balanced suspension (see p. 766) under 10-15 lb. of skeletal traction on the tibial tubercle for about 6 weeks or until healing of the acetabular fracture is sound. Full weight-bearing is not permitted for 6 months or more.

Anterior Hip Dislocation.

In anterior hip dislocation the head of the femur may lie medially on the obturator membrane, beneath the obturator externus muscle (obturator or thyroid dislocation), or, in a somewhat more superior direction, beneath the iliopsoas muscle and in contact with the superior ramus of the pubis (pubic dislocation). The thigh is classically in flexion, abduction, and external rotation, and the head of the femur is palpable anteriorly and distal to the inguinal flexion crease. Anteroposterior and lateral films are required; films prepared by transpelvic projection are likely to be helpful.

Closed manipulation with general anesthesia is usually adequate. Postreduction treatment may be by balanced suspension or by immobilization in a plaster spica with the hip in extension and the extremity in neutral rotation. Active hip motion is permitted after 3 weeks.

Central Dislocation of the Hip With Fracture of the Pelvis.

Central dislocation of the head of the femur with fracture of the acetabulum may be caused by crushing injury or by an axial force transmitted through the abducted extremity to the acetabulum. Comminution is commonly present. There are usually 2 fragments: superiorly, the ilium with the roof of the acetabulum; inferiorly and medially, the remainder of the acetabulum and the obturator ring. Fracture occurs near the roof of the acetabulum, and the components of the obturator ring are displaced inward with the head of the femur. Extensive soft tissue injury and massive bleeding into the soft tissues are likely to be present. Intra-abdominal injury must not be overlooked. Initially, stereoanteroposterior and oblique x-rays are required.

In the absence of complicating injury or immediately after such an injury has received priority attention, closed treatment of the fracture-dislocation by skeletal traction is required. Open reduction is hazardous and technically difficult; it should not be attempted except by the expert. Bidirectional traction is likely to achieve the most satisfactory results in all but the exceptional case. For the average adult, approximately 20 pounds of force are applied axially to the shaft of the femur, in neither abduction nor adduction, through a Kirschner wire placed preferably in the supracondylar region. A second Kirschner wire is inserted in the anteroposterior plane between the greater and lesser trochanters (in substantial cortical bone). Force is applied at a right angle to the direction of axial traction and the magnitude is the same. The extremity is placed in balanced suspension. Progress of reduction is observed by portable x-rays made 3 times a day until adequate positioning is manifested by relocation of the head of the femur beneath the roof of the acetabulum. Bidirectional traction is maintained for 4-6 weeks. Thereafter, the transverse traction component is gradually diminished under appropriate x-ray control until it can be discontinued. Axial traction is maintained until stabilization of the fracture fragments by early bone healing has occurred, usually about 8 weeks after injury. During the next 4-6 weeks, while balanced suspension is continued, gentle active exercises of the knee and hip are encouraged. After discontinuation of balanced suspension, more elaborate exercises designed to aid recovery of maximal hip function are performed frequently during the day. Full and unprotected weight bearing should not be advised before 6 months.

Sequelae are common and the patient should be warned of their probable occurrence. Anatomic reduction is an unattainable goal in most severely comminuted and widely displaced fractures of this type. Scarring within and around the hip joint, with or without ectopic bone and exuberant callus formation, is incidental to the healing process and can be a significant factor in restriction of motion in varying degrees. Osteonecrosis of the femoral head and post-traumatic degenerative arthritis are common sequelae that appear somewhat later.

FRACTURE OF THE SHAFT OF THE FEMUR

FRACTURE OF THE SHAFT OF THE FEMUR IN ADULTS

Fracture of the shaft of the femur usually occurs as a result of severe direct trauma. Indirect violence, especially torsional stress, is likely to cause spiral fractures that extend proximally or, more commonly, distally into the metaphyseal regions. These fractures are likely to be encountered in bone that has become atrophic as a result of disuse or senescence. Most are closed fractures; open fracture is often the result of compounding from within. Extensive soft tissue injury, bleeding, and shock are commonly present.

If the fracture is through the upper third of the shaft, the proximal fragment is apt to be in flexion, external rotation, and abduction, with proximal displacement or overriding of the distal fragment. In midshaft fracture the direction of displacement is not constant, but the distal fragment is almost always displaced proximally if the fracture is unstable; and angulation is commonly present with the apex directed anterolaterally. In complete fracture of the lower third of the shaft the distal fragment is often displaced proximally; the upper end of the distal fragment may be displaced posteriorly to the distal end of the upper fragment.

The most significant features are severe pain in the thigh and deformity of the lower extremity. Surgical shock is likely to be present. Careful x-ray examination in at least 2 planes is necessary to determine the exact site and configuration of the fracture cleft. Splints should be removed either by the surgeon or by a qualified assistant so that manipulation will not cause further damage. The hip and knee should be examined for associated injury.

Injuries to the sciatic nerve and to the superficial femoral artery and vein are not common but must be recognized promptly. Surgical shock and secondary anemia are the most important early complications. Later complications are essentially those of prolonged recumbency, e.g., the formation of renal calculi.

Treatment.

Treatment depends upon the age of the patient and the site and configuration of the fracture. Displaced, oblique, spiral, and comminuted fractures are unstable, and can rarely be treated successfully by closed manipulation and external plaster fixation. Traction followed by closed manipulation should be tried. Skeletal traction is generally the most effective form of closed treatment.

After preliminary traction, biplane x-rays are made to determine the progress of correction of overriding. If alignment and apposition of fragments are not satisfactory, closed manipulation, preferably under general anesthesia, should be carried out while traction is continued.

If soft tissue interposition prevents reduction by closed methods, open reduction may be required in the adult to avoid delay of bone healing.

A. Fracture of the Upper Third: The treatment of subtrochanteric fracture is discussed on p. 771. If a comminuted subtrochanteric fracture extends into the upper third of the femoral shaft, it may be necessary to use skeletal traction through the supracondylar region of the femur and suspend the extremity with hip and knee at a right angle (see p. 770). Otherwise, skeletal traction can be through either the lower femur or the tibial tubercle with the extremity at a less acute angle in balanced suspension. Russell's traction can be used if the patient is small and muscular development is not great. External rotation and abduction of the extremity are usually required to bring the lower fragment into alignment with the proximal fragment.

B. Fracture of the Middle Third: The deformity caused by fracture at this level is not constant. Angulation is commonly present with the apex directed anterolaterally. Treatment may be by skeletal traction through the tibial tubercle or the lower end of the femur (see p. 766). Traction in the transverse plane by a swathe around the thigh may be necessary to prevent recurrence of angulation.

C. Fracture of the Lower Third: In transverse and comminuted fractures, the proximal end of the distal fragment is likely to be displaced posterior to the distal end of the proximal fragment. The same displacement is likely to be encountered in supracondylar fracture. Russell's traction should not be used for comminuted or widely displaced fractures since it may injure the femoral or popliteal vessels. Simultaneous skeletal

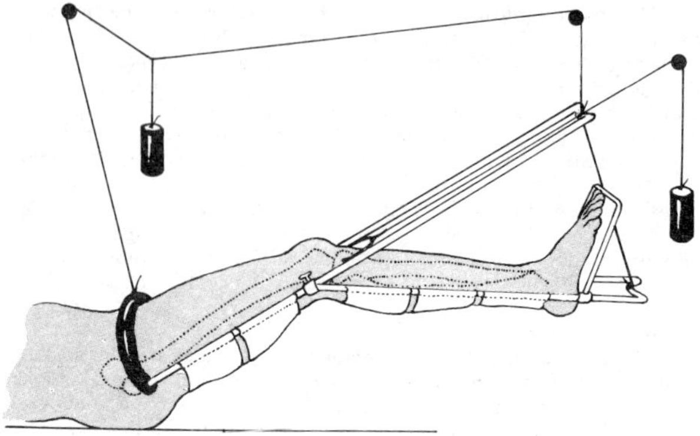

Method of Suspension of Lower Extremity With Biplane Skeletal Traction for Supracondylar Fracture

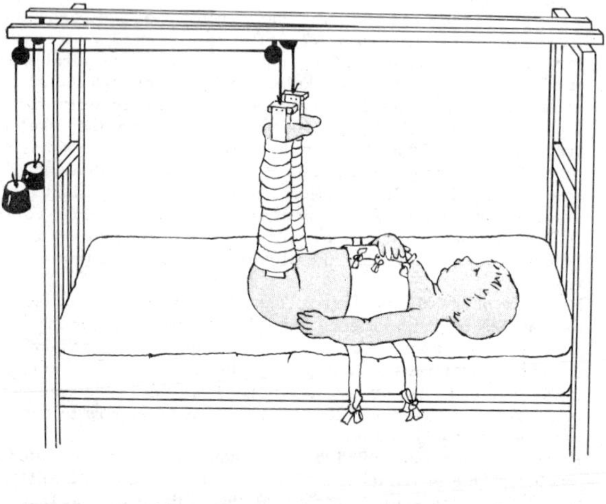

Bryant's Traction

traction through the distal femur at right angles to the tibial tubercle can correct displacement of the distal fragment. The same mechanism of traction is used for supracondylar fracture (see p. 776).

After reduction has been accomplished by traction, biplane x-ray examination should be repeated at least weekly to determine maintenance of reduction and the progress of healing. When sufficient callus has formed to assure stabilization of the fragments, generally after 12 weeks or more, further immobilization can be given by a one and one half plaster spica. Prior to application of the spica, there should be a period of observation in balanced suspension without traction to determine whether displacement of the fracture fragments by overriding will occur. Angulation can generally be corrected in plaster by appropriate wedging.

Elective indications for open reduction and internal fixation may be based upon the desire to avoid prolonged recumbency in bed and hospitalization. Some mandatory indications include inability to obtain adequate reduction by closed technics and delay of bone healing. The purpose of open reduction is generally to provide anatomic reposition and clinically rigid fixation that will permit the patient to be ambulatory without such external supportive apparatus as casts, splints, or braces. Unprotected weight-bearing without crutches until restoration of bone continuity should not be a goal of open operation of most fractures.

FRACTURE OF THE SHAFT OF THE FEMUR IN INFANTS AND CHILDREN

Femoral fracture at birth occurs most often in the middle third. Comminution is usually not present.

Skin traction (see p. 776) and plaster immobilization are adequate, although skeletal traction may be necessary in older children. Open reduction is rarely necessary.

Fracture of the proximal or middle third of the femur in a child under 5 years of age can be treated with Bryant's traction. Adhesive strips are applied to both extremities from the upper thirds of the thighs to the supramalleolar regions, and held firm by circular bandages. Both hips are flexed to a right angle, and the knees are maintained in full extension. Sufficient traction force is applied to raise the buttocks free of the bed. Circulatory adequacy must be observed carefully, and another method substituted if swelling, cyanosis or pallor of the foot, or obliteration of pedal pulsations cannot be managed by adjustment of dressings.

As a rule, sufficient callus is present at the fracture site after 3-4 weeks so that traction can be discontinued. If callus formation is adequate, infants who have not yet begun to walk need no further protection; walking infants may require a single plaster hip spica for an additional 4-6 weeks.

Preliminary treatment of unstable fracture of the femur in children over 5 years of age can be by Russell's traction. If the child is uncooperative, or if adequate correction (see p. 766) cannot be obtained, it may also be necessary to place the sound extremity in traction. Traction should be continued until the fracture is stabilized; if traction is discontinued before the reparative callus is sufficiently mature, the deformity (especially angulation) may recur even though the extremity is protected by a plaster spica. Correction of angulation and torsional displacement around the long axis of the femur are mandatory. Slight shortening (1-2 cm.) can be compensated by growth. Close apposition of fragments is not necessary, since healing will take place in spite of minimal soft tissue interposition.

It is usually necessary to continue traction for 6-8 weeks or until sufficient callus has formed to prevent recurrence of the deformity. Immobilization in a plaster spica should be maintained for another 2 months. Weight-bearing must not be resumed until x-rays show that healing is sound.

INJURIES OF THE KNEE REGION

FRACTURES OF THE DISTAL FEMUR

Supracondylar Fracture of the Femur.

This comparatively uncommon fracture (at the junction of cortical and cancellous bone) may be transverse, oblique, or comminuted. The distal end of the proximal fragment is apt to perforate the overlying vastus intermedius, vastus medialis, or rectus femoris muscles, and may penetrate the suprapatellar pouch of the knee joint to cause hemarthrosis. The proximal end of the distal fragment is usually displaced posteriorly and slightly laterally.

Since the distal fragment may impinge upon the popliteal vessels, circulatory adequacy distal to the fracture site should be verified as soon as possible. Absence of pedal pulsations is an indication for immediate reduction. If pulsation does not return promptly after reduction, immediate exploration and appropriate treatment of the vascular lesion is indicated.

A less frequent complication is injury to the peroneal or tibial nerve.

If the fracture is transverse or nearly so, closed manipulation under general anesthesia will occasionally be successful. Stable fractures with minimal displacement can be immobilized in a single plaster hip spica with the hip and knee in about 30° of flexion. Frequent x-ray examination is necessary to make certain that redisplacement has not occurred.

Stable or unstable uncomplicated supracondylar fracture is best treated with biplane skeletal traction if soft tissue interposition does not interfere with reduction (see p. 776). If adequate reduction cannot be obtained, it may be necessary to manipulate the fragments under general anesthesia, using skeletal traction to control the distal fragment.

Traction must be continued for about 6 weeks or until stabilization occurs. The wires can then be removed and the extremity immobilized in a single plaster spica for an additional 2-3 months.

An alternative method of treatment (applicable only to stable fractures) is to incorporate the wires into a plaster spica after reduction.

Supracondylar fracture is likely to be followed by restriction of knee motion due to scarring and adhesion formation in adjacent soft tissues.

Intercondylar Fracture of the Femur.

This uncommon comminuted fracture, which occurs only in older patients, is classically described as "T" or "Y" according to the x-ray configuration of the fragments. Closed reduction is difficult when the proximal shaft fragment is interposed between the 2 main distal fragments. Maximal recovery of function of the knee joint requires anatomic reduction of the articular components. If alignment is satisfactory and displacement minimal, immobilization for about 4 months in a plaster spica will be sufficient. If displacement is marked, skeletal traction through the tibial tubercle (with the knee in flexion) is required. Manual molding of the distal fragments may be necessary. Open reduction and bolt fixation of the distal fragments may be indicated to restore articular congruity. Further treatment is as described for supracondylar fracture.

Condylar Fracture of the Femur.

Isolated fracture of the lateral or medial condyle of the femur is a rare consequence of severe trauma. Occasionally only the posterior portion of the condyle is separated. The cruciate ligaments or the collateral ligament of the opposite side of the knee are often injured.

The objective of treatment is restoration of anatomic intra-articular relationships. If displacement is minimal, the knee can be manipulated into varus or valgus (opposite the position of deformity). If anatomic reduction cannot be obtained by closed manipulation, open reduction and fixation of the minor fragment with 2-3 bone screws is recommended. The ligaments must be explored, and repaired if found to be injured.

Separation of the Distal Femoral Epiphysis.

Traumatic separation of the distal femoral epiphysis in children is the counterpart of supracondylar fracture in the adult. The direction of displacement of the epiphysial fragment is most commonly anterior. Torsional displacement around the long axis of the femur may be associated.

Reduction of anterior displacement can be achieved by closed manipulation. After reduction is complete, the knee is flexed to a right angle and a tubular plaster cast is applied from the inguinal region to the toes. If the thigh is obese, the plaster should be extended proximally to include the pelvis in a single hip spica.

Peripheral circulation must be observed carefully. After 4 weeks the plaster is changed and flexion of the knee reduced to 135°. At the end of the second month the patient may be permitted to be free in bed until he regains complete knee extension.

FRACTURES OF THE PROXIMAL TIBIA

Fracture of the Lateral Tibial Condyle.

Fracture of the lateral condyle of the tibia is commonly caused by a blow on the lateral aspect of the knee with the foot in fixed position, producing an abduction strain. Hemarthrosis is always present, as the fracture cleft involves the knee joint. Soft tissue injuries are likely to be present also. The tibial collateral and anterior cruciate ligaments may be torn. A displaced free fragment may tear the overlying lateral meniscus. If displacement is marked, fracture of the proximal fibula may be present also.

The objective of treatment is to restore the articular surface and normal anatomic relationships, so that torn ligaments can heal without elongation. In cases of minimal displacement where ligaments have not been extensively damaged, treatment may be by immobilization for 6 weeks in a tubular plaster cast extending from the toes to the inguinal region with the knee in slight flexion. Reduction of marked displacement can be achieved by closed manipulation unless comminution is severe. After x-ray verification of reduction, the extremity can be immobilized in a tubular plaster cast extending from the inguinal region to the toes, preferably with the knee in full extension.

Many fractures of the lateral condyle of the tibia, especially comminuted fractures, cannot be reduced adequately by closed methods. Open reduction and stabilization with a bolt or multiple bone screws may be necessary.

Fracture of the Medial Tibial Condyle.

Fracture of the medial condyle of the tibia is caused by the adduction strain produced by a blow against the medial aspect of the knee with the foot in fixed position. The medial meniscus and the fibular collateral ligament may be torn. Severe comminution is not usually present, and there is only 1 major free fragment.

Treatment is by closed reduction to restore the articular surface of the tibia so that ligamentous healing can occur without elongation. After reduction the extremity is immobilized for 10-12 weeks in a tubular plaster cast extending from the inguinal region to the toes with the knee in full extension. Weight-bearing is not permitted for 4 months at least.

Fracture of Both Tibial Condyles.

Axial force, such as may result from falling on the foot or sudden deceleration with the knee in full extension (during an automobile accident), can cause simultaneous fracture of both condyles of the tibia. Comminution is apt to be severe. Swelling of the knee due to hemarthrosis is marked. Deformity is either genu varum or genu valgum. X-ray examination should include oblique projections.

Severe comminution makes anatomic reduction difficult to achieve by any means and difficult to maintain following closed manipulation alone. Sustained skeletal traction is usually necessary. When stability has been achieved, the extremity can be immobilized for another 4-6 weeks in a tubular plaster cast extending from the toes to the inguinal region with the knee in full extension. Unassisted weight-bearing is not permitted before the end of the fourth month.

If closed methods are not effective, open reduction must be attempted.

Instability and restriction of motion of the knee are common sequelae. If reduction is not adequate, post-traumatic arthritis will appear early.

Fracture of the Tibial Tuberosity.

Violent contraction of the quadriceps muscle may cause avulsion of the tibial tuberosity. Avulsion of the anterior portion of the upper tibial epiphysis, uncommon in childhood, must be differentiated from Osgood-Schlatter disease (osteochondrosis of the tibial tuberosity).

When avulsion of the tuberosity is complete, active extension of the knee is not possible.

If displacement is minimal, treatment is by immobilization in a tubular plaster cast extending from the inguinal to the supramalleolar region with the knee in full extension. Immobilization is maintained for 8 weeks or until stabilization occurs.

A loose fragment which has been displaced more than 0.5 cm. can be treated either by closed reduction and percutaneous fixation, with plaster immobilization, or by open reduction.

Fracture of the Tibial Tubercle.

This injury usually occurs in association with comminuted fracture of the condyles. The medial intercondyloid tubercle may be avulsed with adjacent bone attached to the anterior cruciate ligament, and injury to that structure is of greater importance. In addition to avulsion of the anterior cruciate ligament, there may also be injury to the tibial collateral ligament and the medial knee joint capsule (see p. 785). Hemarthrosis is always present.

Isolated and undisplaced fracture may be treated by immobilization of the extremity for 6 weeks in a tubular plaster cast extending from the inguinal region to the toes with the knee in slight flexion. The treatment of displaced fracture is the same as that of rupture of the anterior cruciate ligament (see p. 786).

Separation of the Proximal Tibial Epiphysis.

Complete displacement of the proximal tibial epiphysis is rare; partial separation due to forceful hyperextension of the knee is more common. The distal metaphysial fragment is displaced posteriorly.

If no circulatory or neurologic deficit is present, immediate treatment by closed manipulation is indicated. Reduction can be accomplished by forced flexion of the knee. Anteroposterior films are then exposed by holding the plate against the anterior surface of the leg with the beam directed through the lower thigh. A lateral film is also prepared. If x-rays show that reduction is adequate, a heavy anterior plaster splint is applied from the inguinal region to the bases of the toes, with the knee in acute flexion. The splint is maintained in position with circular bandages around the foot, ankle, and upper thigh. The bandages are wrapped in figure-of-eight fashion around the thigh and leg (as is done for supracondylar fracture of the humerus). Peripheral circulation must be observed frequently for at least 72 hours. After 3 weeks the knee may be brought to a right angle and a tubular plaster cast applied from the inguinal region to the toes for another 3-4 weeks. Even guarded weight-bearing must be avoided until the end of the second month.

Injury to the proximal tibial epiphysial plate as a result of a blow on the lateral aspect of the knee causes compression but only minor displacement. This lesion, analogous to fracture of the lateral condyle in the adult, is apt to retard or arrest the growth of the lateral aspect of the tibia and thus cause tibia valga, or knock-knee. Surgical arrest of the growth of the medial tibial epiphysis may be necessary to prevent this deformity.

FRACTURE OF THE PROXIMAL FIBULA

Isolated fracture of the proximal fibula is uncommon; this fracture is usually associated with fracture of the femur or of the tibia or fracture-dislocation of the ankle joint. The apex of the fibular head may be avulsed by the activity of the biceps femoris muscle or detached with the fibular collateral ligament by an adduction strain of the knee.

The fracture usually requires no treatment, but avulsion of the apex of the head may necessitate operative repair of the ligament or tendon.

Fracture in this region may be associated with paralysis of the common peroneal nerve.

DISLOCATION OF THE PROXIMAL TIBIOFIBULAR JOINT

This extremely rare lesion is caused by the activity of the biceps femoris muscle. Displacement is posterior, and can be reduced by digital pressure over the head of the fibula in the opposite direction.

FRACTURE OF THE PATELLA

Transverse Fracture of the Patella.

Transverse fracture of the patella is the result of indirect violence, usually with the knee in semiflexion. Fracture may be due to sudden voluntary contraction of the quadriceps muscles or sudden forced flexion of the leg when these muscles are contracted. The level of fracture is most often in the middle. The extent of tearing of the patellar retinacula depends upon the degree of force of the initiating injury. The activity of the quadriceps muscles causes displacement of the proximal fragment; the magnitude of displacement is dependent upon the extent of the tear of the quadriceps expansion.

Swelling of the anterior knee region is caused by hemarthrosis and hemorrhage into the soft tissues overlying the joint. If displacement is present, the defect in the patella can be palpated and active extension of the knee is lost.

Open reduction is indicated if the fragments are separated more than 2-3 mm. The fragments must be accurately repositioned to prevent early post-traumatic arthritis of the patellofemoral joint. If the minor fragment is small (no more than 1 cm. in height), it may be excised and the rectus or patellar tendon (depending upon which pole of the patella is involved) sutured directly to the major fragment. If the fragments are approximately the same size, repair by wire cerclage is preferred.

Removal of 50% of the patella causes incongruity of joint surfaces, and post-traumatic arthritis may occur early.

Comminuted Fracture of the Patella.

Comminuted fracture of the patella is caused only by direct violence. Little or no separation of the fragments occurs because the quadriceps expansion is not extensively torn. Severe injury may cause extensive comminution of the articular cartilages of both the patella and the opposing femur. If comminution is not severe and displacement is insignificant, plaster immobilization for 8 weeks in a cylinder extending from the groin to the supramalleolar region is sufficient.

Severe comminution requires excision of the patella and repair of the defect by imbrication of the quadriceps expansion.

TEAR OF THE QUADRICEPS TENDON

Tear of the quadriceps tendon occurs most often in patients over 40 years of age. Preexisting attritional disease of the tendon is apt to be present, and the causative injury may be minor. The tear commonly results from sudden deceleration, such as stumbling, or slipping on a wet surface. A small flake of bone may be avulsed from the superior pole of the patella, or the tear may occur entirely through tendinous and muscle tissue.

Pain may be noted in the anterior knee region. Swelling is due to hemarthrosis and extravasation of blood into the soft tissues. The patient is unable to extend his knee completely. X-rays may show avulsion of a bit of bone from the superior patella.

Operative repair is required for complete tear. If treatment is delayed until partial healing has occurred, the suture line can be reinforced by transplantation of the iliotibial band from the upper extremity of the tibia.

TEAR OF THE PATELLAR LIGAMENT

The same mechanism which causes tears of the quadriceps tendon, transverse fracture of the patella, or avulsion of the tibial tuberosity may also cause tear of the patellar ligament. The characteristic clinical finding is proximal displacement of the patella. A bit of bone may be avulsed from the lower pole of the patella if the tear takes place in the proximal patellar tendon.

Operative treatment is necessary for complete tear. The ligament is resutured to the patella and any tear in the quadriceps expansion is repaired. The extremity should be immobilized for 8 weeks in a tubular plaster cast extending from the inguinal to the supramalleolar region. Guarded exercises may then be started.

DISLOCATION OF THE PATELLA

Traumatic dislocation of the patellofemoral joint may be associated with dislocation of the knee joint. When this injury occurs alone it may be due to direct violence or muscle activity of the quadriceps, and the direction of dislocation of the patella may be lateral. Spontaneous reduction is apt to occur if the knee joint is extended; if so, the clinical findings may consist merely of hemarthrosis and localized tenderness over the medial patellar retinaculum. Gross instability of the patella, which can be demonstrated by physical examination, indicates that injury to the soft tissues of the medial aspect of the knee has been extensive. Recurrent episodes require operative repair for effective treatment.

DISLOCATION OF THE KNEE JOINT

Traumatic dislocation of the knee joint is uncommon in adults and extremely rare in children. It is caused by severe trauma. Displacement may be transverse or torsional. Complete dislocation can occur only after extensive tearing of the supporting ligaments, and is apt to cause injury to the popliteal vessels or the tibial and peroneal nerves.

Signs of neurovascular injury below the site of dislocation are an absolute indication for prompt reduction under general anesthesia, since failure of circulation will undoubtedly result in gangrene of the leg and foot. Axial traction is applied to the leg and a shearing force is exerted over the fragments in the appropriate direction. If pedal pulses do not return promptly, the popliteal fossa should be explored at once for treatment of any vascular injury.

Anatomic reduction of uncomplicated dislocation should be attempted. If impinging soft tissues cannot be removed by closed manipulation, arthrotomy is indicated. After reduction the extremity is immobilized in a tubular plaster cast extending from the inguinal region to the toes with the knee in slight flexion. (In the obese patient a single hip spica should be applied.) A window should be cut in the plaster over the dorsum of the foot to allow frequent determination of dorsalis pedis pulsation. After 8 weeks' immobilization the knee can be protected by a long leg brace. Intensive quadriceps exercises are necessary to minimize functional loss.

INTERNAL DERANGEMENTS OF THE KNEE JOINT

Internal derangements of the knee joint mechanism may be caused by trauma or attritional disease. Although ligamentous and cartilaginous injuries are discussed separately, they may occur as combined lesions.

Injury to the Menisci.

Injury to the medial meniscus is the most frequent internal derangement of the knee joint. Any portion of the meniscus may be torn. A marginal tear permits displacement of the medial fragment into the intercondylar region ("bucket-handle tear"). A fragment of cartilage displaced between the articular surfaces of the femur and tibia prevents either complete extension or complete flexion.

The significant clinical findings after acute injury are swelling (due to hemarthrosis) and varying degrees of restriction of flexion or extension. Motion may cause pain over the anteromedial or posteromedial joint line. Tenderness can often be elicited at the point of pain. Forcible external rotation of the foot with the knee flexed to a right angle may cause pain over the medial joint line. If symptoms have persisted for 2-3 weeks, weakness and atrophy of the quadriceps femoris may be present.

Injury to the lateral meniscus less often causes mechanical blockage of joint motion. Pain and tenderness may be present over the lateral joint line. Pain can be elicited by forcible rotation of the leg with the knee flexed to a right angle.

Initial treatment may be conservative. Swelling and pain caused by tense hemarthrosis can be relieved by aspiration. If pain is severe, the extremity should be immobilized in a posterior plaster splint with the knee in slight flexion. Younger patients usually prefer to be ambulatory on crutches, but immediate weight-bearing must not be permitted. As long as acute symptoms persist, isometric quadriceps exercises should be performed frequently throughout the day with the knee in maximum extension (as a "straight leg lift"). Unrestricted activity must not be resumed until complete motion is recovered and healing is complete.

Exploratory arthrotomy is advisable for recurrent "locking," recurrent effusion, or disabling pain. Isometric quadriceps exercises are instituted immediately after the operation and gradually increased in frequency. As soon as the patient is able to perform these exercises comfortably, graded resistance maneuvers should be started. Exercises must be continued until all motion has been recovered and the volume and competency of the quadriceps are equal on both sides.

Injury to the Collateral Ligaments.

The collateral ligaments prevent excursion of the joint beyond normal limits. When the knee is in full extension, the collateral ligaments are taut; in flexion, only the anterior fibers of the tibial collateral ligament are taut.

A. Tibial Collateral Ligament: Forced abduction of the leg at the knee, which is frequently associated with torsional strain, causes injury varying from tear of a few fibers to complete rupture of the ligament. A bit of bone may be avulsed from its femoral or tibial attachment.

A history of a twisting injury at the knee with valgus strain can usually be obtained. Pain is present over the medial aspect of the knee joint. In severe injury joint effusion may be present. Tenderness can be elicited at the site of the lesion. When only an isolated ligamentous tear is present, x-ray examination may not be helpful unless it is made while valgus stress is applied to the extended knee. Under local or general anesthesia the extremities are bound together in full extension at the knee joint, and an anteroposterior film is made with the legs in forced abduction. Widening of the medial joint cleft suggests complete rupture.

Treatment of incomplete tear consists of protection from further injury while healing progresses. Painful hemarthrosis should be relieved by aspiration. The knee may be immobilized in a posterior plaster splint or a tubular cast extending from the inguinal to the supramalleolar region.

Complete rupture should be repaired immediately so that healing will take place without ligamentous elongation and subsequent instability of the knee joint. Tear of the medial collateral ligament is frequently associated with other lesions, such as tear of the medial meniscus, rupture of the anterior cruciate ligament, or fracture of the lateral condyle of the tibia.

B. Fibular Collateral Ligament: Tear of the fibular collateral ligament is often associated with injury to surrounding structures, e.g., the popliteus muscle tendon and the iliotibial band. Avulsion of the apex of the fibular head may occur, and the peroneal nerve may be injured.

Pain and tenderness are present over the lateral aspect of the knee joint, and hemarthrosis may be present. X-rays may show a bit of bone avulsed from the fibular head. If severe injury is suspected, x-ray examination under stress, using local or general anesthesia, is required. A firm, padded nonopaque object about 8-12 inches in diameter is placed between the knees and the legs are forcibly adducted while an anteroposterior exposure is made. Widening of the lateral joint cleft indicates severe injury.

The treatment of partial tear is similar to that described for partial tear of the medial collateral ligament. If complete tear is suspected, and especially if the peroneal nerve has been injured, exploration is indicated. The extremity is protected for 8 weeks in a plaster cylinder extending from the inguinal region to above the ankle.

Injury to the Cruciate Ligaments.

The function of the anterior and posterior cruciate ligaments is to restrict anterior and posterior gliding of the tibia when the knee is flexed. If the tibia is rotated internally on the femur, the ligaments twist around themselves and become taut; if the tibia is rotated externally, they become lax.

A. Anterior Cruciate Ligament: Injury to the anterior cruciate ligament is usually associated with injury to the medial meniscus or the tibial collateral ligament. The cruciate ligament may be avulsed with a part of the medial tibial tubercle or may rupture within the substance of its fibers.

The characteristic clinical sign of tear of either cruciate ligament is a positive ''drawer'' sign: the knee is flexed at a right angle and pulled forward; if excessive anterior excursion of the proximal tibia (in comparison with the opposite normal side) can be noted, a tear of the anterior ligament is likely.

Complete recent rupture of the anterior cruciate ligament within its substance can occasionally be repaired with stout sutures. When manifest by avulsed tibial bone that is displaced, attachment of the fragment in anatomic position by arthrotomy is necessary. When the fragment of bone is large, displaced, and not treated until 4 weeks or more after injury, excision of the fragment and reinsertion of the ligament may be necessary to eliminate the blocking effect of the bone fragment and to permit recovery of function. Old tears may require reconstructive procedures.

B. Posterior Cruciate Ligament: Tear of the posterior ligament may occur within its substance or may be manifest by avulsion of a fragment of bone of variable size at its tibial attachment. Tear of the posterior cruciate ligament can be diagnosed by the "drawer" sign: the knee is flexed at a right angle and the upper tibia is pushed backward; if excessive posterior excursion of the proximal tibia can be noted, tear of the posterior ligament is likely.

Treatment is directed primarily at the associated injuries and maintenance of the competency of the quadriceps musculature. Primary repair of tears within the fibers is difficult and of dubious value. Open reduction and fixation of a fragment of tibia with the attached ligament is feasible and is likely to restore functional competency of the ligament.

FRACTURE OF THE SHAFTS OF THE TIBIA AND FIBULA

Fracture of the shaft of the tibia or fibula occurs at any age but is most common during youth and active adulthood. In general, open, transverse, comminuted, and segmental fractures are caused by indirect violence. Fracture of the middle third of the shaft (especially if comminuted) is apt to be complicated by delay of bone healing.

If fracture is complete and displacement is present, clinical diagnosis is not difficult. However, critical local examination is of utmost importance in planning treatment. The nature of the skin wounds which may communicate with the fracture site often suggests the mechanism of compounding, whether it has occurred from within or from without. A small laceration without contused edges suggests that the point of a bone fragment has caused compounding from within. A large wound with contused edges, especially over the subcutaneous surface of the tibia, suggests compounding from without. The presence of abrasions more than 6 hours old, blebs, pyoderma, and preexisting ulcers precludes immediate open treatment of closed fracture. Extensive swelling due to hemorrhagic exudate in closed fascial compartments may prevent complete reduction immediately. Extensive hemorrhagic and edematous infiltration can complicate and make difficult satisfactory closure of the subcutaneous tissue and skin incidental to elective open reduction. Neurovascular integrity below the level of the fracture must be verified before definitive treatment is instituted.

X-rays in the anteroposterior and lateral projection of the entire leg, including both the knee and ankle joints, are always necessary, and oblique projections are often desirable. The surgeon must know the exact site and configuration of the fracture, the severity of comminution, and the direction of displacement of fragments. Inadequate x-ray examination can lead to an incomplete diagnosis.

FRACTURE OF THE SHAFT OF THE FIBULA

Isolated fracture of the shaft of the fibula is uncommon and is usually caused by direct trauma. Fibular shaft fracture is usually

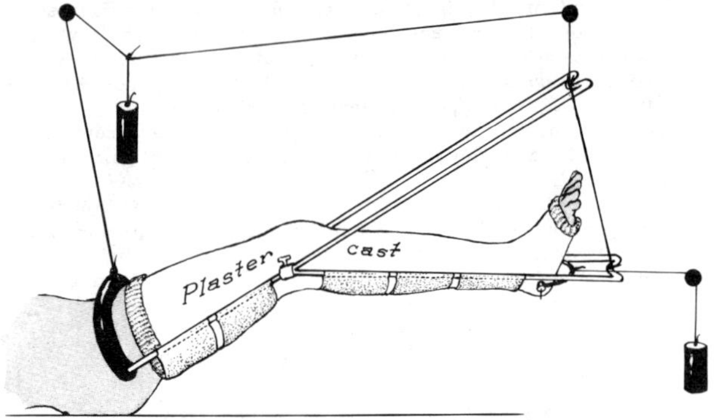

Calcaneal Skeletal Traction and Full Lower Extremity Plaster for Unstable Fracture of Tibia and Fibula

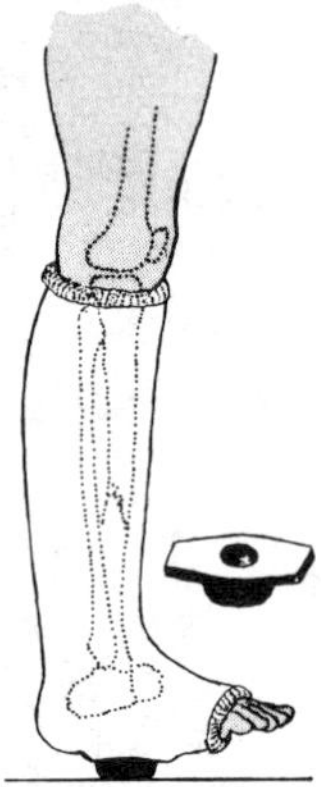

Left: Weight-Bearing Plaster Boot

Right: Gibney Ankle Strapping

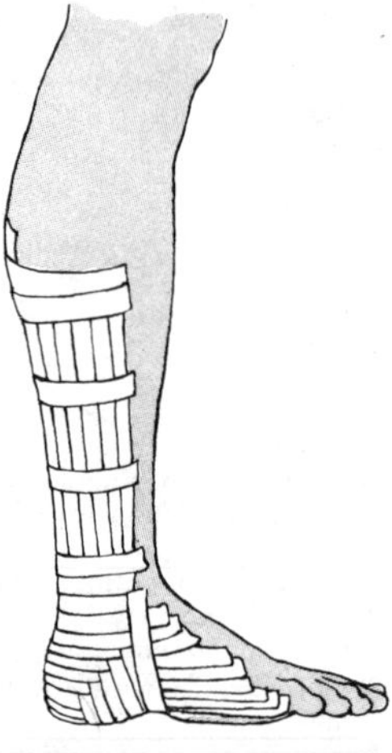

associated with other injury of the leg, such as fracture of the tibia or fracture-dislocation of the ankle joint. If no other lesion is present, immobilization for 4 weeks in a plaster boot (equipped with a walking surface) extending from the knee to the toes is sufficient for displaced, painful fractures. Undisplaced fractures require no immobilization, but discomfort can be minimized during the early days after injury by the use of crutches or a cane. Complete healing of uncomplicated fracture can be expected.

FRACTURE OF THE SHAFT OF THE TIBIA

Isolated fracture of the shaft of the tibia is likely to be caused by indirect injury, such as a torsional stress. Such a fracture is mechanically stable.

Fracture of the shaft of the tibia is comparatively stable unless the fibula is fractured also. Marked displacement does not usually occur, and overriding is not significant unless there is associated dislocation of either tibiofibular joint.

If the fragments are not displaced, treatment may be by immobilization in a tubular plaster cast extending from the inguinal region to the toes with the knee in about 30° of flexion and the foot in neutral position. The plaster should be changed 2-4 weeks after the injury to correct the loosening which will occur as a result of absorption of hemorrhagic exudate and atrophy of the thigh and calf muscles. Immobilization should be continued for at least 10 weeks, or until early bone healing is demonstrated by x-ray.

If the fragments are displaced, manipulation under anesthesia may be necessary. Fractures with a comparative transverse cleft tend to be stable after reduction. Oblique and spiral fractures tend to become displaced unless the fragments are locked.

A tubular plaster cast is applied as for undisplaced fracture. If x-rays do not show satisfactory apposition of fragments, alternative methods of treatment should be used (see below).

FRACTURE OF THE SHAFTS OF BOTH BONES IN ADULTS

Fracture of the shafts of the tibia and fibula are unstable lesions which tend to become displaced following reduction. Treatment is directed toward reduction and stabilization of the tibial fracture until healing takes place. For adequate reduction the fragments must be apposed almost completely, and angulation and torsional displacement of the tibial fracture must be corrected.

If reduction by closed manipulation is anatomic and angular and torsional displacement are corrected, transverse fractures tend to be stable. Repeated x-rays are necessary to determine whether displacement has recurred. The plaster must remain snug at all times. Recurrent angular displacement can be corrected by dividing the plaster circumferentially and inserting wedges in the appropriate direction. If apposition is disturbed, another type of treatment must be substituted.

If oblique and spiral fractures are unstable following manipulation and immobilization, internal fixation or skeletal traction is usually required (see p. 788). This can be accomplished by closed reduction and skeletal distraction. While traction is continued, a tubular plaster cast with pins or wires incorporated is applied.

An alternative method is continuous skeletal traction. Traction must be continued for about 6 weeks until preliminary healing causes stabilization. The extremity is then immobilized in plaster for at least 12 weeks until bone continuity has been restored.

If adequate apposition and correction of the deformity cannot be achieved by closed methods, open reduction and internal fixation are required.

The blood supply to intermediate fragments is likely to be disturbed in comminuted and segmental fractures. These unstable fractures can usually be treated successfully only by closed reduction and external immobilization. If the patient wishes to remain ambulatory, percutaneous fixation of the major fragments with Steinmann pins or Kirschner wires will maintain reduction and alignment. However, continuous skeletal traction in plaster with a Kirschner wire inserted through the calcaneus is usually preferred until stabilization occurs (see p. 788).

FRACTURE OF THE SHAFTS OF THE TIBIA AND/OR FIBULA IN CHILDREN

Open reduction and internal fixation of closed fractures of the tibia or fibula in children are rarely necessary. If a tibial fracture is stable because of the configuration of the ends of the fragments, or if the fibular shaft is intact, closed reduction of axial displacement (overriding) is desirable; angular and torsional displacement must be corrected also. If proper alignment is secured, 1 cm. of overriding is acceptable.

Comminuted or oblique tibial fractures with displacement or fractures of both bones require continuous skeletal traction by means of a Kirschner wire inserted through the calcaneus until early bone healing stabilizes the fragments. Further immobilization in a tubular plaster cast is necessary until bone healing is sufficiently well along to permit weight bearing.

INJURIES OF THE ANKLE REGION

ANKLE SPRAIN

Sprain of the ankle joint during childhood is rare. In the adult, ankle sprain is most often caused by forced inversion of the foot, as may occur in stumbling on uneven ground. Pain is usually maximal over the anterolateral aspect of the joint; greatest tenderness is apt to be found in the region of the anterior talofibular and talocalcaneal ligaments. Eversion sprain is less common; maximal tenderness and swelling are usually found over the deltoid ligament.

Sprain is differentiated from major partial or complete ligamentous tears by anteroposterior, lateral, and 30° internal oblique x-ray projections; if the joint cleft between either malleolus and the talus is greater than 4 mm., major ligamentous tear is probable. Occult lesions can be demonstrated by x-ray examination under inversion or eversion stress after infiltration of the area of maximal swelling and tenderness with 5 ml. of 2% procaine.

If swelling is marked, elevation of the extremity and avoidance of weight-bearing for a few days is advisable. The ankle can be supported with a Gibney strapping (see p. 788). Adhesive support for another 2 weeks will relieve pain and swelling. Further treatment may be by warm foot baths and elastic bandages. Continue treatment until muscle strength and full joint motion are recovered. Tears of major ligaments of the ankle joint are discussed on p. 793.

FRACTURES AND DISLOCATIONS OF THE ANKLE JOINT

Fractures and dislocations of the ankle joint may be caused by direct injury, in which case they are apt to be comminuted and open; or by indirect violence, which often causes typical lesions (see below).

Pain and swelling are the prominent clinical findings. Deformity may or may not be present. X-rays of excellent technical quality must be prepared in a sufficient variety of projections to demonstrate the extent and configuration of all major fragments. Special oblique projections may be required.

Fracture of the Medial Malleolus.

Fracture of the medial malleolus may occur as an isolated lesion of any part of the malleolus (including the tip), or may be associated with (1) fracture of the lateral malleolus with medial or lateral dislocation of the talus, and (2) dislocation of the inferior tibiofibular joint with or without fracture of the fibula. Isolated fracture does not usually cause instability of the ankle joint.

Undisplaced isolated fracture of the medial malleolus should be treated by immobilization in a plaster boot extending from the knee to the toes with the ankle flexed to a right angle and the foot slightly inverted to relax the tension on the deltoid ligament (see p. 788). Immobilization must be continued for 6-8 weeks or until bone healing is sound.

Displaced isolated fracture of the medial malleolus may be treated by closed manipulation under general or local anesthesia. The essential maneuver consists of anatomic realignment by digital pressure over the distal fragment, followed by immobilization in a plaster boot (as for undisplaced fracture) until bone healing is sound (see p. 788). If anatomic reduction cannot be obtained by closed methods, open reduction and internal fixation with 1-2 bone screws are required.

Fracture of the Lateral Malleolus.

Fracture of the lateral malleolus may occur as an isolated lesion, or may be associated with fracture of the medial malleolus, tear of the deltoid or posterior lateral malleolar ligament, or avulsion of the posterior tibial tubercle. If the medial aspect of the ankle is injured, lateral dislocation of the talus is apt to be present. The tip of the lateral malleolus may be avulsed by the calcaneofibular and anterior talofibular ligaments. Transverse or oblique fracture may occur. Oblique fractures commonly extend downward and anteriorly from the posterior and superior aspects.

If swelling and pain are not marked, isolated undisplaced fracture of the lateral malleolus may be treated by Gibney ankle strapping (see p. 788). Otherwise, a plaster boot should be applied for 6 weeks and an elastic bandage worn thereafter until full joint motion is recovered and the calf muscles are functioning normally.

Isolated displaced fracture of the lateral malleolus should be treated by closed manipulation. The foot should be immobilized in slight inversion, which tautens the ligaments over the lateral aspect of the ankle joint and tends to prevent displacement.

If anatomic reduction cannot be achieved by closed methods, open reduction is required.

Combined Fracture of the Medial and Lateral Malleoli.

Bimalleolar fracture may be accompanied by medial or lateral dislocation of the talus, generally medial or lateral. In unstable fractures, displacement is apt to recur after closed reduction.

Bimalleolar fracture may be treated by closed manipulation. A tubular plaster cast is then applied from the inguinal region to the toes with the knee in about 45° of flexion and the foot in neutral position. Immediate open reduction must be resorted to if x-rays show that perfect anatomic reduction has not been achieved by closed manipulation.

Fractures of the Distal Tibia.

Fracture of the distal tibia is usually associated with other lesions.

A. Fracture of the Posterior Margin: Fracture of the posterior articular margin may involve part or all of the entire posterior half and is apt to be accompanied by fracture of either malleolus and posterior dislocation of the talus. It must be differentiated from fracture of the posterior tibial tubercle, which is usually caused by avulsion with the attached posterior lateral malleolar ligament.

   Anatomic reduction by closed manipulation is required if the fracture involves more than 25% of the articular surface. The extremity is immobilized in a plaster cast extending from the inguinal region to the toes with the knee in about 40° of flexion, the ankle at a right angle, and the foot in neutral position.

   Frequent x-ray examination is necessary to make certain that redisplacement does not occur. The plaster should be changed as soon as loosening becomes apparent. Immobilization must be maintained for at least 8 weeks. Weight-bearing must not be resumed until bone healing is sound, usually in about 12 weeks.

B. Fracture of the Anterior Margin: Fracture of the anterior articular margin of the tibia (rare) is likely to be caused by forced dorsiflexion of the foot. If displacement is marked and the talus is dislocated, tear of the collateral ligaments or fractures of the malleoli are likely to be present.

   Reduction is by closed manipulation. If comminution is present, the extremity should be immobilized for about 12 weeks. Healing is apt to be slow.

C. Comminuted Fractures: Extensive comminution of the distal tibia ("compression type" fracture) presents a difficult problem of management. The congruity of articular surfaces cannot be restored by closed manipulation, and satisfactory anatomic restoration is usually not possible even by open reduction. The best form of treatment for extensively comminuted and widely displaced fractures is closed manipulation and skeletal traction (see p. 788). After traction has been applied and impaction of fragments has been disrupted, displacement in the transverse plane is corrected by manual molding with compression. A tubular plaster cast is applied from the inguinal region to the toes with the knee in 10-15° of flexion and the foot in neutral position. With the extremity immobilized in plaster, continuous skeletal traction can be maintained for 8-12 weeks or until stabilization by early bone healing occurs. An alternative is distraction with a wire or pin in the calcaneus and one or 2 wires or pins in the shaft of the tibia.

Healing is likely to be slow. If the articular surfaces of the ankle joint have not been properly realigned, disabling post-traumatic arthritis is likely to occur early. Early arthrodesis is indicated to shorten the period of disability.

Dislocation of the Ankle Joint.

A. Complete Dislocation: The talus cannot be completely dislocated from the ankle joint unless all ligaments are torn. This lesion is rare.

B. Incomplete Dislocation: Major ligamentous injuries in the region of the ankle joint are usually associated with fracture.

1. Tear of the deltoid ligament - Complete tear of the talotibial portion of the deltoid ligament can permit interposition of the posterior tibial tendon between the medial malleolus and the talus. Associated injury is usually present, especially fracture of the lateral malleolus with lateral dislocation of the talus.

   Pain, tenderness, swelling, and ecchymosis in the region of the medial malleolus without fracture suggest partial or complete tear of the deltoid ligament. If fracture of the lateral malleolus or dislocation of the distal tibiofibular joint is present, the cleft between the malleolus and talus is likely to be widened. If significant widening is not apparent, x-ray examination under stress is necessary.

   Interposition of the deltoid ligament between the talus and the medial malleolus often cannot be corrected by closed manipulation. If widening persists after closed manipulation, surgical exploration is indicated so that the ligament can be removed and repaired by suture.

   Associated fracture of the fibula can be treated by fixation with a coaxial intramedullary standard bone screw or a bone nail to assure maintenance of anatomic reduction.

2. Tear of the talofibular ligament - Isolated tear of the anterior talofibular ligament is caused by forced inversion of the foot. X-ray examination under stress may be necessary, using local or general anesthesia. Both feet are forcibly inverted and internally rotated about 20° while an anteroposterior film is exposed. If the tear is complete, the talus will be seen to be axially displaced from the tibial articular surface.

   Rupture of the anterior talofibular ligament may be associated with tear of the calcaneofibular ligament. Tear of both ligaments may be associated with fracture of the medial malleolus and medial dislocation of the talus.

Instability of the ankle joint, characterized by a history of recurrent sprains, may result from unrecognized tears of the anterior talofibular ligament.

Recent isolated tear of the anterior talofibular ligament or combined tear of the calcaneofibular ligament should be treated by immobilization for 4 weeks in a plaster boot. Associated fracture of the medial malleolus creates an unstable mechanism. Unless anatomic reduction can be achieved and maintained by closed methods, open reduction of the malleolar fragment is indicated, followed by internal fixation of the fracture and repair of the ligamentous injury.

Dislocation of the Distal Tibiofibular Joint.

Both the anterior and posterior lateral malleolar ligaments must be torn before dislocation of the distal tibiofibular joint can occur. Lateral dislocation of the talus is also an essential feature, and this cannot occur unless the medial malleolus is fractured or the deltoid ligament is torn. The distal fibula is commonly fractured, but it may remain intact, and dislocation may be caused by a tear of the interosseous ligament.

Anatomic reduction by closed manipulation is difficult to achieve, but should be tried. Under general anesthesia, the foot is forced medially by a shearing maneuver and a snug plaster cast is applied from the inguinal region to the toes. If immediate and repeated x-ray examinations do not demonstrate that anatomic reduction has been achieved and maintained, open reduction and internal fixation should be performed as soon as possible.

Separation of the Distal Tibial and Fibular Epiphyses.

The most common injury of the ankle region of children is traumatic separation of the distal tibial and fibular epiphyses. Sprain is rare in children. Separation of the distal fibular epiphysis may occur as an isolated injury, or may be associated with separation of the tibial epiphysis.

If displacement has occurred, treatment is by closed manipulation and plaster immobilization. Open reduction is seldom justifiable. If injury has been severe, disturbance of growth is likely to follow.

INJURIES OF THE FOOT

FRACTURE AND DISLOCATION OF THE TALUS

Dislocation of the Subtalar and Talonavicular Joints.

Dislocation of the subtalar and talonavicular joints without fracture occasionally occurs. The talocrural joint is not injured. Displacement of the foot can be either in varus or valgus. Reduction by closed manipulation is usually not difficult. Incarceration of the posterior tibial tendon in the talonavicular joint may prevent reduction by closed manipulation. After reduction the extremity should be immobilized in a plaster boot for 4 weeks.

Fracture of the Talus.

Major fracture of the talus commonly occurs either through the body or through the neck; the uncommon fracture of the head involves essentially a portion of the neck with extension into the head. Indirect injury is usually the cause of closed fracture as well as most open fractures; severe comminution is not commonly present. Compression fracture or infraction of the tibial articular surface may be caused by the initial injury or may occur later in association with complicating avascular necrosis. The proximal or distal fragments may be dislocated.

A. Fracture of the Neck: Forced dorsiflexion of the foot may cause this injury. Undisplaced fracture of the neck can be treated adequately by a non-weight-bearing plaster boot for 8-12 weeks. Dislocation of the body or the distal neck fragment with the foot may complicate this injury. Fracture of the neck with anterior and frequently medial dislocation of the distal fragment and foot can usually be reduced by closed manipulation. Subsequent treatment is the same as that of undisplaced fracture.

   Dislocation of the proximal body fragment may occur separately or may be associated with dislocation of the distal fragment. If dislocation of the body fragment is complete, reduction by closed manipulation may not be possible. If reduction by closed manipulation is not successful, open reduction should be done as soon as possible to prevent or to minimize the extent of the avascular necrosis. Bone healing is likely to be retarded since some degree of avascular necrosis is probable.

   Complete dislocation of the neck fragment from the talonavicular and subtalar joints is rare, but if it does happen avascular necrosis of the fragment is to be expected even though anatomic reduction is promptly accomplished. If satisfactory reduction by closed manipulation is not possible, immediate open operation with reduction of the fragment or its removal is advisable since delay may cause necrosis of overlying soft tissues.

B. Fracture of the Body: Closed uncomminuted fracture of the body of the talus with minimal displacement of fragments is not likely to cause disability if immobilization is continued until bone continuity is restored. If significant displacement occurs, the proximal fragment is apt to be dislocated from the subtalar and ankle joints. Reduction by closed manipulation can be achieved best by traction and forced plantar flexion of the foot. Immobilization in a plaster boot with the foot in equinus for about 8 weeks should be followed by further casting with the foot at a right angle until the fracture cleft has been obliterated by new bone formation as evidenced by x-ray examination. Even though prompt adequate reduction is obtained by either closed manipulation or by open operation, extensive displacement of the proximal body fragment is likely to be followed by avascular necrosis. If reduction is not anatomic, delayed healing of the fracture may follow and post-traumatic arthritis is a likely sequel. If this occurs, arthrodesis of the ankle and subtalar joints may be necessary to relieve painful symptoms.

Compression fracture or infraction of the dome of the talus from the initial injury (which is likely to have been violent) cannot be reduced. When this lesion occurs as a separate entity or in combination with other fractures of the body, prolonged protection from weight-bearing is the major means of preventing the further collapse that is so likely to occur in the area of healing.

FRACTURE OF THE CALCANEUS

Fracture of the calcaneus is commonly caused by direct trauma. Since this fracture is likely to occur as a result of a fall from a height, fracture of the spine may also be present. Comminution and impaction are general characteristics. Minor infractions or impactions and fissure fractures are easy to miss on clinical examination, and x-rays must be prepared in multiple projections to demonstrate adequately some fracture clefts. In some instances, minor impactions of articular surfaces will be evident only by tomography.

Various classifications have been advocated. Fractures that are generally comminuted and disrupt the subtalar and calcaneocuboid articulations should be distinguished from those that do not; this differentiation has important implications for treatment and prognosis.

Fracture of the Tuberosity.

Isolated fracture of the tuberosity is not common. It may occur in a vertical or a horizontal direction.

A. Horizontal Fracture: Horizontal fracture may be limited to the superior portion of the region of the former apophysis and represents an avulsion by the Achilles tendon. Where the superior minor fragment is widely displaced proximally with the tendon, open reduction and fixation with a stout wire suture may be necessary to obtain the most satisfactory functional result.

   Further extension of the fracture cleft toward the subtalar joint in the substance of the tuberosity creates the "beak" fracture. The minor fragment may be displaced proximally by the action of the triceps surae. If displacement is significant, reduction can be achieved by skeletal traction applied to the proximal fragment with the foot in equinus. Immobilization is obtained by incorporation of the traction pin or wire in a full extremity plaster with the knee flexed 30° and the foot in plantar flexion. If adequate reduction cannot be accomplished in this way, open reduction is advised.

B. Vertical Fracture: Vertical fracture occurs near the sagittal plane somewhat medially through the tuberosity. Because the minor medial fragment normally is not widely displaced, plaster immobilization is not required. Comfort can be enhanced by limitation of weight-bearing with the aid of crutches.

Fracture of the Sustentaculum.

Isolated fracture of the sustentaculum tali is a rare lesion which may be caused by forced eversion of the foot. Where displacement of the larger body fragment occurs, it is lateral. Incarceration of the tendon of the flexor hallucis longus in the fracture cleft has been reported. Generally this fracture occurs in association with comminution of the body.

Fracture of the Anterior Process.

Fracture of the anterior process is caused by forced inversion of the foot. It must be differentiated from midtarsal and ankle joint sprains. The firmly attached bifurcate ligament (calcaneonavicular and calcaneocuboid components) avulses a bit of bone. Maximum tenderness and slight swelling occur midway between the tip of the lateral malleolus and the base of the fifth metatarsal. The lateral x-ray view projected obliquely is the most satisfactory to demonstrate the fracture cleft. Treatment is by a non-weight-bearing plaster boot with the foot in neutral position for 4 weeks.

Fracture of the Body.

Fracture of the body may occur posterior to the articular surfaces, in a general vertical but somewhat oblique plane, without disruption of the subtalar joint. Most severe fractures of the calcaneal body are comminuted and extend into the subtalar and frequently the calcaneocuboid joints. Fissure fractures without significant displacement cause minor disability and can be treated simply by protection from weight-bearing, either by crutches alone or in combination with a plaster boot until bone healing is sufficiently sound to justify graded increments of loading.

A. Nonarticular Fracture: Where fracture of the body with comminution occurs posterior to the articular surface, the direction of significant displacement of the fragment attached to the tuberosity is proximal, causing diminution of the tuber joint angle. Since the subtalar joint is not disrupted, symptomatic post-traumatic degenerative arthritis is not an important sequel even though some joint stiffness persists permanently. Marked displacement should be corrected by skeletal traction applied to the main posterior fragment to obtain an optimal cosmetic result, especially in women. Success of reduction can be judged by the adequacy of restoration of the tuber joint angle.

B. Articular Fracture: Articular fractures are of 3 general types:

1. Noncomminuted - Fracture of the body without comminution may involve the posterior articular facet. Where displacement of the posterior fragment of the tuberosity occurs, the direction is lateral. Fractures of this category with more than minimal displacement should be treated by the method advocated for nonarticular fracture of the body.
2. With minor comminution - In fractures with minor comminution, the main cleft occurs vertically, in a somewhat oblique lateral deviation from the sagittal plane. From emergence on the medial surface posterior to the sustentaculum it is directed forward and rather obliquely laterally through the posterior articular facet. The sustentaculum and the medial portion of the posterior articular facet remain undisplaced with relation to the talus. The body below the remaining lateral portion of the posterior articular facet with the tuberosity are impacted into the lateral portion of the posterior articular facet. Since anatomic reduction cannot be achieved by closed technics, Palmer has advocated open reduction and bone grafting. Lack of precise reduction, determined in part by restoration of the normal tuber joint angle, causes derangement of the subtalar joint, and symptomatic post-traumatic arthritis is a frequent sequel.
3. With extensive comminution - Fracture with extensive comminution extending into the subtalar joint may involve the calcaneocuboid joint as well as the tuberosity. The multiple fracture clefts involve the entire posterior articular surface, and the facet is impacted into the substance of the underlying body. There are many variants; the clefts may extend across the calcaneal groove into the medial and anterior articular

surfaces, and detachment of the peroneal tubercle may be a feature. This serious injury may cause major disability in spite of the best treatment since the bursting nature of the injury defies anatomic restoration.

Some surgeons advise nonintervention. Displacement of fragments is disregarded. Initially, a compression dressing is applied and the extremity is elevated for a week or so. Warm soaks and active exercises are then started, but weight-bearing is avoided until early bone healing has taken place. In spite of residual deformity of the heel, varying degress of weakness of the calf, and discomfort in the region of the subtalar joint (which may be intensified by weight-bearing), acceptable functional results can be obtained, especially among vigorous men who are willing to put up with the discomforts involved.

Other surgeons, notably Hermann and Böhler, advocate early closed manipulation which can partially restore the external anatomic configuration of the heel region, a cosmetic goal particularly desirable for women.

Persistent and disabling painful symptoms originating in the deranged subtalar joint may require arthrodesis for adequate relief. Concomitant involvement of the calcaneocuboid joint is an indication for the more extensive triple arthrodesis.

FRACTURE OF THE TARSAL NAVICULAR

Minor avulsion fractures of the tarsal navicular may occur as a feature of severe midtarsal sprain and require neither reduction nor elaborate treatment. Avulsion fracture of the tuberosity near the insertion of the posterior tibialis muscle is uncommon and must be differentiated from a persistent, ununited apophysis (accessory scaphoid) and from the supernumerary sesamoid bone, the os tibiale externum.

Major fracture occurs either through the middle in a horizontal or, more rarely, in the vertical plane, or is characterized by impaction of its substance. Only noncomminuted fractures with displacement of the dorsal fragment can be reduced. Closed manipulation by strong traction on the forefoot and simultaneous digital pressure over the displaced fragment can restore it to its normal position. If a tendency to redisplacement is apparent, this can be counteracted by temporary fixation with a percutaneously inserted Kirschner wire. Comminuted and impacted fractures cannot be anatomically reduced. Some authorities offer a pessimistic prognosis for comminuted or impacted fractures. It is their contention that even though partial reduction has been achieved, post-traumatic arthritis supervenes, and that arthrodesis of the talonavicular and cuneonavicular joints will be ultimately necessary to relieve painful symptoms.

FRACTURE OF THE CUNEIFORM AND CUBOID BONES

Because of their relative protected position in the midtarsus, isolated fracture of the cuboid and cuneiform bones is rarely encountered. Minor avulsion fractures occur as a component of severe midtarsal sprains. Extensive fracture usually occurs in association with other injuries of the foot and often is caused by severe crushing. Simple classification is impractical because of the complex character and the multiple combinations of the whole injury.

MIDTARSAL DISLOCATIONS

Midtarsal dislocation through the cuneonavicular and the calcaneocuboid joints or, more proximally, through the talocalcaneonavicular and the calcaneocuboid joints may occur as a result of twisting injury to the forefoot. Fractures of varying extent of adjacent bones are frequent complications. When treatment is given soon after the accident, closed reduction by traction on the forefoot and manipulation is generally effective. If reduction is unstable and displacement tends to recur upon release of traction, stabilization for 4 weeks by percutaneously inserted Kirschner wires is recommended.

FRACTURES AND DISLOCATIONS OF THE METATARSALS

Fractures of metatarsals and tarsometatarsal dislocations are likely to be caused by direct crushing or indirect twisting injury to the forefoot. Besides osseous and articular injury, complicating soft tissue lesions are often present. Tense subfascial hematoma of the dorsum of the forefoot, if not relieved, may cause necrosis of overlying skin or may even lead to gangrene of the toes by interruption of the arterial supply.

Tarsometatarsal Dislocations.

Possibly because of strong ligamentous support and relative size, dislocation of the first metatarsal at its base occurs less frequently than similar involvement of the lesser bones. If dislocation occurs, fracture of the first cuneiform is likely to be present also. More often, however, tarsometatarsal dislocation involves the lesser metatarsals, and associated fractures are to be expected. Dislocation is more commonly caused by direct injury but may be the result of stress applied indirectly through the forefoot. The direction of displacement is ordinarily dorsal, lateral, or a combination of both.

Attempted closed reduction should not be deferred. Skeletal traction applied to the involved bone by a Kirschner wire or a stout towel clamp can be a valuable aid to manipulation. Even though persistent dislocation may not cause significant disability, the resulting deformity can make shoe fitting difficult for men and the cosmetic effect undesirable to women. Open reduction with evacuation of dorsal subfascial hematoma and Kirschner wire stabilization is a preferred alternative to unsuccessful closed treatment. When effective treatment has been deferred 4 weeks or even longer, early healing will prevent satisfactory reduction of persisting displacement by closed technics. Under such circumstances, it is better to defer open operation and to direct treatment toward recovery of function. Extensive operative procedures and continued immobilization can increase joint stiffness. Reconstructive operation can be planned more suitably after residual disability becomes established.

Fractures of the Shafts.

Undisplaced fractures of the metatarsal shafts cause no permanent disability unless failure of bone healing is encountered. Displacement is rarely significant where fracture of the middle metatarsals is oblique, and the first and fifth are uninjured since they act as splints. Even fissure fractures should be treated by a stiff-soled shoe (with partial weight-bearing) or, if pain is marked, by a plaster walking boot.

Great care should be taken in displaced fractures to correct angulation in the longitudinal axis of the shaft. Persistent convex dorsal angulation causes prominence of the head of the involved metatarsal on the plantar aspect with the implication of concentrated local pressure and production of painful skin callosities. Deformity of the shaft of the first metatarsal due to convex plantar angulation can transfer weight-bearing stress to the region of the head of the third metatarsal. After correction of angular displacement, the plaster casing should be molded well to the plantar aspect of the foot to minimize recurrence of deformity and to support the longitudinal and transverse arches.

If reduction is not reasonably accurate, fractures through the shafts near the heads (the "neck") may cause great discomfort from concentrated pressure beneath the head on the plantar surface and reactive skin callus formation. Every effort should be made to correct convex dorsal angulation by disrupting impaction and appropriate manipulation. Unstable fracture can be treated by sustained skeletal traction using a Kirschner wire inserted through the distal phalanx and traction supplied by an elastic band attached to a "banjo" bow. The efficacy of closed treatment should be determined without delay, and, where it is lacking, open operation should be substituted.

Fatigue Fracture of the Shafts.

Fatigue fracture of the shafts of the metatarsals has been described by various terms, e.g., march, stress, and insufficiency fracture, and by a variety of other terms in the French and German literature. Its protean clinical manifestations cause difficulty in precise recognition, even to the point of confusion with osteogenic sarcoma. Commonly, it occurs in active young adults, such as military recruits, who are unaccustomed to vigorous and excessive walking. A history of a single significant injury is lacking. Incipient pain of varying intensity in the forefoot which is accentuated by walking, swelling, and localized tenderness of the involved metatarsal are cardinal manifestations. Depending upon the stage of progress, x-rays may not demonstrate the fracture cleft and extracortical callus formation may ultimately be the only clue. More striking findings may vary from an incomplete fissure to an evident transverse cleft. Persistent, unprotected weight-bearing may cause arrest of bone healing and even displacement of the distal fragment. The second and third metatarsals are most frequently involved near the junction of the middle and distal thirds. The lesion can occur more proximally and in other lesser metatarsals. Since weight-bearing is likely to prolong and aggravate symptoms, treatment is by protection in either a plaster walking boot or a heavy shoe with the sole reinforced by a steel strut. Weight-bearing should be restricted until painful symptoms subside and restoration of bone continuity has been demonstrated by x-ray examination.

Fracture of the Tuberosity of the Fifth Metatarsal.

Forced adduction of the forefoot may cause avulsion fracture of the tuberosity of the fifth metatarsal, and, where supporting soft tissues have been torn, activity of the peroneus brevis muscle may increase displacement of the avulsed proximal fragment. If displacement of the minor fragment is minimal, adhesive strapping or a stiff-soled shoe is adequate treatment. If displacement is significant, treatment should be by a walking boot until bone healing occurs (see p. 788). Rarely does healing fail. Fracture should be differentiated from a separate ossific center of the tuberosity in adolescence and the supernumerary os vesalianum pedis in adulthood.

FRACTURES AND DISLOCATIONS OF THE PHALANGES OF THE TOES

Fractures of the phalanges of the toes are caused most commonly by direct violence such as crushing or stubbing. Spiral or oblique fractures of the shafts of the proximal phalanges of the lesser toes may occur as a result of indirect twisting injury.

Comminuted fracture of only the proximal phalanx of the great toe, alone or in combination with fracture of the distal phalanx, is the most disabling injury. Since wide displacement of fragments is not likely, correction of angulation and support by an adhesive dressing and splint usually suffices. A weight-bearing plaster boot may be useful for relief of symptoms arising from associated soft tissue injury. Spiral or oblique fracture of the proximal phalanges of the lesser toes can be treated adequately by binding the involved toe to the adjacent uninjured member. Comminuted fracture of the distal phalanx is treated as a soft tissue injury.

Traumatic dislocation of the metatarsophalangeal joints and the uncommon dislocation of the proximal interphalangeal joint usually can be reduced by closed manipulation. These dislocations are rarely isolated and usually occur in combination with other injuries to the forefoot.

FRACTURE OF THE SESAMOIDS OF THE GREAT TOE

Fracture of the sesamoid bones of the great toe is rare, but may occur as a result of crushing injury. It must be differentiated from partite developmental lesions. Undisplaced fracture requires no treatment other than a foot support or a metatarsal bar. Displaced fracture may require immobilization in a walking plaster boot with the toe strapped in flexion. Persistent delay of bone healing may cause disabling pain arising from arthritis of the articulation between the sesamoid and the head of the first metatarsal. If a foot support and metatarsal bar do not provide adequate relief, excision of the sesamoid may be necessary.

INFECTIONS OF BONES AND JOINTS

OSTEOMYELITIS

Osteomyelitis is an acute or chronic inflammation of bone caused by infection. It may be accompanied by general manifestations of toxemia. Osteomyelitis may be classified according to mechanism of introduction of infection (i.e., as primary or secondary) and on the basis of microbial etiology.

Primary osteomyelitis is caused by direct implantation of microorganisms into bone. Penetrating wounds, especially those caused by firearms and military missiles, are commonly followed by bone infections. Compound or open fractures are another frequent route of contamination. Primary osteomyelitis may also occur as a sequel to a surgical operation on bone. Intramedullary infusions or injections of drugs account for an occasional infection.

Infection is usually localized to the site of inoculation. Clinical features are variable and somewhat dependent upon circumstances.

In addition to antimicrobial therapy, operative treatment is usually necessary. Because the selection of a particular operative technic depends in part upon the associated bone lesion, primary osteomyelitis is usually discussed in conjunction with open fractures or postoperative wound infections.

The route of infection of **secondary osteomyelitis** is usually through the arterial system. A notable exception is spread from the genitourinary system through veins to the bony pelvis or vertebral column. Infection via the lymphatic system is probably rare. Osteomyelitis occasionally results from direct extension of an infection in contiguous soft tissues or joints.

Acute Pyogenic Osteomyelitis (Secondary or Hematogenous).

About 95% of cases of acute secondary osteomyelitis are caused by pyogenic organisms, usually a single pathogen. Secondary contamination by other organisms during open wound management may complicate treatment. "Superinfection" with a different organism during antibiotic treatment may also occur.

The incidence of acute pyogenic osteomyelitis has decreased markedly since the antibiotics came into widespread use, but subacute and chronic infections still occur and present difficult therapeutic problems.

Hematogenous osteomyelitis is encountered predominantly during the period of skeletal growth. About 8 out of 10 cases of acute pyogenic osteomyelitis occur in children; about one out of 10 occurs in infants under 2 years of age; and about one out of 10 occurs in adults. In children, about three-fourths of all cases are caused by staphylococci. Group A hemolytic streptococci are the next most common pathogen, and the remainder of cases are caused by a wide variety of organisms including other species of streptococci, gram-negative bacilli, and pneumococci. Culture studies are necessary for precise identification and for rational selection of the most effective antibiotics.

Pre-existing infections such as furuncles, infected cutaneous abrasions, acute exanthematous infections, and infections of the respiratory, gastrointestinal, and genitourinary tracts can be identified as sources of the bone infection in about half of cases. Males are affected 4 times as frequently as females. The tibia and the femur are the most commonly involved long bones. A history of localizing trauma is frequently given. Malnutrition and poor hygiene are other significant predisposing factors.

In infants the onset is most often precipitous, with alarming systemic symptoms of toxicity; though it may be insidious, characterized only by irritability and followed, usually within a few hours, by fever and significant local findings. The infant tends not to move the involved extremity and adjacent joints. Tenderness is usually present before swelling appears. Redness and edema of soft tissues usually indicate the presence of an extracortical abscess. Significant changes in bone cannot be identified by x-ray examination before the end of the first week. Soft tissue thickening adjacent to the involved bone may suggest underlying osseous disease.

In children the onset may be with high fever, chills, prostration, and other evidence of general toxicity; or it may be less dramatic, especially if antibiotic therapy has been given for a predisposing infection. Local pain in at least one site may lead the examiner to an area of localized tenderness and possibly limited soft tissue swelling. The erythrocyte sedimentation rate is commonly elevated. Leukocytosis is often present, but a normal or low white count does not rule out the diagnosis. X-ray changes usually appear later in children than in infants, often not before the tenth to fourteenth days. If antimicrobial therapy has been given, x-rays may show no abnormality before 3 to 5 weeks have elapsed. Soft tissue thickening adjacent to the osseous focus may be the earliest significant x-ray finding. Later, alteration of architectural patterns of cancellous bone and destruction of compact bone are indications of processes that have been active for days or even weeks.

In adults the onset may be much less striking than in children and infants. High fever, general prostration, and other systemic symptoms of toxicity may be absent, and vague, shifting, or evanescent pains or aches that gradually increase in severity may be the only early manifestations. Subsequently, localized tenderness and joint stiffness with muscle guarding may draw one's attention to the local lesion. Depending upon the duration of symptoms and the type of treatment given, x-ray examination may or may not be useful. Recurrent (even minor) elevation of temperature, acceleration of the sedimentation rate, and localizing pain with tenderness are suggestive of the disease. Primary involvement may appear in the x-ray to be in the periosteum or medulla, or in cancellous bone of either the metaphysis or epiphysis.

The precise diagnosis at any age depends upon recovery and identification of the causative organism. Early in the disease, and especially during the stage of invasion, blood cultures are likely to be positive, but repeated cultures may be necessary. Aspiration of tender areas may disclose subperiosteal or extra-osseous abscesses. If exploratory puncture is unsuccessful and localizing symptoms persist, puncture of the metaphysial cortex with a small trocar and aspiration of the medullary cavity may be necessary. Careful culture studies should always be made of any tissue or exudates recovered at operation.

Acute hematogenous osteomyelitis may be confused with suppurative arthritis, rheumatic fever, and cellulitis. The pseudoparalysis associated with acute osteomyelitis of infancy may simulate poliomyelitis at the onset, and mild acute osteomyelitis of the proximal femur may mimic transient synovitis of the hip or Legg-Perthes disease at the onset. The subacute forms must be differentiated from tuberculosis, mycotic infections, and Ewing's sarcoma.

Treatment: Although the antibiotics have provided new concepts of treatment of this serious disease, particularly during the early stages, rational treatment continues to rest upon the established surgical principles of drainage of exudates, removal of sequestra, obliteration of cavities, avoidance of secondary microbial contamination, and subsequent wound closure. The selection of treatment depends somewhat upon the type of infecting organism, the stage of progress of the lesion, and the general response of the patient. Treatment must be individualized, and only broad guides can be suggested. The severity of systemic symptoms determines in a measure the general management. Attention must be given to fluid balance of the acutely toxic patient. Immobilization of the affected extremity by splinting, plaster encasement, or suspension is probably necessary for maximal relief of pain and prevention of complications such as pathologic fracture or joint dislocation. Secondary anemia is likely to occur and must be corrected by whole blood replacement. Care must be taken not to prescribe such large doses of analgesics or sedatives that pain is completely abolished, since the presence or absence of pain is an important clue to the effectiveness of treatment.

Rational **antibiotic treatment** is based upon an understanding of the pathologic changes and laboratory isolation of the pathogen followed by antibiotic sensitivity studies. However, in the seriously ill patient antibiotic therapy should be instituted at once, as soon as culture material has been collected and without waiting for laboratory reports. The most common pathogen is the staphylococcus. Because so many strains of staphylococci produce penicillinase, semisynthetic penicillins resistant to the action of that enzyme or cephalothin (Keflin®) should be used until indicative laboratory studies have been completed. When the patient is known to be allergic to those drugs, vancomycin (Vancocin®) is an alternative for use in children and adults and bacitracin for infants. Because treatment should be continued for at least 2-3 weeks and the possibility of emergence of resistant mutants, "broad-spectrum" antibiotics should be avoided as initial treatment. Treatment can be started with sodium methicillin (Staphcillin®, Dimocillin®), 2 Gm. I.V. every 4 hours for adults or 25 mg./Kg. I.V. for infants and children. Although methicillin resistance of staphylococci does occur, it is not commonly encountered at this time. Infections of the pelvis or spine in adults may be caused by gram-negative bacilli originating in the genitourinary tract. Gram-negative bacilli have widely different drug sensitivities, and combinations of drugs that are likely to provide high concentrations in the serum must be given until the causative microorganism has been isolated and its precise drug sensitivities determined. Various drug combinations have been advocated to initiate treatment at this stage on an empirical basis. Kanamycin (Kantrex®) plus polymyxin B (Aerosporin®) may be given I.V. Recent studies have indicated that gentamicin (Garamycin®), with or without cephaloridine (Keflordin®, Loridine®), may be effective for acute severe infections presumably caused by gram-negative enteric bacilli.

Rational drug therapy is based upon drug sensitivity tests. As soon as the pathogen is isolated, a rapidly growing culture can be titrated against the patient's serum to obtain an index of the efficacy of initial antibiotic treatment. The serum assay indicates the antimicrobial concentration of drugs for a particular strain in vivo. To provide an adequate opportunity for tissue saturation by the drug, the serum sample should not be taken until 24-48 hours after starting treatment.

Properly executed disk sensitivity studies will give early guidance concerning the probable efficacy of drugs that might be selected for the treatment of infections due to staphylococci or group A streptococci. The disk sensitivity technic does not indicate the likely effective dosage which should be in the bactericidal range. This test cannot be relied upon for optimal help when enteric bacilli or enteric cocci are involved. Tube dilution sensitivity studies are more reliable under these circumstances. Other advantages of the tube dilution methods include a more realistic indication of drug dosage, determination of drug combinations, and indications of effective drug selections when the flora are mixed.

During the first 48-72 hours after the onset of acute infection open **surgical treatment** can be avoided in most cases. If vigorous general care and appropriate antibiotic therapy are promptly instituted, the local lesion may be controlled and its progress halted before significant tissue destruction and suppuration have occurred. If an abscess forms in the soft tissues or beneath the periosteum, it should be aspirated at least daily in children and infants. Persistent fever and pain 24-72 hours after initiating aspiration along with recurrent collection of exudates suggest that more effective drainage should be instituted and should include decompression of the medullary cavity, preferably by multiple drill holes. The wound need not be packed open, although this is commonly done; it can be closed and continuous suction drainage used in an effort to prevent further bacterial contamination. Closed wound treatment with tube drainage also provides a mechanism for local instillation of antibiotics. If the diagnosis is not made promptly or if treatment has been inadequate or ineffective, extensive destruction of bone may have occurred. Decompression of abscesses and vigorous antibiotic therapy are required since necrosis of bone and subsequent sequestration will lead to chronic infection.

The more radical surgical technics formerly used in the treatment of acute osteomyelitis, such as extensive fenestration, guttering, and diaphysectomy, should be abandoned in the treatment of the acute disease and reserved only for treatment of the chronic phase.

The mortality rate from acute infection is probably no more than 1% at this time. Morbidity, however, continues to be high. If effective treatment can be instituted within the first 48 hours after onset, full recovery can be expected in about two-thirds of cases.

Salmonella Osteomyelitis.

Salmonella infection of the bones and joints occurs as a complication in less than 1% of cases of typhoid fever. Bone and joint infection with all strains of Salmonella are rare in the United States at this time. The infections usually consist of periostitis involving the shafts of long bones without extensive destruction of bone or significant abscess formation. Intervertebral disk space infection is the usual manifestation of spine involvement in typhoid fever. Spontaneous resolution is the rule, but chronic bone abscess occasionally develops.

The onset of bone and joint infection may occur during the acute stage of the primary disease or during convalescence. The late appearance of bone infection is associated with return of fever, local pain, and tenderness. X-rays may show a bone lesion. Even without specific treatment there is no tendency toward extensive abscess formation, and previous antibiotic treatment may modify the process further and make recovery of the organism difficult. It may be necessary to make a presumptive diagnosis based upon serologic agglutination titers (Widal).

Acute symptoms respond favorably to chloramphenicol (Chloromycetin®). The chronic lesion may require evacuation of the abscess and removal of necrotic bone and soft tissue in addition to antibiotics. Eradication of all organisms probably is effected by immune defenses.

Brucella Osteomyelitis.

Brucella infection of the skeletal system is not common, but it may occur as a complication or sequel of undulant fever. Infections both by Brucella melitensis and Br. abortus have been reported. Spondylitis is the most commonly recognized skeletal lesion. The subchondral bone of the intervertebral disk in the lumbar spine is most frequently affected. The lesion is usually a granuloma, although suppuration may take place with extensive abscess formation. Destruction of subchondral bone and disk cartilage may cause angulation and provoke anterior osteophyte formation relatively early in the course of the disease. These large osteophytes adjacent to the intervertebral disk may coalesce and cause spontaneous fusion of the spine.

It may not be possible to recover organisms from blood cultures except during acute phases of the systemic infection, in which case the diagnosis will depend upon serologic agglutination tests or brucellergen skin tests.

Chronic Pyogenic Osteomyelitis.

Chronic pyogenic osteomyelitis is the result of failure of early diagnosis or ineffective treatment of either the acute primary or the acute secondary infection. Symptoms may be so mild and the onset so insidious that the patient experiences little or no disability and ignores the prodromal manifestations. Precipitating trauma or spontaneous exacerbation of symptoms may be the reason for seeking medical care. The infection may remain quiescent for many years without causing any significant symptom. At the other extreme, it may cause a constant foul-smelling discharge and chronic pain that make the life of the patient miserable and even unbearable. A small nidus of infection such as an abscess or a sequestrum surrounded by granulation tissue may communicate through a sinus to the skin surface. Periodic discharge of pus causes no great disability, and the patient compensates by daily dressing changes. Another manifestation of chronicity is recurrent swelling, fever, and local pain. Rest, local heat, or antibiotic therapy causes remission without the necessity for surgical treatment. The infection may then remain dormant for days, weeks, or years before a similar exacerbation occurs.

The causative organism should be determined by culture, and sensitivity studies performed.

Chronic osteomyelitis may uncommonly act as a focus of infection for seeding other areas. During acute exacerbations, involvement of adjacent joints, manifested as sympathetic effusions or frank purulent arthritis, may occur. Constant erosion and progressive involvement of the bone occasionally leads to pathologic fracture. **Periostitis albuminosa** is a chronic infection of periosteum that may be the sole residual manifestation of osteomyelitis. Chronic infections in the region of the epiphysial cartilage may cause hyperemia and overgrowth of bone, resulting in a long extremity. Prolonged drainage, usually after many years, from a sinus or an ulcer extending to bone may on rare occasions be associated with neoplastic transformation, such as squamous cell carcinoma or fibrosarcoma.

Chronic infection may cause general deterioration of health manifested by anemia, weight loss, weakness, and evidence of amyloid disease.

Treatment: No rigid rules of treatment can be outlined because of the varied clinical and pathologic manifestations of this disease. During the quiescent phase, no treatment is necessary and the patient can live an essentially normal life. Minor exacerbations with drainage may be managed satisfactorily with changes of dressings and nothing more. More acute episodes may require rest with local heat and mild analgesics. Persistent sinuses with copious drainage usually imply abscess formation or sequestration and require more aggressive treatment.

(1) Operative Treatment: Soft tissue abscesses occasionally form without sequestra and can then be treated adequately by operative exploration, excision of necrotic soft tissue, and open or closed drainage. (Such treatment generally suffices also for **Brodie's abscess**, a unique type of chronic bone infection which usually occurs in the cancellous extremity of a long bone.) Simple removal of a sequestrum, when present, often permits rapid healing. Removal of necrotic bone that has not separated from the main mass may require extensive cortical guttering and resection of underlying cancellous bone. Diaphysectomy, which consists of subperiosteal resection of the shaft with preservation of the extremities of the bone, should be performed in the chronic stage only when the segment of bone is necrotic. Regeneration of the excised segment is unlikely in older children and adults.

Before antibiotic therapy became available, primary closure of a wound was generally followed by persistent drainage and most surgeons preferred open wound treatment. With local and systemic antibiotic therapy, it is now possible to close the wound and drain it intermittently by tube suction. Meticulous removal of necrotic and infected bone and obliteration of cavities are essential for successful early wound closure. Where the bone is subcutaneous and there is loss of overlying soft tissue, this can be accomplished following saucerization by the early application of a temporary thin split skin graft. Some deep cavities can be obliterated by transferring the belly of an adjacent muscle into the cavity. In other circumstances, the conversion of a deep cavity with vertical walls into a more shallow, saucer-like configuration will permit obliteration by collapse of overlying soft tissues. Attempts to obliterate cavities by filling them with bits of cancellous bone may be successful when performed by the experienced surgeon but are likely to cause persistent infection.

Amputation is no longer a favored method of management. Amputation may occasionally be necessary to sacrifice a functionless extremity or to cope with a complication such as secondary malignant disease.

(2) Antibiotic Therapy: Rational antibiotic therapy is based upon careful sensitivity studies of material cultured from the wound. Antimicrobial drugs in high concentration can be introduced intermittently into the wound for topical therapy. Although the systemic use of a single antibiotic is often successful for the treatment of staphylococcic and beta-hemolytic streptococcic infections, optimal treatment of gram-negative infections often necessitates combinations of drugs. The principle of combined antibiotic action can also be applied by using poorly absorbed, more toxic agents such as kanamycin, neomycin, vancomycin, bacitracin, or polymyxin B locally, and well absorbed, less toxic drugs systemically. Periodic cultures of wound secretions are necessary to determine the effectiveness of treatment. Concentrations of systemically administered drugs are determined by means of periodic serum assays.

Mycotic Infections of Bones and Joints.

Fungus infections of the skeletal system are usually secondary to a primary infection, frequently of the lower pulmonary tract. Although skeletal lesions have a predilection for the cancellous extremities of long bones and the bodies of the vertebrae, the predominant pathologic lesion - a granuloma with varying degrees of necrosis and abscess formation - does not produce a characteristic clinical picture.

Differentiation from other chronic infections depends upon culture studies of synovial fluid or tissue obtained from the local lesion. Serologic and skin tests provide presumptive support of the diagnosis.

Coccidioidomycosis is endemic in the southwestern U. S. and is caused by Coccidioides immitis. Infection of bones and joints is usually secondary to primary pulmonary infection. The focus in the lungs may not be visible by x-ray examination when the skeletal lesion appears. During the initial phase of pulmonary infection, arthralgia with periarticular swelling, especially in the regions of the knee and ankle, should be differentiated from organic bone and joint involvement. Osseous lesions commonly occur in cancellous bone of the vertebrae or near the ends of long bones. Because of a predilection for the latter sites, redness and swelling of the skin over bony prominences may be the first to call attention to the local process; abscess and sinus formation follow. Joint infection may be due to direct spread via the blood stream, or it may be caused by extension from a nearby osseous focus. The granulomatous lesions of bone or the villonodular synovitis of the joints cannot be differentiated microscopically from other mycotic infections. Histologic demonstration of spherules containing endospores supports the diagnosis but is not pathognomonic. Changes in bone seen in x-rays simulate those of tuberculosis. Local atrophy of bone progresses to focal destruction, which may appear cystic, indicating coalescence of granulomas or abscess formation. Subperiosteal new bone formation and sclerosis characterize the healing response. Sequestration is uncommon.

Diagnosis depends upon the recovery of the causative fungus from the lesion by culture. The organism may not be recovered from synovial fluid, especially after systemic treatment with amphotericin B. Under this circumstance, culture of synovia obtained by open biopsy may be rewarding.

Systemic treatment with amphotericin B (Fungizone®) should be tried for bone and joint infections. It may also be of value for instillation into joints during early stages of infection or after synovectomy. Immobilization of joints by plaster casts and avoidance of weight-bearing provide beneficial rest. Chronic infection of bone may respond to operative treatment by curettage or saucerization. Amputation may be the only solution for stubbornly progressive infections which do not respond to less drastic measures. Synovectomy and joint debridement are reserved for more advanced joint infections. Contaminated dressings and plaster casts should be carefully handled to prevent spread of infection to others.

North American blastomycosis (Gilchrist's disease) is a chronic granulomatous and suppurative cutaneous or systemic infection caused by the yeast-like fungus, Blastomyces dermatitidis. It uncommonly involves the skeletal system. Lesions may occur in any part of the skeletal system, but appear most frequently in the cancellous extremities of long bones and the bodies of the vertebrae. The clinical picture is essentially that of chronic osteomyelitis. The diagnosis depends upon microscopic demonstration of the yeast-like organism in tissue specimens and specific identification by culture methods. The prognosis is very poor even with treatment. The care of the local lesion is limited to conservative measures except when destruction is extensive, in which case amputation may be necessary. The only systemic drug that offers any hope is amphotericin B (Fungizone®).

Cryptococcosis (torulosis) or European blastomycosis is an uncommon but world-wide chronic granulomatous pulmonary disease caused by the yeast-like fungus Cryptococcus neoformans. The organisms may be disseminated from the pulmonary tract to the nervous system or to the bones. The lesions in bone are granulomatous, with a gelatinous consistency. The microscopic appearance of the organism is not characteristic, and the diagnosis depends upon recovery of the organism from infected tissues by culture. Agglutination tests for the specific antigen and antibody, when positive, give presumptive support to the diagnosis.

Surgical removal of diseased bone is believed to enhance healing and minimize further dissemination. Systemic treatment with amphotericin B (Fungizone®) is recommended.

Disseminated histoplasmosis may involve the skeletal system, but focal bone or joint lesions are rare and generally represent dissemination from a primary focus in the lungs. The granuloma is not characteristic, and the diagnosis depends upon culture studies of biopsy material recovered from the skeletal focus. Complement fixation tests may provide presumptive support of a diagnosis. Skeletal lesions may be single or multiple.

Surgical debridement of the focal lesion has been recommended. Amphotericin B (Fungizone®) has been useful for treatment of some patients.

PYOGENIC ARTHRITIS

Pyogenic arthritis is an acute or chronic inflammation of joints which may be caused by a variety of microorganisms, especially cocci or enteric gram-negative bacilli. The acute or chronic stage may be of primary or secondary origin. Primary pyogenic arthritis can be the result of direct implantation of microorganisms into joints through penetrating traumatic wounds or can complicate open surgical operations. Secondary pyogenic arthritis is generally blood-borne through the arterial system but occasionally through the veins. It can also result from direct extension from an adjacent focus of osteomyelitis or from an extra-articular soft tissue infection. Chronic pyogenic arthritis may be the result of failure of early diagnosis or ineffective treatment of the acute infection.

Acute Pyogenic Arthritis.

Pyogenic cocci - staphylococci (S. aureus and S. epidermidis), streptococci (alpha and beta, and occasionally S. faecalis), pneumococci, and meningococci - are frequent pathogens. (Although the gonococcus is pyogenic, the clinical picture of the arthritis it causes deviates from other pyogenic arthritides in some respects, and it will be discussed separately.) Enteric gram-negative bacilli, especially Escherichia coli and less frequently members of the Enterobacter (Aerobacter)-Klebsiella-Serratia group or Pseudomonas aeruginosa, may be isolated from acutely infected joints in adults. In children 6 months to 2 years of age, Haemophilus influenzae is a frequent pathogen.

In the hematogenous variety of acute pyogenic arthritis, larger joints (knee, hip, elbow, shoulder, and ankle) are more commonly involved. The presence of acute or chronic infection of bone or soft tissue near a joint should arouse suspicion of spread of infection to the joint. Overt or occult infections of remote organ systems, especially of the skin or respiratory tract in both children and adults and the genitourinary tract in adults, are possible sources of blood-borne infections. Although a single joint is generally involved in adults, multiple joint infections may occur in children when the mechanism of infection is hematogenous. Antecedent trauma may obscure subtle prodromal symptoms.

The initial reaction within the joint is that of acute synovitis. The intra-articular fluid may show only a modest rise in white cell count with an insignificant increase in polymorphonuclear cells. With the passage of time and a virulent pathogen, the character of the synovia rapidly changes to purulency with concomitant edema and cellular infiltration of the subsynovial soft tissues. Gross destruction of the cartilage follows, especially at the point of contact of opposing joint surfaces. Untreated or inadequately treated infections may progress to the stage of destruction of synovia and capsular components as well as cartilage and bone. Following mild or adequately treated early infections, the healing reaction may obliterate all vestiges of the inflammatory process. Extensive destruction of tissue during the active phase can only be partially repaired; fibrous or complete bony ankylosis may be the end result.

Systemic symptoms include fever, which may be accompanied by chills, malaise, and lack of a feeling of well-being. The intensity of pain varies but is generally progressive and accentuated by active or passive joint motions. The patient tends to inhibit motion. Increase in skin temperature about the joint accompanies soft tissue swelling and joint effusion. As the inflammatory response continues, local symptoms tend to become accentuated.

During the incipient stage of infection, synovial fluid may be grossly clear or slightly turbid, but it tends to become purulent as the infection progresses. The white cell count is likely to be greater than 50,000/cu. mm., with more than 90% of polymorphonuclear neutrophils. The fasting blood glucose level is likely to be more than 50 mg./100 ml. greater than that of the synovial fluid. The acid mucin tends to fragment or disintegrate. The erythrocyte sedimentation rate is almost invariably accelerated.

Thorough search of a gram-stained smear of sediment may suggest drug selections that are likely to be effective.

Culture of the blood and synovial fluid exudates establishes a definitive diagnosis and provides a basis for drug treatment. Disk sensitivity determinations are likely to be adequate for selection of drugs to combat gram-positive cocci; tube dilution tests provide reliable information in the treatment of gram-negative bacillary infections.

X-ray changes lag behind the pathologic process. The initial radiologic change is distention of the joint capsule by effusion. As the inflammation spreads, especially in the subsynovial fatty areolar tissues, normal fascial lines and the demarcation between capsule and fat become obliterated. Increase in intra-articular pressure from effusion does not usually cause significant widening of the joint cleft except in the hip and especially in infants, where subluxation can occur. In this case, x-rays of the opposite normal joint aid in identification of subtle changes. As the lesion progresses, persistent hyperemia and lack of use abet demineralization, which starts in the subchondral bone adjacent to the joint cleft and extends centrifugally. As trabecular detail is lost, the more compact subchondral bone becomes accentuated. Destruction of cartilage is reflected by narrowing of the joint cleft until subchondral bone is in apposition. This latter manifestation tends to appear rapidly when Staphylococcus aureus is the causative pathogen.

The severity of systemic symptoms and the presence of other disease partly determine the method of **treatment.** Drugs should not be relied upon for total relief of joint pain because large doses of narcotics may obscure symptoms indicative of the course of the disease. Splinting of the involved joint in the position of maximum comfort (usually semiflexion) alleviates pain. When pain is caused by increased intra-articular pressure, intermittent aspiration or surgical drainage affords dramatic relief. Bilateral suspension of the lower extremities in abduction with traction may prevent subluxation or dislocation of a septic hip joint, especially in infants and children.

Optimal treatment continues to be based on surgical principles and effective drug therapy. The selection of specific measures depends in part upon the virulence of the infecting agent, the stage of the infection, and patient response. Treatment must be individualized, and only the principles are emphasized here. During the first 48-72 hours, intermittent aspiration may be substituted for open or percutaneous drainage of the joint to relieve intra-articular tension and evacuate cytotoxic exudates. When the infection is due to S. aureus, continuous or frequent intermittent evacuation of exudates by open or tube drainage is preferable because of the chondrolytic nature of the altered synovial secretions. If infection is not recognized or not treated effectively within the first 72 hours, establishment of drainage by open or closed tube method is advocated for most cases.

Drug therapy is based upon the sensitivities of the isolated pathogens. The general principles outlined in the treatment of acute osteomyelitis (see p. 803) also pertain to the treatment of acute pyogenic arthritis.

If effective treatment can be instituted within the first 48-72 hours, a prompt response can be expected provided there is no underlying basic factor such as alteration of the normal immune response of the host. Defervescence, disappearance of pain, return of uninhibited joint motion, resorption of joint effusion, and a falling erythrocyte sedimentation rate indicate desirable response to treatment.

Gonorrheal Arthritis.

Gonorrheal arthritis (gonococcal arthritis, gonorrheal rheumatism) is an acute inflammatory disease caused by Neisseria gonorrhoeae which is almost always secondary to infection of the genitourinary tract. At one time, joint involvement occurred in 2-5% of all gonococcic infections. Since the advent of modern chemotherapy, the incidence has decreased to the point that it has become a rarity in the ordinary orthopedic practice. Currently it is encountered more frequently in women who have occult genitourinary infections and occasionally in children. Symptoms related to the musculoskeletal system are likely to appear during the third week of inadequately treated infection.

Joint infection is via the blood stream. Clinical evidence of involvement of multiple joints is often present at onset, but symptoms are likely to be transient in all joints except one. Large weight-bearing joints are affected most frequently. Systemic symptoms may accompany the essential clinical features of the local lesion, which are those of acute arthritis. Initially, the process may only consist of synovitis with effusion, but as it progresses the exudate becomes purulent and destruction of cartilage follows which may lead to fibrous or bony ankylosis.

The precise diagnosis is established by recovery of the causative microorganism from the involved joint by culture. A positive complement fixation test of joint exudate is said to be more significant than a positive reaction in the blood. Identification of gonococcic antibody in serum by the fluorescent technic is more reliable than the complement fixation test. Other presumptive evidence is obtained from positive cultures from the lower genitourinary tract.

Gonorrheal arthritis must be differentiated from rheumatoid arthritis even though there may be a concomitant gonococcic infection of the genitourinary system; from pyogenic arthritis caused by other organisms; from acute nonspecific synovitis; and from Reiter's disease.

Treatment: Gonococcal infection responds promptly in at least 90% of cases to a wide variety of antibiotics. Penicillin, tetracycline, and chloramphenicol are generally effective and should be given systemically in adequate doses. Nonspecific local measures include immobilization of the joint by splinting or plaster, bed rest, and analgesics as necessary for pain. In severe infections, and especially in those in which the organism is demonstrable in the synovial fluid, penicillin should be instilled into large joints in doses of 25-50 thousand units twice daily. Local treatment is given until the joint fluid becomes clear and sterile.

The prognosis for preservation of joint function is good if the diagnosis is established promptly and treatment is vigorous.

Chronic Pyogenic Arthritis.

Chronic pyogenic arthritis follows untreated or unsuccessfully treated acute primary or secondary pyogenic arthritis. Inadequacy of treatment can be manifest by persistence of infection, but the course is either intermittent or continuous at a slow rate. One or more pathogens may produce a purulent inflammatory response within a joint; pyogenic cocci and enteric gram-negative rods are more common. Although a previously identified pathogen is likely to persist, superinfection can occur, especially with open surgical treatment and antibiotics. The original bacterial strain may be eliminated by treatment only to be supplanted by another, or it may persist with the new invader to cause a mixed infection.

Chronic pyogenic arthritis is likely to produce variable but characteristic clinical pictures. An overt or manifest infection can be continuously or recurrently active. Uninterrupted progress from the acute stage is characterized by continued local pain and swelling, restriction of joint motion, sinus formation, and increasing deformity. X-rays show progressive destruction of cartilage manifest by narrowing of the joint cleft, erosion of bone, and even infarction or cavitation. Even though the course is indolent, it is that of continued deterioration. Apparent abatement may follow in the recurrent type; but these episodes of comparative clinical quiescence only reflect temporary dormancy. Occult or covert infections are characterized by insidiousness and indolency. They may be unrecognized for long periods since they do not produce striking clinical findings. They may occur concomitantly with other joint lesions or complicate surgical operations on joints, especially after the use of surgical implants or antibiotic prophylaxis of postoperative infection.

Chronic pyogenic arthritis must be differentiated from all chronic nonpyogenic microbial infections of joints, gout, rheumatoid arthritis, and symptomatic degenerative arthritis.

Treatment is based on the principles of eradication of infection and restoration of maximum joint function. Bacterial sensitivity tests provide a basis for selection of antimicrobial drugs to be used as an adjunct to surgical operations. Operative destruction of the joint by arthrodesis or resection is often necessary to eliminate chronic infection.

SYPHILIS OF BONES AND JOINTS

Syphilitic arthritis or osteitis may occur during any stage of the congenital or acquired systemic disease. The incidence of bone and joint manifestations has decreased in the United States since the advent of antibiotic therapy. The recent increase in the incidence of primary infections may cause a proportionate rise of bone and joint manifestations if the diagnosis is not made promptly and vigorous treatment is not given.

In **infancy**, syphilitic epiphysitis is a typical lesion which is characterized radiologically by a zone of sclerosis adjacent to the growth plate but separated from another similar zone by one of rarefaction. The zone of rarefied bone may become partially replaced by inflammatory tissue, and suppuration and abscess formation may ensue. This explains why epiphysial displacement may occur. Focal periosteal thickening about the anterior fontanel during infancy causes Parrot's nodes.

Periostitis and osteoperiostitis are common manifestations of congenital syphilis in **childhood and adolescence.** Bone involvement is frequently symmetric, and when the tibia is affected along the crest the classical "saber shin" is produced. A painless bilateral effusion of the knees (Clutton's joints) is a rare manifestation which is said to be accompanied by other stigmas of the congenital disease.

In **adulthood**, gumma formation causes localized destruction of bone with surrounding areas of sclerosis and subperiosteal new bone formation. Periostitis in the adult is likely to occur in bones of the thorax and in the shafts of long bones of the extremities. The x-ray picture of syphilitic osteitis in the adult is not diagnostic, but bone production is generally more pronounced than bone destruction.

Since syphilis can mimic so many diseases, clinical suspicion is diagnostically useful. When localized clinical symptoms with compatible x-ray studies are supported by a history of congenital or acquired infection, thorough serologic studies will probably provide confirmatory diagnostic evidence. Biopsy is not necessary to establish a direct diagnosis, but it may differentiate a gumma from other granulomatous and caseating lesions. A favorable response of the local lesion to antibiotic therapy supports the diagnosis.

Treatment: In general, the only local treatment necessary is temporary immobilization to provide comfort and protection during the initial stages of systemic therapy. Operative treatment is necessary only rarely to evacuate an abscess. Lesions of the bones and joints respond to appropriate chemotherapy of the systemic disease.

TUBERCULOSIS OF BONES AND JOINTS

Tuberculosis of the skeletal system is caused by Mycobacterium tuberculosis. Practically all tuberculous infections in the United States are caused by the human strain. Infection of the musculoskeletal system is commonly caused by hematogenous spread from a primary lesion elsewhere. Clinical infection probably occurs only in persons with inadequate immunologic defenses following massive exposure to this ubiquitous organism. In the United States the incidence of tuberculous infection of the musculoskeletal system is diminishing as pulmonary tuberculosis becomes increasingly less common. It is a disease of childhood, occurring most commonly in persons between 3 and 5 years of age. Three-fourths of all infections occur before puberty.

The clinical features of tuberculous arthritis are essentially the same as those of any subacute or chronic joint infection. Pain in the region of the involved joint may be accentuated at night. Restriction of motion, a sensation of stiffness, and limping are due to local swelling caused by effusion into the joint and soft tissue edema. As the disease progresses, muscle atrophy and deformity become apparent.

X-ray manifestations are not characteristic. There is a latent period between the onset of symptoms and the initial positive x-ray finding. The earliest changes in tuberculous arthritis are those of soft tissue swelling and distention of the capsule by effusion. Subsequently, bone atrophy causes thinning of the trabecular pattern, thinning of the cortex, and enlargement of the medullary canal. As the disease progresses, destruction of cartilage is manifested by narrowing of the joint cleft and focal erosion of the articular surface, especially at the margins. Extensive destruction of joint surfaces leads to deformity. As healing takes place, sclerosis becomes apparent around areas of necrosis and sequestration. Where the lesion is limited to bone, especially in the cancellous portion of the metaphysis, the x-ray picture may be that of single or multiple cysts surrounded by sclerotic bone. As the lesion expands toward the cortex, subperiosteal new bone formation follows.

The precise diagnosis of tuberculosis rests upon the recovery of the acid-fast organisms from joint fluid or from an abscess by artificial culture methods or animal inoculation. Biopsy of the lesion or lymph node may demonstrate the characteristic histologic picture of acid-fast bacillary infection but does not differentiate tuberculosis from other nontuberculous mycobacterial lesions. A presumptive diagnosis can be established from clinical and x-ray examination when other lesions have been properly identified. Cutaneous reaction to protein derivatives of various mycobacteria is of presumptive diagnostic value only in so far as the local lesion is concerned.

In people with inadequate defense mechanisms, children, and elderly people with other systemic disease, tuberculosis of the skeletal system is likely to have an accelerated rate of progress. Destruction of bones or joints may occur in a few weeks or months if adequate treatment is not provided. Deformity due to joint destruction, abscess formation with spread into adjacent uninfected tissues, and sinus formation are common. Paraplegia is the most serious complication of spinal tuberculosis. As healing of severe joint lesions takes place, spontaneous fibrous or bony ankylosis follows.

Tuberculosis of the musculoskeletal system must be differentiated from all subacute and chronic infections, rheumatoid arthritis, gout, and occasionally osseous dysplasia. Infections caused by nontuberculous mycobacteria can be differentiated only by laboratory procedures which require expert knowledge.

The modern treatment of tuberculosis of the skeletal system consists of 3 phases: general care, chemotherapy, and surgery.

A. General Care: This is especially important when prolonged recumbency is necessary, and includes skillful nursing care, adequate diet, and appropriate treatment of associated lesions (pulmonary, genitourinary, etc.).
B. Chemotherapy: Modern chemotherapy is based essentially on the systemic administration of drugs to which the strain of pathogen is susceptible. The protection offered by these agents

permits direct surgical attack on local lesions without the likelihood of miliary dissemination. According to current concepts, chemotherapy should be continued for one year or more. Administration is usually systemic, but this route has the disadvantage that the agent must cross an inflammatory or fibrocaseous barrier to reach the organism. Local administration is occasionally feasible and has the advantage of bringing comparatively high concentrations of the drug into direct contact with the surface of the lesion. Combinations of drugs are more effective than the use of a single agent.

1. Streptomycin is effective, but resistant strains are likely to emerge during administration. It is especially valuable for protection against hematogenous dissemination following surgical procedures. It has been used topically in joints and in abscess cavities.
2. Aminosalicylic acid (PAS) appears to increase the effectiveness of streptomycin and isoniazid by preventing the rapid emergence of resistant strains of bacteria.
3. Isoniazid (INH) should be administered with at least one of the other drugs since it may become ineffective when used alone because of development of bacterial resistance. It appears to potentiate the activity of streptomycin. Vitamin B deficiency is likely to occur as a complication of prolonged therapy and should be prevented by administration of pyridoxine.
4. Other useful but more toxic drugs include viomycin, capreomycin, pyrazinamide, cycloserine, ethionamide, and ethambutol.

C. Surgical Treatment: No rigid recommendations can be made for the operative treatment of tuberculosis since the stage of the infection and the character of the lesion are the determining factors. In **acute** infections where synovitis is the predominant feature, treatment can be conservative, at least initially: immobilization by splint or plaster, aspiration, and chemotherapy may suffice to control the infection. This treatment is especially desirable for the management of infections of large joints of the lower extremities in children, and may also be used in adults either as definitive treatment or preliminary to more extensive operative management. Synovectomy may be valuable for less acute hypertrophic lesions which involve tendon sheaths, bursae, or joints.

Various types of operative treatment are necessary for **chronic or advanced** tuberculosis of bones and joints depending upon the location of the lesion and the age and general condition of the patient. The availability of chemotherapy has broadened the indications for synovectomy and debridement. Even though all infected tissue cannot be removed by operation, supplemental chemotherapy seems to afford protection in some cases so that useful function can be retained in weight-bearing joints, whereas arthrodesis was formerly necessary. In general, arthrodesis of weight-bearing joints is preferred when useful function cannot be salvaged by more conservative operative procedures. The technic of reconstructive arthroplasty to restore useful function has not proved reliable in eradicating disease, and is not recommended at present for widespread clinical use.

Special Considerations (Specific Sites).

The treatment of certain lesions requires individual comment.

A. About one-half of cases of tuberculosis of the musculoskeletal system involve the **spine**; the highest incidence is in the thoracolumbar area. At least 2 segments are usually involved, and the initial focus is most often in the body adjacent to the growth plate or intervertebral disk. Three-fourths of cases occur in children less than 5 years of age. Arthrodesis is still the most valuable operative procedure, but Ito's concept of direct attack on the local lesion by radical debridement via an anterior or anterolateral surgical approach in addition to arthrodesis has been successful in a high percentage of cases. Paraplegia is the most serious complication of spinal tuberculosis and is most likely to occur with lesions in the thoracic region.

B. About 25% of cases involve the **hip joint**, principally in children. Although the primary infection may be synovial, the favored osseous foci are the metaphysial side of the head of the femur and the ilium or ischium adjacent to the acetabular cartilage. The clinical features are essentially those of acute or chronic hip joint disease. In addition to general care and chemotherapy, operative treatment is usually required at some stage. It may be deferred in children in whom the most prominent feature is synovitis until the infection becomes quiescent. Extensive bone involvement may so impair function that arthrodesis will be required. Arthrodesis of the hip in childhood is generally associated with disturbance of growth of the lower extremity.

C. Infection of the **knee joint** is frequently manifest as synovitis without significant involvement of either the adjacent femur or the tibia. For this reason, initial treatment frequently can be nonoperative.

D. Lesions of other joints and anatomic structures are encountered less frequently. Tuberculous tenosynovitis usually involves the hand. Tuberculous dactylitis occurs usually in the hand, but occasionally in the foot. It is rare, is characterized by fusiform swelling of the soft tissues of the involved digit, and is referred to as spina ventosa. X-ray examination may show thickening of the bone caused by a periosteal reaction or cyst-like changes with surrounding sclerosis in the cancellous or medullary interior.

E. A solitary and apparently primary tuberculous abscess of muscle without apparent bone or joint involvement occurs rarely.

20...

Organ Transplantation

IMMUNOBIOLOGIC PRINCIPLES

Tissue grafts between individuals of the same species (**homografts or allografts**) are rejected with a vigor proportionate to the degree of genetic disparity between them. Grafts between individuals of different species (**heterografts or xenografts**) are rejected with even greater rapidity. Grafts between identical twins (**isografts**) survive indefinitely.

Rejection of allografts and xenografts is due to an immune response of the recipient against antigens present on the tissues of the donor and absent in the host (primary response). If the host has been previously exposed to the same antigens present in the graft, an accelerated rejection response (second set response) will take place. These immune responses appear to be mediated by both cellular and humoral immunity.

The tissue transplantation antigens by which individuals differ are called histocompatibility antigens. A large variety of antigens localized primarily on the surface of the cell have been chemically identified as proteins or lipoproteins. These antigens are genetically determined by a number of chromosomal loci, but a single major locus (human leukocyte antigen, HLA) governs the development of the strongest antigens. Theoretically, if major antigens of donors and recipients can be matched at this locus, the strength of rejection can be minimized. Consequently, grafts between siblings or between parents and children are far more successful than grafts between unrelated donors. In addition, the best donor from among potential sibling donors can now be selected by tests which determine leukocyte histocompatibility antigens.

In addition to the special histocompatibility antigens on leukocytes, the ABO antigens normally present on tissue cells are also strong transplantation antigens. No graft should be attempted in defiance of the blood group barriers normally observed in clinical blood transfusion.

Immunosuppression.

Despite advances in tissue typing to minimize the antigenic disparity between donors and recipients, clinical organ transplantation depends on immunosuppressive drugs to minimize graft rejection. These drugs do not lessen the need for proper tissue matching, since immunosuppression is much more successful when weaker histocompatibility barriers are present. Nevertheless, even strong histocompatibility barriers between unrelated individuals can be partially overcome by immunosuppressive treatment. Except in the case of isografts, immunosuppressive therapy can rarely be stopped following allograft transplantation.

Azathioprine (Imuran®), a derivative of mercaptopurine (Purinethol®), is the primary immunosuppressant used in man. It is usually administered a few days before transplantation, in progressively lower doses to avoid bone marrow depression. Prednisone is the other major drug used in immunosuppressive therapy. It is usually given in high doses at the time of transplantation and its dosage gradually reduced to more easily tolerated levels. When allograft rejection occurs, the prednisone dosage is increased.

More recently, antisera made in horses against human lymph node, thymus, or spleen cells have been utilized during the early days following transplantation. Such antilymphocyte sera (ALS) and purified antilymphocyte globulins (ALG) are excellent immunosuppressive agents in animals. In man, ALG appears to be an effective adjunctive agent in producing a degree of immunosuppression which can be maintained by lower doses of prednisone and azathioprine than are usually required. Thus, toxicity can be minimized without reducing the effectiveness. Naturally, the administration of any heterologous protein is associated with those complications, i.e., anaphylactic reactions and serum sickness, which appear after the use of any foreign protein. However, these reactions have been lessened by the immunosuppressive drugs. Unfortunately, ALG is less effective than prednisone in reversing graft rejection episodes.

Local irradiation of the graft is also being used to prevent and to treat graft rejection episodes. Other immunosuppressive agents that have been used on occasion include cactinomycin (actinomycin C) and azaserine. Thoracic duct fistulas have been constructed to reduce circulating lymphocyte levels, and splenectomy has been utilized to reduce the mass of potentially reactive lymphoid tissue.

KIDNEY TRANSPLANTATION

Selection of Recipients.

Since there are limited facilities compared to need, criteria of selection have had to be devised as a means of deciding who should receive transplants. The patient must be free of infection or malignancy. The ideal patient is young, emotionally stable, and has no life-threatening disease other than terminal uremia. More recently, patients of any age and with a number of complicating factors (e.g., lupus erythematosus, diabetes, myocardial infarction, peptic ulcer) have received transplants with success. Even patients requiring urinary diversion can be accepted.

Selection of Living Donors.

Only one donor death has been reported as a direct result of nephrectomy. It is possible that other deaths will occur, and the consequences of reducing the renal reserve of a healthy person should not be lightly regarded. Nevertheless, transplantation into related recipients gives so much better results than transplantation between unrelated persons that related volunteer donors should not be discouraged. The living donor should have compatible ABO antigens, normal bilateral renal function, and must be free of all other systemic disease. Either kidney may be used, but it is technically simpler to use a kidney with a single renal artery. If more than one living related donor is available, histocompatibility typing should be done to determine the best possible donor. However, even poorly matched related donors give better long-term renal function than do cadaver donors. A routine work-up of potential donors may be outlined as follows:

(1) CBC, platelet count, prothrombin time, BUN, serum creatinine, serum glutamic-oxaloacetic transaminase, serum sodium, potassium, chloride, calcium, phosphorus, and uric acid, and two-hour postprandial blood glucose.
(2) Urinalysis and urine culture (twice).
(3) Twenty-four-hour creatinine clearance.
(4) Serologic test for syphilis.
(5) Blood typing with minor group typing.
(6) Chest x-ray.
(7) Electrocardiogram.
(8) Intravenous urogram.
(9) Renal arteriogram.
(10) Histocompatibility typing of leukocytes.
(11) Leukocyte cross-match for recipient antidonor leukocyte antibodies.

Selection of Cadaver Donors.

Most cadaver organ donors have sustained fatal brain damage. Neurologic death should be determined by the attending neurologist or neurosurgeon or by a committee designated for the purpose. The donor must have been otherwise healthy. Patients who have had malignancies should not be used since tumors have been inadvertently transplanted along with the kidney in several instances. Under ideal circumstances a creatinine clearance test should have been done during the expectant period before death. ABO compatibility is necessary. The leukocyte cytotoxicity cross-match must be performed to detect antibodies in the recipient directed against the donor, and histocompatibility testing should be done to determine the best recipient in the pool of patients awaiting transplantation. Following determination of neurologic death, the organs should be removed as quickly as possible to minimize ischemic time. Both kidneys should be used whenever 2 compatible recipients are available.

Preoperative Care of the Renal Transplant Recipient.

No patient with terminal renal failure should be kept on medical management to the point of severe malnutrition, anemia, infection, or malignant hypertension. As soon as dietary means of controlling uremia have failed and normal ambulatory functions are no longer possible, intermittent hemodialysis should be started. (Peritoneal dialysis is too cumbersome and potentially hazardous for routine use over an extended time.) The frequency of hemodialysis varies with each case. Nephrectomy is usually best done several weeks prior to the transplantation procedure. Splenectomy is usually done at the same time in order to reduce the total lymphoid mass. Dialysis should be performed more frequently in the week prior to transplantation.

Since dialysis frequently produces a chronic hypovolemic state, the blood volume is determined and restored to normal before transplantation. Serum electrolytes, serum creatinine, BUN, serum calcium and phosphorus, and serum protein electrophoresis should be done. Cultures of the nose, throat, and umbilicus should be done within several days before transplantation, since infecting organisms are usually endogenous. A voiding cystogram should be taken to determine the integrity of the lower urinary tract. An upper gastrointestinal series is useful because gastrointestinal complications often result from prolonged prednisone therapy following transplantation. In patients who have been nephrectomized, bladder irrigation with neomycin-bacitracin solution is indicated because the bladder may become infected in the absence of urinary flow. During dialysis, supplementary folic acid and vitamins B and C should be given since symptomatic deficiencies of these vitamins may develop. On occasion it is necessary to anticoagulate the patient's blood in order to maintain patency of the hemodialysis shunts before transplantation. Anticoagulant therapy should be stopped and a normal prothrombin time reestablished prior to transplantation. Daily hexachlorophene scrubs of the abdomen should be given before transplantation to maintain the utmost cleanliness of the skin. Although the need for antihypertensive drug therapy is reduced following nephrectomy, some antihypertensive therapy is usually necessary until the transplantation operation.

The following immunosuppressive protocol has been used with good results:

(1) Two days before transplantation, treatment with antilymphocyte globulin, 15-30 mg./Kg./day, is started.

(2) Thirty-two hours before operation, begin prednisone, 1 mg./Kg./day, and azathioprine (Imuran®), 2.5 mg./Kg./day.

(3) At 5 a.m. on the morning of the operation, give azathioprine, 5 mg./Kg., and draw blood for a complete blood count, platelet count, and BUN as a baseline for future studies.

Transplantation Operation.

The kidney and a length of ureter are removed from the donor and transplanted into the retroperitoneal space of the recipient pelvis by anastomosis of the recipient hypogastric artery to the renal artery of the donor kidney and the iliac vein of the recipient to the renal vein of the donor kidney. Utilizing a submucosal tunneling technic, the ureter is then implanted into the bladder.

Postoperative Management.

Postoperative vital signs, temperature, and central venous pressures are continually monitored. Urinary output, specific gravity, and pH are measured every hour. The Foley catheter is placed to straight drainage but is not irrigated unless there are signs of obstruction by clot.

Intravenous fluids are administered hourly and in an amount equivalent to the previous hour's urine output (at least 30 ml./hour). The solution utilized consists of half-normal saline in 5% dextrose in water with 10 mEq/L. $NaHCO_3$ added. Creatinine clearance is determined during a two-hour period immediately after operation and again 6 hours after operation. Blood is drawn for serum electrolytes, creatinine, BUN, white count, and platelet count several hours after operation and again on the night of the operation.

The immunosuppressive regimen consists of giving azathioprine (Imuran®), 5 mg./Kg./day initially, reducing dosage during the first week to about 3 mg. /Kg. /day. The amount of azathioprine required thereafter is determined daily on the basis of the white count and platelet count. A maintenance dose of 1.5-2.5 mg. /Kg. is usual. Prednisone is also given daily in an initial dose of 1 mg. /Kg., reduced over the first 3 weeks after operation to levels of approximately 0. 3 mg. /Kg. /day. The exact maintenance dose required is determined by the function of the recipient kidney and the degree of toxicity. ALG is continued for 14 consecutive days postoperatively and then may be discontinued.

Antihypertensive drugs such as methyldopa (Aldomet®) and hydralazine (Apresoline®) are occasionally required in patients with long-standing hypertension and should be given early following operation.

Isolation precautions are no longer required after renal transplantation. Foley catheter drainage is discontinued after 3 days. The diet should be moderately low in sodium, with vitamin supplementation. In order to determine optimal maintenance levels of immunosuppressive agents and detect rejection early, the patient should be kept in the hospital for about 2 weeks. After discharge, he is followed 3 times weekly with urinalysis, serum and urine creatinine, BUN, hematocrit, blood pressure, and weight determinations.

Complications of Renal Transplantation.

A. Rejection: The most common complication of renal allotransplantation is rejection. There are varying intensities of rejection depending upon the degree of histoincompatibility; the rejection process is rarely complete and irreversible, progressing to total graft destruction. The classical rejection picture includes oliguria, swelling of the graft, tenderness, fever, leukocytosis, mononuclear cells in the urine, proteinuria, hypertension, and azotemia. However, in the presence of prophylactic immunosuppression, there is usually only a slight elevation in creatinine and fall in creatinine clearance.

An intravenous urogram and I^{125}-Hippuran® renogram will rule out urinary obstruction or renal vascular insufficiency, respectively. The mildest functional change thus becomes presumptive evidence of immunologic rejection of the graft. Treatment with high doses of prednisone, local graft irradiation (150 r every other day for 3 doses) should be instituted immediately to reverse the rejection process with minimum change in renal function. Seldom, however, does renal function return to preexisting levels; some degree of permanent renal impairment usually persists following each episode of rejection.

Most rejection episodes occur 2-8 weeks after transplantation, but "hyperacute" rejection has been noted immediately after grafting. The graft becomes cyanotic and soft; the vessels appear to be occluded by intravascular thrombi. Such hyperacute rejection episodes are most frequently associated with preexisting cytotoxic antibodies in the recipient directed against donor tissue.

In contrast to the hyperacute rejection episode, subclinical rejection may occur without prompt decline in creatinine clearance. A tendency to gain weight, slight recurrent fever without other signs of systemic infection, and hypertension suggest progressive rejection.

B. Other Complications: In the early postoperative period, massive diuresis or oliguria may appear. Both may represent damage to the kidney during the ischemic period. In patients with oliguria, clots in the Foley catheter, vascular accidents, and hyperacute rejection should be ruled out before assuming that this is acute tubular necrosis. Acute tubular necrosis with oliguria usually corrects itself spontaneously 2-3 weeks after transplantation and may be followed by a diuretic phase. The azathioprine dosage should be reduced during the oliguric phase in order to avoid toxicity since the drug is partially excreted by the kidney.

The complications of prednisone administration include upper gastrointestinal bleeding despite the prophylactic use of antacids. Cushingoid changes, increased susceptibility to infection, diabetes, and aseptic necrosis of the femoral heads have been seen.

Azathioprine toxicity is characterized primarily by leukopenia and thrombocyotpenia, which are best treated by withdrawal of the drug for brief periods. Pancreatitis, stomatitis, skin ulcerations, loss of hair, and an increased susceptibility to infection have all been related to azathioprine administration.

Death following renal transplantation is usually due to overwhelming infection accompanying the use of azathioprine and prednisone. Bacterial infections predominate, but candida, nocardia, pneumocystis, and cytomegalovirus have all been implicated in fatal infections following renal transplantation.

Pulmonary insufficiency is the most common cause of death after transplantation and is usually of infectious origin. A syndrome called "transplant lung," consisting of progressive hypoxemia with minimal clinical findings and variable x-ray findings, has been described. An immunologic etiology has been ascribed to this disease, but its pathogenesis is probably related to interstitial pulmonary edema secondary to renal allograft rejection.

In recipients of twin isografts, recurrent glomerulonephritis has been a frequent concomitant of prolonged survival. This is less of a problem following allotransplantation because of the effect of immunosuppressive agents in preventing the development of this "autoimmune" disease. Low doses of azathioprine will usually prevent recurrent glomerulonephritis in isografts.

Surgical complications include thrombosis of the renal artery, bleeding, and breakdown of the ureteral anastomosis. Small urinary leaks usually close without surgical intervention, but larger leaks require surgical repair.

Prognosis.

The most recent results compiled by the Kidney Transplant Registry in sibling, parental, and cadaver donor-recipient combinations are tabulated below. It is apparent that a large percentage of recipients of sibling and parental kidneys will survive for prolonged periods and that these results are improving.

Functional survival of cadaver kidney transplants is less likely. These patients are frequently subject to repeated rejection crises with the ultimate result of transplant failure. Such patients can be placed on chronic dialysis and receive second transplants with results similar to a first transplant. These results can be expected to improve somewhat as histocompatibility matching is improved and as more experience is obtained in immunosuppressive management.

Estimated Transplant Survival at Two Years (Kidney Transplant Registry)

Donor	Percentage
Monozygotic twin	100
Sibling	75
Parent	70
Other relative	60
Cadaver	45
Unrelated living donor	23

TRANSPLANTATION OF OTHER ORGANS

The transplantation of vital organs other than the kidney entails the use of cadaver donors exclusively. Consequently, the problems of histocompatibility matching between donor and recipient are multiplied. In addition, there are no artificial organs to sustain patients in severe heart failure, hepatic failure, or respiratory failure for prolonged periods while donors are being sought for transplantation. Thus, these patients may die while awaiting a suitable cadaver donor. Cooperative regional and national programs for typing and matching recipients and donors are now being set up in order to minimize these problems.

1. HEART TRANSPLANTATION

Heart transplantation is discussed in Chapter 10. The immunologic problems are similar to those of organ transplantation in general.

2. LIVER TRANSPLANTATION

Both orthotopic replacement of the diseased liver and auxiliary transplantation of livers have been carried out in man. Auxiliary livers tend to atrophy when excluded from the portal circulation and have never functioned well as transplants. Orthotopic transplants, i.e., transplantation of the liver into its normal site with anastomoses of the vena cava, portal vein, hepatic artery, and biliary tract, have been carried out in a number of patients with hepatoma or biliary atresia. The technical problems are formidable and not all have been overcome. Such patients do not tolerate large doses of azathioprine well. In addition, a recurrent problem has been septic infarction of large segments of liver tissue which are dependent on a limited blood supply. It is not known whether such infarction represents intravascular coagulation secondary to a vascular rejection phenomenon or whether it is due to mechanical vascular problems. Most characteristically, however, segmental infarction is heralded by fever, bacteria in the peripheral blood, the appearance of ischemia on liver scan, and elevations of hepatocellular enzymes 24-48 hours following the fever. On occasion, such areas of infarction can be debrided and drained. Despite these hazards, a number of patients are now well several years after hepatic allotransplantation.

3. PANCREATIC TRANSPLANTATION

More than a dozen patients have received pancreaticoduodenal transplants. All have had severe diabetes, and some have required simultaneous renal transplantation. The pancreas is generally transplanted by anastomosis of the celiac axis and superior mesenteric arteries to the iliac vessels of the recipient; the duodenum is anastomosed to a Roux-en-Y segment of jejunum. All pancreases have functioned well with respect to insulin and exocrine secretion, and there is some evidence that the rejection process in these grafts is less than that in simultaneous renal grafts. Rejection of the duodenum progresses insidiously, however, and necrosis may occur without warning. All of the grafts have had to be removed or the patients have died, although several transplants were successful for 6 months to 1 year. It is doubtful that many indications for pancreatic transplantation exist, although the unmanageable juvenile diabetic may represent one such instance.

4. ENDOCRINE TRANSPLANTATION

There are few indications for transplantation of endocrine organs in which one can justify the substitution of immunosuppressive drugs for endocrine replacement therapy. A number of patients have received parathyroid transplants without convincing evidence of successful function. Similarily, allografts of adrenal tissue, thyroid tissue, and ovarian tissue have been carried out without prolonged useful results.

5. LUNG TRANSPLANTATION

Lung transplantation has been performed in more than 20 patients without long-term success. In addition to the usual immunologic problems and those involving donor selection, pulmonary venous thrombosis, disruption of the bronchial anastomosis, bronchial stenosis, disruption of the bronchial arterial supply, interruption of the pulmonary nerves, and impairment of pulmonary compliance seem to play significant roles in pulmonary dysfunction in the early post-transplant period. Thus far, these factors have militated against serious attempts at lung transplantation.

6. BONE MARROW TRANSPLANTATION

Allogeneic transplants of bone marrow can be done in animals following lethal irradiation. Attempts have been made to transplant bone marrow into patients who received accidental lethal irradiation. A number of infusions of marrow were successful, but success is not uniform. Early deaths due to irradiation are common. In addition to the problem of graft survival, the marrow itself is immunocompetent and tends to react against the host in a graft-versus-host immunologic reaction. This is characterized by hepatic dysfunction, dermatitis, diarrhea, weight loss, aplasia of the marrow, and death.

More recently, attempts at bone marrow transplantation have been carried out following massive chemotherapy of patients with leukemia or Hodgkin's disease. In some cases, the marrow of carefully matched related donors has been used. In a few recipients, the graft-versus-host reaction has been minimized, and thus far the bone marrow transplantation has been a success. The most successful application of this technic is in patients with congenital immunologic deficiency states where immunocompetent cells are required to prevent recurrent infections which characterize these conditions. Thymus transplants are also useful in certain cases of thymic aplasia.

Appendix: Drug Dosages

The rational use of drugs demands that the physician anticipate the wide variations in response that may occur when a fixed dosage is prescribed without consideration of individual differences among patients as well as day to day variations in response in the same patient. Individualization of drug dosage for the pediatric and geriatric patient and the importance of various pathologic states (particularly of the cardiovascular and respiratory systems, the liver, and the kidneys) must also be considered before instituting any form of drug therapy.

Several formulas based on proportions of the adult dose have long been used for calculation of pediatric drug dosage. Three of these formulas are reproduced below. The surface area formula probably is most accurate. These formulas may be erroneous in premature infants and neonates because certain enzymes necessary for drug conjugation are not yet active.

Surface area:

$$\text{Child dose} = \frac{\text{Surface area of child in } M^{2*} \times \text{adult dose}}{1.75}$$

Clark's rule: (Based on weight, for children over 2 years)

$$\frac{\text{Weight of child (lb.)}}{150} \times \text{Adult dose} = \text{Child's dose}$$

Young's Rule: (Based on age)

$$\frac{\text{Age (in years)}}{\text{Age} + 12} \times \text{Adult dose} = \text{Child's dose}$$

DRUGS FOR GENERAL USE

Nonnarcotic Analgesics.

Most of these compounds are able to produce a definite antipyretic and antiinflammatory effect in addition to a mild analgesic effect.

A. Aspirin, 0.3-0.6 Gm. (5-10 gr.) every 3-4 hours p.r.n., best taken with 1/2-1 glass of water or with food. Often causes

---

*Derived from standard nomograms (see pp. 828-829).

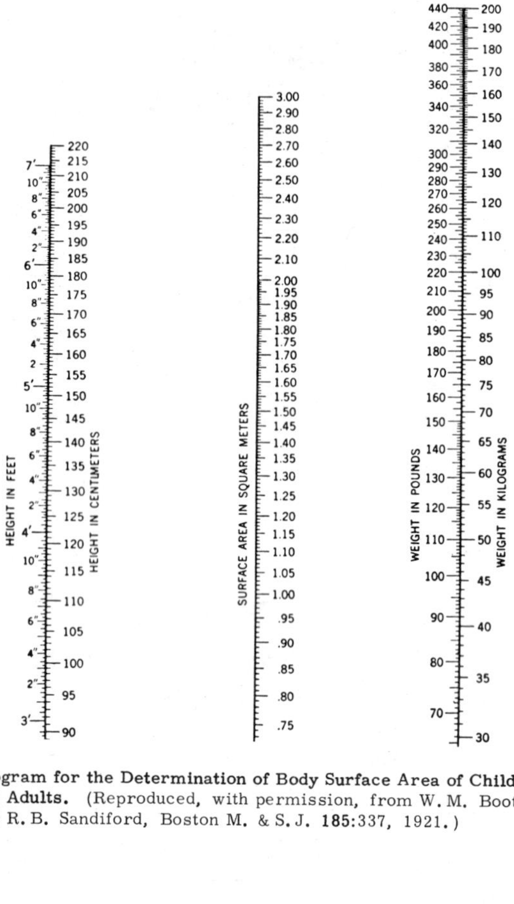

Nomogram for the Determination of Body Surface Area of Children and Adults. (Reproduced, with permission, from W. M. Boothby and R. B. Sandiford, Boston M. & S. J. **185**:337, 1921.)

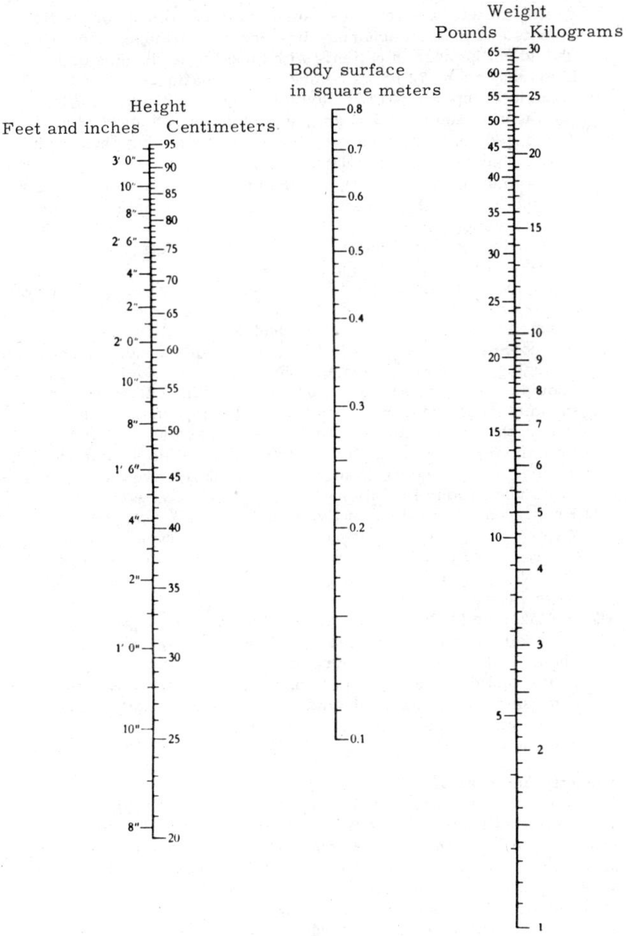

Nomogram for the Determination of Body Surface Area of Children.
(Reproduced, with permission, from E.F. DuBois, Basal Metabolism in Health and Disease. Lea & Febiger, 1936.)

gastric upset. Large doses cause tinnitus. Blood coagulation defects and platelet abnormalities occur; therefore, aspirin should not be used in patients with bleeding tendencies or in blood donors 48-72 hours before blood donation.

B. Aspirin Compound (APC): Contains aspirin, 225 mg. (3½ gr.), phenacetin, 150 mg. (2½ gr.), and caffeine, 30 mg. (½ gr.). Prolonged, excessive use of compounds containing phenacetin may cause serious renal damage.

C. Acetaminophen (Tylenol®), 325-650 mg. orally 3-4 times daily, has the same analgesic potency and antipyretic action as aspirin. It has no appreciable anti-inflammatory action. The drug does not produce gastric irritation or coagulation defects and may be used in patients with aspirin allergy.

D. Phenylbutazone (Butazolidin®) and Oxyphenbutazone (Tandearil®): 100 mg. orally 3-4 times daily. These drugs possess a more potent anti-inflammatory action than do the salicylates. They are potentially dangerous in that serious side actions may occur, including peptic ulceration and blood dyscrasias. Their use should be restricted to a period not exceeding one week.

E. Indomethacin (Indocin®): A nonsteroid compound used for various arthritic conditions. It possesses analgesic and anti-inflammatory effects. Gastrointestinal side-effects commonly occur. The dosage is 25 mg. 2-4 times daily given with food to reduce gastric irritation.

F. Propoxyphene and Aspirin Compound (Darvon® Compound): Aspirin compound with propoxyphene HCl (Darvon®), 30 mg. (½ gr.), 1-2 capsules every 6 hours p.r.n. In doses less than 65 mg. (1 gr.), the analgesic effect of Darvon® alone is quite doubtful.

G. Pentazocine (Talwin®), 50 mg. orally, is about equal to 60 mg. of codeine in analgesic effect. A dose of 30 mg. subcut. is about equal to 10 mg. of morphine. Pentazocine will not suppress abstinence symptoms in morphine-dependent subjects, and, since it is a narcotic antagonist, it can actually induce severe withdrawal reactions. The drug is subject to abuse and can cause addiction.

Narcotic Analgesics.

The narcotic analgesics are capable of producing significant analgesia, but not without causing significant effects on other organ systems. All are respiratory depressants. The main differences between the various agents seem to be related to their potency and duration of action. These agents are contraindicated in respiratory insufficiency, bronchial asthma, Addison's disease, myxedema, and hepatic disease and in the presence of increased intracranial pressure or coma.

Although morphine and the synthetic substitutes have a high addiction potential in addiction-prone individuals, their judicious use is warranted for the relief of severe pain. Potent narcotics may obscure matters in undiagnosed, acute surgical problems (e.g., acute surgical abdomen).

A. Morphine and Morphine Equivalents:

1. Morphine sulfate - The average dose is 8-15 mg. (1/8-1/4 gr.) orally or subcut. every 3 hours p.r.n. The oral route is only about one-tenth as effective as the parenteral. An

I. V. dose of 2-4 mg. (1/30-1/15 gr.) may be given slowly in 5 ml. saline solution for rapid effect. A very useful drug; the advantages of the synthetic "substitutes" over morphine have probably been exaggerated.

2. Morphine equivalents - A number of drugs are available which are equal to morphine in potency but offer no advantages. The following subcut. doses are equivalent in analgesic effect to 10 mg. (1/6 gr.) of morphine: dihydromorphinone (Dilaudid®), 2 mg.; levorphanol (Levo-Dromoran®), 2 mg.; oxymorphone (Numorphan®), 1.5 mg.; and phenazocine (Prinadol®), 2 mg.
3. Methadone (Dolophine®) is as potent as morphine but has a more prolonged effect. It is highly addictive and is rarely used except in the institutional treatment of addicts. The usual dosage range is 5-10 mg. (1/12-1/6 gr.) subcut.

B. Meperidine and Others of Intermediate Potency:
1. Meperidine (Demerol®) - The analgesic properties and side effects of this drug at a dose of 75-100 mg. are equivalent to those which occur with 10 mg. of morphine. The usual dosage range is 50-150 mg. orally or I. M. **(not subcut.)**. It may be given I. V. in urgent situations.
2. Meperidine congeners - Alphaprodine (Nisentil®), 60 mg., and anileridine (Leritine®), 50 mg., subcut., are equivalent to meperidine, 100 mg.
3. Dihydrohydroxycodeinone is available as Percodan®, which also contains APC and homatropine. Two or 3 tablets represent 10-15 mg. (1/6-1/4 gr.) of the narcotic, equivalent to 10 mg. (1/6 gr.) of morphine. The average adult dose is 1 tablet every 6 hours.

C. Codeine: Codeine, 8-60 mg. (1/8-1 gr.) orally or subcut. every 3-4 hours p. r. n., is a less potent analgesic than the drugs listed above, but it is also less addictive and causes fewer side reactions. For convenience in prescribing it is most often given in combination with aspirin. If 60 mg. (1 gr.) are not effective, a more potent analgesic is indicated.

Narcotic Antagonists.

The following drugs immediately counteract the effects of overdosage with morphine and other narcotic analgesics. They may produce withdrawal symptoms in addicts currently using narcotics. These agents may act as depressants when given alone in large doses.

A. Nalorphine (Nalline®), 5-10 mg. subcut., I. M., or I. V., repeated if necessary every 15-20 minutes to a total of 40 mg.

B. Levallorphan (Lorfan®), 0.5-1 mg. I. V. If necessary, one or 2 additional doses of 0.5 mg. may be given.

Antiallergic Agents.

A. Antihistamines:
1. Diphenhydramine (Benadryl®) - 50 mg. orally 3-4 times daily, or 5-20 mg. I. V. May be given with drug to which allergic reaction is anticipated. May cause drowsiness.
2. Chlorpheniramine (Chlor-Trimeton®), 4 mg. orally 3-4 times daily.

B. Adrenergic Drugs:
1. Epinephrine (adrenaline) - For immediate response, give

0.3-0.5 ml. of 1:1000 solution subcut. or I. M. In emergencies, give 0.2-0.5 ml. of 1:1000 solution I. V. For prolonged action, give 0.2-1 ml. of 1:500 solution in oil I. M. every 10-14 hours. Epinephrine is used in acute allergic reactions such as serum sickness, severe bronchial asthma, and anaphylaxis.

2. Ephedrine, 25-50 mg. ($^3/_8$-$^3/_4$ gr.) orally q. i. d.

C. Corticotropin (ACTH) and Corticosteroids: For use in acute or chronic allergic reactions which fail to respond to more conservative measures.

1. Prednisone and prednisolone - These derivatives of hydrocortisone have a greater degree of antiinflammatory and antiallergic activity than the parent compound. They have less sodium-retaining effect than the cortisones but potentially have the same hazardous effects. Prolonged administration of high doses may cause profound abnormalities (e.g., hypokalemia, hyperglycemia, hyperuricemia, peptic ulceration, glaucoma, psychiatric disturbances). Sudden withdrawal may cause adrenal insufficiency.

   a. Oral preparations - Prednisone (Deltasone®, Meticorten®) or prednisolone (Delta-Cortef®, Hydeltra®), 5-50 mg. (avg. 10-20 mg.) daily orally in divided doses every 4-8 hours. The following congeners differ from prednisone and prednisolone only in absolute potency and offer no advantages: methylprednisolone (Medrol®), triamcinolone (Aristocort®, Kenacort®), dexamethasone (Decadron®, Deronil®), betamethasone (Celestone®), paramethasone (Haldrone®), and fluprednisolone (Alphadrol®).

   b. Parenteral preparations (for I. M. or I. V. use) -

      (1) Prednisolone hemisuccinate (Meticortelone®), 50-100 mg. daily I. M. or I. V.

      (2) Prednisolone-21-phosphate (Hydeltrasol®), 40-100 mg. daily I. M. or I. V.

      (3) Methylprednisolone sodium succinate (Solu-Medrol®), 40-120 mg. daily I. M. or I. V.

2. Hydrocortisone sodium succinate (Solu-Cortef®) - 100-250 mg. I. V. in not less than 30 seconds for immediate effect. May be repeated p. r. n. at increasing intervals (1, 3, 6, 10 hours, etc.). The same precautions must be observed as with prednisone and prednisolone. May also be used in the treatment of adrenal insufficiency.

3. Corticotropin (ACTH) - 20-40 U. S. P. units in any I. V. fluid over 8-12 hours; or 40-200 U. S. P. units I. M. in saline solution every 6 hours; or 10-200 U. S. P. units of corticotropin gel (repository injection) once or twice daily I. M.

Sedatives and Hypnotics.

A. Short-Acting:

1. Pentobarbital sodium - 30 mg. orally 3-4 times daily, or 100-200 mg. h. s. Use cautiously in hepatic insufficiency. May be given I. V. or I. M.: 100-250 mg.
2. Secobarbital sodium (Seconal®) - 15-30 mg. orally every 4 hours, or 100-200 mg. h. s. Use cautiously in hepatic insufficiency.
3. Chloral hydrate - 0.25-1 Gm. orally. Use cautiously in hepatic insufficiency.

4. Paraldehyde - 4-16 ml. orally in milk or fruit juice. May also give rectally, 16-32 ml. in 30-60 ml. of oil. The stock solution is sterile but unstable.

B. Intermediate-Acting:
1. Amobarbital sodium (Amytal®) - 15-30 mg. orally 3-4 times daily, or 200-300 mg. h.s. Use cautiously in hepatic insufficiency. May be given I.M. or I.V. (as anticonvulsant), 65-500 mg. Stat. More rapid anticonvulsant action may be obtained with thiopental (Pentothal®), 50-100 mg. I.V.
2. Meprobamate (Miltown®, Equanil®) - 400 mg. 3-4 times daily.

C. Long-Acting:
1. Phenobarbital - 15-30 mg. (1/4-1/2 gr.) orally 2-4 times daily, or 100-200 mg. (1 1/2-3 gr.) h.s. Use cautiously in renal insufficiency. Phenobarbital sodium, 65-100 mg. (1-1 1/2 gr.), may be given subcut. or I.M.
2. Chlordiazepoxide (Librium®) - 5-10 mg. 3-4 times daily, or diazepam (Valium®), 2-10 mg. 1-3 times daily.

CARDIORESPIRATORY DRUGS

Coronary Dilator Drugs.

A. Nitroglycerin: Place one 0.3, 0.4, or 0.6 mg. (1/200, 1/150, or 1/100 gr.) tablet under the tongue and allow to dissolve. Begin with 0.3 mg. (1/200 gr.) and increase p.r.n. effectiveness. Undesirable side-effects include flushing, pounding pulse, dizziness, and headache.

B. Amyl Nitrite: 1 pearl, crushed and inhaled (about 3 inhalations), acts in about 10 seconds. Side effects as for glyceryl trinitrate, above.

Digitalis.

See table on p. 835.

Anticoagulants.

Anticoagulant therapy is most frequently employed in the prevention of intravascular clotting following venous thrombosis or arterial embolism and during periods of bed rest following myocardial infarction. Heparin is usually given for immediate and prothrombin depressants for prolonged effect. Contraindications to anticoagulant therapy include severe hepatic disease, renal failure, recent gastrointestinal hemorrhage, severe hypertension, and recent brain, prostatic, or other surgery in which delayed hemorrhage may occur. **Caution:** Determine Lee-White clotting time and prothrombin level before anticoagulant therapy is started. The use of salicylates should be avoided.

A. Heparin Sodium: The optimal dose is that which prolongs the Lee-White clotting time to 20-30 minutes. Anticoagulant action can be counteracted promptly with protamine sulfate, I.V., mg. for mg. of heparin. Each mg. of dried heparin contains 100 U.S.P. units of anticoagulant activity.
1. I.V. - For immediate effect, give 2500-7500 units and repeat every 6 hours, determining the Lee-White clotting time before each dose. Concomitantly with the first I.V.

PROTHROMBIN DEPRESSANTS*

	DOSAGE (ORAL)†			Approximate Time to Peak Effect (Days)	Approximate Duration of Effect (Days)
	1st Day	2nd Day	Usual Daily Maintenance and Range		
Dicumarol	200-400 mg. (3-6 gr.)	100-200 mg. (1 1/2-3 gr.)	100 mg. (25-150 mg.)	2-3	4
Warfarin (Coumadin®, Panwarfin®, Athrombin®)	30-50 mg. (1/2-3/4 gr.)	10-15 mg. (1/6-1/4 gr.)	7 mg. (5-15 mg.)	1-2	2-3
Diphenadione (Dipaxin®)‡	40-60 mg. (2/3-1 gr.)	10-20 mg. (1/6-1/3 gr.)	7 mg. (2.5-10) mg.)	2-3	10
Phenindione (Danilone®, Hedulin®)‡	100-250 mg. (1 1/2-4 gr.) b.i.d.	25-75 mg. (3/8-1 1/4 gr.) b.i.d.	50 mg. (12.5-75 mg.) b.i.d.	1-2	4
Anisindione (Miradon®)‡	300 mg. (5 gr.)	200 mg. (3 gr.)	75 mg. (25-250 mg.)	1-2	4
Phenprocoumon (Liquamar®)	30 mg. (1/2 gr.)	10 mg. (1/6 gr.)	3 mg. (1-6 mg.)	1-2	4
Acenocoumarol (Sintrom®)	16-28 mg. (1/4-1/2 gr.)	8-16 mg. (1/8-1/4 gr.)	6 mg. (2-10 mg.)	1-2	2
Ethyl biscoumacetate (Tromexan®)	750-900 mg. (12-14 gr.) b.i.d.	150-300 mg. (2 1/2-5 gr.) b.i.d.	300 mg. (150-450 mg.) b.i.d.	1	2

*Reproduced, with permission from Krupp and Chatton (editors), Current Diagnosis & Treatment 1973. Lange, 1973.

†Only warfarin may be given I.V. The oral route is almost always used. Dosages given are single daily doses unless otherwise specified.

‡Indandione derivative. Allergic reactions, including agranulocytosis, occur. Hepatitis may occur with phenindione.

Oral Administration of Digitalis Drugs*

Urgency	Drug	Dosage
Moderate	Digitalis	0.4 Gm. (6 gr.) every 8 hours for 3 doses
	Digitoxin	0.4 mg. (1/150 gr.) every 8 hours for 3 doses
	Digoxin	1 mg. (1/60 gr.) every 8 hours for 3 doses
Interme-diate	Digitalis	0.2 Gm. (3 gr.) 3 times daily for 2 days or 0.1 Gm. (1 1/2 gr.) 4 times daily for 3 days
	Digitoxin	0.2 mg. (1/300 gr.) 3 times daily for 2 days
	Digoxin	0.5-0.75 mg. (1/120-1/80 gr.) 3 times daily for 2 days or 0.25-0.5 mg. (1/240-1/120 gr.) 4 times daily for 3 days
Least	Digitalis	0.1 Gm. (1 1/2 gr.) 3 times daily for 4-5 days
	Digitoxin	0.1 mg. (1/600 gr.) 3 times daily for 4-6 days
	Digoxin	0.25-0.5 mg. (1/240-1/120 gr.) 3 times daily for 4-6 days

*When digitalization is urgent, or if the patient is unable to take oral medication, give deslanoside (Cedilanid-D®), 1.2 mg. (6 ml.) I.M or I.V., and follow with 0.2-0.4 mg. I.M. or I.V. every 3-4 hours until the effect is maintained. Special precautions to avoid digitalis toxicity are necessary when giving rapid-acting I.V. digitalis preparations in patients who have hypokalemia or in those whose history of recent digitalis therapy is uncertain.

injection, administer heparin subcut. (see below) and discontinue I. V. dosage when the subcut. dose becomes effective (as indicated by persistent prolongation of clotting time).

2. Subcut. - Inject a concentrated aqueous solution of heparin (200 mg./ml.) through a No. 25 needle just below the posterior iliac crest. Average doses are as follows:
   a. 100 lb. (45.5 Kg.) patient - 10,000 units every 12 hours.
   b. 150 lb. (68 Kg.) patient - 12,500 units every 12 hours.
   c. 175-200 lb. (80-91 Kg.) patient - 12,500-15,000 units every 12 hours.

   Determine Lee-White clotting time before each dose. If the clotting time exceeds 18 minutes, defer the next injection until the clotting time falls below this level. The above dosage is usually repeated every 12 hours, but the effect may last 18-36 hours and the schedule should be modified accordingly. After heparin requirements have become stabilized, daily clotting time determinations may be sufficient for control.

   Heparin is generally used for the first few days of anticoagulant therapy until an oral prothrombin depressant becomes effective. However, subcutaneous heparin may be used alone for long-term therapy.

B. Prothrombin Depressants: (See table on p. 834.) The various prothrombin depressants differ in rapidity and duration of effect. Dicumarol and warfarin are the most widely used. The indandiones cause an appreciably greater incidence of side-effects. The physician should select one drug and use it consistently to become familiar with its action.

   The objective of therapy is to maintain a prothrombin activity of 10-30%. Initially, the prothrombin activity is determined daily and dosage adjusted accordingly. In well-stabilized patients, weekly or even monthly determinations may be adequate. Spontaneous hemorrhages may occur with prothrombin activities below 10-20% and should be treated in one of the following ways:

1. Phytonadione (vitamin K, Mephyton®), 50-200 mg. I.V. slowly (at a rate of not over 10 mg./minute by syringe or added to venoclysis of dextrose or saline); repeat every 6 hours as necessary.
2. Menadione sodium bisulfite, 50-100 mg. I.V. Stat. and repeat 2-3 times the first day (acts more slowly than phytonadione).
3. Fresh whole blood transfusions if hemorrhage is severe.

The usual starting doses and maintenance doses of the common antiprothrombin drugs are shown in the chart on p. 676. Patients with initial prothrombin activities below 80-100% should receive smaller doses.

Diuretics.

A. Thiazide Diuretics: Example: Hydrochlorothiazide (Esidrix®, Hydro-Diuril®, Oretic®), 25-50 mg. orally once or twice daily. The thiazides produce sodium diuresis accompanied by potassium loss, and supplementary potassium may be required (especially early in treatment). They are useful in all fluid retention states, but must be used with great caution in cirrhotic patients. They are contraindicated in acute renal failure.

B. Ethacrynic acid (Edecrin®), 25-50 mg. orally 2-4 times daily, is a rapid-acting diuretic. Initial doses should be small, and because of the marked sodium and potassium depletion which may occur, the drug should be used with caution in patients with renal insufficiency and those taking digitalis. Ototoxicity has been reported. Potassium supplements are necessary if the drug is used for long periods.

C. Furosemide (Lasix®), 20 mg. orally 1-4 times daily, produces diuretic effects similar to those of ethacrynic acid. If the drug is ineffective orally - or if oral use is not possible - a single dose of 20-40 mg. may be given slowly I.V. Precautions are the same as for ethacrynic acid.

D. Mercurial Diuretics: The mercurial diuretics are potent, and cause less potassium depletion than the thiazides. No satisfactory oral preparation is available. Since the advent of potent oral diuretic drugs, the mercurials are now used only in an occasional patient with congestive heart failure. The dose of the available mercurials (e.g., meralluride [Mercuhydrin®]) is 0.5-2 ml. of the prepared solution, no oftener than once daily.

E. Aldosterone Antagonist: Spironolactone (Aldactone®) causes sodium loss but some potassium retention. The initial dose is 25 mg. (3/8 gr.) 4 times daily, and the response is slow to develop.

F. Triamterene (Dyrenium®), 50-100 mg. orally twice daily after meals, is frequently used for its additive diuretic effect in combination with the thiazide diuretics or mercurial diuretics. This may be especially desirable because triamterene prevents hypokalemia. It is necessary to determine periodically the blood potassium and BUN to prevent possible hyperkalemia and renal insufficiency.

G. Acidifying Diuretics: Ammonium chloride, 1-2 Gm. (15-30 gr.) q.i.d. for no more than 3 days without interruption is occasionally used mainly to potentiate the effect of mercurial diuretics.

Expectorants.

A. Potassium Iodide Solution: 0.5 ml. q.i.d. (p.c. and h.s.), gradually increasing to 1-2 ml. q.i.d. Gastric intolerance or symptoms of iodism (coryza, acneform eruptions, etc.) occasionally occur.

B. CO_2 at intervals by face mask.

Cough Depressant Drugs.

A. Codeine: 8-15 mg. (1/8-1/4 gr.) orally every 4 hours p.r.n. Most effective when given in small doses at frequent intervals. Codeine is most conveniently prescribed as a mixture, e.g., with elixir of terpin hydrate.

B. Dextromethorphan Hydrobromide (Romilar®): 15-30 mg. orally 1-4 times daily. Equivalent in antitussive effect to codeine (mg. for mg.). Nonnarcotic and nonaddictive.

C. Noscapine (Nectadon®): 15-30 mg. orally 1-4 times daily. Nonnarcotic and nonaddictive. Doses as high as 90 mg. daily may be tolerated for 4-6 weeks.

GASTROINTESTINAL DRUGS

Laxatives and Cathartics.

A. Lubricants: Liquid petrolatum (mineral oil), alone or with agar, 15-45 ml. h.s., p.r.n. Should not be used for prolonged periods. Particularly useful for patients who have painful defecation (e.g., posthemorrhoidectomy).

B. Saline Cathartics: Observe caution in the use of sodium salts in cardiac patients.
   1. Sodium phosphate - 5-10 Gm. in a glass of water before breakfast. Phosphate salts are more palatable than the salts listed below.
   2. Magnesia magma (milk of magnesia) - 15-30 ml. h.s., p.r.n.
   3. Sodium or magnesium sulfate, 4-8 Gm. in a glass of warm water before breakfast.

C. Colloid or "Bulk" Laxatives: Psyllium hydrophilic mucilloid (Metamucil®), 1-3 tsp. 2-3 times daily p.c. mixed in a full glass of water and followed by a second glass of water.

D. Irritants:
   1. Aromatic cascara sagrada fluidextract - 4-8 ml. h.s., p.r.n. Frequently given in combination with 30 ml. of milk of magnesia or mineral oil.
   2. Castor oil - 15-60 ml. as a single dose in late afternoon. Capsules and emulsions also available. Emulsions contain 50% of the oil, and twice the dose must be given. Liquid preparation should be served cold and mixed with syrup or carbonated beverages to partially disguise the taste.
   3. Bisacodyl (Dulcolax®) - (Supplied as 5 mg. tablets or 10 mg. rectal suppositories.) 1-3 (usually 2) tablets h.s., or 1

suppository at the time a bowel movement is desired. Tablets are not to be chewed or taken with antacid.

E. Fecal Softeners: Dioctyl sodium sulfosuccinate (Colace®, Doxinate®) - 50-100 mg. 2-3 times daily, or 240-480 mg. once daily. Liquid preparations also available. A surface wetting agent for stool softening. No action on the bowel. Available also as Peri-Colace®, which contains casanthranol, a mild laxative.

Antidiarrheal Agents.

A. Pectin-kaolin Compound (Kaopectate®): 30-60 ml. q.i.d. (a.c. and h.s.) or after each liquid bowel movement. Often combined in proprietary preparations with antimicrobial agents, e.g., neomycin, or with paregoric.

B. Bismuth Magma (Bismuth Hydroxide and Bismuth Subcarbonate): 4 ml. q.i.d. or after each liquid bowel movement.

C. Paregoric: 4-8 ml. after each liquid bowel movement p.r.n. Often combined with equal parts bismuth magma. Contraindicated in diarrhea associated with undiagnosed abdominal pain.

D. Bismuth Magma and Paregoric: 8-15 ml. q.i.d. or after each liquid bowel movement.

E. Codeine: 15-30 mg. (1/4-1/2 gr.) orally or subcut. after each liquid bowel movement p.r.n. Contraindicated in diarrhea associated with undiagnosed abdominal pain.

F. Diphenoxylate Hydrochloride With Atropine Sulfate (Lomotil®): Contraindicated in patients with hepatic disease and in the presence of undiagnosed abdominal pain. The dose is 5 mg. 3-4 times daily.

Antiemetics.

A. Chlorpromazine Hydrochloride (Thorazine®): 10-50 mg. (avg. 25 mg.) orally every 4-6 hours p.r.n.; 25-50 mg. I.M. every 4-6 hours p.r.n. Many other phenothiazine tranquilizers are used.

B. Dimenhydrinate (Dramamine®): 50-100 mg. (avg. 50 mg.) orally q.i.d. Available also as rectal suppositories, 100 mg. for insertion once nightly. Less effective in prevention of vomiting than phenothiazine derivatives such as chlorpromazine, but effective against motion sickness.

C. Meclizine Hydrochloride (Bonine®): 25-50 mg. daily. May be taken 1 hour before travel or radiation as antiemetic prophylaxis. Cyclizine (Marezine®), 50 mg. every 4-6 hours orally or I.M., is an equivalent drug.

Antacids.

A. Absorbable (Systemic) Antacids: Sodium bicarbonate, 1 Gm. (15 gr.) in one-half glass of water. This agent is convenient and readily available, but it causes an "acid rebound" and can produce gaseous distention.

B. Nonabsorbable Antacids: Aluminum hydroxide gel and magnesium trisilicate, alone or in combination, liquid or tablets, 4-8 ml. or 1-2 tablets (0.5 Gm. each) with one-half glass of water every 2-4 hours p.r.n., preferably 30-90 minutes before meals.

Anticholinergic Drugs.

The anticholinergic drugs are of principal value in the treatment of pain due to smooth muscle spasm. They also decrease excessive salivary secretion. In the doses ordinarily employed, they do not exert significant gastric antisecretory effect in peptic ulcer, and they prolong the gastric emptying time. The relative advantages of the large number of synthetic preparations available, other than for those which may be required for parenteral use, are debatable.

A. Belladonna Alkaloids:
1. Belladonna tincture, 0.3-0.6 ml. (5-10 drops) in one-half glass of water orally, t. i. d., 30 minutes before meals and at bedtime p. r. n. (0.6 ml. of the tincture equals about 0.2 mg. of atropine). Available with phenobarbital.
2. Belladonna extract, 8-15 mg. (1/8-1/4 gr.), tablets or capsules, orally t. i. d., 30 minutes before meals and at bedtime p. r. n. (15 mg. equals about 0.2 mg. of atropine alkaloid). Available with phenobarbital.
3. Atropine sulfate tablets, 0.3-0.6 mg. (1/200-1/100 gr.) may be administered orally or subcut. The usual dose is 0.3 mg. (1/200 gr.) t. i. d.

B. Synthetic Anticholinergic Drugs: A few are listed below.
1. Methantheline bromide (Banthine®), 50-100 mg. every 6 hours around the clock as initial dosage, reduced to one-half for maintenance. Ampuls of 50 mg. are available for I. V. or I. M. use.
2. Propantheline bromide (Pro-Banthine®), 15 mg. with each meal and 30 mg. at bedtime. Available in parenteral form for I. V. or I. M. use.
3. Tridihexethyl chloride (Pathilon®), 25 mg. t. i. d. before meals and 50 mg. at bedtime. Parenteral dose (I. V., I. M., or subcut.) is 10-20 mg. every 6 hours.

CANCER CHEMOTHERAPY

See table on pp. 840-841.

• • •

HYPERBARIC OXYGENATION

During the past 2 decades there has been a revival of interest in the study of the therapeutic effects of oxygen breathing at increased pressure. The partial pressure of breathed oxygen at 3 atmospheres is approximately 2200 mm. Hg (760 × 3) or about 15 times the partial pressure of oxygen in air when breathing under normal atmospheric pressure (150 mm. Hg). This enables the plasma to carry an amount of oxygen comparable to that ordinarily carried by hemoglobin. The result is a high tissue content of oxygen and a high diffusing capacity which permits oxygen to reach relatively ischemic areas in therapeutically significant amounts.

Medical hyperbaric chambers have been installed in a number

CANCER CHEMOTHERAPEUTIC AGENTS USEFUL AGAINST SOLID TUMORS*

	Principal Usefulness	Dosage	Toxicity
Alkylating Agents.			
Mechlorethamine (nitrogen mustard, HN2, Mustargen®)	Hodgkin's disease, neoplastic effusions.	0.4 mg./Kg. I.V. as single dose every 4-6 weeks; 0.4 mg./Kg. by intracavitary injection.	Nausea and vomiting, marrow depression, ulcer if extravasated, hypogonadism, fetal anomalies, alopecia.
Cyclophosphamide (Cytoxan®)	Burkitt's lymphoma, Hodgkin's disease, other lymphomas.	40-60 mg./Kg. I.V. every 3-5 weeks; 5 Gm./Kg./day orally for 10 days, then 1-3 mg./Kg./day as maintenance.	Nausea and vomiting, marrow depression, alopecia, hemorrhagic cystitis.
Chlorambucil (Leukeran®)	Hodgkin's disease.	0.1-0.2 mg./Kg./day orally.	Marrow depression, gastroenteritis.
Phenylalanine mustard (Melphalan, Alkeran®)	Myeloma, ovarian carcinoma.	0.25 mg./Kg./day orally for 4 days every 6 weeks; 2-4 mg./Kg./day as maintenance	Marrow depression (occasionally prolonged), gastroenteritis.
Thiotepa	Ovarian carcinoma, neoplastic effusions.	0.8 mg./Kg. I.V. as single dose every 4-6 weeks; 0.8 mg./Kg. by intracavitary injection.	Marrow depression.
Structural Analogues.			
Methotrexate (amethopterin)	Choriocarcinoma, Burkitt's lymphoma.	20-40 mg. I.V. twice weekly; 5-15 mg. intrathecally weekly; 2.5-5 mg./day orally.	Ulcerative mucositis, gastroenteritis, dermatitis, marrow depression, hepatitis, abortion.
Fluorouracil (5-FU, Efudex®)	Breast carcinoma, colon and rectal cancer.	15-20 mg./Kg. I.V. weekly for at least 6 weeks; 15 mg./Kg. orally weekly.	Atrophic dermatitis, gastroenteritis, mucositis, marrow depression, neuritis.

Cytotoxic Antibiotics.			
Dactinomycin (actinomycin D, Cosmegen®)	Wilms's tumor, choriocarcinoma.	0.01 mg./Kg./day for 5 days every 4-6 weeks.	Nausea and vomiting, stomatitis, gastroenteritis, proctitis, marrow depression, ulcer if extravasated, alopecia; radiation potentiator.
Mithramycin (Mithracin®)	Hypercalcemia of malignancies.	0.05 mg./Kg. I.V. every other day to toxicity or 8 doses per course.	Marrow depression, nausea and vomiting, complex coagulopathies, hepatotoxity.
Bleomycin (Blenoxane®)	Lymphomas, testicular carcinoma.	15 mg. twice weekly I.V., I.M., or subcut.; total cumulative dose should not exceed 300 mg.	Allergic dermatitis, pulmonary fibrosis, fever, mucositis.
Vinca Alkaloids.			
Vinblastine (Velban®)	Hodgkin's disease.	0.1-0.2 mg./Kg. I.V. weekly.	Marrow depression, alopecia, ulcer if extravasated, nausea and vomiting, neuropathy.
Vincristine (Oncovin®)	Hodgkin's disease, other lymphomas, Wilms's tumor, neuroblastoma, medulloblastoma, choriocarcinoma.	Give I.V., 1.5 mg./sq. M. (or less) weekly. No one dose should exceed 2 mg.	Alopecia, neuropathy (peripheral and autonomic), ulcer if extravasated; rarely, marrow depression.
Miscellaneous Agents.			
Mitotane (Lysodren®; o, p´DDD)	Hypersecretion in adrenocortical carcinoma.	5-12 Gm. orally daily.	Gastroenteritis, dermatitis, CNS abnormalities.
Procarbazine (Matulane®)	Hodgkin's disease.	50-150 mg./sq. M. orally daily to toxicity or response; maintain with 50-100 mg./day orally.	Marrow depression, gastroenteritis, dermatitis, CNS abnormalities.

*Modified from Spivack in Dunphy and Way (editors), Current Surgical Diagnosis and Treatment. Lange, 1973. [Investigational agents and hormones not included. - Ed.]

of medical centers. Much of the treatment being conducted under hyperbaric oxygenation (usually at 2-3 atmospheres) is on an experimental basis. The usefulness of hyperbaric therapy is currently limited by the expense and complexity of hyperbaric chambers and by the complications of compression, which include inert gas narcosis, decompression sickness, and oxygen toxicity. In certain conditions, however, the response to hyperbaric oxygenation has already proved sufficiently impressive to warrant its recommendation in their management where facilities are available. These conditions include the following:

Gas Gangrene. (See p. 210.)

Infection by clostridial organisms often shows dramatic improvement following hyperbaric oxygen therapy. Systemic toxicity and local tissue destruction are reported to be rapidly controlled. Encouraging responses have also been noted in tetanus and in infections with bacteroides and anaerobic streptococci (Wallyn and others, S. Clin. North America **44**:107, 1964; Davis, J. C. and others, JAMA **224**:205-209, 1973).

Carbon Monoxide Poisoning. (See p. 46.)

The release of carbon monoxide from the blood is markedly accelerated in the hyperbaric environment. Exposure to 2.5 atmospheres of oxygen will decrease the clearance time of body carbon monoxide from 4 hours to 1 hour. An alternative and simpler means of clearing carbon monoxide from the blood has been described by Linder et al. (Surg. Forum **14**:277, 1963), who found that carbon monoxide dissociates rapidly from blood in the presence of strong light and oxygen in an extracorporeal oxygenator.

Other Uses.

Hyperbaric oxygenation is of proved value in the treatment of decompression sickness. Some success with hyperbaric oxygenation has been recorded in air embolism, acute coronary artery occlusion, acute cerebral vascular accident, acute peripheral ischemia, radiotherapy of tumors, cardiac surgery in infants with congenital heart disease, and preservation of tissue for transplantation. In these and various other conditions, the indications for hyperbaric oxygenation and its relative merit compared with other methods have yet to be established (Saltzman and others, Monographs in the Surgical Sciences 2:1, 1965).

VASOPRESSORS AND THEIR USE IN ANESTHESIA*

	Levarterenol Bitartrate (Levophed®)	Ephedrine Hydrochloride or Sulfate	Methoxamine Hydrochloride (Vasoxyl®)	Metaraminol Bitartrate (Aramine®)	Phenylephrine Hydrochloride (Neo-Synephrine®)
Dosage and Duration					
Intramuscular		20-50 mg. 40-90 min.	10-20 mg. 30-60 min.	2-5 mg. 20-60 min.	2-5 mg. 30-60 min.
Intravenous single dose	Not used	10-25 mg. 20 min.	4-10 mg. 10-30 min.	0.25-0.5 mg. 20-60 min.	0.25-0.50 mg. 20 min.
Intravenous continuous drip	Usual method, 4 mg./1000 ml.	Not usually employed	Not usually employed	May be used	1-2 mg./100 ml.
Effects					
Myocardial stimulation	Yes	Yes	Slight	Yes	Slight
CNS stimulation	Slight	Marked	None	Slight	Slight
Cardiac rate	Increased or decreased	Increased	Reflex slowing effect	Increased, or reflex slowing effect	Reflex slowing effect
Peripheral vessels	Constricts	Constricts	Constricts	Constricts	Constricts
Use with cyclopropane, chloroform, trichloroethylene, halothane	Dangerous, may cause ventricular fibrillation	Yes, but causes supraventricular arrhythmias	Yes	Arrhythmias may occur.	Yes

*Epinephrine is not employed during anesthesia as a systemic vasopressor.

MUSCLE RELAXANTS COMMONLY USED IN ANESTHESIA

	Tubocurarine Chloride	Gallamine Triethiodide (Flaxedil®)	Decamethonium Bromide (Syncurine®)	Succinylcholine Chloride (Anectine®, Quelicin®, Sucostrin®)
How supplied	10 ml. vials, 3 mg. (1/20 gr.)/ml.	10 ml. vials, 20 mg. (1/3 gr.)/ml.	10 ml. vials, 1 mg. (1/60 gr.)/ml.	10 ml. vials, 20 mg. (1/3 gr.)/ml. 10 ml. ampuls, 100 mg. (1 1/2 gr.)/ml.
Dose				
Initial	3-15 mg. (1/20-1/4 gr.) I. V.	40-100 mg. (2/3-1 1/2 gr.) I. V.	1-4 mg. (1/60-1/15 gr.) I. V.	20-60 mg. (1/3-1 gr.) I. V.
Subsequent	1/2-1/3 previous I. V. dose	1/2 previous I. V. dose	0.5-1 mg. I. V.	Same as initial I. V.
Continuous drip	Not used	Not used	Not used	0.1-0.2% solution
Onset of action	3-5 minutes	2-5 minutes	3-5 minutes	1-3 minutes
Duration of action of single paralyzing dose	30-60 minutes	25-30 minutes	20 minutes	2-5 minutes
Side effects	Histamine release, hypotension.	No histamine effect; tachycardia.	May show tachyphylaxis. Effect erratic.	Muscle fasciculations with rapid injection. Salivation. Increases intraocular tension.
Other effects	Cumulative action. Additive with ether and certain antibiotics, e.g., neomycin.	Same as tubocurarine chloride.	Usually no cumulative effect. Not additive with ether.	Not additive with ether. Bradycardia. May produce anti-depolarizing type block.
Contraindications	Myasthenia gravis.	Myasthenia gravis.		Severe liver disease. Increased intraocular tension.
Antidote	(1) Edrophonium chloride (Tensilon®): 10-20 mg. (1/6-1/3 gr.) I. V., may be repeated once. (2) Neostigmine (Prostigmin®): 0.5-2.5 mg. (1/120-1/25 gr.) I. V. slowly. Bradycardia caused by neostigmine should be prevented or treated with atropine sulfate, 0.4-1 mg. (1/150-1/60 gr.) I. V.		None	After large total dosage a prolonged apnea may be reversed by neostigmine (Prostigmin®). Transfusion.

TABLES OF APPROXIMATE EQUIVALENTS

Weight Equivalents			Volume Equivalents		
Apothecary		Metric	Apothecary		Metric
1/320 gr.	=	0.2 mg.	1 min.	=	0.06 ml.
1/210 gr.	=	0.3 mg.	3 min.	=	0.18 ml.
1/160 gr.	=	0.4 mg.	5 min.	=	0.3 ml.
1/120 gr.	=	0.5 mg.	8 min.	=	0.5 ml.
1/100 gr.	=	0.6 mg.	10 min.	=	0.6 ml.
1/60 gr.	=	1.0 mg.	12 min.	=	0.75 ml.
1/30 gr.	=	2.0 mg.	15 min.	=	0.9 ml.
1/16 gr.	=	4.0 mg.	16 min.	=	1.0 ml.
1/12 gr.	=	5.4 mg.	20 min.	=	1.2 ml.
1/10 gr.	=	6.5 mg.	30 min.	=	1.8 ml.
1/8 gr.	=	8.0 mg.	50 min.	=	3.0 ml.
1/6 gr.	=	11.0 mg.	1 fl.dr.	=	3.7 ml.
1/4 gr.	=	16.0 mg.	65 min.	=	4.0 ml.
1/3 gr.	=	22.0 mg.	80 min.	=	5.0 ml.
3/8 gr.	=	24.0 mg.	2 fl.dr.	=	7.5 ml.
1/2 gr.	=	32.0 mg.	2-2/3 fl.dr.	=	10.0 ml.
3/4 gr.	=	50.0 mg.	4 fl.dr.	=	15.0 ml.
1 gr.	=	65.0 mg.	5-1/2 fl.dr.	=	20.0 ml.
1-1/2 gr.	=	0.1 Gm.	8 fl.dr.	=	1.0 fl.oz.
2 gr.	=	0.13 Gm.	1 fl.oz.	=	30.0 ml.
3 gr.	=	0.2 Gm.	1-2/3 fl.oz.	=	50.0 ml.
5 gr.	=	0.32 Gm.	2 fl.oz.	=	60.0 ml.
7-1/2 gr.	=	0.5 Gm.	3-3/8 fl.oz.	=	100.0 ml.
10 gr.	=	0.65 Gm.	4 fl.oz.	=	120.0 ml.
15 gr.	=	1.0 Gm.	8 fl.oz.	=	240.0 ml.
1 dr.	=	4.0 Gm.	16 fl.oz.	=	480.0 ml.
1 oz.	=	30.0 Gm.			

Household Measures		Apothecary		Metric
1 teaspoon	=	1 fl.dr.	=	4 ml.
1 tablespoon	=	1/2 fl.oz.	=	15 ml.
1 teacup	=	4 fl.oz.	=	120 ml.
1 glass (tumbler)	=	8 fl.oz.	=	240 ml.
1 measuring cup	=	8 fl.oz.	=	240 ml.
1 pint	=	16 fl.oz.	=	480 ml.

CENTIGRADE TO FAHRENHEIT TEMPERATURES

C.°	F.°	C.°	F.°	C.°	F.°
35 =	95	37.5 =	99.5	40 =	104
35.5 =	95.9	38 =	100.4	40.5 =	104.9
36 =	96.8	38.5 =	101.3	41 =	105.8
36.5 =	97.7	39 =	102.2	42 =	107.6
37 =	98.6	39.5 =	103.1	43 =	109.4

MILLIEQUIVALENT CONVERSION FACTORS

To determine mEq./L. of:	Divide mg./100 ml. or Vol.% by:
Calcium	2.0
Chlorides (from Cl)	3.5
(from NaCl)	5.85
CO_2 combining power	2.22
Magnesium	1.2
Phosphorus	3.1 (mM.)
Potassium	3.9
Sodium	2.3

CLINICAL CHEMISTRY VALUES*

Determination	Material Required†	Normal Values
Ammonia‡	Blood, 2 ml.	40-70 μg./100 ml. (Conway).
Amylase	Serum, 2 ml.	80-180 units/100 ml. (Somogyi).
Base, total serum	Serum, 2 ml.	145-160 mEq./L.
Bilirubin	Serum, 2 ml.	Direct: 0.1-0.4 mg./100 ml. Indirect: 0.2-0.7 mg./100 ml.
Blood volume (Evans blue dye method)		Adults: 2990-6980 ml. (Men: 66.2-97.7 ml./Kg. Women: 46.3-85.5 ml./Kg.)
Calcium	Serum, 2 ml. (fasting)	9-10.6 mg./100 ml.; 4.5-5.3 mEq./L. (varies with protein concentration).
Cephalin flocculation	Serum, 1 ml.	Up to ++ in 48 hours.
CO_2 content	Serum or	24-29 mEq./L.; 55-65 Vol. %.
CO_2 combining power	plasma, 1 ml.	55-75 Vol. %.
Chloride (as chloride) (as NaCl)	Serum, 1 ml.	100-106 mEq./L.; 350-375 mg./100 ml. 580-620 mg./100 ml.
Cholesterol, total	Serum, 1 ml.	150-280 mg./100 ml.
Cholesterol esters	Serum, 1 ml.	50-65% of total cholesterol.
Congo red test		More than 60% in serum after 1 hour.
Creatinine	Blood or serum, 1 ml.	0.7-1.5 mg./100 ml.
Creatinine clearance test		116-148 L./24 hours (100-120 ml./min.) corrected to 1.73 sq. M. surface area.
Fat, fecal		Less than 30% of dry weight.
Glucose (Folin)	Blood, 1 ml.	80-120 mg./100 ml. (fasting).
Glucose (true)	Blood, 1 ml.	60-100 mg./100 ml. (fasting).
Icterus index	Serum, 1 ml.	3-8 I.I. units.
Iodine, butanol-extractable	Serum, 10 ml.	3-6.5 μg./100 ml.
Iodine, protein-bound	Serum, 5 ml.	4-8 μg./100 ml.
Iron	Serum, 2 ml.	65-175 μg./100 ml.
Iron-binding capacity, unsaturated	Serum, 2 ml.	250-410 μg./100 ml.
Lipase	Serum, 2 ml.	0.2-1.5 units (ml. of N/10 NaOH).
Magnesium	Serum, 2 ml.	1.5-2.5 mEq./L.; 1-2 mg./100 ml.
Nonprotein nitrogen‡	S or B, 1 ml. (fasting)	15-35 mg./100 ml.
Oxygen: Capacity	Blood, 5 ml.	16-24 Vol. % (varies with Hgb. concen.).
Arterial content		15-23 Vol. % (varies with Hgb. concen.).
Arterial % sat.		94-100% of capacity.
Venous content		10-16 Vol. % (varies with Hgb. concen.).
Venous % sat.		60-85% of capacity.
A-V difference		4.5-7 Vol. %.
pH (reaction)	Arterial blood, 2 ml.	7.35-7.45
Phenolsulfonphthalein (PSP) excretion	Total voiding of urine	25% or more in first 15 min., 40% or more in 30 min., 55% or more in 2 hours.
Phosphatase, acid	Serum, 2 ml.	0.5-2 units (Bodansky). 1-5 units (K-A).
Phosphatase, alkaline	Serum, 2 ml.	2-4.5 units (Bodansky). 5-13 units (King-Armstrong).
Phosphorus, inorganic	Serum, 1 ml. (fasting)	3-4.5 mg./100 ml. (Children, 4-7 mg.); 0.9-1.5 mM./L.
Phospholipid	Serum, 2 ml.	145-200 mg./100 ml.
Potassium	Serum, 1 ml.	3.5-5.3 mEq./L.; 14-21 mg./100 ml.
Protein: Total	Serum, 1 ml.	6-8 Gm./100 ml.
Albumin	Serum, 1 ml.	3.5-5.5 Gm./100 ml.
Globulin	Serum, 1 ml.	1.5-3 Gm./100 ml.
Fibrinogen	Plasma, 1 ml.	0.2-0.6 Gm./100 ml.

*Values vary with technics used and in different laboratories.

†Blood = Whole blood (without anticoagulant). Collect 5 ml. blood/ml. of serum required.

‡Do not use anticoagulant containing ammonium oxalate.

CLINICAL CHEMISTRY VALUES* (Cont'd.)

Determination	Material Required†	Normal values
Prothrombin clotting time	Plasma, 2 ml.	By control.
Sodium	Serum, 1 ml.	136-145 mEq./L.; 310-340 mg./100 ml. (as NaCl).
Sulfobromophthalein (Bromsulphalein®, BSP) retention	Serum, 1 ml.	< 5% retention 30 min. after injection of 2 mg./Kg. I.V. or 45 min. after injection of 5 mg./Kg. I.V.
Thymol turbidity	Serum, 1 ml.	Maximum 5 units.
Transaminase tests		
SGOT	Serum, 2 ml.	5-40 units (6-25 IU/L.).
SGPT	Serum, 2 ml.	5-35 units (3-26 IU/L.).
SLDH (serum lactate dehydro genase)	Serum, 2 ml.	215-450 units.
Urea clearance test	Urine and plasma	Standard: 40-65 ml./min. Maximal: 60-100 ml./min.
Urea nitrogen‡	S or B, 1 ml. (fasting)	8-20 mg./100 ml.
Uric acid	Serum, 1 ml.	3-7.5 mg./100 ml.
Urobilinogen	Urine	0-4 mg./24 hours. Semi-quantitative, positive 1:20; negative 1:30.
	Feces	40-280 mg./24 hours.
Vanillylmandelic acid (VMA)	Urine	Up to 9 mg./24 hours.
Zinc turbidity (gamma globulin)	Serum, 1 ml.	Maximum 12 units.

*Values vary with technics used and in different laboratories.

†Blood = Whole blood (without anticoagulant). Collect 5 ml. blood/ml. of serum required.

‡Do not use anticoagulant containing ammonium oxalate.

NORMAL HEMATOLOGIC VALUES

White blood cells: 4500-11,000/μl.
Differential: band neutrophils, 0-5%; segmented neutrophils, 40-60%; lymphocytes, 20-40%; eosinophils, 1-3%; basophils, 0-1%; monocytes, 4-8%

Platelets: 200,000-400,000/μl.

Red blood cells: Men, 4.5-6.2 million/μl.
Women, 4.5-5.5 million/μl.

Reticulocytes: 0.5-1.5% of red cells.

Hemoglobin (Hgb.): Men, 14-18 Gm./100 ml.
Women, 12-16 Gm./100 ml.

Hematocrit (Hct.) or packed cell volume (PCV):
Men, 40-54% Women, 37-47%

Bleeding time: 1-7 minutes (Ivy).

Coagulation time: Lee and White, 6-18 minutes.

Clot retraction: Begins in 1-3 hours; complete in 24 hours.

Fragility of red cells: Begins 0.45-0.38% NaCl. Complete, 0.36-0.3% NaCl.

Sedimentation rate: Cutler, 2-10 mm./hour. Wintrobe, 0-10 mm./hour.
Westergren, less than 20 mm./hour.

Index

-C-

-D-

-E-

-F-

-I-

-Q-

-R-

-S-

-T-

-W-

-X-

-Y-

-Z-

X2548